Immunology in Medicine

A comprehensive guide to clinical immunology

Immunology in Medicine

A comprehensive guide to clinical immunology

Edited by

E. J. HOLBOROW *and* W. G. REEVES

Head MRC Immunology Group,
The Bone and Joint
Research Unit,
London Hospital Medical
College, London, England

Consultant Immunologist,
Nottinghamshire Area Health
Authority (Teaching),
Senior Lecturer,
Nottingham University
Medical School, England

ACADEMIC PRESS . London

GRUNE & STRATTON . New York

U.K. edition published and distributed by
ACADEMIC PRESS INC. (LONDON) LTD.
24/28 Oval Road
London NW1

United States Edition published and distributed by
GRUNE & STRATTON INC.
111 Fifth Avenue
New York, New York 10003

Library of Congress Catalog Card Number: 76-016974
ISBN (Academic Press): 0–12–352250–1
ISBN (Grune & Stratton): 0–8089–1054X

Text set in 11/12½ pt Monophoto Times New Roman
and printed and bound in Great Britain by
William Clowes & Sons Limited
London, Beccles and Colchester

Contributors

D. D. ADAMS, Director *Immunopathology Research Unit, Medical Research Council of New Zealand, Otago University Medical School, Box 913, Dunedin, New Zealand*

B. R. ALLEN, Consultant Dermatologist *Department of Dermatology, Nottingham General Hospital, Nottingham NG1 6HA, England*

J. BRADLEY, Associate Professor and Unit Head *Department of Clinical Immunology, Flinders Medical Centre, Flinders University of South Australia, Bedford Park, South Australia 5042*

M. A. BRAY, Research Scientist *Department of Clinical Pharmacology, Cardiothoracic Institute, Fulham Road, London SW3 6HP, England*

D. L. BROWN, Consultant Immunologist *Immunology Division, Addenbrooke's Hospital, Hills Road, Cambridge, England*

E. G. L. BYWATERS, Emeritus Professor of Rheumatology *Royal Postgraduate Medical School, Du Cane Road, London W12, England*

J. S. CAMERON, Professor in Renal Medicine *Department of Medicine, Guy's Hospital, London SE1 9RT, England*

P. M. CARTER, Assistant Director *Biochemistry Department, Royal Melbourne Hospital, Parkville, Melbourne, Victoria, 3050, Australia*

P. J. COLE, Senior Lecturer in Medicine and Honorary Consultant Physician *Host Defence Unit, Department of Medicine, Cardiothoracic Institute, Brompton Hospital, Fulham Road, London SW3 6HP, England*

G. A. CURRIE, Senior Lecturer and Honorary Consultant Physician *Department of Tumour Immunology, Institute of Cancer Research and The Royal Marsden Hospital, Sutton, Surrey, England*

R. L. DAWKINS, Head, Department of Clinical Immunology *Hospital and University Pathology Services, Perth Medical Centre, Nedlands, Western Australia 6009*

A. M. DENMAN, Consultant Immunologist *Clinical Research Centre, Northwick Park Hospital, Watford Road, Harrow, Middx. HA1 3UJ, England*

O. E. EADE, Lecturer in Medicine *Professorial Medical Unit, South Laboratory and Pathology Block, Southampton General Hospital, Tremona Road, Southampton SO9 4XY, England*

W. PAGE FAULK, Professor and Vice Chairman *Department of Basic and Clinical Immunology and Microbiology, Medical University of South Carolina, 80 Barre Street, Charleston, South Carolina 29401 USA*

B. M. GREENWOOD, Senior Lecturer in Medicine *Department of Medicine, Ahmadu Bello University, Zaria, Nigeria*

E. J. HOLBOROW, Head, MRC Immunology Group *The Bone and Joint Research Unit, London Hospital Medical College, London E1 2AD, England*

R. A. C. HUGHES, Consultant Neurologist, *Department of Neurology, Guy's Hospital, London SE1 9RT, England*

E. R. HURD, Associate Professor of Internal Medicine *Department of Internal Medicine, Southwestern Medical School, The University of Texas Health Science Center at Dallas, 5323 Harry Hines Boulevard, Dallas, Texas, 75235, USA*

K. A. JOHANSEN, Consultant in Obstetrics and Gynaecology *St David's and Llandough Hospitals, University Hospital of Wales, Heath Park, Cardiff CF4 4XW, Wales*

G. D. JOHNSON, Research Scientist *Bone and Joint Research Unit, London Hospital Medical College, Turner Street, London E1 2AD, England*

J. V. JONES, Director *Department of Rheumatology, Rush-Presbyterian—St Luke's Medical Center, 1753 West Congress Parkway, Chicago, Illinois 60612, USA*

S. LEIBOWITZ, Reader in Immunopathology *Department of Pathology, Guy's Hospital Medical School, London Bridge, London SE1 9RT, England*

J. MORLEY, Director *Department of Clinical Pharmacology, Cardiothoracic Institute, Fulham Road, London SW3 6HP, England*

M. PAPAMICHAIL, Scientific Director *The National Research and Training Centre in Immunology, 48 Vassileos Constantinou Avenue, Athens, Greece*

W. G. REEVES, Consultant Immunologist and Senior Lecturer *Department of Immunology, University Hospital, Nottingham, England*

A. J. SWANNELL, Consultant in Rheumatology and Rehabilitation *Department of Rheumatology and Rehabilitation, Nottingham City Hospital, Hucknall Road, Nottingham NG5 1PD, England*

R. A. THOMPSON, Consultant Immunologist *Regional Immunology Laboratory, East Birmingham Hospital, Bordesley Green East, Birmingham N9 5ST, England*

M. W. TURNER, Senior Lecturer *Department of Immunology, Institute of Child Health, University of London, 30 Guilford Street, London WC1N 1EH, England*

J. WATKINS, Principal Scientific Officer *Department of Immunology, Hallamshire Hospital Medical School, Sheffield S10 2RX, England*

A. D. B. WEBSTER, Consultant Physician *Division of Immunological Medicine, Clinical Research Centre, Northwick Park Hospital, Watford Road, Harrow, Middx. HA1 3UJ, England*

P. C. WILKINSON, Senior Lecturer and Honorary Consultant *Bacteriology and Immunology Department, University of Glasgow, Western Infirmary, Glasgow G11 6NT, Scotland*

D. G. WILLIAMS, Senior Lecturer and Consultant Physician *Department of Medicine, Guy's Hospital, London SE1 9RT, England*

D. V. WILSON, Research Scientist *Immunology Division, Addenbrooke's Hospital, Hills Road, Cambridge, England*

R. WRIGHT, Professor of Medicine *Professorial Medical Unit, South Laboratory and Pathology Block, Southampton General Hospital, Tremona Road, Southampton SO9 4XY, England*

Foreword

It is nowadays widely recognized that the activities of the immune system not only protect against microbial invasion and maintain the integrity of higher organisms, but that exaggeration or aberration of these activities can lead to disease. Much of the knowledge on which this recognition is based has been gained only within the last twenty years, and its application in medicine is even more recent. Although concepts in immunology are by no means static, and the mechanisms whereby the immune response is regulated are still far from clear, the use of an immunological approach has produced plausible experimental models of and possible explanations for a wide variety of human disease processes whose pathogenesis was previously obscure. In some instances, the explanations have proved nearly enough correct to guide therapy or even to indicate new therapeutic approaches. In others, the application of immunological techniques has suggested that immunological factors may play a part in production or control of the disease processes but has left their aetiology tantalizingly unsolved, and has revealed *inter alia* that there is still much to learn about fundamental aspects of the immune response, in respect not only of the part played by lymphocytes but also by mononuclear cells, granulocytes and the complement system. In others still, immunological investigations, even when negative, are important for differential diagnosis.

Because the ramifications of immunology are very wide, and the relevant primary information or review articles are scattered throughout many journals, clinicians, pathologists and students badly need critical compilations of existing knowledge. In a rapidly expanding subject, it is difficult to decide when is the right time to make such a compilation, but to my mind, the present is as near to a nodal point as is likely to occur in the forseeable future. Clinical immunologists, during the last year or two, have reached a fair degree of agreement about what should be their scope and function, and good manuals have been published lately describing most of the basic techniques in their armamentarium. "Immunology in Medicine" sets out to give an account of the relevance of immunological concepts and of information obtained with these techniques in the whole field of clinical practice, using language which is intelligible to the non-specialist and attempting to assess critically the significance of the observations described. Insofar as these have implications for treatment, this is also indicated. The editors and their fellow authors have succeeded in their aim. Because they write from practical experience, the information which they provide has been predigested sufficiently to inform rather than to confuse the reader. Nevertheless, plenty of facts and raw data are included when these are appropriate, backed up by suitable references to the literature. Although this is a multi-author book, the editors have avoided serious overlap or repetition. The volume is large, but so is its subject matter, and it can properly be regarded as a magnum opus.

April, 1977

J. H. HUMPHREY M.D., F.R.S.
Professor of Immunology,
Royal Postgraduate Medical School,
Hammersmith Hospital,
London

Preface

"Immunology in Medicine" is primarily designed for the practising clinician, be he physician, surgeon or pathologist. The large majority of doctors in practice today escaped any specific training in immunology and many find its unfamiliar jargon and growing complexity formidable. Books abound on the more fundamental and specialized aspects, but there is a dearth of texts which communicate the practical importance of immunological developments across the breadth of clinical medicine. Twenty-three of the 34 contributors to this book are actively involved in day-to-day problems of medical care as well as contributing to immunological advances in their own field.

In an initial chapter we have attempted to give an overview of immunology: its history, jargon, cardinal features and mechanisms. The following eight chapters review the important basic aspects and the highlighted keywords in the general index refer back, predominantly, to this section for important definitions. Chapters 10–12 discuss the means by which immunological mechanisms cause disease, with particular emphasis on auto-immune processes in Chapters 11 and 12. Although the basic defect underlying auto-immune reactivity is poorly understood, clinical observation has almost as many clues to offer as have the various animal models which fascinate immunologists.

The traditional *raison d'être* of the immune response—defence against infection—is emphasized in chapters on infective disease and immunodeficiency. The largest section deals with the immunology of individual system disorders and is followed by contributions on malignancy and transplantation. Although therapy is mentioned wherever relevant, the last two chapters categorize the various means by which untoward immunological responses may be controlled. Apart from improved methods of diagnosis and increasing knowledge of mechanisms, the immunological manipulation of disease processes offers an exciting prospect for the future. Various non-pharmacological manoeuvres have already proved successful and the growth of disease-specific or antigen-specific treatment will add significantly to the skills required of the clinical immunologist in the future.

Guidelines and training programmes are now established for the various personnel necessary for the pursuit of clinical immunology, i.e., physician, pathologist, technologist and non-medical scientist.[1] We hope that this book will prove of value to each of these. Little space has been devoted to the finer details of laboratory technique which are covered by several recent publications.[2,3,4]

The complexities of producing and collating a multi-author work such as this are exponentially related to the number of authors involved. We owe a special debt to our wives and families for their acceptance and support of the role of immunological medicine within the domestic scene.

March, 1977 *E. J. HOLBOROW*
W. G. REEVES

---

1. Reeves, W. G. (1976). Clinical immunology. *Lancet*, **11**, 459.
2. Rose, N. R. and Friedman, H. (Eds.) (1976). "Manual of Clinical Immunology". American Society for Microbiology, Washington.
3. Thompson, R. A. (Ed.) (1977). "Techniques in Clinical Immunology". Blackwell Scientific Publications, Oxford.
4. Weir, D. M. (Ed.) (1977). "Handbook of Experimental Immunology". Third edition. Blackwell Scientific Publications, Oxford.

Contents

II. Mediator Systems

VI. Malignancy and Transplantation

VII. Therapeutic Aspects

1

General Introduction

W. G. REEVES and E. J. HOLBOROW

HISTORICAL DEVELOPMENT OF IMMUNOLOGY

Origins in Microbiology

The proposal of the germ theory of infectious disease by Louis Pasteur in 1847 and the confirmation that many important life-threatening diseases are caused by microorganisms, soon led to a search for factors which might protect individuals from the dire consequences of infection (Reid, 1974). Two of the early investigators in this field were Eli Metchnikoff, first in Messina and later in Pasteur's laboratory in Paris, and Paul Ehrlich, working with von Behring and Kitasato in Koch's institute in Berlin.

Metchnikoff became impressed with the ability of migratory cells, present in most multi-cellular organisms, to detect and defend against the invasion of foreign material. On the basis of experiments on water-fleas and starfish larvae he propounded a genera theory which gave pride of place to his wandering "phagocytes". Von Behring and Kitasato on the other hand, found that serum taken from animals or patients who had recovered from diphtheria or tetanus was able to confer specific protection when passively transferred to another host. Paul Ehrlich painstakingly continued this work and proposed his "side-chain" theory of immunity to explain these biological events. There seemed to be no way of reconciling these two opposing points of view until Almroth Wright described the enhancing effect of antibody on phagocytosis in 1903; a process which he called "opsonization". Although this work shed important light on the process of defence against bacterial infection, his unbridled enthusiasm for "stimulating the phagocytes" led to derision by Bernard Shaw in his play "The Doctor's Dilemma" (1908). In addition to the serum constituents already described by Ehrlich and his colleagues, Jules Bordet discovered in 1899 that a further heat labile serum factor—soon to be known as complement—was necessary for the lysis of infecting microorganisms.

The detection of the appropriate antibodies in the sera of patients recovering from infectious disease and the elaboration of specific antisera for use in their treatment was followed by a rest phase in the development of immunological knowledge. The general view was that infecting organisms were "bad" and the host response essentially "good". In support of this was work performed almost a hundred years before by the Gloucestershire general practitioner Edward Jenner on the protection against smallpox which could be conferred by inoculating material from cowpox vesicles. His unethical but courageous experiment on an eight-year-old boy—James Phipps—yielded an effective immunological means of controlling a disease which had previously affected 60% of the population in the United Kingdom. Such has been the success of this procedure that some authorities now speak with confidence of the world wide eradication of smallpox.

Soon after 1900, several lines of evidence began to suggest that the host response to the ingress of foreign material might not always be favourable and could cause serious harm. While cruising on the Prince of Monaco's yacht, Portier and Richet decided to study the effect of injecting jelly fish extracts into various animals. On their return they experimented with an extract prepared from sea anemone tentacles and made the surprising discovery that dogs which survived a first injection were more severely affected upon subsequent exposure to this antigenic material. This caused these workers to propose the term "anaphylaxis" in contra-distinction to the state of prophylaxis brought about by the use of bacterial antisera. At about the same time, Von Pirquet and Schick working at the Royal and Imperial Paediatric Clinic in Vienna found that "immune antisera" did not always produce the desired effect. They had cause to inject horse anti-diphtheria serum into a large number of children during an epidemic of the disease and soon found that a condition characterized by fever, urticarial rash, lymphadenopathy, arthritis and proteinuria was liable to ensue approximately eight days after the injection. This was most commonly seen following a second injection but in a few instances was provoked by the initial treatment. This response gave rise to the term "serum sickness", a condition now known to be mediated by circulating immune complexes.

Arthus described a similar phenomenon occuring locally in the skin after the repeated injection of foreign serum and Robert Koch became particularly interested in the nature of the host response to tuberculin, describing the phenomenon of delayed hypersensitivity. Although several workers became interested in the nature of "bacterial allergy" it was not until 1945 that

Landsteiner and Chase demonstrated the importance of cellular responses in the tuberculin reaction (Turk, 1975) and little thought was given to the relative contribution of "seed" and "soil" in the pathogenesis of infectious diseases until relatively recently.

Studies on lymphocytic choriomeningitis (LCM) in mice have provided dramatic evidence of the role of host factors in the production of immunologically-determined tissue damage (Cole *et al.*, 1971). Adult animals inoculated intracerebrally with the virus die from an acute encephalitis within 6–8 days. If inoculation is performed neonatally then the animals do not succumb and become life-long carriers of the virus. A similar effect can be produced by pretreating the adult animal with cyclophosphamide although either form of "carrier state" can be rapidly terminated by the administration of compatible spleen cells from a normal animal. Studies in man on hepatitis B, various forms of glomerulonephritis and other conditions such as dengue haemorrhagic fever have confirmed the importance of host factors in disease.

Although answers to many questions have emanated from work on microbial disease, it has mostly been a combination of interests in auto-immune disease, tissue transplantation and the development of techniques in protein chemistry that has fostered immunological enquiry to its present level.

The Recognition of Auto-immunity

Ehrlich and Morgenroth had anticipated the prospect of auto-immune disease in 1901 when they suggested the term "horror autotoxicus" for this possibility. Donath and Landsteiner described the first red cell auto-antibody in 1904 but it was not until 1938 that Dameshek and Schwartz re-discovered auto-immune haemolytic anaemia and proposed that auto-reactivity might be a more general phenomenon. Various experimental models were developed by Witebsky and others: the commonest means of production being to inject animals with tissue extracts in the presence of Freund's adjuvant. That a number of human diseases are characterized by the presence of auto-antibodies was soon established following the development of the technique of immunofluorescence by Coons in 1955. More recently, the story has come full circle with the knowledge that viruses have an important role in the development of several spontaneously occurring auto-immune diseases in animals and possibly in man. This adds a further dimension to the role of host factors in the pathogenesis of infectious disease.

Immunological Individuality and Transplantation

The existence of genetically determined tissue antigens was first established by Gorer in the 1930s. The further observation was made (Owen, 1945) that di-zygotic twin cattle sharing a placenta possess red cells with blood group antigens of both parental types. It was also shown that these non-identical twin animals would tolerate skin grafts exchanged between them. This led to work by Burnet's group in 1950 and Billingham, Brent and Medawar in 1953 in an attempt to discover whether the introduction of "foreign" material before an animal was immunologically mature would result in that material becoming recognized as "self". The latter group found that this was feasible in newborn mice receiving foreign cells and this phenomenon was termed "actively acquired tolerance".

Human organ grafting became a reality in the early 1960s with the advent of renal allo-transplantation. Although elegant animal experiments have suggested the possibility of inducing specific unresponsiveness to foreign antigens, this has not yet proved to be widely applicable as a means of immunosuppression in man and transplanted patients still have to be maintained on relatively large doses of non-specifically "immunosuppressive" drugs. It now appears that "immunological enhancement" or some other form of antibody-mediated immunosuppression may be more likely to achieve satisfactory results than antigen-induced tolerance (see Chapter 31).

Protein Chemistry and Antibody Structure

The presence of an unusual protein—now recognized as free antibody light chains—in the urine of a patient with myelomatosis was described as long ago as 1847 (Clamp, 1967). Little progress was made toward a clearer understanding of the nature of serum antibody until the development of plasma protein electrophoresis by Tiselius and Kabat in 1938. Antibodies were then characterized as γ-globulins and in 1948 Fagraeus demonstrated their synthesis by plasma cells. Porter showed in 1959 that the antigen combining sites of antibody molecules could be chemically separated from the biologically active sites that trigger the various effector systems such as serum complement. Soon after, Edelman discovered that antibody molecules contain four protein subunits—two "heavy" and two "light". These two lines of evidence enabled the asymmetrical four-chain structure of antibody molecules to be elucidated (see Chapter 4).

The development of gel diffusion methods for studying antigen–antibody interactions by Elek, Oudin and Ouchterlony in the late 1940s as well as the application of immunoelectrophoresis by Grabar and Williams in 1953 enabled great strides to be made in the analysis of antibody reactivity.

IgG (γG) and IgM (β2M) were early recognized to be two different kinds of antibody molecule but it was not until 1961 that Heremans identified IgA (β2A) as a separate class of antibody synthesized predominantly in the gastrointestinal tract. The recognition of myelomatosis as a condition associated with the neoplastic proliferation of a single clone of antibody-producing plasma cells and the discovery of "atypical" myeloma proteins made possible the identification of two further classes of antibody molecule—IgD in 1965 by Rowe and Fahey, and IgE in 1967 by Johansson and Bennich.

Cellular Immunology

Studies of cellular aspects of immunology had a much more leisurely start. Rudolf Virchow had noted as long ago as 1858 that circulating mononuclear cells could be either large or small, and was aware that "the more the glands become enlarged . . . the larger and more perfectly developed are the individual colourless cells of the blood wont to be". There was little addition to this state of knowledge until Gowans and his group described the heterogeneity and recirculation of lymphocytes in the 1960s (Gowans, 1966). Since then the study of the cells and tissues of the lymphoid system has been one of the most prolific areas of development. Glick and his colleagues described the accidental discovery of the importance of the bursa of Fabricius in antibody production in the chicken in 1956 and Miller drew attention to the key role of the thymus in immunological development in 1961. Cell mediated responses and their clinical counterpart "delayed hypersensitivity" had already been shown to function independently of antibody and in the 1960s it was found that some lymphocytes are capable of synthesizing soluble factors of their own—now known as lymphokines—which are responsible for many of the phenomena seen in cellular responses (Turk, 1975). It was not until 1970 that the presence of surface immunoglobulin was detected on those lymphocytes (B-cells) that are destined to transform into plasma cells and secrete antibody (Raff, 1976) and other "markers" were identified for the lymphocytes (T-cells) involved in cell mediated responses.

Evidence from various immunodeficiency states has given adequate confirmation of the compartmentation of the immune system into T- and B-cell components but the 1970s have also brought much work elucidating the phenomenon of "co-operation" between these two kinds of lymphocyte. Initially, this was thought only to operate in terms of T-cells providing help toward optimal B-cell function but evidence has now accumulated for suppressor activities as well. More recently, work in the mouse utilizing the Ly system of lymphocyte surface antigens suggests that there are different subpopulations of T-lymphocyte subserving the different biological roles that these cells may have i.e. helper cells, suppressor cells and killer cells (Feldmann *et al.*, 1975).

The Problem of Diversity

Each individual immunological response is remarkably specific in its reactivity but yet there are potentially millions of different responses. The means by which such a wide range of specificity of response could be elaborated within a single multi-cellular organism has produced various explanatory theories. In 1932 Haurowitz proposed an "instructive" theory of antibody formation in which the reactivity and specificity of the resultant antibody was largely determined by the nature of the immunizing antigen in so far as the latter acted as a "template" for the synthesis of the antibody molecules. The rival view that pre-existing clones of cells with their "ready-made" specific receptors are "selected" by antigen still holds sway (Burnet, 1959), but there is a long way to go before it satisfactorily explains how so much diversity is generated in the immune response. The differential contribution of the three possible sources of variation, i.e. germ-line genes, somatic mutation and, possibly, refinement of antibody specificity following antigen stimulation, is still under active investigation.

Genetic Aspects

In addition to the chemical and immunological uniqueness of the individual, evidence is accumulating concerning individual variation in the quality of immunological responses to defined antigens (Benacerraf and Katz, 1975). The genes which control the degree of reactivity are known as "immune response genes" and are closely linked with the histocompatibility genes in the mouse and perhaps also in man. Munro and Taussig (1975) emphasize how important the immune response gene products are in the co-operative process between T- and B-lymphocytes and suggest that there are two separate kinds of molecule involved: the one functioning as a co-operative factor released from the T-lymphocyte; the other functioning as an "acceptor" molecule on the surface of the B-lymphocyte. The exact nature of the specific antigen receptor on T-lymphocytes is still a matter for speculation, the choice lying between a molecule of immunoglobulin type or an immune response gene product.

THE LANGUAGE OF IMMUNOLOGY

The science of immunology is now readily divisible into immunochemistry, immunobiology and immunopathology. Much of the fundamental work which has been achieved in the last decade has been performed in academic departments embracing several basic disciplines other than immunology *per se* e.g. cell biology, protein chemistry, genetics and microbiology—with a recent accent on virology. It is not too surprising, therefore, that this spectrum of academic advancement should have brought with it a complex jargon of its own which may seem strange and unintelligible to the doctor with an enquiring interest in immunology. In some respects the language of immunology has become unnecessarily duplicated and this multiplies the potential confusion. Despite this, it is possible to understand most immunological nomenclature once a minimum vocabulary is mastered. A few immunological terms used to convey the more important ideas are discussed here and the meanings of some others can be located by reference to the index at the end of this book. For other definitions recourse should be had to the particularly useful "Dictionary of Immunology" recently published in a second edition (Herbert and Wilkinson, 1975).

Autologous or Allogeneic?

One of the commonest causes of confusion is the collection of words that are used to describe the immunological relationship between tissues or sera derived from animals of different genetic origins. Some of these are listed in Table 1 and it will be seen that there are four degrees of relationship for which there have arisen two different sets of terms. This is unfortunate but as both sets of terms are used frequently and synonymously they are listed here in parallel. Tissue or tissue fluid, e.g. serum, which has been returned to the organism from whence it came is described as *autologous* or *autochthonous* (the latter term was introduced initially by tumour immunologists). A transfer between two genetically identical members of the same species e.g. identical twins or two members of an inbred strain, is described as an *isologous* or *syngeneic* relationship. Where the relationship is between two different

TABLE 1
Parallel terms used to describe immunological relationships

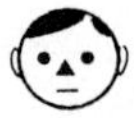	Autologous	Autochthonous
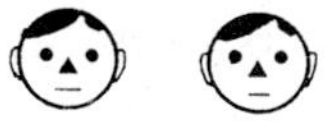	Isologous	Syngeneic
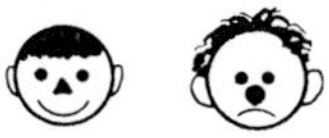	Homologous	Allogeneic
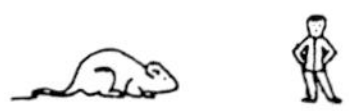	Heterologous	Xenogeneic

members of the same species it is described as *homologous* or *allogeneic*, and transfer between two entirely different species is described as *heterologous* or *xenogeneic*. The established tendency is to use the first set of terms to describe sera and the second to describe cells or whole organ grafts.

Antigen or Immunogen?

There is also a surfeit of words to describe foreign materials which elicit or interact with an immunological response. The most commonly used word is, simply, "antigen" which is best thought of as any material which when introduced into a whole organism is capable of inducing a specific immunological change in the reactivity of that organism. This change can take positive or negative forms and for this reason antigens have been subdivided into *immunogens* and *tolerogens* (Table 2). The word "tolerogen" has become more widely used as methods, mostly experimental at present, have been developed for inducing states of specific immunological unresponsiveness—often referred to as tolerance. This nomenclature has been widely adopted in a recent symposium on this subject (Dresser, 1976). An alternative, and more traditional, way of looking at antigen molecules is in terms of their small chemical determinants or *haptens* that are recognized by the relevant antibodies, and the surrounding or remaining part of the molecule, the *carrier*, which has to be covalently linked to individual haptens before the production of anti-hapten antibody can be induced (Table 2).

TABLE 2

Two different ways of assessing and describing antigenic material with reference to its biological properties

A.		
	Specific responsiveness	Specific unresponsiveness
IMMUNOGEN	+	−
TOLEROGEN	−	+
B.		
	EFFECT ON ANTI-HAPTEN ANTIBODY	
	Production	Neutralization
HAPTEN	−	+
HAPTEN-CARRIER	+	+

The term "antigenic determinant" is often used to refer to any definable part of an antigenic structure and usually one of an haptenic nature. More recently it has acquired the synonym *epitope*, with the term *paratope* denoting the complementary specific combining site on the antibody molecule. In certain circumstances antibodies can be raised against antigenic determinants occurring exclusively within the paratope of an antibody molecule and such determinants are referred to as *idiotypic*. As recent chemical and crystallographic studies suggest that the paratope is a cleft formed by the juxtaposition of three "hypervariable" regions (see Chapter 4) of the antibody molecule it is likely that anti-idiotypic antibodies are only able to recognize shallow or convex regions at the edge of the paratopic cleft.

A term which we have avoided throughout this book is *allergen*, which we take to be entirely synonymous with antigen. The word allergen is sometimes used to indicate foreign material that tends to elicit an immunological response which gives rise to an untoward effect within the host rather than conferring protection or benefit. We do not consider that there is sufficient evidence to indicate that chemical differences between antigens are themselves the primary reason for an untoward rather than a beneficial immune response in the host. Such considerations are reminiscent of the view alluded to above, and extant until relatively recently, that "bugs are bad" and the "host response is good". Antigens and related substances are dealt with in more detail in Chapter 5.

Allergy versus Immunity

The use of the word allergen is closely related to the interpretation of the word allergy. The majority of the lay public would consider the terms "allergy" and "allergic" to imply an unfortunate circumstance. When von Pirquet coined the term "allergy" he defined it simply as "altered reactivity", on the basis of his experience with Schick in the treatment of diphtheria with foreign immune sera. Others have argued (Gell and Coombs, 1963) that the term allergy should still be kept, among immunologists, to describe the whole breadth of immunological activity, whether beneficial or otherwise. This necessitates the use of terms such as "auto-allergy" and "allergized cells", a usage which has not gained general acceptance although, in terms of the original definition, it is more correct. It now seems too late to turn the clock back and restore the terms allergy and allergic to their originally intended use and meaning. For this reason we prefer to use the words immune, immunity and immunological in the most general sense so that immunological responses against self are referred to as auto-immunity and responses against foreign antigens as hetero-immunity. While not semantically ideal this usage, we feel, will be understood by a larger proportion of readers than the alternative nomenclature.

THE NATURE OF IMMUNOLOGICAL RESPONSES

Immunological responses are distinguishable from other recognition processes that occur in biological systems in their possession of three cardinal features. Firstly the recognition part of the response is remarkably *specific*, e.g. antibody can distinguish even between *l*- and *d*-forms of an isomeric antigen. Secondly, the acquisition of *memory* for the primary or first experience of a particular antigen enables subsequent responses to that antigen to occur over a shorter time scale. Subsequent responses also show *amplification* in both the quantity and quality of the response, although a plateau of reactivity may be reached after repeated challenge.

Specificity, alone, is a feature of various other recognition systems e.g. enzyme-substrate reactions and nucleotide interactions as well as many intercellular recognition events e.g. the re-aggregation of primitive multi-cellular organisms (such as slime moulds) and the entire process of embryogenesis. The strength of binding or affinity, and its range, varies widely among different systems (Fig. 1). Where the binding is homogeneous e.g. that between haem and globin, and between avidin and biotin, there is little spread around the mean but where a wide variety of molecules and their respective *ligands* exist, as with enzymes and their substrates and antibodies and their antigens, a broad range of heterogeneity is found.

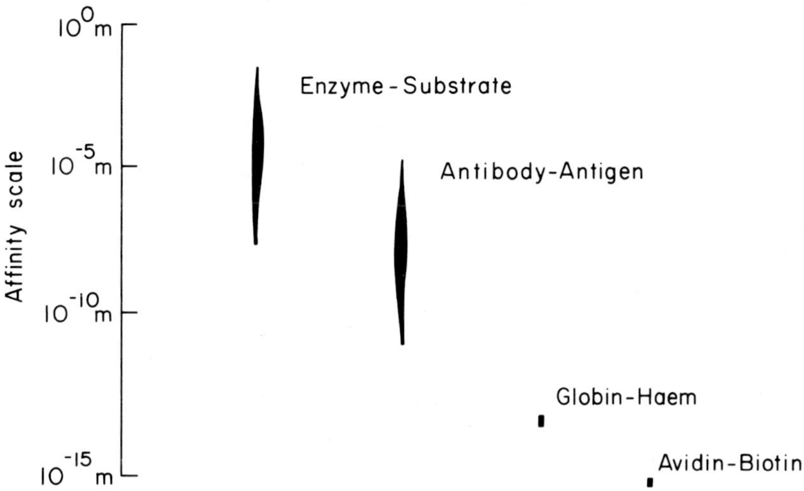

Fig. 1. A comparison of the contrasting affinity values and their ranges for different biological systems. The affinity value is the concentration of ligand at which half the binding sites are occupied. (Modified from Mitchison, 1968.)

The accurate identification of self is an intriguing example of the phenomenon of specific recognition and is likely to have been the evolutionary requirement which led to the immunological system becoming so highly specialized, both in phylogeny and ontogeny (Vitetta *et al.*, 1975). A similar discrimination is seen in the way in which individual members of some species are able to distinguish each other by the detection of olfactory stimuli or pheromones. There is evidence to suggest that although tracking dogs are able to discriminate between individual human beings they are unable to distinguish the scents of identical twins (Thomas, 1974).

Amplification might be thought to be a unique feature of immunological responses but a parallel is seen in the quantitative indication of enzyme activity that can occur e.g. in the liver, following the administration of significant amounts of substrates such as certain drugs. In the latter event, however, there is not the qualitative change in the reactive material seen with antibody responses, e.g. the switch from IgM to IgG production, and this, with the attribute of specific and long-lasting memory—the "altered reactivity" of von Pirquet—attests the distinctive nature of immunological responses.

It may not always be possible to demonstrate these three cardinal features in every response which is putatively immunological but a serious attempt should be made to do so before an immunological cause is ascribed to a particular clinical problem. Otherwise there is a real danger that "cause unknown"—often hallowed in medical jargon as "idiopathic"—may be replaced almost automatically by the word "immunological". When favism was first described, the haemolytic anaemia which followed the ingestion of broad beans (as well as other unrelated substances) in susceptible subjects was thought to be due to immunological hypersensitivity. This was only disproved when the deficiency of glucose-6-phosphate dehydrogenase was discovered in the red cell membrane. Likewise, the very severe exacerbations of asthma that are sometimes seen after the administration of relatively small amounts of aspirin have also been attributed to an immunological mechanism. These patients show the same kind of reaction to various other drugs and the abnormality is now thought to be one of prostaglandin metabolism. In both these examples the lack of chemical specificity was always a pointer to a non-immunological event.

On the other hand the reaction occurring in the lungs of certain individuals exposed to thermophilic *actinomycetes* found in mouldy hay is not only a specific phenomenon, at both the clinical and serological level, but can lead to progressive lung damage and fibrosis if exposure to the provoking antigen is not prevented. The more severe but fortunately rare reactions to bee stings, characterized by urticaria, nausea, vomiting, dyspnoea, cardiovascular collapse and unconsciousness, are not only specific, but the interval between the bite and the onset of unconsciousness is a guide to the degree of hypersensitivity and the likelihood of a fatal outcome (Frankland, personal communication).

LYMPHOID AND RETICULO-ENDOTHELIAL SYSTEMS

There has often been confusion concerning the distinction and interrelationship between the lymphoid and reticulo–endothelial systems. The latter term was coined by Aschoff to describe a system of cells that would take up and retain various dyes and particles. The *mononuclear phagocyte system* is a more common term today (see Chapter 8). The larger and more active phagocytic cells or *macro*phages fall into two categories:

i. *fixed macrophages*, which are usually found in intimate relationship with an extracellular reticular meshwork in tissues such as liver, spleen, lymph node, thymus, bone marrow and connective tissue in general. They are also referred to as reticular cells and play a part in the synthesis and maintenance of reticular fibres.

ii. *free macrophages*, which are the monocytes of the blood as well as the freely motile cells present in tissues and often referred to as histiocytes.

There is a constant interchange between both kinds of cell whose function is non-specific in immunological responses, except that specificity may be secondarily acquired by the passive uptake of antibody molecules and possibly other antigen-specific lymphokines (q.v.).

It is only very recently that the real functional activity of lymphocytes has been studied in any detail, but we know enough about their specific role in immunological responses and their unique pattern of recirculation to justify their collective consideration as "the lymphoid system". This term includes all tissue aggregations of lymphocytes, be they in lymph nodes, spleen, thymus and gut-associated lymphoid tissue or the freely circulating cells of the lymph or blood. The complex topography of lymphoid organs is gradually being defined in more accurate detail (Weiss, 1972), but what we already know of the differential aggregation of T- and B-lymphocytes into identifiable zones, and of their relationship with both categories of phagocytic cell, has provided an anatomical basis for the biological events of the immune response discussed in the following chapter.

A BIRD'S EYE VIEW OF THE IMMUNE SYSTEM

Subsequent chapters deal in some detail with the lymphoid system, immunoglobulins and various non-specific cells and mediators of relevance to the immune response. Nevertheless, in this introductory chapter, it may be useful to put a relatively simplified view of the immune system as a whole. Figure 2 presents a diagrammatic outline of the various components of the immune system and the way in which they react together to provide the highly specialized humoral and cellular responses characteristic of all mammalian organisms.

The primitive stem cells soon become committed to one of two progenies of lymphoid cell which differentiate in the *primary lymphoid organs* independently of the presence of antigen. These T- or B-lymphocytes emerge and

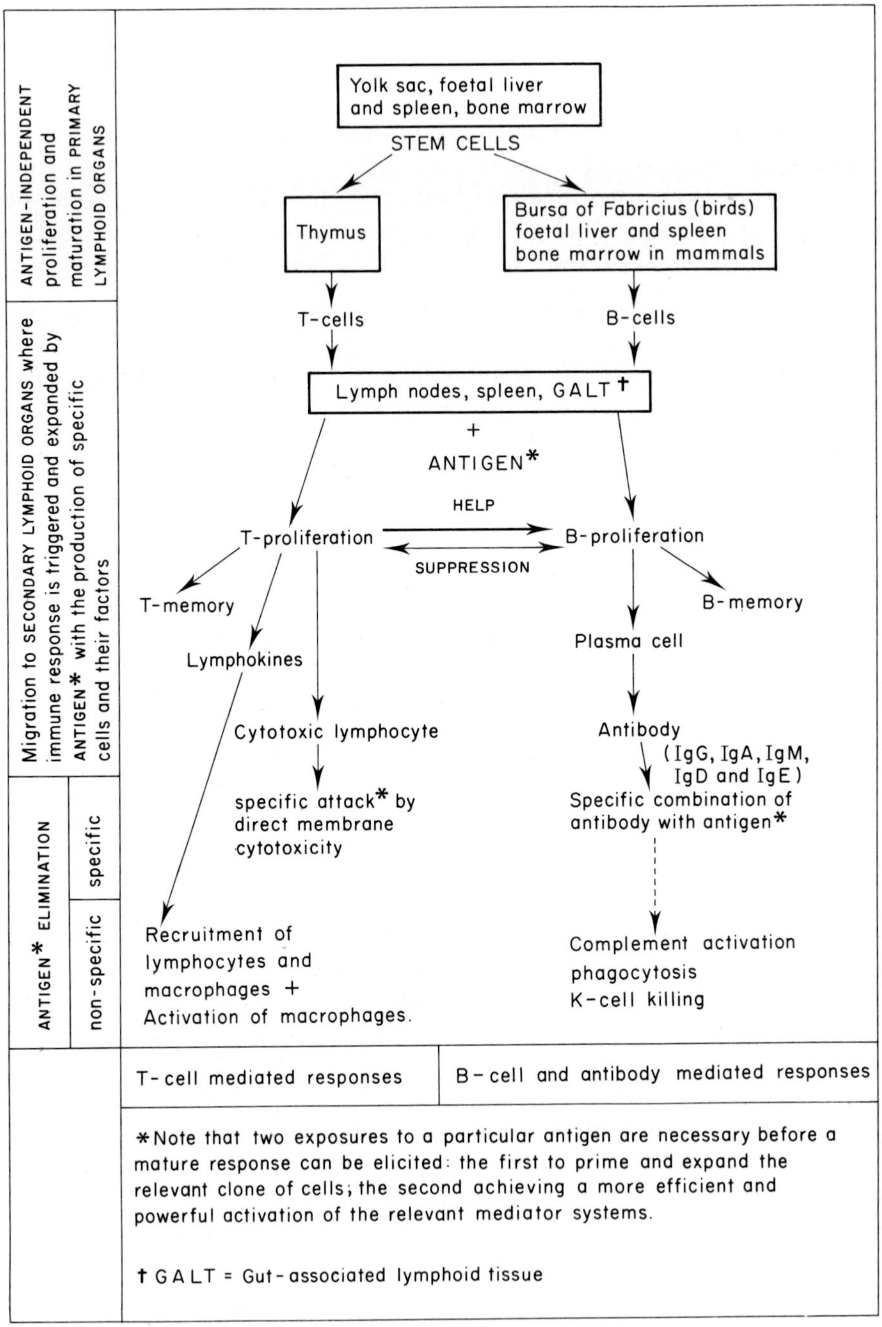

Fig. 2. A diagrammatic view of the interrelating components of the immune system.

migrate to various loci, the *secondary lymphoid organs*, where they are triggered and proliferate in response to contact with antigenic material. Studies of B-cell development in the avian bursa of Fabricius have helped to establish the two-compartment system of lymphocyte development, and studies on the nature of the thymic micro-environment have confirmed the view that the majority of the differentiation process occurs independently of antigen (Greaves *et al.*, 1973).

The lymph nodes, white pulp of the spleen and other secondary lymphoid organs, act as much more than filters of particulate and microbiological material. It is in these complex meeting places that T- and B-lymphocytes come into intimate contact with each other and with fixed and free macrophages and, in addition, it is here that antigen is localized in the early stages of the immune response. Antibody is first synthesized in plasma cells in the medulla of the lymph node and the red pulp of the spleen.

The structure of a typical lymph node is outlined in Figure 3. The lymphoid follicles occupy most of the cortex and consist predominantly of B-cells. The adjacent or "paracortical" area is that through which most of the T-cells circulate. The follicles become more prominent during an active local response and are then often referred to as germinal centres.

Lymphocytes have two routes of entry into the lymph node:

i. via the afferent lymphatics into the marginal sinus, and,
ii. direct entry from the blood stream across the post-capillary venules (p.c.v.s).

The p.c.v.s have become highly specialized in lymphoid tissue and occur at the cortico–medullary junction of the lymph node. The passage of lymphocytes across the p.c.v. is increased when a local response is taking place. This rapid and more direct route of lymphocyte ingress into the node can be seen as a means of disseminating the process of sensitization as efficiently as possible. Lymphocytes pass out of the node via the single efferent lymphatic and return to the blood via the thoracic duct. The relative lack of microscopical landmarks in lymph nodes has often caused their structure to be over-simplified but their functional anatomy is intricate (de Sousa, 1974).

The spleen is more complex in that it shares haematological and immunological functions and lacks lymphatic vessels. Despite this the white pulp shows similar lymphoid follicles and germinal centres and antigen localizes promptly after gaining access to the blood stream.

When T- and B-lymphocytes are successfully triggered by antigen they both respond initially in a similar way by transforming into blast cells. These cells are larger; they have a lower nuclear–cytoplasmic ratio; a vacuolated

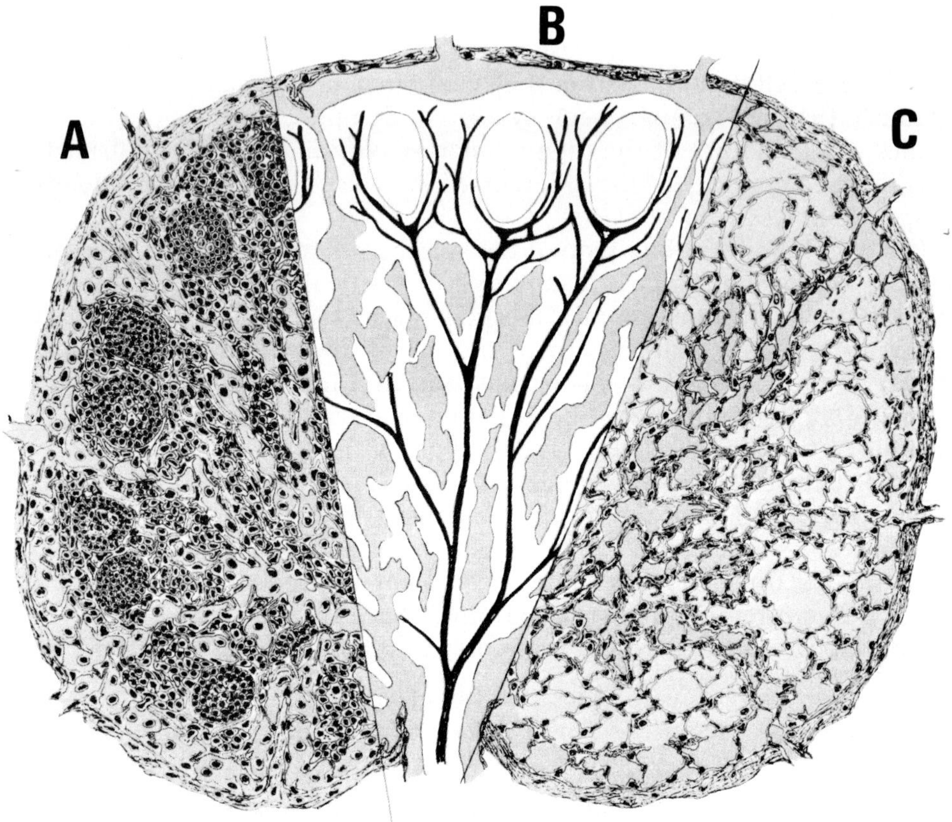

Fig. 3. Three aspects of lymph node structure:
A. lymphocytes are present in follicles in the cortex as well as within sinuses which extend into the medulla;
B. the venous network originates from the post-capillary venules situated around the lymphoid follicles;
C. the reticular meshwork extends throughout the node from the marginal sinus to the hilum and forms the structural basis for the follicles and sinuses.
(Modified from Weiss, 1972.)

and more basophilic cytoplasm; a lighter and more granular nucleus often with identifiable nucleoli; an outline which is less circular and a tendency to aggregate together, when compared with resting "small" lymphocytes (Fig. 4). On methyl green pyronin staining both T- and B-blasts show a bright pink "pyroninophilic" cytoplasm indicating an increase in its RNA content. In the electron microscope the two kinds of blast cell can be distin-

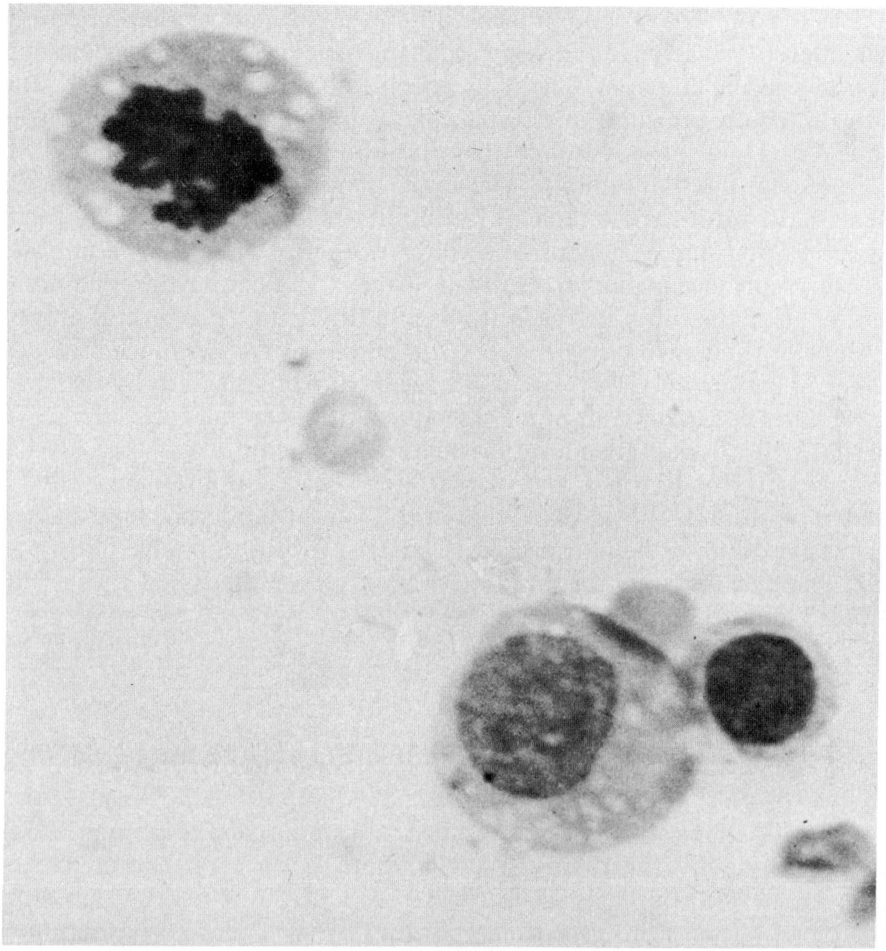

Fig. 4. Blast transformation of lymphocytes. A small resting lymphocyte is seen bottom right with a large stimulated or "blast" cell on its left-hand side. Another stimulated cell is seen proceeding to cell division (upper left). (Courtesy of Dr Joan Parker).

guished, for the T-cell cytoplasm contains many polyribosomes whereas B-cell blasts are characterized by a well developed endoplasmic reticulum. It is these latter cells which will give rise to mature plasma cells each capable of secreting *c.* 2,000 antibody molecules per hour during its brief life span of a few days. The T-blasts divide and give rise to daughter lymphocytes of like specificity which may function as helper, suppressor or killer cells (see above and Chapter 2).

It is as the afferent or recognition limb of the immune response hands over to the efferent or defence pathways that the specificity of the system merges with non-specific effectors. The truly specific components are T-cells, B-cells and the antibody products of plasma cells, although at least one of the soluble products of T-cells, the lymphokine migration inhibition factor, may exhibit a degree of antigen specificity. The large majority of the efferent mediator systems have no inherent recognition ability of their own but rely for their activation upon signals generated by one or other of the specific components. These non-specific mediators are responsible for creating the inflammatory component of the immune response and in doing so have several amplification steps of their own (see Chapters 7, 8 and 9). It is their inaccurate aim or unchecked action which is responsible for the host tissue damage which often occurs during a hetero-immune response. In auto-immune disease their efforts are misdirected by a faulty recognition system.

In the centre of Figure 2 the words "help" and "suppression" have been included to indicate the ways in which the T- and B-compartments have been shown to modulate their respective activities, in both positive and negative ways. These aspects of the immune response are discussed more fully in Chapter 2.

IMMUNOLOGICAL MECHANISMS IN DISEASE

Soon after Portier and Richet subdivided immunological responses into those with "prophylactic" and "anaphylactic" consequences, it became clear that there were several patterns of untoward response. For many years different kinds of reactions were grouped according to the speed of development of the pathological event e.g. erythema or oedema, and this gave rise to such terms as "immediate" and "delayed" hypersensitivity. The former category soon required subdivision, and it often proved difficult to assess the exact chronology of an individual response in tissues not amenable to direct observation. In 1963 Gell and Coombs proposed a classification of mechanisms of immunologically mediated tissue damage based on the kind of effector event that was giving rise to the inflammatory process. This has been used widely and has considerably enhanced understanding of immunological processes in disease. Their classification is currently expressed as follows:

Type I (anaphylactic, reagin-dependent)
Type II (cytotoxic or cell stimulating)

Type III (damage by antigen–antibody complexes)
Type IV (delayed, tuberculin-type, cell mediated).

It has become customary to refer to each of these four types by the appropriate Roman numeral and this, as well as a lack of a single unambiguous name for each of these mechanisms can cause confusion to those who are not using this classification in everyday speech. Furthermore, it is becoming increasingly difficult to include all the documented immunopathological phenomena within this framework. Antibody-dependent K-cell cytotoxicity does not fit clearly into this scheme as it can occur in the absence of complement and is an effective means of target cell damage. The classical "Type IV" reaction still rests upon the clinical phenomenon of delayed hypersensitivity for which various components of the immune system may be required e.g. T-cells, macrophages and lymphokines. Yet macrophages and T-cells can produce tissue damage when activated independently of each other. It is for these reasons that we propose an extended form of this classification which allows each well-documented immunopathological process to stand alone without prejudging its contribution to any particular clinical entity (Table 3).

We have chosen to define six mechanisms of immunological damage, three "antibody" and three "cellular", each with its own self-explanatory title. The first three (antibody) mechanisms are exactly comparable to those of Gell and Coombs' classification except that we have opted for a nomenclature that describes and thus reminds the reader of the nature of the mechanism concerned.

We have used the term "reaginic" in preference to anaphylactic for two reasons. Firstly, "reaginic" allows inclusion of any class of antibody e.g. IgG_4, which sensitizes the appropriate mediator cells. Secondly, the term "anaphylactic" is sometimes used loosely to describe a particular clinical picture which may not always be mediated by basophil or mast cell degranulation e.g. endotoxin shock. The term "anaphylatoxin" which is still used collectively for active fragments of C3 and C5, confuses this usage further.

The term "cytotoxic" seems to have out-lived its usefulness for complement mediated damage to cell-surface or basement membranes and excludes the stimulating effect that some antibodies may have when interacting with antigen on cell-surfaces. Thus we have chosen the term "membrane-reactive" as the least ambiguous for describing this mechanism.

"Immune-complex" mediated damage is self-explanatory and widely understood. The term immune is used here in its most general sense as discussed on p. 10.

The subdivision of "cell mediated" reactions into three mechanistic components is the more adventurous part of our classification. Now that the particular kind of cell involved in antibody-independent target cell killing has been more clearly defined as a thymus-processed or T-lymphocyte it seems reasonable to let this stand alone as a separate T-cell mechanism in which the damage may be brought about by direct membrane cytotoxicity or inflammatory lymphokines or a combination of both.

TABLE 3
Mechanisms of immunological damage

	Title	Triggering device	Mediators
ANTIBODY MECHANISMS	Reaginic	Reaginic antibody (IgE or possibly IgG_4)	Histamine, SRS-A,[a] ECF-A,[b] etc.
	Membrane-reactive	Antibody (IgG, IgM or IgA) with specificity for membrane bound antigen	Complement, polymorphs and their lysosomal enzymes
	Immune complex	Cell-free antigen–antibody complexes	Complement, polymorphs and their lysosomal enzymes
CELLULAR MECHANISMS	T-cell	T-Lymphocytes	Lymphokines ± membrane effects
	K-Cell	Other cytotoxic mononuclear cells plus membrane-fixed antibody	Soluble factors ± membrane effects
	Macrophage	Macrophages plus antibody, antigen–antibody complexes or other activating factors	Lysosomal enzymes ± membrane effects

[a] SRS-A = slow-reacting substance of anaphylaxis
[b] ECF-A = eosinophil chemotactic factor of anaphylaxis

It is now well established that certain mononuclear cells having Fc receptors are able to destroy antibody coated target cells (Seligmann *et al.*, 1975). These are most often referred to as K (or killer) cells and probably achieve their effect via direct membrane damage or release of soluble factors. This mechanism, which has been shown to be of importance in various clinical situations e.g. thyroiditis, graft rejection and the response to tumours, we call K-cell damage.

Lastly, macrophages may acquire cytotoxic properties in the presence of antibody of classes IgG_1 and IgG_3, especially when complexed to antigen, and in the presence of specific macrophage arming factor which may itself be antibody-like (Evans *et al.*, 1972), as well as other non-specific factors. Much of the damage seen in this macrophage mechanism is due to direct membrane contact although the release of lysosomal enzymes can produce abundant tissue injury.

Table 3 contrasts the six mechanisms in terms of their triggering devices and mediators. It is important to realize that practically any combination of these mechanisms may be operating in a particular clinical situation and there is certainly much more to be learned about their interrelationships in disease. Jones-Mote (cutaneous basophil) hypersensitivity (Turk, 1975) represents an interesting link between reaginic and T-cell mechanisms. Reaginic and immune-complex mechanisms seem to have an interdependent relationship in some patients with asthmatic responses to foreign antigens (Pepys *et al.*, 1968).

This six-fold classification of immunologically-mediated tissue damage is discussed further in Chapter 10 and has been adopted throughout this book. Time alone will determine its usefulness but we hope it may help to communicate to the uninitiated the various immunopathological possibilities at present defined.

In a clinical context such classifications obviously emphasize the pathological aspects of the immune response but it is important to consider the physiological roles of the individual mechanisms. Chapter 7 discusses the importance of complement mediated mechanisms in host defence. The gross and, often systemic, manifestations of "immune complex" disease need to be considered in terms of extreme overload of normal (and sometimes abnormal) processes by which complexed material is disarmed and eliminated. Chapter 11 takes up the question why such overload should occur, permitting the development of what is often widespread tissue damage. Chapter 9 deals with the physiological aspects of T-cell functions; K-cells are discussed further in Chapter 3 although their physiological role, as yet ill-defined, and macrophages are covered in Chapter 8. The raison d'etre of the reaginic mechanism is still a major enigma. Several possibilities are discussed briefly in Chapter 22.

The Immunological Balance Sheet

This introduction has tended to emphasize the debit side of the immune response only because the potential for host damage has often been overlooked in the past. Man has attained his relative freedom from microbial and parasitic disease as well as his expectation of longevity only in the last hundred years or so and it is not improbable that for most of his evolutionary history, ecological survival has been won at a considerable price.

In addition, the continual intrusion of foreign genetic material e.g. viruses, may have an important role in the expansion and heterogeneity of the host genome and it has even been postulated that our cellular energy-producing organelles, the mitochondria, may have a microbial ancestry.

TABLE 4

States of host responsiveness

Response state	Examples
Specific reactivity: *Hetero-immunity* without host damage	Response to oral polio vaccine Graft rejection
Specific reactivity: *Hetero-immunity* with host damage	Post-primary tuberculosis Drug hypersensitivity
Specific reactivity: *Auto-immunity*	Idiopathic Addison's disease Auto-immune haemolytic anaemia
Non-specific reactivity:	Auto-immune disorders e.g. SLE Some bacterial and viral infections Atopic disease
Specific non-reactivity:	"Enhancement" of renal allografts Response to some tumours
Non-specific non-reactivity: i.e. "anergy"	Primary immunodeficiency Sarcoidosis Hodgkin's disease Lepromatous leprosy

Although a significant part of the ontogenetic development of the immune system occurs independently of antigenic stimulation the latter is required for a degree of immunological maturity to be reached which will equip the normal organism to cope adequately with most likely antigenic experiences. When the mature organism comes into contact with a particular antigen there are several possible ways in which it may respond, each having a different potential for host benefit or damage (Table 4). These different states of host responsiveness include all the patterns of reactivity that may be seen in health and disease. They are discussed more fully in Chapter 31 in relation to the desirability of a particular response and its manipulation by therapeutic means.

It is toward limiting or preventing the damaging effects of immune responses that much effort is now directed in clinical immunology. Nonspecific measures for blotting out immune responses have been with us for some time and have given rise to a steady flow of iatrogenic disease, especially opportunistic infection. The development of more specific methods of modulating the powerful effects of antigenic stimulation is likely to transform many aspects of medical care in the future.

REFERENCES

Benacerraf, B. and Katz, D. H. (1975). The nature and function of histocompatibility-linked immune response genes. *In* "Immunogenetics and Immunodeficiency". (Ed. B. Benacerraf), MTP. Lancaster.

Billingham, R. E., Brent, L. and Medawar, P. B. (1953). "Actively acquired tolerance" of foreign cells. *Nature* **172**, 603.

Burnet, M. (1954). The clonal selection theory of acquired immunity. Cambridge University Press, London and Cambridge.

Clamp, J. R. (1967). Some aspects of the first recorded case of multiple myeloma. *Lancet* **2**, 1354.

Cole, G. A., Gilden, D. H., Monham, A. A. and Nathanson, N. (1971). Lymphocytic choriomeningitis virus pathogenesis of acute central nervous system disease. *Fed. Proc.* **30**, 1831.

Dresser, D. W. (Editor) (1976). Immunological tolerance. *Brit. Med. Bull.* **32**, 99–192.

Evans, R., Grant, C. K., Cox, H., Steele, K. and Alexander, P. (1972). Thymus-derived lymphocytes produce an immunologically specific arming factor. *J. Exp. Med.* **136**, 1318.

Feldman, M., Beverley, P. C. L., Dunkley, M. and Kontiainen, S. (1975). Different Ly antigen phenotypes of *in vitro* induced helper and suppressor cells. *Nature* **258**, 614.

Gell, P. G. H. and Coombs, R. R. A. (1963). "Clinical Aspects of Immunology." Blackwell, Oxford.

Glick, B., Chang, T. S. and Jaap, R. G. (1956). The bursa of Fabricius and antibody production. *Poultry Sci.* **35**, 224.

Gowans, J. L. (1966). Life-span, recirculation and transformation of lymphocytes. *Int. Rev. exp. Path.* **5**, 1.

Greaves, M. F., Owen, J. J. T. and Raff, M. C. (1973). "T and B Lymphocytes: Origins, Properties and Roles in Immune Responses." *Excerpta Med.* Amsterdam.

Herbert, W. J. and Wilkinson, P. C. (Editors) (1975). "A Dictionary of Immunology." Second edition. Blackwell, Oxford.

Miller, J. F. A. P. (1961). Immunological function of the thymus. *Lancet* **2**, 748.

Mitchison, N. A. (1968). *Symp. Int. Soc. Cell. Biol.* **7**, 29.

Munro, A. J. and Taussig. M. J. (1975). Two genes in the major histocompatibility complex control immune response. *Nature* **256**, 103.

Owen, R. D. (1945). Immunogenetic consequences of vascular anastomoses between bovine twins. *Science* **102**, 400.

Pepys, J., Hargreave, F. E., Chan, M. and McCarthy, D. S. (1968). Inhibitory effects of disodium cromoglycate on allergen-inhalation tests. *Lancet* **2**, 134.

Porter, R. R. (1962). The structure of gamma-globulin and antibodies. *In* "Basic Problems in Neoplastic Disease". (Eds. A. Gellhorn and E. Hirschberg.) Columbia University Press, New York.

Raff, M. C. (1976). Cell-surface immunology, *Scient. Amer.* **234**, 30.
Reid, R. (1974). "Microbes and Men." BBC Publications, London.
Seligmann, M., Preud'Homme, J. L. and Kourilsky, F. M., (Eds.). (1975). Membrane receptors of lymphocytes. North-Holland Publishing Co., Amsterdam and Oxford.
de Sousa, M. (1974). Lymphocyte traffic. *Progr. Immunol.*, II, **2**, 353.
Thomas, L. (1974). Biological signals for self-identification. *Progr. Immunol.* II, **2**, 239.
Turk, J. L. (1975). "Delayed Hypersensitivity." Second edition, North-Holland Publishing Co., Amsterdam.
Virchow, R. (1858). "Cellular Pathology."
Vitetta, E. S., Artzt, K., Bennett, D., Boyse, E. A. and Jacob, F. (1975). Structure similarities between a product of the T/t-locus isolated from sperm and teratoma cells, and H-2 antigens isolated from splenocytes. *Proc. Nat. Acad. Sci. (U.S.A.)* **72**, 3215.
Weiss, L. (1972). "The Cells and Tissues of the Immune System." Prentice-Hall, New Jersey.

I

The Immune System

2

The Lymphoid System

E. J. HOLBOROW and W. G. REEVES

ADAPTIVE IMMUNITY

The evolution of multi-cellular organisms brought with it even at a very primitive stage a vital need for an internal system of defence against invasive foreign organisms. The basic requirements for success in such a defence system are the ability to distinguish foreign cells from the individual's own body cells, combined with the ability to destroy or in some other way inactivate them. A means of recognition evolutionarily to hand was the array of macromolecules at the surface of cell membranes whose molecular configurations were already providing recognition patterns between cells, and contributing to cell ordering and growth regulation both in the organism as a whole and in differentiated organs and tissues within it. It is possible that as well as regulating cell association in a general way, such inter-cell reactions based on the fit or lack of fit of surface conformations may have also been playing an important role in reproduction by discouraging self-fertilization between the gametes of a single individual. At any rate, it appears that the primitive development of defences against microbial infection along Metchnikovian lines by the differentiation of scavenger cells with phagocytic properties was based upon molecular recognition patterns already operating at the surface of the phagocytic cell membrane.

The effectiveness of a non-specific defence system of this cell-based sort is limited, and with the increasing complexity and size of multi-cellular organisms evolutionary pressure called for its amplification. To some degree this need was met by the development of complement-like and other enzymically activated non-specific humoral systems and by further refinement of the recognition properties of phagocytic cells, even to the point of allowing a degree of self/non-self discrimination, as seen in the coelomocytes of some invertebrate species. With vertebrate development, however, further amplification along purely phagocytic lines proved inadequate and evolution of more versatile mechanisms of tissue defence against microorganisms and their products became a pre-condition of survival. Table 1 (taken from Manning, 1975) lists some of the steps in vertebrate evolution which have had important consequences for immunological development.

It has been plausibly argued that another reason for the development of a more sophisticated system of immunity was the relatively marked tendency of vertebrate tissues to undergo malignant changes. Malignant cells may express new surface components, and a sensitive tissue surveillance system capable of fine discrimination between normal and malignant cells might have developed in response to the need to keep this tendency in check. The hard evidence for such a tumour surveillance role for the immune system is however lacking, and it now seems more likely that the oft-quoted increased incidence of lymphoid tumours in immunodeficient patients represents a failure of defence against oncogenic viruses, rather than deficient surveillance of neoplasia.

Whether from one or more such root causes, vertebrates evolved a second defence system on an altogether different scale of versatility, a system of immunity based upon the lymphocyte. The versatility and the enhanced immune potential inherent in the lymphoid immune system stem from its adaptiveness, which contrasts strongly with the limited and more rigidly constitutive character of more primitive phagocytic systems. The lymphoid system exploits a different property, the ability of lymphocytes not merely to recognize a general foreignness in macromolecules, but to distinguish with marked specificity quite small differences in chemical composition between them, for example the insertion of a different amino acid in a polypeptide sequence or a change in a terminal sugar in a polysaccharide side-chain. This property of each individual lymphocyte, a genetically directed ability to recognize one of a very large number of possible chemical determinants (not only such as occur naturally in biological macromolecules, but even chemical groupings artificially synthesized and incorporated into appropriate carrier molecules) is the basis of the adaptive immunity of vertebrates. Recognition at this specific level of chemical determinants depends upon a fundamental biological event, the binding at the lymphocyte surface of the molecule (antigen) carrying the specific determinant in question. The specific binding sites on the lymphocyte surface have a three-dimensional cleft-like configuration which for each cell precisely fits the shape of a particular antigenic determinant and fits less well a few others which bear a more or less close relationship to it. The binding-sites or antigen-receptors of lymphocytes thus have the same specificity properties as antibody, and it is not surprising that they have turned out to be immunoglobulin or immunoglobulin-like in nature. The closer the fit the higher the binding affinity generated by non-covalent intermolecular forces of the van der Waal type, and under appropriate conditions this close binding triggers lymphocyte mitosis and proliferation, generating from each cell so stimulated a clonal progeny of like binding affinity.

TABLE 1

Steps in vertebrate evolution with possible immunological implications (Manning, 1975)

Evolutionary step	Significance to immune system
Increased body size and longer life span	Requirement for efficient self-surveillance
Loss of free-living larval stages	Amniotic protection from environmental antigens; this may permit prolongation of immune differentiation
More efficient circulation of body fluids	Lymphocytic circulatory pathways may become more specialized
Homoiothermy	Affects internal environment for growth of micro-organisms
Placentation	Maternal-foetal interactions

Macromolecules able to stimulate certain genetically programmed lymphocytes to mitosis on this specific basis are antigens, or immunogens, by definition (see Chapter 1, and Index). Their triggering effect is thus clonal, and contrasts with the action of non-specific lymphocyte mitogens such as phytohaemagglutinin and bacterial lipopolysaccharide, which by binding to a different category of cell-surface receptors stimulate broad subpopulations of lymphocytes in polyclonal fashion irrespective of the specific antigen receptors they also carry.

The effects of antigenic stimulation are thus to enlarge by clonal proliferation the population of lymphocytes with high binding affinity for the antigen in question. Some of these lymphocyte clones are launched on the pathway to maturation as immunoglobulin-synthesizing and immunoglobulin-secreting cells (plasma cells), the secreted immunoglobulins produced by the latter being antibodies which carry binding sites identical with those represented on the parent lymphocyte surface. These newly generated lymphocytes, together with antibody molecules of identical specific binding affinity, between them deploy a markedly enhanced potential for activating existing non-specific defence mechanisms, a potential which is released (and at the same time focussed) on interaction with antigen wherever they encounter it in the body. The lymphoid immune system is thus truly adaptive, its specific biological reactivity with antigenic material leading to recruitment of cellular and humoral specific effectors of defence both distantly and locally, and bringing them to bear where needed in augmented numbers and concentration.

An important corollary of the specific responsiveness of an adaptive immune system of this sort is that as well as providing for a rapid primary increase in specific effectors against antigen, it creates also a reserve of new lymphocytes of the same specificity—memory cells—which persists after the immediate need for specific effectors has passed, and is in turn able to mount a further enhanced response—the classical secondary response—on subsequent antigenic encounter. Meanwhile the effector potential of the system as a whole remains unimpaired and may be readily expanded and refocussed by similar processes of clonal proliferation against successive invasive immunogenic materials of completely different specificities.

LYMPHOCYTES AND ANTIBODIES

The existence of specific antibodies in immune serum had been unequivocally demonstrated, and many of their properties studies in depth long before immunoglobulin proteins were biochemically characterized or their cellular origin demonstrated. In 1900, Ehrlich proposed that the specificity of cell surface receptors must reflect that of circulating antibodies, and that antibodies are in fact specific receptors whose production at the cell surface has been stimulated to such a degree by the binding of antigen that many are shed free into the tissue fluids and blood. Except that Ehrlich did not think the cells in question were lymphocytes, his theory adumbrated modern views on the clonal basis of antibody production with remarkable verity. Since it was first shown that plasma cells produce and secrete antibody (Fagraeus, 1948), the ontogeny of these unicellular immunoglobulin factories has been gradually sketched in, and we now know that they are end cells differentiating from a distinct subpopulation of precursor lymphocytes as a result of antigenic stimulation. The prior maturation of this precursor subpopulation in the bone marrow and elsewhere after an earlier mitotic sequence still ill-defined but demonstrably independent of antigen, has equipped them with specific antigen-binding receptors which are readily identifiable by immunofluorescence as immunoglobulin in nature. These precursor lymphocytes belong to the B-cell subpopulation.

CELL MEDIATED IMMUNITY

Lymphocytes play a central role in immune responses not only in antibody production but also in the different types of specific cell mediated response, including immune reactions to viruses, delayed hypersensitivity and graft rejection. Clinical evidence of this comes from the rare immune deficiencies consequent upon congenital thymic aplasias such as diGeorge's and Nézelof's syndromes (Chapter 14). Clear cut experimental evidence was provided by J. L. Gowans and his colleagues, who studied the effects of manipulating the small lymphocyte population of the lymph in the thoracic ducts of rats. These experiments showed (i) that depletion of the lymphocyte population of thoracic duct lymph by chronic drainage impairs the ability to reject grafts, (ii) that intravenous injection of thoracic duct lymphocytes obtained from a given donor induces graft-versus-host reactions in appropriately chosen recipients, unless the donor has been previously rendered tolerant to the recipient strain in question, (iii) that as well as mediating these cellular immune reactions, thoracic duct lymphocytes also play a part in antibody production, and (iv) that they belong to a mobile population of small lymphocytes that recirculates from blood to lymph and back again.

Another major step confirming the central immunological role of lymphocytes was Miller's notable demonstration that neonatal thymectomy in mice not only reduces the subsequent count of circulating lymphocytes as compared with that of normal mice, but leads both to runting and to a striking impairment of the ability of the treated animals to reject skin grafts from other strains. Mouse thymocytes carry a particular surface antigen (θ) which is readily identifiable by fluorescent staining with anti-θ serum or by the cytotoxic effect of the latter (Raff and Wortis, 1970). The θ-antigen is also present on cells which form part of the lymphocyte population present in normal mouse spleen and blood. These θ-positive cells are a distinct subpopulation, however, and do not carry readily demonstrable surface immunoglobulin; the B-cells have the latter, but no θ-antigen. In neonatally thymectomized mice, while serum immunoglobulin levels remain unaffected or even increase, θ-positive peripheral lymphocytes are absent; but when a thymus graft from another mouse is implanted as a replacement, chromosome marker studies have shown that the thymus graft becomes repopulated with the *recipient's* lymphocytes, and that θ-positive peripheral lymphocytes also of recipient type re-appear. Both these events depend upon the presence of intact bone marrow.

The implication of these findings is that there must be at least two major functional subpopulations of lymphocytes in the spleen, blood and peripheral lymphoid organs of the mouse. The lymphocytes belonging to one of these subpopulations have readily detectable surface Ig, and are the precursors of plasma cells and the progenitors of memory cells with antibody producing potential; the lymphocytes of the other subpopulation require the presence of the thymus for their maturation, and although also carrying antigenic-specific receptors do not possess readily demonstrable surface Ig. The lymphocytes of this latter subpopulation function as immune effectors in their cellular capacity.

The presence of these two subpopulations of lymphocytes, thymus dependent (T-cells) and thymus independent (B-cells), appears to be a general characteristic at least of mammalian immune systems. In man, a thymus cell marker antigen comparable with mouse θ is not so readily demonstrable and a completely different surface property, the ability to form rosettes with sheep red cells, is commonly used as a distinguishing T-cell feature (see Chapter 3).

THE ORIGIN OF B-CELLS

The precursors of antibody forming cells were first identified as a separate subpopulation of lymphocytes in chickens, where the development of these cells takes place in the microenvironment of the bursa of Fabricius, an epithelial organ situated in the cloaca at the junction of endoderm and ectoderm. In the embryo chick, haemopoietic stem cells infiltrate the proliferating epithelium of the bursa and initiate formation of follicles from which the precursors of antibody-forming cells (the term B-cell indicates their bursal origin) are exported to mature in the lymphoid tissue of the spleen and gut. No plasma cells develop in the bursa itself, and in the adult bird the latter atrophies. Nevertheless its essential role as a *primary lymphoid organ* is demonstrated by the effects of treating the developing embryo with testosterone; this inhibits bursal development by changing the character of its epithelium in such a way as to prevent infiltration of haemopoietic cells, with the result that the hatched bird is permanently depleted not only of B-cells, but of serum immunoglobulins and plasma cells, although its cellular immunity responses remain effective.

In the developing chick embryo, Ig-receptor-bearing B-cells appear in the peripheral lymphoid tissues and blood at the time of peak infiltration of the bursa with haemopoietic stem cells. Initially these B-cells carry IgM surface immunoglobulin only. IgG follows, and soon most cells have both IgM and IgG. Early administration of specific anti-chicken IgM antiserum prevents not only the appearance of IgM cells and their acquisition of IgG, but also suppresses the subsequent appearance of IgM, IgG and IgA immunoglobulins in the serum.

The bursal analogue which in mammals produces the Ig-receptor-bearing B-lymphocytes was for long in doubt. Haemopoietic stem cells in the mouse embryo initially migrate into the developing liver, and later into the developing spleen and bone marrow. The first cells identifiable as B-lymphocytes appear in the liver, and very soon afterwards in the marrow, spleen and peripheral blood. B-cell precursors have no convenient marker antigen comparable with θ on mouse thymocytes. Conclusions about their lineage are largely based on studies of cell clones developing from haemopoietic tissues under appropriate culture conditions (Metcalf and Moore, 1971). Cells capable of giving rise to such colonies of B-lymphocytes are present in the foetal liver, spleen and bone marrow, and in the bone marrow of adult mice. If the mouse embryo may be taken as a model, it seems that in mammalian lymphoid systems there is no single organ which is the bursal analogue, but rather that haemopoietic tissue, especially in the foetal liver, as well as elsewhere, plays the primary lymphoid role of inducing B-cell progenitor cells. In adult mammals, B-lymphocyte formation takes place in the bone marrow but it has not been excluded that it is also occurring in the spleen and lymph nodes.

THE ORIGIN OF T-CELLS

As we have seen, a functionally distinct subpopulation of lymphocytes recirculates in the blood and lymph, and traverses the lymphoid tissues of the spleen, gut and lymph nodes; these are T-cells, depending upon prior passage through the thymus for their maturation. For the essential part it plays in producing T-cells in effective functional form, the thymus is also classed as a primary lymphoid organ; without it, cell-mediated immune function does not develop and the deprived infant is immunologically crippled. In contrast, the lymphoid tissues of the spleen, gut and lymph nodes play no such primary role in T-cell physiology. The stem cells ancestral to T-cells arise, like those of B-cells, in the yolk sac of the embryo and initially localize in the bone marrow, from which they are released into the blood and pass to the thymus.

The thymus thus provides an inductive microenvironment for differentiation of these bone marrow precursor cells into T-lymphocytes, the inductive stimulus arising from its epithelial cells. This epithelium is, like that of the bursa, derived from a junctional region of ectoderm and endoderm. In the case of the thymus it arises from the third branchial pouch, epithelium from which it buds off, migrates into the thorax, and differentiates further under mesenchymal influence. The T-cell precursors enter the thymus anlage, and their maturation begins, a process which again has been more closely studied in the mouse than in man. In the foetal mouse, T-cell precursors are large blast-like cells, which rapidly acquire the "θ-antigen", now known as Thy-1. These precursor cells proliferate vigorously and differentiate into two distinct types of small lymphocytes. The major class, accounting for 90% of thymus lymphocytes, carries large amounts of Thy-1 antigen and is sensitive to injury by both cortisone and irradiation. These cells are immunologically non-functional, and are mostly located in the thymic cortex. The majority apparently never leave the thymus, and die within it. A minor class, less than 10% of the total thymocytes, are small lymphocytes which carry less Thy-1 antigen, are cortisone resistant, and are immunocompetent (Droege and Zucker, 1975). They are located primarily in the medulla, and more closely resemble peripheral T-cells in their properties. It is postulated from the results of challenge experiments with alloantigens that differentiation of cells in the thymus, as well as producing precursors of the T-cells destined for peripheral circulation, at the same time eliminates by modification or death the cells which have recognized antigen intrathymically—that is to say, auto-reactive cells—and that this may in part explain how the peripheral T-cell population becomes tolerant of self-antigens.

Thymic Hormone

The thymus produces a number of soluble factors which influence differentiation and maturation of T-cells. A low molecular weight acidic polypeptide isolated from calf or human thymus, known as thymosin, has the properties of a hormone, since it appears to act at sites distant from the thymus on stem cells already committed to the pathways of T-cell differentiation. The thymus thus behaves as an endocrine gland, and to this extent thymosin can substitute for it. Administration of thymosin *in vivo* prevents or modifies the sequelae of neonatal or adult thymectomy in mice, and incubation with thymosin *in vitro* converts T-cell precursors from the spleens or bone-marrow of congenitally athymic ("nude") mice into functional T-cells.

Thymosin is present in human blood, and may be assayed by an ingenious rosette method. Nucleated cells from mouse lymphoid tissues form rosettes on mixing with sheep red blood cells, but in the presence of the drug azathioprine, rosette formation is inhibited. If thymosin is also present, the minimal inhibitory concentration of azathioprine is reduced in proportion to the concentration of thymosin. With this assay method it has been shown that thymosin levels in the blood in young people are high, and that the thymosin content of human blood falls significantly between 20 and 40 years of age. Blood levels of thymosin are low in patients with Hodgkin's disease, chronic lymphatic leukaemia, and some primary immunodeficiency states (Goldstein *et al.*, 1974). Exposure to thymosin *in vitro* increases the number of blood lymphocytes forming E-rosettes in primary immunodeficiency (Wara *et al.*, 1975) and reverses the apparent T-cell lymphopenia in patients with acute influenza virus infection (Scheinberg *et al.*, 1976). What useful role thymosin may have in the diagnosis and treatment of T-cell deficiency conditions remains to be defined.

CELLULAR INTERACTIONS IN IMMUNE RESPONSES

Although lymphocytes fall into at least two subpopulations, one equipped for antibody formation and the other for direct cellular action, the two do not function independently. The central feature of the immune response is the interaction of antigen and the immunocompetent cell; but for full implementation of the response a variety of cellular interactions is necessary, not only between different classes of lymphocytes but also between lymphocytes and accessory cells such as macrophages, monocytes and polymorphonuclear leucocytes.

These interactions have again been identified predominantly on the basis of information from mouse experiments, where the development of highly inbred strains has allowed detailed studies of the effects of selective cell depletion and transfer in genetically defined stock. Similar interactions occur in man, although supporting evidence is predictably more difficult to come by, and we may be sure that normal human immune function likewise depends on a complex system of precise and distinct cellular interactions which link and control the afferent or recognition and efferent or defence limbs of the immune system.

Co-operation Between T- and B-cells

Two types of experiment initially made clear the fundamental fact that interaction between T- and B-cells is necessary for a full antibody response to most antigens. Firstly, irradiated thymectomized mice reconstituted with either thymus cells or bone marrow cells proved capable of making only a weak antibody response to injection of sheep red cells, but when given both cell types together they responded normally. Secondly, it had long been known that when an artificially prepared hapten-carrier conjugate is used as antigen to produce specific anti-hapten antibody, a classical secondary response is obtained only when the same protein carrier is used for the secondary as for the primary stimulus. It was now shown that if with the primary injection of hapten-carrier (h-C_1) a second different carrier protein (C_2) is given at the same time, then a secondary stimulus with hapten conjugated to the latter (h-C_2) is as effective as h-C_1 in producing a characteristic secondary antibody response to the hapten in question (Mitchison *et al.*, 1970).

These results could only mean that two different cell populations, both carrying antigen-specific, though not necessarily identical, receptors interact to produce a secondary type of antibody response. Cell-transfer and cell culture experiments have since amply confirmed that, at any rate for a major group of antigens, thymus derived lymphocytes acts in a specific way as "helper" cells, allowing B-cells to realize their full specific antibody forming potential. Such antigens are styled "thymus-dependent" and are usually protein in nature. Most proteins carry a heterogeneous range of different antigenic determinants, or epitopes, but there is another class of immunogens, which includes some antigenic polysaccharides and glycans, in which the epitope density tends to be high but is of much more restricted heterogeneity. Such antigens often have the ability independently to activate complement by the alternative pathway (Chapter 7), are poorly metabolized and hence persistent in the body, and are often mitogenic for B-cells. In normal animals and in man they induce IgM but not IgG antibody responses, and do not elicit a classical secondary type of humoral response on repeated administration. Furthermore they do not induce delayed hypersensitivity, and indeed elicit a good, even augmented, antibody response in thymectomized animals. They are thus "T-independent", and presumed capable of stimulating B-cells directly. The modulatory influence of T-cells on B-cell responses is seen in the switch from IgM to IgG antibody production, in the rise in affinity of antibody which occurs with continued immunization, and in the establishing of immunological memory, all features of the immune response to T-dependent antigens.

The Role of Macrophages

How T- and B-cell cooperation takes place is still not clearly understood. It was initially thought of as a simple bridging between T-cell and B-cell, to provide a stimulus to the latter by concentrating antigen, but evidence was soon forthcoming that responses to T-dependent antigens are to a large extent also macrophage-dependent. A proportion of foreign antigenic material gaining access to the tissues undergoes phagocytosis by macrophages, and for many antigens immunogenicity is dependent upon or at least enhanced by this process. A small fraction of the ingested antigen escapes intracellular degradation and becomes associated with cell membranes, either of cytoplasmic organelles, or at the macrophage surface. Its presentation to the lymphocyte in the latter form in some way favours stimulation of antibody production, the macrophage surface serving as a focal point for the meeting and interaction of the relatively rare pairs of T- and B-lymphocytes that carry the appropriate antigen receptors. The experimental induction of helper T-cells *in vitro* certainly requires the presence of macrophages, for in their absence lymphoid cell cultures otherwise responsive to known T-dependent antigens are unable to produce antibody.

Another important function of macrophages in the immune response is to reduce by uptake and digestion the size of the extracellular antigen pool which would otherwise strongly tend to block antigen receptors and hence reduce opportunities for clonally selected lymphocytes to meet under the guidance of antigen localized predominantly at the macrophage surface. Such direct random interaction of excess antigen with lymphocytes probably produces the unresponsiveness seen in "high dose" tolerance.

How the macrophage fosters T-B cooperation is still a matter for debate. It has been proposed that the T-cell's antigen receptors are immunoglobulin-like molecules peculiar to T cells (IgT) and cytophilic for macrophages, binding antigen by its "carrier"-like determinants to the macrophage surface in multiple fashion, and thus presenting a stimulatory matrix of "hapten"-like determinants to the B-cell. Alternatively, a non-Ig antigen specific T-cell factor has been postulated which might have the effect of stimulating B-cells, supplementing the lack of repeating, i.e. stimulating, determinants that characterizes T-independent antigens. Another idea, based on the observation that graft versus host responses in experimental mice activate B-cells to respond to unrelated haptens, is that T-cells under macrophage influence produce a short range non-specific B-cell triggering factor. For at least some antigens T-B co-operation has proved to be complement-dependent, and this might argue that complement binding sites on the macrophage are instrumental in antigen binding, or B-cell binding, or both.

IMMUNE RESPONSE GENES

The T-cell antigen receptor appears to have a dual specificity which is directed both at antigenic determinants and at a special macrophage surface structure separately coded for by immune response (Ir) genes (Rosenthal *et al.*, 1975).

Ir genes are closely linked to the genes of the major histocompatibility complex (MHC), at any rate in the mouse. Inbred strains of mice show strain variation in response to a wide variety of antigens. Low or high responses to well-defined polypeptide antigens in such strains show a regular correlation with the type expressed by the MHC (Shreffler and David, 1975).

The MHC is a "supergene" which controls the classical murine H-2 transplantation antigens (detected by graft rejection) and the corresponding antigens present on all nucleated cell surfaces which are detected by anti-H-2 antisera. In addition the MHC controls a number of other traits, including the immune responses to specific antigens already mentioned, susceptibility to viral oncogenesis, and stimulation in mixed leucocyte culture (MLC), in which lymphocytes are stimulated to proliferate on exposure to allogeneic lymphocytes *in vitro*. Strain crossing between high and low responder mice shows that their immune responses to specific antigens are controlled by dominant autosomal immune response (Ir) genes which display a high degree of polymorphism due to multiple alleles, multiple genetic loci, or both (McDevitt and Sela, 1965). The identification of Ir genes was the initial step towards defining a new region within the MHC supergene, denoted the I-region, controlling traits detected by non-serological means e.g. specific antibody production following immunization, MLC proliferation, graft-versus-host reactions, and graft rejection, all involving specific responses by lymphocytes. For this reason the I-region traits were designated lymphocyte-defined (LD) in contrast to the serologically detected (SD) products of other genes within the MHC.

The next developments followed Benacerraf and McDevitt's (1972) suggestion that Ir genes code for antigen-recognition structures on T-cell surfaces, since the products of the MLC stimulating genes seemed likely to be cell-surface antigens. Cross-immunization between pairs of recombinant mouse strains differing only in their I-regions produced antisera that reacted specifically with cell membrane allo-antigens genetically controlled by the I-region. Such antigens, termed immune-associated or Ia, thus became serologically detectable. Unlike the SD determinants previously recognized as coded for by the MHC, which are present on all nucleated cells, Ia antigens seem to be restricted to lymphocytes, macrophages, epidermal cells and spermatozoa (Hammerling, 1976). The genes controlling these cell-membrane structures are thus likely to be closely implicated in the cell–cell interactions involved in immune mechanisms. For example, the MHC matching known to be a requirement for the effective interaction of T-cell and macrophage in the immune response is partly dependent on I-region matching, as mentioned above, indicating a role for the Ia molecule in the recognition of antigen by the macrophage and in the presentation of antigen to the T-cell receptor (Niederhuber and Frelinger, 1976). It soon transpired, however, that it is the B-cells that have to express Ia antigens before they reach full immunological competence (Sachs and Cone, 1973) and that subsets of T-lymphocytes (see below) differ in the amounts of Ia antigen they carry, according to their helper or suppressor function in T-T or T-B co-operation. In the MLC reaction the presence of the Ia molecule is critical for the stimulating cell activity, but not for the responder cell (Niederhuber and Frelinger, 1976). It begins to look as if the macrophage, the helper T-cell, the suppressor T-cell, and the B-cell—the cells involved in the regulation of the immune response—may all express Ia antigens (McDevitt *et al.*, 1976).

In man, the MHC is the HLA supergene, within which map the HLA-A, HLA-B and HLA-C genes coding for the serologically detected transplantation antigens present on all nucleated cells. The HLA-D locus controls determinants recognized in the MLC tests (the LD determinants). In addition, the HLA supergene codes for properdin and complement factors, and for some red cell and serum protein allotypes, but although claims have been made that genes controlling IgE responses map with HLA (Levine *et al.*, 1972) it is still a matter for speculation whether human Ir genes exist in this region.

Nevertheless, antibodies have been demonstrated in the sera of pregnant women which block MLC stimulation between otherwise HLA identical cell combinations; these appear to be recognizing an allo-antigen system preferentially expressed in B-cells and coded for by loci closely linked to the MLC or HLA-D locus (van Rood *et al.*, 1976). These antibodies appear to be the human equivalent of mouse Ia antibodies, reacting with Ia-like determinants, but it is premature to denote them as such, since little is yet known of the localization of Ia genes in the HLA system.

The clinical importance of these B-cell allo-antigens is not yet clear, but their recognition may help to clarify some of the associations now increasingly noted between HLA types and disease states. In multiple sclerosis, for example, more than half the patients are of HLA type DW2, but with B-cell allo-antigen 7a the association is near 100% (Wernet, 1976).

CONTROL OF THE IMMUNE RESPONSE

The benefits for survival that flowed from the evolution of adaptive immunity were conditional upon the simultaneous development of intrinsic checks and balances within the system—checks to prevent inapposite stimulation of damaging auto-immune responses to self-antigens present in the tissue environment, and balances to restrain what might otherwise become runaway responses to the first foreign antigens encountered which proved capable of triggering the full clonal potential of the system. Mechanisms regulating the immune response are being identified, among the different cellular and humoral products generated as parts of it, and they reflect its complexity. Suppressor effects are being increasingly recognized as natural corollaries of immune stimulation, and their relevance to tolerance and unresponsiveness is becoming increasingly obvious.

Feedback Inhibition by Antibody

Removal of antibody from the circulating plasma by exchange transfusion increases the total antibody produced, and conversely passive administration of antibody inhibits its active production in response to a primary antigenic stimulus. This is an antigen-specific effect, and its best known clinical application is in the prevention of rhesus iso-immunization. Passive administration of anti-D antibody of IgG, though not of IgM class appears to cause sequestration of the red cell iso-antigen, diverting it from contact with lymphocytes and preventing sensitization (with high affinity antibody quite small doses are effective). Another role postulated for antibody is simply a competitive one, blocking antigenic determinants and thus preventing further stimulation of antigen-specific lymphocytes. A more critical regulatory effect of IgG antibody, however, seems to arise from its ability to bind to Fc receptors which are present at the macrophage surface, altering the interaction between macrophage and antigen so that the latter is presented to the T-cell in the form of an antigen-antibody complex. This appears to induce in the T-cell a "suppressor" rather than a "helper" role in B-cell activation.

Allotype suppression

We have already noted that antibody to chicken IgM suppresses the appearance of plasma cells and serum immunoglobulins in the developing chick. A more selective effect of antibody is that produced by the perinatal exposure of hybrid mice of certain strains to antibody against one of the parental immunoglobulin allotypes, a manoeuvre which specifically and completely suppresses subsequent production of that allotype in the recipient. This is the experimental counterpart of the naturally-occurring suppressive effect in rabbits of maternally transmitted iso-antibodies, which delete expression of gammaglobulin allotype specificities contributed to the offspring's genome by the male parent. Another type of antibody-mediated suppression of antibody production is seen in the restricted response of young mice to antigens against which the mother has been immunized.

Suppressor T-cells

The antibody response of mice to sheep RBC is thymus dependent—that is to say, thymus deprived mice do not respond, but mice with normal thymuses do. Thymus deprived mice which have been reconstituted with small numbers of syngeneic thymocytes and then given a large dose of sheep RBC are rendered tolerant—i.e., they make no detectable antibody response to this or to subsequent doses of the antigen. They differ from thymus deprived mice which have not been so reconstituted with thymus cells in that a supplementary injection of fresh thymocytes from a normal mouse does not restore their ability to respond. This can only mean that the responsiveness of the normal thymocytes administered in the second injection has been suppressed by the presence of thymocytes which have experienced a "tolerizing" dose of the antigen.

This important experimental result showed that antigen induced unresponsiveness, or tolerance, can just as well result from an induced suppressor effect of T-cells upon B-cell responses as from clonal deletion, although in many cases it is difficult in practice to distinguish so readily between the absence of specifically reactive cells and the presence of specifically non-reactive cells.

This type of experiment also gave rise to the idea that T-cells, as well as mediating some types of tolerance, might also regulate antibody production in normal immune responses, a concept that derived support from the observation that animals depleted of T-cells by various means actually make enhanced antibody responses to T-independent antigens such as pneumococcal polysaccharide. Experiments on *in vitro* antibody production, moreover, showed that the addition of small numbers of immune cells can suppress the response of cultured normal cells to antigen. Such suppressor effects appear to be predominantly the result of interactions between different subsets of T-cells e.g. virgin T-cells not yet stimulated by antigen are induced as suppressors by feedback from immune T-cells. Immune B-cells can also signal normal T-cells to act as suppressors through the effects of immune complexes on T-cell surface receptors. This type of blocking effect of immune complexes on cytotoxic T-cells may explain some forms of transplantation tolerance and the enhancement of tumour growth by antibody (Humphrey, 1976).

The suppressor T-cell activity operating in antigen-induced unresponsiveness of the type described above is multi-clonal in its effect, reducing the total antibody response to characteristically multi-determinant T-dependent antigens. A somewhat different state of affairs exists in the allotype suppression experiments already mentioned, where suppressor T-cell activity directed at a particular antigenic species within the sum of the recipients' own immunoglobulin molecules is generated in the absence of foreign antigen. The suppression is chronic, lasting long after the administration of the anti-allotype serum, and presumably reflects a loss of T-cell tolerance to the allotype in question, so that B-cells bearing it are suppressed as if by a graft versus host reaction. This implies the existence of a different type of mechanism by which T-cells may control immune responsiveness—direct reactivity against antigen-receptors (immunoglobulins, allotypes) at the B-cell surface. Such specific interactions between the immune system and its autogenous components are in effect auto-immune reactions. Further, the conformational individuality which gives the immunoglobulin antigen-receptor on the B-cell its specificity for a particular antigenic determinant, confers on each receptor itself (and on the specific antibody molecule subsequently secreted) an antigenic specificity of its own, a specificity, known as the idiotype, which is even more highly individual than that of the allotype. The existence of idiotypic antigenic determinants on Ig molecules has been demonstrated by making guinea-pigs tolerant to mouse IgG, and then injecting purified mouse antibody of known single-determinant specificity. The guinea-pigs produce anti-mouse IgG antibody of anti-idiotypic specificity. Furthermore, injection of such anti-idiotypic antibody at appropriate dose into recipient mice eventually induces a chronic inability to make antibody of precisely the same single specificity, a result which, moreover, like allotype suppression, requires the presence of cells belonging to the T-subpopulation. The implication is strong that these T-cells are producing their suppressive effect through an auto-anti-idiotypic or self-recognizing property. Anti-idiotype antibody can be raised in animals of the same species and of the same allotype, but it is not yet known whether it can be autogenously produced. If initial activation of the B-cell led to the production of such anti-idiotypic antibody reactive with the immunoglobulin product of the cell in question, this would activate suppressor T-cells with consequent regulatory effects on the immune response originally initiated by antigen.

These are but a few examples of a large number of *in vivo* and *in vitro* animal experiments which have been carried out to elucidate the nature of control mechanisms within the immune system. There seems to be little doubt that regulator effects are exerted by T-cells on other T-cells, by T-cells (directly, or indirectly through macrophages) on B-cells, and even by B-cells on T-cells. Disturbances of such regulatory mechanisms may well be important causes of immunological abnormalities in man. Evidence has been reported that in common variable hypogammaglobulinaemia the peripheral blood cells inhibit mitogen stimulated immunoglobulin production by B-cells taken from at least some normal donors (Waldmann *et al.*, 1974), but that this is due to abnormally suppressive T-cells is in doubt (Platts-Mills, 1976).

Functional Subsets of T-cells

In their capacity as effectors of the immune response, T-cells provide immunity mechanisms against certain bacteria, fungi and viruses and against foreign grafts. By producing lymphokines in response to the antigenic stimuli in question, they initiate the various inflammatory reactions of delayed hypersensitivity, and by their direct cytotoxic activities destroy cells antigenically marked as targets by viral products or by histoincompatibility.

In addition to these effector functions, T-cells, while unable to produce antibody themselves, assist B-lymphocytes to do so; and, as we have seen, they at the same time exert a powerful controlling influence on immune responses. The existence of these various functions—helper, delayed hypersensitivity, cytotoxic or killer, and suppressor—raises the question whether distinct types of T-cell subserve each, or whether T-cells are functionally versatile. In the present state of knowledge derived from mouse experiments it appears that T-cells are divisible on a basis of maturity into T1 (immature) and T2 (mature) subsets. T1-cells are short-lived, do not recirculate and are spleen-seeking, while T2-cells are long-lived, recirculate and on injection seek the lymph nodes preferentially. Consequently thymus and spleen are rich in T1-cells, and blood, thoracic duct lymph and lymph node tissue rich in T2-cells. While T2-cells seem to mediate helper, killer and delayed hypersensitivity functions, both T1- and T2-cells manifest suppressor activity, and it looks as if the regulatory effects of T1-cells may be superimposed on a self-regulatory mechanism inherent in T2-cells.

The recent elaboration of lymphocyte allo-antisera of the Ly system has confirmed the functional division of labour between discrete T-cell subpopulations in the mouse (Feldmann *et al.*, 1975). This work suggests that these various subsets do not represent different stages of maturation but their immunopathological significance in man is not yet clear. Methods are required for identifying and enumerating T-cell subsets before assessment of their relevance to immune disorders such as Hodgkin's disease and sarcoidosis is possible.

Self-tolerance and Auto-immunity

Among the most important mechanisms controlling the activities of the immune system are those concerned with suppressing auto-immune responses. The ideas underlying present understanding of these mechanisms derive from Burnet's explanation of the absence of an immune response to self in terms of self-recognition based on clonal selection, and the cognate experiments on acquired transplantation tolerance of Medawar and his colleagues (Burnet, 1959; Billingham *et al.*, 1953).

Transplantation tolerance was initially regarded as a central failure of the immune response resulting from clonal deletion of those lymphocytes genetically endowed with the capability of reacting specifically against the antigenic determinants of the foreign graft. Alternatively it was thought that these cells might be irreversibly inactivated rather than deleted.

The subsequent discovery of the existence of distinct T- and B-lymphocyte subpopulations, the realization that lymphocytes of both types often need to cooperate in specific fashion if antigenic stimuli are to produce a full immune response, and, later, the conclusion that intercellular co-operation is as closely involved with control and indeed suppression of the immune response as with its activation, raises the question whether the simple interpretation of tolerance in all its forms as clonal deletion is still tenable. Since auto-immunity undoubtedly occurs in a clinical context, the question is also relevant to suggested mechanisms of self tolerance. Pointers to the nature of self-tolerance came from experiments on the induction of tolerance to serum proteins used as hetero-antigens. These are T-dependent antigens powerfully immunogenic under appropriate conditions of administration in other species, but never (if we exclude the auto-anti-idiotypic possibility in the case of immunoglobulin discussed on page 42) auto-immunogenic.

The upshot of such experiments (Taylor, 1969; Chiller *et al.*, 1971) was that administration of a foreign serum protein such as albumin or immunoglobulin in low dosage produces tolerance or unresponsiveness to the protein in question. This was shown by various cell transfer experiments to be a tolerance purely due to T-cell unresponsiveness, the B-cells of the tolerant animals retaining their ability to respond with antibody production, and indeed actively doing so as soon as the possibility of cooperating with normal T-cells was restored. Administration of antigen at high dosage, on the other hand, produced an unresponsiveness which affected both T- and B-cells. The unresponsiveness of T-cells is rapidly induced at either dose level but persistent, while B-cell unresponsiveness is more slowly induced and transient.

The finding that tolerance to T-dependent antigens is thus capable of operating solely through an unresponsiveness of T-cells, while B-cell responsiveness is unimpaired, suggested that tolerance induced by low doses of a given protein might be bypassed by further immunization with a different but cross-reacting protein. By virtue of its antigenic differences this would stimulate other (non-tolerant) T-cells, which in turn would act as helpers for B-cells reactive to the determinants on the second antigen, including those it shared with the first. This proved to be the case. Rabbits made tolerant to bovine serum albumin and challenged with pig serum albumin produced antibodies reactive with both.

The implied analogy with self-tolerance was pointed out by Allison (1971) and by Weigle (1971). Proteins present in the blood and tissues in low concentration, like thyroglobulin, might be expected to induce a low dose tolerance of T-cells only; proteins present in high concentration, like serum albumin, should make both T- and B-cells tolerant. The implication is that where tolerance of T-dependent self-antigens is of low dose, the individual is vulnerable to development of auto-immunity against these antigens since immunocompetent B-cells are presumably present and responsive if the required T-cell help is forthcoming. By analogy with the tolerance-breaking experiments above, this help could be provided by a cross-reacting antigen—in infection, for example, gaining access to the body as a microbial constituent (see Chapter 13). Virus proteins may appear in the membranes of infected cells, and complexes of virus with host antigens or host antigenic determinants incorporated in virions would have a similar auto-immunizing potential (Allison and Denman, 1971). Proved instances of this role for virus in auto-immunity, however, are scarce in human disease; the smooth muscle antibody of infectious mononucleosis is a possible example.

Thus for T-dependent self antigens, clonal deletion need not extend to the B-cell component to produce tolerance. The possibility also has to be considered however, that control over B-cell activation and perhaps also over T-cell activation by antigen is mediated not through deletion but through suppressor activity. There are indications of T-cell defects in several animal models of auto-immunity. The development of the lupus-like auto-immune condition of New Zealand B × W hybrid mice is preceded by marked changes in T-cell function (Talal, 1974). Further, the auto-immunity that appears in the older mice is transferable with their spleen cells to young unaffected mice of this strain, but the effect is only transient; if the young recipients have been previously depleted of T-cells with anti-thymocytic globulin, however, it persists (Denman *et al.*, 1970). Another example is seen in the spontaneous auto-immune thyroiditis of obese strain Leghorn chickens where neonatal thymectomy leads to earlier onset of the thyroiditis, and increases its severity (Welch and Rose, 1973). Both these animal models exemplify genetic influences on auto-immune responsiveness. In a third animal model, certain mice that make antibody responses to injections of mouse thyroglobulin and develop thyroiditis, a controlling gene linked to the major histocompatibility locus at or near the immune response gene locus, has been identified (Tomazic *et al.*, 1974). The fact that normal mouse thymocytes reduce the response to mouse thyroglobulin made by irradiated recipients of bone marrow from high responder mice, draws attention to the possibility that the high responder mice have a genetically determined defect in suppressor T-cell function.

REFERENCES

Allison, A. C. (1971). Unresponsiveness to self antigens. *Lancet* **2**, 1401.

Allison, A. C. and Denman, A. M. (1976). Self-tolerance and auto-immunity. *Brit. Med. Bull.* **32**, 124.

Benacerraf, B. and McDevitt, H. O. (1972). Histocompatibility-linked immune response genes. *Science* **175**, 273.

Billingham, R. E., Brent, L. and Medawar, P. B. (1953). "Actively acquired tolerance" of foreign cells. *Nature* **172**, 603.

Burnet, F. M. (1959). "The Clonal Selection Theory of Acquired Immunity." Cambridge University Press, London and Cambridge.

Chiller, J. M., Habicht, G. S. and Weigle, W. O. (1971). Kinetic differences in unresponsiveness of thymus and bone marrow cells. *Science* **171**, 813.

Denman, A. M., Russell, A. S. and Denman, E. J. (1970). ALG and a model for autoimmunity. *In* "International Symposium on Antilymphocyte Serum. Versailles, 1970". Symp. Series Immunobiol. Standard. Vol. 16, p. 253, Karger, Basel.

Droege, W. and Zucker, R. (1975). Lymphocyte subpopulations in the thymus. *Transpl. Rev.* **25**, 1.

Fagraeus, A. (1948). *Acta. Med. Scand.* **130**, Suppl. 204, 3.

Feldmann, M., Beverley, P. C. L., Dunkley, M. and Kontiainen, S. (1975). Different Ly antigen phenotypes of *in vitro* induced helper and suppressor cells. *Nature* **258**, 614.

Goldstein, A. L., Hooper, J. A., Schulof, R. S., Cohen, G. H., Thurman, G. B., McDaniel, M. C., White, A. and Dardenne, M. (1974). Thymosin and the immunopathology of aging. *Fed. Proc.* **33**, 2053.

Hammerling, G. J. (1976). Tissue distribution of Ia antigens and their expression on lymphocyte subpopulations. *Transpl. Rev.* **30**, 64.

Humphrey, J. H. (1976). Some reflections on principles and mechanisms of immunological tolerance. *Brit. Med. Bull.* **32**, 182.

Levine, B. B., Sternber, R. H. and Fottino, M. (1972). Ragweed hayfever: genetic control and linkage to HL-A haplotypes. *Science* **178**, 1201.

McDevitt, H. O. and Sela, M. (1965). Genetic control of the antibody response. I. Demonstration of determinant-specific differences in response to synthetic polypeptide antigens in two strains of inbred mice. *J. Exp. Med.* **122**, 517.

McDevitt, H. O., Delovitch, T. L., Press, J. L. and Murphy, D. B. (1976). Genetic and functional analysis of the Ia antigens; their possible role in regulating the immune response. *Transplant Rev.* **30**, 197.

Manning, M. J. (1975). The phylogeny of thymic dependence. *Am. Zool.* **15**, 63.

Metcalf, D. and Moore, M. A. S. (1971). "Haemopoietic Cells" (ed. E. L. Tatum and A. Neuberger) North Holland Publishing Co., Amsterdam and Oxford.

Mitchison, N. A., Taylor, R. B. and Rajewsky, K. (1970). *In* "Developmental Aspects of Antibody Formation and Structure" (ed. J. Sterzl), p. 547, Czechoslovak Academy of Science, Prague.

Niederhuber, J. E. and Frelinger, J. A. (1976). Expression of Ia antigens on T and B cells, and their relationship to immune-response functions. *Transplant Rev.* **30**, 101.

Platts-Mills, T. A. E. (1976). Suppressor cells in immunodeficiency. 3rd European Immunology Meeting, Copenhagen.

Raff, M. C. and Wortis, H. H. (1970). Thymus dependence of θ-bearing cells in the peripheral lymphoid tissues of mice. *Immunology* **18**, 931.

Rosenthal, A. S., Lipsky, P. E. and Shevach, E. M. (1975). Macrophage lymphocyte interaction and antigen recognition. *Fed. Proc.* **34**, 1743.

Sachs, D. H. and Cone, J. L. (1973). A mouse B cell alloantigen determined by gene(s) linked to the major histocompatibility complex. *J. Exp. Med.* **138**, 1289.

Scheinberg, M. A., Blacklow, N. R., Goldstein, A. L., Parrino, T. A., Rose, F. B. and Cathcart, E. S. (1976). Influenza: response of T-lymphopenia to thymosin. *New Eng. J. Med.* **294**, 1208.

Shreffler, D. C. and David, C. S. (1975). The H-2 major histocompatibility complex and the I immune response region: genetic variation, function and organization. *Adv. Immunol.* **20**, 125.

Talal, N. (1974). *In* "Progress in Clinical Immunology" (ed. R. S. Schwartz), Vol. 2, p. 101, Grune and Stratton, New York.

Taylor, R. B. (1969). Cellular cooperation in the antibody response of mice to two serum albumins: specific function of thymus cells. *Transplant Rev.* **1**, 114.

Tomazic, V., Rose, N. R. and Shreffler, D. C. (1974). Autoimmune murine thyroiditis. IV. Localization of genetic control of the immune response. *J. Immunol.* **112**, 965.

van Rood, J. J., van Leeuwen, A., Termijtelen, A. and Keuning, J. J. (1976). B-cell antibodies, Ia-like determinants, and their relation to MLC determinants in man. *Transplant Rev.* **30**, 122.

Waldman, T. A., Durm, M., Broder, S., Blackman, M., Blaese, M. and Strober, W. (1974). Role of suppressor T cells in pathogenesis of common variable hypogammaglobulinaemia. *Lancet* **2**, 609.

Wara, D. W., Goldstein, A. L., Doyle, N. E. and Ammann, A. J. (1975). Thymosin activity in patients with cellular immunodeficiency. *New Eng. J. Med.* **292**, 70.

Weigle, W. O. (1971). Recent observations and concepts in immunological unresponsiveness and auto immunity. A review. *Clin. Exp. Immunol.* **9**, 437.
Welch, P. and Rose, N. R. (1973). Neonatal thymectomy increases spontaneous autoimmune thyroiditis. *J. Immunol.* **110**, 575.
Wernet, P. (1976). Human Ia-type allo-antigens: methods of detection, aspects of chemistry and biology, markers for disease states. *Transplant Rev.* **30**, 271.

3

Lymphocyte Subpopulations in Health and Disease

M. PAPAMICHAIL and E. J. HOLBOROW

The existence of separate T- and B-subpopulations of lymphocytes was originally inferred from results of depletion-and-challenge experiments in mice and other animal species (Chapter 2), and from observation of gross forms of human immunodeficiency (Chapter 14). It was not long before a cell surface iso-antigen (θ) distinguishing mouse thymocytes was discovered, the first of a number of surface antigens and receptors on lymphocytes which have since become known. Techniques for their rapid identification by immunofluorescence or rosette formation have been developed, by the use of which cells belonging to different lymphoid cell subpopulations present in the blood, body fluids or tissues may be recognized and enumerated. The relevance of such tests to clinical immunology has been demonstrated for a number of conditions in which the disturbance of lymphocyte ecology is gross, and the possibility of developing methods of detecting lesser and commoner degrees of lymphocyte derangement is being widely explored.

In this chapter some tests for lymphocyte markers, the validity of their current interpretations, and some of their applications in human disease will be discussed.

SURFACE RECEPTORS OF HUMAN LYMPHOCYTES

Identification and Separation of Blood Lymphocytes

Several of the methods for detecting surface receptors depend upon formation of rosettes with added red cells, so that to study such receptors on lymphocytes from the peripheral blood, it is necessary first to separate the leukocytes from the accompanying red cells, and the mononuclear white cells from the polymorphonuclear cells which carry related receptors. Both results can be achieved at once by use of a density method, layering defibrinated or heparinized blood, diluted with an equal volume of buffered saline, over Ficoll-Na metrizoate and centrifuging. The red cells and the polymorphs go to the bottom of the tube and the interface cell population of mononuclear cells may be removed by careful aspiration. These are then washed in medium containing 10% foetal calf serum to remove most of the human serum or plasma proteins. With defibrinated blood, this population is free from platelets, which makes the results of E-rosette testing (described below) more reproducible, and also eliminates possible errors in subsequent immunofluorescent examination due to staining of platelets which may be coated with antibody. Such cell preparations usually contain less than 1% polymorphs, but up to 40% of the mononuclear cells may be monocytes, identifiable morphologically by examination of Romanovsky-stained cytocentrifuged preparations, or by other methods described below.

Monocyte Contamination

By direct immunofluorescence, some monocytes show surface staining with anti-IgG fluorescent conjugates, due to prior binding of serum IgG to their Fc receptors ("cytophilic" antibody) or to the presence of surface-bound immune complexes. Monocytes do not stain with anti-IgM fluorescent conjugates (in which the antibody is usually of IgG class) by the direct method, so it appears that their Fc receptors do not bind enough conjugated IgG to produce a visible density of fluorescent molecules. In the indirect method, however, where sheep or rabbit IgG antibody with activity against human IgG, IgA, IgM or IgD constitutes the first layer, non-specific binding of any of these by Fc receptors on the cells under test is rendered visible as surface fluorescence through the amplifying effect of the second layer of fluorescent antibody against sheep or rabbit IgG.

The presence of monocytes is a potent cause of discrepant results between preparations of normal lymphocytes obtained in different ways and from different subjects. The following experiment illustrates how their contribution may falsify enumeration of Ig-bearing lymphocytes.

After separation of mononuclear cells from a sample of normal human blood by the density method, a BSA gradient (0·2–2·0%) was used to obtain three cell fractions (Papamichail and Temple, 1975). The first (heaviest) cell fraction contained 70% monocytes and 30% lymphocytes, the second 15%

monocytes and 85% lymphocytes, and the third 100% lymphocytes. Direct fluorescence with specific anti-IgG and anti-IgM conjugates gave the following results:

	IgG	IgM
1st fraction	40%	4%
2nd fraction	12%	6%
3rd fraction	4%	17%

Although some selection of lymphocytes by size may have occurred, these results show that monocytes can make a major contribution to the IgG surface-positive human peripheral blood cell population separated by a commonly used method. It is necessary, therefore, to check separated mononuclear cell preparations for monocyte contamination before proceeding to test for surface receptors.

Identification of Monocytes

Incubation of the separated mononuclear cell suspension with latex particles assists in identification and enumeration of monocytes in which ingested latex particles are readily seen on microscopy (Winchester *et al.*, 1974).

Removal of Monocytes

The number of monocytes present in a separated cell population may be reduced by the use of added carbonyl iron and a magnet, or by layering 0·1 ml quantities of the cell suspension (in culture medium containing 40% foetal calf serum) on clean sterile glass coverslips and incubating at 37°C for 25 minutes in a moist chamber (Papamichail and Temple, 1975). The non-adherent cells, removed by repeated gentle washing with medium 199, are more than 95% lymphocytes, and more than 98% of the adherent cells are monocytes as judged by the presence of cytoplasmic peroxidase activity. If the procedure is repeated a second time, the purity of the recovered lymphocytes approaches 100%. The period of incubation with coverslips is critical; longer than 25 minutes leads to adherence of an increasing number of B-cells.

Effect of Manipulating Cell Suspensions to Remove Unwanted Cells

Manipulation of blood and of cell suspensions changes the relative proportions of the different cell populations. Procedures based upon sedimentation and density increase the relative proportion of B-cells, while methods based upon adherence favour recovery of T-cells. Brown and Greaves (1974a), have pointed out that a lymphocyte yield of over 70% is essential if estimates of the T-B proportion are to be accurate enough to permit extrapolation to the blood lymphocyte level and to absolute T- and B-cell numbers, and for this reason they favour the use of whole unseparated blood to measure the latter directly. The method they describe however, requires specific fluorescent anti-T-cell antibody, and demands positive identification as such of every stained lymphocyte seen; it is perhaps too exacting for routine use.

Percentages or Absolute Numbers?

The relationship between the numbers of T-cells and the numbers of B-cells should be expressed in percentages only if both populations have been estimated independently and the total number of lymphocytes in the suspension is also stated. Percentage values alone can be misleading, as in chronic lymphatic leukaemia, where the percentage of lymphocytes that are T-cells may be very low, although their absolute number in the blood may be within normal limits or even raised. It should be remembered that enumeration of cells in the peripheral blood gives no information about the make-up of the total lymphocyte pool.

Immunoglobulins on Lymphocyte Surfaces: B-lymphocytes

The demonstration of surface immunoglobulin is the most widely used test for identifying and enumerating B-cells in human lymphocyte preparations. That human Ig-bearing cells are of bone marrow origin was inferred from study of conditions with thymus (and hence T-cell) deficiency, such as diGeorge's and Nezélof's syndromes, and conditions of bone marrow deficiency, such as X-linked hypogammaglobulinaemia, where increased and decreased proportions respectively of Ig-bearing lymphocytes in the peripheral blood are the rule. The combined use of a test separately identifying T-cells confirmed that in normal human blood cells bearing readily identifiable surface Ig constitute a separate population (Papamichail *et al.*, 1972).

Different classes and subclasses of Ig are identifiable on human lymphocytes. Where the immunoglobulin detected is a product of the cell and not of

TABLE 1

Some methods of detecting surface Ig on human lymphocytes

Immunofluorescence	(Papamichail *et al.*, 1971; Froland and Natvig, 1971; Preud'homme *et al.*, 1973)
Autoradiography	(Wilson and Nossal, 1971)
Mixed antiglobulin reaction	(Coombs *et al.*, 1969; Hutteroth *et al.*, 1972)
Reversed cytoadherence	(Paraskevas *et al.*, 1971)
Stimulation with anti-Ig	(Abdou *et al.*, 1973)
Cytotoxic effect of anti-Ig	(Wernet *et al.*, 1972)

extrinsic origin, it is of one allotype, in accordance with allelic exclusion; the simultaneous presence of IgM and IgD is discussed below. There are several methods of detecting surface Ig on human lymphocytes, as shown in Table 1. The most commonly used at present is direct immunofluorescence with anti-Ig antisera conjugated with the fluorochromes fluorescein or rhodamine.

Immunofluorescence

The staining of surface antigenic determinants is usually observed by examining cell suspensions. The essential requirements are fluorescent reagents of known specificity and reactivity, and efficient fluorescence microscopy. Conjugate specificity is important, since as discussed above, the direct staining method is preferable, and this limits the effective dilution of the conjugate. The use of living cell suspensions favours specificity, since only dead cells show non-specific (usually cytoplasmic) staining propensities. Living cell suspensions, furthermore, permit observation of "capping"—the cross-linking by antibody of antigen molecules favourably distributed and mobile in the cell surface and thus capable of being aggregated at one pole of the cell to form a cap or patch.

Lymphocytes Bearing Surface Ig

The percentage of peripheral blood lymphocytes in healthy human subjects initially reported to carry surface Ig varied widely, ranging from 12–34% in different laboratories. The first section of Table 2 shows the results of differential staining for IgG and IgM classes of immunoglobulin among the Ig-bearing lymphocytes in normal human blood, as reported by ten different laboratories between 1971 and 1973. In three out of four laboratories where the proportion of IgM-positive lymphocytes seen exceeded the proportion of IgG positive cells, only small lymphocytes morphologically identified as such (for example by phase contrast appearances) were admitted to the count, all

TABLE 2

Some reported mean percentages of Ig-bearing lymphocytes in normal human blood, determined by immunofluorescence

<table>
<tr><th></th><th>IgG</th><th>IgM</th><th>IgD</th></tr>
<tr><td>Papamichail et al. (1971)</td><td>16</td><td>7</td><td>n.d.</td></tr>
<tr><td>Grey et al. (1971)</td><td>14·5</td><td>8</td><td>n.d.</td></tr>
<tr><td>Siegal et al. (1971)[a]</td><td>2·7</td><td>9·3</td><td>n.d.</td></tr>
<tr><td>Aisenberg and Bloch (1972)</td><td>4</td><td>10</td><td>n.d.</td></tr>
<tr><td>Lawton et al. (1972)</td><td>17·3</td><td>8·9</td><td>n.d.</td></tr>
<tr><td>Preud'homme and Seligmann (1972b)[a]</td><td>4</td><td>13</td><td>n.d.</td></tr>
<tr><td>Froland and Natvig (1973)[a]</td><td>5</td><td>10</td><td>n.d.</td></tr>
<tr><td>Gajl-Peczalska et al. (1973b)</td><td>14·3</td><td>8·8</td><td>n.d.</td></tr>
<tr><td>Nicod et al. (1973)</td><td>15·3</td><td>8·2</td><td>n.d.</td></tr>
<tr><td>Williams et al. (1973)</td><td>12</td><td>7</td><td>n.d.</td></tr>
<tr><td colspan="4">Effect of Fc of fluorescent antibody (Winchester et al., 1975a)</td></tr>
<tr><td>Whole anti-heavy chain</td><td>4·8</td><td>6·7</td><td>4·8</td></tr>
<tr><td>F(ab′)₂ anti-heavy chain</td><td>0·36</td><td>4·6</td><td>4·6</td></tr>
<tr><td>Whole anti-(μ+δ)</td><td></td><td colspan="2">7·3</td></tr>
<tr><td>F(ab′)₂ anti-(μ+δ)</td><td></td><td colspan="2">5·9</td></tr>
<tr><td colspan="4">Double-staining for IgM/IgD (Rowe et al., 1973)</td></tr>
<tr><td>Whole anti-heavy chain—Adults</td><td>n.d.</td><td>5·6 (82% also IgD+)</td><td>5·3 (75% also IgM+)</td></tr>
<tr><td>Whole anti-heavy chain—Newborns</td><td>n.d.</td><td>13·0 (86% also IgD+)</td><td>14·6 (86% also IgM+)</td></tr>
<tr><td colspan="4">Effect of pretreatment at 37°C (Lobo et al., 1975)</td></tr>
<tr><td></td><td></td><td></td><td>Ig+</td></tr>
<tr><td colspan="3">Lymphocytes with surface stable (37°C) Ig</td><td>8·9%</td></tr>
<tr><td colspan="3">Lymphocytes with surface labile Ig (difference between number + at 4° and number + at 37°)</td><td>22%</td></tr>
</table>

[a] Only small lymphocytes morphologically identified as such were counted.

larger cells, whether monocytes or large lymphocytes, being excluded. The strong likelihood of monocyte contamination of separated cells has been mentioned above.

Causes of Error in Enumerating Lymphocytes Bearing Intrinsic Surface Ig

An important cause of surface staining of lymphocytes for Ig is the presence of extrinsic IgG bound by Fc determinants to receptors for the latter on the cell surface. When lymphocytes separated from whole blood were washed at room temperature before staining with anti-Ig conjugate the mean percentage of Ig positive cells in 17 normal bloods was 18%. When the cells were washed at 37°C in medium containing foetal calf serum this value decreased to 9%, while washing at 4°C increased it to 32% (Lobo *et al.*, 1975). This variation with temperature proved to be due to changes in the number of IgG-bearing cells; the number of IgM cells did not change, as might be expected from the apparent lack of receptors for IgM on lymphocytes. A similar reduction of IgG positive cells from 20% to less than 5% is produced by preliminary incubation of the cell suspension at 37°C for 30 mins or by brief pretreatment at pH 5·0 (Kumagi *et al.*, 1975).

The indications are that blood lymphocytes may carry two sorts of immunoglobulin, "surface stable" and "surface labile", the former intrinsic to the cell, the latter extrinsic IgG bound by receptors for IgG Fc which are present on the cell surface.

An additional cause of error in identifying lymphocyte surface Ig is the presence of Fc determinants on fluorochrome conjugated anti-IgG antibody molecules which are themselves of IgG class. Immune complexes may form during staining, either with minute quantities of IgG remaining in the fluid phase of the washed cell suspension, or with monomeric IgG bound to cell Fc receptors. In such complexes, the Fc regions of the labelled antibody molecules, possibly with increased affinity, become bound to cells which have Fc receptors, so that they give positive membrane staining for IgG irrespective of whether intrinsic surface IgG is actually present. Binding of conjugated anti-IgG by its Fc region is eliminated if the conjugate is prepared from an IgG fraction isolated from the anti-IgG antiserum and digested with pepsin before conjugation with fluorochrome. In this way it is converted to an $F(ab')_2$ reagent with anti-IgG specificity but lacking the Fc determinants which may bind it to Fc receptors on the cell surface. Winchester *et al.* (1975a) have shown that with such conjugated $F(ab')_2$ reagents prepared from IgG antibodies specific for human μ, γ and δ chains, the percentage of normal human blood lymphocytes carrying surface IgG after incubation for 1 hour at 37°C is less than 1%. With whole Ig anti-IgG conjugate more than 10 times as many cells showed surface staining (Table 2). The percentage of cells staining for surface IgM, however, was much less affected by substitution of the $F(ab')_2$ anti-IgM reagent for whole Ig anti-IgM, and remained at about 5%. A similar percentage of blood lymphocytes positive for surface IgM is reported in normal adults by Rowe *et al.* (1973).

Table 2 summarizes the reported effects that IgG bound in different forms to lymphocyte receptors for IgG Fc may have on the enumeration of Ig-bearing lymphocytes. It is apparent that when this cause of error is excluded, the percentage of Ig-bearing lymphocytes in normal adult blood is no more than 5–10% of the total lymphocytes, and that most of these are IgM cells, IgG cells constituting less than 1%.

IgM and IgD Cells

A finding of particular theoretical interest is that IgM and IgD occur together on the same lymphocyte (Table 2). Both components are intrinsic products of the cell, share light chains of the same κ- or λ-type, and even show similar idiotype specificity, although they are evidently independent structures in the cell membrane as shown by their separate capping with specific anti-μ and anti-δ antisera on double fluorochrome labelling. It thus seems probable that when both are present on a given cell both are antigen receptors with the same combining site. IgD may be the primary antigen receptor, not secreted, and the appearance of IgM, potentially a secreted immunoglobulin, may indicate the first step in differentiation towards a plasma cell (Rowe *et al.*, 1973). New evidence, however, favours a primary role for IgM (Seligmann, 1975). The significantly higher proportion of IgD positive cells in newborn (cord) blood (15%) is striking, but here too IgD mostly shares its cellular location with IgM.

Surface immunoglobulins are antigen receptors in the cell membranes of B-cells, and in each clone of B-cells they are coded for by the same V-genes that determine the combining specificity of the antibody molecules subsequently synthesized and secreted by the plasma cells that are the lineal progeny of the clone in question. Whether the antigen receptors of T-cells are likewise immunoglobulin molecules is still controversial. The IgM membrane immunoglobulin of B-cells is present in a monomeric (7S) form, and an immunoglobulin-like protein, similar to but distinguishable from IgM has also been demonstrated in T-cell membranes by a sensitive method (Marchalonis, 1975). Lymphocytes with surface immunoglobulin readily detectable by immunofluorescence, however, are identifiable, with the technical provisos discussed above, as B-cells.

Non-Ig Lymphocyte Surface Receptors

As well as receptors for antigen, lymphocytes have other surface receptors, or the potential to produce them, which play as yet only partly understood roles in lymphocyte function. Among these are receptors for the Fc portions of IgG molecules already mentioned, receptors for complement components, and the various different receptors for xenogeneic and other erythrocyte membrane determinants.

Fc Receptors

Red blood cells coated with specific antibody (EA) are a form of antigen complex whose interaction with Fc receptors on mononuclear cell surfaces is readily observable as rosette formation.

There is disagreement, however, about both the results this method gives with human blood lymphocytes and their interpretation. Some have been unable to obtain EA-rosettes (Shevach *et al.*, 1973), and others have reported positive but conflicting findings. Thus 18–35% of lymphocytes from different subjects tested by Brain and Marston (1973) gave EA-rosettes, in most of which the central cell was Ig-bearing by immunofluorescence. Jondal *et al.* (1973) likewise found that about 50% of the Ig-bearing cells in the blood form EA-rosettes. On the other hand, Froland and Natvig (1973) found a mean incidence of 14·5% EA-rosettes in the mononuclear cells separated from human blood, and that the proportion of EA-rosetting cells was not reduced, but increased, when both Ig-bearing cells and monocytes were removed by prior passage through nylon-fibre columns.

As we have seen, Ig bearing cells in the blood include a population of cells carrying Ig bound through Fc receptors (surface labile Ig) which is considerably more numerous than the population of true B-cells defined by their possession of intrinsic surface Ig. B-cells undoubtedly carry receptors for IgG, since like monocytes, they readily bind heat-aggregated human gamma globulin (Agg HGG) and soluble immune complexes (Dickler and Kunkel, 1972). We have found, however, that the presence of 7S IgG does not inhibit such binding of AggHGG, nor does AggHGG displace bound 7S IgG from the lymphocyte surface.

The population of non-B-lymphocytes carrying Fc receptors appears to be heterogeneous. It includes cells that both bind AggHGG and form EA-rosettes, others that only form EA-rosettes (Papamichail *et al.*, 1976) and cells that can act as effectors in antibody-mediated cytoxicity (Papamichail and Temple, 1975). Dickler (1974) has shown that the presence of AggHGG does not entirely inhibit the activity of the latter, and Ferrarini *et al.* (1975) report that the same is true for EA-rosetting. They also find that some human T-cells may show Fc receptors of this sort, probably as a result of stimulation. The picture is thus somewhat confusing, but it seems that different subpopulations of lymphocytes in normal human blood are identified by different methods of detecting Fc receptors. When monocytes and B-lymphocytes with intrinsic surface Ig are excluded, the remaining blood lymphocytes with Fc receptors are a mixed population which includes activated T-cells, and cells ("killer" or K-cells) that are cytotoxic towards antibody-coated target cells. Whether these cytotoxic cells are immature cells that will eventually become Ig-bearing B-cells is at present unknown.

K-cell Cytotoxicity (Antibody-mediated Cytotoxicity-AMC)

Non-immune human lymphoid cells have a lytic effect on antibody-coated target cells (Perlmann and Holm, 1969), which is mediated through the Fc part of the antibody (Moller and Svehag, 1972) but is independent of complement, and is inhibited by the presence of soluble immune complexes (MacLennan, 1972). The exact mechanism of cytolysis is not clear but intimate contact between lymphoid cells and target cells is a prerequisite.

The effector or killer cells (K-cells) are not thymus-derived (Harding *et al.*, 1971; Van Boxel *et al.*, 1972) but their identification amongst the heterogeneous population of bone marrow-derived lymphocytes and monocytes which carry Fc receptors is controversial. Patients with X-linked agammaglobulinaemia, lacking B-cells bearing surface Ig, show normal antibody-mediated cytotoxicity (Wisloff and Froland, 1973) and removal of Ig bearing lymphocytes from lymphoid cell suspensions causes no decrease in AMC (Greenberg *et al.*, 1973).

A subpopulation of lymphocytes exists—"null cells"—which has Fc receptors but no detectable surface Ig (Froland and Natvig, 1973) and this subpopulation contains effector cells participating in AMC, as we have seen (Papamichail and Temple, 1975; Wisloff *et al.*, 1974). There is no correlation, however, between the percentage of EA rosette-forming cells and the degree of AMC activity in cell suspensions from various lymphoid tissues, and although treatment with the enzymes trypsin, pronase or phospholipase-C, markedly diminishes the number of EA rosettes formed, the AMC activity remains unimpaired (Kedar *et al.*, 1974). Thus AMC may be mediated by cells with fewer Fc receptor sites per unit surface area than are required for rosette formation. Chess *et al.* (1974a) however, suggest that AMC is ascribable to lymphocytes in both the B- and "null" cell populations. Such differences probably reflect differences in sensitivity in the systems used for detection.

The importance of AMC as an *in vivo* mechanism producing tissue damage in human disease is not yet clear. Human peripheral blood mononuclear cells can kill a microorganism, *Cryptococcus neoformans*, in the presence of specific antibody, by a non-phagocytic mechanism (Diamond, 1974), and the presence of anti-cryptococcal antibody in the serum of patients with cryptococcosis has been correlated with eventual cure (Bindschadler and Bennett, 1968). A serum factor in a patient with transitional-cell carcinoma of the urinary tract which induced lymphocyte-mediate cytotoxicity against the carcinoma cells was an IgG immunoglobulin, possibly an antibody against an antigen associated with the tumour (Hakala *et al.*, 1974). In auto-immune thyroid disease Calder *et al.* (1976) find a marked elevation of K-cell cytotoxic activity in the peripheral blood lymphoid cells. The fact that this was most marked in patients with little or no goitre, and inversely related to goitre size, might suggest that K-cells are sequestered in the enlarged thyroids.

It is postulated by Campbell *et al.* (1976) as a result of a study carried out in ulcerative colitis that the immunosuppressive drug azathioprine selectively diminishes antibody dependent K-cell activity on prolonged administration. In patients receiving azathioprine (2·5 mg/kg weight/day) the total blood lymphocyte count fell by 36% after a year, but a much greater (25 fold) fall in K-cell activity was noted. Azathioprine produced little clinical benefit in the disease—perhaps not surprisingly, since K-cell activity was sometimes very low during acute exacerbations—but these observations suggest that measurement of AMC might provide a useful pointer to the individual dose requirements of patients receiving azathioprine for conditions where it has more obvious beneficial effects.

Receptors for Complement (C3 Receptors)

Sheep erythrocytes coated with antibody and complement (EAC) bind to certain human lymphocytes, forming rosettes. These EAC-rosetting lymphocytes belong to the B-cell population (Jondal *et al.*, 1972). Many other human cells have C3 receptors, namely, monocytes, polymorphonuclear cells, platelets and red blood cells; the ability of primate red cells to promote immune adherence of microorganisms and other particulate antigens in the presence of antibody and complement is due to their C3 receptors.

The formation of EAC-rosettes is not inhibited by pretreatment of lymphocytes with anti-Ig antisera, nor by the presence of antigen-antibody complexes, so that antigen receptors, Fc receptors and C3 receptors are distinct.

When mononuclear cells separated from normal human blood by a density gradient method are tested for C3-rosette formation about 15–20% of the cells form rosettes. When phagocytic cells are eliminated, the percentage of EAC falls to less than 10% (Pincus *et al.*, 1972) a figure which is in good agreement with the expected incidence of B-cells. The difference draws attention to the fact that monocytes carry C3 receptors as well as Fc receptors, but it is not yet clear that all B-cells form EAC-rosettes. With this proviso, EAC-rosetting can be used as an independent test for B-cells.

Human lymphocytes have different receptors for mouse C3 and human C3. Further, there are two different receptors on human lymphocytes for human complement, one specific for C3b and one specific for C3b-inactivator-cleaved C3b or C3d (Ross *et al.*, 1973). C3 receptors are present on granulocytes as well as on B lymphocytes but differ in specificity, granulocytes binding only C3b (Eden *et al.*, 1973). Recently a receptor for C4b has been demonstrated on human peripheral B-lymphocytes and polymorphonuclear leukocytes (Ross and Polley, 1974) which co-operates with the C3b receptor in the binding of complexes of antigen-antibody and complement to lymphocytes. The binding of EAC to complement receptors is firm, and has been successfully used to indicate by adherence to cryostat sections the anatomical distribution of B-cell populations in human lymphoid tissues, for example in germinal centres and in the marginal zone of the white pulp in spleen (Silveira *et al.*, 1972). This method has also been used to demonstrate the B-cell origin of malignant lymphomas (Jaffe *et al.*, 1974) leukaemic infiltrates in the skin (Eddelson *et al.*, 1973) and mononuclear cell infiltrates in lip biopsies from patients with Sjögren's syndrome (Chused *et al.*, 1974).

Another rosetting indicator for B-lymphocytes bearing C3 receptors is zymosan particles which have been incubated with fresh serum and have absorbed activated C3 (Mendes *et al.*, 1974).

Other Methods of Identifying B-lymphocytes

Spontaneous Rosettes with Mouse Erythrocytes

Under conditions similar to those for forming E-rosettes (see below) mouse red blood cells form spontaneous rosettes with a proportion of normal human blood lymphocytes. The mean percentage of cells forming mouse RBC-rosettes is 8·5% (Stathopoulos and Elliot, 1974). Tests combining immunofluorescent staining of surface Ig and mouse RBC-rosetting show that mouse-rosetting cells have surface Ig (Catovsky *et al.*, 1975). This is a useful simple alternative method for B cells.

B-cell Antigens

Antisera raised in rabbits by injection of chronic lymphocytic leukaemia lymphocytes with B-cell characteristics have been successfully rendered specific for B-lymphocytes by fluorescence after absorption with human red cells, liver, IgG and thymus cells. Specificity has been established by the concordant results of staining for surface Ig, and by an inverse relationship with E-rosette formation (Greaves and Brown, 1973). An antiserum against human tonsil cells depleted of T-cells, and similarly absorbed, was likewise specific for B-cells (Ishii *et al.*, 1975). This antiserum was non-toxic for thymocytes but lysed the majority of chronic lymphocytic leukaemia cells, and tonsil and blood lymphocytes carrying complement receptors. In frozen sections of tonsil it stained by immunofluorescence the membranes of cells in germinal centres, while the plasma cells and cells located in thymus-dependent areas were negative.

Markers for Thymus-derived Lymphocytes (T-cells)

Rosette-formation with Sheep Erythrocytes (E-rosettes)

In mixtures of human thymocytes and sheep erythrocytes virtually all the thymus cells form rosettes (Lay *et al.*, 1971). The proportion of human blood lymphocytes forming E-rosettes (Brain *et al.*, 1970) varies according to the conditions of the test, but up to 65–80% of separated blood mononuclear cells may do so. These cells constitute a clearly defined separate population which does not overlap with that bearing surface Ig (Papamichail *et al.*, 1972). On sedimentation and recovery the E-rosetting cells have the properties of T-cells, and lack both C_3 receptors and, unless activated, Fc receptors. Monocytes do not form E-rosettes.

The nature of the E-rosette phenomenon is not clearly understood. Dead cells do not rosette, and anti-human Ig antisera do not inhibit rosette formation. Reagents which interfere with cell respiration, glycolysis and microfilament movement, though not microtubule structure, inhibit rosette formation, as do drugs that elevate intracellular levels of cyclic AMP. Neuraminidase treatment of the sheep red cells increases their binding affinity, and hence facilitates separation of rosetting cells by density gradient methods.

The E-rosette test provides a ready means of enumerating T-cells, but its significance for T-cell function is obscure. A so called "active rosette test" has been described which is performed without incubation (Wybran and Fudenberg, 1973). Under these conditions a mean of 28·4% of human peripheral lymphocytes are reported to form rosettes and these presumably have a higher affinity for SRBC. It is possible that this test distinguishes two T-cell subpopulations with different immunological functions.

In patients treated with transfer factor, an increased number of E-rosettes has been found and the number of E-rosettes correlates well with the clinical status of patients with cancer (Wybran and Fudenberg, 1973). Lymphocytes forming E-rosettes have been found to kill tumour cells from the same individual.

Lowering of the minimal *in vitro* concentration of anti-lymphocyte serum (ALS) inhibiting E-rosette formation has been used as a measure of the effect of immunosuppressive drugs on patients' lymphocytes, but Chapel and Batchelor (1974), testing the lymphocytes of patients with spontaneous immunosuppression following severe burns were unable to show any increase in the minimal inhibitory concentration of ALS at a time when skin grafts were being rejected after prolonged survival.

T-lymphocytes activated by mitogen stimulation make rosettes with human group O red cells (H-rosettes) and increased numbers of blood lymphocytes forming such H-rosettes are reported in T-cell proliferative conditions such as infectious mononucleosis (Sheldon and Holborow, 1975).

Anti-T-cell Specific Antisera

Numerous anti-T-cell antisera have been produced in rabbits by injection of either human thymocytes or peripheral blood lymphocytes from patients with X-linked agammaglobulinaemia. Absorption of these antisera with chronic lymphocytic leukaemia cells, or lymphocytes from cell lines positive for surface Ig has been used to make them specific for human T-cells, as judged by immunofluorescent staining, or by cytotoxicity in the presence of complement. Anti-brain antiserum raised in rabbits and absorbed with human red cells, liver homogenates and cell lines with B-cell characteristics has also been reported to react specifically with T-cells (Brown and Greaves, 1974b).

Such antisera, though difficult to render specific, are additional reagents for detecting T-cells, probably most useful for identifying the origin of blast cells, for example in cases of acute lymphoblastic leukaemia where other tests for T- and B-cells are negative.

Other Markers for T-cells

Infectious mononucleosis sera may contain IgM antibody which reacts with T-lymphocytes (Thomas, 1972). This detects only about 30% of T-cells and the need to use the indirect method with fluorescein-labelled anti-human Ig (which of course also detects the B-cells) has not encouraged its use.

Sera from patients with cold agglutinin disease, systemic lupus erythematosus and cryoglobulinaemia may contain cold IgM antibodies cytotoxic for a subpopulation of normal lymphocytes (Thomas, 1973). By separation of Ig-positive lymphocytes it has been found that these antibodies are specific for human T-cells, the percentage of peripheral blood lymphocytes reactive with them ranging from 29–50%.

Neuraminidase-treated human lymphocytes are agglutinated by a purified haemagglutinin from the snail *Helix pomatia* (Hammerstrom *et al.*, 1973). Immunofluorescence tests show that approximately 65% of peripheral blood lymphocytes react in this way, and an inverse relationship with results of tests for Fc and complement receptors and for cells bearing surface Ig, suggests that it is a reagent specific for T-lymphocytes.

β_2-microglobulin has been shown by immunofluorescent staining and by the mixed antiglobulin reaction to be present on the surface of both T- and B-human peripheral blood lymphocytes. Although β_2-microglobulin is detectable on the surface of all peripheral blood lymphocytes, a proportion (18%) stains more brightly than the rest (Fanger and Bernier, 1973). This minority does not bear detectable surface Ig and may constitute a part of the T-lymphocyte subpopulation.

Specific Markers for Blast Cells

An antiserum raised against human thymocytes after appropriate absorption with Ig-bearing cell lines and normal peripheral lymphocytes was specific for thymocytes and T-lymphoblasts (PHA stimulated cells) but did not react with normal resting lymphocytes (Thomas and Phillips, 1973a).

In mice 80% of T-lymphoblasts but only 8% of B-lymphoblasts stain with the periodic acid Schiff (PAS) reagent after stimulation with pokeweed mitogen (Greaves and Janossy, 1972), and this is attributed to cytoplasmic glycogen content. We have found that 60% of human peripheral lymphocytes after PHA stimulation are PAS positive. In a patient with a T-cell leukaemia we investigated (Stathopoulos *et al.*, 1974) the number of PAS positive cells was 30%, but these were only very weakly positive. After PHA stimulation the percentage increased to 90% by the third day. This suggests that PAS staining might be a useful histochemical marker for T-cell lymphoblasts.

Antisera against B-cell blasts have been produced by injecting rabbits with Burkitt's lymphoma cells and rendered specific by absorption with thymocytes and normal peripheral lymphocytes (Thomas and Phillips, 1973a). These antisera react with all lymphoblastoid cell lines having surface Ig and with B cell blasts, but not with normal peripheral blood lymphocytes.

IgM antibodies found in the sera of 20% of cases of infectious mononucleosis are directed against surface antigen present on B-lymphoblasts (Thomas and Phillips, 1973b). This B-blast antigen is present in a subpopulation of the blast cells induced by PHA stimulation and is also present in B-cell lines.

STIMULATION BY POLYCLONAL MITOGENS

The ability of these to stimulate T- or B-cells selectively, although extensively studied in mice, was initially investigated in man in patients with selective immunodeficiency diseases. In the absence of the thymus (di George syndrome) PHA responsiveness is absent; there is a progressive increase of PHA response after thymus transplantation, together with a decrease in the proportion of Ig-bearing lymphocytes in the peripheral blood (Gajl-Peczalska *et al.*, 1973a).

Nevertheless, Phillips and Roitt (1973) showed that 30% of blast cells in a human peripheral blood lymphocyte suspension stimulated with PHA were stained by immunofluorescence with anti-light-chain sera. Further, using a digestible Sephadex column coated with anti-Fab to separate B-cells, they showed that 86% of the cells thus obtained gave staining blast forms when cultured with PHA. These results were confirmed by staining with a specific antiserum against B-lymphoblasts (Thomas and Phillips, 1973a), but contrasted with the fact that pretreatment of the lymphocytes with cytotoxic anti-T-cell serum abolishes the capacity to respond to PHA (Aiuti and Wigzell, 1973a). Later experiments (Greaves *et al.*, 1974), in which the two main lymphocyte sub-populations were separated in different ways and in which the surface properties of the blast cells produced were studied (Jondal, 1974), verified that PHA is predominantly a selective T-cell mitogen and that B-lymphocytes alone are not stimulated by PHA, but also showed that in a mixture of T- and B-cells from 5% to 15% of the B-cells undergo stimulation. Concanavalin A produces a similar effect (Lohrmann *et al.*, 1974a). Pokeweed mitogen, in contrast, stimulates T- and B-cells independently (Greaves *et al.*, 1974).

A "non-specific" mitogen for human B-cells is still lacking. The only stimulant so far found which unequivocally acts on human B-cells but not on T-cells is anti-human Ig antiserum (Abdou and Abdou, 1972). Levan, bacterial lipopolysaccharide and dextran are mitogenic for mouse B-cells (Andersson *et al.*, 1973) but appear to require phagocytic cells to produce this effect on human B-cells. They may thus be releasing endogenous macrophage mitogen rather than acting directly.

MIXED LYMPHOCYTE REACTION (MLR)

Mixed leukocyte culture has been used chiefly in studies of the recognition aspect of the homograft reaction, where skin graft survival correlates inversely with MLC reactivity, in evaluating cellular responsiveness, and in histocompatibility testing. There is general agreement that the responder cells in the MLR are T-lymphocytes, based on evidence from experiments with cell suspensions either depleted of T-cells with specific anti-T-sera and complement (Aiuti and Wigzell, 1973b) or enriched by passage through columns coated with anti-Ig to remove B-cells (Jondal *et al.*, 1973). Such activation of T-cells by allogeneic cells requires the presence of monocytes (Lohrmann *et al.*, 1974a).

Both T- and B-target cells are capable of inducing proliferation of allogeneic T-cells (Chess *et al.*, 1974) but the major stimuli in the human MLR appear to be B-cell alloantigens, human T-cells possessing only weak stimulatory capacity (Lohrmann *et al.*, 1974a).

Although the MLR thus appears to be a good way of assessing the responsiveness of T-cells it should be remembered that the presence of auto-antibodies directed against surface antigen(s) of T-cells may have an inhibitory effect (Wernet and Kunkel, 1973).

LYMPHOCYTE MARKER TESTS IN DISEASE

The markers described above have been used for the identification and characterization of lymphocytes in a variety of infections, connective tissue diseases, malignancies and other human disorders.

Lymphoproliferative Disorders

The introduction of reliable recognition tests for human B- and T-lymphocytes has greatly helped to characterize the predominant lymphoid cells in various lymphoproliferative disorders. These provided good models for initial studies in human disease because the presence of large numbers of abnormal lymphoid cells in the peripheral blood or lymphoid tissues of patients allowed clear-cut observations and unambiguous conclusions.

In *chronic lymphatic leukaemia* (*CLL*), tests for B-cell markers show that in the majority of cases the leukaemic cells belong to the B-cell subpopulation (Papamichail *et al.*, 1971; Wilson and Nossal, 1971; Froland and Natvig, 1971; Pernis *et al.*, 1971; Preud'homme *et al.*, 1971; Pincus *et al.*, 1972; Ross *et al.*, 1973b). In *Waldenstrom's macroglobulinaemia* (Preud'homme and Seligmann, 1972a) and in *plasma cell leukaemia* likewise, the B-cell series is affected. The percentage of lymphocytes bearing surface IgM is usually high in Waldenstrom's macroglobulinaemia and in some cases near 100%. In other patients, however, low numbers of IgM bearing cells are present and they may even be absent. No influence of treatment on the percentage of cells with membrane bound IgM has been found (Knapp *et al.*, 1974).

These three conditions thus appear to be B-cell neoplasias occurring at different stages of differentiation. Lymphocytes from fresh biopsy samples or cell lines from Burkitt's lymphoma patients also carry intrinsic surface IgM (Klein *et al.*, 1968) and are classed as B-lymphocytes.

A low proportion of T-lymphocytes has been reported in many studies of chronic lymphocytic leukemias. This reflects the dilution of the T-cell population by the much larger number of B-cells. Assessment of the T-cell population as a percentage of the total lymphocytes is thus misleading. A normally reactive T-cell population is present in CLL patients and the lack of responsiveness in CLL to mitogens is due to the dilution of normally responding cells (Wybran *et al.*, 1973). Further, the absolute number of T-lymphocytes is reported to correlate with the clinical pattern in CLL patients (Catovsky *et al.*, 1974a). A significantly greater absolute number of circulating T-lymphocytes was observed in untreated patients with clinically stable disease, as compared with a treated group of patients with evidence of active disease.

Although the abnormal lymphoid cells in most patients with the foregoing conditions have B-cell characteristics, in some patients it is the T-cells that are selectively affected by malignancy. The first of these to come to light was a malignant mediastinal lymphoid tumour (Smith *et al.*, 1973), and subsequently cases of chronic lymphatic leukaemia have been reported where the abnormal cells were negative for B-cell markers but gave a large number of E-rosettes (Lille *et al.*, 1973; Dickler *et al.*, 1973) and positive staining with anti-T antisera. We have studied such a case where all the B-cell markers (Fc receptor, C3, Ig, reactivity with specific anti-B antisera) were negative and the T-cell markers positive (95% E-rosettes, staining with anti-T-cell antisera). The response to T-cell mitogens (phytohaemagglutinin, concanavalin A) in this patient was normal, but the base-line incorporation of labelled thymidine was very high (Stathopoulos *et al.*, 1974). Such T-cell leukaemias may prove to have a worse prognosis than leukaemias of B-cell type, since two out of three such patients reported have had concomitant carcinoma, while none of 23 B-cell leukaemias concurrently studied had second neoplasms (Russell and Cochran, 1973).

Bizarre results of lymphocyte identification are sometimes obtained in chronic lymphatic leukaemia. Two patients are reported whose lymphocytes bore monoclonal Ig on their surface and formed rosettes with sheep erythrocytes (Brouet and Prieur, 1974). In one, the rosette formation was due to an anti-erythrocyte activity of surface bound Ig, and in the other the surface Ig could not be shown to be a product of the cells. In another patient with a lymphoproliferative disorder, reported by Sandilands *et al.* (1974) the tumour cells formed spontaneous rosettes with sheep erythrocytes and also EA-rosettes but did not have detectable surface Ig. A third example is a patient with CLL whose leukaemic lymphocytes bore the receptor for sheep erythrocytes characteristic of human T-lymphocytes and the receptor for antigen-antibody-complement complexes characteristic of human B-lymphocytes (Shevach *et al.*, 1974). It is of interest that a small number (2%) of normal human lymphocytes appear to bear both of these receptors so that the CLL lymphocytes in this case may represent a clone originating from this subpopulation.

Ig Class of CLL Cells

The predominant class of Ig on the surface of CLL cells is IgM (Grey *et al.*, 1971; Pernis *et al.*, 1971; Aisenberg and Bloch, 1972). Cases have been reported however where more than one heavy chain class of surface Ig was found on CLL lymphocytes (Papamichail *et al.*, 1971; Holborow and Papamichail, 1973; Piessens *et al.*, 1973; Preud'homme and Seligman, 1972b). After enzymatic digestion, these dual-staining cells resynthesize only one class of Ig i.e. they are presumably monoclonal as far as the Ig they synthesize is concerned. This is confirmed by experiments in which incorporation of radioactive amino acids by CLL cells in short-term culture was used to analyse their Ig product (Nies *et al.*, 1973). The surface density of Ig on CLL lymphocytes varies from case to case, but it is not known whether this is a prognostic feature.

Receptors for aggregated HGG are consistently present on CLL lymphocytes, even in the absence of detectable surface Ig (Dickler *et al.*, 1973). Our own observations confirm this. C3 receptors on CLL cells have been looked for, but conflicting results are reported (Pincus *et al.*, 1972; Shevach *et al.*, 1972; Michlmayr and Huber, 1970; Nishioka, 1971) perhaps because of the different sources of complement used. It is known that mouse complement is better than human complement for detecting receptors on human CLL lymphocytes (Ross *et al.*, 1973b).

Much work still remains to be done in CLL to determine whether the presence or absence of any of the known B-cell markers is related to prognosis or the effects of therapy.

The origin of the malignant cells in *leukaemic reticuloendotheliosis* (*hairy-cell leukaemia*) has been the subject of some controversy. It was first reported (Shevach *et al.*, 1973) that the cells are probably of monocytic origin since they possess a receptor for 7S immunoglobulin and do not form EAC-rosettes. Subsequently it was shown that hairy cells have similarities to B-lymphocytes, namely, they bear surface Ig of one (Aisenberg *et al.*, 1973) or sometimes two or more Ig classes (Catovsky *et al.*, 1974b); and form spontaneous rosettes with mouse erythrocytes (Catovsky *et al.*, 1975). Unlike monocytes, they do not form rosettes with human red cells coated with traces of C_3 (Catovsky *et al.*, 1974). From the foregoing it seems that hairy cells are closely related to B-cells. The possibility of passive absorption of immunoglobulin on the surface of those cells, however, has not been entirely ruled out.

Tests for T-cells have been positive with lymphoblast forms in some cases of *acute lymphoblastic leukaemia* (*ALL*) both with specific anti-T sera (Smith *et al.*, 1973) and by E-rosetting (Kersey *et al.*, 1973). Occasionally the lymphoblasts in ALL have apparently been like B-cells in character (Gajl-Peczalska *et al.*, 1974) but in the majority of cases neither T- nor B-receptors have been demonstrated. Allo-antibodies in pregnancy sera with specificity for Ia-like antigens preferentially expressed on B-cells (p. 39) identify a proportion of ALL cases as probably of B-cell origin (Fu *et al.*, 1975).

Lymphoma and Lymphosarcoma

Table 3 shows some reported frequencies of T- and B-cells in normal human lymphoid tissues for comparison.

TABLE 3

T- and B-cells in normal human lymphoid tissues

	Ig-bearing cells	EAC-rosettes	E-rosettes	References
Bone marrow	6%	—	—	Klein *et al.*, 1970
Thoracic duct	18%	24%	—	Ross *et al.*, 1973b
Lymph node	23%	—	—	Verma *et al.*, 1971
Lymph node	—	31%	—	Pincus *et al.*, 1972
Lymph node	20·7%	—	57·4%	Stathopoulos *et al.*, 1977a
Spleen	—	58%	26%	Visakorpi and Repo, 1973
Spleen	24–35%	18–30%	23–32%	Fiorelli *et al.*, 1974
Spleen	35%	—	—	Kaur *et al.*, 1975
Spleen	34%	—	50·7%	Stathopoulos *et al.*, 1977a
Spleen	31%	—	40%	Belpomme *et al.*, 1974
Tonsils	—	59·6%	40%	Pincus *et al.*, 1972
Tonsils	42·4%	—	53·4%	Brown and Greaves, 1974b

Most cases of lymphoma and lymphosarcoma are probably B-cell malignancies (Seligmann *et al.*, 1973, Jaffe *et al.*, 1974), but according to Kaplan *et al.* (1974) lymph node lymphocytes from childhood lymphoblastic lymphoma possess T-cell characteristics. Lymph node lymphocytes from nine patients with non-Hodgkin's lymphomas were tested for T- and B-cell markers and it was found that in six the cells resembled B-cells, in two there was T-cell proliferation and in one the cells had no detectable receptors (Peter *et al.*, 1974). In fresh lymph node biopsy material from 24 patients with non-Hodgkin's malignant lymphomas, we found that the lymphocytic lymphomas, either nodular or diffuse, were of B-cell type, while in the histiocytic lymphomas and immunoblastic lymphadenopathies there were more lymphocytes forming E-rosettes than bearing Ig (Stathopoulos *et al.*, 1977a). Unlike CLL cells, lymphocytic lymphoma cells do not usually rosette with mouse erythrocytes (Stathopoulos and Davies, 1976).

Hodgkin's Disease

Some have found depleted numbers of T-cells in the blood (Aiuti and Wigzell, 1973b) especially where the histological picture is one of mixed cellularity rather than nodular sclerosis (Andersen, 1974); others report normal numbers of both T- and B-cells (Froland, 1972; Cohnen *et al.*, 1973). T-cell depletion might result from preferential sequestration in the spleen and lymph nodes, and Kaur *et al.* (1974) found that the mean percentage of T-lymphocytes in the spleens of Hodgkin's disease patients was higher (67%) than in non-malignant spleens (23%), although the T-cell/B-cell proportion in the blood was normal.

In a comparison of lymph nodes infiltrated with Hodgkin's tissue and tumour free lymph nodes, we have also found that the lymphocytes from lymph nodes removed from Hodgkin's patients were 70% E-rosetting cells and 17·3% Ig-bearing. In lymph nodes from patients without malignant disease the percentages were 57·3% and 20·7% respectively (Stathopoulos *et al.*, 1976). This does not necessarily mean that the malignant cell in Hodgkin's disease is a T-cell, since the increase in T-cells numbers may be due to proliferation against the Hodgkin's cells (Kay, 1975).

In summary, it seems that malignant proliferation may occur in any of the lymphocyte subpopulations, though with proportionately different frequencies. Studies in more patients are needed to identify the origins of the abnormal cells in the different lymphoproliferative disorders and to determine whether the presence or absence of given cell receptors correlates with prognosis or responses to treatment.

Leprosy

Two studies (Gajl-Peczalska *et al.*, 1973b; Dwyer *et al.*, 1973) have revealed a disturbed ratio of T- to B-lymphocytes in leprosy, with increased B-cell numbers and decreased T-cells with a low PHA response. This is consistent with the reported depletion of T-cells in the paracortical areas of the lymph nodes in such patients (Mendes *et al.*, 1974). Recently it was found (Nath *et al.*, 1974) that a subpopulation of T-cells is reduced in lepromatous leprosy cases with high bacillary load. Tuberculoid and treated lepromatous patients who were bacillus-negative, had normal levels of these cells. Again, a high number of B-lymphocytes was found in lepromatous patients irrespective of treatment and bacillary load.

Infectious Mononucleosis

Increased numbers of T-cells in the peripheral blood are the rule and the majority of atypical cells form E-rosettes and are thus of thymic origin (Sheldon *et al.*, 1973; Pattengale *et al.*, 1974). Rosette formation is not attributed to the presence of heterophile antibody on the surface of the lymphocytes since pretreatment of the cell with anti-Ig serum did not inhibit it (Papamichail *et al.*, 1974). While the atypical lymphocytes have T-cell characteristics, lymphoid cell lines established from infectious mononucleosis blood leukocytes show the surface properties of B-cells (Yata *et al.*, 1973). A minority (about 10%) of the atypical cells in infectious mononucleosis do not form rosettes, and may be B-cells infected by EB virus (Papamichail *et al.*, 1974; Denman and Pelton, 1974). T-cells evidently play an important part in the immune response to the EB virus and therefore in the progress of the disease.

The presence of increased numbers of IgM bearing lymphocytes is reported in the blood during the early phase of the disease (Piessens *et al.*, 1973), but we have not been able to confirm this. A possible explanation is that in some cases T-cells are coated with auto-antibodies directed against their surface antigens (Thomas, 1972) so that they stain as B-cells by immunofluorescence. In one patient we have studied, for example, 40% of the peripheral blood mononuclear cells gave surface fluorescence with anti-Ig but when a combined test was done 40% of these Ig-bearing cells formed E-rosettes, thus revealing their T-cell nature.

Hashimoto's Thyroiditis and Graves's Disease

A greatly increased proportion of T-cells was found in the blood in Hashimoto's thyroiditis and in Graves' disease by Farid *et al.* (1973) using a dextran sedimentation method for lymphocyte separation, but in another study, when a Ficoll-triosil gradient was used, the numbers of T- and B-cells were not significantly different from controls (Urbaniak *et al.*, 1974). This is a reminder that where absolute numbers of blood lymphocytes are not grossly abnormal, different methods of lymphocyte separation and different degrees of contamination with monocytes have to be especially considered as causes of discrepant findings.

Connective Tissue Diseases

In initial studies (Papamichail *et al.*, 1971) we found a raised proportion of B-cells in the blood of rheumatoid arthritis patients but this was not confirmed in a larger series of patients (Sheldon *et al.*, 1974). Winchester *et al.* (1975b) have drawn attention to the effect of anti-lymphocyte antibodies in rheumatoid arthritis in simulating surface Ig in immunofluorescence. Decreased numbers of T-cells have been reported in the blood of some patients with severe forms of the disease (Williams *et al.*, 1973), but usually a majority of the lymphocytes in the synovial fluid in rheumatoid joints are T-cells (Sheldon *et al.*, 1974). An unusually high number of "null" cells, neither T nor B, has also been noted (Winchester *et al.*, 1973) and K-cell activity has been demonstrated in the synovial effusion cells at about the level present in the blood (Scheinberg and Cathcart, 1976a).

In systemic lupus erythematosus (SLE) and in Felty's syndrome low numbers of B-cells have been found in the blood and in SLE an increased number of "null" cells (Williams *et al.*, 1973). As discussed above, there is evidence to suggest that a "null" cell population participates in antibody mediated cytotoxicity (Greenberg *et al.*, 1973), but K-cell activity in the blood is reported to be reduced in SLE (Schneider *et al.*, 1975). Scheinberg and Cathcart (1976b) have confirmed this, and have demonstrated in addition a blocking effect of serum from active SLE on the K-cell activity of normal lymphocytes, presumably due to the presence of soluble immune complexes. They found, however, that overnight incubation of SLE blood lymphocytes failed to restore K cell activity, and concluded that there is a real depletion of K cells in active SLE, rather than a functional blocking by complexes. The increase in "null" cells, which they also confirm, they attribute to an influx of immature T-cells. The reported effect of azathioprine on K-cell activity is described on p. 59.

Changes in B-lymphocytes as measured by Ig and C3 receptors, and in T-lymphocytes as measured by T-cell-specific antiserum and E-binding techniques, were studied during the course of SLE (Messner *et al.*, 1973). Both relative and absolute decreases in T-lymphocytes and in cells bearing a receptor for complement were found in active lupus. Absolute numbers of cells bearing surface Ig were decreased to a lesser extent, while the proportion of these cells was increased. From these data it was postulated that the reduction of delayed hypersensitivity and the increase of autoantibody formation in lupus may be due to a partial loss of T-lymphocyte function. Absolute numbers and the proportions of B- and T-lymphocytes were also determined in 16 active and 11 inactive patients with SLE by Scheinberg and Cathcart (1974). The total number of T- and B-lymphocytes was significantly reduced compared with normal subjects, the T-lymphocytes being predominantly affected. These abnormalities improved in patients in remission, and it was concluded that serial T- and B-cell enumeration may be of value in assessing the clinical activity of the disease.

Sézary's Syndrome

The atypical mononuclear cells in the peripheral blood and in the skin infiltrates have the properties of T-cells (Preud'homme and Seligmann, 1972b; Brouet *et al.*, 1973).

Immunodeficiencies (See Chapter 14)

T-cell Defects

Di George's syndrome is characterized by congenital absence of the thymus with normal serum levels of immunoglobulins. A high proportion of Ig bearing lymphocytes is found in the peripheral blood (Cooper and Lawton, 1972) and lymph nodes (Gajl-Peczalska *et al.*, 1973a). High numbers of B-cells (Froland *et al.*, 1974) and very few E-rosettes (Wybran *et al.*, 1973a) are seen in Nezélof's syndrome, another congenital thymic dysplasia.

After thymus transplant in a patient with di George's syndrome the high levels of B-lymphocytes found before treatment decreased to normal, and restoration of a normal PHA response was achieved (Gajl-Peczalska *et al.*, 1973a). In a patient with severe immunodeficiency, an absent thymus shadow and lymphocyte unresponsiveness to PHA, a very high percentage (94%) of B-cells was found in the peripheral blood (Preud'homme *et al.*, 1973).

Bone Marrow Deficiency

Results of tests for surface Ig show two main patterns; i) absence or very low numbers of Ig-bearing lymphocytes, and ii) normal or increased numbers of Ig-bearing cells but low levels of corresponding serum Ig and absence of plasma cells in the lymphoid tissues. These two patterns probably represent arrest of bone marrow lymphocyte maturation at different stages of differentiation. Most cases of X-linked agammaglobulinaemia show the first pattern, Ig-bearing lymphocytes being scanty or absent (Grey *et al.*, 1971; Gajl-Peczalska *et al.*, 1973a; Froland and Natvig, 1972; Cooper *et al.*, 1971). Three out of six cases in one study, however, had Ig-bearing lymphocytes in numbers above the lower limit of normal (Siegal *et al.*, 1971). In another proved case of X-linked agammaglobulinaemia, and in two further probable cases, numbers of B-lymphocytes as judged by immunofluorescence were normal (Geha *et al.*, 1973). The numbers of EAC-rosettes are usually within normal limits (Schiff *et al.*, 1974; Luckasen *et al.*, 1974).

When pokeweed mitogen is used to stimulate B-lymphocytes in culture to undergo terminal differentiation, lymphocytes from normal people synthesize and secrete IgM, IgG and IgA, as may be shown by immunofluorescence and by incorporation of ^{14}C-amino acids in the immunoglobulins produced. Cultures from cases of X-linked agammaglobulinaemia without Ig-bearing cells stimulated in this way do not synthesize immunoglobulins. Cultures from agammaglobulinaemia patients with normal numbers of B-lymphocytes usually, on stimulation with pokeweed, produce the different Ig classes in ratios reflecting the frequencies of the different surface Ig classes on the B-lymphocytes (Wu *et al.*, 1973). However lymphocytes from a boy with low IgG and IgA serum levels, but normal number of lymphocytes bearing surface IgM, IgG and IgA could not be stimulated by pokeweed mitogen to make IgG and IgA. On the other hand synthesis and secretion of IgA as well as IgM and IgG was detected in cell cultures from patients with isolated IgA deficiency. Normal or increased numbers of IgA bearing lymphocytes may be present in the latter condition (Gajl-Peczalska *et al.*, 1973a; Lawton *et al.*, 1972). Thus identification of lymphocyte surface markers may provide a means of separating patients with variable immunodeficiency and panhypogammaglobulinaemia into distinct groups which differ in the nature of their fundamental defect.

REFERENCES

Abdou, N. I. and Abdou, N. L. (1972). Bone marrow: the bursa equivalent in man? *Science* **175**, 446.

Abdou, N. I., Zweiman, B. and Casella, S. R. (1973). Effects of azathioprine therapy on bone marrow-dependent and thymus-dependent cells in man. *Clin. Exp. Immunol.* **13**, 55.

Aisenberg, A. C. and Bloch, K. J. (1972). Immunoglobulins on the surface of neoplastic lymphocytes. *New Eng. J. Med.* **287**, 272.

Aisenberg, A. C., Bloch, K. J. and Long, J. C. (1973). Cell-surface immunoglobulins in chronic lymphocytic leukemia and allied disorders. *Am. J. Med.* **55**, 184.

Aiuti, F. and Wigzell, H. (1973a). Function and distribution pattern of human T lymphocytes. II. Presence of T lymphocytes in normal humans and in humans with various immunodeficiency disorders. *Clin. Exp. Immunol.* **13**, 183.

Aiuti, F. and Wigzell, H. (1973b). Function and distribution pattern of human T lymphocytes. I. Production of anti-T lymphocyte specific sera as estimated by cytotoxicity and elimination of function of lymphocytes. *Clin. Exp. Immunol.* **13**, 171.

Andersen, E. (1974). Depletion of thymus dependent lymphocytes in Hodgkin's disease. *Scand. J. Haemat.* **12**, 263.

Andersson, J., Melchers, F., Galanos, C. H. and Luderitz, O. (1973). The mitogenic effect of lipopolysaccharide on bone marrow derived mouse lymphocytes. Lipid A as the mitogenic part of the molecule. *J. Exp. Med.* **137**, 943.

Belpomme, D., Joseph, R., Navares, L., Gerard-Marchant, R., Huchet, R., Botto, I., Grandjon, D. and Mathé, G. (1974). T lymphocytes and Reed-Sternberg cells in spleen of Hodgkin's disease. *New Eng. J. Med.* **291**, 1417.

Bindschadler, D. D. and Bennett, J. E. (1968). Serology of human cryptococcosis. *Ann. Intern. Med.* **69**, 45.

Brain, P. and Marston, R. H. (1973). Rosette formation by human T and B lymphocytes. *Europ. J. Immunol.* **3**, 6.

Brain, P., Gordon, J. and Willetts, W. A. (1970). Rosette formation by peripheral lymphocytes. *Clin. Exp. Immunol.* **6**, 681.

Brouet, J. C. and Prieur, A. M. (1974). Membrane markers on chronic lymphocytic leukemia cells; a B cell leukemia with rosettes due to anti sheep erythrocytes antibody activity of the membrane bound IgM and a T cell leukemia with surface Ig. *Clin. Immunol. Immunopath.* **2**, 481.

Brouet, J. C., Flandrin, G. and Seligmann, M. (1973). Indications of the thymus-derived nature of the proliferating cells in six patients with Sézary's syndrome. *New Eng. J. Med.* **289**, 341.

Brown, G. and Greaves, M. F. (1974a). Enumeration of absolute numbers of T and B lymphocytes in human blood. *Scand. J. Immunol.* **3**, 161.

Brown, G. and Greaves, M. F. (1974b). Cell surface markers for human T and B lymphocytes. *Europ. J. Immunol.* **4**, 302.

Calder, E. A., Irvine, W. J., Davidson, N. McD., Wu, F. (1976). T, B and K cells in autoimmune thyroid disease. *Clin. Exp. Immunol.* **25**, 17.

Campbell, A. C., Skinner, J. M., MacLennan, I. C. M., Hersey, P., Waller, C. A., Wood, J., Jewell, D. P. and Truelove, S. C. (1976). Immunosuppression in the treatment of inflammatory bowel disease. II. The effects of azathioprine on lymphoid cell populations in a double blind trial in ulcerative colitis. *Clin. Exp. Immunol.* **24**, 249.

Catovsky, D., Miliani, E., Okos, A. and Galton, D. A. G. (1974a). Clinical significance of T-cells in chronic lymphocytic leukaemia. *Lancet* **2**, 751.

Catovsky, D., Pettit, J. E., Galetto, J., Okos, A. and Galton, D. A. G. (1974b). The B-lymphocyte nature of the hairy cell of leukaemia reticuloendotheliosis. *Brit. J. Haemat.* **26**, 29.

Catovsky, D., Papamichail, M., Okos, A., Miliani, E. and Holborow, E. J. (1975). Formation of mouse red cell rosettes by "hairy" cells. *Biomedicine* **23**, 81.

Chapel, H. M. and Batchelor, J. R. (1974). The rosette inhibition test in skin-grafted patients. *Brit. Med. J.* **2**, 636.

Chess, L., MacDermott, R. P., Sondel, P. M. and Schlossman, S. F. (1974). *In* "Progress in Immunology II". (eds. L. Brent and E. J. Holborow), Vol. 3, p. 125, North Holland Publishing Co., Amsterdam and Oxford.

Chused, T. M., Hardin, J. A., Frank, M. M. and Green, I. (1974). Identification of cells infiltrating the minor salivary glands in patients with Sjogren's syndrome. *J. Immunol.* **112**, 641.

Cohnen, G., Augener, W., Konig, E., Brittinger, G. and Douglas, S. D. (1973). B Lymphocytes in Hodgkin's disease. *New Eng. J. Med.* **288**, 161.

Coombs, R. R. A., Feinstein, A. and Wilson, A. B. (1969). Immunoglobulin determinants on the surface of human lymphocytes. *Lancet* **2**, 1157.

Cooper, M. D. and Lawton, A. R. (1972). Circulating B-cells in patients with immunodeficiency. *Am. J. Path.* **69**, 513.

Cooper, M. D., Lawton, A. R. and Bockman, D. E. (1971). Agammaglobulinaemia with B lymphocytes. Specific defect of plasma-cell differentiation. *Lancet* **2**, 791.

Denman, A. M. and Pelton, B. K. (1974). Control mechanisms in infectious mononucleosis. *Clin. Exp. Immunol.* **18**, 13.

Diamond, R. D. (1974). Antibody-dependent killing of Cryptococcus neoformans by human peripheral blood mononuclear cells. *Nature* **247**, 148.

Dickler, H. B. (1974). Studies of the human lymphocyte receptor for heat-aggregated or antigen-complexed immunoglobulin. *J. Exp. Med.* **140**, 508.

Dickler, H. B. and Kunkel, H. G. (1972). Interaction of aggregated γ-globulin with B lymphocytes. *J. Exp. Med.* **136**, 191.

Dickler, H. B., Siegal, F. P., Bentwich, Z. H. and Kunkel, H. G. (1973). Lymphocyte binding of aggregated IgG and surface Ig staining in chronic lymphocytic leukaemia. *Clin. Exp. Immunol.* **14**, 97.

Dwyer, J. M., Bullock, W. E. and Fields, J. P. (1973). Disturbance of the blood T:B lymphocyte ratio in lepromatous leprosy. *New Eng. J. Med.* **288**, 1036.

Edelson, R. L., Smith, R. W., Frank, M. M. and Green, I. (1973). Identification of subpopulations of mononuclear cells in cutaneous infiltrates. I. Differentiation between B cells, T cells, and histiocytes. *J. Invest. Dermatol.* **61**, 82.

Eden, A., Miller, G. W., Nussenzweig, V. (1973). Human lymphocytes bear membrane receptors for C3b and C3d. *J. Clin. Invest.* **52**, 3239.

Fanger, M. W. and Bernier, G. M. (1973). Subpopulations of human lymphocytes defined by ß2-microglobulin. *J. Immunol.* **111**, 609.

Farid, N. R., Munro, R. E., Row, V. V. and Volpe, R. (1973). Peripheral thymus-dependent (T) lymphocytes in Graves's disease and Hashimoto's thyroiditis. *New Eng. J. Med.* **288**, 1313.

Ferrarini, M., Moretta, L., Abrile, R. and Durante, M. L. (1975). Receptors for IgG molecules on human lymphocytes forming spontaneous rosettes with sheep red cells. *Europ. J. Immunol.* **5**, 70.

Fiorelli, G., Fargion, S., Capellini, M. D. and Salerno, F. (1974). T and B lymphocytes in human spleen. *Lancet* **1**, 99.

Froland, S. S. (1972). Binding of sheep erythrocytes to human lymphocytes. A probable marker of T lymphocytes. *Scand. J. Immunol.* **1**, 269.

Froland, S. S. and Natvig, J. B. (1971). *In* "Progress in Immunology". (Ed. B. Amos), p. 107, Academic Press, New York and London.

Froland, S. S. and Natvig, J. B. (1972). Surface-bound immunoglobulin on lymphocytes from normal and immunodeficient humans. *Scand. J. Immunol.* **1**, 1.

Froland, S. S. and Natvig, J. B. (1973). Identification of three different human lymphocyte populations by surface markers. *Transplant. Rev.* **16**, 114.

Froland, S. S., Natvig, J. B. and Michaelsen, T. E. (1974). Binding of aggregated IgG by human B lymphocytes independent of Fc receptors. *Scand. J. Immunol.* **3**, 375.

Fu, S. M., Winchester, R. J., Kunkel, H. G. (1975). The occurrence of the HL-B alloantigens on the cells of unclassified acute lymphoblastic leukemias. *J. exp. Med.* **142**, 1334.

Gajl-Peczalska, K. J., Park, B. H., Biggar, D. and Good, R. A. (1973a). B and T lymphocytes in primary immunodeficiency disease in man. *J. Clin. Invest.* **52**, 919.

Gajl-Peczalska, K. J., Lim, S. L., Jacobson, R. R. and Good, R. A. (1973b). B lymphocytes in lepromatous leprosy. *New Eng. J. Med.* **288**, 1033.

Gajl-Peczalska, K. J., Bloomfield, C. D., Nesbit, M. E. and Kersey, J. H. (1974). B-cell markers on lymphoblasts in acute lymphoblastic leukaemia. *Clin. Exp. Immunol.* **17**, 561.

Geha, R. S., Rosen, F. S. and Merler, E. (1974). Unresponsiveness of human B lymphocytes to phytohaemagglutinin. *Nature* **248**, 426.

Greaves, M. F. and Janossy, G. (1972). Elicitation of selective T and B lymphocyte responses by cell surface binding ligands. *Transplant Rev.* **11**, 87.

Greaves, M. F. and Brown, G. (1973). A human B lymphocyte specific antigen. *Nature, New Biol.* **246**, 116.

Greaves, M. F., Janossy, G. and Doenhoff, M. (1974). Activation of human T and B lymphocytes by polyclonal mitogens. *Nature* **248**, 698.

Greenberg, A. H., Shen, L. and Roitt, I. M. (1973). Characterization of the antibody-dependent cytotoxic cell. A non-phagocytic monocyte? *Clin. Exp. Immunol.* **15**, 251.

Grey, H. M., Rabellino, E. and Pirofsky, B. (1971). Immunoglobulins on the surface of lymphocytes. IV. Distribution in hypogammaglobulinemia, cellular immune deficiency, and chronic lymphatic leukemia. *J. Clin. Invest.* **50**, 2368.

Hakala, T. R., Lange, P. H., Castro, A. E., Elliott, A. Y. and Fraley, E. E. (1974). Antibody induction of lymphocyte-mediated cytotoxicity against human transitional-cell carcinomas of the urinary tract. *New Eng. J. Med.* **291**, 637.

Hammarstrom, S., Hellstrom, U., Perlmann, P. and Dillness, M. L. (1973). A new surface marker on T lymphocytes of human peripheral blood. *J. Exp. Med.* **138**, 1270.

Harding, B., Pudifin, D. J., Gotch, F. and MacLennan, I. C. M. (1971). Cytotoxic lymphocytes from rats depleted of thymus processed cells. *Nature, New Biol.* **232**, 80.

Holborow, E. J. and Papamichail, M. (1973). Observations on lymphocytes bearing surface immunoglobulin in health and in disease. *Int. Arch. Allergy* **45**, 210.

Hutteroth, T. H., Litwin, S. D. and Cleve, H. (1972). Cultured lymphoid cell lines from normal subjects: membrane associated immunoglobulins studied by the mixed antiglobulin reaction. *Cell Immunol.* **5**, 446.

Ishii, Y., Koshiba, H., Ueno, H., Maeyama, I., Takami, T., Ishibashi, F. and Kikuchi, K. (1975). Characterization of human B lymphocyte specific antigens. *J. Immunol.* **114**, 466.

Jaffe, E. S., Shevach, E. M., Frank, M. M., Berard, C. W. and Green, I. (1974). Nodular lymphoma; evidence for origin from follicular B lymphocytes. *New Eng. J. Med.* **290**, 813.

Jondal, M. (1974). Surface markers on human B and T lymphocytes. V. Characterization of the lymphoproliferative response to three different lectins and allogeneic lymphocytes by surface markers. *Scand. J. Immunol.* **3**, 749.

Jondal, M., Holm, G. and Wigzell, H. (1972). Surface markers on human T and B lymphocytes. I. A large population of lymphocytes forming non immune rosettes with sheep red blood cells. *J. Exp. Med.* **136**, 207.

Jondal, M., Wigzell, H. and Aiuti, F. (1973). Human lymphocyte subpopulations: classification according to surface markers and-or functional characteristics. *Transplant Rev.* **16**, 163.

Kaplan, J., Mastrangelo, R. and Peterson, W. D. (1974). Childhood lymphoblastic lymphoma, a cancer of thymus-derived lymphocytes. *Cancer Res.* **34**, 521.

Kaur, J., Catovsky, D., Spiers, A. S. D. and Galton, D. A. G. (1974). Increase of T lymphocytes in the spleen in Hodgkin's disease. *Lancet* **2**, 800.

Kaur, J., Spiers, A. S. D. and Galton, D. A. G. (1975). T and B lymphocytes in spleens of patients with malignant diseases. *Lancet* **1**, 747.

Kay, M. M. B. (1975). Surface characteristics of Hodgkin's cells. *Lancet* **2**, 459.

Kedar, E., Ortiz de Landazuri, M. and Fahey, J. L. (1974). Comparative studies on immunoglobulin receptors and antibody-dependent cell cytotoxicity (ADCC) in rat lymphoid organs. *J. Immunol.* **112**, 37.

Kersey, J. H., Sabad, A., Gajl-Peczalska, K., Hallgren, H. M., Yunis, E. J. and Nesbit, M. E. (1973). Acute lymphoblastic leukemic cells with T (thymus-derived) lymphocyte markers. *Science* **182**, 1355.

Klein, E., Klein, G., Nadkarni, J. S., Nadkarni, J. I., Wigzell, H. and Clifford, P. (1968). Surface IgM-kappa specificity on a Burkitt lymphoma cell in vivo and in derived culture lines. *Cancer Res.* **28**, 1300.

Knapp, W., Schuit, H. R. E., Bolhuis, R. L. H. and Hijmans, W. (1974). Surface immunoglobulins in chronic lymphatic leukaemia, macroglobulinaemia and myelomatosis. *Clin. Exp. Immunol.* **16**, 541.

Kumagai, K., Abo, J., Sekizawa, T. and Sasaki, M. (1975). Studies of surface immunoglobulins on human B cell. I. Dissociation of cell bound immunoglobulin with acid pH or at 37°C. *J. Immunol.* **115**, 982.

Lawton, A. R., Royal, S. A., Self, K. S. and Cooper, M. D. (1972). IgA determinants on B-lymphocytes in patients with deficiency of circulating IgA. *J. Lab. Clin. Med.* **80**, 26.

Lay, W. H., Mendes, N. F., Bianco, C. and Nussenzweig, V. (1971). Binding of sheep red blood cells to a large population of human lymphocytes. *Nature, New Biol.* **230**, 531.

Lille, I., Desplaces, A., Meens, L., Saracino, R. T. and Brouet, J. C. (1973). Thymus-derived proliferating lymphocytes in chronic lymphocytic leukaemia. *Lancet* **2**, 263.

Lobo, P., Westervelt, F. B. and Horwitz, D. A. (1975). Identification of two populations of immunoglobulin bearing lymphocytes in man. *J. Immunol.* **114**, 116.

Lohrmann, H-P., Novikovs, L. and Graw, R. G. (1974a). Cellular interactions in the proliferative response of human T and B lymphocytes to phytomitogens and allogeneic lymphocytes. *J. Exp. Med.* **139**, 1553.

Lohrmann, H-P., Novikovs, L. and Graw, R. G. (1974b). Stimulatory capacity of human T and B lymphocytes in the mixed leukocyte culture. *Nature* **250**, 144.

Luckasen, J. R., Sabad, A., Gajl-Peczalska, K. J. and Kersey, J. H. (1974). Lymphocytes bearing complement receptors, surface immunoglobulins and sheep erythrocyte receptors in primary immunodeficiency diseases. *Clin. Exp. Immunol.* **16**, 535.

MacLennan, I. C. M. (1972). Competition for receptors for immunoglobulin on cytotoxic lymphocytes. *Clin. Exp. Immunol.* **10**, 275.

Marchalonis, J. J. (1975). Lymphocyte surface immunoglobulins. *Science* **190**, 20.

Mendes, N. F., Kopersztych, S. and Mota, N. G. S. (1974). T and B lymphocytes in patients with lepromatous leprosy. *Clin. Exp. Immunol.* **16**, 23.

Messner, R. P., Lindstrom, F. D. and Williams, R. C. (1973). Peripheral blood lymphocyte cell surface markers during the course of systemic lupus erythematosus. *J. Clin. Invest.* **52**, 3046.

Michlmayr, G. and Huber, H. (1970). Receptor sites for complement on certain human peripheral blood lymphocytes. *J. Immunol.* **105**, 670.

Moller, G. and Svehag, S-E. (1972). Specificity of lymphocyte-mediated cytotoxicity induced by *in vitro* antibody-coated target cells. *Cell. Immunol.* **4**, 1.

Nath, I., Curtis, J., Bhutani, L. K. and Talwar, G. P. (1974). Reduction of a subpopulation of T lymphocytes in lepromatous leprosy. *Clin. Exp. Immunol.* **18**, 81.

Nicod, I., Girard, J. P. and Cruchaud, A. (1973). Membrane-associated immunoglobulins of human lymphocytes in immunologic disorders. *Clin. Exp. Immunol.* **15**, 365.

Nies, K. M., Oberlin, M. A., Brown, J. C. and Halpern, M. S. (1973). Immunoglobulin biosynthesis by normal and leukemic human peripheral blood lymphocytes. *J. Immunol.* **111**, 1236.

Nishioka, K. (1971). Complement and tumor immunology. *Adv. Cancer Res.* **14**, 231.

Papamichail, M. and Temple, A. (1975). Characterization of the human effector cell causing antibody-mediated cytotoxicity. *Clin. Exp. Immunol.* **20**, 459.

Papamichail, M., Brown, J. C. and Holborow, E. J. (1971). Immunoglobulins on the surface of human lymphocytes. *Lancet* **2**, 850.

Papamichail, M., Sheldon, P. J. and Holborow, E. J. (1974). T- and B-cell subpopulations in infectious mononucleosis. *Clin. Exp. Immunol.* **18**, 1.

Papamichail, M., Gutierrez, C. and Holborow, E. J. (1976). The use of nylon fibre as a method of separating human lymphocytes. *J. Immunol. Meth.* **11**, 225.

Papamichail, M., Keith, H. L., Currey, H. L. F. and Holborow, E. J. (1972). Subpopulations of human peripheral blood lymphocytes distinguished by combined rosette formation and membrane immunofluorescence. *Lancet* **2**, 64.

Paraskevas, F., Lee, S-T. and Israels, L. G. (1971). Cell surface associated gamma globulins in lymphocytes. I. Reverse immune cytoadherence: a technique for their detection in mouse and human lymphocytes. *J. Immunol.* **106**, 160.

Pattengale, P. K., Smith, R. W. and Perlin, E. (1974). Atypical lymphocytes in acute infectious mononucleosis. Identification by multiple T and B lymphocyte markers. *New Eng. J. Med.* **291**, 1145.

Perlmann, P. and Holm, G. (1969). Cytotoxic effects of lymphoid cells *in vitro*. *Adv. Immunol.* **11**, 117.

Pernis, B., Ferranini, M., Forni, L. and Amante, L. (1971). *In* "Progress in Immunology" (ed. B. Amos), p. 95, New York.

Peter, C. R., MacKenzie, M. R. and Glassy, F. J. (1974). T or B cell origin of some non-Hodgkin's lymphomas. *Lancet* **2**, 686.

Phillips, B. and Roitt, I. M. (1973). Evidence for transformation of human B lymphocytes by PHA. *Nature, New Biol.* **241**, 254.

Piessens, W. F., Schur, P. H., Moloney, W. C. and Churchill, W. H. (1973). Lymphocyte surface immunoglobulins. Distribution and frequency in lymphoproliferative diseases. *New Eng. J. Med.* **288**, 176.

Pincus, S., Bianco, C. and Nussenzweig, V. (1972). Increased proportion of complement-receptor lymphocytes in the peripheral blood of patients with chronic lymphocytic leukemia. *Blood* **40**, 303.

Preud'homme, J. L. and Seligmann, M. (1972a). Immunoglobulins on the surface of lymphoid cells in Waldenstrom's macroglobulinemia. *J. Clin. Invest.* **51**, 701.

Preud'homme, J. L. and Seligmann, M. (1972b). Surface bound immunoglobulins as a cell marker in human lymphoproliferative diseases. *Blood* **40**, 777.

Preud'homme, J. L., Klein, M., Verroust, P. and Seligmann, M. (1971). Immunoglobulines monoclonales de membrane dans les leucemies lymphoide chroniques. *Rev. Eur. Etud. Clin. Biol.* **16**, 1025.

Preud'homme, J. L., Griscelli, C. and Seligmann, M. (1973). Immunoglobulins on the surface of lymphocytes in fifty patients with primary immunodeficiency diseases. *Clin. Immunol. Immunopath.* **1**, 241.

Ross, G. D. and Polley, M. J. (1974). Human lymphocyte and granulocyte receptors for the fourth component of complement (C4) and the role of granulocyte receptors in phagocytosis. *Fed. Proc.* **33**, 759 (Abstr.).

Ross, G. D., Rabellino, E. M., Polley, M. J. and Grey, H. M. (1973). Combined studies of complement receptor and surface immunoglobulin-bearing cells and sheep erythrocyte rosette-forming cells in normal and leukemic human lymphocytes. *J. Clin. Invest.* **52**, 377.

Rowe, D. S., Hug, K., Forni, L. and Pernis, B. (1973). Immunoglobulin D as a lymphocyte receptor. *J. Exp. Med.* **138**, 965.

Russell, M. J. and Cochran, J. A. (1973). Concurrent malignancy in T-cell chronic lymphocytic leukaemia. *Lancet* **2**, 1215.

Sandilands, G. P., Gray, K., Cooney, A., Browning, J. D., Grant, R. M., Anderson, J. R., Dagg, J. H. and Lucie, N. (1974). Lymphocytes with T and B cell properties in a lymphoproliferative disorder. *Lancet* **1**, 903.

Scheinberg, M. A. and Cathcart, E. S. (1974). B cell and T cell lymphopenia in systemic lupus erythematosus. *Cell. Immunol.* **12**, 309.

Scheinberg, M. A. and Cathcart, E. S. (1976a). Antibody dependent direct cytotoxicity of human lymphocytes. II. Studies on peripheral blood lymphocytes, synovial fluid cells and sera from patients with rheumatoid arthritis. *Clin. Exp. Immunol.* **24**, 323.

Scheinberg, M. A. and Cathcart, E. S. (1976b). Antibody dependent direct cytotoxicity of human lymphocytes. I. Studies on peripheral blood lymphocytes and sera of patients with systemic lupus erythematosus. *Clin. Exp. Immunol.* **24**, 317.

Schiff, R. I., Buckley, R. H., Gilbertsen, R. B. and Metzgar, R. S. (1974). Membrane receptors and *in vivo* responsiveness of lymphocytes in human immunodeficiency. *J. Immunol.* **112**, 376.

Schneider, J., Chin, W., Friou, G. J., Cooper, S. M., Harding, B., Hill, R. L. and Quismorio, F. P. (1975). Reduced antibody dependent cell mediated cytotoxicity in systemic lupus erythematosus. *Clin. Exp. Immunol.* **20**, 187.

Seligmann, M. (Ed) (1975). Membrane receptors of Lymphocytes. North Holland, Amsterdam.

Seligmann, M., Preud'homme, J. L. and Brouet, J. C. (1973). B and T cell markers in human proliferative blood diseases and primary immunodeficiencies, with special reference to membrane bound immunoglobulins. *Transplant Rev.* **16**, 85.

Sheldon, P. J. and Holborow, E. J. (1975). H-rosette formation in T-cell proliferative diseases. *Brit. Med. J.* **4**, 381.

Sheldon, P. J., Papamichail, M. and Holborow, E. J. (1974). Studies on synovial fluid lymphocytes in rheumatoid arthritis. *Ann. Rheum. Dis.* **33**, 509.

Shevach, E. M., Jaffe, E. S. and Green, I. (1973). Receptors for complement and immunoglobulin on human and animal lymphoid cells. *Transplant Rev.* **16**, 3.

Shevach, E. M., Herberman, R., Frank, M. M. and Green, I. (1972). Receptors for complement and immunoglobulin on human leukemic cells and human lymphoblastoid cell lines. *J. Clin. Invest.* **51**, 1933.

Shevach, E. M., Edelson, R., Frank, M. M., Lutzner, M. and Green, I. (1974). A human leukemia cell with both B and T cell surface receptors. *Proc. Nat. Acad. Sci.* (U.S.A.) **71**, 863.

Siegal, F. P., Pernis, B. and Kunkel, H. G. (1971). Lymphocytes in human immunodeficiency states: a study of membrane-associated immunoglobulins. *Europ. J. Immunol.* **1**, 482.

Silveira, N. P. A., Mendes, N. F. and Tolnai, M. E. A. (1972). Tissue localization of two populations of human lymphocytes distinguished by membrane receptors. *J. Immunol.* **108**, 1456.

Smith, J. L., Barker, C. R. Clein, G. P. and Collins, R. D. (1973). Characterisation of malignant mediastinal lymphoid neoplasm (Sternberg sarcoma) as thymic in origin. *Lancet* **1**, 74.

Stathopoulos, G. and Davies, A. J. S. (1976). Human lymphocytes and mouse red cells. *Lancet* **1**, 1078.

Stathopoulos, G. and Elliot, E. V. (1974). Formation of mouse or sheep red blood cell rosettes by lymphocytes from normal and leukaemic individuals. *Lancet* **1**, 600.

Stathopoulos, G., Papamichail, M., Sheldon, P., Catovsky, D., Davies, A. J. S., Holborow, E. J. and Wiltshaw, E. (1974). Immunological studies in a case of T-cell leukaemia. *J. Clin. Path.* **27**, 851.

Stathopoulos, G., Papamichail, M., Wiltshaw, E., Holborow, E. J. and Davies, A. J. S. (1976a). Description of the cells from the lymph nodes of patients with non-Hodgkin's lymphoma according to some B and T cell characteristics (in preparation).

Stathopoulos, G., Papamichail, M., Peckham, M. J., Davies, A. J. S. and Holborow, E. J. (1976b). T and B lymphocyte distribution in lymph nodes and spleen of patients with Hodgkin's disease (in preparation).

Thomas, D. B. (1972). Antibodies to membrane antigen(s) common to thymocytes and a subpopulation of lymphocytes in infectious mononucleosis sera. *Lancet* **1**, 399.

Thomas, D. B. (1973). Antibodies specific for human T lymphocytes in cold agglutinin and lymphocytotoxic sera. *Europ. J. Immunol.* **3**, 824.

Thomas, D. B. and Phillips, B. (1973a). Membrane antigens specific for human lymphoid cells in the dividing phase. *J. Exp. Med.* **138**, 64.

Thomas, D. B. and Phillips, B. (1973b). Evidence for membrane antigen(s) specific for human B lymphoblasts. *Clin. Exp. Immunol.* **14**, 91.

Urbaniak, S. J., Penhale, W. J. and Irvine, W. J. (1974). Peripheral blood T and B lymphocytes in patients with thyrotoxicosis and Hashimoto's thyroditis and in normal subjects. A comparison of lymphocyte separation methods. *Clin. Exp. Immunol.* **18**, 449.

Van Boxel, J. A., Stobo, J. D., Paul, W. E. and Green, I. (1972). Antibody-dependent lymphoid cell-mediated cytotoxicity: no requirement for thymus-derived lymphocytes. *Science* **175**, 194.

Verma, R. C., Balakrishnan, K., Vasudevan, D. M. and Talwar, G. P. (1971). Lymphocytes bearing immunoglobulin determinants in normal human lymph nodes and in patients with lepromatous leprosy. *Int. J. Lepr.* **39**, 20.

Visakorpi, R. and Repo, H. (1973). T-lymphocytes in human spleen. *Lancet* **2**, 740.

Wara, D. W., Reiter, E. D., Ammans, J. A. and Kaplan, S. L. (1973). T-cell rosettes in thyrotoxic Graves disease. *New Eng. J. Med.* **289**, 1145.

Wernet, P. and Kunkel, H. G. (1973). Antibodies to a specific surface antigen of T cells in human sera inhibiting mixed leukocyte culture reactions. *J. Exp. Med.* **138**, 1021.

Wernet, P., Feizi, T. and Kunkel, H. G. (1972). Idiotype determinants of immunoglobulin M detected on the surface of human lymphocytes by cytotoxicity assays. *J. Exp. Med.* **136**, 650.

Williams, R. C., DeBoard, J. R., Mellbye, O. J., Messner, R. P. and Linstrom, F. D. (1973). Studies of T- and B-lymphocytes in patients with connective tissue diseases. *J. Clin. Invest.* **52**, 283.

Wilson, J. D. and Nossal, G. J. V. (1971). Identification of human T and B lymphocytes in normal peripheral blood and in chronic lymphocytic leukaemia. *Lancet* **2**, 788.

Winchester, R. J., Siegal, F. P., Bentwich, Z. H. and Kunkel, H. G. (1973). Alteration in the proportion of B and T lymphocytes in rheumatoid arthritis joint fluids with low complement and increased complexes. *Arthr. Rheum.* **16**, 138.

Winchester, R. J., Winfield, J. B., Siegal, F., Wernet, P., Bentwich, Z. and Kunkel, H. G. (1974). Analyses of lymphocytes from patients with rheumatoid arthritis and systemic lupus erythematosus. Occurrence of interfering cold-reactive antilymphocyte antibodies. *J. Clin. Invest.* **54**, 1082.

Winchester, R. J., Fu, S. M., Hoffman, T. and Kunkel, H. G. (1975a). IgG on lymphocyte surfaces: technical problems and the significance of a third cell population. *J. Immunol.* **114**, 1210.

Winchester, R. J., Fu, S. M., Hoffman, J. B., Winfield, J. B. and Kunkel, H. G. (1975b). Delineation of peripheral lymphocyte populations: analysis of some interfering factors. *In* "The Immunological Basis of Connective Tissue Disorders" (ed. L. G. Silvester), p. 209, North Holland Publishing Co., Amsterdam and Oxford.

Wisloff, F. and Froland, S. S. (1973). Antibody-dependent lymphocyte-mediated cytotoxicity in man: no requirement for lymphocytes with membrane-bound immunoglobulin. *Scand. J. Immunol.* **2**, 151.

Wisloff, F., Froland, S. S. and Michaelsen, T. E. (1974). Antibody-dependent cytotoxicity mediated by human Fc-receptor-bearing cell lacking markers for B- and T-lymphocytes. *Int. Arch. Allergy* **47**, 139.

Wu, L. Y. F., Lawton, A. R. and Cooper, M. D. (1973). Differentiation capacity of cultured B lymphocytes from immunodeficient patients. *J. Clin. Invest.* **52**, 3180.

Wybran, J. and Fudenberg, H. H. (1973). Thymus-derived rosette-forming cells in various human disease states: cancer, lymphoma, bacterial and viral infections, and other diseases. *J. Clin. Invest.* **52**, 1026.

Yata, J., Desgranges, C., The, G de and Tachiband, T. (1973). Lymphocytes in infectious mononucleosis. Properties of atypical cells and origin on the lymphoblastoid lines. *Biomedicine* **19**, 479.

4

The Immunoglobulins

M. W. TURNER

All higher vertebrates have a sophisticated adaptive immune system which includes various types of cell and an array of specialized protein molecules. These proteins constitute the humoral limb of the system and include a heterogeneous group of molecules which have structural features enabling them to bind firmly to a wide spectrum of foreign antigens. Following such interactions one or more secondary biological events, directed towards removal of the complexed antigen, may occur; for example phagocytosis, complement mediated cell lysis and inflammation. These antigen-binding proteins comprise a family of structurally and functionally related molecules to which the name "immunoglobulins" was given by Heremans in 1959. Their antibody nature had, however, been recognized some twenty years previously when Tiselius and Kabat (1938) demonstrated an association between antigen binding activity and the electrophoretic gamma-globulin fraction of serum. The hallmark of antibodies is heterogeneity and this became apparent at a very early stage when the proteins were studied by electrophoresis and ultracentrifugation. By 1959 there were three clearly recognized groups of proteins differing in size and charge characteristics and yet all having antibody activity. These groups were later designated the IgG, IgA and IgM classes (Ig = Immunoglobulin). Two more classes have now been added to the family of human immunoglobulins (IgD and IgE) and it is probable that all five classes occur in most higher mammals. Table 1 shows the recommended present nomenclature and some of the synonyms which have been used in the past.

Electrophoretically the proteins show a unique range of heterogeneity and are found in the γ-, β- and α-fractions of normal serum. In general it is the IgG class which exhibits most charge heterogeneity, the other classes having a more restricted electrophoretic mobility in the slow β- fast-γ region (see Fig. 1). Predictably, the heterogeneity of immunoglobulins has made characterization of normal polyclonal antibodies an extremely difficult task and much of our understanding of these proteins has come from studies on the homogeneous immunoglobulins found in the blood and urine of patients with myelomatosis and Waldenström's macroglobulinaemia (see Chapter 27). These proteins are the products of a neoplastic, proliferating plasma cell clone and are usually present in large amounts so that their isolation, purification and characterization is relatively simple. The existence of the IgD and IgE classes was only definitively established after the description of "untypable" myeloma proteins of each class.

TABLE 1
The human immunoglobulins

Present nomenclature	Shorthand	Previous nomenclature
Immunoglobulin G	IgG	γ-G globulin, 7Sγ-globulin
Immunoglobulin A	IgA	γ-A globulin, β_2A-globulin
Immunoglobulin M	IgM	γ-M globulin, 19Sγ-globulin γ_{IM}, γ-macroglobulin
Immunoglobulin D	IgD	γ_{SJ}
Immunoglobulin E	IgE	Reagin, IgND

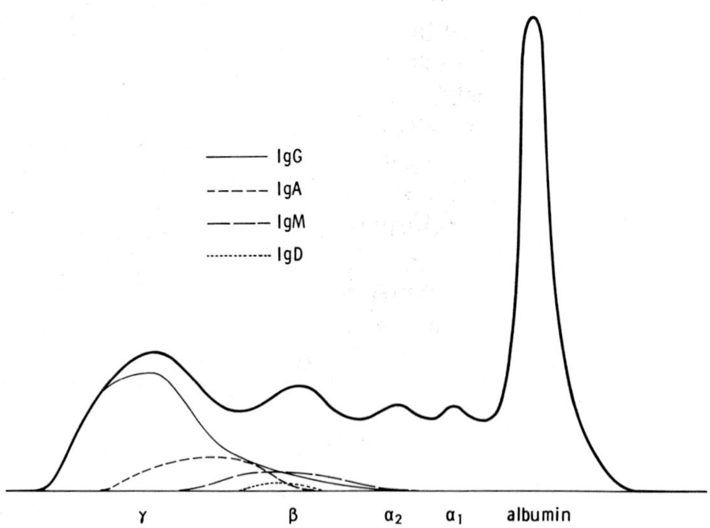

Fig. 1. Distribution of four human immunoglobulins on electrophoresis of serum. The IgE class has a similar mobility to IgD but cannot be represented quantitatively because of its low level in serum.

This chapter will describe the main structural features, biosynthesis and biological activity of these proteins. The emphasis will naturally be on human immunoglobulins but examples from other mammals, particularly the mouse, will be used for those areas in which there is a paucity of data for man (e.g. biosynthesis).

STRUCTURE OF HUMAN IMMUNOGLOBULINS

In the last fifteen years impressive advances have been made in our understanding of immunoglobulin structure.

The stimulus to this work was provided by the experiments of Porter in 1959. Porter showed that rabbit (IgG) antibody molecules could be split by the plant proteolytic enzyme papain into three major fragments which were separable by ion-exchange chromatography. Two of these fragments, known as Fab (fragment antigen binding), were identical and the third, known as Fc (fragment crystalline) was quite different (see Fig. 2). Porter found that each Fab fragment possessed one antigen combining site so that the two together in the intact molecule would account for the known divalency of IgG molecules. The Fc fragment was subsequently found to be responsible for several effector functions of IgG including C_{1q} binding, macrophage binding and membrane transmission (e.g. across the placenta).

Shortly after the demonstration of proteolytic cleavage of antibody molecules chemical methods of separating the constituent peptide chains were described and applied to the different classes. These studies showed that all

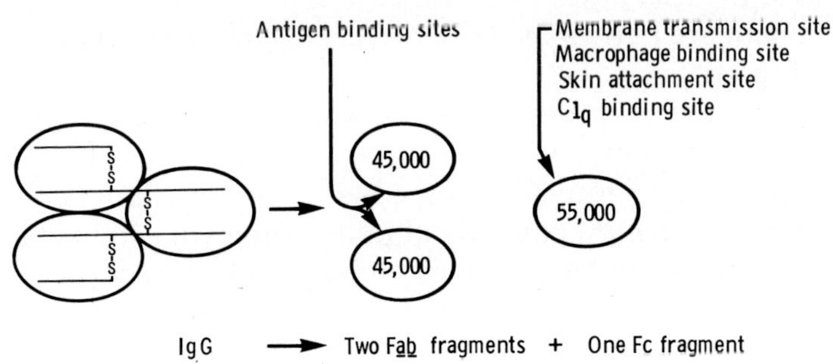

Fig. 2. Schematic diagram illustrating papain cleavage of the IgG molecule to give two Fab fragments (mol. wt. 45,000) and one Fc fragment (mol. wt. 55,000). Method according to Porter (1959).

immunoglobulins have a similar structure based on two distinct types of polypeptide chain. The smaller (light) polypeptide chain has a molecular weight of 25,000 and is common to all classes of immunoglobulin whereas the larger (heavy) chain has a molecular weight of 50–77,000 and is structurally distinct for each class.

Thus the heavy chain characteristic of the IgG class (the γ-chain) is antigenically distinguishable, by both chemical and immunological methods, from the heavy chains of IgA (α-chains), IgM (μ-chains), IgD (δ-chains) and IgE (ε-chains).

Immunoglobulin polypeptide chains are linked together by both covalent and non-covalent bonds to give a four-chain structure based on pairs of identical heavy and light chains. Each light chain is linked to a heavy chain and the two heavy chains are in turn linked to each other (see Fig. 8). IgG, IgD and IgE occur as monomers of this four-chain unit but IgA can occur (especially in secretions) in a polymeric form and IgM mainly exists as a pentameric structure with five of the four-chain subunits linked together.

Light chains are common to all the immunoglobulin classes but exist in two forms called kappa (κ-type) and lambda (λ-type). In any one molecule light chains are of the same type and hybrid molecules do not occur. Thus IgG molecules exist in two forms which may be written as $\gamma_2\kappa_2$ and $\gamma_2\lambda_2$ (see Table 2).

Primary amino acid sequencing of immunoglobulin molecules began with the light chains (mainly Bence-Jones proteins) but has now been extended to several heavy chains of different classes. When the first light chain sequences were examined it was found that amino acid residues 1–108 (approximately) frequently varied from protein to protein within a group of κ-chains or λ-chains whereas residues 109–215 of the same proteins were remarkably constant, with the exception of certain allotypic markers. These two regions of the light chain are known as the V or variable region and the C or constant region (see Fig. 3).

Heavy chains are also composed of variable and constant regions but while the variable region is of similar length to that found in light chains the constant region is much longer than the light chain constant region. As shown in Fig. 3 there are two *intra* chain disulphide bridges in a light chain, but there are four such bridges in each γ- and α-chain and five (or more) in each μ-, ε- and δ-chain. Each bridge encloses a peptide loop of 60–70 amino acid residues and if the amino acid sequences of these loops are compared within a given heavy chain a striking degree of homology is revealed. Each loop represents the central portion of what is known as a homology region comprising some 110 amino acid residues. In the γ heavy chain the amino terminal

TABLE 2

Physiochemical characteristics of the five known classes of human immunoglobulin

Class	Sedimentation coefficient	Molecular weight	Carbo-hydrate (%)	Type of heavy chain	Molecular formula	Molecular weight of heavy chain	Approx. number of residues in heavy chain	Number of heavy chain domains
IgG	7S	160,000	2·9	γ	$\gamma_2\kappa_2$ and $\gamma_2\lambda_2$	53,000	446	4
IgA	7S	170,000	9·9	α	$(\alpha_2\kappa_2)_n$ and $(\alpha_2\lambda_2)_n$	56,000	470	4
	(9, 11, 13S)							
IgM	19S	900,000	11·8	μ	$(\mu_2\kappa_2)_5$ and $(\mu_2\lambda_2)_5$	65,000	576	5
IgD	7S	184,000	12–14	δ	$\delta_2\kappa_2$ and $\delta_2\lambda_2$	69,000	?	5(?)
IgE	8S	188,000	11·6	ε	$\varepsilon_2\kappa_2$ and $\varepsilon_2\lambda_2$	72,000	550	5

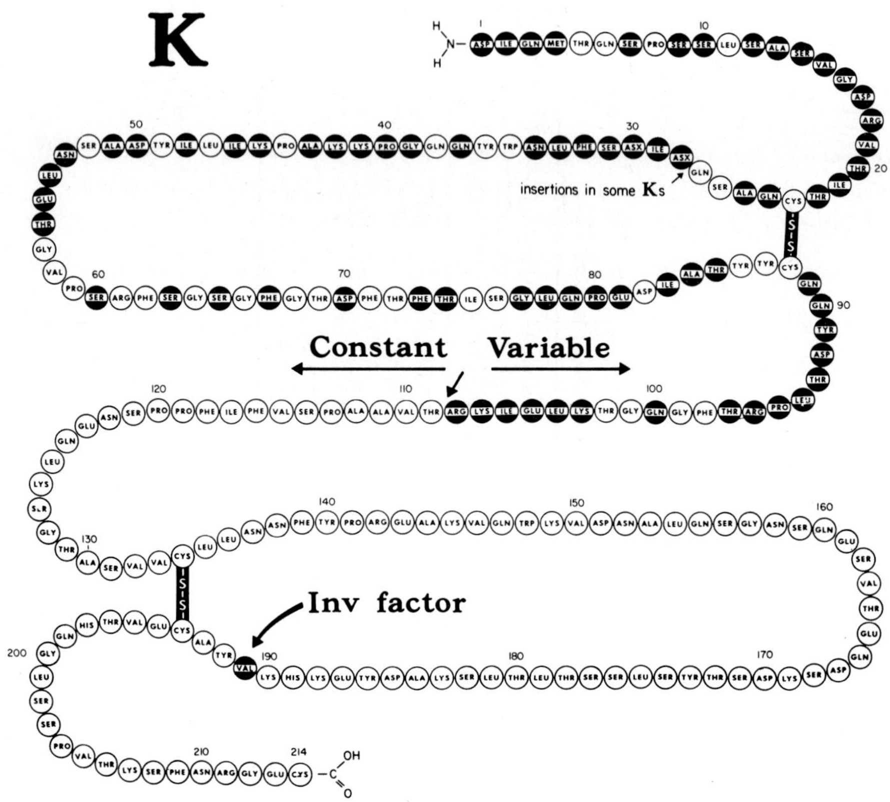

Fig. 3. Amino acid sequence of a human kappa Bence-Jones protein. The black circles indicate variable residues where different amino acids have been found in other human kappa Bence-Jones proteins. Courtesy of Dr F. W. Putnam.

homology region is called the V_H-region and there are three homology regions in the constant part of the chain. These are called the $C_\gamma1$-, $C_\gamma2$- and $C_\gamma3$-regions and it has been suggested that each region (or "domain") is associated with a specific biological property, e.g. macrophage binding may be a function of the $C_\gamma3$-region and complement binding of the $C_\gamma2$-region (see Fig. 16).

At the time of the recognition of a variable region in each immunoglobulin molecule it was suggested that this might constitute the basis of antibody specificity and this view is now generally accepted. However, not every variable residue is involved in the process of antigen binding and in the variable regions of light chains three regions stand out as hypervariable (see Fig. 4).

These regions are located between residues 25 to 35, 50 to 56 and 89 to 96. Similar hypervariable regions are present in heavy chains and the X-ray diffraction data (see later) supports the view that the hypervariable regions of a heavy chain and its linked light chain come together to create the contact residues of the antigen binding site. The variability observed in other parts of heavy and light chain V-regions is more restricted and follows definite patterns which are recognized as subtypes (see next section).

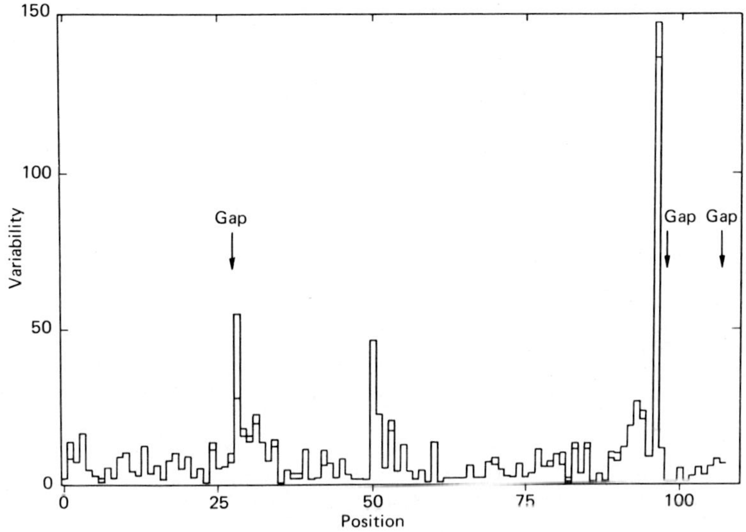

Fig. 4. Amino acid sequence variability in the variable region of immunoglobulin light chains. In some sequences extra amino acids occur and to maximize the comparison these have been excluded as indicated by the arrows. Reproduced from Wu and Kabat (1970) with permission.

Subclasses of human IgG and IgA exist and are thought to be likely for IgM and IgD. Most mammals studied appear to have at least two subclasses of IgG but such subclasses appear to be relatively recent evolutionary events which have arisen independently in each species. The four subclasses of human IgG (IgG1, IgG2, IgG3 and IgG4) are antigenically distinguishable, differ in their serum concentration and have different biological properties (see Table 4).

All healthy individuals have the subclass variants of IgG in their serum but certain genetic markers are also identifiable which are inherited as autosomal co-dominant factors. These *allotypic markers* are the Gm antigens found on γ-chains, the Am antigens of α-chains and InV antigens of κ-chains.

A series of Gm factors has been described, each confined to a single subclass. The segregation and properties of the Gm markers have provided useful information on the genetic control of immunoglobulin production.

Genetic Basis of Immunoglobulin Diversity

The variability in amino acid sequence of immunoglobulin V-regions is not random but of two kinds. There is, firstly, a wide range of variation in each so-called hypervariable region (see Fig. 4) and this occurs against a background of more limited variation. The latter became apparent from sequence studies on many different Bence-Jones and myeloma proteins and we now recognize several distinct V-region subgroups, Figure 5 shows the amino-terminal sequences of the three V-region subgroups of kappa chains ($V_{\kappa I}$–$V_{\kappa III}$) and of the five V-region subgroups of lambda chains ($V_{\lambda I}$–$V_{\lambda V}$). Four subgroups of heavy chain V-regions have also been identified and it is of considerable interest that identical heavy chain V-regions may be associated with different heavy chain C-regions. It is now generally accepted that the unorthodox suggestion, first proposed by Dreyer and Bennett in 1965, that two genes are involved in the synthesis of each immunoglobulin chain is correct. According to this view one structural gene controls the constant carboxy terminal part of the chain and the other gene controls the variable, amino terminal part of the chain. Studies of allotypic markers on the immunoglobulins of man, mouse and rabbit suggest that there are three linkage

SUB GROUPS	SEQUENCE
	κ-CHAINS
$V_{\kappa I}$	Asp - Ile - Gln - Met - Thr - Gln - Ser - Pro - Ser - Ser - Leu - Ser - Ala - Ser - Val - Gly - Asp - Arg - Val - Thr
$V_{\kappa II}$	Glu - Ile - Val - Leu - Thr - Gln - Ser - Pro - Gly - Thr - Leu - Ser - Leu - Ser - Pro - Gly - Glu - Arg - Ala - Thr
$V_{\kappa III}$	Asp - Ile - Val - Met - Thr - Gln - Ser - Pro - Leu - Ser - Leu - Pro - Val - Thr - Pro - Gly - Glu - Pro - Ala - Ser
	λ-CHAINS
$V_{\lambda I}$	*Glp - Ser - Val - Leu - Thr - Gln - Pro - Pro - ( ) - Ser - Val - Ser - Gly - Ala - Pro - Gly - Gln - Arg - Val - Thr
$V_{\lambda II}$	Glp - Ser - Ala - Leu - Thr - Gln - Pro - Ala - ( ) - Ser - Val - Ser - Gly - Ser - Pro - Gly - Gln - Ser - Ile - Thr
$V_{\lambda III}$	( ) - Tyr - Val - Leu - Thr - Gln - Pro - Pro - ( ) - Ser - Val - Ser - Val - Ser - Pro - Gly - Gln - Thr - Ala - Ser
$V_{\lambda IV}$	Glp - Ser - Ala - Leu - Thr - Gln - Pro - Pro - ( ) - Ser - Ala - Ser - Gly - Ser - Pro - Gly - Gln - Ser - Val - Thr
$V_{\lambda V}$	( ) - Ser - Glu - Leu - Thr - Gln - Pro - Pro - ( ) - Ala - Val - Ser - Val - Ala - Leu - Gly - Gln - Thr - Val - Arg

* The symbol Glp indicates the residue derived from pyrrolid - 2 - one - 5 - carboxylic acid

Fig. 5. Amino acid sequences at the amino terminus of κ- and λ-chains belonging to different variable region subgroups.

groups of structural genes. The data for man is summarized schematically in Fig. 6. There appear to be two distinct light chain linkage groups, one coding for κ-chains and the other for λ-chains and the numbers of genes shown are minimum numbers for both constant and variable regions. Within any linkage group any V-region subgroup gene can associate with any C-region gene but this poses the question of how this association is achieved.

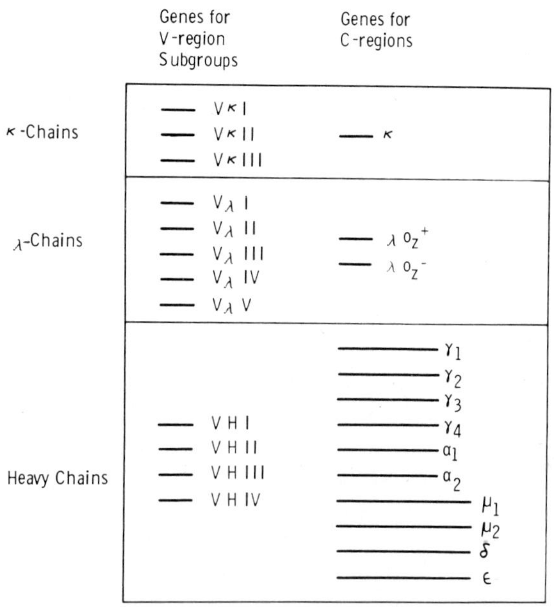

Fig. 6. Schematic representation of minimum number of genetic systems for human immunoglobulin genes. Each box encloses a set of genes (represented by bars) which are probably linked. One V-region gene and one C-region gene contribute to each immunoglobulin chain. Genes are labelled by the name of their protein product.

It could occur at one of three levels; DNA, messenger RNA or protein. Most investigators favour fusion at the DNA level but controversy still exists about the nature of the mechanism. Similarly, there has been much discussion of the generation of antibody diversity, which requires a large number of amino acid variants in the hypervariable regions. Is there a separate V-gene for each variant so that the genome of each individual has a full complement of appropriate V-genes for antibodies of widely different specificity? Or is there a somatic mechanism which operates on a much smaller number of V-genes (basically the V-region subgroups) and generates the required number of variants for that individual? Arguments for and against both points of view have enlivened the field of immunogenetics for more than five years. The issue is still unresolved and a full discussion of this field is outside the scope of this chapter. Recent reviews by Smith (1973) and Cohn (1974) present the opposing arguments in detail.

X-Ray Diffraction Studies of Immunoglobulins

In recent years the three dimensional structure of immunoglobulins has been under investigation in several laboratories and high resolution data are available for the Fab region of human IgG1, human λ-Bence-Jones dimer and the Fab region of mouse IgA.

The structure of the Fab fragment of the human myeloma protein IgG1 New has been determined to a resolution of 2 Å (Amzel *et al.*, 1974). The fragment consists of two structural domains with two homology subunits within each domain (see Fig. 8). There is a similar pattern of polypeptide chain folding in each subunit (the so-called "immunoglobulin fold") with two roughly parallel β-pleated sheets surrounding a tightly coiled internal structure of hydrophobic side chains. The two β-sheets are covalently linked by the intrachain disulphide bridge and there appears to be no major helical structure present in any of the subunits. From an analysis of the primary sequence of this protein it appears that many of the constant residues in the two variable regions (i.e. V_H and V_L) occur at hairpin bends, or contribute to intra and intersubunit bonds thereby enhancing overall structural stability. In these positions only specific combinations of amino acids are compatible with the requirements of the constant three-dimensional structure of the homology subunits. In contrast, the hypervariable regions occur at the end of the molecule and appear not to be subject to structural constraints. These hypervariable regions occur in close spatial proximity to form a shallow groove of dimensions 15 × 6 Å with a depth of approximately 6 Å. This is regarded as the antigen binding site of the molecule since studies at 3·5 Å resolution have shown that the hapten vitamin K_1OH binds to this site. The quinone moiety of the hapten has been shown to make close spatial contact with the phenolic ring of tyrosine 90 in the light chain, with the backbone and side chain of residue 101 of the heavy chain and with the backbone of residues 29 and 30 of the light chain. Other points of contact with residues of both heavy and light chains have been demonstrated.

Segal *et al.* (1974) studied the binding of phosphorylcholine to the Fab fragment of a mouse IgA myeloma (see Fig. 7) and identified a large wedge shaped binding cavity (12 Å × 15 Å × 20 Å). These authors suggest that

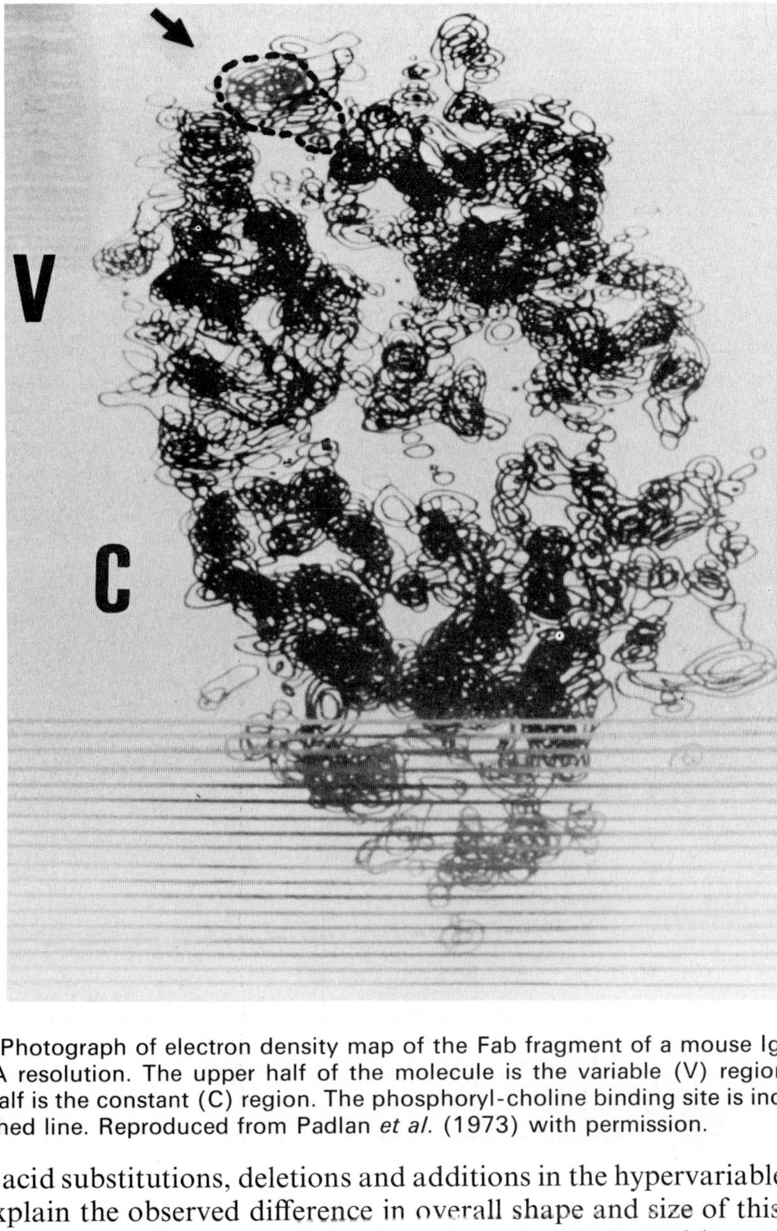

Fig. 7. Photograph of electron density map of the Fab fragment of a mouse IgA protein at 4·5°A resolution. The upper half of the molecule is the variable (V) region and the lower half is the constant (C) region. The phosphoryl-choline binding site is indicated by the dashed line. Reproduced from Padlan *et al.* (1973) with permission.

amino acid substitutions, deletions and additions in the hypervariable regions may explain the observed difference in overall shape and size of this antigen binding site and that reported by Amzel *et al.* (1974). Neither group has obtained any evidence to suggest a significant conformational change following hapten binding such as might be necessary to initiate complement fixation and other Fc-region functions. However, these possibilities cannot be ruled out on the basis of our present relatively crude knowledge.

Structure of IgG

The gross structure of human IgG1 is shown in Fig. 8. Both partial and complete amino acid sequences of several such proteins are now available and have provided much of the basic data on V-region subgroups and allotypic antigens. Although this structure provided the model four-chain subunit it is rather unusual in one respect; the linkage of light chains to heavy chains usually occurs close to the V–C junction of the heavy chain and not between the first and second constant region domains. For example, in the IgG2, IgG3 and IgG4 subclasses linkage is at the V–C junction. Another major structural difference between the subclasses is to be found in the number of interchain disulphide bridges which varies from two in IgG1 to a possible fifteen in IgG3. These interchain bonds occur in a region of the γ-chain which is sometimes called the "hinge" or bridge region. This section of the molecule is extremely susceptible to proteolytic cleavage and is thought to play a role in the transmission of conformational changes from the Fab regions to the Fc region following antigen binding.

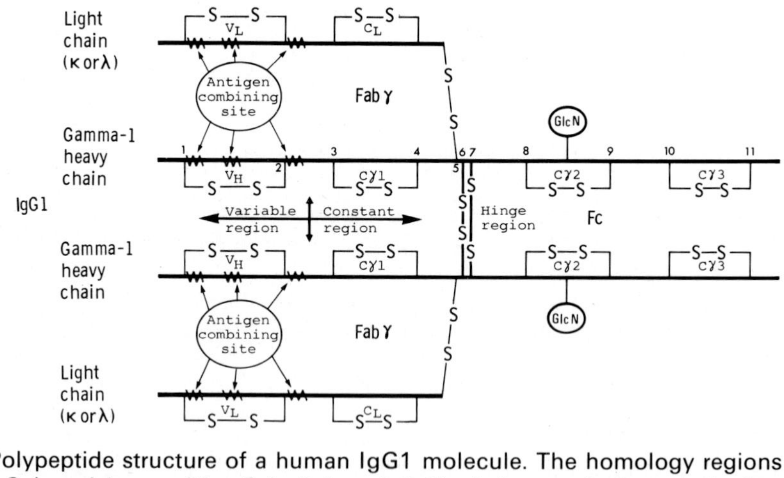

Fig. 8. Polypeptide structure of a human IgG1 molecule. The homology regions of light (V_L and C_L) and heavy (V_H, $C_\gamma 1$, $C_\gamma 2$ and $C_\gamma 3$) chains are indicated. A glucosamine (GlcN) oligosaccharide is attached to the γ-chain in the $C_\gamma 2$ homology region. The half-cysteine residues of the γ-chain are numbered from the amino-terminus. Modified from Putnam (1974) with permission.

All IgG subclasses have a single oligosaccharide attached to an asparagine residue in the Cγ2-domain and in this respect differ from all other immunoglobulin classes which are relatively rich in carbohydrate.

Structural analysis of the human IgG subclasses has shown that the proteins differ mainly in their Cγ2-regions with IgG3 showing the greatest differences. Attempts to correlate functional properties with different structural regions have so far met with limited success (see later).

Structure of IgA

The complete amino acid sequence of an IgA molecule has yet to be described and the structure shown in Fig. 9 for a human IgA1 molecule must at this stage be regarded as tentative. It is probable that there are three constant region domains as in IgG but there appear to be two additional intrachain bridges in the hinge region of the molecule. Furthermore it is in the hinge region that the greatest differences between IgA1 and IgA2 molecules are seen. As in IgM, oligosaccharides are attached at multiple sites and the penultimate cysteine residue is linked to J-chain in polymeric forms of IgA. An unusual feature of IgA is its tendency to occur in different molecular sizes, e.g. 7S, 10S, 13S, 15S and 17–18S. Most commonly serum IgA occurs in man

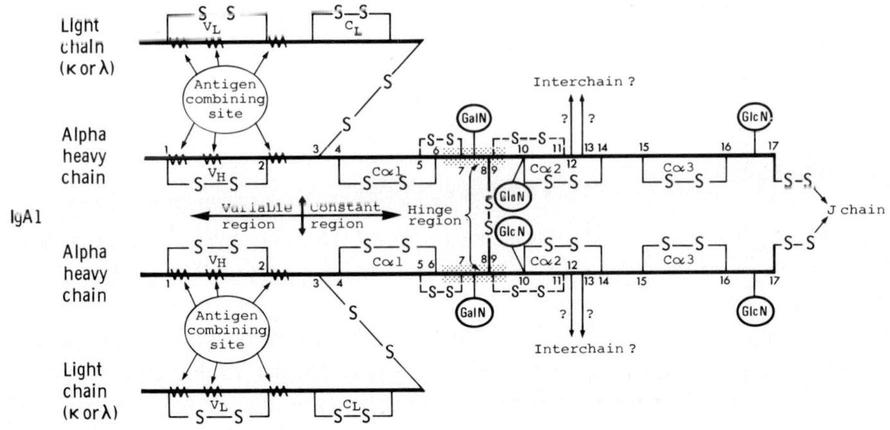

Fig. 9. Tentative polypeptide structure of human IgA1 molecule. The approximate location of galactosamine (GalN) and glucosamine (GlcN) oligosaccharides are indicated and the possible site of interchain S–S bridges of polymeric IgA are shown. Half cysteine residues on the α-chains are numbered from the amino-terminus. Modified from Putnam (1974) with permission.

as the 7S monomeric form but this is not true of most other mammalian species in which the 10S dimer predominates. On electron microscopy the dimeric form of IgA appears as two Y-shaped structures opposed stem to stem (see Fig. 10).

The IgA found in exocrine secretions differs from serum IgA in that it is associated with an additional polypeptide chain called secretory component. The latter is added to the molecule after secretion from the plasma cell and is thought to confer a degree of protection against proteolysis. It is now generally agreed that the secretory component is a single polypeptide chain with a molecular weight of approximately 70,000. In man it is covalently linked to the α-chains in the Fc region but the site of attachment is still unclear. Electron microscopic studies of secretory IgA have shown similar structures to that illustrated in Fig. 10.

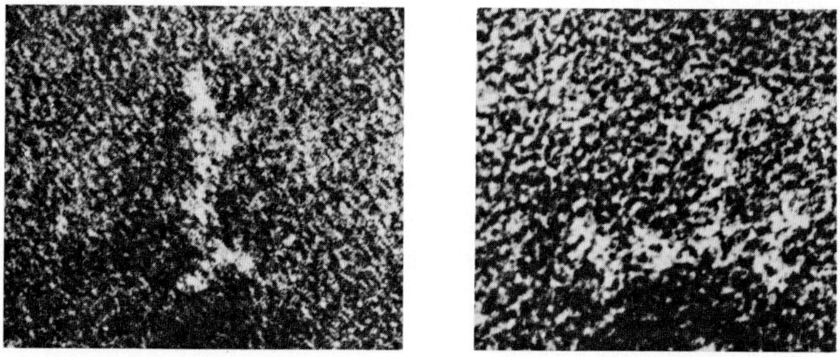

Fig. 10. Electron micrograph of murine IgM (×880,000). Reproduced from Parkhouse *et al.* (1970) with permission.

Structure of IgM

Two IgM proteins have now been sequenced and the overall structure of the IgM subunit is shown in Fig. 11. As previously noted the μ-chain has five domains and the single interchain bridge is located between the $C_\mu 2$ and $C_\mu 3$ homology regions (cf. IgE structure). The protein is rich in carbohydrate having five oligosaccharide groups on each μ-chain. These oligosaccharides are of two types, simple and complex. Both types contain glucosamine and the complex side chains terminate in sialic acid. The function of the oligosaccharides has yet to be established although they are known to increase the solubility of the molecule and influence its conformation.

The site of attachment of the J-chain to IgM (see p. 95) is through the penultimate cysteine and the intersubunit bridge which stabilizes the pentameric structure is formed between adjacent $C_\mu 3$ domains (see Fig. 11). The fully assembled IgM molecule has a stellate structure when viewed in the electron microscope with the Fab regions of the subunits arranged around the periphery of the molecule. An electron micrograph of murine IgM is shown in Fig. 12.

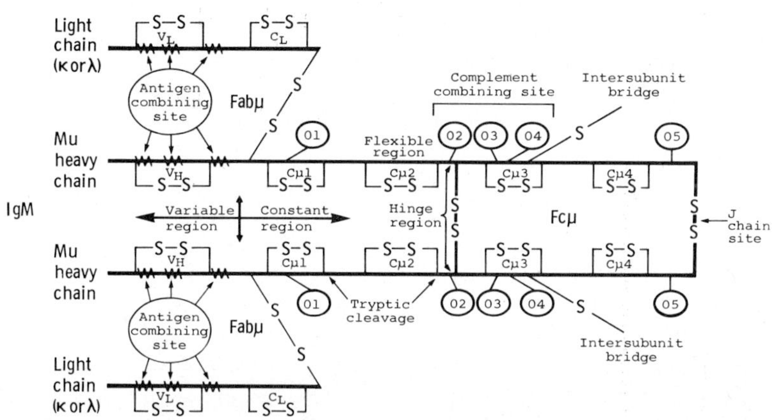

Fig. 11. Polypeptide structure of a human IgM subunit (IgMs). The attachment points of five oligosaccharides (01–05) are indicated as are the locations of the intersubunit bridge and J-chain attachment. Modified from Putnam (1974) with permission.

Structure of IgD

To date comparatively little work has been done on the structure of IgD, partly because the isolated protein tends to undergo spontaneous proteolytic cleavage in the presence of traces of plasmin or trypsin.

There is evidence that the δ-chain is of similar size to the μ- and ε-chains and therefore that the whole molecule has an extra homology region (see Fig. 13). The extra domain is associated with a galactosamine residue but the other oligosaccharide groups are located in the C-terminal Fc region domains. The δ-chains appear to be linked to each other by a single S–S bridge and each δ-chain is linked to a light chain through a cystcine near the V–C junction. There is some evidence that λ-light chains are disproportionately represented in the IgD class unlike all other classes where κ light chains predominate.

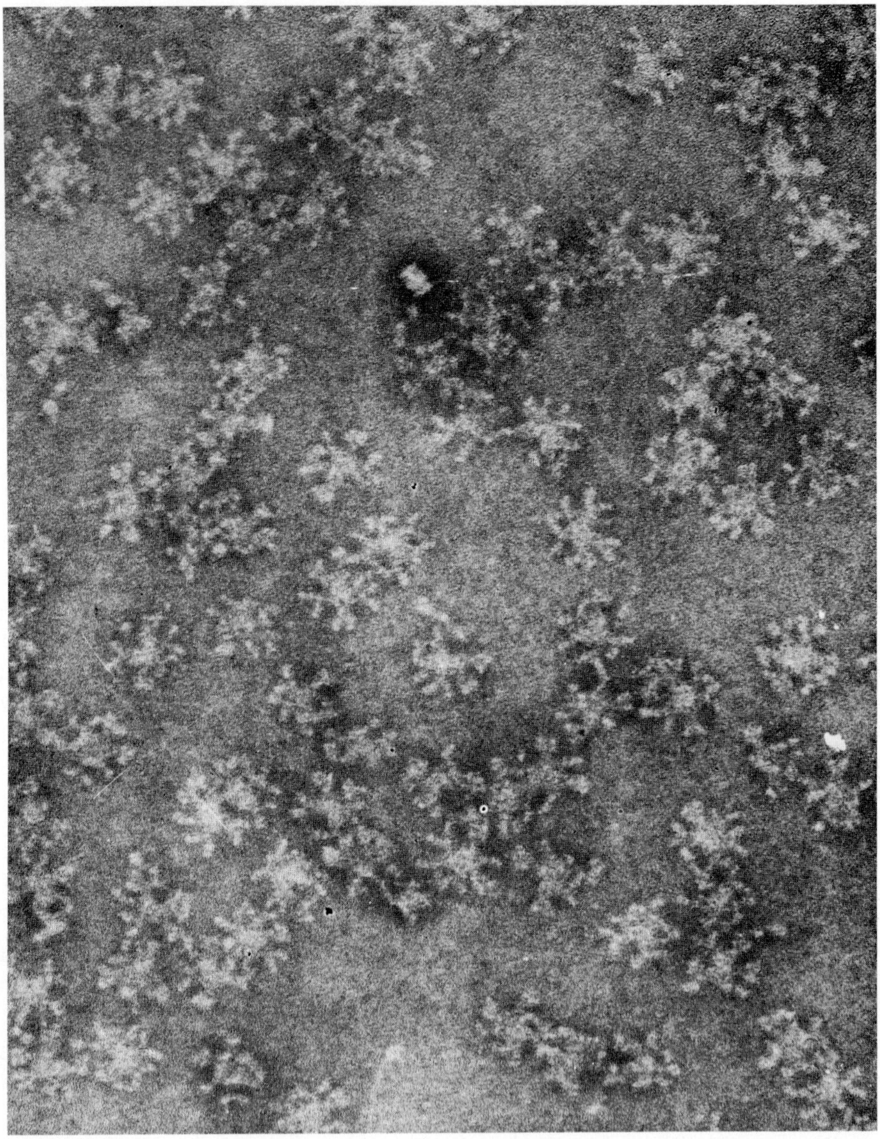

Fig. 12. Electron micrographs of dimeric (10S) human IgA (× 270,000). Reproduced from Parkhouse, *et al.* (1971) with permission.

Recent amino acid sequence studies on the Fc fragment of IgD have shown that the protein is more closely related to IgE (41% homology) and IgG (34% homology) than to IgM (23% homology). This has been interpreted as indicative of the early evolution of this class but further evidence is required before this can be regarded as established.

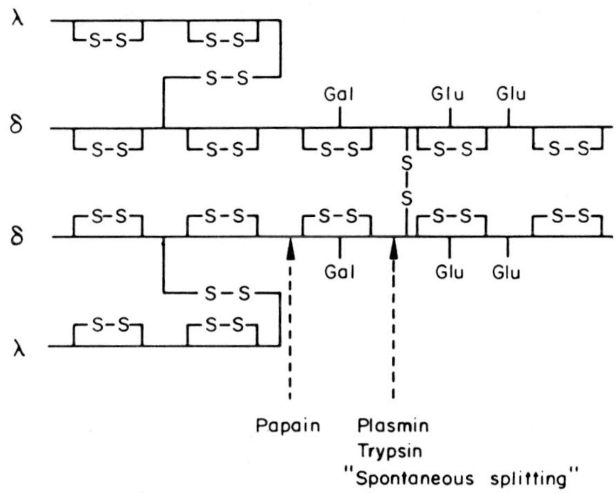

Fig. 13. Tentative polypeptide structure of human IgD showing possible location of oligosaccharide units and the single interchain disulphide bond. Reproduced from Stanworth and Turner (1973) with permission.

Structure of IgE

A total of seven human IgE myeloma proteins have now been identified and studies on two of these (ND and PS) have provided most of our knowledge on the primary structure of this protein. In common with monomeric IgA, IgD and IgG the IgE molecule consists of a single four-chain unit and, as shown in Table 2, has a molecular weight of 188,000 and a carbohydrate content of 12%.

The complete amino acid sequence of the ε heavy chain of IgE (ND) has now been determined by Bennich and von Bahr-Lindström (1974) and partial sequences of the IgE (PS) protein are also available. There is no evidence from such studies that the V-regions of ε-chains are in any way different from the V-regions of other immunoglobulin heavy chains. Comparison of constant region sequences from μ-, γ- and α-chains with the ε-chain sequence suggests that IgE has marked homology with IgG (33%) but as mentioned above recent work on IgD points to even greater homology (41%).

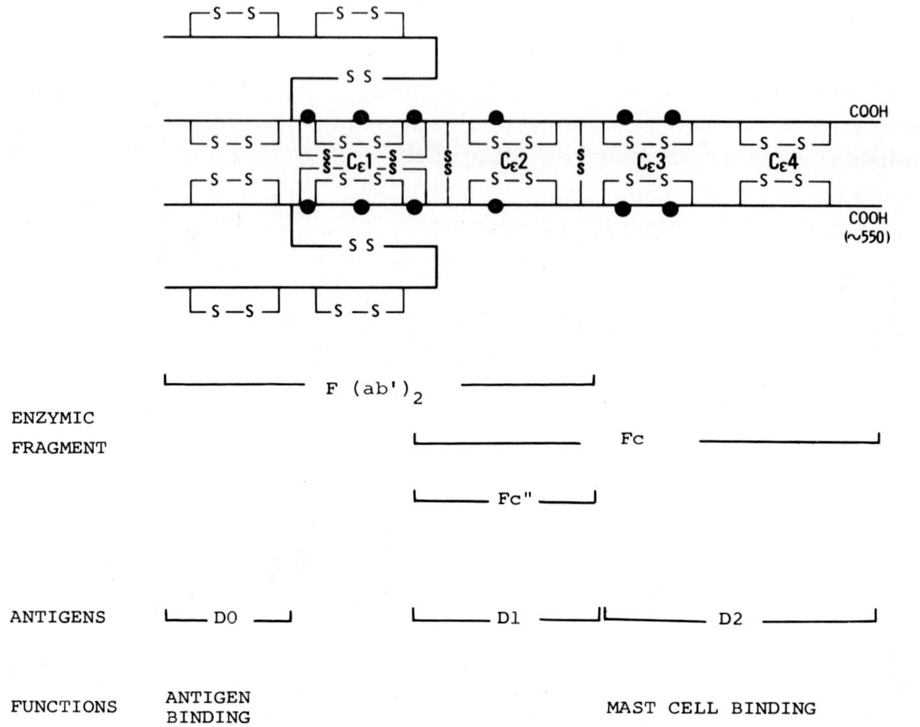

Fig. 14. Polypeptide structure of human IgE. Oligosaccharides are indicated by black circles. The location of various enzymic fragments, antigenic determinants and biological activities are indicated below. Data from Bennich and von Bahr-Lindström (1974).

An unusual feature of the structure of IgE (ND) is the presence of an extra intrachain disulphide bridge in the $C_\varepsilon 1$ homology region (see Fig. 14). This has not been found in any other human immunoglobulin, although it is seen in the rabbit γ-chain. Another structural feature of IgE is unique to this protein; there are two interchain S–S bridges separated by a complete domain (i.e. there is an interchain S–S bridge between $C_\varepsilon 1$ and $C_\varepsilon 2$ and also between $C_\varepsilon 2$ and $C_\varepsilon 3$).

Various fragments of the IgE molecule can be obtained by peptic and papain treatment and such fragments have been used to localize antigenic characteristics, biological activity and various physical properties of the molecule. For example, mast cell binding activity (the most significant property of IgE) is associated with the Fc fragment but not with the Fc″ and $F(ab')_2$ fragments (see Fig. 14). This suggests that one or both of the homology regions $C_\varepsilon 3$ and $C_\varepsilon 4$ might be involved in such interactions. To date, fragments consisting of a single domain have not been successfully isolated and this has prevented a more precise submolecular localization of cytotropic activity. Nevertheless, Bennich and von Bahr-Lindström (1974) have put forward the following working hypothesis. The binding of an IgE molecule to a mast cell (or basophil) membrane may involve two distinct sites which are presumed to be in the $C_\varepsilon 3$–$C_\varepsilon 4$ region of the molecule. One type of site, which they term "primary", has a recognition function, interacts with a membrane receptor on the basophil or mast cell and may be located in the $C_\varepsilon 4$ domain. "Secondary" binding sites may be present in either the $C_\varepsilon 3$ or $C_\varepsilon 4$ domains and show no particular cell specificity for basophils and mast cells, but interact with cell membrane receptors after antigen binding.

BIOSYNTHESIS, SECRETION AND METABOLISM OF IMMUNOGLOBULINS

Synthesis of Light and Heavy Polypeptide Chains

The detailed elucidation of immunoglobulin structure posed problems of genetic control which could not be answered by conventional concepts based on other gene–protein systems. The old dogma of molecular biology "one gene–one polypeptide" first proposed more than thirty years ago, breaks down with the immunoglobulins because the V- and C-regions are clearly under separate genetic control, yet both the heavy and light polypeptide chains are synthesized sequentially from amino terminus to carboxy terminus just as with other proteins. Most investigators now agree that the integration of V- and C-gene information takes place at the DNA level and not during transcription or translation of L- and H-chains (see p. 91).

Lymphoid cells actively secreting immunoglobulins have a network of rough endoplasmic reticulum and nascent light and heavy chains are found only on the membrane bound ribosomes. The polyribosomes synthesizing light and heavy chains are distinct and differ in size. L-chain synthesis occurs on polyribosomes sedimenting at about 200S whereas H-chains are synthesized on larger polyribosomes sedimenting at about 300S. As might be expected separate messenger RNA molecules code for H- and L-chains and several studies have shown that the first translation product of the L-chain mRNA is a precursor of L-chain which is a little longer than native L-chain. It has also been shown that the major L-chain mRNA fraction contains about 850 nucleotides which is about 200 nucleotides more than is required to code for the complete L-chain. Similarly the H-chain mRNA appears to be about 2,000 nucleotides in length which is about 650 nucleotides in excess of the necessary coding length for H-chain. Evidence from other eukaryotic cells suggests that large nuclear mRNA is a precursor of cytoplasmic mRNA and this has now been demonstrated for H-chain mRNA.

Synthesis of J-Chain and Secretory Component

Polymeric forms of IgA and IgM have an additional polypeptide chain called J-chain. This is a single chain (mol. wt. 15,000) associated with each polymeric molecule whether it be dimeric IgA or pentameric IgM; monomeric forms of IgA lack the J-chain. These observations suggest that J-chain plays a role in polymerization. Since intracellular IgA and IgM exist predominantly in the monomeric form, J-chain is apparently added to the immunoglobulin molecule at the time of polymerization and is indeed an essential requirement for the process (see below).

Secretory component is a glycopeptide (mol. wt. 70,000) which is covalently linked to the dimeric IgA of secretions. Unlike H-, L- and J-chains the secretory component is not a product of lymphoid cells but is probably synthesized in the epithelial cells of the secretory organ.

Assembly and Secretion of Complete Immunoglobulin Molecules

In the assembly of four-chain immunoglobulin molecules various intermediates are produced and play a role in the control of synthesis. Freshly synthesized light chains are released from the polyribosomes and contribute to an intracisternal pool of free L-chains which is a common feature of all Ig synthesizing cells thus far examined. This L-chain pool provides the light chains for assembly of H_2L_2 molecules via various covalent intermediates such as H_2, H_2L or HL. The intermediates formed vary from immunoglobulin class to class depending on the order of disulphide bond formation between H-chains or between H- and L-chains. It has been postulated that the intracellular pool of H_2L_2 molecules controls H-chain production by a feedback mechanism in which the interaction between H_2L_2 molecules and H-chain mRNA is a critical step.

After the H_2L_2 molecules are released into the cisternae of the endoplasmic reticulum they pass to the exterior via the Golgi apparatus. As this occurs oligosaccharides are added in a definite sequence by membrane bound glycosyl transferases and, in the case of polymeric IgA and IgM, J-chain is also incorporated before polymerization takes place. The process of polymerization has been studied in detail by Parkhouse (1974). An essential prerequisite appears to be a disulphide interchange enzyme which is present at high concentrations in the Golgi apparatus. There is evidence that J-chain is covalently bonded to only two monomer subunits of either IgA or IgM. In the case of the latter further polymerization to give a pentamer is achieved by non-covalent interactions of monomer subunits with the dimer whereas with IgA such interactions are thought to be infrequent and thus the formation of higher polymers is relatively rare.

Completely assembled immunoglobulin molecules are either secreted from the cell or become incorporated into the plasma membrane. Dimeric IgA secreted from plasma cells in the submucosa of serous glands acquires a further addition of peptide when the immunoglobulin is transported through the epithelial cell layer. It has been suggested that the dimeric IgA enters the epithelial cell in pinocytotic vacuoles which fuse with vesicles containing freshly synthesized secretory component so that conjugation takes place. The initial combination of dimeric human IgA with secretory component depends on non-covalent forces and subsequent covalent stabilization probably takes place by disulphide exchange. The completed secretory IgA molecules are then released from the external mucin-coated surface of the cell (see Fig. 15).

IgM is also able to bind secretory component, although the association is weak and only 60–70% of isolated secretory IgM contains bound SC. In contrast, when IgG and IgE occur in local secretions it is not in association with SC. IgE is particularly interesting in that many IgE producing plasma cells are located in the submucosa of the upper respiratory tract. Thus abundant local production occurs but in healthy individuals IgE is rarely detected in secretions (see Fig. 15). In atopic individuals with hyperpermeable mucosae the protein is more readily demonstrated.

Defective Biosynthesis

Much of the data on immunoglobulin biosynthesis has been obtained by studying neoplastic plasma cell tumours maintained in long-term culture or serially transplanted in mice. Many defective products have arisen spontaneously which are identical or analogous to some unusual, naturally occurring, paraproteins. However, the most frequent aberration is unbalanced production of heavy and light chains. Almost invariably there is an excess of light chain production and in many clinical cases of myelomatosis this extra light chain is secreted and appears in the urine as Bence Jones protein.

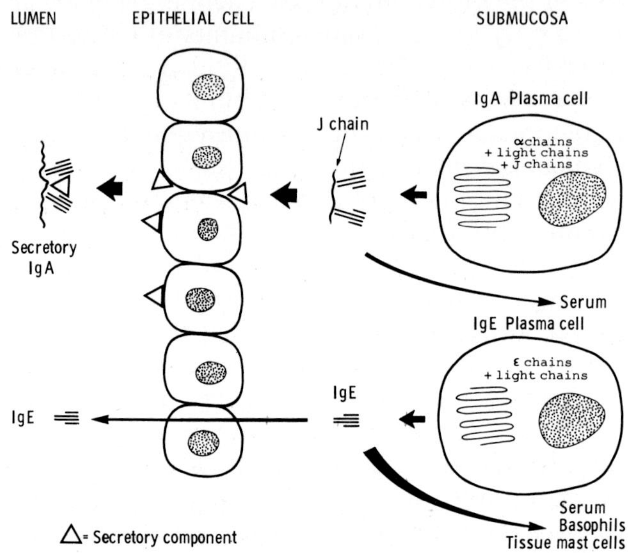

Fig. 15. Schematic illustration contrasting the synthesis and secretion of IgA and IgE in submucosal sites. The major portion of such locally produced IgA is dimeric and passes through the epithelial cell layer where it binds to secretory component. The fully assembled secretory IgA molecule may then be released into the secretions or perhaps remain firmly bound to the mucinous layer of the epithelial cell (see Fig. 17). In the case of IgE synthesized in the submucosa there is no selective transport to the secretions and most of the production is probably taken up by tissue mast cells and blood basophils. Except when the mucosal membranes are damaged only small amounts of IgE reach the secretions.

Heavy chain disease (HCD) proteins are interesting examples of aberrations of immunoglobulin biosynthesis. The original cases described were all examples of γ-chain disease but both μ- and α-chain disease proteins have now been reported (see Franklin, 1970)

Patients with γ-chain disease present with recurrent fever, lymphadenopathy and hepatosplenomegaly. On electrophoresis of serum and urine an abnormal peak is found in the β-γ region and characteristically lacks light chain antigenic determinants. Several proteins have now been studied in detail and all appear to have deletions of various parts of the heavy chain. Thus a protein designated *Cra* consists of the $C_\gamma 2$ and $C_\gamma 3$ homology regions of IgGl, lacking both the V_H and $C_\gamma 1$-regions. Protein *Hal* is an IgG4 protein of similar structure whereas protein *Gif* is an IgG2 molecule with the $C_\gamma 1$-region only deleted. These findings suggest that the proteins arise as a result of abnormalities of gene expression. The deletions observed in these pathological proteins may also be present in a small number of molecules secreted by healthy individuals.

Alpha-chain disease has generally been described in patients with abdominal lymphoma but has also been reported in association with respiratory tract disease. Immunoelectrophoresis of serum reveals a heterogeneous IgA band and, as with γ-HCD, light chain antigenic determinants are apparently absent. The data available suggests that α-HCD proteins have deletions from the amino terminal end of the α-chain. Polymerization frequently occurs and hence little protein is detectable in the urine (unlike γ-HCD disease).

The first case of μ-HCD was described by Forte *et al.* in 1970. The associated clinical picture in the small number of cases reported is hypogammaglobulinaemia, chronic lymphocytic leukaemia and hepatosplenomegaly. On immunoelectrophoresis of serum with anti-μ antiserum a strong reaction is obtained in the α_2-region. As with the other HCD proteins the μ-chain is a fragment of the normal chain. The protein exhibits a marked tendency to polymerize and polymers ranging in molecular weight from 110,000 to 330,000 have been noted. *In vitro* biosynthetic studies indicate that μ-HCD proteins arise by faulty biosynthesis rather than by degradation.

The structural abnormalities of the HCD proteins distinguish them from the monoclonal proteins found in myelomatosis and macroglobulinaemia which are the normal products of an abnormally proliferating clone of plasma cells.

Catabolism of Immunoglobulins

Turnover studies using purified radiolabelled immunoglobulin preparations have provided most of the information on the metabolism of these proteins (Table 3). Each class of immunoglobulin appears to be metabolically distinct with different synthetic and different fractional catabolic rates. It is the balance between these two parameters which determines the serum concentration of a particular protein. The synthetic rate for IgG is approximately 32 mg/kg/day which is similar to that for IgA but the serum concentration of the latter is much less because of its higher fractional catabolic rate. In addition to the differences among the major classes there are probably differences among the subclasses. For example it has been found that IgG1, IgG2 and IgG4 have similar fractional catabolic rates (7% of i.v. pool degraded/day) and half-lives of about 12 days whereas IgG3 has a fractional catabolic rate of 17% and a half-life of 8 days. However, such data must be interpreted with caution since they were obtained by injecting myeloma proteins into patients with neoplastic disease. Similar studies performed in a healthy volunteer gave considerably longer half-lives (e.g. 15–19 days for IgG1 and 24 days for IgG2).

TABLE 3

Metabolic characteristics of human immunoglobulins

	Distribution (% intravascular)	Half-life (days)	Fractional catabolic rate (% intravascular pool catabolized per day)	Synthetic rate (mg/kg/day)
IgG	45	7–23	6·7	33
IgA	42	6	25·0	24
IgM	80	5	18	6·7
IgD	75	3	37	0·4
IgE	51	2·3	71	0·002

In contrast to the increasing level of knowledge about immunoglobulin biosynthesis we know very little about the catabolism of these proteins. Even the site of catabolism is unknown. The liver, the gastrointestinal tract and the kidney have been implicated but it has also been suggested that diffuse catabolism occurs in the endothelial system all over the body.

The most important factor influencing immunoglobulin synthesis is antigenic stimulation. In germ free animals the rate of immunoglobulin synthesis is extremely low and in humans exposed to constant, prolonged antigenic stimulation with a wide spectrum of viral, protozoal and helminthic disease the levels are often very high. The serum level of immunoglobulin may, in turn, influence the catabolism of the protein. Thus, in the case of IgG the fractional catabolic rate is directly proportional to the serum concentration. In patients with IgG myeloma proteins there is accelerated catabolism and the protein has a short half-life whereas in patients with sex-linked hypogammaglobulinaemia the fractional catabolic rate is reduced. In the case of IgD and IgE there appears to be an inverse relationship between serum concentration and catabolic rate. Thus in patients with high serum levels of these proteins the fractional catabolic rate is low. For IgM and IgA the fractional catabolic rate is independent of the serum concentration.

To explain the observed concentration-catabolism effects Brambell *et al.* (1964) proposed a saturable protein protection system specific for IgG molecules. In this model a constant fraction of the IgG molecules is isolated, possibly within pinocytotic vacuoles, in a catabolic pool separate from the circulating protein pool. It is suggested that these IgG molecules become attached to specific receptors from which they are ultimately returned to the circulation. The remaining unbound IgG molecules are degraded by proteolytic enzymes (cathepsins and neutral proteases). There is evidence that in IgG the site controlling catabolism is located in the C_H2 domain near the hinge region (i.e. N-terminal end) and requires both heavy chains for its expression (Waldmann and Hemmings, 1974).

Disorders of immunoglobulin catabolism occur but are probably rare. A condition of familial idiopathic hypercatabolic hypoproteinaemia has been described in which the levels of IgG and albumin are markedly low. Synthetic rates are normal but the fractional catabolic rate of IgG is increased five-fold to 35% of the intravascular pool per day. A more common disease involving hypercatabolism of immunoglobulins is dystrophia myotonica. This is an inherited progressive, muscular abnormality characterized by muscle wasting and weakness, myotonia, personality changes, electromyographic and electrocardiographic changes and low serum levels of immunoglobulins G and M. IgG has been isolated from patients with the disease, labelled with a radioactive isotope and injected into both control subjects and patients. The controls catabolized the myotonic IgG at normal rates but the patients with myotonic dystrophy catabolized it at accelerated rates. The exceptionally long half-life of IgG make the detection of metabolic abnormalities in this immunoglobulin much easier than in IgA and IgM with their short half lives and further work is required before it can be asserted that the abnormality is confined to the IgG class.

BIOLOGICAL FUNCTION OF HUMAN IMMUNOGLOBULINS

The primary function of the immunoglobulins is that of binding to relevant antigens—foreign substances, pathogenic or otherwise, which have gained access to the body. The striking features of any antibody response are 1) specificity and 2) memory. The antibodies produced immediately following primary exposure to an antigen are generally of "poor fit" or low affinity but eventually there occurs a shift towards the production of high affinity antibodies which bind to the antigen with a high degree of specificity. The combination of antibody with antigen is discussed more fully in Chapter 6 but here we can say that the immunoglobulin molecules which are selected for proliferation as "specific" antibodies are those which make the closest contact at the atomic level with the chemical groupings constituting the antigenic determinant. Once this selection has occurred some of the population of antibody producing cells become memory cells. These cell lines persist for many years and can be stimulated on re-exposure to the antigen to proliferate rapidly and so provide a secondary response of specific antibody.

Since light chains and V_H-regions are common to all immunoglobulin classes there are theoretical grounds for expecting any particular antibody response to involve antibody production in all classes and subclasses of immunoglobulins. This maybe generally true but some exceptions seem to exist and certain IgG antibodies, for example, occur preferentially in one subclass only (see p. 109).

The classes and subclasses of the immunoglobulins provide a diversity of expression of antibody activity in different body fluids and compartments, on cell membranes and in association with other proteins such as complement, lysozyme and α_1-anti-trypsin. This section reviews the main features of this expression and Table 4 provides a summary of the biological characteristics associated with each class. Various aspects of immunoglobulin effector functions have been reviewed by Spiegelberg (1974).

TABLE 4

Some biological properties of human immunoglobulins

	Mean serum concentration (mg/ml)[a]	Classical complement fixation	Alternative pathway complement activation	Placental transfer	Binding to mononuclear cells	Binding to mast cells and basophils	Reactivity with Staphylococcal protein A
IgG 1	9	++	+	+	+	−	+
IgG 2	3	±	+	+	−	−	+
IgG 3	1	+++	+	+	+	−	−
IgG 4	0·5	−	(?)	+	−	(?)	+
IgA 1	3	−	+	−	−	−	−
IgA 2	0·5	−	+	−	−	−	−
IgM	1·5	+++	+	−	−	−	−
IgD	0·03	−	−	−	−	−	−
IgE	0·00005	−	+	−	(?)	++	−

[a] Approximate values for healthy adult Caucasians

Biological Function of IgG

Quantitatively, IgG is the most important serum immunoglobulin and after prolonged exposure to most antigens antibody activity is mainly associated with this class. Nevertheless, there is evidence that certain antigens preferentially stimulate production of a single IgG subclass and not, as might be expected, a polyclonal response from all four subclasses. Most IgG antibodies produced in response to immunization with dextrans are of the IgG2 subclass, antibodies to the blood clotting factor VIII (which occur in some patients with haemophilia) are mainly of the subclass IgG4 and most anti-Rh antibodies appear to belong to the IgG1 and IgG3 subclasses. It is not clear why such restriction should occur but it may indicate an indirect role of the constant region of the molecule in the expression of antibody activity.

IgG is synthesized by the foetus at an early stage of gestation ($\sim$20 weeks) but the level is insignificant compared to that in the mother until IgG is transferred to the foetus during the last trimester of pregnancy. At parturition the infant usually has an IgG level equal to or even greater than that of its mother. Despite some initial controversy it is now generally agreed that all four of the human IgG subclasses cross that placenta (see Table 4) thus providing the newborn infant with a spectrum of molecules differing in both antibody specificity and expression of effector function.

The IgG1 and IgG3 subclasses of human IgG are both able to bind the C_{1q} component of complement for activation of the classical pathway (Table 4). Although binding of C_{1q} has long been recognized as a function of the Fc region of the molecule the exact structural location of this activity (and indeed of other effector functions) is not known. It is now generally thought that the $C_{\gamma}2$ homology region is critical for this activity since work with a murine IgG myeloma protein has shown that a 62 residue fragment from this region (occupying positions 253–314) binds complement when adsorbed on polystyrene latex particles.

Several observed activities of IgG are incompletely understood at present. For example, unaggregated IgG1 and IgG3 proteins bind to both lymphocyte and neutrophil cell membranes but the significance of these reactions has still to be evaluated. Furthermore, the Fc regions of IgG1, IgG2 and IgG4 proteins can bind to staphylococcal protein A but whether this enhances immunity in staphylococcal infections is unclear.

IgG antibodies promote phagocytosis not only by their ability to generate the C3b fragment of complement, which has binding affinity for a specific receptor on the cell membrane of macrophages, but also by direct binding to another receptor on the macrophage surface. There is evidence that the macrophage binding site of IgG is located in the $C_{\gamma}3$ homology region of the IgG1 and IgG3 subclasses (see Fig. 16 and Table 4). The association of complement binding with the $C_{\gamma}2$-region and macrophage binding with the $C_{\gamma}3$-region supports the so-called "domain hypothesis" of Edelman (1970) which postulates that each homology region of the immunoglobulin molecule has evolved to fulfil a specific function.

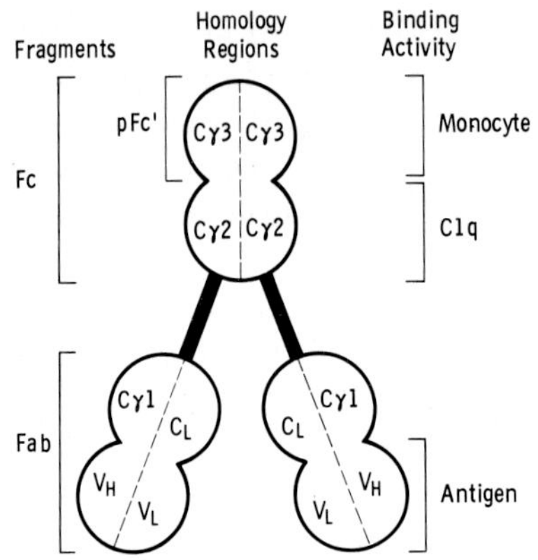

Fig. 16. Schematic model of human IgG showing the binding activities associated with the different homology regions. Reproduced from Okafor *et al.* (1974) with permission.

A major function of IgG is the neutralization of bacterial exotoxins. Since the majority of such toxins are relatively small rapidly diffusing molecules the ability of IgG to reach the extravascular spaces of the body is clearly advantageous in efficient toxin neutralization. Moreover, the rapid secondary response characteristic of the IgG class enables large amounts of specific antitoxin to be mobilized quickly in an individual previously exposed to the toxin.

IgG can be isolated in high yield from large volumes of serum by ethanol fractionation (the so-called Cohn fractionation procedure) and most commercially available γ-globulin is IgG prepared in this manner. Such material prepared from a pool of serum donated by healthy individuals contains IgG with multiple antibody specificities, whereas that obtained from individuals who have had a specific infection is enriched in a particular type of antibody. Thus preparations with high levels of IgG antibodies to vaccinia, varicella-zoster, mumps and hepatitis B are available from the Central Public Health Laboratory, Colindale, London, as also is pooled normal human immunoglobulin containing significant levels of antibodies to rubella, measles and hepatitis type A. In addition stocks of human anti-tetanus immunoglobulin are held at several hospitals throughout the country.

Another major application of gammaglobulin therapy is in the prevention of haemolytic disease of the newborn. It is well known that it is difficult to induce sensitization to an antigen in the presence of inhibiting specific antibody (e.g. the failure of attempts to immunize newborn infants having high levels of maternal antibody) and this effect is exploited in preventing sensitization due to materno-foetal Rh incompatibility. Rh-negative mothers who have given birth to Rh-positive infants will probably have received small doses of foetal red cells and therefore may develop anti-Rh antibodies which can endanger any subsequent Rh-positive foetus. It is now common practice to immunize passively Rh-negative mothers at risk, within three days of delivery, by giving high titre anti-Rh antibody (usually obtained from Rh-negative males immunized with Rh-positive red cells). In the vast majority of cases the injected IgG antibody inhibits a maternal response to Rh antigen although the exact reason for its effectiveness is still not clear. Further aspects of this important clinical application are considered in Chapter 20.

Biological Function of IgA

IgA accounts for about 20% of the serum immunoglobulin pool and a wide range of antibodies to bacterial and viral antigens has been identified in this class. Man appears to be unusual in that the major part of human serum IgA is monomeric. In most other mammals studied the serum IgA is dimeric and present in lower concentration than human serum IgA. These differences may reflect different sites of synthesis of the protein. In the dog there is evidence that 80% of the serum IgA is derived from gut associated lymphoid tissue but in man a different situation appears to obtain and there is no evidence that the gut is an important source of human serum IgA.

The IgA found in serum may not be of great importance since it merely duplicates some of the antibody roles of IgG and IgM (although lacking most of their effector functions). The discovery by Tomasi and Zigelbaum (1963) that IgA is the main immunoglobulin of exocrine secretions (milk, colostrum, saliva, nasal secretions, tracheobronchial secretions, gastrointestinal secretions, bile and urine) stimulated re-appraisal of the biological significance of this immunoglobulin class. Most of the secretory IgA is produced by a population of IgA plasma cells found in large numbers beneath the epithelial surface of the mucosa. IgA containing cells occur at a density approaching 400,000/mm^3 in the lamina propria of the human small intestine. In general, there appears to be a direct correlation between the IgA cell population density in a mucosal tissue and the absolute concentration of IgA in the corresponding secretions.

The human gastrointestinal tract may contain up to 50 g of immunoglobulin secreting lymphoid tissue producing about 3 g of IgA per day. Fifty per cent of this production is excreted, but a large proportion is always detectable (e.g. by immunofluorescence) on mucosal surfaces. Although it has yet to be established that IgA binds specifically to such surfaces it is possible that this may occur through covalent interactions between the secretory component or the J-chain on the IgA dimer and free SH groups of cysteine residues in the mucinous layer (see Fig. 17). Such interactions would provide a protective immune blanket for mucosal surfaces and facilitate the exclusion of potentially harmful antigens. Recent experiments in my laboratory have demonstrated the ability of IgA to prevent absorption of antigen

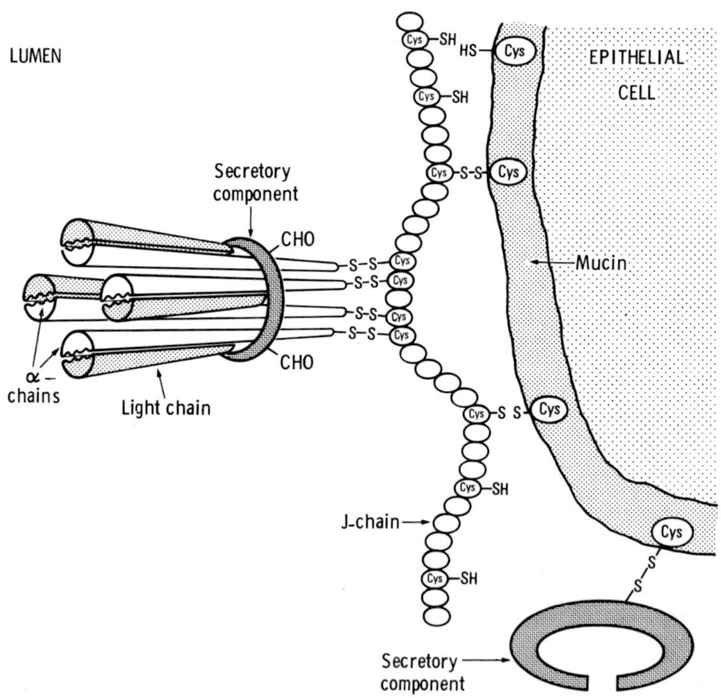

Fig. 17. Possible mechanism for binding secretory IgA to the mucinous coat of mucosal epithelial cells. Heremans (cited by Bienenstock, 1974) has shown that mucin possesses cysteine residues available for protein interactions and this may provide a mechanism for covalent binding of secretory IgA through either the J-chain or the secretory component.

across the respiratory mucosae of rats and support the suggestion that immune exclusion is a primary function of IgA. There is also evidence that secretory IgA antibody inhibits bacterial adherence to mucosal surfaces (thereby preventing colonization) and other studies have shown that specific secretory antibodies are produced following oral feeding with a variety of antigens. Such antibody is able to prevent further absorption of antigen and extends the concept of "immune exclusion" to the gut.

Secretory IgA has antibody activity towards a variety of different organisms but in general the production of such antibody appears to be anatomically restricted to the site where antigenic stimulation occurred. Several studies have now been reported which show that such secretory immunoglobulins play a role in maintaining immunity.

Figure 18 shows the results of one such study. An isolated local antibody response was induced in the nasopharynx of a group of children following intranasal inoculation with inactivated polio-vaccine. Each child was then challenged with live attenuated polio-vaccine administered orally. The child with the lowest level of secretory antibody before challenge showed the least significant antibody effect in terms of the magnitude and duration of virus

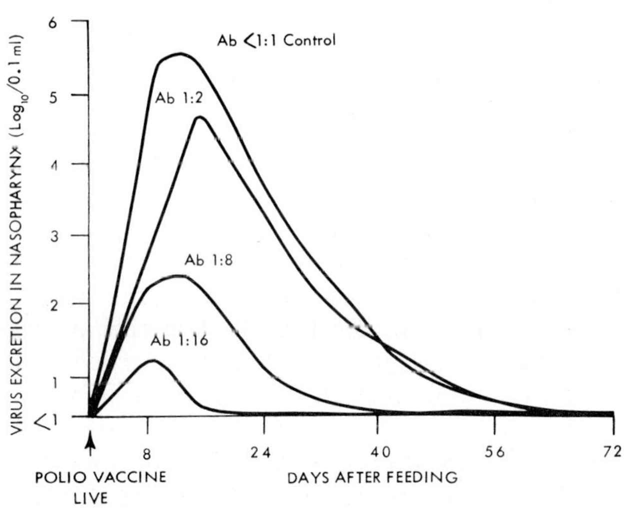

Fig. 18. Effect of pre-existing nasal IgA poliovirus antibody on poliovirus replication in the nasopharynx. Three infants were previously inoculated with inactivated polio-vaccine and subsequently fed live attenuated polio-vaccine on day 0 when the nasopharyngeal antibody titres were 2, 8 and 16. The control infant without IgA antibody had received no prior immunization. Reproduced from Ogra and Karzon (1969) with permission.

excretion. In contrast, in the children with higher levels of pre-existing secretory antibody the level and duration of virus excretion were significantly reduced.

Aggregated serum IgA has been shown to activate the alternative complement pathway and thus theoretically the molecule should be able to promote phagocytosis and intracellular killing of organisms by peritoneal macrophages. However, there is no convincing evidence of IgA mediated opsonization by either peripheral blood phagocytes or alveolar macrophages. Recently, it has been reported that secretory IgA completely devoid of IgM contamination is unable to activate complement by either pathway but doubts about possible denaturation during lengthy isolation and purification steps remain. There is, nevertheless, agreement among several workers that IgA antibodies can be bacteriolytic in the presence of complement and lysozyme although whether such a mechanism is biologically significant in the harsh environment of the gut is open to doubt.

Recent reviews of secretory IgA include that of Tomasi (1972) and the Workshop report of Brandtzaeg (1974). Various aspects of the biological role of secretory IgA particularly with reference to the gastrointestinal tract have also been discussed by Bienenstock (1974).

Biological Function of IgM

The level of IgM in serum is relatively low (about 7–10% of the total immunoglobulin pool) but antibodies in this class are frequently the first to be demonstrated following exposure to antigen. Moreover the development of the IgM system seems to occur more rapidly than that of any other class of immunoglobulin (see later). There is also evidence from structural analyses of immunoglobulins in many species that IgM is the most primitive of all classes; among lower orders of vertebrates a macroglobulin analogous to IgM is the only immunoglobulin detectable in the serum.

When bound to cell membrane antigens IgM is particularly effective in activating complement by the classical pathway and thereby generating immune lysis of cells. It has been estimated that IgM antibodies are 1,000 times as efficient at lysing red cells as IgG antibodies. Despite this impressive lytic efficiency a more important biological function of IgM is complement mediated immune adherence to phagocytic cells. In man there appears to be no specific receptor for IgM on phagocytic cell membranes and thus IgM cannot function alone as an opsonizing or cytophilic antibody. It is, however, able to promote phagocytosis through the generation of the C3b fragment of C3 and subsequent binding of such fragments to specific C3b receptors on macrophage membranes.

As well as being a potent activator of complement, the IgM molecule, with its polymeric structure and potentially multivalent binding capacity, is an extremely efficient agglutinating antibody. Even when the affinity between a single IgM binding site and an antigenic determinant is low (thereby increasing the probability of antigen–antibody dissociation) there is an increased possibility of binding to identical antigenic determinants elsewhere on the surface of a microorganism with one of the other nine Fab regions. This enhanced facility is known as *avidity* and differs from *affinity* which is a quantitative measurement of the strength of binding at a single binding site.

Taken together, the characteristics of good complement fixation, efficient agglutination and the predominantly intravascular location of the protein suggest that this class of immunoglobulin plays a special role in the elimination of particulate antigens and large microorganisms from the blood stream. Levels of IgM are frequently high following prolonged exposure to parasites with a blood phase e.g. in trypanosomiasis and malaria.

IgM is synthesized by the foetus and low levels of this foetally produced protein are usually demonstrable at birth (see Table 7). High levels of serum IgM in the newborn usually indicate an intra-uterine infection such as rubella, syphilis, toxoplasmosis or with cytomegalovirus.

Although no placental transmission of maternal IgM occurs, colostrum is known to be rich in this immunoglobulin and it is possible that small amounts of such maternal IgM is absorbed intact across the relatively permeable neonatal gut. After birth the level of serum IgM rises very rapidly (see Table 7) presumably as a response to antigenic stimulation; indeed infants delivered into germ free isolators do not show a rise in their IgM level until they leave the protected environment. By the age of one year most healthy infants have an IgM level approximately 90% of the adult value.

Despite its predominantly intravascular location IgM occurs in many external secretions, frequently in association with secretory component. Generally the level of such secretory IgM is less than that of IgA except in cases of IgA deficiency when IgM seems able to take over the role of major secretory immunoglobulin, both in animals and in man. Thus, although numerically inferior to IgG and unable to cross the placenta, IgM molecules may be regarded as functionally the most flexible of all the immunoglobulins.

Biological Function of IgD

IgD has been recognized for 10 years but there is still no clear evidence of a major antibody specificity associated with this class. Using sensitive techniques IgD class specific binding to penicillin-G and diphtheria toxoid has been demonstrated in certain sera but the levels of such activity were very low. IgD secreting plasma cells have been found in tonsillar and adenoid tissue but occur rarely in the spleen, peripheral lymphoid tissue or the gut.

In adult Caucasians the protein accounts on average for only 0·2% of the total serum immunoglobulin pool and in about 10% of the population it cannot be detected at all by gel methods. IgD levels in Gambians living in West Africa are higher during childhood and early adolescence than in comparable subjects in Britain, and elevated levels have also been noted in some Ugandan children with kwashiorkor, but the significance of this is not clear.

In addition to the apparent absence of a major antibody function for IgD there is no known effector function mediated by this class of immunoglobulin. It does not cross the placenta and does not appear to activate complement by either the classical or the alternative pathway. Furthermore, the protein does not have the capacity *in vitro* to bind (in a cytophilic sense) to monocytes, neutrophils or lymphocytes.

In view of the low serum levels of IgD, the finding that circulating B-lymphocytes frequently have IgD on their surface membranes was somewhat surprising. Nevertheless, its presence has been confirmed in several independent laboratories and the observations may be summarized as follows. In both cord blood from patients with chronic lymphocytic leukaemia IgD is the predominant class of surface immunoglobulin found on B-lymphocytes (approximately 60%) whereas in adults only 20% of circulating lymphocytes bear surface IgD. Usually IgD bearing lymphocytes also have IgM on the surface and in patients with Sjögren's syndrome the lymphocytes have IgG, IgA and IgM in addition to IgD. Recent work shows that lymphocytes produce the IgD found on their surface membranes and confirms that it is not acquired by cytophilic process.

It has been suggested that the predominance of IgD bearing lymphocytes in the neonatal period indicates involvement of this immunoglobulin class in induction of immunological tolerance (Rowe *et al.*, 1973). Recent structural evidence suggests that this protein arose early in evolution, and the fact that it has persisted for 250 million years seems to support the view that it fulfils a critical function as a membrane receptor.

Biological Function of IgE

The demonstration that the IgE class of immunoglobulin accounts for many of the (reaginic) antibodies mediating allergic reactions (Bennich and

Johansson, 1971; Ishizaka and Ishizaka, 1971) and the development of methods for estimating both total protein and specific antibody have provided a respectable scientific basis for the study of reaginic disease.

The concentration of IgE in serum is minute and rarely detectable by gel-techniques. In any individual the bulk of the protein is bound to the surface membranes of blood basophils and tissue mast cells. It has been calculated that 10,000–40,000 molecules of IgE bind to the surface of a single basophil and that even this is not saturation level since *in vitro* most cells can be induced to take up more. The binding of IgE to the basophil membrane takes place through Fc_{ε} receptors, does not involve covalent interactions and is reversible:

$$\text{Cell receptor} + \text{IgE} \overset{\text{K}}{\rightleftharpoons} \text{Cell-bound IgE}$$

where the affinity constant (K) has been calculated to be 10^8–10^9 L/mole. The IgE bound to the basophil surface is presumed to present its antigen binding sites to the microenvironment of the cell and biologically significant events occur only if an antigen molecule interacts independently with two adjacent IgE molecules thereby forming a bridge (IgE–antigen–IgE). This implies repeating antigenic sites (with a minimum of two) on each antigen molecule and there is presumptive evidence in favour of this. Once the IgE–antigen–IgE interaction has occurred on the cell surface a complex series of biochemical events takes place which culminate in the release of vaso-active amines from the cell. Principally these are histamines, slow reacting substance (SRS-A) and eosinophil-chemotactic factor (ECF-A) and between them these pharmacological mediators are responsible for most of the clinical features of immediate hypersensitivity (see Chapter 10).

The basal serum IgE level of a non-atopic individual seems to be stable over long periods of time whereas significant fluctuations in level can occur in atopic subjects. Pollen sensitive individuals frequently show increased levels at the beginning of the pollen season and a gradual decline in levels during the non-pollen season.

A correlation between elevated IgE levels and atopic disease has now been confirmed in several studies (Bennich and Johansson, 1971; Johansson *et al.*, 1974). Although modest elevations of the serum IgE may occur in allergic rhinitis and in extrinsic asthma, the highest levels are usually observed in patients with atopic eczema (in association with asthma or rhinitis) and broncho-pulmonary aspergillosis. High IgE levels are also associated with various parasitic (especially helminthic) diseases, e.g. ascariasis, visceral larva migrans, capillariasis, fascioliasis, paragonimiasis, trichinosis, hookworm and schistosomiasis. However, worms confined to the alimentary tract (e.g. tapeworms) do not appear to stimulate synthesis of IgE.

Low levels of serum IgE have been found in association with various types of immunodeficiency and ataxia telangiectasia but isolated serum IgE deficiency is apparently not incompatible with a healthy life (Polmar *et al.*, 1972).

It has long been recognized that atopic disease is familial and several attempts have been made recently to study the genetic control of IgE levels. This is a controversial issue which is difficult to resolve at present. There is general agreement that basal IgE levels are under genetic control and some evidence points to X-chromosome linkage since a mother's serum IgE concentration is more closely related to that of her son than of her daughter. Another level of genetic control may involve specific immune responsiveness to particular antigens (yet to be demonstrated in man although known to be associated with autosomal dominant Ir genes linked to a histocompatibility locus in mice). Superimposed on both types of genetic control is the degree of environmental exposure to various antigens. The combined genetic and environmental effects produce serum IgE levels in humans which range from 1 unit/ml to $>$40,000 units/ml.

IgE is present in nasal and tracheobronchial secretions, in colostrum and in urine. Such secretory IgE appears to be of similar size to its counterpart in serum and there is no evidence that any additional peptide moiety is added to the molecule during its transport into the secretions (Fig. 15). Indeed the evidence seems to point to a "passive" origin for most secretory IgE. It is probably of local origin and represents a minor fraction of the output. Only when the adjoining mucosal surfaces are made hyperpermeable (by infection or an allergic reaction) is a large amount of IgE found in the external secretions.

The "nuisance value" of overstimulation of the IgE system poses an immunologic enigma. What, if any, is the protective role of IgE? At the present time there is surprisingly little direct evidence on this subject but a popular idea is that IgE antibodies protect against certain parasites, perhaps by locally inducing an increase in vascular permeability with consequent migration of antibody and phagocytic cells from the blood. Recent work with rats infected with schistosomiasis suggests that IgE antibodies complexed with schistosomulae are able to bind to membrane receptors on macrophages, presumably through an Fc_{ε} receptor. Whether IgE promotes immune adherence in human parasitic disease remains to be elucidated.

QUANTITATION OF IMMUNOGLOBULINS

With present understanding of the complexities of the immunoglobulin system it is clearly desirable that the clinician should be able to obtain quantitative information about these proteins and be in a position to interpret the findings in terms of data from healthy individuals. There are four main methods of quantitation currently in use and these will be briefly described and contrasted in terms of cost, reproducibility and sensitivity. Unfortunately the choice of method is merely the first of several problems which bedevil this field at the present time. By their very nature immunoglobulins are heterogeneous and a diverse range of standard preparations have been used in different laboratories. Furthermore the antisera used for assay, although usually monospecific, can be assumed to be heterogeneous both in affinity and in the range of antigenic determinants with which they react. Some of these problems and some suggested solutions are discussed in the section on *Standards and Units* (p. 123). In the final section immunoglobulin values for healthy individuals of all ages are presented for ready reference.

Methods for Quantitation of IgG, IgA, IgM and IgD

Single Radial Diffusion

This remains the most popular method of quantitation in any laboratory doing less than one hundred determinations per week. The method was first described by Mancini *et al.* (1965) and has been modified by Fahey and McKelvey (1965). It is performed as follows: an appropriate dilution of a monospecific antiserum (i.e. absorbed to remove all antibodies reactive with light chains or the V_H-region) is mixed with molten agar or agarose at 56–60° and the mixture poured on to a glass plate or into a petri-dish. After gelling, holes are punched in the gel and the samples added. A series of standards are included and the plate is then incubated in a humid atmosphere. As diffusion proceeds a halo of precipitate is produced and once this becomes stationary the diameter or area of the halo is measured. If the halo is difficult to read flooding the plate with 4% tannic acid may increase the opacity of the precipitate. The area of the halo shows a linear relationship to the concentration of the antigen and the concentration of antigen in the unknowns can be read off a standard curve. This linear-linear plot was used in the original

Mancini procedure and gives the most accurate results. Unfortunately it is time consuming and it is frequently many hours before migration ceases (e.g. 120 hours for IgG). In order to obtain reasonably accurate values after 24 hours Fahay and McKelvey introduced a modification in which the log of the concentration of antigen is plotted against ring diameter or area. There is naturally some loss of accuracy but it is claimed (Hobbs, 1970) that experts can achieve 95% reproducibility of ±3% (twice the coefficient of variation). In a routine laboratory an error of ±9% is acceptable. The single radial diffusion procedure is simple and cheap and requires very little specialized equipment.

Electroimmunoassay ("Rocket" Electrophoresis)

This technique has been reviewed in detail by Laurell (1972) who first described it. Like single radial diffusion it provides a simple and reproducible method for determination of a single protein in a protein mixture. An agarose gel containing an appropriately diluted monospecific antiserum is prepared and diluted samples are applied in circular wells side by side. Electrophoresis of the antigen into the agarose gel produces rocket-shaped precipitates which can be quantitated by measuring the height of the peak and comparing this with appropriate standard dilutions.

Most plasma proteins migrate towards the anode in this technique but polyclonal IgG gives double precipitation cones pointing both towards the anode and the cathode (Laurell, 1972). The enclosed area is a measure of the antigen content and may, under standardized conditions, enable quantitative estimations to be performed. Although the precision of the method is acceptable, antigenic heterogeneity gives rise to intrabatch variability. Successful quantitation of immunoglobulins by electroimmunoassay has been reported following carbamylation, performed as follows: one volume of 2M KOCN and one volume of serum are mixed and incubated at 70° for 30 min. After cooling in an ice bath, dilutions of the serum are prepared and applied to the plate. The standard serum is treated in a similar manner. Laurell (1972) has described a further modification in which carbamylated IgM is reduced to 7S subunits before the electrophoresis. The precipitate tips reach a final height related to the IgM content but the rocket is usually not contiguous with the well. Laurell (1972) has compared in detail the single radial diffusion and electroimmunoassay procedures and his conclusions may be summarized as follows. The accuracy and sensitivity of the two techniques are similar although radial diffusion is preferable for quantitation of proteins with molecular weights of less than 50,000. In the molecular weight range 50–250,000 radial diffusion may give the same or slightly higher precision if the diffusion time is prolonged for several days or a week. With a short diffusion time (1–2 days) the errors are greater than for electroimmunoassay. With electroimmunoassay, results are obtained much more quickly and this is a major advantage in routine clinical work. On the other hand, radial diffusion requires less equipment.

Automated Immunoprecipitation

An automated immunochemical procedure for the determination of plasma proteins was introduced in 1970 and subsequently applied to immunoglobulins G, A and M by Killingsworth and Savory (1971). In this procedure samples of serum are aspirated through a continuous flow manifold and diluted with saline. An aliquot of this dilution is then resampled and rediluted with saline before mixing (at a final dilution of 1:760 for IgG and 1:120 for IgA and IgM, in the original description of the method) with monospecific antiserum to IgG, IgA or IgM (at a dilution of 1:25 in the original method). The reaction mixture is then passed through a mixing coil and the light scattering produced by the antigen–antibody complex measured using a fluorimeter as a nephclometer. The concentration of immunoglobulin in the serum sample is then determined using a standard curve. It is essential to work in the antibody excess position of the curve if significant results can be obtained.

A comparison of the automated method and single radial diffusion for the quantitation of immunoglobulins gives correlation coefficients between 0·881 (for IgM) and 0·960 (for IgA). The coefficients of variation obtained with the automated method are better than those for single radial diffusion (3·6% for IgG, 5·1% for IgA and 6% for IgM). The speed with which results can be obtained and the improved precision suggests that this method should be seriously considered in any laboratory with a large through-put of samples. Unfortunately the commercial equipment for automated immunoprecipitation is expensive and should probably be used for the quantitation of a range of plasma proteins to make it cost-effective. A laboratory responsible for less than one hundred estimations per week can obtain satisfactory results with the gel techniques particularly if care and attention is paid to sample loading and manual dilution techniques.

Radioimmunoassay for IgE

The levels of IgE in most sera are too low to be measured by classical gel procedures and special radioimmunoassay procedures have been developed for this class of immunoglobulin. A radioimmunosorbent test (sometimes called RIST) is commercially available which uses a sephadex particle chemically treated and linked to anti-IgE molecules. Radiolabelled IgE is then allowed to compete with unknown IgE for the sephadex coupled antibody. This competitive capacity is then compared with that of standard IgE preparations of known concentration. For samples containing more than 80 International Units of IgE (1 I.U. = 2·4 ng of IgE) this assay is satisfactory in routine clinical use, but for serum samples with a lower IgE content, and for most secretions, a significant error is introduced by an unidentified macromolecule which blocks the binding of the labelled IgE to the sephadex coupled antibody. A more accurate and sensitive assay for low IgE levels is the double antibody procedure which can be modified to measure concentrations of IgE as low as 0·1 ng per ml. In this procedure the IgE of the sample competes with radiolabelled IgE for extremely dilute rabbit anti-IgE and the resultant antigen–antibody complexes are precipitated in a second antibody stage using a goat or donkey anti-rabbit globulin. Unknowns are again compared with a range of standards of known IgE concentration. At the time of writing a low-level assay kit is not available commercially.

Standards and Units

IgG, IgA and IgM

It has been the practice of most laboratories to use a locally prepared (or acquired) immunoglobulin standard for quantitative estimations. Thus many different standards, often consisting of isolated myeloma proteins, came into common use and this contributed greatly to the observed inter-laboratory variability. In an attempt to overcome some of these problems an International Reference Preparation has been established and made available for general use. Originally this preparation was described as the British Research Standard for Immunoglobulins G, A and M (Rowe *et al.*, 1970) but part of this material subsequently became established as the International Reference Preparation of Human Immunoglobulins G, A and M (Rowe *et al.*, 1972). The preparation and testing of the standard are fully described in these references.

Units of potency of the three immunoglobulins were assigned to the British Research Standard and the W.H.O. Expert Committee subsequently defined international units of the same size for the International Reference Preparation. Each ampoule of the International Reference Preparation contains an average of 100 arbitrarily defined units of IgG, IgA and IgM and it is recommended that individual laboratories calibrate their own internal standards (preferably pooled normal serum) against the Reference Preparation. Ideally, for comparative purposes, all laboratories should adopt the International Standard and unitage but although the International Standard is now widely used there has been some reluctance to accept the use of arbitrarily defined units. For this reason Humphrey and Batty (1974) recommended that concentrations should continue to be estimated relative to the International Preparation but that the values be calculated in terms of weight based on the best available estimates. This recommendation has been challenged on the grounds that gravimetric standardization of such heterogeneous proteins is impossible. The problems of assigning a weight equivalent to the International Reference Preparation was investigated in depth by Rowe *et al.* (1972). Ten different laboratories took part in a collaborative investigation in which the immunoglobulin content of the Reference Preparation was estimated by comparison with solutions of purified immunoglobulin. Myeloma proteins or Waldenström's macroglobulins were sometimes used as calibrating proteins but most preparations of IgG came from normal or pathological sera from which myeloma proteins were absent. The concentration of protein in the isolated "laboratory preparation" was usually estimated from its content of nitrogen or from optical density measurements at 280 nm. The immunoglobulins were usually quantitated by single radial diffusion and in most cases the diffusion of antigen proceeded until completion. The estimates of immunoglobulin concentration in the reconstituted International Reference Preparation showed a wide range of values. The IgG level ranged from 5·3 to 11·5 mg ml^{-1}, the IgA level from 0·98 to 3·19 mg ml^{-1} and the IgM level from 0·19 to 0·95 mg ml^{-1} (see Table 5). Thus even laboratories specializing in immunoglobulin preparation and in quantitative immunochemical measurement failed to achieve close agreement between themselves. In general, estimates made in one laboratory (using a single batch of calibrating protein and a single antiserum) were homogeneous, whereas highly significant inter-laboratory heterogeneity was the rule. This heterogeneity was probably due to

i. the use of different calibrating proteins;
ii. the use of different antisera;
iii. other aspects of the assay system.

TABLE 5

Mean IgM concentration in reconstituted International Reference Preparation obtained using the calibrating proteins of different laboratories

Laboratory Code number	Number of estimates	Mean concentration of IgM (mg/ml)
3	4	0·95
5	2	0·87
6[a]	2	0·28
6[b]	2	0·22
6[a]	5	0·50
6[a]	5	0·19
7[b]	2	0·82
7[b]	2	0·68
10	3	0·69

[a] Four different calibrating proteins
[b] Two different calibrating proteins

TABLE 6

International Reference Preparation for human serum IgG, IgA and IgM. Content of ampoule by weight and approximate weight of immunoglobulin corresponding to one I.U.

Immunoglobulin	Code No. of preparation	International Units per ampoule	mg/ml per ampoule[a]	Weight (μg) per unit and confidence interval
IgG	67/86	100	7·58	80·5(69·2–93·3)
IgA	67/86	100	1·34	14·2(12·1–16·6)
IgM	67/86	100	0·80	8·47(6·99–10·1)

[a] Concentration of immunoglobulin in a solution prepared by dissolving the contents of one ampoule of the International Reference Preparation by the addition of 1 ml of distilled water

In some laboratories the calibrating proteins were themselves heterogeneous and it further appears that the various calibrating proteins were more heterogeneous between themselves than the immunoglobulins of normal sera. Variability between antisera is also a significant cause of heterogeneity.

Since these studies have clearly shown that precise determination of immunoglobulin concentration by weight is not possible it is recommended that such concentrations be expressed in International Units (I.U.) per ml and not in mg per ml. Occasionally, however, it may be necessary to compare results with previous work and for this purpose weight equivalents of the International Units have been reported by Rowe *et al.* (1972) and Humphrey and Batty (1974). This data is summarized in Table 6.

IgE An International Reference Preparation for IgE has been prepared by the National Institute for Biological Standards and Control in London and is code numbered 68/341. Unfortunately it has given a positive reaction in screening tests for hepatitis B antigen and another standard is being prepared to replace it. Further information may be obtained from NIBSC, Holly Hill, London NW3 6RB.

Immunoglobulin Levels

Table 7 gives means and ranges of IgG, IgA and IgM for healthy British individuals of different ages. Values are given in both g/L and IU/ml and were obtained using the W.H.O. International Reference Preparation as a standard.

Note that human serum immunoglobulin levels do not have a normal Gaussian distribution and should always be analysed by log-normal statistics. As a result, ranges of average concentration do not have symmetric confidence intervals about the mean concentration.

Although not shown in Table 7 slight but statistically significant sex differences exist for IgG and IgA. Males generally have a lower IgG and a higher IgA than females. In the case of IgM there is a more marked sex difference with females having a higher mean at all ages after five years. Studies of larger groups of individuals in the USA have shown that IgG and IgA concentrations increase progressively with age but that IgM levels do not change with age.

There is still controversy regarding the most appropriate assay method for IgE (see p. 122) and there is little reliable information concerning IgE levels

TABLE 7

IgG, IgA and IgM levels in healthy British subjects (means and range)
(Hobbs, 1975 personal communication)

Age	Number of subjects studied		IgG		IgA		IgM	
			g/L	I.U./ml	g/L	I.U./ml	g/L	I.U./ml
Cord blood		+2SD	18·0	224			0·20	24
	36	Mean	10·0	124	>0·02	>1·4	0·10	12
		−2SD	5·0	62			0·02	2
0–2 weeks		+2SD	18·0	224	0·08	6	0·20	24
	40	Mean	9·5	118	0·02	1·4	0·10	12
		−2SD	5·0	62	0·01	0·7	0·05	6
2–4 weeks		+2SD	13·1	163	0·15	11	0·30	35
	36	Mean	7·2	90	0·05	4	0·15	18
		−2SD	3·9	48	0·02	1	0·05	6
4–6 weeks		+2SD	13·1	163	0·15	11	0·50	59
	36	Mean	7·2	90	0·05	4	0·20	24
		−2SD	3·9	58	0·02	1	0·10	12
6–12 weeks		+2SD	7·8	97	0·40	28	0·70	83
	36	Mean	4·0	50	0·15	11	0·35	41
		−2SD	2·1	26	0·05	4	0·15	18
3–6 months		+2SD	8·9	111	0·60	42	0·90	106
	20	Mean	4·6	57	0·25	18	0·50	59
		−2SD	2·4	30	0·10	7	0·20	24
6–9 months		+2SD	9·0	112	0·70	49	1·50	177
	12	Mean	3·0	65	0·30	21	0·70	83
		−2SD	5·2	37	0·15	11	0·35	41
9–12 months		+2SD	11·0	137	0·75	53	2·00	236
	18	Mean	5·8	72	0·40	28	0·90	106
		−2SD	3·1	39	0·25	18	0·45	53
1–2 years		+2SD	13·9	173	1·30	92	2·00	236
	18	Mean	6·5	81	0·70	49	0·90	106
		−2SD	3·1	39	0·30	21	0·45	53
2–3 years		+2SD	15·8	197	1·40	99	2·00	236
	16	Mean	7·0	87	0·85	60	0·90	106
		−2SD	3·7	46	0·35	25	0·45	53
3–6 years		+2SD	15·8	197	2·20	155	2·00	236
	40	Mean	7·0	87	1·00	70	0·90	106
		−2SD	3·7	46	0·40	28	0·45	53
6–9 years		+2SD	15·8	197	2·50	176	2·00	236
	52	Mean	7·0	87	1·35	95	0·90	106
		−2SD	3·7	46	0·55	39	0·45	53
9–12 years		+2SD	15·8	197	2·60	183	2·00	236
	48	Mean	7·0	87	1·45	102	0·90	106
		−2SD	3·7	46	0·07	49	0·45	53
12–15 years		+2SD	15·8	197	3·00	211	2·00	236
	44	Mean	7·0	87	1·75	123	0·90	106
		−2SD	3·7	46	0·80	56	0·45	53
>15 years		+2SD	14·0	174	3·00	211	1·90	224
	280	Mean	9·4	117	1·80	127	1·10	130
		−2SD	5·0	62	0·50	35	0·50	59
>45 years		+2SD	16·0	199	4·00	282	1·90	224
	80	Mean	9·4	110	1·80	99	1·10	130
		−2SD	5·0	62	0·50	35	0·50	59

at different ages in the general population. However, the data obtained by Gerrard *et al.* (1974) for Canadian individuals constitutes a useful guide for each group (Fig. 19). The adult median level reported in this study (75 I.U./ml) is high according to recent estimations using the double antibody procedure (log mean of ~20 I.U./ml for non-atopic adults). Nevertheless it

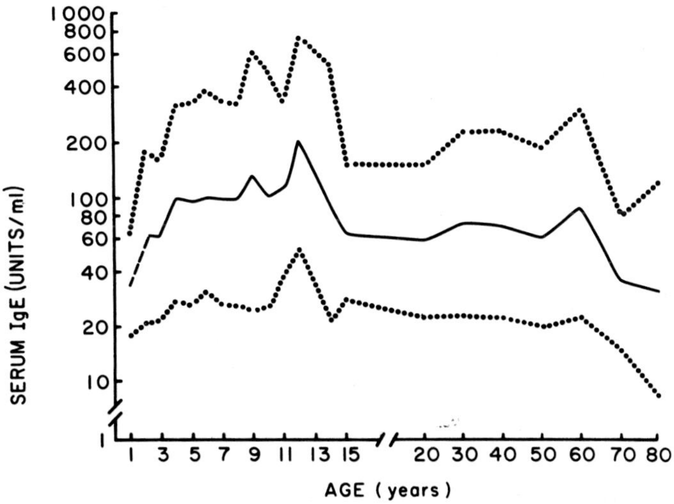

Fig. 19. Serum IgE levels in members of 80 families from 2 years to 80 years of age. (Solid line: geometric mean, dotted line: ±S.D. of $\log_{10}$ IgE). Reproduced from Orgel (1975) and derived from Gerrard *et al.* (1974), with permission.

is anticipated that the general pattern of development will be similar for a British population with adult values reached by 4 years of age. In the case of IgE the level of the protein is greatly influenced by environmental factors, such as helminthic infcstations and allergen exposure. In part, this accounts such as helminthic infestations and antigenic exposure. In part, this accounts for the wide scatter of IgE levels observed in clinical practice.

REFERENCES

Amzel, L. M., Chen, B. L., Phizackerley, R. P., Poljak, R. J. and Saul, F. (1974). High resolution X-Ray diffraction studies of the Fab' fragment of IgG New. "Progress in Immunology II. Vol. 1. (Eds. L. Brent and J. Holborow), p. 85. North Holland Publishing Co., Amsterdam and Oxford.

Bennich, H. and Johansson, S. G. O. (1971). Structure and function of human immunoglobulin E. *Adv. Immunol.* **13**, 1.

Bennich, H. and von Bahr-Lindström, H. (1974). Structure of Immunoglobulin E (IgE). "Progress in Immunology II." Vol. 1. (Eds. L. Brent and J. Holborow), p. 49. North Holland Publishing Co., Amsterdam and Oxford.

Bienenstock, J. (1974). The physiology of the local immune response and the gastrointestinal tract. "Progress in Immunology II." Vol. 4. (Eds. L. Brent and J. Holborow), p. 197. North Holland Publishing Co., Amsterdam and Oxford.

Brambell, F. W. R., Hemmings, W. A. and Morris, I. G. (1964). A theoretical model of γ-globulin catabolism. *Nature* **203**, 1352.

Brandtzaeg, P. (1974). Secretory immunoglobulins. "Progress in Immunology II." Vol. 1. (Eds. L. Brent and J. Holborow), p. 238. North Holland Publishing Co., Amsterdam and Oxford.

Cohn, M. (1974). A rationale for ordering the data on antibody diversification. "Progress in Immunology II." Vol. 2. (Eds. L. Brent and J. Holborow), p. 261. North Holland Publishing Co., Amsterdam and Oxford.

Dreyer, W. J. and Bennett, J. C. (1965). The molecular basis of antibody formation: a paradox. *Proc. Nat. Acad. Sci. (U.S.A.)* **54**, 864.

Edelman, G. M. (1970). The covalent structure of a human γG immunoglobulin. XI. Functional implications. *Biochemistry* **9**, 3197.

Fahey, J. L. and McKelvey, E. M. (1965). Quantitative determination of serum immunoglobulins in antibody–agar plates. *J. Immunol.* **94**, 84.

Forte, F. A., Prelli, F., Yount, W. J., Jerry, L. M., Kochwa, S., Franklin, E. C. and Kunkel, H. G. (1970). Heavy chain disease of the μ (γM) type: report of the first case. *Blood* **36**, 137.

Franklin, E. C. (1970). Heavy chain diseases. *New Eng. J. Med.* **19**, 1098.

Gerrard, J. W., Horne, S., Vickers, P., MacKenzie, J. W. A., Goluboff, N., Garson, J. Z. and Maningas, C. S. (1974). Serum IgE levels in parents and children. *J. Pediatrics* **85**, 660.

Heremans, J. F. (1959). Immunochemical studies on protein pathology. The immunoglobulin concept. *Clin. Chim. Acta* **4**, 639.

Hobbs, J. R. (1970). Simplified radial immunodiffusion. Appendix. Association of Clinical Pathologists Broadsheet 68.

Humphrey, J. H. and Batty, I. (1974). International Reference Preparation for Human Serum IgG, IgA, IgM. *Clin. Exp. Immunol.* **17**, 708

Ishizaka, K. and Ishizaka, T. (1971). Mechanisms of reaginic hypersensitivity: a review. *Clin. All.* **1**, 9.

Johansson, S. G. O., Foucard, T. and Dannaeus, A. (1974). IgE in human disease. Progress in Immunology II. Vol. 4. (Eds. L. Brent and J. Holborow), p. 61. North Holland Publishing Co., Amsterdam and Oxford.

Killingsworth, L. M. and Savory, J. (1971). Automated immunochemical procedures for measurement of immunoglobulins IgG, IgA, and IgM in human serum. *Clin. Chem.* **17**, 936.

Laurell, C-B. (1972). Electroimmunoassay. *Scand. J. Clin. Lab. Invest.* **29**, suppl. 124, 21.

Mancini, G., Carbonara, A. O. and Heremans, J. F. (1965). Immunological quantitation of antigens by single radial diffusion. *Immunochemistry* **2**, 235.

Ogra, P. L. and Karzon, D. T. (1969). Poliovirus antibody response in serum and nasal secretions following intranasal inoculation with inactivated poliovaccine. *J. Immunol.* **102**, 15.

Okafor, G. O., Turner, M. W. and Hay, F. C. (1974). Localisation of monocyte binding site of human immunoglobulin G. *Nature* **248**, 228.

Orgel, H. A. (1975). Genetic and developmental aspects of IgE. *Pediat. Clin. N. Amer.* **22**, 17.

Padlan, E. A., Segal, D. M., Rudikoff, S., Potter, M., Spande, T., and Davies, D. R. (1973). Structure at 4·5Å resolution of a phosphoryl-choline-binding Fab. *Nature New Biol.* **245**, 165.

Parkhouse, R. M. E. (1974). Biosynthesis of polymeric immunoglobulins. "Progress in Immunology II." Vol. 1. (Eds. L. Brent and J. Holborow), p. 119. North Holland Publishing Co., Amsterdam and Oxford.
Parkhouse, R. M. E., Askonas, B. A. and Dourmaskin, R. R. (1970). Electron microscopic studies of mouse immunoglobulin M; structure and reconstitution following reduction. *Immunology* **18**, 575.
Parkhouse, R. M. E., Virella, G. and Dourmashkin, R. R. (1971). Structural characterization of a human monoclonal IgA protein. *Clin. Exp. Immunol.* **8**, 581.
Polmar, S. H., Waldmann, T. A. and Terry, W. D. (1972). IgE in immunodeficiency. *American J. Path.* **69**, 499.
Porter, R. R. (1959). The hydrolysis of rabbit γ-globulin and antibodies with crystalline papain. *Biochem. J.* **73**, 119.
Putnam, F. W. (1974). Comparative structural study of human IgM, IgA and IgG immunoglobulins. "Progress in Immunology II." Vol. 1. (Eds. L. Brent and J. Holborow), p. 25. North Holland Publishing Co., Amsterdam and Oxford.
Rowe, D. S., Anderson, S. G. and Grab, B. (1970). A research standard for human serum immunoglobulins IgG, IgA and IgM. *Bull. Wld Hlth Org.* **42**, 535.
Rowe, D. S., Grab, B. and Anderson, S. G. (1972). An international reference preparation for human serum immunoglobulins G, A and M: content of immunoglobulins by weight. *Bull. Wld Hlth Org.* **46**, 67.
Rowe, D. S., Hug, K., Forni, L. and Pernis, B. (1973). Immunoglobulin D as a lymphocyte receptor. *J. Exp. Med.* **138**, 965.
Segal, D. M., Padlan, E. A., Cohen, G. H., Silverton, E. W., Davies, D. R., Rudikoff, S. and Potter, M. (1974). The structure of McPC 603 Fab and its hapten complex. "Progress in Immunology II." Vol. 1. (Eds. L. Brent and J. Holborow), p. 93. North Holland Publishing Co., Amsterdam and Oxford.
Smith, G. P. (1973). The variation and adaptive expression of antibodies. Harvard University Press, Cambridge, Massachusetts, U.S.A.
Spiegelberg, H. L. (1974). Biological activities of immunoglobulins of different classes and subclasses. *Adv. Immunol.* **19**, 259.
Stanworth, D. R. and Turner, M. W. (1973). Immunochemical analysis of immunoglobulins and their subunits, Chapter 10. *In* "Handbook of Experimental Immunology", (2nd edition), Blackwell Scientific Publications, Oxford.
Tiselius, A. and Kabat, E. A. (1938). Electrophoresis of immune serum. *Science* **87**, 416.
Tomasi, T. B. (1972). Secretory immunoglobulins. *New Eng. J. Med.* **287**, 500.
Tomasi, T. B. and Zigelbaum, S. (1963). The selective occurrence of gamma-1A globulins in certain body fluids. *J. Clin. Invest.* **42**, 1552.
Waldmann, T. A. and Hemmings, W. A. (1974). Transport and catabolism of immunoglobulins. "Progress in Immunology II." Vol. 1. (Eds. L. Brent and J. Holborow), p. 230. North Holland Publishing Co., Amsterdam and Oxford.
Wu, T. T. and Kabat, E. A. (1970). An analysis of the sequences of the variable regions of Bence Jones proteins and myeloma light chains and their implications for antibody complementarity. *J. Exp. Med.* **132**, 211.

5

Antigens and Antigenicity

D. V. WILSON

The term "antigen" incorporates two distinct ideas each of which may be described and studied separately although both are closely related at a molecular level. Firstly, an antigen is a substance that has the capacity to produce an immunological response (mediated by antibody and/or sensitized cells) with specificity related to its own structure. This aspect of antigenicity is often referred to as "immunogenicity". Clearly it is not a property of the antigen alone but must take into account the animal in which the phenomenon is observed. For example, poly-L-proline is immunogenic in guinea pigs but not in several other species studied; certain dextrans produce excellent antibodies in rabbits but only a poor response in man and, moreover, even within a species it is possible to obtain responder and non-responder strains to a particular antigen. Secondly, an antigen is a molecule which will react specifically at the combining site of an antibody. This *antigenic specificity* is in many ways analogous to the binding of substrate to the active site of an enzyme; reversible binding occurs in both cases but subsequent making or breaking of covalent chemical bonds is not a feature of antigen–antibody reactions.

The term antigen is also applied in a rather imprecise way to complex biological materials such as bacteria, viruses, cells, multi-component mixtures of proteins and many less well defined substances, especially when they provoke an immunological response in an animal. These are really mixtures containing many different antigens.

It is important to distinguish between immunogenicity and the capacity to react with an existing antibody because these two properties do not always coincide. An isolated capsular polysaccharide of molecular weight 33,000 from *Bacillus anthracis* is non-immunogenic but it will react with certain of the antibodies produced against the whole organism. Penicilloyl-ε-amino-caproic acid will inhibit the reaction between anti-penicilloyl antibodies and a penicilloylated protein but does not itself produce any immunological response when injected into an animal which has not previously received a penicillin injection.

GENERAL PROPERTIES OF AN EFFECTIVE IMMUNOGEN

Size

All the major classes of macromolecular substances—that is proteins, polysaccharides, polynucleotides, and complex lipids—are capable of producing an antigenic response in at least one species but whether they will do so in a particular set of circumstances depends on many factors; the host, the physical form in which they are administered, the site and frequency of administration and, most important, their detailed molecular structure. There is a certain minimum molecular size below which a molecule is incapable of showing immunogenicity. A molecular weight of about 1,000 is on the borderline but most antigens are a great deal larger than this. A few apparent exceptions to this generalization have been reported but these are explicable in some cases by the formation of a larger antigen *in vivo* (Frey *et al.*, 1969). However, smaller molecules may initiate the synthesis of specific antibodies provided they are first attached (conjugated) to a larger molecule. The small molecule is described as the *hapten*, the larger molecule as the *carrier* (Fig. 1). Hapten carrier systems are important in adverse immunological reactions to drugs (discussed below) and in procedures used to prepare antisera to small molecules for immuno-assay purposes (Playfair *et al.*, 1974). In this latter case the objective is to produce antisera with high affinity and great specificity for use in quantitative assays of substances of physiological importance. Unfortunately it has been found that many peptide hormones are poorly immunogenic. For example, early attempts to raise antisera to angiotensin 1 (Asp Arg Val Tyr Ileu His Pro Phe His Leu OH) were unsuccessful, probably because of its small size and susceptibility to enzymic degradation, but after conjugation to carriers good antibodies were obtained. Antibodies to free angiotensin may also be raised by injecting the aspartic acid β-amide of angiotensin II (Asp Arg Val Tyr Ileu His Pro Phe OH) physically adsorbed on to microparticles of carbon, an example where the physical form in which the antigen is administered influences the response.

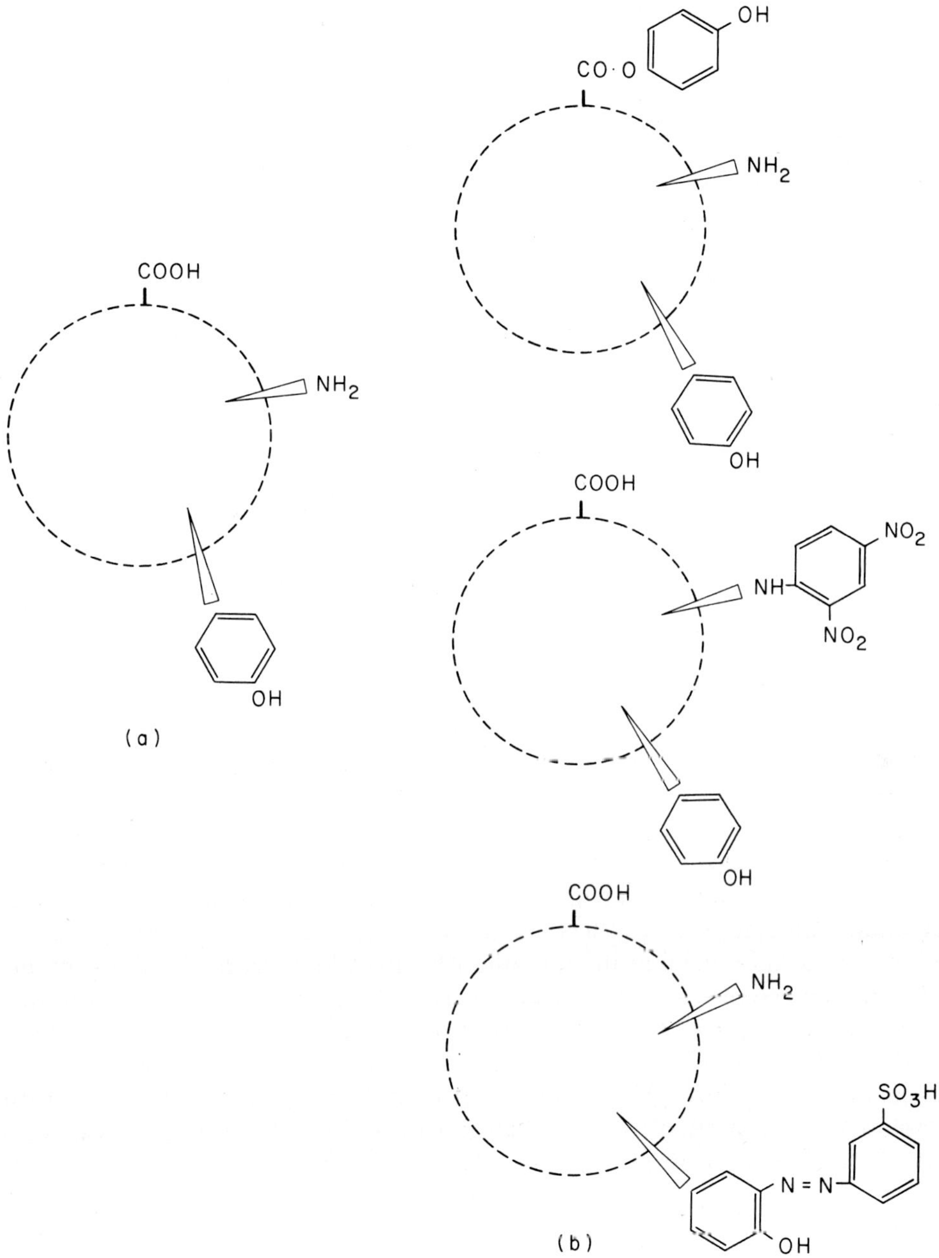

Fig. 1. Hapten and carrier systems. (a) Protein molecule showing various surface groups to which an hapten may be attached. (b) Three examples of hapten-carrier systems. In each case the carrier is the protein molecule illustrated in (a) but the hapten is different.

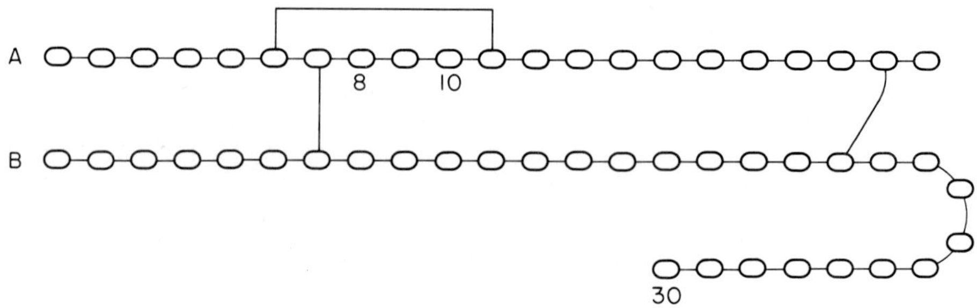

	8	10	30
Human :	Threonine	Isoleucine	Threonine
Bovine :	Alanine	Valine	Valine
Pig :	Threonine	Isoleucine	Alanine

Fig. 2. Structure of insulin derived from different species. Those amino acids which vary between species are listed in the table. All the other positions are filled with the same amino acids in these three species.

"Foreignness"

To be immunogenic a molecule must be dissimilar in structure to all of the natural constituents of the animal which is to be challenged. The foreignness may be obvious, for example injection of a bacterial dextran into a rabbit, or may involve only a subtle variation in the primary amino acid sequence of a peptide or protein which naturally occurs in the animal to be treated. Beef and pig insulins differ only slightly in structure from human insulin (Fig. 2) but elicit detectable antibodies of clinical significance in a proportion of diabetic patients receiving insulin therapy. It follows from the requirement of foreignness that a constituent taken from an animal will not be immunogenic when re-injected. It may, however, be converted *in vitro* into an antigen for the same species by almost any modification which changes its three dimensional structure. Mild heat treatment causing partial denaturation, attachment of a hapten, or modification of a single amino acid side chain may be all that is required.

Stability

An antigen must persist for a certain time after injection for it to be recognized by the appropriate cellular mechanisms at the commencement of an immunological response. This demands a resistance to chemical and enzymic change. The observation that some antigens which are not immunogenic when injected in a solution in saline are effective when co-precipitated with alum may be related in part to this requirement for stability.

Three-dimensional Structure

The three-dimensional structure of an antigen, which is in turn related to its chemical composition and the arrangement of atoms within it, has an overriding influence on the nature and magnitude of any antibody or cellular response. Sela and his co-workers (Sela, 1969) used chemically defined antigens to demonstrate that the more heterogeneous the composition, the better the response. Polymers of 2, 3, 4 or more amino acids gave antibodies with good affinity and specificity whereas homopolymers generally did not. The response is usually directed towards certain restricted areas of an antigen molecule known as antigenic determinants which may be haptens but more commonly are inherent structural features of the molecule itself. Several determinants may be present on the surface of the same molecule, each with a different composition and structure but all giving rise to responses. There are also present regions which do not usually exhibit immunogenicity. These have been described as *immunodominant* and *immunosilent groups* respectively, and are shown diagramatically in Fig. 3. However, it is not possible to say with certainty that a particular molecular feature could not under any circumstances give rise to antibodies or sensitized cells.

MOLECULAR FEATURES OF ANTIGENIC DETERMINANTS

Information derived from the fragmentation of antigens followed by investigation of the immunological properties of such fragments; from experiments with hapten carrier systems; from inhibition experiments, and from the analysis of responses to chemically synthesized antigens has led to a partial description of antigenic determinants in molecular terms, at least for antigens in which the main determinants are protein-like. In one case, that of sperm whale myoglobin, the complete antigenic structure has been worked out in great detail and generalizations from this example appear to be valid for

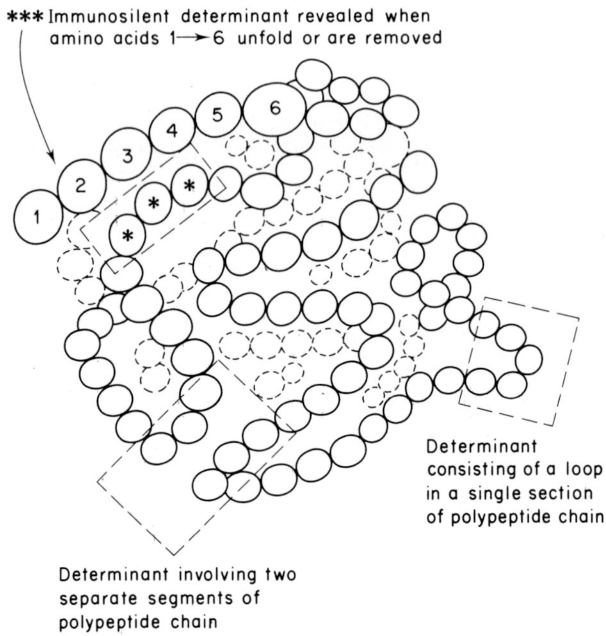

Fig. 3. Nature and location of determinants. A stylized view of a protein molecule showing the polypeptide chain folded and looped to form a roughly spherical structure. Certain regions will be specific determinants. Major determinants will be on the surface. They may be *immunodominant* because of special structural features or their easily accessible position, or they may be *immunosilent* because of masking or steric hindrance.

many other molecules. Figure 4 shows the intricate way in which the polypeptide chain of myoglobin is coiled and folded into a globular three dimensional structure with a recognizable "surface", an "interior" and several loops and clefts. The native protein contains five *antigenic reactive regions* (amino acid sequences 16–21; 56–62; 94–99; 113–119 and 146–151). Thus not every bend or loop is immunodominant.

From the final form of the antigenic structure advanced for myoglobin and the strategy by which it was deduced, Atassi and co-workers (Atassi, 1975) have derived a number of important generalizations which will be applicable to other proteins and their early course antisera. They conclude:

i. determinants occupy surface locations on native proteins. This implies that antigens are not degraded or altered in a significant way before the machinery for antibody production recognizes them. An *area* of the

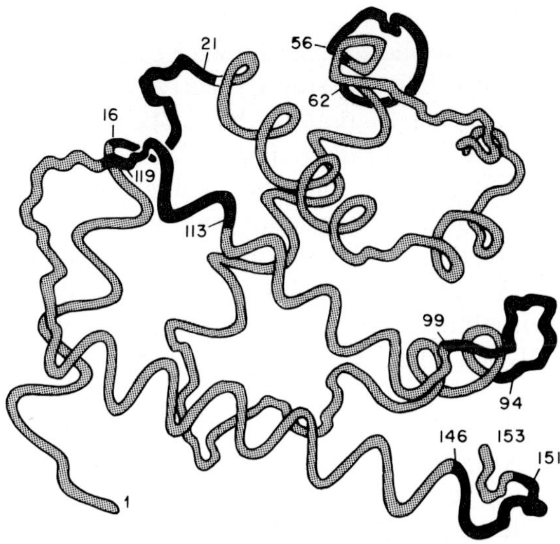

Region	Structure and Location *	No. of Residues
Region 1	16 Lys-Val-Glu-Ala-Asp-Val 21	6
Region 2	56 Lys-Ala-Ser-Glu-Asp-Leu-Lys 62	7
Region 3	94 Ala-Thr-Lys-His-Lys-Ile 99	6
Region 4	113 His-Val-Leu-His-Ser-Arg-His 119	7
Region 5	146 Tyr-Lys-Glu-Leu-Gly-Tyr 151	6

* These are shaded black in the diagram above. Certain sera react as if another (adjacent) amino acid is also included in the antigenic reactive region

Fig. 4. The antigenic structure of myoglobin. Modified from Atassi, 1975.

surface of the molecule is involved which may be made up from amino acid side chains of two or more sections of the primary sequence (*antigenic reactive regions*). Present techniques do not allow the detailed molecular interactions in the whole determinant to be studied and most conclusions relate to single reactive regions only;

ii. antigenic reactive regions have well defined boundaries. Thus in a series of antisera raised in different animals against the same protein, antibodies will be present against the same segments of primary sequence, although perhaps one additional amino acid residue might be involved in the reaction with certain of the sera, one fewer with others. When multiple determinants are present on the same molecule the contribution from each to the total response may differ in different animals but all determinants will be represented to some extent in every case;

iii. antigenic reactive regions are usually small (6 or 7 amino acid residues) and oligopeptides of the correct structure which are even shorter should be able to react although less efficiently than the complete sequence.

iv. No amino acid side chain appears in every antigenic reactive region but because of the surface location of determinants it is to be expected that amino acids with hydrophilic side chains (lysine, aspartic acid, serine, histidine, etc.) will predominate. Binding of antibody by these residues will involve ionic interactions. Hydrophilic groups may also be present and hydrophobic interactions will then occur;

v. the conformation of a protein dominates its reactivity. Even minor changes in three dimensional arrangement will change the ability to bind to a particular antibody. A major rearrangement as in denatured material may completely prevent reaction. A convincing demonstration of the importance of conformation was provided by Arnon and Sela (1969). Antibodies were raised against a fragment of the molecule of hen egg white lysozyme which had been prepared in such a way that it retained the rigid three-dimensional structure it possessed in the native protein. These antibodies bound the native protein and binding was inhibited by the fragment itself. A polypeptide of identical sequence but without such a rigid structure was not inhibitory.

   It is possible that conformational changes brought about by binding of a metal ion or small organic molecule generate a determinant where none existed before. Allergic reactions to beryllium metal involve this type of conformational determinant (Jones and Amos, 1975);

vi. If two different proteins have similar (but not necessarily identical) antigenic reactive regions then antibodies raised against one will react with the other (Fig. 5). It is necessary only that a similarity exists in a single determinant, all others may be different. Naturally, the more antigenic reactive regions there are in common, the greater the extent of cross-reaction. This type of immunochemical cross-reaction is seen in the pattern of reactions of many anti-globulins which will react with immunoglobulins of the same class from two or more different species.

The same general conclusions relating to the antigenic determinants of myoglobin should be applicable to most oligopeptides, enzymes and other macromolecules containing substantially similar sections of polypeptide chain provided that their three dimensional structure is also similar. Fibrous

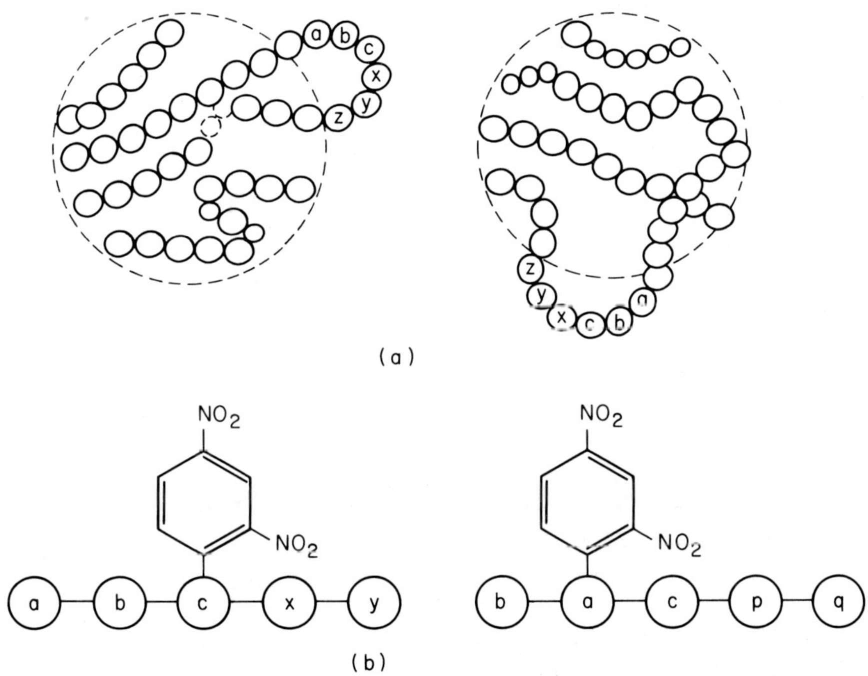

Antibodies to these two determinants could be expected to show cross-reactions

Fig. 5. Structural basis of cross-reaction. (a) Two different macromolecules with a single common identical determinant (the x, y, z, a, b, c, loop). Elsewhere they differ in structure. (b) Antibodies to an immunodominant group (possibly a hapten) may react with determinants containing the immunodominant structure although nearby features are different.

proteins, cyclic peptides and polypeptides with unusual conformations will differ in their overall immunogenicity but here again, similar determinants may be expected.

Other classes of natural macromolecules which do not have amino acids as monomers will differ. Polysaccharides, and to a lesser extent polynucleotides are the most important.

Polysaccharide Antigens

The most striking feature of most polysaccharides is their regular repeating structure in which monosaccharide units are linked in long chains which may be branched. As the antigenic determinant embraces about five monosaccharide units, polysaccharides may be regarded as chains of repeating antigenic determinants, possibly with extensive overlap between one determinant and the next (Fig. 6). Despite their repeating structure, polysaccharides possess an antigenic fine structure which is at least as complex as that of a protein antigen. For example, the capsular polysaccharide of Type 3 pneumococcus (Fig. 7) is a polymer of cellobiuronic acid and the whole organism or

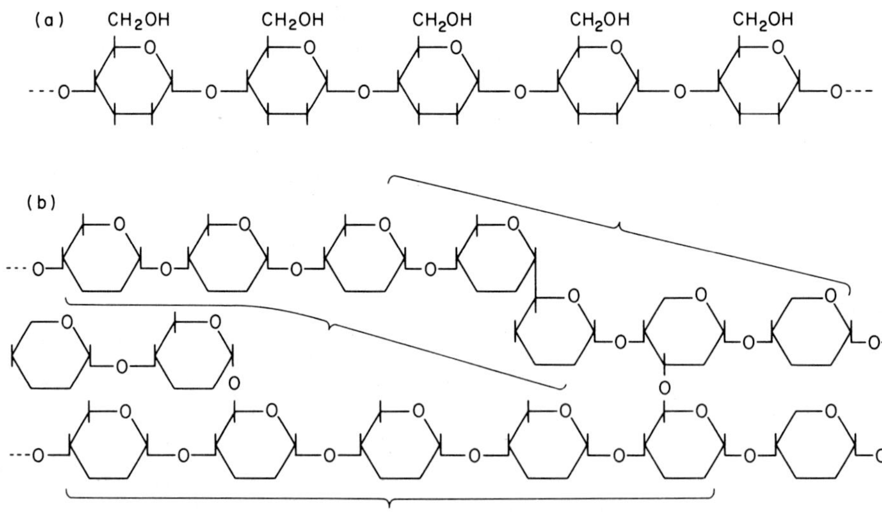

Fig. 6. The size and general nature of determinants in polysaccharides. Part of a polysaccharide chain is illustrated to show, in (a), a region of about the size expected for a determinant and, in (b), the way in which extensive overlaps may be seen in branched chains. Possible determinants are bracketed.

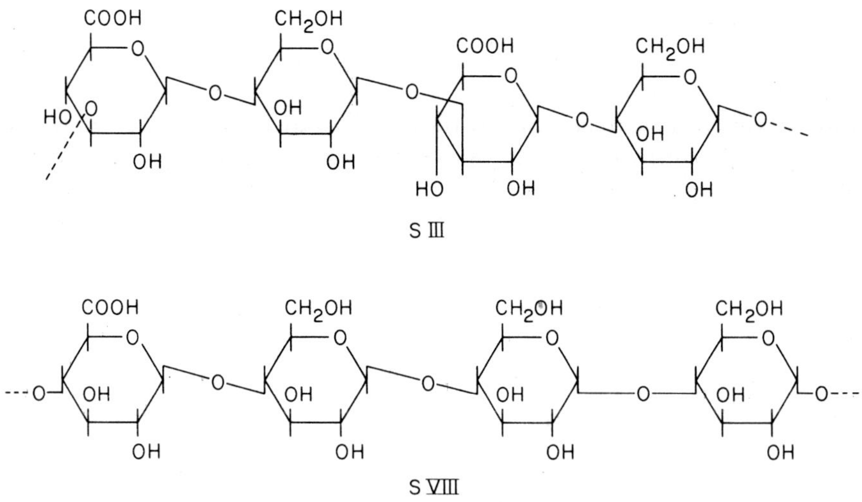

Fig. 7. Chemical structures of polysaccharide antigens from Type 3 (SIII) and Type 8 (SVIII) pneumocci.

capsular material derived from it will provoke the production of antibodies which react with this structure. These sera will also react with the capsular material from Type 8 pneumococcus but not with many other polysaccharides which differ only in the position of one hydroxyl in the cellobiuronic acid moiety. Although most types of bacteria elicit antibodies against their cell wall components when they are injected without any pretreatment, isolated polysaccharides derived from them may be non-immunogenic unless attached as hapten to a suitable carrier. Carbohydrates need to be larger than proteins to evoke similar responses.

Polynucleotide Antigens

Stollar (1973) has recently reviewed this group of antigens. Nucleic acids or their components will react with naturally occurring antibodies but are only very weakly immunogenic in their own right. In order to prepare antibodies against natural polynucleotides it is necessary to complex them with a peptide or protein (both chemical coupling and binding by non-covalent mechanisms have been used) or to inject a performed complex like a ribosome. With these techniques it has been possible to raise antisera against denatured DNA, ribosomal RNA, artificial double helical polynucleotides (which often do not require complexing to a carrier) and a few others; but not against DNA + histone or DNA + poly-L-lysine complexes. Antibodies against *native* DNA are known only in their spontaneous appearance in the serum of SLE patients.

Many different arrangements of four or five nucleotides (the size expected to occupy an antibody combining site) are possible in a single strand of RNA, depending on base sequence and which aspect of the chain (base residues or sugar-phosphate support) is exposed. Adjacent portions of different chains could contribute to the determinant as is the case with proteins and the unique stacking properties of bases could produce unusual three-dimensional arrangements and hence antibody specificities.

A summary of the nature and properties of the vast number of known antigens is outside the scope of this chapter. Instead, the properties of a few representative substances will be described, grouped for convenience under the headings of antigens of known chemical structure; cell-related antigens; and complex antigens of ill-defined structure.

Antigens of Known Chemical Structure

Synthetic Antigens

The inherent complexity of most natural polypeptides and proteins may be a disadvantage when particular areas of the immune response are to be investigated. A simpler molecule is required to avoid multiple responses which are difficult to interpret. The obvious choice would be a homopolymer of a single amino acid, for example poly-L-lysine, but homopolymers of α-amino acids are not usually immunogenic. However, effective immunogens may be synthesized from them by attaching other homopolypeptides. This approach has been used to great effect by Sela (1969) who has synthesized a wide range of multi-chain co-polymers and examined their reactivity. This has helped in the delineation of many structural and conformational features important in determining immunogenicity. For example, the co-polymer depicted in Fig. 8a is a potent and specific antigen in rabbits whereas the analogue in Fig. 8b is unreactive, showing that in order to elicit biosynthesis of antibody the antigenic reactive region must be readily accessible and not buried within the interior of the molecule.

A further important use of synthetic antigens is in the investigation of the so-called T-independent immune response (Sela *et al.*, 1972). Other synthetic antigens have been employed in studies of antigenic competition and genetic

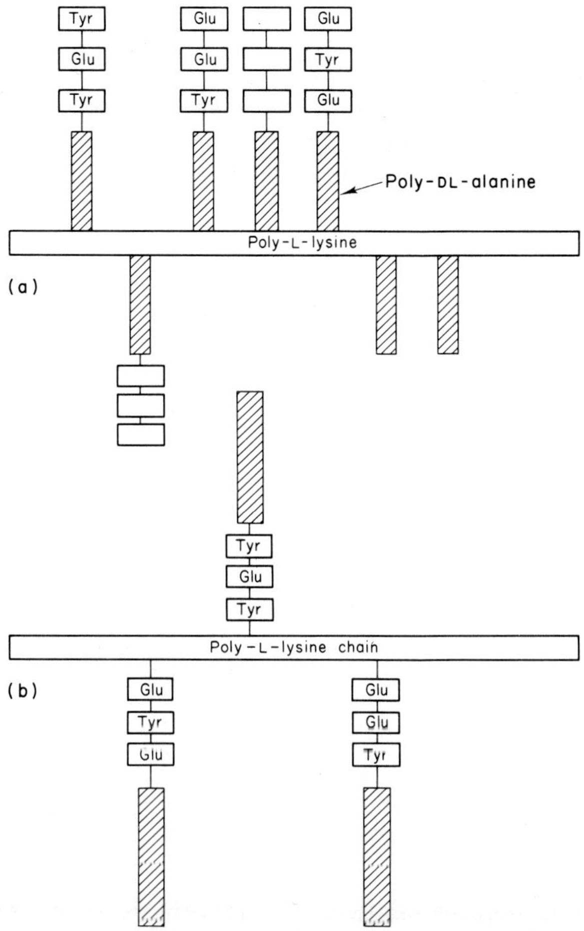

Fig. 8. Synthetic co-polymers with accessible (a) and buried (b) antigenic reactive regions.

control of the immune response (Taussig *et al.*, 1973). Three synthetic polymers were used as antigens (Fig. 9a). In a highly responsive strain of mice it was found that intramolecular competition with the (Phe Glu)-Pro-Lys molecule and intermolecular competition with mixtures of (Tyr Glu)-Pro-Lys and (Phe Glu)-Ala-Lys could both occur. (Pro-Lys) was the dominant determinant and suppressed the response to (Phe Glu). In another strain of mice with a low response to (Pro-Lys), intramolecular competition was absent but intermolecular competition could still be demonstrated. These

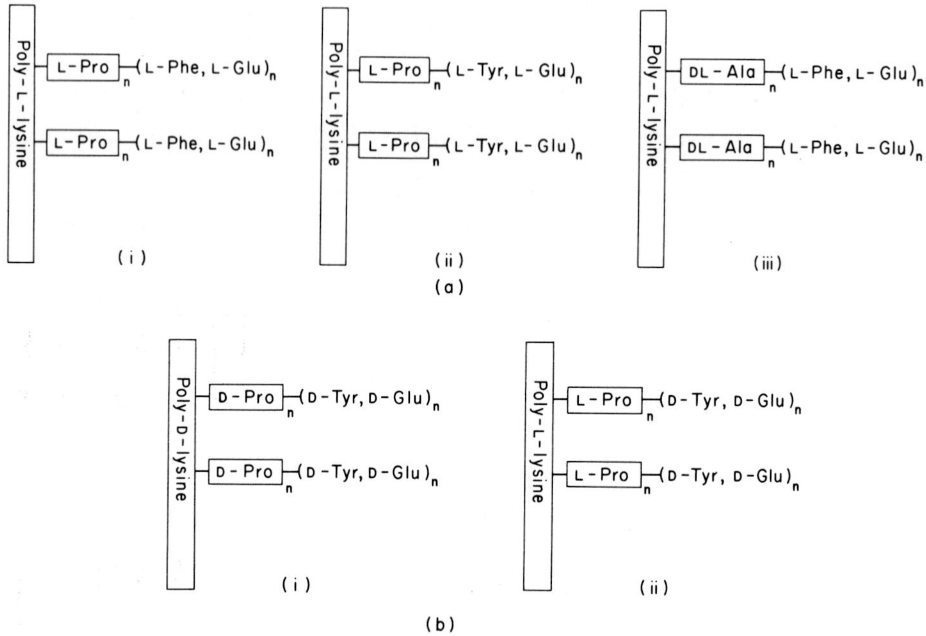

Fig. 9. Synthetic co-polymers of related structure which exhibit widely different immunological properties. (a) All three compounds are based on a poly-lysine backbone. When present, Pro-Lys is the dominant determinant. It suppresses the response to Phe Glu when compound (i) is injected alone into suitable strains of mice (intramolecular antigenic competition) and also when (ii) and (iii) are injected together (intermolecular antigenic competition). (b) Threshold dose for high zone tolerance in mice to the enantiomer (i) is about 100 pg whereas for (ii) it is only 1 pg.

findings resulted in the formulation of a hypothesis for intramolecular competition. Somewhat similar antigens (Fig. 9b) were used by the same workers to show the importance of optical configuration in an immune response. The threshold dose for high zone tolerance for the two antigens differed by two orders of magnitude although the structural variations were minor, involving only a reversal of optical configuration in the amino acids of the supporting chain.

Immunogenic Conjugates of Drugs and other Small Molecules

It is an apparent paradox that many of the adverse reactions to therapeutically useful drugs of low molecular weight are regarded by the clinician as allergic although it is known that small molecules do not themselves elicit immunological reactions. The explanation is that the drug participates in the formation of a macromolecular complex which is the functional antigen. This causes production of antibodies and sensitized cells. Later encounters between the drug, either complexed or free, and receptors on antibody molecules or cells initiate the observed reactions.

It has proved surprisingly difficult to gain information on the structure of the drug-containing antigen *in vivo* because the carrier molecule to which the drug becomes attached as hapten is not known. However, synthetic drug-carrier conjugates may be synthesized and used to investigate the specificity of circulating cells and antibodies in patients showing a drug reaction. This approach has revealed that the small molecule may be linked in various ways to give immunodominant groups of differing specificity. Penicillin is the most widely investigated example. It elicits antibodies against one or more of the determinants shown in Fig. 10. Other drugs (Fig. 11) undoubtedly form conjugates but their precise mode of attachment is not known. Some of them, like penicillin, form conjugates by straightforward chemical reactions. Aspirin (or an impurity in commercial preparations of acetylsalicylic acid) could probably form an acetylsalicyloyl protein; but other drugs may need to be activated enzymically or be partially metabolized before they are bound, and the structure of the hapten may then be difficult to identify. A recent monograph (Amos, 1976) discusses in more detail the present state of understanding of allergic drug reactions and the methods available for their investigation.

Another quite separate development—radioimmunoassay—has stimulated the chemical synthesis of antigens made up from a protein carrier (commonly bovine serum albumin or another readily available plasma protein) and a drug or other small molecule. Although originally an endocrinological technique, radioimmunoassay is now an important tool in many areas of diagnosis and medical investigation and in numerous non-medical research areas. Whatever the final application it is always necessary to make antisera of high avidity and specificity. When an antiserum against a small molecule is sought the molecule or a derivative must be attached as a hapten to a suitable carrier before injection. Figure 12 lists a selection of molecules against which antisera have been raised and are available commercially.

Complex Antigens of Ill-defined Structure

Naturally occurring materials of foreign animal or vegetable origin which are capable of stimulating production of reaginic antibody are sometimes referred

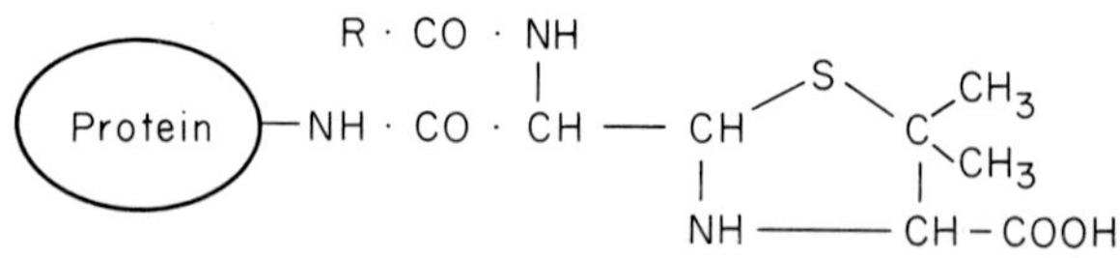

Penicilloyl-

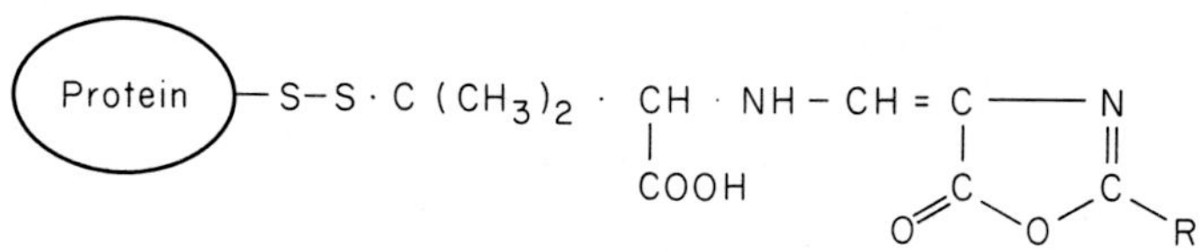

Penicillenate-

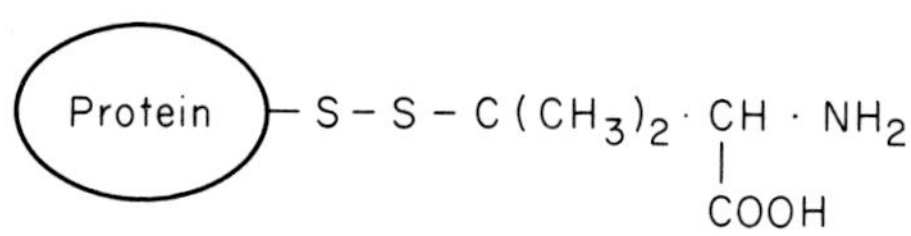

Penicillamine derivative

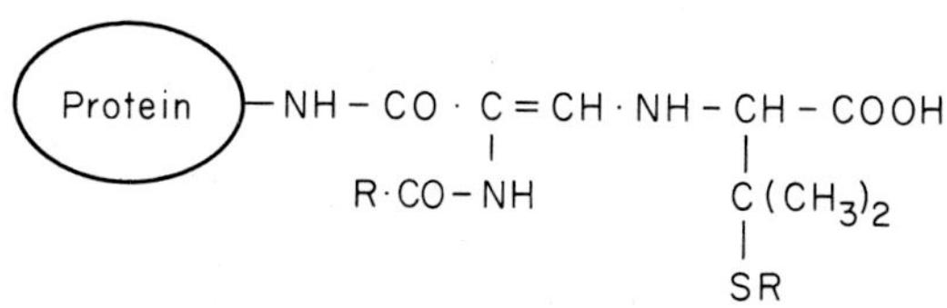

Penamaldoyl

Fig. 10. Haptens which may be formed during reaction of penicillin with a carrier protein. The penicilloyl groups occur most commonly but may not always have the greatest significance in eliciting adverse immunological reactions to the drug.

to as "allergens". Such antigens which are capable of triggering hypersensitivity reactions in sensitized individuals have been studied intensively for more than half a century but precise structural information is available for only a few examples. There appears to be no consistent chemical feature that will identify an "allergen". They may be protein, glycoprotein or carbohydrate of high molecular weight—although it has been claimed (Marsh, 1975) that

Penicillins	Amidopyrine
Aspirin	D-Penicillamine
α-Methyldopa	Rifampicin
Quinine	Streptomycin
Sedormid	Insulin
Novobiocin	

Fig. 11. Some drugs known to elicit specific antibodies in man.

Insulin	Thyroxine
Human growth Hormone	Triiodothyronine
ACTH	Digoxin
HCG	Testosterone
HCS	Cortisol
Gastrin	Progesterone
	17β - Oestradiol
	Cyclic-AMP

Fig. 12. Antigens and haptens for which antisera suitable for radioimmunoassay are available commercially.

they are usually "at the lower end of the molecular weight range, <40,000 daltons, and frequently seem to contain acidic glycoproteins".

Grass Pollen Antigens

There are at least 14 antigenic components in extracts of common grass pollens. In some cases these have been isolated and partially purified. Often the antigenic activity is remarkably resistant to heat treatment. Perennial rye grass (*Lolium perenne*) yields distinct groups of antigens designated I, II, III and IV each of which may be further fractionated. Subfractions I-B and I-C derived from Group I are both proteins of molecular weight 27,000. They contain about 5% carbohydrate which does not appear essential for the main antigenic activity.

Substances which cross-react with rye grass group I antigens occur in pollen of many other grasses and in one study of 250 individuals with grass pollen sensitivity almost all were sensitive to the group I antigens. Thus it appears that some feature of the structure of group I substances is unusually potent. If identified it may well lead to improved hyposensitization therapy as well as a greater understanding of the basic mechanism of pollen hypersensitivity.

Ragweed Antigens

Pollen of the short ragweed (*Ambrosia elatior*) which is the commonest cause of hayfever in the United States is known to contain 14 antigens including what may be the major one, AgE, of molecular weight about 40,000 daltons, which exists in a number of closely related variants. AgE is atypical in the way it loses activity when subjected to mild heating, 8M urea, or buffers with pH values outside the range 6–8·5. It readily dissociates into two non-identical inactive fragments (α and β) which re-associate without regaining biological activity. It is possible that the antigenic reactive region embraces components of both subunits. Alternatively the active area may be confined to one unit but may be made ineffective by steric hindrance in the re-combined aggregate.

In addition to the large antigens, a small basic antigen Ra5 has been isolated from ragweed and in this case the complete amino acid sequence is known (Fig. 13). Two forms exist differing at a single position and the molecule is unusually rigid because of cross linking disulphide bridges between the various half cystine residues. This rigid configuration and the high proportion of hydrophilic amino acids may contribute to its immunogenicity.

Codfish Antigens

A number of glycoproteins from cod which are potent antigens in codfish-hypersensitive patients have been isolated, purified and subjected to detailed structural investigation. The antigenic reactive region appears from enzymic studies to consist of carbohydrate-free determinants.

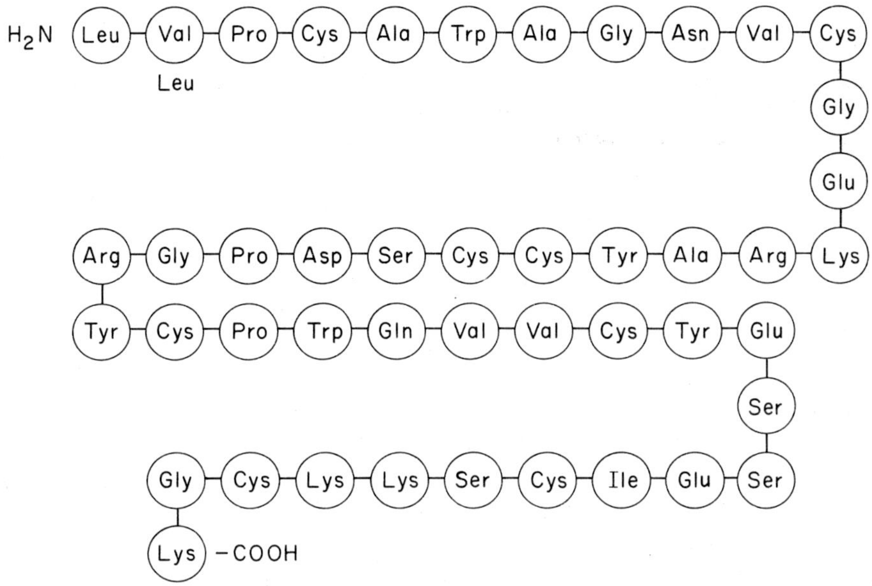

Fig. 13. Amino acid sequence of allergen Ra5 from ragweed. From Mole *et al.*, 1974.

Castor Bean Antigens

Components of the seed of the castor bean (*Ricinus communis*) may give rise to reactions in individuals who live or work in an environment where the beans are processed. Hypersensitivity, which can be severe, is mainly respiratory, and serum from sensitive individuals can be shown to contain IgE antibodies against extracts of the bean (Coombs *et al.*, 1968). The active constituent is a mixture which has been partly separated by electrophoresis but the nature of the separate components has not been worked out in detail. It seems likely that glycoproteins are involved.

Mite and House Dust Antigens

Patients with asthma and rhinitis attributable to house dust usually give a positive skin test to extracts of house mites (*Dermatophagoides pteronyssinus* or *D. farinae*) and since hypersensitivity to house dust is one of the most important causes of asthma there is considerable interest in the nature of the antigens involved. However the belief that mite antigens are the principle antigen in all cases has been questioned and other components of house dust may be of greater significance depending on circumstances of climate, house construction and living patterns.

Theories of "Allergenicity"

Despite the paucity of data on the fine structure of the most important "allergens" there have been many attempts to formulate a detailed structure—activity hypothesis to explain "allergenicity". Berrens (1971) believes the key factor to be the presence of sugars linked *N*-glycosidically to the ε-amino groups of lysine residues but this theory fails to explain the activity of many pollen and food antigens which are devoid of carbohydrate and of the protein-free polysaccharides, for example dextrans, which are capable of inducing hypersensitivity reactions but do not contain protein.

Marsh (1975) has pointed out that whatever the mechanism, factors which enhance immunogenicity must be involved and must do so by making the conditions for immunization less limiting. It seems likely that a fuller understanding of "allergenicity" will only emerge when immunogenicity is better understood.

Cell-related Antigens

There is no reason to doubt that the same fundamental chemical structures that are determinants of relatively simple soluble macromolecules also constitute the determinants of cells. Glycoproteins, lipoproteins lipopolysaccharides, and even small haptenic molecules can form part of cell surfaces and the same rules of "foreignness", "size", and "stability" apply for immunogenicity. The antibodies are capable of the same types of reaction and cross-reaction as antibodies to non-cellular antigens. Some differences may occur in steric aspects of antigenicity, for example in the degree to which access to a particular determinant is hindered by neighbouring groups but this is no more than an extreme form of a phenomenon observable in other systems. The main immunochemical difference between cell-related and soluble antigens is in the range of experimental methods by which they are investigated. Antigens on cells are easy to detect but difficult to isolate and characterize, whereas the reverse is true of non-particulate antigens.

The ease of detection of antigens on cells arises from the simplicity, convenience, and high sensitivity of agglutination tests and of reactions in which the biological consequences of binding antibody to a particular cell-related antigen are measured (for example, cytotoxicity reactions). However, isolation of a defined antigen in active form from a cell membrane is almost always difficult, the chemical procedures which have to be used to release the antigen often denaturing or disrupting it at the same time.

Despite these limitations, the clinical importance in man of cell-related antigens has provided sufficient incentive for the formidable problems of characterization to be tackled and a great deal of data exists on the chemical nature of blood group antigens (Hakamori and Kobata, 1974), histocompatibility antigens (Ferrone *et al.*, 1975), and microbial antigens. Tumour antigens and basement membrane antigens have been studied less extensively.

Blood Group Antigens in Man

Investigation of the chemistry of the main blood group antigens was helped by the discovery that water soluble substances which are serologically identical with the antigens on red cell membranes are present in fairly high concentration in saliva and other secretions in many individuals. They are large mucopeptides with molecular weights up to 1,000,000 and appear to be assembled from five simple sugars and about 15 amino acids (Kabat, 1956).

H-antigen derived from Group O individuals, and A-substance and B-substance secreted by Group A, Group B and Group AB individuals are all known in highly purified form; they are closely related. A-substance is split by a specific enzyme into H-substance and *N*-acetylgalactosamine, B-substance with a different enzyme gives H-substance plus galactose, and H-substance itself is degradable to a molecule related to the Lewis blood group system. Thus the principle determinants which define the main blood groups are carried on the same macromolecular precursor.

A, B and H-substances are not confined to red blood cells but are detectable on many human epithelial and endothelial cells.

Histocompatibility Antigens

Histocompatibility antigens exist on cells of every mammalian species (although they differ in structure in different species), and as they are capable of persisting in long term tissue culture they are likely to be an important feature of membrane structure. Chemically, they are polypeptides. Human HLA antigens have a molecular weight of 31,000, are relatively stable, and when isolated are associated with β_2-microglobulin—a protein present also in urine.

The involvement of HLA antigens in organ transplantation is discussed in Chapter 29. Other indications of the importance of this extensively polymorphic antigen is the growing realization of correlations between HLA antigen type and the incidence of particular diseases.

Microbial Antigens

Diffusible exotoxins of gram-positive bacteria; complex endotoxins extractable from gram-negative bacteria; substances upon which the serological classifications of microorganisms are based, and numerous other macromolecules that are external components of microorganisms or are released by them may be considered under this classification. Not surprisingly, the most extensively studied are those related to organisms pathogenic for man.

All those exotoxins which have been extensively purified are proteins. They vary in size—Type A botulinus toxin has a molecular weight above 1,000,000; tetanus toxin is much smaller with a molecular weight of about 67,000—but all are large enough to exhibit several distinct antigenic determinants. Bacterial exotoxins are amongst the most poisonous substances known but their toxicity is lost on any one of a number of treatments including chemical modification of amino groups by exposure to formaldehyde or ketene, controlled treatment with denaturing agents (heat or mineral acid) or partial digestion with proteolytic enzymes.

It is possible to regulate the inactivation process and halt it at the stage where toxicity has been destroyed but many antigenic determinants remain. These modified exotoxins are known as toxoids; they exhibit considerable immunological cross-reactivity with the parent toxin and when administered to man in an appropriate way they are capable of inducing an immune response which protects against the pharmacological effects of the original toxin.

Endotoxins differ from exotoxins in being heat stable and in their composition. They are exceedingly complex lipopolysaccharides and normally exist as an integral part of the outer membrane of the organism. Other polysaccharides are found in the capsules surrounding certain bacteria.

The lipopolysaccharides from many different sources show a regularity of structure, which may be regarded as consisting of three main regions:

O-specific chain — Core polysaccharide — LIPID A

Apparently the lipid-A section is identical in structure even when lipopolysaccharides from a large number of different organisms are compared. This is the region by which the complete antigen is linked to the cell membrane. O-specific chains are constructed from oligosaccharide repeating units but the fine structure varies in different chemotypes: different sugars are immunodominant leading to many variations in determinants.

Capsular polysaccharides of bacteria are generally carbohydrates of high molecular weight. They are highly immunogenic and show considerable immunological heterogeneity. More than 75 serologically distinct types of pneumococci may be distinguished by means of antisera against capsular antigens. A recent review (Jann and Westphal, 1975) describes in some detail the chemical basis of this variation. It also deals with lipopolysaccharides and with many related polysaccharide antigens.

DETECTION AND MEASUREMENT OF ANTIBODIES

The whole range of immunological procedures designed to monitor the interaction of an antigen with its antibody is capable in theory of detecting antigens, and often can give quantitative information on the amount present in a sample. Chapter 6 lists some of these. However, a method which is ideal for *antibody* measurements may be unsuitable for antigens and *vice versa*.

Precipitation reactions in liquid media or in gels are cheap and convenient but relatively insensitive, complement fixation tests are capable in favourable cases of detecting as little as 0·5 μg of antigen in a sample, and even more sensitive is the technique of reverse passive haemagglutination (Fig. 14). The most sensitive of current methods for antibody quantitation are probably radioimmunoassays or related methods using labelled antibodies (Wilson *et al.*, 1976); whereas the most convenient for antigen detection is the fluorescent antibody technique.

In addition to numerous research applications, techniques for antigen detection and measurement have an important role in the diagnosis of infectious diseases. The presence of microbial antigen may be taken as an indication of the presence of the microorganism from which it is derived, in contrast to positive detection of specific antibody, which merely indicates a current or previous infection. Soluble bacterial capsular antigens have been

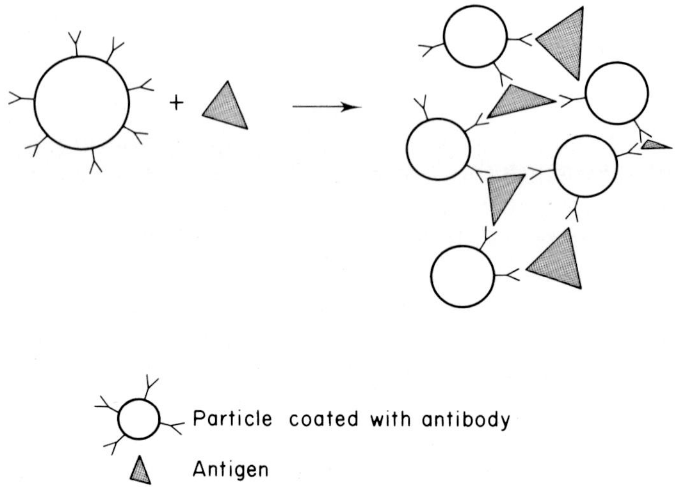

Fig. 14. Principle of reverse passive haemagglutination. A particle (e.g. an erythrocyte) is coated with specific antibody by chemical means. If antigen is added, agglutination results.

detected in the body fluids (including urine) of patients infected with the organisms causing trichinosis and schistosomiasis. Identification of the specific polysaccharide of either *pneumoccus*, *meningococcus* or *Haemophilus influenzae* may be used to identify the causative organism in the CSF of patients with meningitis. Both radioimmunoassay and reverse passive haemagglutination have their advocates for screening blood for hepatitis B antigen. Increased knowledge of antigens and their structure is likely to lead to further useful diagnostic tests, as well as aiding the development of new vaccines against infectious agents and improvement of those already in use.

REFERENCES

Amos, H. E. (1976). "Allergic Drug Reactions." Edward Arnold, London.

Arnon, R. and Sela, M. (1969). Antibodies to unique region in lysozyme by a synthetic antigen conjugate. *Proc. Nat. Acad. Sci. (U.S.A.)* **62**, 163.

Atassi, M. A. (1975). Antigenic structure of myoglobulin: the complete immunochemical anatomy of a protein and conclusions relating to the antigenic structure of a protein. *Immunochemistry* **12**, 423.

Berrens, L. (1971). "The Chemistry of Atopic Allergens." Karger, Basel.

Coombs, R. R. A., Hunter, A., Jonas, W. E., Bennich, H., Johansson, S. G. O. and Panzani, R. (1968). Detection of IgE (IgND) specific antibody (probably reagin) to castor bean allergen by the Red Cell Linked Antigen Antiglobulin Reaction. *Lancet* **i**, 1115.

Ferrone, S., Pellegrino, M. A. and Reisfeld, R. A. (1975). A biologic and chemical profile of histocompatibility antigens. *In* "The Antigens" Vol. III (ed. Sela), p. 362. Academic Press, London and New York.

Frey, J. R., De Weck, A. L., Geleick, H., Lergier, W. (1969). The immunogenicity of dinitrophenyl amino acids. *J. Exp. Med.* **130**, (5), 1123.

Hakamori, S. and Kobata, A. (1974). Blood group antigens. *In* "The Antigens" Vol. II (ed. Sela), p. 79. Academic Press, London and New York.

Jann, K. and Westphal, O. (1975). Microbial polysaccharides. *In* "The Antigens" Vol. III (ed. Sela), p. 1. Academic Press, London and New York.

Jones, J. M., and Amos, H. E. (1975). Antigen formation in metal contact sensitivity. *Nature* **256**, 499.

Kabat, E. A. (1956). "Blood Group Substances: Their Chemistry and Immunochemistry." Academic Press, New York and London.

Marsh, D. G. (1975). Allergens and the genetics of allergy. *In* "The Antigens" Vol. III (ed. Sela), p. 271. Academic Press, London and New York.

Mole, L. E., Goodfriend, L., Lapkoff, C. B., Kehoe, J. M. and Capra, J. D. (1975). The amino acid sequence of ragweed pollen allergen Ra5. *Biochemistry* **14**, 1216.

Playfair, J. H. L., Hurn, B. A. L. and Schulster, D. (1974). Production of antibodies and binding agents. *Brit. Med. Bull.* **30**, (1), 24.

Sela, M. (1969). Antigenicity: some molecular aspects. *Science* 1365.

Sela, M., Mozes, E. and Shearer, G. M. (1972). Thymus independence of slowly metabolized immunogens. *Proc. Nat. Acad. Sci. (U.S.A.)* **69**, 2696.

Stollar, D. (1973). Nucleic acid antigens. *In* "The Antigens" Vol. I (ed. Sela, M.), p. 2. Academic Press, London and New York.

Taussig, M. J., Mozes, E., Shearer, G. M. and Sela, M. (1973). Antigenic competition and genetic control of the immune response. An hypothesis for intramolecular competition. *Cell. Immunol.* **8**, 299.

Wilson, D. V., Thornley, M. J. and Coombs, R. R. A. (1976). A solid phase assay using radioactively labelled antibody for the detection of *Brucella abortus*. *J. Med. Microbiol.* (in press).

6

Antigen–Antibody Interaction

G. D. JOHNSON and J. WATKINS

GENERAL FEATURES

Reactions between antigens in solution and their corresponding antibodies occur in two stages. In the first stage primary binding between individual molecules takes place, usually rapidly, with the production of complexes which remain initially in solution. Subsequent contact between these complexes results in their aggregation to large size and possible insolubilization.

Primary binding may be detected by radioimmunoassay, by measurement of antigen binding capacity, and with insoluble antigens by immunofluorescence. Depending on the nature of the antigen and/or antibody involved, secondary interactions in solution are recognized by the development of visible precipitate formation—directly, or under the influence of an electrical charge—and in the case of particular antigens by agglutination and by complement fixation. All these have applications in clinical immunology.

It is useful to bear in mind the following general properties of immunological reactions in assessing the significance of results obtained with a particular serological method.

Specificity

This is the characteristic property of antigen–antibody reactions, providing the basis for identification of reactants involved. Immunological specificity may be manifest to a high degree and enables distinctions to be made that would otherwise be possible only by elaborate chemical analysis. For example the sera of most patients with systemic lupus erythematosus (SLE) display marked reactivity with various combinations of single purine or pyrimidine bases, with the analogous nucleosides and nucleotides and with oligonucleotides containing mixed purine–pyridine sequences. All these distinct specificities are related to reactivity with single-stranded DNA molecules, but in addition many SLE sera react specifically with double-stranded DNA. Antibodies to antigens present in cell nuclei may react with nuclei in a variety of tissues by immunofluorescence, but antinuclear antibodies in some sera show a predilection for nuclei of particular cells such as granulocytes or cells of parts of renal tubules.

Cross-reactivity is a different manifestation of specificity and reveals the ability of antibodies to combine with common determinants present in heterologous material. Precipitation reactions performed in gel by the double diffusion method provide a means of identifying such cross-reactions (Fig. 1).

Sensitivity

Although immunological reactions have a high degree of sensitivity it should not be assumed that similar levels of sensitivity obtain in different technical procedures; modification of a method may have a significant effect on its

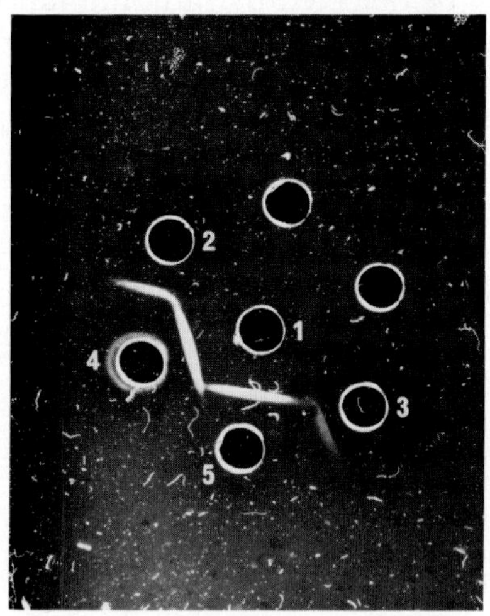

Fig. 1a. Double diffusion in agarose gel. In well 1, IgG: in wells 2, 3, IgM; in well 4, anti-kappa light chain antiserum; in well 5, anti-lambda light chain antiserum. The precipitation lines each antiserum gives with IgG and IgM are continuous with each other, showing identity of light chains between the two classes. The "spurring" of the line with anti-κ over the line with anti-λ reflects some of the antigenic differences between the two light chain types.

overall sensitivity. Thus *direct* immunofluorescence is a more sensitive procedure than precipitation; but the indirect technique with an antiglobulin step further enhances its sensitivity by a factor of about seven (Johnson, 1971). Similarly, precipitation by double diffusion is ten times more sensitive when carried out by the countercurrent electrophoretic method, in which movement of the reactants is directed towards each other, than with simple diffusion in which the diffusing reactants are distributed radially in the medium.

Affinity

The ability of antigens to combine with antibodies is dependent on the closeness of fit of the respective specific determinants and combining sites. Antibodies of high affinity readily produce complexes with low dissociation constants which manifest themselves as rapidly-formed precipitates. Low affinity antibodies on the other hand, may not be detectable by such second-stage phenomena and there may even be difficulties in detecting their primary

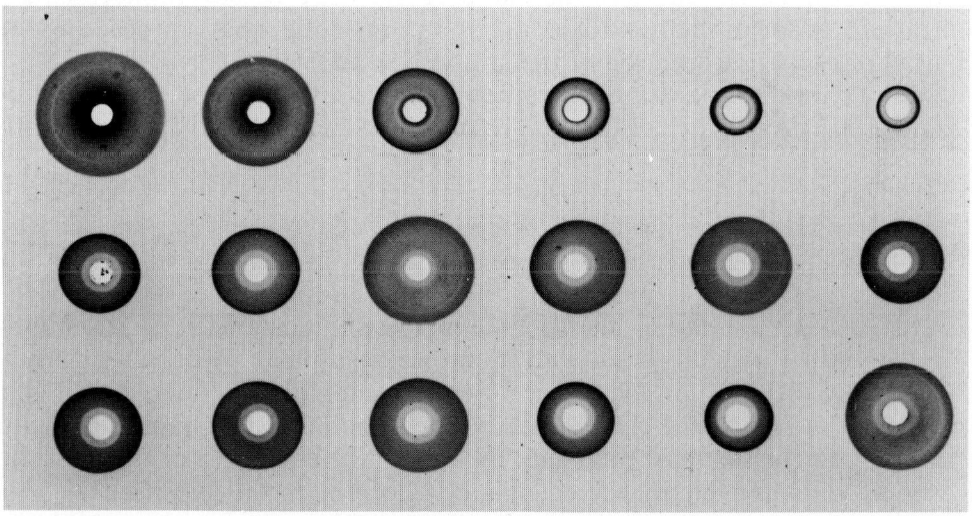

Fig. 1b. Estimation of C_3 by single radial immunodiffusion (Mancini method). Wells in 1% agarose gel containing anti-C_3 antiserum are filled as follows: top row—serial dilutions of a standard serum of known C_3 content; 2nd and 3rd rows—each well contains a dilution of an unknown serum. The diameters of the standard precipitation zones are plotted on linear graph paper against their C_3 contents. The C_3 concentrations in the unknown sera are read from the resulting curve and corrected for dilution.

reactions. Antibody affinity may be especially relevant to the fate and immunopathogenicity of soluble immune complexes formed in the circulation (Steward *et al.*, 1975).

DETECTION OF PRIMARY INTERACTIONS

Radioimmunoassay

Procedures based on the original saturation assay method of Yalow and Berson (1960) for the measurement of insulin levels, are widely used for measuring substances of immunological significance in body fluids including other hormones, microbiological antigens, tumour antigens and drugs.

Radioimmunoassay requires (1) radioactively-labelled material corresponding to the substance to be measured and added to compete with the test material for combination with specific antibody (2) specific antiserum of known binding capacity and (3) a means of separating free from bound material; methods employed include chromatography, electrophoresis, gel filtration, adsorption, fractional precipitation, solid phase procedures or immunological precipitation of the antibody used in the assay.

Many clinical applications of radioimmunoassay are based on the use of commercial test kits which include reactants of known potency as controls.

Measurement of Antigen Binding Capacity (ABC)

Here the test serum is incubated with radioisotope-labelled antigen. Uncombined antigen is separated from the mixture by precipitation of immunoglobulin either by salting-out with ammonium sulphate (Minden and Farr, 1977) or by the addition of antiserum to immunoglobulin (double antibody method). By comparing the radioactivity contained in the immunoglobulin precipitate with the total radioactivity added to the test the capacity of the serum to bind antigen may be calculated according to the formula:

$$\text{ABC per cent} = \frac{\text{Activity of precipitate}}{\text{Total activity}} \times 100$$

A useful clinical application of this test is the detection and measurement of antibodies to DNA in the diagnosis and management of systemic lupus erythematosus. Published results show considerable variation in sensitivity and specificity and underline the need for reference standard reagents in order to establish comparability between different laboratories carrying out the test. Standardization needs especially to take into account the influence of the reaction conditions, including ionic strength and pH, and also the effect of size, structure and molecular weight of the DNA antigen and the possibility of reactions attributable to the binding of non-antibody protein, especially C1q (Aarden *et al.*, 1975a,b). Since binding capacity is influenced by the ratio of serum to antigen in the reaction mixture, the level of electrostatic binding of protein to DNA, the reaction volume and antibody avidity it is not surprising that the reported upper limits of normal from different laboratories cover a wide range so that results can at present be interpreted only in the light of local experience of the test.

Immunofluorescence

Immunofluorescence provides a simple visual method of identifying antibodies which may be present in patients' sera (or body fluids), and also of using specific antisera to identify microorganisms in human or culture material. It is one of the essential techniques of clinical immunology, differing from most other immunological procedures in that it does not require separated or extracted antigens for its performance, but depends solely upon observation under the microscope of the selective distribution of antigen–antibody reactions as rendered visible by fluorescence, whether in tissue sections or in cell preparations, including those containing or consisting of microorganisms (Johnson *et al.*, 1973). The method combines the specificity and sensitivity of immunology with the precision of topographical localization obtainable by microscopy (Nairn, 1969). Its success depends upon the sensitivity obtained by labelling antibody molecules with a fluorescent dye visually detectable in extremely small amounts.

The clinical value of immunofluorescence also is significantly enhanced by the use of reference standards. An international standard "antinuclear factor" is available from W.H.O. sources which provides direct comparability between results in different laboratories (Anderson *et al.*, 1971). Reference standards for conjugated specific antiglobulin antibodies are in preparation.

Indirect Immunofluorescence

Tests for antibodies in patients' sera are usually carried out by the indirect staining procedure. In this a preparation containing the antigen in question—smear, imprint, tissue section, cell suspension—is treated with the patient's serum to allow combination of antibody, if present. After a standard time for reaction, non-immunologically bound protein is removed by washing. Sites of antibody–antigen reaction are revealed by applying anti-globulin chemically conjugated with a fluorochrome, usually fluorescein, less often rhodamine. The preparation is finally washed to remove non-specifically bound conjugate. When viewed in the fluorescence microscope the sites where the initial immunological reaction has occurred appear as apple-green (fluorescein) or red (rhodamine) fluorescence. Extensive studies of the immunological and fluorescent characterization of conjugates, and developments in microscope technology have led to the commercial availability of highly reliable conjugates of precise specification and the production of high performance components for fluorescence microscopy.

The most widely employed application of immunofluorescence in microbiology is the test for syphilitic antibodies—the fluorescent treponemal antibody (FTA) test, which has proved to be highly sensitive and specific (Deacon and Hunter, 1962). The relevance of auto-immunity to the immunopathology of connective tissue disease, and the association of auto-antibodies with a wide range of other diseases has made it necessary for clinical laboratories to provide a routine service for detecting a variety of tissue-reactive antibodies (Fig. 2) including those reactive with nuclei (Holborow *et al.*, 1957), mitochondria (Doniach *et al.*, 1966), both smooth (Johnson *et al.*, 1965) and striated muscle fibres (Strauss *et al.*, 1960), reticulin (Seah *et al.*, 1971), gastric parietal cells (Taylor *et al.*, 1962) thyroid epithelium (Holborow *et al.*, 1959) and other endocrine tissues (Doniach, 1975). To reduce the labour involved in testing large numbers of sera, many laboratories use cryostat sections taken from composite frozen tissue blocks containing a range of different tissues so that each serum may be tested for several antibodies at once on a single section.

A recently-developed application of immunofluorescence is based upon the fact that the DNA content of a giant mitochondrion present in a non-pathogenic flagellate, Crithidia luciliae, provides a substrate for detecting antibody specific for double-stranded DNA. This provides a simple routine test useful in the diagnosis and management of systemic lupus erythematosus (Aarden *et al.*, 1975c).

Direct Immunofluorescence

Direct immunofluorescence employing immunoglobulin class-specific anti-globulin conjugates has several applications in the clinical laboratory.

Identification of Paraproteins in Myeloma Cells

In this procedure fresh myeloma marrow cells are separated, washed and spread on slides by means of a cytocentrifuge (van Furth *et al.*, 1966). By staining the preparations with conjugates specific for heavy and light chain determinants respectively the class and type of immunoglobulin contained in myeloma cells may be readily established. The reverse application of this—the use of myeloma cells from the bone marrow of patients in whom monoclonal paraprotein has been characterized, to test the specificity of antiglobulin conjugates—is a useful procedure for testing the staining specificity of fluorescent conjugates.

Identification of Lymphocytes Carrying Surface Immunoglobulins

For this purpose suspensions of cells obtained from whole blood by density gradient sedimentation are treated with anti-immunoglobulin conjugates, washed and examined as suspensions in the fluorescence microscope, preferably by incident illumination. Surface staining in its various forms is readily detected on immunoglobulin-bearing lymphocytes, but there are pitfalls which are discussed in Chapter 4.

Tissue-bound Ig and Complement

Direct immunofluorescence is also used to demonstrate the presence of bound immunoglobulin or complement components in biopsies, particularly of skin and kidney. Positive staining is obtained when antibody bound to a component of the tissue examined is present, and also when the tissue contains deposited complexes of antibody and antigen, e.g. anti-DNA and DNA in lupus glomerulonephritis. It may be possible to demonstrate also the presence of bound complement in the complex by applying a fluorescent conjugate specific for components of complement such as C_3, C_4 or C1q.

Immunoenzyme Methods

An alternative to fluorescent compounds as labels for proteins is provided by enzymes which yield a microscopically detectable reaction product on ex-

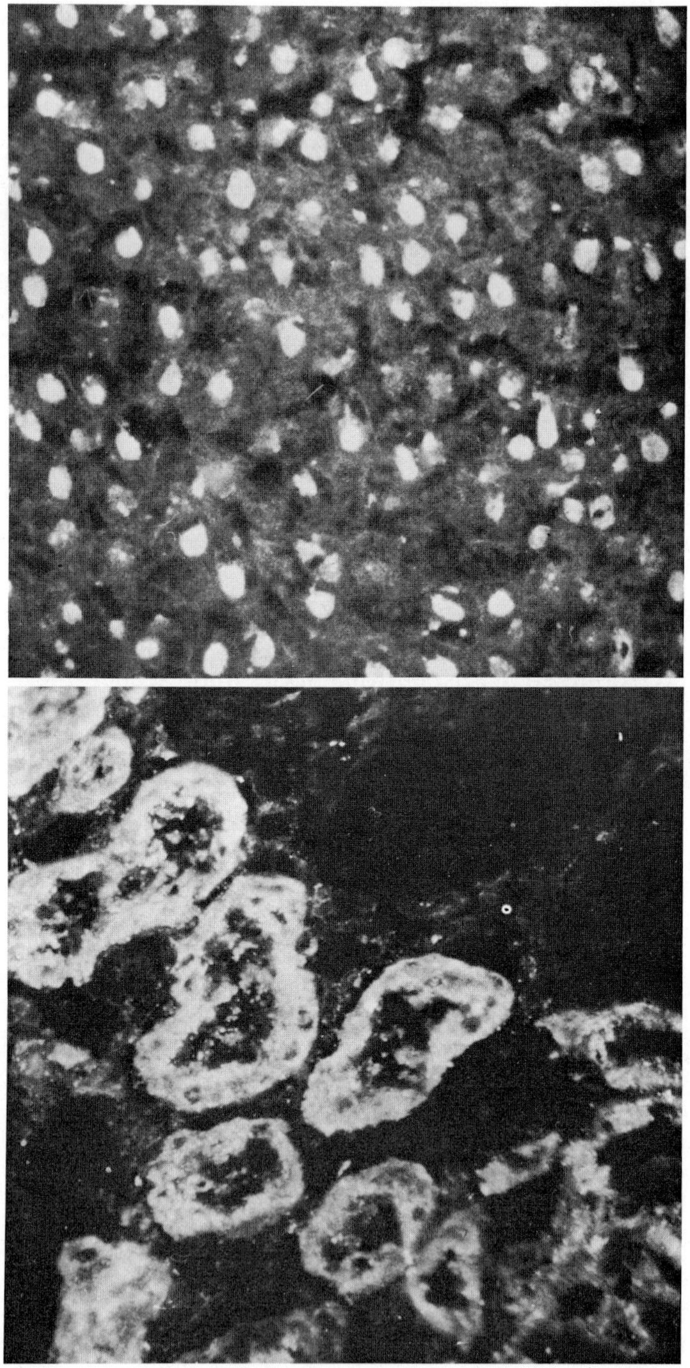
(a)
(b)

Fig. 2a, b. See caption p. 166.

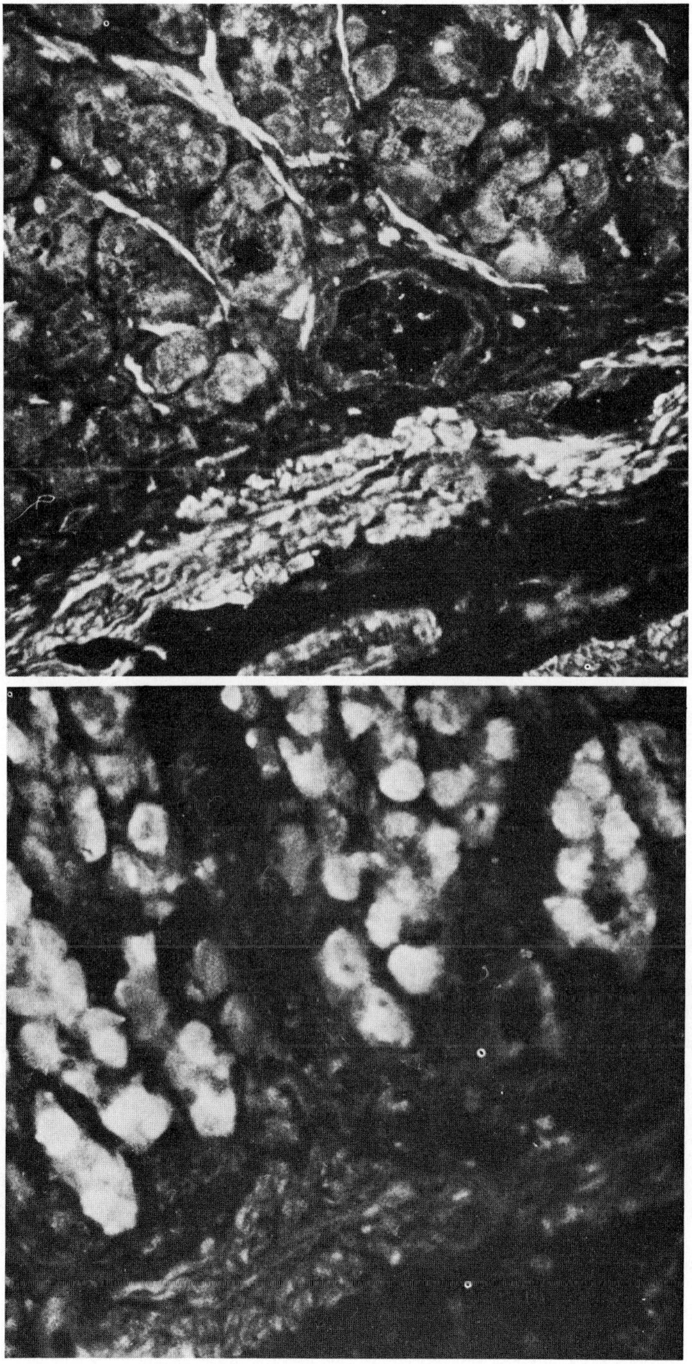
(c)
(d)

Fig. 2c, d. For caption see p. 166.

(e)

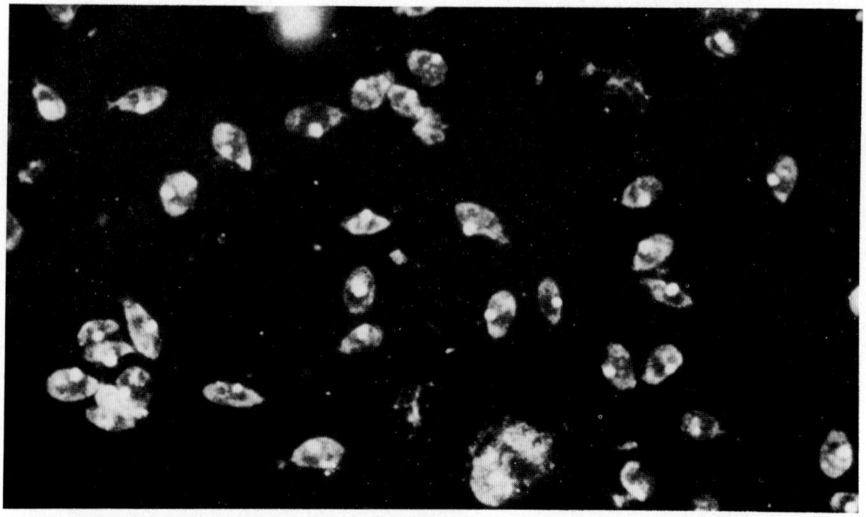

Fig. 2. Detection of auto-antibodies by immunofluorescence: a–d cryostat sections of rat tissues (microscope magnification ×252; Agfa CT-18). (a) Antinuclear antibody: Homogeneous staining of nuclei in liver. (b) Mitochondrial antibody: Cytoplasmic staining of epithelial cells of distal tubules in renal cortex. (c) Smooth muscle antibody: Staining of intergastric gland fibres and muscularis mucosae. (d) Gastric parietal cell antibody: Staining of the cytoplasm of parietal cells in the stomach. (e) Antibody to native DNA: Staining of the kinetoplast of Crithidia luciliae.

posure to their specific substrates. Horseradish peroxidase (HRP) may be coupled to antibody protein by a simple procedure to give stable conjugates which retain immunological reactivity and can be used for tracing. Sites of uptake are made visible by treatment with hydrogen peroxide and diaminobenzidine which yields a coloured and insoluble reaction product at the site of the antiglobulin reactions (Nakane and Pierce, 1966). The HRP method has a sensitivity similar to that of immunofluorescence (Dorling *et al.*, 1971). It has considerable additional potential for precise identification of tissue components since the relative electron density of its reaction product permits its ultrastructural localization in the electron microscope (Nakane, 1975).

Horseradish peroxidase is itself immunogenic and immune complexes of HRP and anti-HRP antibody can be used to localize the sites of attachment of test antibody to a tissue section by a binding reaction with antiglobulin, provided the test antibody and the anti-HRP antibody are from the same species.

The advantages of the immuno-enzyme method as compared with immunofluorescence are permanence of the stained preparations, absence of bleaching, and lack of requirement for special microscopy.

Enzyme-labelled antiglobulin serum has also been applied in a solid-phase assay procedure for measurement of nanogram quantities of immunoglobulins. The antisera are labelled with alkaline phosphatase. After the immune reaction has taken place the coloured reaction product following addition of substrate is dissolved and measured by spectrophotometry (Engvall and Perlmann, 1972).

DETECTION OF SECONDARY REACTIONS

Precipitation

In the quantitative precipitin reaction a range of dilutions of antigen solution are added to tubes containing a constant amount of antiserum (Maurer, 1971). As originally postulated by Marrack (1934), visible precipitation depends on the formation of a lattice resulting from the linking together of antigen–antibody complexes on which free antibody combining sites and antigenic determinants are present. Maximal and rapid precipitation occurs when antigen and antibody are present in optimal combining proportions. Excess antigen or excess antibody both result in reduction or even absence of precipitation, some or all of the immune complexes initially formed remaining in solution. Tube precipitation tests are little used now in the clinical laboratory, except for microbiological purposes, e.g. grouping of streptococci, where the specific antiserum is layered on a culture extract in a precipitin tube. As the reactants diffuse into each other a ring of precipitation develops in the zone where microbial antigen and corresponding antibody are present in optimal combining ratio. Gel diffusion techniques based on the same principle of obtaining maximum precipitation by mutually diffusing the reactants are widely used.

Precipitation in Gels

Antigen solutions and antisera placed in wells are allowed to diffuse towards each other through an inert solid matrix such as agar or agarose which is sufficiently transparent to allow any precipitate that develops to be seen.

Diffusion occurs at a rate largely determined by the molecular weight of the reactants relative to the pore size of the matrix, and in such double diffusion reactions the position of the precipitation arc formed is at the equivalence region determined by the relative concentrations of antigenic components and specific antibodies in the respective wells. As precipitates are usually more soluble in excess of antigen than of antibody the reactions usually appear as arcs concentric with the source of antigen. A feature of double diffusion, described originally by Ouchterlony (1958), is its ability to detect and identify cross-reacting antigens or antibodies in adjacent wells by the specific solubilization of precipitates by excess concentrations of related antigens (Fig. 1a).

In mycology double-diffusion tests are useful for detecting antibodies to fungal antigens in suspected cases of pulmonary aspergillosis and farmer's lung (Longbottom and Pepys, 1964; Pepys and Jenkins, 1965).

Single diffusion of antigen in gel is the basis of the widely-used Mancini method of quantifying serum proteins (Mancini *et al.*, 1965). Specific antibody to the protein to be measured is incorporated in the gel. The radial distance travelled by the corresponding antigen diffusing from a well through the gel before its concentration becomes low enough to permit precipitate formation, is proportional to its initial concentration. The diameter of the ring of precipitation around the antigen-containing well may then be compared with diameters obtained with solutions of antigen of known concentration (Fig. 1b). Precipitation techniques depending on electrophoretic migration of reactants are described below.

Agglutination

This occurs when antibodies react with antigen present on the surface of insoluble particles—red blood cells, microorganisms or inert materials. The test is carried out in round-bottomed tubes or in wells formed in plastic plates, and semi-quantitative results are obtained by using serial dilutions of serum containing antibodies with a constant amount of particle suspension. The highest dilution of serum that gives a visible reaction in the form of clumping or agglutination is the titre.

The direct agglutination of bacteria as in the Widal reaction and of red blood cells in blood group serology are well known procedures. Agglutination tests with erythrocytes are not limited to detecting reactions involving antigens native to the cells themselves, since the red cell envelope has the capacity to adsorb a wide range of antigenic substances and become agglutinated in the presence of the corresponding specific antibody—so called passive haemagglutination. The adsorptive capacity may be considerably enhanced by chemical modification of the cell surface. Tannic acid has been often used for this purpose since Boyden (1951) showed its efficacy in preparing red cells coated with an extract of *M. tuberculosis* for haemagglutination, and it is used for sensitizing cells with thyroglobulin for use in thyroid antibody tests. Another use of tanned cells is in the test for antibody to extractable nuclear antigen (ENA), found in the serum of patients with "mixed connective tissue disease" (Sharp *et al.*, 1972). An alternative to tannic acid as a coupling agent is chromium chloride (Faulk and Houba, 1973). This gives less non-specific agglutination and the coupling procedure is simpler and more rapid than with tannic acid. Cells treated in this way are satisfactory in tests with both ENA and DNA (Johnson *et al.*, 1975) as antigen. The sensitivity of these passive haemagglutination tests compares favourably with that of other serological methods, and with the development of automated techniques they provide convenient, readily standardized clinical tests.

The tests for rheumatoid factors are further examples of passive agglutination, with gamma-globulin as antigenic reactant. In the Rose-Waaler and differential agglutination tests (Fig. 3) the latter takes the form of a non-agglutinating dose of anti-sheep erythrocyte serum coating the sheep cells with antibody (Rose *et al.*, 1948), in the latex test the polystyrene particles adsorb human IgG protein (Singer and Plotz, 1956).

Inhibition of latex agglutination can be used as an assay method for antigen, and commercial kits measuring inhibition by urine of antibody-induced agglutination of gonadotropin-coated particles are widely employed in pregnancy diagnosis.

Complement Fixation

Activation of the complement sequence by the classical pathway via C142 (see Chapter 8) is brought about by antibody altered by reaction with its antigen, but not by native immunoglobulins. The classical complement fixation test is typified by the Wasserman reaction. The presence of complement remaining free in a mixture containing antigen, antibody and complement is determined by adding to the mixture a suspension of red blood cells sensitized with specific red cell antibody. Free complement in the mixture results in the development of lesions in sensitized red cell membranes leading to visible haemolysis; under appropriate quantitative conditions an antigen–antibody reaction occurring in the initial stage of the test binds the complement so that none is available to participate in the haemolytic reaction. Immune

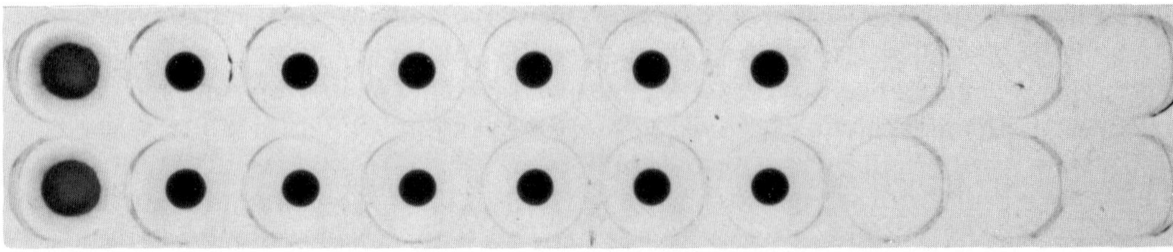

Titration of Haemolysin. End point of agglutination 1/200 - subagglutinating dose 1/800

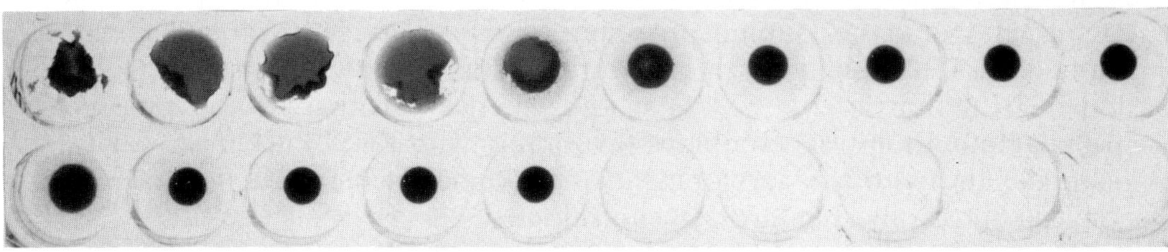

S.S.C. = Agglutination with R.A. serum to 1/128   N.S.C. = 1/8   DAT = 1/16

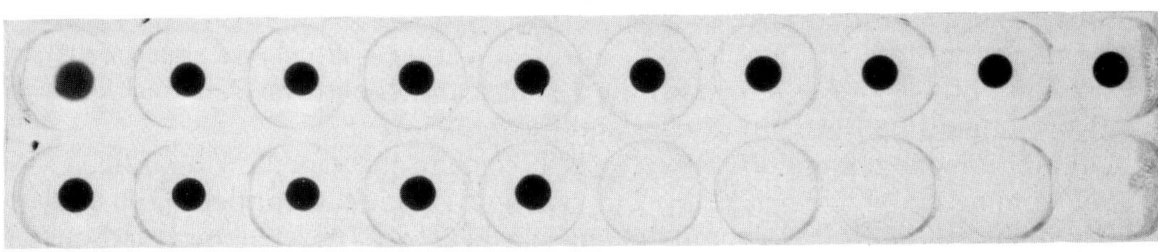

S.S.C. = 1/8   N.S.C. = 1/8   DAT = 1/1

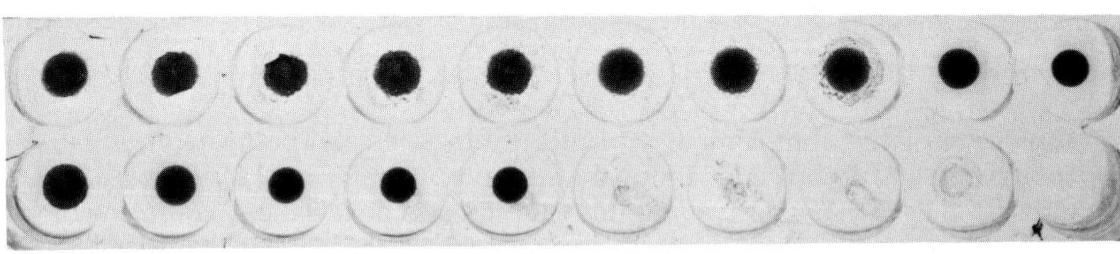

S.S.C. = 1/1024   N.S.C. = 1/8   DAT = 1/128

Key: S.S.C. = Sensitized sheep cells
N.S.C. = Non-sensitized sheep cells

Fig. 3. Differential agglutination test (DAT) for rheumatoid factor. Top two rows: determination of subagglutinating dose of sensitizing anti-sheep red cell antibody. Doubling dilutions start at 1/200. Below: Results with 3 sera. Starting dilution—1/8.

complexes formed in gross excess of antigen are less efficient at fixing complement than those formed in the equivalence region.

All classes of antibody molecules do not mediate complement fixation via the classical pathway with the same efficiency (see Chapter 7). IgM is the most efficient, on a weight for weight basis, among human immunoglobulins and of the four subclasses of IgG, IgG-1, IgG-2 and IgG-3 all fix complement whereas IgG-4 does not.

The sensitivity of complement fixation tests is enhanced if small amounts of complement are used, producing less than complete haemolysis of the antibody-sensitized erythrocytes (Mayer, 1961). This permits detection of low levels of antibodies, but requires careful control to yield useful results.

The development of quantitative complement fixation methods in which the amount of haemoglobin released from a standard number of erythrocytes under precisely defined conditions is accurately measured, has widened the scope of the procedure as an analytical tool for studying antigenic relationships, for example in detecting single amino-acid differences in haemoglobin molecules (Wasserman and Levine, 1961) and the relationship of the antigen: antibody ratio to complement fixation. As in quantitative precipitation three zones of reactivity are detectable, and maximum binding of complement occurs in the equivalence region where neither antigen nor antibody is in marked excess.

Immunofluorescence may be used to test the complement-fixing properties of tissue-reactive antibodies. Antibodies to gastric parietal cell antigen, thyroid microsomes and non-organ-specific mitochondria, for example, when applied to appropriate tissue sections in the presence of fresh normal serum as a source of active complement give their characteristic patterns of staining when a fluorescent conjugate specific for complement is used in place of the usual antiglobulin conjugate; the reaction is abolished by previously heat-inactivating the complement-containing serum.

DETECTION OF CIRCULATING IMMUNE COMPLEXES

In many drug reactions and infections, and in some auto-immune conditions, soluble immune complexes form in or gain access to the circulation, and their dispersal and deposition in sites remote from their formation are implicated in complications such as glomerulonephritis, arthritis, and vasculitis. Their detection may be important for diagnosis and in determining therapy and management. Several methods are in use, but their relative merits are not yet fully established.

Where the antigen is known and has a recognizable morphology, such as a virus, electron microscopy provides a simple and sensitive means of identifying virus–antibody complexes. The method has been most successfully used in demonstrating by negative staining the presence of morphologically typical aggregates of HB Ag in certain sera from patients with hepatitis Type B, or with HB Ag-positive chronic hepatitis (Almeida and Waterson, 1969).

Ultracentrifugation is a physical method of measuring soluble immune complexes under mild conditions and yields accurate information about their size. Two procedures in use are (1) free solution analysis, by methods measuring rapidly dispersing high molecular weight aggregates, and based on absorption measurements on runs at low speed and at high speed and (2) sedimentation in isokinetic gradients, providing sedimentation co-efficients as $S^{\circ}_{20,w}$ values (Stanworth and Johns, 1976).

Polyethylene glycol (PEG) is a water-soluble polymer (mol. wt. 6,000 daltons) which precipitates plasma proteins according to their molecular size. Addition of PEG to serum at a final concentration of 4% leads to precipitation of high molecular weight proteins as well as macromolecular immune complexes. It does not precipitate the latter selectively, and its proper use is in concentrating immune complexes from serum as a preliminary to purification and characterization (Zubler *et al.*, 1976).

A number of methods for immune complexes depend upon their reactions with complement. Sera containing immune complexes are often anti-complementary, and Mowbray *et al.* (1973) have reported a method based on the binding of C1 to circulating complexes, after heat inactivation at 56° of C1 which may have been bound in the blood, with subsequent back titration of added guinea-pig complement. IgG complexes are more efficient than IgM in producing an anticomplementary result. In terms of the amount of antigen in the complex, this method is sensitive, being able to detect a minimum complexed antigen concentration of 0·5 ng/ml.

The ability of immune complexes to bind C1q is the basis of a double diffusion precipitation method in agarose, with partially purified human C1q in a central well and the test sera in surrounding wells (Winchester and Agnello, 1976). C1q gives a precipitin line with the large IgG complexes present in joint fluids from rheumatoid arthritis, but not with the intermediate size complexes present in rheumatoid patients' blood. Selected rheumatoid factors isolated from blood can be used as precipitants for immune complexes in a similar way (Winchester *et al.*, 1971).

A more sensitive method for immune complexes is the ^{125}I-C1q binding test, which is based on the higher binding affinity of C1q for polymeric as compared with monomeric immunoglobulins. The serum under test is first incubated with EDTA in order to dissociate the intrinsic C1qrs complex, and then incubated with ^{125}I-C1q and 3% polyethylene glycol. Free C1q remains soluble under these conditions, but C1q bound to macromolecular complexes is precipitated. The amount of radioactivity in the precipitate indicates the C1q binding activity (Zubler and Lambert, 1976). The possibility that other biological substances such as DNA and bacterial lipopolysaccharide, may interfere by binding C1q has to be considered in interpreting results.

A solid phase radioassay method for C1q binding has been devised in which C1q is immobilized on the surface of a plastic tube, and complexes in the patients' serum compete with radio-labelled aggregated IgG for binding to it (Hay *et al.*, 1976).

Activation of the complement system by immune complexes produces binding of C_3 to the complex. This results in bound C_3 in serum being separable from free C_3 by fractionation on G200 Sephadex, the bound ("macromolecular") C_3 appearing in the first protein peak on elution with phosphate buffered saline, the free C_3, of mol. wt. 185,000 daltons, eluting in the second protein peak. Activation of the complement system either by the classical or the alternative pathway increases the amount of C_3 in the first peak (Williams and Slaney, 1976).

The ability of macrophages to bind aggregated human IgG (HAGG) is the basis of a radiobioassay for complexes in which ^{125}I-labelled HAGG and immune complexes compete for Fc receptor sites on guinea pig macrophages (Mohammed *et al.*, 1976). Sera from systemic lupus erythematosus patients usually contain immune complexes which inhibit the uptake of HAGG by the macrophages. Quantitatively, this method has about the same sensitivity as the C1q-binding test, and is capable of detecting 25 µg/ml of HAGG. An interesting feature is that sera containing both rheumatoid factor and immune complexes enhance rather than inhibit the uptake of HAGG by the macrophages (Onyewotu *et al.*, 1975). An essentially similar method uses human lymphoblastoid cells (Raji cells), which bind complexes by means of Fc surface receptors (Theofilopoulos *et al.*, 1974). Another biological assay method for complexes measures the capacity of immune complexes to compete with IgG bound to target cell antigens for Fc receptors on mononuclear cells (K-cells) which act as effectors in antibody-mediated cytotoxicity (Panayi *et al.*, 1976). The reaction of immune complexes with Fc receptors is also the basis of a platelet aggregation test. Platelet receptors show a preference for IgG_1 and IgG_3, and like K-cell receptors are independent of complement (Penttinen *et al.*, 1976).

The complement receptors on B-lymphocytes have also been used to indicate the presence of complexes. Lymphocyte-bearing complement receptors form rosettes with sheep erythrocytes sensitized with antibody and complement (EAC). EAC-rosette formation is inhibited by addition of sera containing activated C_3, either free or bound to complexes, and such inhibition has been noted with sera from patients with steroid-sensitive nephrotic syndrome in relapse, with Henoch-Schönlein purpura with nephritis, and with acute post-streptococcal glomerulonephritis and also in Crohn's disease, lepromatous leprosy, and membranoproliferative glomerulonephritis (Hayward *et al.*, 1976).

ELECTROPHORETIC AND NEPHELOMETRIC METHODS FOR ASSAY OF IMMUNOPRECIPITATION REACTIONS

Immunoelectrophoretic Techniques

Since its introduction in 1953 by Grabar and Williams "immunoelectrophoresis" has become one of the most useful and simple tools available for the resolution of biological fluids. The technique depends on both the electrophoretic mobility and the antigenic specificity of the components. Its application to human plasma analysis soon revealed both the existence of several immunoglobulin classes and their remarkable degree of electrophoretic heterogeneity. For routine screening of sera or plasma for suspected monoclonal gammopathies its simplicity and sensitivity is unequalled by any other technique (Fig. 4). Unfortunately the technique is essentially qualitative.

Fig. 4. (a) Immunoelectrophoretic patterns produced by serum from a patient with multiple myeloma (MM). The patterns produced by a normal serum (NS) are included for comparison. The troughs in the agar gel contain respectively (from the top) anti whole human serum (AHS), anti IgG, anti IgA, anti IgM, anti Kappa light chain and anti Lambda light chain. The antigen wells were filled alternately with normal serum and with patient serum as indicated on the photograph. The monoclonal component is clearly revealed as an IgG lambda protein (see arrows). These patterns may be contrasted with those in (b) which illustrates limited clone involvement in an immune response. This pattern can sometimes be confused with that of a malignant monoclonal gammopathy. The troughs are filled with antisera as in (a) with the exception that the extra trough (second from top) contains a thyroid extract (antigen). The IgG antibodies in the patient's serum (PS) produce an immune precipitin arc against thyroglobulin in this extract (see arrow).

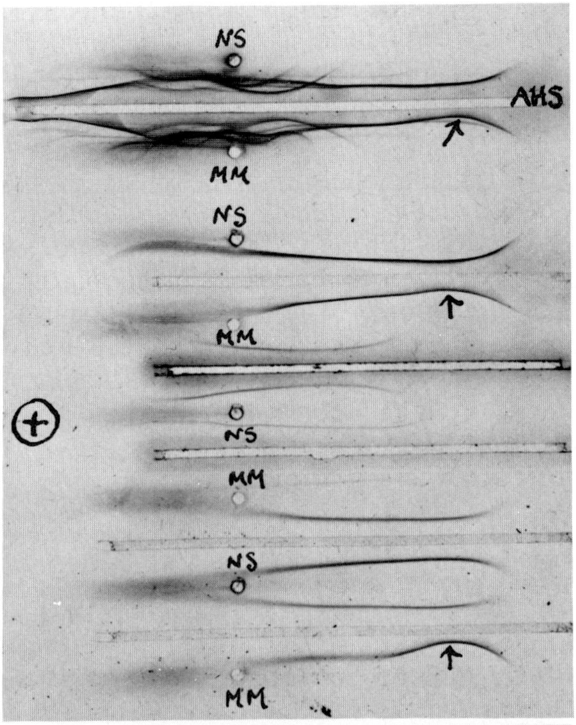
NS
AHS
MM
NS
MM
NS
MM
NS
MM

(a)

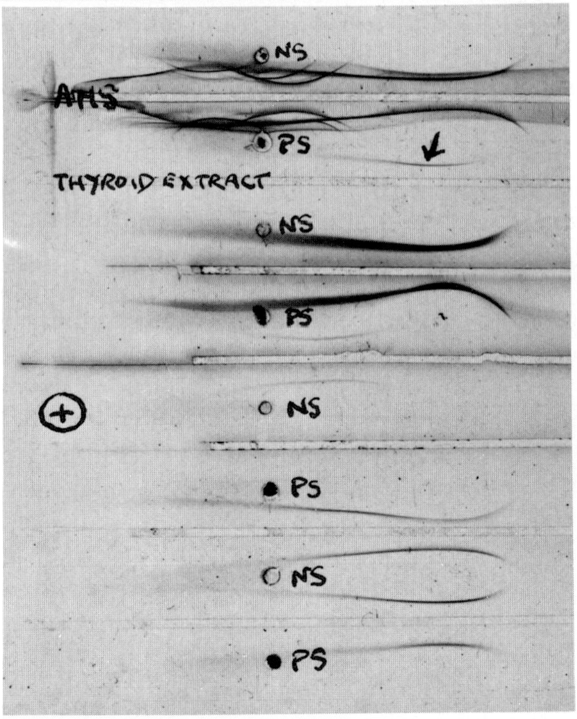
NS
AHS
PS
THYROID EXTRACT
NS
PS
NS
PS
NS
PS

(b)

The first practical methods for the quantitation of proteins by electrophoresis through specific antibody-containing agarose gels were described by Laurell in 1965. The names given to these techniques "crossed immunoelectrophoresis, two-dimensional immunoelectrophoresis" and "rocket immunoelectrophoresis" are now familiar in the literature. Various modifications have been described which increase the resolution of the original techniques. Although widely recommended for the quantitation of protein antigens, with the exception perhaps of albumin "rockets", such immunochemical quantitations are generally more readily carried out either by radial immunodiffusion methods or by automated nephelometric assay of the specific antibody–antigen complexes in solution. However, some specific quantitative requirements are emerging which can only be satisfactorily achieved by crossed immunoelectrophoresis.

Principles in Quantitative Immunoelectrophoresis

In two dimensional immunoelectrophoresis the plasma proteins are first separated by conventional electrophoresis in agarose gel supported on a glass plate. The agarose is then cut away with a razor blade a few mm distant from the loading origin and parallel to the electrophoretic migration. This agarose is replaced with molten agarose containing either mono- or multi-specific antiserum at a predetermined concentration. After allowing the agarose to set the proteins are electrophoresed into the antibody-containing gel at right angles to the direction of their original migration. Conditions are chosen such that the antibodies do not migrate appreciably in the gel. The antigens, however, migrate through the antibody population forming soluble complexes which eventually fuse to form a visible non-soluble precipitate outlining a peak or peaks (Fig. 5). The latter does not change in position during continued electrophoresis and the area enclosed by the precipitate depends only on the concentration of antigen and antibody in the system. Quantitation of a specific protein may be made by comparison with the area produced by a reference protein solution under identical experimental conditions. Measurement of the enclosed area can be achieved by any of the usual techniques, e.g. planimetry.

Rocket immunoelectrophoresis is restricted to quantitation of a single protein in a mixture. The samples to be compared are applied side by side in circular wells cut in agarose gel containing a monospecific antiserum. Electrophoresis then produces the characteristic rocket shaped precipitate

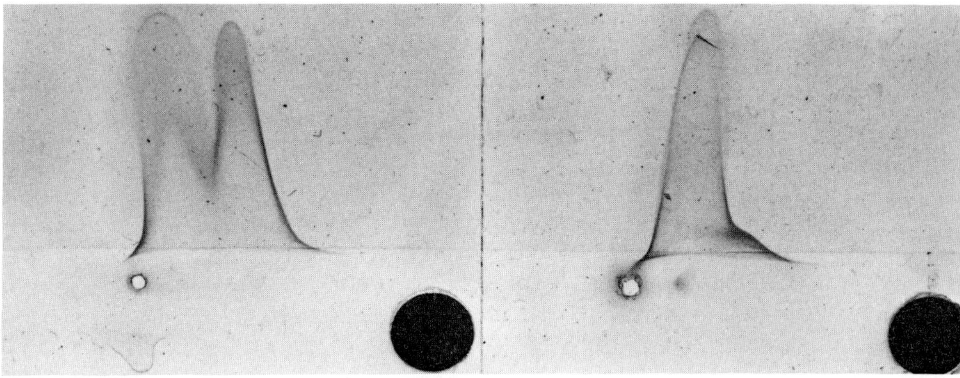

Fig. 5. Two dimensional immunoelectrophoresis of complement component C3 in the serum of a patient who exhibited an apparent anaphylactic response to an intravenous anaesthetic agent. The first sample was taken from the patient two minutes after induction, at the height of the response. This (left) shows two immunologically related peaks, the more mobile of these electrophoretically is the C3 conversion product, C3c. After 24 hr (right) this functionally inactive protein has been eliminated and only a single peak due to native C3 is present in the now recovered patient's serum. The electrophoretograms were produced by electrophoresis of 2 µl samples of the patient's serum. The second dimension gel contained 7·5 µl Behringwerke anti human C3/ml agarose gel.

(Fig. 6) and quantitation is based simply upon measurement of the height of the rocket instead of the area.

Although electroimmunodiffusion methods yield excellent results with proteins possessing α_1 or α_2 globulin-like mobility, proteins with lower mobility pose special problems in defining the enclosed area and it is often necessary to modify these chemically e.g. by acetylation or by carbamylation, to increase their anodic mobility.

Experimental Procedures

For practical details of the various quantitative immunoelectrophoretic methods the reader is referred to the excellent monograph, edited by Axelsen *et al.* (1973). Although quantitative immunoelectrophoresis is usually carried out at pH 8·6 in 1% agarose gel, a support medium chosen to minimize electroendosmotic flow, several types of cellulose acetate gel are available commercially which give comparable results to agarose (Miller and Mutzelburg, 1973) and also possess certain advantages, particularly for large scale clinical screening. These advantages include immediate availability and considerable economy of antisera. Acetate gels can also be readily used for qualitative immunoelectrophoresis and for radial immunodiffusion quantitation (Vergani *et al.*, 1967).

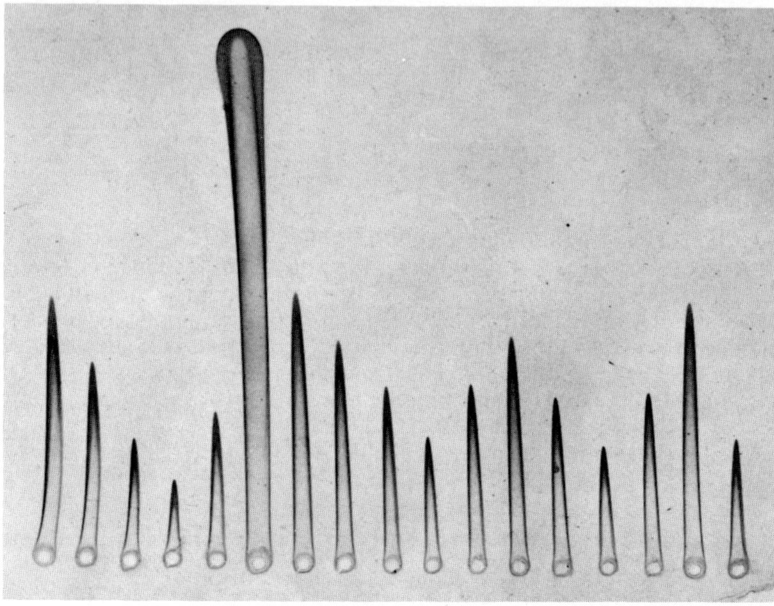

Fig. 6. Albumin in human serum quantitated by means of rocket immunoelectrophoresis. Samples (2 μl) applied from left of photograph, standard serum diluted initially, neat (N), 2N/3, N/3 and N/5 and then diluted 1 : 50 before application, a neat serum illustrating gross antigen excess, and various test sera diluted 1 : 50. The agarose gel contains Behringwerke anti human albumin, 15 μl/ml.

The first-dimension electrophoresis can be carried out in medium other than agar, agarose or acetate gel, if this medium offers an advantage for a particular examination. Resolution in the first dimension may be achieved in terms of molecular size (horizontal starch gel electrophoresis) or by isoelectric charge (isoelectric focusing in acrylamide gel (Fig. 7a)). The unfixed and unstained zone is cut out as a block from the media and embedded in agarose containing the specific antibody. Electrophoresis at right angles to the first dimension then develops a pattern which could not have been resolved by electrophoresis alone. This technique is made use of in Pi phenotyping of α_1 antitrypsin proteins (Fagerhol, 1968) (Fig. 7b) for classifying the rarer

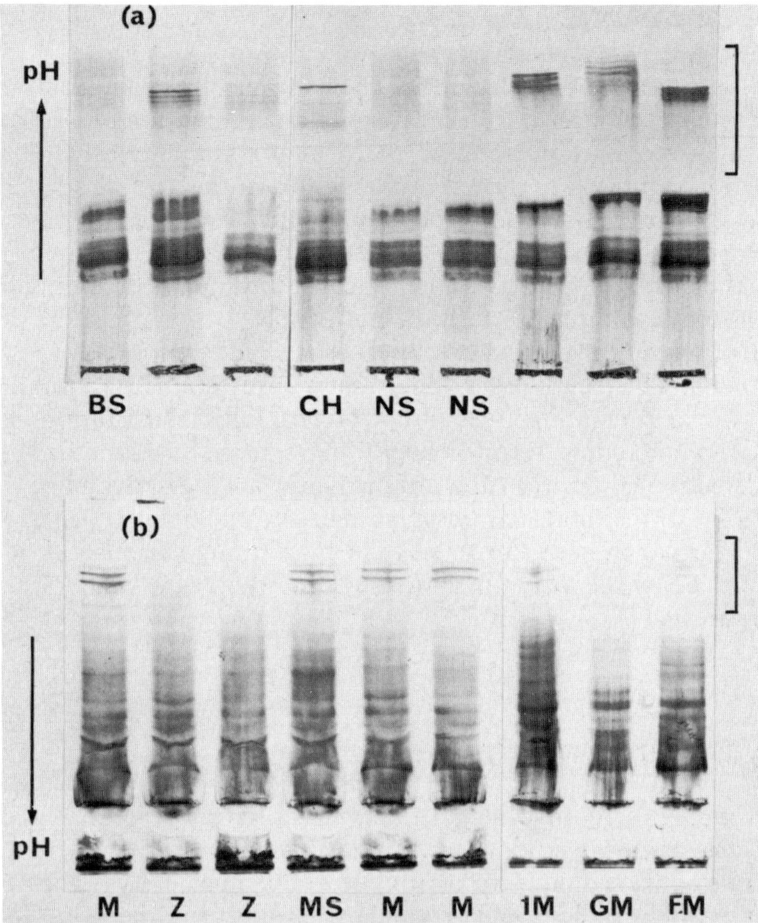

Fig. 7. Isoelectric focusing patterns. (a) Focusing patterns of normal and pathological sera in a pH3–10 gradient. The zone indicated on the photograph encloses the banding spectra of the 7S immunoglobulins. Patient BS, a myeloma patient in remission, shows the extreme microheterogeneity characteristic of normal sera (NS). Patient CH has a IgD monoclonal gammopathy. (b) Focusing patterns of human sera in a pH4–6 gradient showing resolution of the α_1 antitrypsin proteins into the so called Pi phenotype patterns. The usual PiM phenotype is contrasted with the homozygous Pi ZZ α_1 antitrypsin deficiency state. Some rarer heterozygous phenotypes are also shown.

phenotypes whose gene transmission is associated with a number of pulmonary conditions.

Crossing-Over Electrophoresis

Although most media are selected for their low electroendosmotic characteristics the latter can be used to advantage in a combination of electrophoretic and immunoprecipitation analysis performed simultaneously. The antigen and antibody samples are placed in the gel or on the acetate strip a few mm apart and electrophoresis commenced such that the antigen migrates (anodically) towards the antibody "well". The antibody is meanwhile migrating towards the antigen electroendosmotically and an immunoprecipitate is induced as the reactants cross. With agar gel the formation of the precipitate can be clearly seen during the run but fixation and staining is necessary with acetate media. The technique is widely used in screening for a number of important antigens including Australia antigen, anti-DNA antibodies and α_1 foeto-protein (including sera for hepatoma examination and amniotic fluid for the detection of neural tube abnormalities). Its disadvantage lies in the tendency of the precipitate to redissolve in excess of either antigen or antibody. This can be compensated to some extent by running various dilutions of the test samples or by the use of ingenious geometry in the "well" design (Kohn and Morgan, 1971).

Isoelectric Focusing (Fig. 7)

Although not directly involving an antigen-antibody reaction the technique of isoelectric focusing is not out of place in this chapter. This technique exploits the extraordinary resolving power achieved by electrophoresing proteins in a pH gradient and is widely used both routinely and in research for various investigations into antibody diversity. The proteins migrate to the point in the gradient at which their net charge is neutral, i.e. at their isoelectric point, and become sharply focused as visible bands of precipitated protein in either liquid or gel support media. Although the origins of the techniques go back to 1912 it was not until 1961 that the conditions necessary for the establishment of natural pH gradients were defined, and only since 1966, when Vesterberg and Svensson synthesized a mixture of polyamino-polycarboxylic acids, which fulfilled most of the requirements of an ideal carrier ampholyte system, has the technique become a practical research tool. In the same year the Swedish firm LKB Instruments Ltd. started development work based on Vesterberg and Svensson's results which finally led to the product known as Ampholine, first marketed in 1967.

Although first introduced as a preparative technique the potential for the analytical separation of proteins in biological fluids was soon realized and methods for isoelectric focusing in thin layers or rods of polyacrylamide gels appeared. LKB have produced a thin layer apparatus, the "LKB Multiphor" which gives excellent results even in inexperienced hands.

The use of isoelectric focusing in immunology is still in its infancy although its potential in both research and in the diagnosis of immunological abnormalities is being increasingly recognized.

Antibody Diversity

The degree of antibody diversity to an antigen is enormous. Even when antibody is elicited in the experimental animal to a defined haptenic group the resultant hapten-specific antibody is still a heterogeneous population of molecules. Analytical isoelectric focusing is proving to be an invaluable tool in the study of the extent of this heterogeneity. Some current problems are concerned with the need to define the genetic basis of antibody diversity. One problem has been to find suitable phenotypic markers for the variable region (V-region) of the immunoglobulin molecule so that inheritance of the V-genes might be followed. Isoelectric focusing of hapten specific antibodies is providing a powerful tool in these investigations since it can distinguish between different antibodies of similar specificity (see Williamson, 1975).

Homogeneous (Monoclonal) Immunoglobulins

The myeloma tumour arises from a single neoplastic plasma cell clone. Its products, the myeloma proteins, are the most widely studied examples of homogeneous immunoglobulins. It is perhaps surprising to discover that even these monoclonal proteins have a multi-band isoelectric spectrum, although the number of bands is limited (Fig. 7a). Experiments by Awdeh *et al.* (1970) with a mouse plasma cell tumour demonstrated that the initial intracellular synthesis was of an IgG protein showing only a single band on isoelectric focusing, whereas the secreted protein could be resolved into three components. This suggests that the heterogeneous pattern arises as a result of post synthetic charge alterations. However, the relationship between molecular heterogeneity and multiple electrophoretic bands is complex (Ressler, 1973). Charge alterations in proteins arising solely by intramolecular rearrangements would be unlikely to be resolved by purely electrophoretic techniques but nevertheless a number of reports have described multi-banding patterns of some myeloma proteins resolved by starch gel electrophoresis. Some of these starch gel patterns appear to be identical with the patterns produced by the protein when subjected to isoelectric focusing and it seems possible that this represents a second type of charge heterogeneity, conceivably related to differences in protein bound oligosaccharide residues. There are some indications that this type of charge heterogeneity correlates either with benign, or with early malignant paraproteinaemia (Cwynarski *et al.*, 1975).

Nephelometric Techniques

With the increasing importance of the measurement of serum protein levels as an accurate procedure for determining a variety of disease states and genetic abnormalities, a need has arisen for a rapid quantitative methodology. The conventional immunochemical techniques are rather slow and are not suitable for automation. As a solution to the problem a turbidometric procedure was first described by Libby (1938) and later modified by Ritchie (1967, 1972). A more sensitive modification of this approach was the detection of antigen–antibody complexes by light scattering and Kahan and Sundblad (1967) were able to develop an automated immunochemical system for β-lipoprotein assay. This principle has now been applied to a large number of plasma

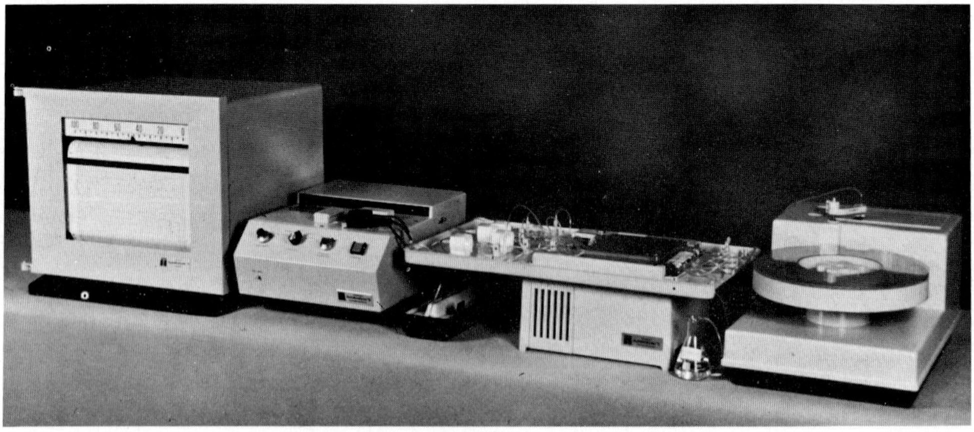

Fig. 8. The Technicon Auto Analyser System II (photograph by courtesy of Technicon Instruments Company Limited, Basingstoke, Hants., England).

proteins following the development of the Technicon Automated Immunoprecipitation System. This is illustrated in Fig. 8.

Immunoprecipitation Method (A.I.P.)

Technicon Instruments provide concise details and flow diagrams of their apparatus. Briefly, undiluted serum or other biological fluid is aspirated at a rate of 50 or 80 samples/hr into a recipient stream of saline. After initial dilution and mixing the diluted serum is resampled and introduced into a stream of pre-diluted antiserum segmented with air bubbles. Incubation takes place at room temperature for 15 minutes in a reaction coil with the formation of antigen–antibody complexes. These complexes continue along the apparatus manifold to the nephelometer where their light scattering effect is measured quantitatively and displayed on the chart record as individual peaks for each sample. The amount of light scatter in the nephelometer is proportional to the concentration of specific protein in the original sample and is reflected in the recorder peak height (Fig. 9). After correcting the light scattering for the sample background contribution the heights of the recorder peaks are compared with a standard reference curve prepared from dilutions of a standard reference serum (Fig. 9).

Advantages and Disadvantages of A.I.P.

Under optimum conditions the A.I.P. system combines rapid quantitation with a high degree of accuracy and reproducibility. The latter are similar to those obtained from "rocket" electrophoresis and better than those of simple radial diffusion. Its rapidity raises the problem of using it directly or in co-ordination with simple routine methods such as zone and immunoelectrophoresis. However even a cursory examination of routine electrophoretic "strips" may reveal abnormalities not at all obvious by quantitation. This is particularly true when the patient's serum contains a small quantity of a monoclonal immunoglobulin and it would appear wise to use AIP and simple routine methods in co-ordination.

The formation of the antigen–antibody complex imposes special requirements on the antiserum reagent which, in addition to being monospecific, must also show high avidity for the antigen. Consequently many commercial antisera which may be satisfactory for rocket or radial diffusion quantitation give shallow, non-linear, calibration plots with AIP with a corresponding

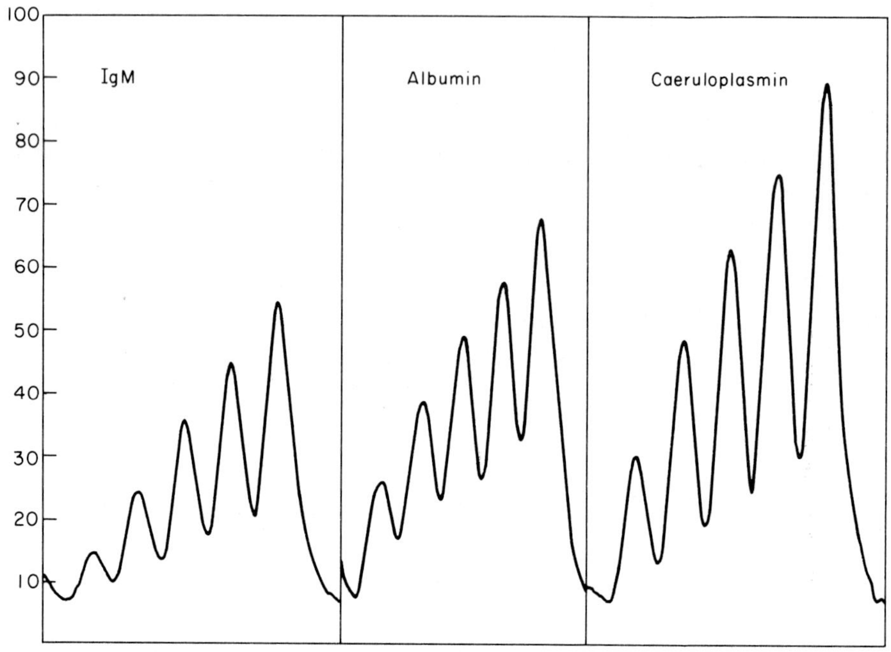

Fig. 9. Calibration peaks recorded on AIP system for (a) IgM, (b) Albumin and (c) Caeruloplasmin. A standard serum was used for calibration: the concentrations used were 20%, 40%, 60%, 80% and 100% respectively of the standard.

loss of accuracy. Nevertheless a large range of antisera are available commercially which satisfy the rigid requirements of the technique. In general antisera raised in goats appear to be suitable.

The formation of the immune complex itself deserves some comment, its formation is almost certainly speeded by the air–liquid interphases of the sample-antisera reaction segment and in 1964 it was observed that polymers added to the system enhanced the precipitin reaction. This enhancing effect can be seen even in agar gels. The use of polyethylene glycol (PEG) in AIP systems is now becoming established since it has been found to increase the sensitivity several fold and to shorten considerably the reaction time with a subsequent increase in the sampling rate and a saving in antisera.

The AIP technique offers particular advantage in the estimation of low protein concentrations in biological fluids such as urine and CSF. Such measurements are gaining importance in clearance or selectivity studies designed to measure the effectiveness of glomerular filtration and the blood-brain barrier respectively. These studies may give a very precise diagnosis of demyelinating disease or neoplasia based on CSF proteins (Ganrot and Laurell, 1979) and of renal lesions based on urinary protein measurements (Cameron and White, 1965). Previously such biological fluids required concentration prior to assessment with the possibility of specific loss of certain proteins during concentration. With the AIP method the original sample may be aspirated directly into the system at the resample point with a tremendous increase in accuracy of quantitation.

In addition to the obvious application of specific protein analysis, methods describing unusual applications of such analysis have appeared. Thus Fletcher *et al.* (1972) have described its use to detect biochemical and biophysical alterations in fibrinogen during thrombotic and other disease states.

REFERENCES

Aarden, L. A., Lakmaker, F. and Feltkamp, T. E. N. (1975a). Immunology of DNA I. The influence of reaction conditions on the Farr assay. *J. Immunol. Meth.* **10**, 27.

Aarden, L. A., Lakmaker, F. and Feltkamp, T. E. N. (1975b). Immunology of DNA II. The effect of size and structure of the DNA antigen on the Farr assay. *J. Immunol. Meth.* **10**, 39.

Aarden, L. A., de Groot, E. R. and Feltkamp, T. E. N. (1975c). Immunology of DNA III. *Crithidia luciliae*, a simple substrate for the determination of anti-ds DNA with the immunofluorescence technique. *Annl. N.Y. Acad. Sci.* **254**, 505.

Almeida, J. D. and Waterson, A. P. (1969). Immune complexes in hepatitis. *Lancet* **ii**, 983.

Anderson, S. G., Addison, I. E. and Dixon, H. G. (1971). Antinuclear-factor serum (homogeneous): An international collaborative study of the proposed Research Standard 66/233. *Annl. N.Y. Acad. Sci.* **177**, 337–345.

Awdeh, Z. L., Williamson, A. R. and Askonas, B. A. (1970). One cell-one immunoglobulin origin of limited heterogeneity of myeloma protein. *Biochem. J.* **116**, 241–248.

Axelsen, N. H., Krøll, J. and Weeke, B. (Eds.) (1973). "A Manual of Quantitative Immunoelectrophoresis". Universitetsforlaget, Oslo-Bergen-Tromsø.

Boyden, S. V. (1951). The absorption of proteins on erythrocytes treated with tannic acid and subsequent haemagglutination by antiprotein sera. *J. Exp. Med.* **93**, 107–120.

Cameron, J. S. and White, R. H. R. (1965). Selectivity of proteinuria in children with the nephrotic syndrome. *Lancet* **i**, 463–465.

Cwynarski, M. T., Watkins, J. and Johnson, P. M. (1975). *In* "Isoelectric Focusing" (eds. J. P. Arbuthnott and J. Beeley), pp. 319–326. Butterworths, London.

Deacon, W. E. and Hunter, E. F. (1962). Treponemal antigens as related to identification and syphilis serology. *Proc. Soc. Exp. Biol.* (*N.Y.*) **110**, 352–356.

Doniach, D. (1975). "Autoimmunity in Endocrine Disease." *Medicine* (2nd series) No. 6, p. 277.

Doniach, D., Roitt, I. M., Walker, J. G. and Sherlock, S. (1966). Tissue antibodies in primary biliary cirrhosis, active chronic (lupoid) hepatitis, cryptogenic cirrhosis and other liver diseases and their clinical implications. *Clin. Exp. Immunol.* **1**, 237–262.

Dorling, J., Johnson, G. D., Webb, Janet A. and Smith, Mavis E. (1971). The use of peroxidase-conjugated antiglobulin as an alternative to immunofluorescence for the detection of serum antinuclear factor; a comparison of the sensitivity of the two procedures. *J. Clin. Path.* **24**, 501–505.

Engvall, E. and Perlmann, P. (1972). Enzyme-linked immunosorbent assay, Elisa. *J. Immunol.* **109**, 129–135.

Fagerhol, M. K. (1968). The Pi-System Genetic variations of serum α_1-antitrypsin. *J. Immunol.* **109**, 129–135.

Faulk, W. P. and Houba, V. (1973). Immunological reactions with chronic chloride treated erythrocytes. *J. Immunol. Meth.* **3**, 87.

Feltkamp, T. E. W. (1975). The significance of the determination of anti-DNA and DNA/anti-DNA complexes. *Scand. J. Rheumatol.* Supplement II.

Fletcher, A. P., Alkjaesig, N., Roy, L. and Owens, O. (1972). Early detection of blood hyper-coagulable states and early thrombo-embolic lesions in man. *In* "A.I.P. Automated Immuno Precipitin Reactions: New Methods, Techniques and Evaluations", p. 1. Technicon Instruments Corp., N.Y.

Ganrot, K. and Laurell, C. B. (1974). Measurement of IgG and Albumin content of cerebro-spinal fluid, and its interpretation. *Clin. Chem.* **20**, 571–573.

Grabar, P. and Williams, C. A. (1953). Méthodes, permettent l'etude conjugée des propriétés electrophorétiques et immunchemiques d'un melange des proteins; applications au sérum sanguin. *Biochim. Biophys. Acta* (Amst.) **10**, 193–194.

Hay, F. C., Nineham, L. J. and Roitt, I. M. (1976). Simple procedure for the estimation of immune complexes of known class using plastic tubes coated with C1q. *Ann. Rheum. Dis.* Suppl.

Hayward, A. R., Ezer, G. and Smith, M. (1976). Inhibition of complement dependent lymphocyte rosette formation. *Ann. Rheum. Dis.* Suppl.

Holborow, E. J., Weir, D. M. and Johnson, G. D. (1957). A serum factor in lupus erythematosus with affinity for tissue nuclei. *Brit. Med. J.* **32**, 732–734.

Holborow, E. J., Brown, P. C., Roitt, I. M. and Doniach, D. (1959). Cytoplasmic localization of "complement-fixing" auto-antigen in human thyroid epithelium. *Brit. J. Exp. Path.* **40**, 583–588.

Jewell, D. P. and MacLennan, I. C. M. (1973). Circulating immune complexes in inflammatory bowel disease. *Clin. Exp. Immunol.* **14**, 219.

Johnson, G. D. (1971). Quantitative aspects of immunofluorescence. Ph.D. thesis, Council for National Academic Awards.

Johnson, G. D., Holborow, E. J. and Dorling, J. (1977). *In* "Handbook of Experimental Immunology", 3rd Edition, (ed. D. M. Weir), Chapter 15. Blackwell Scientific Publications, Oxford and London.

Johnson, G. D., Holborow, E. J. and Glynn, L. E. (1965). Antibody to smooth muscle in patients with liver disease. *Lancet* **ii**, 878–879.

Johnson, G. D., Konice, M. and Holborow, E. J. (1975). Comparison of methods employed for the detection of antibodies to ds-DNA. *Scand. J. Rheum.* Suppl. 8, abst. 42–05.

Kahan, J. and Sunblad, L. (1967). Automated immunochemical determination of β-lipoproteins. Technicon Symposia 1966, Vol. II, Automation in Analytical Chemistry, N.Y. Technicon.

Kohn, J. and Morgan, J. R. (1971). Pitfalls of Australia antigen detection and screening. *J. Clin. Path.* **24**, 673–674.

Laurell, C. B. (1965). Antigen-antibody crossed electrophoresis. *Anal. Biochem.* **10**, 358–361.

Libby, R. L. (1938). New and rapid quantitation techniques for the determination of potency of Types I and Ii antipneumococcal serum. *J. Immunol.* **34**, 269–279.

Longbottom, Joan L. and Pepys, J. (1964). Pulmonary aspergillosis diagnostic and immunological significance of antigens and C-substance in Aspergillus fumigatus. *J. Path. Bact.* **88**, 141–151.

Mancini, G., Carbonara, A. O. and Heremans, J. F. (1965). Immunochemical quantitation of antigens by single radial immunodiffusion. *Immunochem.* **2**, 235–254.

Marrack, J. (1934). Nature of antibodies. *Nature (Lond.)* **133**, 292–293.

Maurer, P. H. (1971). The quantitative precipitin reaction. *In* "Methods in Immunology and Immunochemistry". (Eds. C. A. Williams and M. W. Chase), p. 1. Academic Press, New York and London.

Mayer, M. M. (1961). "Experimental Immunochemistry", by E. A. Kabat and M. M. Mayer, 2nd ed. Thomas. Springfield, Illinois.

Miller, J. N. and Mutzelburg, I. D. (1973). *J. Chromat.* **75**, 165–168.

Minden, P. and Farr, R. S. (1977). "Handbook of Experimental Immunology." 3rd edition, (ed. D. M. Weir), Chapter 13. Blackwell Scientific Publications, Oxford and London.

Mohammed, I., Thompson, B. and Holborow, E. J. (1976). Radiobioassay for immune complexes using macrophages. *Ann. Rheum. Dis.* Suppl.

Mowbray, J. F., Hoffbrand, A. V., Holborow, E. J., Seah, P. P. and Fry, L. (1973). Circulating immune complexes in dermatitis herpetiformis. *Lancet* **1**, 400.

Nairn, R. C. (1969). *In* "Fluorescent Protein Tracing", 3rd edition, p. 3. Livingston, Edinburgh.

Nakane, P. K. and Pierce, G. B. Jr. (1966). Enzyme-labelled antibodies: preparation and application for the localization of antigens. *J. Histochem. Cytochem.* **14**, 929.

Nakane, P. K. (1975). Recent progress in the peroxidase-labelled antibody method. *Ann. N.Y. Acad. Sci. (U.S.A.)* **254**, 203.

Onyewotu, I. I. Johnson, P. M., Johnson, G. D. and Holborow, E. J. (1975). Enhanced uptake by guinea-pig macrophages of radioiodinated human aggregated immunoglobulin G in the presence of sera from rheumatoid patients with cutaneous vasculitis. *Clin. Exp. Immunol.* **19**, 267–280.

Ouchterlony, O. (1958). "Progress in Allergy", Vol. V. (ed. P. Kallos), pp. 1–78. Karger, Basel and New York.

Panayi, G. S., Poston, R. N. and Corrigall, V. (1976). Inhibition of antibody-mediated lymphocyte cytotoxicity by aggregated human immunoglobulin G. *Ann. Rheum. Dis.* Suppl.

Penttinen, K. (1976). The platelet aggregation test. *Ann. Rheum. Dis.* Suppl.

Pepys, J. and Jenkins, P. A. (1965). Precipitin (F.L.H.) test in farmer's lung. *Thorax,* **20**, 21–35.

Ressler, N. (1973). A systematic procedure for the determination of the heterogeneity and nature of multiple electrophoretic bands. *Anal. Biochem.* **51**, 589.

Ritchie, R. F. (1967). A simple direct and sensitive technique for measurement of specific protein in diluted solution.

Ritchie, R. F. (1972). The clinical utilization of specific protein analysis in a large general hospital. A.I.P. Automated Immuno Precipitin Reactions: New Methods, Techniques and Evaluations, p. 27. Technicon Instruments Corp. N.Y.

Rose, H. M., Ragan, C., Pearce, E. and Lipman, M. O. (1948). Differential agglutination of normal and sensitized sheep erythrocytes by sera of patients with rheumatoid arthritis. *Proc. Soc. Exp. Biol. (N.Y.)* **68**, 1, 6.

Seah, P. P., Fry, L., Hoffbrand, A. V. and Holborow, E. J. (1971). Tissue antibodies in dermatitis herpetiformis and adult coeliac disease. *Lancet* **1**, 834.

Sharp, G. C., Irvin, W. S., Tan, E. M., Gould, R. G. and Holman, H. R. (1972). Mixed connective tissue disease – an apparently distinct rheumatic disease syndrome associated with a specific antibody to an extractable nuclear antigen (ENA). *Am. J. Med.* **52**, 148–159.

Singer, J. M. and Plotz, C. M. (1956). The latex fixation test. *Am. J. Med.* **21**, 888.

Stanworth, D. R. and Johns, P. (1976). Ultracentrifugal methods of detecting soluble immune complexes. *Ann. Rheum. Dis.* Suppl.

Steward, M. W., Katz, F. E. and West, N. J. (1975). The role of low affinity antibody in immune complex disease. The quantity of anti-DNA antibodies in NZB/W Fl hybrid mice. *Clin. Exp. Immunol.* **21**, 121.

Strauss, A. J. L., Seegal, B. C., Hsu, K. C., Burkholder, P. M., Nastuk, W. L. and Osserman, K. E. (1960). Immunofluorescence demonstration of a muscle binding, complement fixing serum globulin fraction in myasthenia gravis. *Proc. Soc. Exp. Biol.* (*N.Y.*) **105**, 184–191.

Taylor, K. B., Roitt, I. M., Doniach, D., Couchman, K. G. and Shapland, C. (1962). Autoimmune phenomena in pernicious anaemia: gastric antibodies. *Brit. Med. J.* **2**, 1347–1352.

Theofilopoulos, A. N., Wilson, C. B., Bokisch, I. A. and Dixon, F. J. (1974). Binding of soluble immune complexes to human lymphoblastoid cells. II. Use of Raji cells to detect circulating immune complexes in animal and human sera. *J. Exp. Med.* **140**, 1230.

Vergani, C., Stabilini, R. and Agostoni, A. (1967). Quantitative determination of serum immunoglobulins by single radial immunodiffusion on cellulose acetate. *Immunochemistry* **4**, 233.

Vesterberg, O. and Svennson, H. (1966). Isoelectric fractionation analysis and characterization of ampholytes in natural pH gradients. IV. Further studies on the resolving power in connection with separation of myoglobins. *Acta. Chem. Scand.* **20**, 820.

Van Furth, R., Schuit, H. R. E. and Hijmans, W. (1966). The formation of immunoglobulins by human tissues *in vitro*. 1. The methods and their specificity. *Immunology* **II**, 1–11.

Wasserman, E. and Levine, L. (1961). Quantitative micro-complement fixation and its use in the study of antigenic structure by specific antigen–antibody inhibition. *J. Immunol.* **87**, 290.

Williams, B. P. and Slaney, J. M. (1976). Macromolecular C3 – an indirect marker of circulating immune complexes. *Ann. Rheum. Dis.* Suppl.

Williamson, A. R. (1975) Antibody isoelectric spectra. *In* "Isoelectric Focusing". (Eds. J. P. Arbuthnott and J. Beeley), p. 291. Butterworth, London.

Winchester, R. J. and Agnello, V. (1976). Detection of Immune Complexes by direct precipitation with Clq or IgM rheumatoid factors. *Ann. Rheum. Dis.* Suppl.

Winchester, R. J., Kundel, H. G. and Agnello, V. (1971). Occurrence of γ-globulin complexes in serum and joint fluid of rheumatoid patients: use of mono-clonal rheumatoid factors as reagents for the demonstration. *J. Exp. Med.* **134**, 286–295.

Yalow, R. S. and Berson, S. A. (1960). Immunoassay of endogenous plasma insulin in man. *J. Clin. Invest.* **39**, 1157.

Zubler, R. H. and Lambert, P. (1976). ^{125}I–Clq binding test for the detection of soluble immune complexes. *Ann. Rheum. Dis.* Suppl.

Zubler, R. H., Perrin, L. H., Creighton, W. D. and Lambert, P. (1976). The use of polyethylene glycol (PEG) to concentrate immune complexes from serum or plasma samples. *Ann. Rheum. Dis.* Suppl.

II

Mediator Systems

7

Complement in Perspective

R. A. THOMPSON

Complement was the name given by Bordet (1898) to the heat-labile activity in fresh serum which caused the lysis of red blood cells in the presence of specific antibody. The same activity had previously been shown to be present in the serum of goats immunized with *Vibrio cholerae*. These organisms were destroyed by fresh serum, but not by serum heated at 58°C for 60 minutes. Fresh non-immune guinea-pig serum, while without effect on its own, could restore the bactericidal power of the heated immune serum.

The lysis of sheep erythrocytes (E) coated with specific antibody (A) has since been the reaction by which complement has been identified, estimated and analysed. Bordet showed that this activity of fresh serum was also lost on prior incubation with other antigen–antibody systems, even those employing soluble antigens, and this gave rise to the complement fixation test, which has been widely exploited in basic and applied immunology.

That complement is a multi-component system was first appreciated by Ferrata (1907) who showed that there were at least two components, one in the water-insoluble (euglobulin) fraction of the plasma proteins and the other in the water soluble (pseudoglobulin) fraction. In the first two decades of this century four components were described, and it became apparent that they acted sequentially during the process of cell lysis, the order of action being C1, C4, C2 and finally C3. Moreover during this process the early acting components attached to the cell, and could be separated from the other serum factors, yet remaining in an active state, thereby forming red cell-complement intermediates (EAC).

The ability of early workers to isolate the various components was technically limited and most studies employed the so-called R reagents. These were made from whole serum, modified by various procedures aimed at eliminating one component, but leaving the others intact; thus R1 was serum less C1, R2 was serum less C2, and so on. Although the use of these relatively crude reagents produced a considerable body of information, their use has been abandoned in recent years with the advent of more efficient protein separation methods and the availability of reagents from individuals and animals with congenital deficiencies of individual components.

The refinements of the techniques for kinetic studies of cell lysis and the analysis of components, and the correct requirements of hydrogen ion concentration, tonicity, temperature, etc., were elucidated in the 1940s and early 1950s. Mayer (1961) proposed the "one-hit" theory of red cell lysis by complement in which it was postulated that reactions at a single site on the membrane of the cell caused lysis. This contrasted with the older "multi-hit" theory, where cell lysis was considered to be the consequence of the development of a finite number of complement lesions, the cumulative effect of which was to lyse the cell. The application of the one-hit theory allowed the critical biochemical analysis of the reaction mechanisms, and led to a considerable understanding of the sequence of events, particularly those in the early stages of the reaction. It allowed extension of the kinetic analysis to the interaction of complement with other antigen–antibody systems and the demonstration that similar reactions were taking place during complement activation however it was initiated. The one-hit theory was validated subsequently by electron microscopic studies (Borsos *et al.*, 1964).

Purification and characterization of the early complement components in the late 1950s and 1960s was paralleled by the observation by several groups that the third component was really multiple (Rapp, 1958; Klein and Wellensiek, 1965; Nilsson, 1967; Vroon *et al.*, 1970), leading to the identification of five further factors C5, C6, C7, C8 and C9, operating during the terminal stages of immune haemolysis of red cells.

While research concentrated on the nature and biochemistry of the components and the reactions involved in lysis, it became evident that activation of the components by any antigen–antibody complex engendered other biological activities of considerable importance, particularly anaphylaxis, chemotaxis and opsonization for phagocytosis and removal by the reticulo-endothelial system. Appreciation of the biological role of complement has been modified in the last five years or so by the observation that the latter components C5–C9 which interact with the cell membrane and produce cell lysis, can do so independently of the early components (Gotze and Muller-Eberhard, 1969; Lachmann and Thompson, 1970). The important physiological event in the handling of extrinsic antigens is the fixation of C3 and the generation of the relevant chemotactic and anaphylactic factors. One of the consequences of C3 fixation is the priming of the "attack mechanism" (Muller-Eberhard, 1971), resulting in the activation of the lytic components.

This second stage is, however, not apparently essential in defence against microorganisms, since strains of laboratory animals and some humans have been reported with genetic deficiencies of these later components in whom no defect in antigen-handling or increased susceptibility to infection can be detected, although their sera cannot lyse sensitized erythrocytes.

The priming, or C3 fixation stage on the other hand, is essential, and there are at least two mechanisms by which it can be achieved. Both processes require the generation of a C3-fixing enzyme (called C3 convertase), which causes activated C3 to adhere to the initiating antigen–antibody complex. One convertase is formed by the sequential action of the classical components C1, C4 and C2, and the other is generated by the factors of the alternative pathway of complement activation. This latter system was first postulated by Pillemer and his associates (1954) as important for the complete activation of C3 in serum, and necessary for non-specific defence against bacteria and viruses. It fell into disrepute in the 1960s, at a time when discovery of the nature and reaction mechanisms of the complement sequence was proceeding rapidly, and interest was centred on cell lysis. However, as a result of a number of independent lines of investigation, it became apparent that an alternative system exists for the activation of complement, entering at the C3 stage and bypassing the early components C1, C4 and C2. The elements of the system and the reaction mechanisms are still under investigation, but part of the alternative pathway appears to operate as a positive feed-back mechanism, re-inforcing C3 fixation however initiated.

Recent research has elucidated a number of interesting additional biological roles for complement, including interaction with the clotting and fibrinolytic systems, and interaction with B-lymphocytes in the initiation of the immune response; so that a system which was once considered almost a laboratory artefact and investigated from a biochemical standpoint, now attracts the attention of immunologists with a wide range of interests.

Clinical interest in complement was largely empirical and arose from the fact that changes in circulating complement levels occurs in certain diseases. However, the more recent elucidation of its role in the pathogenesis of many auto-immune and hypersensitivity diseases, and observations on the pathological consequences of complement deficiencies, has led to an intensification of interest, and the need to study complement in many disease situations.

DEFINITION OF COMPLEMENT

Complement has been defined as the system of large molecular weight proteins in plasma or tissue fluid, which is activated by antibody in combination with its specific antigen, and under special circumstances by other agents, and which subsequently mediates a series of biological events. If the antigen is on the surface of the red cell, the end result of this chain of activation is that the cell is lysed. The components exist as inactive precursors and become activated as enzymes in sequence; individual components once activated acting on the next component, and so on. There is thus a cascade effect, with considerable expansion in the number of molecules successively involved at each stage. This process is similar to that seen in other enzyme systems in the plasma, such as the clotting system and the fibrinolytic and kinin systems. The concept of complement as comprising only components leading to the lysis of antibody-coated red cells (EA) has broadened with recent knowledge.

Nomenclature

The components leading to red cell haemolysis have been clearly defined (Bull W.H.O. 1968) and are designated numerically in the order of their action, C1, C2 etc. to C9, with the exception of C4, which is so-called for historical reasons as the fourth component to be described, although it acts second in the sequence (Table 1). Whenever the first component is activated, be it by antibody coated red cells, or by other antigen–antibody complexes, or by certain other substances capable of activating it directly *in vitro*, it sets off the same chain of interrelated reactions.

An activated component is designated with a bar over the number, e.g. C1 is activated to C$\overline{1}$. Fragments are designated by arabic letters after the number, e.g. C3 is split by the enzyme C3 convertase into two fragments C3a and C3b. Complement intermediates are indicated by the stage in the sequence which has been reached, e.g. EAC$\overline{1}$ $\overline{4b2a}$.

In addition to the rapid decay of active sites, there are a number of specific inhibitors acting at various stages in the sequence to modulate the progress of the complement cascade. These are designated by the active component they inhibit. The most well recognized of these are the C1 esterase inhibitor (Pensky *et al.*, 1961), the C3b inactivator, a C6 inhibitor, described by Tamura and Nelson (1967), and inhibitory activity to the C567 stage of reactive lysis (McLeod *et al.*, 1974).

The components of the alternative pathway have not yet been fully defined, but those that have been are designated by capital letters following the system originally used by Pillemer and his colleagues. Recognized at present are factors P (properdin), B and D (Table 2), and these will be considered in more detail later. In this system, activated components are indicated by a

TABLE 1

Complement components (classical activation pathway)

Component	Electrophoretic mobility	S value	Mol. wt.	Approx. serum concentration (μg/ml)	Consequences of binding to Ag/Ab complex or Ab—sensitized cell/particle
PRIMING MECHANISM					
C1					Inhibits viral activity; Inhibits spontaneous E-rosettes with anti-lymphocyte globulin.
C1q	γ-2	11	400,000	100	
C1r	β	7	170,000	?	
C1s	α-2	4·5	80,000	120	
C4	β-1	10	240,000	250	Inhibits spontaneous E-rosettes with anti-lymphocyte globulin. Forms immuno-conglutinogen.
C2	β-2	6	100,000	30	Forms C3 convertase with C4; releases kinin-like peptides.
C3	β-2	9·5	185,000	1,200	Forms immuno-conglutinogen; interacts with phagocytes and B lymphocytes; activates alternative pathway; releases C3a chemotactic and anaphylactic peptide; forms C5 convertase to trigger "attack" mechanism.
ATTACK SYSTEM					
C5	β-1	8·5	170,000	100	Release C5a chemotactic and anaphylactic peptide; ?opsonizes bacteria for killing by polymorphs.
C6	β-1	6·0	100,000	20	Forms stable $C\overline{56}$ complex which can be released.
C7	β-1	5·5	110,000		Forms stable $E\overline{C567}$; releases $C\overline{567}$ chemotactic factor.
C8	γ-1	8·0	160,000	10	Forms EC5678—subject to slow spontaneous lysis.
C9	α-2	4·5	70,000	2	Forms E*—subject to rapid spontaneous lysis.

bar over the latter and fragments by small arabic letters, as with the classical complement system.

TABLE 2
Alternative pathway components

Factor	Synonyms	Physico-chemical characteristics
Properdin		5·5S γ-globulin
A	C3	9·5S β-globulin
B	Glycine rich β-globulin (GBG) C3 pro-activator (C3PA) Cobra venom factor co-factor	5 S β-globulin
D	GBG-ase, C3PA-ase	3 S α-globulin

PRINCIPLE OF ACTION

Activation of a component usually results in its proteolytic cleavage into two or more fragments of varying sizes and differing biological activities. One of these, usually the largest, has two functional sites revealed, a hydrophobic site for the attachment to cell membranes or to the initiating antigen–antibody complex, and an enzymatic site usually for the next component in the sequence. There may also be sites for interaction with other effector cells, e.g. phagocytes and lymphocytes, so that the biological fate of the complex to which the component attaches is altered, and the potential increases as successive components become attached. However, only a small proportion of activated molecules actually attaches, the remainder being released into the surrounding fluid, where their attachment site decays rapidly and the enzyme site decays or is inactivated by inhibitors. These activities cannot be regenerated, and components once activated are unable to participate in the reaction sequence again; activation is followed immediately by inactivation. The smaller fragments generated during the sequences may have other biological activities at a distance from their point of generation, i.e. anaphylaxis or chemotaxis. The rapid decay and inhibition of active sites ensures that the potentially harmfully consequences of opsonization and lysis are confined to the antigen–antibody complex that initiates them, without affecting bystander host cells.

ACTIVATION (PRIMING) PATHWAYS

A more appropriate view of complement is to consider it as a system for activating the third component C3, generating phlogistic peptides and coating the initiating complex or agent with C3 so as to opsonize it for phagocytosis and removal by the reticulo–endothelial system. This can be achieved by at least two major activation pathways, each of which generates a specific enzyme (C3 convertase) for this purpose (see Fig. 1).

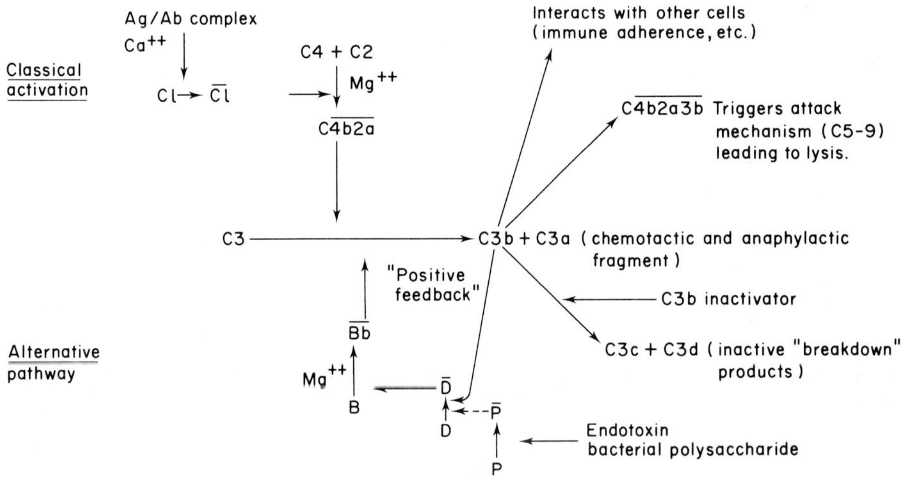

Fig. 1. C3 fixation.

The classical C3 convertase is generated by the early components involved in the immune lysis of sheep red cells. The other convertase is derived from the activation of factors in the alternative pathway, the most directly involved in acting on C3 being activated factor B, previously known as the C3 pro-activator or glycine-rich β-globulin.

With the demonstration that cell lysis was independent of the presence of the early components it was realized that fixed C3, generated by either pathway, could trigger the attack phase of complement by activating the components C5–C9 which on attachment to the cell surface results in cell death. However, the evidence suggests that the assembly on the surface of the classical C3 convertase provides a more efficient triggering mechanism for the attack phase, one that is more likely to lead to cell lysis. As will be discussed, it appears that the C3 convertase itself, together with its product, activated C3, participates in this triggering.

THE CLASSICAL C3 CONVERTASE

This is formed when the system is activated by antibody in combination with its specific antigen. The nature of the antibody is important since not all immunoglobulin classes of antibody can activate complement.

IgM and IgG antibodies from a number of mammalian species (including guinea-pig γ_2- and sheep γ_1-globulins) have been shown to initiate the formation of the classical convertase although the lysis of EA by complement has been generally studied using rabbit IgM antibody to the Forsmann antigen. One IgM molecule can interact with the first component to initiate the events leading to haemolysis, but for IgG antibody two molecules must be in juxtaposition to activate the sequence. The site of binding to C1 is on the Fc portion of the immunoglobulin molecule, revealed in the configurational changes that occur on combination with antigen. Recent work has shown that in the γ heavy chain it is on the C_H2 domain. Using aggregated myeloma immunoglobulins, the human IgG subclasses, IgG1, IgG3 and to a slight extent IgG2, but not IgG4, have been shown to bind to the C1q subcomponent of C1. There are thus differences in the ability of the human IgG subclasses to activate the classical pathway. IgA, IgD and IgE immunoglobulins do not activate this pathway.

First Stage

$$\text{Ag/Ab} + \text{C1} \xrightarrow{\text{Ca}^{++}} (\text{Ag/Ab})\ \overline{\text{C1}}.$$

C1 is a complex of separate proteins or subcomponents, C1q, C1r and C1s, held together by calcium ions, and having a combined molecular weight of approximately 800,000. Recently an additional subcomponent C1t has been described although its role has not been elicidated. C1q is the component which interacts directly with antibody. It is a complex collagen-like protein which consists of six subunits connected non-covalently by strands to a central core, and it is thought that the subunits bind to the site on the immunoglobulin molecule. C1q also interacts with acidic substances with a positive charge, and will form a precipitate with DNA and with lipid A, especially at low ionic strength. It can be activated directly by plasmin, and as has been recently demonstrated, by complexes between bacterial polysaccharide and C-reactive protein. On isolation from serum, C1 undergoes a slow spontaneous activation. On combination of the C1q with antibody, C1r is activated and this in turn activates C1s. Activated C1s possesses esterase activity which can be demonstrated using the synthetic esters acetyl tyrosine ester (ATE) and tosyl arginine methyl ester (TAME). Its preferred substrate is C4; it also acts on C2 but does so with greater efficiency in the presence of C4. Its action is destroyed by heating at 56°C for 30 minutes. Activated C1 has been shown to have vasodilator effects when injected into the skin of guinea-pigs, but this is probably because it activates the complement sequence and releases anaphylactic peptides.

C1 Esterase Inhibitor

There is a specific inhibitor for the first stage, which combines stoichiometrically with activated C1, but not with native C1. It blocks the enzymatic activity either on the cell surface or in free solution, although it is more efficient in blocking C1 esterase in free solution. It is an α-2-neuramino-glycoprotein of approximately 90,000 molecular weight, and is destroyed by heating at 60°C for one hour. It can be estimated functionally by its action in blocking the hydrolysis by C1 esterase of the synthetic ester ATE, thus decreasing the amount of titratable acid released. Besides inhibiting C1 esterase the α-2-neuramino-glycoprotein also inhibits kallikrein, plasmin, PF/dil and factors in other plasma activable enzyme systems (Ratnoff *et al.*, 1969), and this is of significance for the pathological consequences of C1 esterase deficiency.

Second Stage (convertase formation)

$$
\begin{array}{l}
(\mathrm{Ag/Ab})\mathrm{C}\bar{1} + \mathrm{C4} + \mathrm{C2} \xrightarrow{\mathrm{Mg}^{++}} (\mathrm{Ag/Ab})\mathrm{C}\bar{1}\,\overline{\mathrm{4b2a}} + (\mathrm{C4a} + \mathrm{C4b} \\
\qquad\qquad\qquad\qquad\qquad\qquad\qquad\qquad\quad \mathrm{C2b} + \text{Kinin-like peptide} \\
\qquad\qquad\qquad\qquad\qquad\qquad\qquad\qquad\quad \mathrm{C2a} \longrightarrow \mathrm{C2d})^{*}
\end{array}
$$

C4 and C2 are β-globulins which associate in the presence of magnesium ions. Activated C1 acts on both proteins splitting them into a and b fragments;

---

* Brackets denote fragments which can be detected free in the supernatant.

C4b is the major fragment of C4 and has a transient binding site for attachment to cell surfaces and antibodies. It has another site for combination with the C2a fragment to form a bi-molecular product $C\overline{4b2a}$, which is the classical C3 convertase. Unbound C4b soon loses its attachment site and is found in the supernatant, together with C4a, C2b and a kinin-like peptide derived from C2. Other functions of these fragments are unknown. The C2a portion of the convertase is labile, and is subject to spontaneous decay, after which it detaches from the complex and is known as C2d. However, further C2a can be generated from fresh C2 by $C\overline{1}$, and attach to existing C4b, thereby regenerating the enzyme.

The decay of C2 is probably the main mechanism which modulates this stage of the sequence; a C2 decay-accelerating factor in serum has been described, but has not yet been fully characterized.

C4 is a 10S β-globulin of approximately 230,000 molecular weight, also known as β-1-E globulin, and its serum concentration is 0·25 mg per ml. Activated C4 has a slightly more anodal electrophoretic mobility than native C4. The protein is inactivated by treatment of serum with ammonia; of the other components, only C3 is partially inactivated by this treatment, which was used in the preparation of R4 reagents (see above).

Third Stage (C3 Fixation)

$$(Ag/Ab)C\overline{1}\ \overline{4b2a} + C3 \longrightarrow (Ag/Ab)C\overline{1}\ \overline{4b2a3b} + (C3a + C3b)$$

The reactions are independent of divalent cations after the formation of the C3 convertase. C3 is split into a small fragment of 10,000 molecular weight, C3a, with anaphylactic and chemotactic properties, and a major fragment C3b, of approximately 170,000 molecular weight, which binds to the antigen–antibody complex in considerable quantity. One convertase site attaches several hundred C3b molecules, although only 10% of molecules activated actually attach. The remainder rapidly lose their attachment site and are found in the supernatant. C3 is the major component of the complement system, with a serum concentration of 1 mg per ml, i.e. from four to ten times the concentration of any other component. Thus this is the bulk reaction stage of the system, analogous to fibrin formation in the clotting system. As discussed below, there exists also a positive feed-back mechanism utilizing part of the alternative pathway, which further enhances C3 fixation once it has begun.

C3b Inactivator

C3b, both on the cell and in the fluid phase is inactivated by a specific C3b inactivator. This is a β-globulin, originally identified in two different ways; on the one hand by its function in inhibiting the lytic activity of fixed C3 (Tamura and Nelson, 1967; Ruddy and Austen, 1969), and on the other by its function in revealing a site on fixed C3 which reacts with the bovine protein conglutinin(K) for which it was also called conglutinogen-activating factor, or KAF (Lachmann and Muller-Eberhard, 1968). These two factors proved to be identical. The C3b inactivator has no action on native C3, but acts on C3b enzymatically to split it into two further fragments, C3c and C3d. When the inactivator acts on cell- or complex-bound C3b, C3d remains attached, and C3c is released.

THE ALTERNATIVE PATHWAY CONVERTASE

The mode of generation of the alternative pathway convertase has not been fully ascertained. Factors involved are properdin (Factor P), Factor D and Factor B. Pillemer originally characterized an ammonia-sensitive factor, which he termed Factor A, but it is now clear the Factor A is native C3 itself, which takes part in the sequence of reactions that lead to the formation of the alternative pathway C3-splitting enzyme. While the formation of the classical convertase is an efficient process occurring at high serum dilutions, the alternative pathway convertase is formed only at relatively low serum dilutions. There is no requirement for calcium ions, although the formation of the convertase is dependent on magnesium ions, as is formation of the classical $C\overline{42}$ enzyme (Fig. 1).

The activation of the alternative pathway is initiated by certain agents, such as bacterial endotoxins and the solid polysaccharides zymosan and inulin, which interact with properdin, probably in the absence of specific antibody. Properdin becomes activated in the process, although it is not clear what changes occur in the molecule, or what co-factors are involved. Activated properdin, which "fires" the alternative pathway, has a γ electrophoretic mobility, while native properdin is a β-globulin. It is an asymmetrical molecule with a molecular weight of 220,000.

Aggregated human myeloma IgA and some aggregated myeloma IgGs also activate the alternative pathway (and there is a report of slight activation by aggregated IgE) and it is presumed that complexed antibodies of the same classes can do likewise. IgM antibodies cannot activate the alternative pathway. It is not clear to what extent antibody activation utilizes properdin.

Factor D is a 3S α-globulin of 24,000 mol. wt. which is probably activated directly by activated properdin in the presence of native C3 (Factor A). Activated Factor D can then activate the final enzyme, Factor B. This reaction requires Mg^{++}.

Factor B is a 5·5S β-globulin of 93,000 mol. wt. which on activation is cleaved into a small fragment of α mobility, and a larger γ fragment (63,000 mol. wt.). It is this latter fragment which possesses the C3 convertase activity.

Positive C3b Feedback

The C3b fragment formed during the activation of C3 by either pathway can itself again interact with Factor D and cause further activation of Factor B, thus leading to further C3 breakdown, and providing a positive feed-back mechanism. This action of C3b is modulated by the C3b inactivator, which cleaves it into two further fragments, C3c and C3d, and thus inhibits its participation in this feedback (Fig. 1).

It is thought that an initiating factor is involved at an early stage in the activation of properdin, but its identity is uncertain. There is some evidence that the "nephritic factor" found in the sera of some patients with mesangiocapillary glomerulonephritis (see later), may in fact be this initiating factor in an activated form (Muller-Eberhard, 1974).

The assembly of the alternative pathway factors on the cell wall or on the activating complex, the integrity of the attachment sites and the formation of intermediates are by no means as clearly understood as the formation of the EAC intermediates of the classical activation pathway. However, the existence of the alternative pathway evidently ensures massive C3 fixation on the complex, and under appropriate circumstances both pathways trigger the "attack" mechanism leading to cell lysis.

Other Pathways

C3 can be cleaved directly by other enzymes, such as plasmin, trypsin, and lysosomal cathepsins, to release the anaphylactic and chemotactic peptide C3a. It is not clear whether these processes, if occurring at a cell surface, could result in activation of the later components and cell lysis, but it is likely that C3b, derived from such direct enzyme cleavage, has some if not all of the other functional attributes of conventionally-generated C3b, namely immune adherence, ability to activate the alternative pathway, interaction with B lymphocytes, etc. It has been shown that trypsin can substitute for the C5 convertase, in that it acts on C5 in the presence of C6 to form the stable intermediate, C$\overline{56}$ and in the presence of fresh C7, C8 and C9, this will attach to and lyse unsensitized red cells.

Cobra venom has been known since the first decade of this century to inactivate the complement system. But only in the last 10 years has the mechanism been made clear. The investigations concerned helped to furnish part of the evidence re-establishing the validity of the properdin or alternative pathway of complement activation. The complement-fixing activity is distinct from the toxic factors in the venom. It is the property of an 8·5S globulin (cobra venom factor, or CVF), which activates the alternative pathway by combining with factor B in the presence of magnesium ions to form a C3 convertase. There is some evidence that an additional serum factor is necessary for this process. Factor B appears not to dissociate into its α- and γ-fragments, but to form a macromolecular complex with CVF. This convertase is also able, under the appropriate conditions, to trigger the attack mechanism and cause the lysis of cells.

THE "ATTACK" MECHANISM

EAC$\overline{1}$ $\overline{4b2a3b}$ + C5 $\longrightarrow$ EAC$\overline{1}$ $\overline{4b2a3b5b}$ + (C5a chemotactic and anaphylactic factors)

EC$\overline{5b}$ + C6 + C7 $\longrightarrow$ EC$\overline{5b}$67 + (C$\overline{5b}$67 chemotactic factor)

EC5b67 + C8 + C9 $\longrightarrow$ EC$\overline{5b}$6789 $\longrightarrow$ E* (cell which lyses without further serum factors)

The C3 convertase together with activated C3b form an enzyme, C5 convertase, which cleaves C5 into a minor fragment, C5a and a major portion C5b. This new enzyme has peptidase activity.

According to Muller-Eberhard (1974), this is the only enzymatic step in the interaction between the components comprising the attack mechanism. Activated C5b binds weakly to the cell surface, but associates strongly with

C6 to form a complex, C$\overline{5b6}$ and in the presence of C7, interaction occurs to form a C$\overline{5b}$67 complex which has a firm binding site for protein, glycoprotein or lipid surfaces. Unattached C567 complexes soon lose their attachment site and form the macromolecular C567 chemotactic factor. The C$\overline{5b}$67 also has a receptor site for C8 and its co-factor C9, which associate together on the cell surface in a macromolecular protein complex which inserts into the cell membrane. It disrupts the lipid layer causing the release of electrolytes from within the cell and the entry of water from without, so that the cell swells up and bursts. The association of activated C5, C6, C7, C8 and up to four molecules of C9 in a macromolecular complex has been shown also to occur in the fluid phase.

In the absence of C7, activation of the attack mechanism results in the formation of stable C$\overline{5b6}$ complexes which detach from the cell and are released into the supernatant. This occurs more readily on triggering via the alternative pathway. The C$\overline{5b6}$ complexes can be isolated and in the presence of C7, C$\overline{5b}$67 is formed which has a transient attachment site for cell walls. This forms EC$\overline{567}$ with unsensitized cells and on the addition of C8 and C9 the cells will lyse. This process, which occurs following fluid phase interaction between C$\overline{5b6}$ and C7, C8 and C9 in the presence of unsensitized cells and without a requirement for the early complement components, is termed "reactive lysis" (Thompson and Lachmann, 1970; Lachmann and Thompson, 1970). It is a possible means whereby complement activation can result in damage to bystander host cells or particles not primarily a target for the reaction. It has been suggested that this mechanism operates in the complement-mediated lysis of platelets which aggregate in the presence of endotoxin or antigen–antibody complexes.

Its potentially "auto-toxic" effect is kept in check by an inhibitory mechanism recently described by McLeod and his colleagues (1974) and attributed to an α-glycoprotein of considerable size heterogeneity. Inhibition is blocked by polyanions, which suggests that it depends on the existence of strong charge differences between C$\overline{567}$ and the inhibitor, which are mutually attracted so that the attachment of C$\overline{567}$ to the cell is blocked.

The reactions of the attack mechanism are thought to be the same whether the C3 convertase is formed by the classical or alternative pathway, although the nature of the alternative pathway C5 activating enzyme is not as well established as is the classical. Under the electron microscope, the final result is the appearance of circular lesions ("holes") approximately 100 Å in diameter, on the cell surface (Humphrey and Dourmashkin, 1965). With human complement these appear in clusters, while with guinea-pig complement they tend to separate. They are not true holes but are membrane lesions formed by association of the terminal complement components in macromolecular complexes with lipids of the cell surface.

FUNCTIONS OF ACTIVATED C3

Activation of C3 is the key step in the reaction sequence. In addition to the release of chemotactic and anaphylactic factors, C3b is coated on to the complex, and interacts with receptors on a number of effector cells (Fig. 1).

Immune Adherence

This was originally described (Nelson, 1963) as a reaction between complement coated complexes (either particulate or soluble antigen–antibody complexes) and primate red cells or non-primate platelets. It occurs when C3 becomes bound to the complex. This reaction causes the indicator particles to agglutinate and has been used as an alternative to cell lysis for titration of serum complement activity. More recently it has been shown that macrophages possess a site for interaction with bound C3, and it is likely that the adherence phenomenon applies generally to endothelial cells, and is a prelude to phagocytosis.

Opsonization

Antigen–antibody complexes coated with complement to the C3 stage are more readily phagocytosed through attachment to specialized receptors on the phagocytic cells. It is not clear whether engulfment requires any further specific surface activation by C3b or whether it is a "non-specific" consequence of attachment. Experimentally, intravenously injected complement coated red cells are rapidly taken up by Kupffer cells in the liver, and portions of the engulfed red cells are removed, the remainder being extruded as microcytes (Brown *et al.*, 1970). These cells are found to have only C3d on their surface, as a consequence of the *in vivo* action of the C3b inhibitor. The intracellular killing of ingested microorganisms is enhanced in the presence of serum factors which are complement-related, although the precise role of complement in this process is uncertain.

Conglutination

Bound complement on the surface of antigen–antibody complexes presents new "auto-antigenic" determinants, which are capable of stimulating immune responses. The antibodies so formed are called immuno-conglutinins, and are usually detected by their ability to agglutinate complement coated red cells. In humans they are usually of the IgM class although IgG and IgA immuno-conglutinins have been described. C3 provides the major antigenic determinants, but immuno-conglutinins against bound C4 have also been described. Circulating immuno-conglutinins are increased after infections or inflammation, and by agglutinating complement-coated microorganisms are thought to prevent their spread and enhance their removal; they do not react with native C3.

Bound C3 also has a very specific site for interaction with conglutinin(K). This is a large molecular weight non-immunoglobulin protein, found only in the genus *Bovidae*. Conglutinin does not react with native C3, nor with C3b in its freshly formed state. The conglutinogen is only revealed after the action of the C3b inhibitor, and is presumably on C3d. The biological function of this reaction is not clear but presumably in the *Bovidae* conglutinin acts in the same manner as immuno-conglutinins in other species.

Alternative Pathway Activation

As has been mentioned, C3b, either bound to complexes or in the fluid phase, activates the alternate pathway, probably by activating Factor D, and then forming with it an enzyme which activates Factor B. This function augments the important C3-fixing stage of the cascade to a considerable degree. It is modulated by the C3b inhibitor.

Interaction with B-Lymphocytes

B-lymphocytes carry on their surface a receptor specific for bound C3, and interact with C3 coated red cells to form EAC-rosettes. Formation of these rosettes is inhibited by the presence of C3b, C3c, and C3d in free solution. It is thought that this interaction plays some part in the induction of specific immune responses, although the evidence is as yet indirect. Antibody responses to some antigens are impaired in mice in which the circulating C3 levels are depleted (Pepys, 1974). Similarly the localization of immune aggregates in germinal centres in lymphoid tissue is inhibited in the absence of complement. Agents such as endotoxin, which stimulate the alternative pathway, act as effective inducers of B-lymphocyte transformation *in vitro*. In addition, experiments investigating the role of macrophages as intermediaries between T- and B-cells cooperating in production of antibody show inhibition of the latter in the presence of an anti-C3 antiserum, which suggests a requirement for complement in this essential immune process.

CHARACTERISTICS OF C3

C3 is a 9·5S β-globulin which consists of two polypeptide chains, an α-chain of 110,000 mol. wt. and a β-chain of 70,000 mol. wt. The α-chain contains the C3a anaphylactic and chemotactic peptide at its N-terminal end. The C3 concentration in serum and tissue fluids is approximately 1g/litre.

C3 was known as β-1-C globulin before its precise role in the complement sequence was established. It comprises the β-2 band in fresh serum, which alters its electrophoretic mobility on ageing or after inactivation by antigen–antibody complexes, becoming β-1-A globulin.

C3 contains a number of antigenic determinants, antibodies to which are present to varying degrees in anti-C3 antisera. The most antigenic of the determinants are those associated with C3c (called the A antigenic determinants by West *et al.* (1966), who defined the antigenic relationships before the functional activities of the fragments were known) and all anti-C3 antisera react well with these determinants, on native C3 as well as on C3b and C3c. The latter have a more anodal electrophoretic mobility than native C3, and in two-dimensional electrophoresis such an antiserum can determine the degree of C3 conversion or C3 inactivation by antigen–antibody complexes or other agents (Fig. 2).

Native C3 has a configurational determinant called the "B" antigen, which is lost on activation or ageing. Thus antisera raised by injecting animals with complement coated complexes, or purified C3 preparations made from aged serum or plasma, do not contain antibodies to the "B" antigen. An anti-"B" antiserum is made by immunization with C3 prepared from fresh serum under conditions which minimize its spontaneous breakdown. It can be made specific for native "uninactivated" C3 by absorption with fully aged serum. One use of such an antiserum is to measure C3 inactivation by quantitation of the decrease in the "B" antigen.

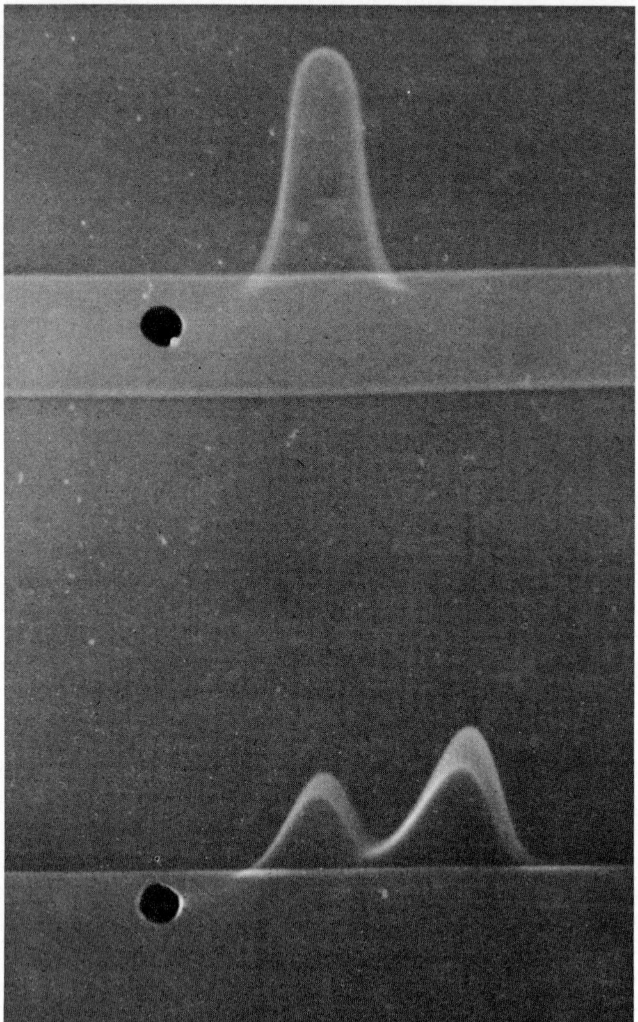

Fig. 2. This shows the crossed electrophoresis of normal serum (top), and serum treated with antigen–antibody complexes for one hour at 37° (bottom). The antiserum in the second phase was anti-C3.

The anaphylactic fragment C3a can also be antigenic when isolated and injected into experimental animals, although few anti-C3 antisera contain antibodies to this peptide. Similarly C3d contains an antigenic determinant (or determinants) called the D antigen, which is not present on C3c. On immunoelectrophoresis of aged serum or serum treated with antigen–antibody complexes this fragment migrates more anodally than C3c, and is known as α-2-D, although it is more heterogeneous than the other major C3 breakdown product. Many anti-C3 antisera fail to show precipitating antibodies to this determinant.

C3 is metabolized relatively rapidly with a fractional catabolic rate of approximately 2% of the plasma pool per hour, and a synthetic rate of approximately 1·5 mg/kg/hr, and a plasma half-life of between two and three days. Activated C3 (C3b or C3c or both) is much more rapidly removed with a clearance of from 5 to 20 times that of native C3. However, there appears to be a more slowly removed component, and it is likely that this is α-2-D or free C3d, since this component is readily observed free in plasma freshly taken in clinical illnesses in which complement deposition and utilization are known to be occurring. Severe falls in circulating C3 levels occur in some diseases, as will be discussed later, and are usually associated with a decrease in synthesis; it has been suggested that this is a result of a negative feedback resulting from an accumulation of C3 breakdown products, probably α-2-D.

Like many plasma proteins, C3 exhibits genetic polymorphism. It occurs in nine genetically-controlled electrophoretic forms, inherited as autosomal co-dominant traits. The major allele in Caucasians is $C3^S$ (slow form), with a gene frequency of 0·77, the other main form being $C3^F$ (fast form) with a gene frequency of 0·22. Difference in gene frequency exist in different ethnic populations.

Site of Synthesis of Complement

Many of the complement components are synthesized in the liver, namely C2, C4, C3 and C6. C4 and C2 are also synthesized by large macrophage-like cells in peritoneal exudates, and even in the liver the cells producing these components are the large phagocytic cells, presumably of reticulo–endothelial origin rather than hepatocytes. Cells derived from lymphoid tissue and spleen have been shown by radio-immune labelling techniques to make C3, but it is not known to what extent this contributes to the body pool. With a functional assay system, C1 has been shown to be synthesized by epithelial cells of the small intestine.

BIOLOGICAL ROLE OF COMPLEMENT

The biological effect of complement is the sum of the biological activities generated at the various stages of activation. The complement system enhances the clearance of antigen–antibody complexes by producing vasodilator peptides, chemotactic factors to attract polymorphs, and by coating the complexes with C3, opsonizes them for ingestion. Sensitized cells or microorganisms can be lysed although for the lysis of bacteria, the final action of lysozyme is required to disrupt the polysaccharide membrane.

The biological role of complement can best be understood by studying animals or individuals with a genetic deficiency. No complete complement deficiency is known, but several strains of laboratory animals and some families of humans are deficient in single components of the system (Alper and Rosen, 1974). Guinea-pigs completely deficient in C4, mice deficient in C5 and rabbits deficient in C6, have been described, and although their sera cannot sustain immune lysis, other complement mediated biological functions are normal, and the animals remain as healthy as their complement sufficient counterparts. In man genetic defects in single components have been described and are considered in more detail later. Provided that a mechanism for C3 activation and fixation is present, the biological effect of a single complement component deficiency is minimal.

Interaction with Other Enzyme Systems

In recent years evidence has been produced of interrelationships between the plasma activable systems. Experiments have shown that some substances activate more than one system, that inhibitors of activated components are shared between systems, and cross-activation can occur between components of different systems.

In the fibrinolytic system, plasmin activates C1, and also splits C3 in a manner similar to the action of C3 convertase. It can also substitute for activated Factor D in splitting Factor B in the presence of C3b to form an effective C3 convertase. Trace amounts of C3 breakdown products are present in most sera, although these are undetectable in plasma samples taken at the same time. Taylor and Muller-Eberhard (1967) showed that the lysis of blood clots could be prevented by antisera to C3. The kinin system also interacts with complement in that kallikrein can activate C1 and increases the efficiency of its action on C4 and C2.

With regard to the clotting system, antigen–antibody complexes can initiate the intrinsic clotting pathway due to activation of Hageman factor. The inactivation of C3 by zymosan is impaired in plasma deficient in Hageman factor so it probably plays a role in alternative pathway activation. C6 deficient rabbits have a defect in clotting which is restored by the addition of fresh C6; this defect has been shown to be the result of an inability to generate platelet Factor 3. When complement is present, the interaction between antigen–antibody complexes, or endotoxin, and leucocytes and platelets, results in the liberation of kinins and clotting factors.

As for inhibitors, the activated C1 inhibitor also inhibits kallikrein, plasmin and P/F dil. The plasma inactivator of the anaphylactic fragments C3a and C5a also inactivates bradykinin, while the chemotactic factor inactivator also destroys the chemotactic activity of kallikrein.

INVOLVEMENT OF COMPLEMENT IN PATHOLOGICAL MECHANISMS

A major biological role of complement is to remove antigen–antibody complexes, and in this it acts non-selectively. The system is directed and activated ("pointed and fired") by antibody. Vasodilator and chemotactic peptides are released during this process. Other non-specific elements, e.g. platelets and neutrophil polymorphs, trapped at or attracted to the site of activation may be lysed as a consequence of the interaction with the initiating complex and the complement system, with the release of further inflammatory substances including vasoactive peptides and lysosomal cathepsins. The resulting inflammatory response is a necessary part of immune defence, a fact which has been recognized clinically for many years; indeed in the pre-chemotherapeutic era the formation of "laudable pus" heralded recovery from infection. Host tissue death and subsequent repair are thus natural accompaniments of immune reactions, and if these are long-standing, repetitive and complement-fixing they produce chronic tissue damage and interference with physiological function.

Immunological reactions which interfere with physiological function are referred to as hypersensitivity reactions. Originally these were taken to represent reactions brought about by non-replicating biological environmental antigens (allergens) other than pathological microorganisms, but recently it has become clear that some of the pathology of infection is related to the immune response of the host, and that in many instances hypersensitivity reactions are implicated. These may be classified into six types (see Chapters 1 and 10). Complement is most involved in membrane-reactive and immune-complex mediated hypersensitivity.

Hypersensitivity Reactions

Reaginic Hypersensitivity

This is mediated by IgE or tissue-bound homocytotropic antibody, which in the presence of antigen results in the degranulation of mast cells and the release of vasoactive amines. Complement is not necessary for this process, but there is some evidence that in rats formation of one of the vasodilator substances, SRS-A, requires an intact complement system, although the role it plays is unknown.

Membrane-reactive Hypersensitivity

This is mediated by antibody directed against cell surface, or surface-bound, antigens. If the antibody can activate complement then lysis will occur. This is seen in the various forms of auto-immune haemolytic anaemia and thrombocytopenia, and in some forms of drug-induced disease, where the drug becomes adsorbed to cells which are passively lysed by anti-drug antibodies and complement. It also occurs in paroxysmal cold haemoglobinuria, due to the Donath–Lansteiner antibody, which fixes C1 and C4 in the relatively low temperatures of the extremities, and then on returning to the central core temperature is eluted leaving the activated components to form C3 convertase, and continue the process to cell lysis. Similarly in paroxysmal nocturnal haemoglobinuria (PNH) the red cells are unusually susceptible to the lytic effects of the later components. These effects are discussed in detail in Chapter 26. Lowering the blood pH, or decreasing the ionic strength, by activating C1 produce sufficient fluid phase activation and generates enough $C\overline{567}$ to lyse the unsensitized PNH red cells in the presence of the C8 and C9 in the plasma. In the active stages of both auto-immune haemolytic anaemia and PNH, C3 turnover is increased; in severe haemolytic disease, temporary amelioration may result if the C3 level falls severely because of decreased synthesis.

In some instances of auto-immune haemolytic anaemia, the C3 convertase does not trigger the attack mechanism, or at least not effectively, so that direct lysis in the circulation does not occur. Antibody and complement coat the cells with C3 so that they are removed in the reticulo–endothelial system. This happens particularly with IgM cold antibody auto-immune haemolytic disease, often seen after infections, especially virus and mycoplasma infections.

Immune Complex Reactions

These occur when antigen–antibody complexes interact with complement in the capillary circulation and in the tissues; this is seen when antigen is introduced locally in the presence of existing antibody (Arthus reaction). Such reactions occur in the lungs on repeated inhalation of fungal or other antigens to which the individual has become sensitized and to which appreciable amounts of precipitating antibody have developed (see Chapter 21). It is also the basis of the severe local reactions which may occur after re-immunization with tetanus toxoid, or during courses of "densensitization" to antigens. Histologically there is a marked vasculitis, and immunofluorescence shows that immunoglobulins and C3 are deposited on the vascular endothelium, and in the tissue spaces.

Soluble Complex Disease

If a large molecular weight protein antigen is introduced systemically in the absence of antibody, then as the antibody response occurs, the antigen–antibody complexes first formed are in antigen excess. These are poorly cleared by the reticulo–endothelial system, since they do not reach sufficient size and fix complement poorly.

Circulating complexes may deposit in the walls of small vessels, often end-arterioles of the skin, joints, kidneys and serous surfaces, where they cause low-grade complement fixation with subacute inflammation and tissue damage. In man this is seen in serum sickness where an injection of hetero-specific serum (e.g. horse anti-tetanus serum) is followed by pyrexia, urticaria, joint pains and proteinuria. At the onset of proteinuria and the other clinical manifestations there is a fall in the serum complement. In animals the development of widespread vasculitis can be prevented by prior decomplementation with cobra venom factor or by inducing a neutropenia. This illustrates the dependence on the complement system of damaging effects of immune complexes.

Cell-mediated Reactions

Complement is not thought to play a role in the inflammatory events that accompany cell mediated reactions, although lymphocytes carry C8 molecules on their surfaces and it has been suggested that these may be activated directly in some mechanisms of lymphocyte cytotoxicity. This has yet to be clarified.

THE ROLE OF COMPLEMENT IN RENAL DISEASE

There are two main types of immunologically mediated renal damage (see Chapter 17). One is due to the presence of anti-basement membrane antibodies, which result in a direct complement-mediated attack. This is seen in Goodpasture's syndrome, rarely in some other types of chronic glomerulonephritis, and occasionally in fulminant acute nephritis. The more common mechanism is produced by the deposition of soluble immune complexes, as in serum sickness, systemic lupus erythematosus (SLE) and malarial nephrosis. The complexes activate both classical and alternative complement pathways, and immunoglobulins, C3 and elements of both the classical and alternative pathways are deposited in irregular aggregates ("lumpy-bumpy" immunofluoresent staining) in the mesangium and on the basement membrane. In many forms of chronic glomerulonephritis, e.g. proliferative, membranous or mesangio–capillary glomerulonephritis, immunoglobulins and complement are also deposited in the glomeruli, and are presumed to be responsible for the damage, although in the vast majority of cases the nature of the antigen involved is obscure. In many cases of glomerulonephritis, activation of complement appears to be almost exclusively by the alternative pathway, since although the serum C3 may be depressed, levels of C1, C4 and C2 may be normal. Also C3, properdin and Factor B, but not C1q or C4 may be demonstrated by immunofluorescence in the glomeruli. This suggests the possibility that the antigens involved are mainly derived from bacterial polysaccharides, although other factors, such as chronic hypercatabolism of C3 via the alternative pathway (see below), and the polysaccharide nature of the basement membrane itself may play some part in the pattern of complement activation seen. In acute post-streptococcal glomerulonephritis immune complexes of streptococcal antigens and antibody are deposited in the kidney, but although there is initial classical and alternative pathway activation, the alternative pathway soon predominates. Some patients with acute nephritis showing characteristic histological lesions and immunofluorescent appearances, never develop a low serum complement, presumably because synthesis, instead of being inhibited, increases to match the increased consumption. The nature of the aetiological agent may be important in this respect and organisms and antigens other than the β-haemolytic streptococcus may be involved.

C3 "Nephritic Factor" (C3 NeF)

Some patients with renal disease, especially those with mesangio–capillary glomerulonephritis, have a factor in their serum which on incubation with normal serum results in inactivation of C3 via the alternative pathway. This has been called the C3 nephritic factor (Spitzer *et al.*, 1969) although it has also been found, in the absence of clinical and histological renal diseases, in children with partial lipodystrophy (Thompson and White, 1973). It is a heat-labile 7S globulin, associated with the IgG fraction of the serum proteins. A report that it could be precipitated by anti-IgG (Thompson, 1972) has not been substantiated and it has been isolated free from immunoglobulins (Vallota *et al.*, 1974). There is some evidence that it is a component of the alternative pathway in an activated form but further characterization is required. During the course of the disease its presence in the circulation can vary, but in general it is unrelated to the clinical state of the patient. It has been reported to persist in serum for several weeks after bilateral nephrectomy and renal transplantation before becoming undetectable. Its presence is associated with very low C3 levels and hypercatabolism of C3. Transient C3 inactivators have been reported in acute nephritis and it is well known that circulating immune complexes can be anti-complementary and activate C3 via the classical pathway.

INHERITED OR PRIMARY COMPLEMENT DEFICIENCIES

Most changes in complement levels are a reflection of immunological processes occurring in diseased organs and tissues. However, in some instances preimary defects in the complement system are present and are a major contributing factor to the pathology.

Immune complex diseases, including SLE, mesangiocapillary glomerulonephritis and chronic anaphylactoid purpura occur with greater frequency than would be expected among the relatively few individuals with known genetic complement deficiencies. These illnesses have been described among kindreds with C2 deficiency, patients with hereditary angioneurotic oedema (in which there are chronically low levels of C4 and C2), and in partial lipodystrophy, in which hypercatabolism and low levels of C3 may be present. It has been postulated that the common factor in these conditions is inadequate antigen clearance due to the defective complement system, allowing immune complexes to circulate and be deposited in the kidneys and other organs, rather than be removed in the reticulo–endothelial system.

Complement defects are relatively rare, and broadly two types of clinical syndrome are recognized. One is angioneurotic oedema, due to a deficiency of the Cl esterase inhibitor, and the other is immune deficiency, with a decreased ability to resist bacterial infection. This may be the consequence of a deficiency of any of a number of complement components, e.g., C3b inhibitor, Clr, C3 or C5.

Complement Inhibitor Deficiencies

Genetic deficiency of inhibitors of the complement system produces characteristic disease patterns.

C1 Esterase Inhibitor Deficiency

This gives rise to the condition of hereditary angioneurotic oedema. This protein inhibits activated components of several systems, including kallikrein, plasmin and PF/dil as well as Cl. All the systems are subject to low-grade continuous activation, and their combined effects may exhaust any limited supplies of the inhibitor. In this disease such deficits occur locally in the body, allowing activated Cl to act on C4 and C2 in the fluid phase, generating the kinin-like peptide, and also producing some C3 convertase to generate C3a anaphylotoxin. Kallikrein becomes activated and generates bradykinin.

The defect occurs as a familial trait and several kindreds have been described. The inheritance is by an autosomal dominant gene, and it is one of the few situations where the heterozygote manifests the disease; this is presumably because the normal level of the inhibitor is critical. Acquired forms and spontaneous, non-familial cases have been described: 10–20% of cases have normal amounts of the protein, but it is defective and does not function.

The clinical syndrome consists of painless swelling of local areas in the limbs, face and trunk, which in children may be preceded by a transient skin rash resembling erythema marginatum. Sometimes the oedema occurs in the mesentery, causing episodes of abdominal pain and vomiting, or watery diarrhoea, and occasionally the vocal cords are affected causing respiratory obstruction, which can be fatal. The swelling disappears spontaneously in 2–3 days. The attacks are relatively infrequent in childhood, but increase in adolescence. Although they can occur without a precipitating cause, they sometimes follow infections, trauma or even psychological stress.

The diagnosis is made by finding low levels of the inhibitor, either functionally or immunochemically. In the active stages of the disease, the uninhibited C1 esterase acts on C4 and C2 causing an increased turnover and low serum levels. Although the turnover of C3 is increased slightly, the serum levels are usually normal. In about 15% of cases, the inhibitor is present, but is functionally defective. This form usually has a slower electrophoretic mobility than the normal inhibitor, but unless electrophoresis or a functional assay are performed the diagnosis may be missed.

The symptoms usually fail to respond to antihistamines, and poorly if at all to steroids. Treatment of an acute attack is by infusion of fresh plasma, while success in prevention has been achieved by long term treatment with ε-amino–caproic acid or its cyclic analogue, tranexamic acid.

C3 Inhibitor Deficiency

This has been recognized in association with Klinefelter's syndrome and life-long tendency to recurrent infections (Alper *et al.*, 1970). Since the inhibitor (also called KAF) modulates the effect of C3b, its absence results in a constant overaction and exhaustion of the alternative pathway. This patient had an increased C3 turnover and a low serum C3 level—all of it in the form of C3b—as well as activated Factor D and a very low level of Factor B. The red cells were Coombs positive for C3 although not for IgG or other auto-antibody. The serum was unable to support phagocytosis and bacterial killing, although normal levels of C1, C4 and C2 were present. These defects were reversed by an infusion of plasma, and also in subsequent tests, by replacement of the C3b inhibitor alone. Changes similar to those seen in this patient have been produced *in vitro*, by immunochemically depleting fresh normal serum of the inhibitor (Nicol and Lachmann, 1973). The discovery of this patient and the results of the study on his serum provided one line of evidence that helped to re-establish the validity of the properdin system.

Complement Related Immunodeficiency

C1r Deficiency and C3 Deficiency

A few individuals with isolated C1r deficiency and a single case of the complete absence of C3 have been described, all of whom show an increased tendency to bacterial infections. The C1r deficiency was reported in two families.

C3 Hypercatabolism

An acquired hypercatabolism of C3 has also been associated with increased infections. This has been reported in some patients with partial lipodystrophy, a condition of unknown aetiology affecting children, in which the upper half of the body loses its subcutaneous fat. The children are often otherwise well, although there is an increased association with chronic mesangio–capillary glomerulonephritis, and some cases have been reported with an increased susceptibility to infections. Their serum may show a low haemolytic complement and C3 level, and a circulating C3 inactivator, which acts via the alternative pathway. The basic defect is unknown, but as mentioned earlier, there is evidence that this is really an activated form of an early component of the alternative pathway, and it is possible that this represents another inhibitor deficiency.

However, not all patients with partial lipodystrophy show the complement abnormality, and only a minority of those who do suffer clinical effects. Nevertheless, the association with nephritis has been used as an argument that the complement defect results in a basic inability to clear immune complexes.

C5 Deficiency

A defect in opsonization has been described in several members of a single family in which the defect was restored by purified C5, although the haemolytic C5 activity was normal. This suggested a functional abnormality of the C5, but the investigation of this defect is still not complete. More recently a case has been described of a complete absence of C5, with a syndrome of recurrent infection.

Complement Defects Without Specific Symptoms

A number of kindreds with defects of C2 production and single cases of C4, C6 and C7 deficiency have been described. While most individuals are healthy, as a group they show an increased incidence of immune complex disease, which may prove to be the real hazard of a defective complement system.

CLINICAL ASSESSMENT OF THE COMPLEMENT SYSTEM

The complement system can be studied functionally or its components can be analysed immunochemically with specific antisera. While single point analyses are of limited value, they are frequently all that is possible in clinical practice since the evaluation of complement metabolism is too complex except as a research procedure. Immunohistological methods can detect complement components bound in pathological lesions, e.g. the kidney and skin.

Functional Tests

Complement components, especially C2, decay rapidly if stored inadequately so that all functional tests are subject to the possibility of artefact. Sera should be tested fresh, or deep frozen at least at −20°C until tested, and if for longer than a week, then at −70°C or below. Refrozen sera are usually unsuitable.

The ability to haemolyse optimally sensitized erythrocytes is still the most widely used functional test of complement. The cells are usually sheep erythrocytes and the antibody is made in rabbit or horses. In research studies the IgM fraction of an anti-Forsmann antiserum is often used but for clinical purposes commercial whole haemolytic antiserum at 2–3 minimum haemolytic doses is satisfactory.

Total haemolytic complement is measured by using EA (antibody-coated erythrocytes), and because of the sigmoid dose-response curve, the end-point of a quantitative complement titration is taken as 50% lysis, i.e. the dilution of serum which will lyse half the sensitized cells in a given suspension (the CH50 titre). This reaction is carried out in veronal buffered saline (VBS) with added Ca^{++} and Mg^{++} and 0·1% gelatin to stabilize the cells.

A method that gives excellent reproducibility and has withstood the test of time is that devised by Mayer (1961). The basis of the method is that a narrow range of dilutions is made on either side of the 50% lysis point. This is achieved by making an initial large dilution of the test serum, e.g. 1 in 100 or 120 and then adding the diluted serum in 0·5 ml increments, from 2·0 to 4·5 ml, to a series of 6 × 20 ml test tubes. The volume in each tube is made up with buffer to 6·5 ml and 1·0 ml of a suspension of optimally sensitized EA, containing 5×10^8 cells per ml, is added, mixed and incubated for 90 minutes at 37°C, with occasional further mixing. A tube containing cells and buffer alone to detect spontaneous lysis is included.

After incubation, the unlysed cells are spun down and the haemoglobin in the supernatant read on a spectrophotometer at 541 nm using the supernatant from the spontaneous lysis tube as a blank. The degree of lysis (y) is calculated by relating the optical density to that of the haemoglobin released from 1 ml of cells lysed by 6·5 ml of distilled water. The relationship between y and the complement in each tube is expressed by the Van Krogh equation and the value $y/1-y$ is plotted on two-cycle logarithmic paper against the volume of diluted serum in each tube. This usually produces a straight line with a slope of 0·2. From this the volume (v) of diluted serum giving a value for $y/1-y$ of 1·0 (i.e. 50% lysis) can be calculated. If n is the reciprocal of the original serum dilution, then the CH50 titre is n/v units per ml.

Sheep erythrocytes of different genetic phenotypes vary in their susceptibility to complement lysis. A standard serum should always be titrated in every series of tests, and a correction applied if there is a significant deviation from the expected value. By this method the normal range varies from 25–40 units per ml. Ideally cells of a standard phenotype should be used although their availability can present problems.

Immune Adherence

The ability of serum to make EA positive in immune adherence tests (i.e. to cause them to fix C3) is another convenient method for assaying complement. Provided a minimum of C3 is present it is a particularly useful assay of early components, especially C4. The immune adherence indicator cell suspension is prepared by mixing 1 volume of 1% EA with 4 volumes of 1% washed human Group O cells. 0·5 ml volumes of this are added to similar volumes of serially diluted test serum from 1/10 to 1/5120, in 5 ml round-bottomed tubes. After mixing and incubation for 30 minutes at 37°C the titre is determined as the highest tube to give an immune adherence settling pattern. Normal sera give values of 1/640–1/2560.

Tests for Individual Components

These can be measured by using complement intermediates, and/or providing an excess of the other components; e.g. functional haemolytic C3 is measured by finding the dilution of serum which will lyse EAC $\overline{142}$ cells in an excess of C5–9. If serum genetically deficient in a single component is available, then this component can be measured by using EA and a relative excess of the deficient serum; e.g. C6 can be measured by finding the highest dilution of test serum which will lyse EA in 10% C6-deficient rabbit serum.

Titration of individual components is time-consuming and expensive in special reagents and purified components. A relatively convenient method using micro-titre plates has been devised for the titration of all the main components by Nelson and his co-workers (Nelson *et al.*, 1966).

Such functional assays are seldom necessary in clinical practice. What is often useful is to determine whether a low haemolytic complement titre is due to consumption of the early classical components (i.e. C1, C4 and C2) or only of components from C3 onwards. The latter occurs in some forms of glomerulonephritis where complement consumption is predominantly via the alternative pathway, sparing the components that generate the classical convertase.

"C142" Test

This is a useful, relatively simple test (Thompson, 1972) which discriminates between complement consumption due to the classical and alternative pathways. It exploits the fact that the stages after C3 are cation independent. Thus whole serum in EDTA can provide the components C3–9 in excess provided that the C$\overline{42}$ convertase has been generated. The test is in two steps, the first of which generates the maximum number of EAC142 sites by reacting

EA with dilutions of the test serum in cation containing buffer. At a predetermined optimum time, an excess of EDTA serum is added to ensure that as many EAC142 sites as possible result in cell lysis.

Immunochemical Assessment of Complement

Quantitation of individual complement components by means of specific antisera is a convenient method of analysis which is widely employed in clinical laboratories. Many clinical specimens are obtained under circumstances which prevent their adequate storage. Due to decay these give falsely low functional levels although normal levels are found as measured immunochemically. There is the rare possibility that a component may exist *in vivo* in a non-functional form not revealed by immunochemical testing, but on the whole, complement components inactivated *in vivo* are rapidly removed by the reticulo–endothelial system, and this is seldom a problem in routine immunochemical analyses. The exception is the non-functional form of the C1 esterase inhibitor, discussed above.

Complement "Breakdown Products"

If complement is activated/inactivated to an appreciable extent *in vivo*, then fragments can be recognized by the differences in their electrophoretic mobility from the parent molecule. This is true especially for C3 breakdown products. The procedure is susceptible to artefact, since natural decay begins soon after blood is removed from the circulation and may be hastened by inadequate storage or handling. C3 breakdown following interaction with the agar can occur during the electrophoretic process. Artefacts are minimized if blood is taken into EDTA, and plasma separated by centrifugation within 30 minutes. If analysis cannot be carried out straight away, the sample may be stored at 4°C for two or three hours, or at −20°C for two or three days, but for longer periods −70°C or below is necessary. Once thawed the sample must be tested immediately. The electrophoresis is preferably carried out in 1% agarose in 0·4 M veronal buffer, pH 8·6 containing 0·005 M EDTA. After electrophoresis, the antiserum used to develop the pattern should contain antibodies to C3d, or alpha-2-D, since this is the component found most commonly in the circulation in complement-consuming diseases.

C3 Inactivators (e.g. C3 NeF)

These are assayed by their ability to inactivate the C3 in fresh normal serum on incubation at 37°C for 30 minutes. Usually one volume of the test serum is mixed with 3 or 4 volumes of normal serum. After the incubation period C3 conversion can be determined by immunoelectrophoresis. It may be quantitated by two-dimensional electrophoresis with an anti-C3c antiserum, or as mentioned above, it may be estimated by single radial diffusion against an antiserum specific for the "B" antigen of C3. The difference in this antigen between the test and control normal serum indicated the amount of C3 inactivator present in the original serum. As previously pointed out, these tests do not discriminate between C3NeF found in some forms of glomerulonephritis, and other C3 inactivating factors, such as immune complexes or activated plasmin, which may also be present in pathological sera.

Alternative Pathway Activation

Activation of the alternative pathway is reflected in the degree of conversion of Factor B from the β- to the γ-form on immunoelectrophoresis. Again, electrophoresis should be carried out in the presence of EDTA to minimize artefactual activation during the procedure. Antisera to Factor B (C3 proactivator, or β-2 glycoprotein II) are available commercially. Some assessment of the overall capability of the alternative pathway mechanism in a single serum can be obtained by incubating the serum for 30 minutes with zymosan (4 mg per ml serum) at 37°C. In normal serum this results in 90% conversion of Factor B and more than 75% conversion of C3. It has been proposed that lysis of unsensitized rabbit erythrocytes by human serum in Mg EDTA is an index of the activity of the alternative pathway, but this has yet to be substantiated.

CLINICAL SIGNIFICANCE OF ALTERATIONS IN COMPLEMENT

Alterations in the levels of circulating complement occur relatively frequently in ill health. Several components behave as acute phase proteins; thus total haemolytic activity and the levels of individual components rise during many acute illnesses and infections e.g. after trauma or myocardial infarction in chronic infections; and during the active stages of many chronic inflammatory diseases such as rheumatoid arthritis or Crohn's disease. The patterns of change in individual components are not particularly useful, although information on this point is relatively scarce. Most published information concerns C3 and to a lesser extent C4. In many instances all components are elevated, although just as often one or more components may be within the normal limits.

Low levels are more likely to be of diagnostic value, and provide presumptive evidence of *in vivo* complement consumption by an immunologically mediated disease process, a decrease in synthesis or an inherited primary deficiency. Some examples of the common patterns seen in disease are given in Table 3.

Complement in Renal Disease

Low levels of haemolytic complement are frequent in certain forms of glomerulonephritis, notably acute post-streptococcal glomerulonephritis, cryoglobulin nephritis, in some patients with proliferative glomerulonephritis, and in chronic mesangio–capillary glomerulonephritis, as well as in most patients with glomerulonephritis secondary to immune complex deposition such as serum sickness, SLE, and malarial and penicillamine nephroses.

The pattern of complement consumption can be helpful diagnostically. In SLE and many forms of immune complex nephropathy there is active consumption and membrane deposition of the early classical components, leading to low levels of these components as well as low C3 levels, and variable changes in the components of the attack mechanism. Alternative pathway components, particularly Factor B, may also be low and there may be evidence of its deposition on the glomerular basement membrane.

In many forms of glomerulonephritis of unknown aetiology, a low complement may be due principally to the activation of the alternative pathway. so that C3, Factor B and properdin may be found deposited in the glomerulus in the absence of C1q, or C4. In the serum C1, C4 and C2 are normal, or nearly so, while C3, and often C5 and later components, are low, together with normal or low normal Factor B, and low properdin levels. However, these distinctions are not absolute.

In acute post-streptococcal glomerulonephritis, C4 may be low in the early stages of the disease but soon returns to normal and may in fact be normal on admission to hospital. The C2, C3 and total haemolytic complement remain low, returning gradually to normal as recovery progresses.

TABLE 3

Complement patterns in disease

	Renal disease		Acute hepatitis		Chronic liver disease[c]	Intravascular complement consumption[d]
	Immune complex[a]	G/Nephritis[b]	Early	Late		
CH50	↓	↓	↓	↔↑	↓↔	↓↔
Components						
C1	↓	↔				↓↔
C4	↓	↔↑	↓	↔↑	↓↔	↓↔
C2	↓					
C3	↓	↓	↓	↔↑	↓↔↑	↓↔
C5	↓	↓	↓			↓↔
C6	↓	↓↔	↓↔	↔	↓↔	↓↔
C7	↓	↓↔	↔↑	↔	↑ ↑↑	↓↔
C8	↔↑					
C9	↔↑					

↓ = below normal; ↑ = above normal; ↔ = normal level.

[a] e.g. SLE, penicillamine nephropathy, cryoglobulin nephritis, and serum sickness.

[b] e.g. proliferative glomerulonephritis, mesangio–capillary glomerulonephritis and after the first few days in acute nephritis.

[c] e.g. chronic active hepatitis and occasionally in "active stages" of portal cirrhosis.

[d] e.g. severe auto-immune haemolytic anaemia, severe malaria, septicaemia and endocarditis (in Gram-negative bacterial endotoxin shock, C3 may be low while C1, C4 and C2 may be normal).

In many forms of the acute nephritic syndrome and in many types of chronic glomerulonephritis the total complement level may be normal, and in fact may be above the normal range, as may individual components. There is seldom any obvious clinical distinction between those with a normal and those with a low complement, and the same components may be deposited in the kidneys in both types. There is a suggestion that patients with a high complement do less well than those with a normal or low level. While this may not reflect a causal relationship, it is possible that the switch-off of synthesis leading to low levels has a beneficial effect by decreasing the complement available for immunological damage.

In SLE and other forms of soluble complex disease, the complement level returns to normal on recovery, and may be used as a parameter of response to treatment, and as an early indicator of relapse. In chronic mesangio–capillary glomerulonephritis, in contrast, complement levels vary independently of the clinical state of the patient and the degree of renal impairment.

In many forms of renal disease, notably in acute and chronic pyelonephritis, obstructive nephropathy, most forms of congenital renal failure, Henoch-Schonlein nephritis, and usually in the haemolytic–uraemic syndrome, complement levels may be normal or elevated.

Complement in Arthritis

In rheumatoid arthritis the complement levels are generally normal or elevated, being decreased only in patients with vasculitis. Levels in the synovial fluid are usually about 50–70% of serum levels, but in active rheumatoid joint fluids complement levels are low, often less than 20% of the serum level, and C3 breakdown products may be detected electrophoretically in freshly obtained synovial fluid. These changes may be of diagnostic value, but since they may result from a high polymorph count with enzyme release in fluid from any acutely inflamed joint, they are not specific.

In SLE with arthritis but without renal involvement, the serum complement may be normal although often the C4 is low. In most forms of arthritis high serum complement levels are found during stages of activity.

Complement in Liver Disease

In severe liver damage low levels of haemolytic complement of some of the components are found. There has been some debate as to whether this indicates consumption as a consequence of immunopathological damage or whether it simply reflects a damaged liver failing to synthesize amounts adequate to maintain normal circulating levels. The latter is the usual explanation for a low serum albumin, for example in liver disease. While studies of complement metabolism in liver disease have not been carried out, many low levels are accompanied by detectable C3 breakdown products, suggesting that complement inactivation is proceeding *in vivo*.

In acute infective hepatitis, the C3 and C4 components are low in the very early stages of the disease, rising to levels above normal soon after the onset of the jaundice, and returning to normal in convalescence. In acute yellow atrophy low levels persist. In chronic liver disease the levels are usually normal or high, although in about a quarter of cases with chronic active hepatitis, and a smaller proportion of those with micronodular cirrhosis, the C4 and often the C3 are below normal. These improve on treatment with steroids. Patients with chronic liver disease often have low levels of C6, which is synthesized in the liver, and for some unknown reason, may have very high C7 levels, sometimes 4 or 5 times the mean normal level.

Complement in Other Conditions

Complement levels are usually raised in infections, except in patients with gram-negative septicaemia, when somewhat low levels of C3 may be found. In acute malaria, especially *P. falciparum* infections in non-indigenous individuals, complement is invariably depressed, usually due to low levels of the classical pathway components and C3, and this is often accompanied by disseminated intravascular coagulation.

In patients with recurrent infections in association with hypogammaglobulinaemia, the total complement is normal, although the C1q component is usually low. In acute asthma, the haemolytic complement is also elevated, but often the C4 is at the lower end of the normal range. Measurement of this component may give a better correlation with extrinsic asthma than IgE levels. Although in most cases of auto-immune haemolytic disease, the complement levels are normal, C3 turnover is increased, and in severe disease C4 and C3 may be low. Complement is also normal in many states of disseminated intravascular coagulation, unless these are associated with an infective cause.

REFERENCES

Alper, C. A. and Rosen, F. S. (1974). The role of complement *in vivo* as revealed by genetic defects. *In* "Progress in Immunology II", Vol. 1 (eds. L. Brent and J. Holborow), p. 201. North Holland Publishing Co., Amsterdam and Oxford.

Alper, C. A., Abramson, N., Johnston, R. B., Jr., Jandl, J. H. and Rosen, F. S. (1970). Increased susceptibility to infection associated with abnormalities of complement mediated functions and of the third component of complement (C3). *New Eng. J. Med.* **282**, 349.

Bordet, J. (1896). Sur l'agglutination et la dissolution des globules rouges par le sérum d'animaux injecties de sang defibriné. *Ann. Inst. Pasteur (Paris)* **12**, 688.

Borsos, T., Dourmaskin, R. R. and Humphrey, J. H. (1964). Lesions in erythrocyte membranes caused by immune haemolysis. *Nature* **202**, 251.

Brown, D. L., Lachmann, P. J. and Dacie, J. V. (1970). The *in vivo* behaviour of complement-coated red cells; studies in C6-deficient, C3 depleted and normal rabbits. *Clin. Exp. Immunol.* **7**, 401.

Bull. Wd. Hth. Org. (1968). **39**, 935.

Ferrata, A. (1907). Die Unwirksamkeit der komplexen Hamolysine in Salzfreien Losungen undihre Ursache. *Berlin Klin. Wschr.* **44**, 366.

Gotze, O. and Muller-Eberhard, H. J. (1969). Mechanism of lysis of non-sensitised cells by complement. *Fed. Proc.* **28**, 818.

Humphrey, J. H. and Dourmashkin, R. R. (1965). Electron microscope studies of immune cell lysis in Complement – Ciba Foundation Symposium (eds. Wolstenholme and Knight), p. 175. Little Brown and Co., Boston.

Klein, P. G. and Wellensiek, H. J. (1965). Multiple nature of the third component of guinea-pig complement. I. Separation and characterisation of the three factors, a, b and c, essential for haemolysis. *Immunology* **8**, 590.

Lachmann, P. J. and Muller-Eberhard, H. J. (1968). The demonstration in human serum of conglutinogen activating factor and its effect on the third component of complement. *J. Immunol.* **100**, 691.

Lachmann, P. J. and Thompson, R. A. (1970). Reactive Haemolysis: the Complement mediated lysis of unsensitised cells. *J. Exp. Med.* **131**, 643.

Mayer, M. M. (1961a). Development of the one-hit theory of immune haemolysis. *In* "Immunochemical Approaches to problems in Microbiology", (ed. Heidelberger and Plescia), p. 268. Rutgers University Press, New Brunswick.

Mayer, M. M. (1961b). Complement and Complement fixation. *In* "Experimental Immunochemistry" 2nd Ed., by Kabat and Mayer, p. 133. Thomas, Springfield, Illinois.

McLeod, B., Baker, P. and Gewurz, H. (1974). Studies on the inhibition of $C\overline{56}$ initiated lysis (reactive lysis) I. Description of the phenomenon and methods of assay. *Immunology* **26**, 1145.

Muller-Eberhard, H. J. (1971). Biochemistry of Complement in Progress. *In* "Immunology I". (Ed. B. Amos), p. 553. Academic Press, New York and London.

Muller-Eberhard, H. J. (1974). Patterns of Complement Activation. *In* "Progress in Immunology II", Vol. 1 (eds. L. Brent and J. Holborow), p. 173. North Holland Publishing Co., Amsterdam and Oxford.

Nelson, D. S. (1963). Immune adherence. *Adv. Immunol.* **3**, 131.

Nelson, R. A. Jr., Jensen, J., Gigli, I. and Tamura, N. (1966). Methods for the separation, purification and measurement of nine components of haemolytic complement in guinea-pig serum. *Immunochemistry* **3**, 111.

Nicol, P. A. E. and Lachmann, P. J. (1973). The alternate pathway of complement activation. The role of C3 and its activator (KAF). *Immunology* **24**, 259.

Nilsson, U. R. (1967). Separation and partial purification of the sixth, seventh and eighth components of human haemolytic complement. *Acta Path. Microbiol. Scand.* **70**, 469.

Pensky, J., Levy, L. R. and Lepow, I. H. (1961). Partial purification of a serum inhibitor of C′1-esterase. *J. Biol. Chem.* **236**, 1674.

Pepys, M. B. (1974). Role of complement in induction of antibody production *in vivo*. *J. Exp. Med.* **140**, 126.

Pillemer, L., Blum, L., Lepow, I. H., Ross, O. A., Todd, E. W. and Wardlaw, A. C. (1954). The properdin system and immunity. I. Demonstration and isolation of a new serum protein, properdin and its role in immune phenomena. *Science* **120**, 279.

Rapp, H. J. (1958). Mechanism of immune haemolysis: recognition of two steps in the conversion of EAC 142 to E*. *Science* **127**, 234.

Ratnoff, O. D., Pensky, J., Ogston, D. and Naff, G. B. (1969). The inhibition of plasmin, plasma kallikrein, plasma permeability factor, and the Clr subcomponent of the first component of complement by serum Cl esterase inhibitor. *J. Exp. Med.* **129**, 315.

Ruddy, S. and Austen, K. F. (1969). C3 inactivator of man: I. Haemolytic measurement of inactivation of cell-bound C3. *J. Immunol.* **102**, 533.

Spitzer, R. E., Vallota, E. H., Forristal, J., Sudora, E., Spitzel, A., Davis, N. C. and West, C. D. (1969). Serum C3 lytic system in patients with glomerulonephritis. *Science* **164**, 436.

Tamura, N., and Nelson, R. A., Jr. (1967). Three naturally occurring inhibitors of components of complement in guinea-pig and rabbit serum. *J. Immunol.* **99**, 582.

Taylor, F. B. and Muller-Eberhard, H. J. (1967). Factors influencing the lysis of whole blood clots. *Nature (London)* **216**, 1023.

Thompson, R. A. (1972). C3 inactivating factor in the serum of a patient with chronic hypocomplementaemic proliferative glomerulo-nephritis. *Immunology* **22**, 147.

Thompson, R. A. and Lachmann, P. J. (1970). Reactive haemolysis: the complement mediated lysis of unsensitised cells I. The characterisation of indicator factor and its identification as C7. *J. Exp. Med.* **131**, 629.

Thompson, R. A. and White, R. H. R. (1973). Partial lipodystrophy and hypocomplementaemic nephritis. *Lancet* **2**, 679.

Vroon, D. H., Schultz, D. R. and Zarco, R. M. (1970). The separation of nine components and two inactivators of components of complement in human serum. *Immunochemistry* **7**, 43.

Vallota, E. H., Gotze, O., Spiegelberg, H. L., Forristal, J., West, C. D. and Muller-Eberhard, H. J. (1974). A serum factor in chronic hypo-complementaemic nephritis distinct from immunoglobulins and activating the alternate pathway of complement. *J. Exp. Med.* **139**, 1249.

West, C. D., Davis, N. C., Forristal, J., Herbst, J. and Spitzer, R. (1966). Antigenic determinants of human Beta-1-C and Beta-1-G globulins. *J. Immunol.* **96**, 650.

8

Non-specific Cells: Granulocytes, Mononuclear Phagocytes and Mast Cells

P. C. WILKINSON

No survey of clinically important immunological phenomena would be complete without consideration of the cells which mediate non-specific effects of immune reactions. These cells do not carry intrinsic receptors with the structural characteristics necessary for antigen recognition nor do they produce antibody, and yet they play an important role in defence of the body against pathogenic microorganisms and in clearance of products of tissue damage and breakdown. Apart from mast cells, the cells to be discussed in this chapter belong to either the myeloid or the mononuclear phagocyte system. Metchnikoff (1893) was the first to study these cells in a systematic way and his book is still worth reading, posing many questions which investigators are still busy trying to answer. Metchnikoff studied the function of phagocytic cells in an extremely wide variety of animal species from the most simple multicellular organisms to mammals. He showed that in all of these species an essential response to injury or infection was migration of phagocytes into the injured site and the subsequent ingestion and digestion of the offending material.

There is clear evidence for specific adaptive immunity only in vertebrates. Since phagocytic responses occur throughout the animal kindgom, it is clear that these responses represent a much earlier form of immunity than that provided by lymphocytes and their antibody products. If carbon particles are injected into the coelomic cavity of the sea urchin, within an hour or so most of the carbon has been cleared and is present as intracytoplasmic inclusions in phagocytic coelomocytes. This reaction is essentially similar in appearance and perhaps in mechanism to what happens when carbon is injected into the peritoneal cavity of the mouse or guinea-pig.

In higher species, macrophages and neutrophils have membrane sites to which antibody, especially of the IgG1 or IgG3 subclasses in man, can become attached, binding by the Fc fragment, or by complement (C3b). These cells can therefore "borrow" the specific recognition capacity of antibody for their own function. Similarly, these cells may be directed into lesions and act there by virtue of their response to lymphokines, which are products released from lymphocytes on contact with specific antigen. These are examples where a specific immune response is harnessed to assist phagocytic function. However, in many other situations where there is no specific immune response, for example in the initial inflammatory response to an invading organism against which the host lymphocytes have not yet been primed, or in the clearance of material which is damaged but still in antigenic terms "self", the phagocytic cells must possess some means of recognizing the invader or the damaged self tissue. There is no evidence that this recognition is specific in the sense that a phagocyte possesses receptors which can discriminate between different bacteria or different macromolecules or can recognize different chemical forms of damage to a host cell. The question in non-specific recognition is how phagocytes (and other non-specific cells) detect many different sorts of abnormality in their environment without having specific receptors to do it. This problem has been rather neglected, and later in this chapter I shall allude to possible mechanisms which these cells use to distinguish between material that requires removal and normal tissue which must not be attacked.

ORIGINS AND FATE OF CELLS WHICH MEDIATE NON-SPECIFIC IMMUNITY

Myeloid Cell System

The mature cells of the myeloid system which circulate in blood are known as *granulocytes* or *polymorphonuclear leucocytes*. The granulocytes are divided into *neutrophil*, *eosinophil* and *basophil* leucocytes on the basis of the affinity of their cytoplasmic granules for Romanowsky stains. Of these cells the neutrophils are both the most numerous and the best studied. While in man their cytoplasmic granules show little affinity for either basic or acidic dyes, in other species such as the rabbit or in birds, these granules are moderately eosinophilic. These cells are often known as *heterophil* leucocytes in those species, but heterophils and neutrophils are functionally alike and can be considered together. The term polymorphonuclear leucocyte (PMN) is frequently used, rather inaccurately, to refer to neutrophils alone. Eosinophil nuclei are often bilobed but sometimes have more than two lobes, so they also can be described as polymorphonuclear.

The myeloid cells arise in the bone marrow from stem cells which are poorly identified because they have not been isolated in purity. It is probable that there are pluripotential stem cells in the bone marrow from which all blood white cells originate. We have seen two patients with combined immunodeficiency in whom defects of T- and B-cell mediated immunity were associated with defects of function of blood neutrophils and monocytes. In one case the marrow was examined and was grossly hypoplastic, and it is possible that such global abnormalities are due to a defect in a stem cell precursor of all the white cells. Probably representing a later stage of development are stem cells in the bone marrow which are precursors of both granulocytes and mononuclear phagocytes but not of lymphocytes. These cells can be demonstrated *in vitro* by addition to marrow cells in semi-solid agar culture of *colony stimulating factor*, a glycoprotein found in normal urine and serum. Single cells treated in this way differentiate into a clone of mixed macrophages and granulocytes. Presumably the myeloblasts and myelocytes which can be confidently identified in the bone marrow as granulocyte precursors represent a still later stage of differentiation at which myeloid maturation has taken a separate pathway from that of the mononuclear phagocytes. Myeloblasts and myelocytes do not normally leave the bone marrow. The ability to migrate develops late in differentiation in the myeloid series—at about the metamyelocyte stage and it is probable that exodus from the bone marrow requires an active migration of cells out of the haemopoietic spaces of the marrow into the vascular sinuses and thence into the circulation. Under normal circumstances the haemopoietic tissue contains a considerable number of mature granulocytes which form a reserve which can be mobilized when needed. Within a few hours of onset of a bacterial infection or following extensive necrosis of tissue, as in a cardiac or renal infarct, the blood neutrophil numbers may rise sharply as this reserve is called upon. The leucocytosis seen in disease states clearly involves two processes (a) mobilization of reserve cells already present in the marrow, which may happen within a few hours; (b) accelerated maturation of leucocyte precursors, a process which probably takes a few days to complete. The detailed mechanisms by which blood granulocyte levels are normally maintained at a constant level, the stimuli for their maturation and release, and the acceleration of these functions in disease states are not at all understood. This is partly because it is difficult to devise satisfactory experiments to study these bone marrow functions, and partly because this is a rather neglected field. One suggestion is that the level of granulocytes in the peripheral blood itself acts as a regulator of marrow release by some form of negative feedback. If so, its mode of operation is obscure.

Neutrophils, having left the marrow, circulate in the blood for a brief period only, about ten hours or so. The total lifespan of the neutrophil is not known accurately. They are certainly short-lived cells, estimates of whose survival vary. The longest I have seen is 13 days. They may leave the bloodstream to migrate into the tissues, particularly in sites of inflammation, or they may simply disappear. When it is considered that there are about 5×10^6 of these cells per ml of normal blood, it will be realized what an enormous turnover this represents. The fate of most of these neutrophils is unknown. They may be removed when effete by healthy phagocytes although there is no evidence that this happens on a large scale, or they may simply disappear. Neutrophils can disappear completely from a sample of blood left in the laboratory overnight leaving hardly a trace of debris and dying neutrophils may simply auto-digest themselves. They have a very efficient armoury of enzymes which would be capable of this self-destructive task.

Neutrophils are end cells incapable of cell division and capable of only limited protein synthesis. Their brief life is devoted primarily to the task of migrating into the site of an inflammatory lesion, performing their phagocytic and digestive functions there and probably exhausting their metabolic reserves in so doing. Neutrophils in the tissues cannot re-enter the bloodstream. However, they may leave inflammatory sites by the afferent lymphatics, arriving at the draining lymph node during the first 24 hours after onset of inflammation. They may also be seen in the efferent lymph at this time, a site where they are not found under normal circumstances. After the first 24 hours the number of neutrophils reaching the lymph nodes declines sharply and they are replaced by macrophages.

If the origin and fate of the neutrophil leucocytes are uncertain, this is still more true of the eosinophil and basophil leucocytes. Both are bone-marrow derived cells of the myeloid line, becoming morphologically distinguishable from one another and from neutrophils at the myelocyte stage. Eosinophils, like neutrophils, circulate in the blood for only a short period, perhaps hours, then migrate into the tissues, where the majority of the body's eosinophils are found. Their lifespan in the tissues is believed to be not more than a few days. Blood eosinophilia is a prominent feature of two types of disease state, conditions such as asthma and hay fever associated with IgE-mediated hypersensitivity, and infestations with metazoan intestinal parasites. A model of the latter which has produced useful information has been Trichinella infection in rats. Basten and Beeson (1970) showed that blood eosinophilia in infected animals was dependent on the presence of recirculating lymphocytes and suggested that the eosinophilia was an immunological phenomenon belonging to the category of cell-mediated immune responses. T-cells activated by parasitic antigens may release a factor which influences eosinophil release from or maturation in the marrow. However, the eosinophilia in other conditions may be due to completely different causes. In any case the lack of parallel between neutrophil leucocytosis and eosinophilia in disease states suggests that release of the two cell types from the marrow is controlled in quite different ways.

Blood basophils are also marrow-derived cells and, in function, they resemble the tissue mast cells. Both possess large basophilic intracytoplasmic granules containing histamine and other vasoactive substances and their membranes both bind IgE. However, it is not known whether the blood basophil and the tissue mast cell have a common source of origin. The source of mast cells is unknown, although they have been classed as arising from undifferentiated mesenchymal cells. There is recurrent interest in the idea that lymphocytes can develop into mast cells.

Mononuclear Phagocyte System

The name "macrophage" was introduced by Metchnikoff to describe the large phagocytes of mammalian blood and tissues, which he wanted to contrast with the smaller phagocytes or "microphages" the name he gave to granulocytes. Macrophages were early recognized as occurring both as fixed cells in tissues and as free forms in both blood and tissues. Aschoff (1924) introduced the term "reticulo-endothelial system" to cover all the cells with macrophage-like properties. Once cells are grouped into a "system", the assumption is encouraged that they all share a common origin, function and fate. There is a fair amount of evidence that this may be largely true of the various forms of macrophage and their precursors. However, there has been some dissatisfaction with the use of the word "reticuloendothelial" to describe these cells and it has recently been decided to replace this term by the name "mononuclear phagocyte system" (van Furth *et al.*, 1972). Both terms are now in circulation and widely used. "Mononuclear phagocyte" used in this context, and as I shall use it here, is a generic term which includes all the cells of the system including marrow promonocytes, blood monocytes, tissue macrophages, hepatic Kupffer cells, splenic macrophages, etc.

As mentioned above, observations *in vitro* of the effect of colony stimulating factor on marrow cells indicate that mononuclear phagocytes and myeloid cells may originate from the same stem cells. The earliest recognizable precursor of macrophages clearly distinguishable from myeloid cell precursors is the bone marrow monoblast. This is the precursor of the promonocyte, which divides and differentiates into monocytes which are released into the blood. The monocytes circulate for a fairly short time, estimated to be about 32 hours in mice, then they leave the circulation to develop into tissue macrophages. Blood monocytes are phagocytic cells although less efficient at killing ingested microorganisms than the macrophages into which they are destined to develop. However, their chemotactic responses are as good as, if not better than, those of macrophages, which is what would be expected since an efficient locomotor apparatus is necessary for them to migrate out of the bloodstream. Tissue macrophages are most easily collected for study from the peritoneal cavity or the pulmonary alveolar spaces in experimental animals although they are obviously present in many other tissues. Macrophage numbers increase greatly in both the peritoneal cavity and the alveolar spaces following local introduction of an inflammatory agent. During the first 24 hours after injection of such agents as casein, glycogen, paraffin oil or BCG, the major cell reaching the site of injection is the neutrophil. By 48 hours neutrophil numbers have declined and are replaced by macrophages, with lymphocytes and some eosinophils.

Macrophages are motile and actively phagocytic cells. Unlike myeloid cells, which are end cells with little regenerative capacity, macrophages are capable of protein synthesis and of cell division. Macrophages stimulated with agents such as BCG or *Bordetella pertussis* may divide rapidly and then form a cell line with a long life, perhaps months, which gives them the possibility of re-entering the circulation via the lymphatics, passing through the draining lymph nodes and on to the thoracic duct, and thus possibly migrating from tissue to tissue and transporting foreign or antigenic material, bringing it into close contact with lymphocytes and co-operating in the induction of immune responses. In certain inflammatory lesions whose type-example is tuberculosis, macrophages may undergo a morphological change to become epithelioid cells which are polygonal palely-staining lysosome-rich cells, or polykaryotic giant cells in which the membranes of a number of macrophages or epithelioid cells have fused to form a large cell which still acts as a phagocyte and whose nuclei continue to show mitoses.

As well as these motile macrophages, a considerable proportion of the functioning cell population of the mononuclear phagocyte system is made up of "fixed" tissue macrophages, so-called because they form constant components of the architecture of the organs in which they appear, are adherent to adjacent cells and are usually non-motile. It is not known how permanent a state this is, nor how great is the turnover between "fixed" and "free" macrophages. There is considerable evidence to suggest that fixed macrophages, like the free macrophages, are derived from blood monocytes. However, it has also been suggested that under conditions of increased demand they may be derived from thoracic duct cells resembling lymphocytes. It is not always easy to tell whether a cell is a macrophage or a lymphocyte. The largest proportion of the fixed tissue macrophages are found in the liver as sinusoidal lining cells, of which the largest and most numerous are the Kupffer cells. These cells form about 15% of the total liver weight and represent an important filter of blood-borne particles in a site of high blood flow. Other sites are the spleen where macrophages are found lining the sinuses and in the reticulum of the red pulp and also in the white pulp where they are in close association with lymphocytes; and in the lymph nodes, again both as sinus-lining cells e.g. in medullary and marginal sinuses, and as stellate macrophages within the node tissue. They are also found in connective tissue (histiocytes) and in specialized sites such as bone (osteoclasts) and the central nervous system (microglia).

The phagocytes of the body thus consist of two specialized groups of cells: the myeloid cells (granulocytes), which can be mobilized rapidly and which reach inflamed sites quickly and in large numbers, and which are highly efficient at dealing with many types of injury and infection but which have no capacity for differentiation and live only a short time; and the mononuclear phagocyte system consisting partly of motile cells which respond initially more slowly than myeloid cells but which can differentiate in sites of inflammation into cells which are more efficient cytotoxic cells than the cells from which they originated. Many mononuclear phagocytes are fixed cells located in tissues where they act as traps or filters for material circulating through the tissue.

THE FUNCTIONS OF MYELOID AND MONONUCLEAR PHAGOCYTES

The essential features of phagocyte function are similar whichever cell-type is being considered, although the details may vary from one cell-type to another. I shall outline in the next section the common functional features of the motile phagocytes, pointing out differences between the different types where necessary. This is essentially a description of what these cells are believed to do in inflammatory foci, although it must be pointed out that a great deal of the information has been derived from studies of cell behaviour *in vitro*.

Margination and Adherence

One of the simplest types of inflammation is the weal and flare response which follows release of histamine. This short-lived inflammation is not associated with cellular infiltration and, in experimental lesions induced with histamine, the vascular endothelium becomes permeable to protein, leading to fluid exudation, but it does not become permeable to leucocytes. However, long-acting permeability factors do increase the permeability of vessels to cells and, in inflammations lasting hours rather than minutes, cellular exudation is usually a major feature.

The way cells leave vessels has been studied for many years by direct observation of living tissues and the effect of injury on them. This can be achieved by observing living tissues directly under the microscope using techniques such as the rabbit ear chamber. With such chambers, a micro-injury, e.g. a burn with a micro-electrode can be made near a blood vessel and the events in the vessel and its surrounding tissue can then be watched. The most striking events are seen in venules. When the vessels dilate the rate of blood flow through them, after a brief initial acceleration, diminishes and when this happens the leucocytes become marginated near the vessel wall while the red cells continue to flow centrally. On contact with the vessel wall, the leucocytes become adherent to it. Florey (1970) has described this process as follows

> "As they begin to adhere more closely, some are pushed slowly along by the blood stream, becoming flattened and elongated in the direction of flow so that they have the appearance of blobs of jelly being pushed along over a sticky surface. Gradually some of the cells adhere more firmly until even a relatively swift stream of plasma and red corpuscles cannot dislodge them."

The early chapters of Florey's book still form an excellent introduction to the subject of inflammation and the role of phagocytic cells, even though it is out-of-date in places.

Since it can be shown that the leucocytes adhere to the vascular endothelial cells on the side of an injury but not on the opposite side, it seems likely that some change has occurred in the relative adhesiveness of the endothelial cell and the leucocyte, and this change is likely to have resulted from a change in the properties of the endothelial cells. This change is not understood and is not easy to investigate experimentally. Plausible hypotheses about what is happening at the molecular level allowing adhesion of the plasma membrane of the endothelial cell to the leucocyte include the suggestion that cation bridges are formed. Both cells normally carry a net negative surface charge. Divalent cations might form ionic links between two negatively charged groups, one on each cell, although there are biophysical objections to a role for divalent cations in binding extensive areas of cell membrane except where the cells contact one another by the extension of fine microvilli. These objections would apply less strongly to the possibility that larger molecules, such as peptides with several basic groups, might form cation bridges, especially since a number of cationic peptides are known to be released at sites of injury. The other hypothesis popular at present is that the glycoproteins of the two contiguous cells might form primitive recognition units and be able to interact with one another. In an inflamed site changes might occur in the outer glycoproteins of the endothelial cell membrane which allow them to interact with the glycoproteins of leucocyte membranes. Glycosyl transferases have been suggested as enzymes which might play a part in interactions of this type by altering the glycoside composition of membrane glycoproteins, a change which might both initiate and terminate cell-cell adhesion.

Chemotaxis

Once they have become adherent to the vascular endothelium, leucocytes frequently migrate out from the vessel into the surrounding tissue. This is achieved by migration between adjacent vascular endothelial cells and electron photomicrographs show that the leucocytes put forward slender processes from their leading edges which penetrate between the endothelial cells and that the whole leucocyte follows this pseudopod-like projection into the space between the two cells. The leucocyte then reaches the extravascular tissue by penetrating the basement membrane. Once in the tissues, the leucocytes home on to the site of tissue injury or of infection, where they phagocytose and digest the material which requires to be removed.

Theodor Leber in 1888 first suggested that the migration of leucocytes into injured tissue was due to chemotaxis and Metchnikoff took up the idea enthusiastically. It has generally been assumed ever since that the migration of leucocytes is chemotactic although this has never really been convincingly demonstrated *in vivo* chiefly because it is not easy to do so. For this reason, progress in the study of leucocyte chemotaxis has relied on *in vitro* techniques. There are two of these which have proved really useful. The first is direct observation, usually with a time-lapse camera, of the locomotion of individual cells in the presence of an attractant. This gives much information about the details of the locomotor process and how it may be activated or modified. The second is the Boyden method (1962) in which a sample of leucocytes is placed on top of a micropore filter and an attractant is placed below. The leucocytes are thus induced to migrate into the filter and after a given time the test is stopped and the migration of the cells can be measured. This method gives an idea of the response of a population of cells to an attractant, but gives less information about the behaviour of single cells or about how they actually reached the attractant. The Boyden method is in wide use because it gives prompt information about the migration of a cell population, and two populations can be compared, so that it can be used to examine the leucocytes of patients. The method has recently been made more accurate and sensitive by using measurement of the distance migrated by the leading front of cells (Zigmond and Hirsch, 1973) as an index of chemotaxis rather than counting the number of cells reaching the lower surface of the filter.

Although leucocyte chemotaxis has been studied for a long time, few people have asked the question whether the migration they were observing was really chemotactic. Chemotaxis has been defined as "a reaction by which the direction of locomotion of cells or organisms is determined by substances in their environment" (McCutcheon, 1946). It is a reaction in which cells orient themselves and move towards a tactic source and to show chemotaxis it is not sufficient to observe accumulation of cells at the source of an attractant. They must be shown to have arrived there by orientated migration towards the source. Leucocytes placed in the presence of a chemical attractant at even concentration on all sides of the cell (no gradient) show accelerated movement but the movement is random.

Chemokinesis

The reaction by which chemical substances control only the speed of movement of cells and not their orientation, is known as chemokinesis. A combination of chemokinesis and trapping, perhaps by increased adhesion, could account for the accumulation of leucocytes in inflammatory sites. However, in a gradient of an attractant, the migration of leucocytes can be shown not only to be accelerated but also to become orientated and directional. This has not been easy to show in Boyden chambers and the best evidence for it has been obtained by direct observation of the migrating cells. On watching leucocytes moving in an unconstrained space, the first thing to be seen is that they put forward a broad anterior hyaline membrane or "lamellipodium". The cell becomes elongated in the plane of migration (Fig. 1) with a knob-like tail. The contents of the cell flow forwards into the lamellipodium but the

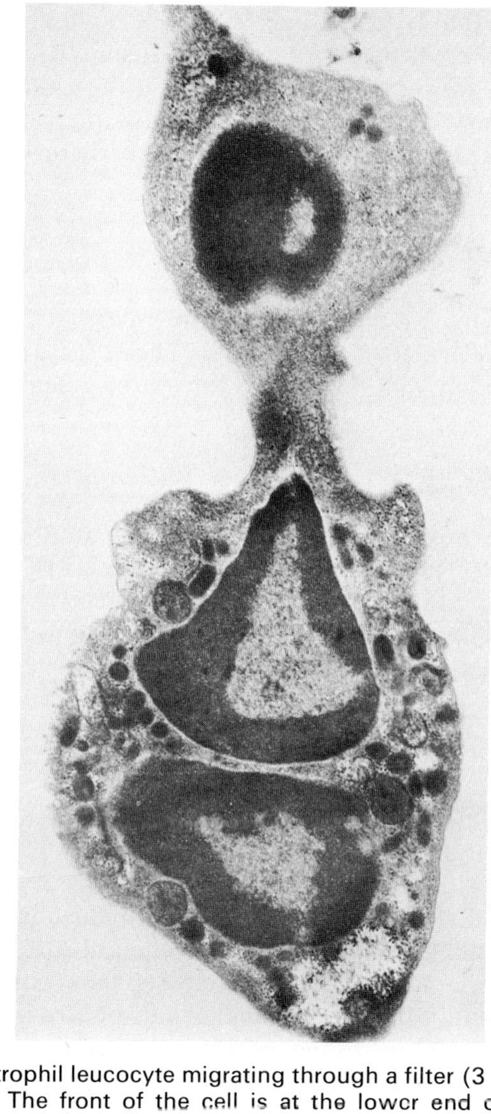

Fig. 1. Human neutrophil leucocyte migrating through a filter (3 μm pore size) towards a chemotactic agent. The front of the cell is at the lower end of the picture. Note the oriented morphology of the cell with the elongated tail disappearing off the top of the picture. Osmium tetroxide fixation. Stain: uranyl acetate and lead citrate ×17,066. From Wilkinson (1974).

tail may remain adherent until forward propulsion detaches it. The cell may then round up and the process starts again. In chemotactic gradients it can be shown that most of the leucocytes become orientated with their anterior membranes facing the source and their tails away from it.

In the tissues it is probably advantageous for leucocytes to be able to migrate by chemotaxis when there is a good gradient diffusing from a source, but also for them to be able to migrate by chemokinesis if the gradient is disturbed as must happen frequently *in vivo*. This would allow them to reach a focus of infection even though the gradient was completely disturbed.

Chemotactic Factors

A lot of interest has been devoted over many years to determining exactly what factors in tissues attract leucocytes. These factors, many of which have now been identified, can be divided into three groups.

Exogenous Factors

Products of invading microorganisms. Although a number of bacteria have been shown to release chemotactic factors, little work has been done to characterize and define these factors. Some act directly, others act by virtue of their capacity to activate complement or other chemotactic systems *in vivo*. Both bacteria and viruses exert an indirect chemotactic effect of this type.

Products of Specific Immune Reactions

a. Products of antigen–antibody reactions released at a distance from the cells. The major factors under this heading are released when complement is activated by immunoglobulin on binding to antigen or by other complement activators. The best documented of the complement chemotactic factors is C5a. C3a and $C\overline{567}$ are also reported to be chemotactic but some workers disagree about this. Chemotactic activity released from complement has been shown to be of importance in many clinical situations, for instance in glomerulonephritis, in arthritides in which immune complexes are present in the joints and in other clinical situations associated with the presence of complement-fixing immune complexes.

Non-complement-fixing antigen-antibody reactions occurring on cell surfaces may cause release of leucocyte chemotactic factors without a requirement for complement. An example is the reaction of IgE with antigen on the mast cell surface which causes release of an eosinophil chemotactic factor from the mast cell.

b. Products of cell-mediated immune reactions released at a distance from the cells. Primed lymphocytes on contact with antigen, or lymphocytes treated with mitogens, release a number of chemotactic factors which are classified as lymphokines. It has been shown that macrophages and neutrophils may be attracted by such factors into lesions where lymphocytes and antigen are present.

c. Antigen–antibody reactions occurring on the surface of the leucocyte itself. Leucocytes coated with cytophilic antibody and placed above a filter in a Boyden chamber can be shown to migrate towards the specific antigen (diffusing from below) against which the cytophilic antibody is specific, but not to other substances. Binding of antigen by the cytophilic antibody appears to initiate locomotion in the cell carrying the cytophilic antibody. This is a recent observation whose general validity has yet to be tested.

Products of Non-specific Tissue Injury

a. Humoral factors released in non-immunological tissue injury. Besides the complement enzyme cascade, other cascade reactions are activated when tissue is injured. These include the coagulation and fibrinolytic cascades and the kinin cascade. Chemotactic factors may be generated in clotted blood and certain fibrinopeptides are believed to be chemotactic. Kallikrein activated in the kinin sequence is chemotactic. Proteins in injured tissues may become denatured and some proteins e.g. serum albumin, IgG or haemoglobin are chemotactic in the denatured or conformationally altered state. Casein is a protein which is frequently used to induce cellular exudates *in vivo*. Casein is not at all chemotactic in its natural milieu, milk, in which it is present in a high molecular weight micellar form, but, at the molarities existing in other body fluids, α-casein and β-casein are in low molecular weight soluble form and are strongly chemotactic.

b. Cellular factors released during non-specific tissue injury. When cells observed in tissue culture by time-lapse cinematography become injured or lysed, leucocytes in the culture migrate towards the damaged cell and digest it. This phenomenon has been called *necrotaxis*. Not only dead or dying cells but also healthy living cells may release chemotactic factors which attract other cells. It has been particularly noted that macrophages or neutrophils engaged in phagocytosis, although themselves immobilized, release substances which attract other leucocytes.

Chemotactic responses are well established in neutrophil and eosinophil leucocytes and in blood monocytes and peritoneal and alveolar macrophages. We have recently observed typical chemotactic responses in lymphocytes, although these were clearly shown only by blast-transformed cells. Some chemotactic factors (C5a for instance) seem to be able to attract all three cell types, neutrophil, eosinophil and mononuclear phagocyte. Other factors are cell-specific or at least attract one cell type much more strongly than the others. The basis for this selectivity is not yet understood, but it is likely to be important in regulating the pattern of phagocyte emigration into different types of tissue lesion.

Phagocytosis

The major phagocytic cells in man are the neutrophil leucocytes in the myeloid series and the macrophages, fixed or free, in the mononuclear phagocyte series. Eosinophils are also phagocytic although it is not certain that this is their major function. Blood monocytes are phagocytic but not so avidly as macrophages. The process of phagocytosis seems to be similar in outline in all these cells, so they will all be considered together.

The phagocytic process consists in the attachment of a particle or particles to the cell surface followed by ingestion of the particle which becomes included within a vacuole in the interior of the phagocyte. Once the particle has become attached to the cell membrane, the cell puts out pseudopodia round it. The pseudopodia join at the opposite side of the particle and membrane fusion takes place so that the particle is completely enclosed in a vacuole—the *phagosome*—bordered on its outside by invaginated plasma membrane. Phagocytosis is a form of endocytosis in which the ingested matter is particulate. In mechanism it may be similar to macropinocytosis, a form of endocytosis in which soluble material is taken into vacuoles (pinosomes) greater than 1 μm in diameter. However, its mechanism is probably different from that of micropinocytosis, the ingestion of small droplets of less than 1 μm diameter, which is a major function in many cell types. Phagocytosis is a major function only of what have been called the "professional" phagocytes, the cells of this chapter, although other cells may occasionally show it. In the professional phagocytes it is linked in an operational sequence with other functions essential to defence, chemotaxis preceding it and intracellular digestion following it.

Although phagocytosis is a fundamental biological phenomenon and can easily be demonstrated, it has proved surprisingly difficult to study quantitatively *in vitro*. Microscopically, it is difficult to distinguish from one another the two stages in phagocytosis, *attachment* of the particle to the cell membrane, and *ingestion* of the particle. Even a particle which appears in an electron photomicrograph to be inside a cell may prove, if serial sections are cut, to be only in an invagination of the plasma membrane. Since particles may become attached to cell surfaces by mechanisms unrelated to phagocytosis, and even attached to dead cells, methods which depend on counting "phagocytosed" particles are open to criticism. Various methods have been developed to overcome this problem and to distinguish ingestion from attachment, either using chemical techniques to distinguish intracellular particles from those outside the cell, or measuring the velocity of particle uptake using "zero time" uptake, or uptake at 4°C or in the presence of metabolic inhibitors, as negative controls.

Many different types of particle are ingested by phagocytes. Gelatin-stabilized carbon particles, saccharated iron oxide, colloidal gold, zymosan or starch, or beads of polystyrene latex and other plastics are commonly used by investigators to study the mechanism of particle uptake. More importantly, in disease invading microorganisms of many types are removed by phagocytosis in the infected tissue as Metchnikoff first conclusively demonstrated. Phagocytosis by neutrophils which have migrated into a site of bacterial infection is exemplified by the familiar appearance of pus from staphylococcal infections containing neutrophils with numerous intracellular gram-positive bacteria (Fig. 2 shows an early stage), or from gonococcal or meningococcal infections in which single cells may contain twenty or thirty intracellular gram-negative diplococci. Phagocytosis is also an important mechanism for clearance of microorganisms from the bloodstream. When an organism such as *Proteus vulgaris* is injected into the circulation of a normal unimmunized animal, almost all the organisms become trapped and ingested by hepatic Kupffer cells within the next half hour. Another important clearance function of the phagocytes, especially the fixed macrophages, is the removal of damaged blood cells from the circulation. The Kupffer cells probably clear the majority of these, but splenic macrophages play a major role in the clearance of antibody-coated red cells and thus in the increased red cell destruction associated with auto-immune haemolytic anaemia.

Although many bacteria are phagocytosed readily, some are remarkably resistant to phagocytosis. These are the capsulated bacteria of which the best

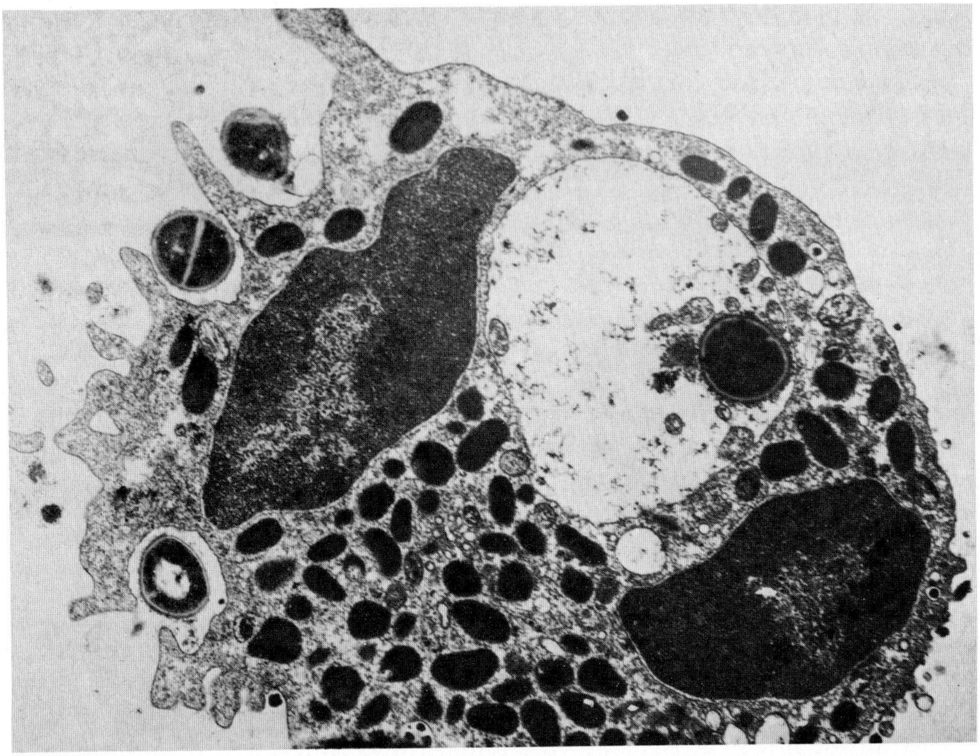

Fig. 2. Neutrophil leucocyte ingesting staphylococci and showing several bacteria at different stages of the ingestion process. From a case of bovine mastitis. ×18,500. Photograph by courtesy of Dr B. Reiter, National Institute for Research in Dairying, Shinfield, Berks.

studied is the pneumococcus, *Streptococcus pneumoniae*, which is not taken up by phagocytes unless the bacteria are first treated with an antibody specific for the capsular polysaccharide. This antibody was named *opsonin* by Sir Almroth Wright, a term he used to describe any antibody or other serum factor which could be used to coat any microorganism or particle and increase its susceptibility to phagocytosis. This opsonic property of antibody is of considerable importance in resistance to certain infections of which pneumococcal lobar pneumonia provides a particularly clear example. In the days before pneumococcal infections were treated with antibiotics, and when the infection could be observed taking its natural course, host resistance in patients with lobar pneumonia leading to clearance of the pneumococci was shown to become effective only at the time when anti-pneumococcus polysaccharide antibody appeared in the circulation, some days after the onset of the infection. A high level of serum antibody was accompanied by a rapid clinical improvement. Before this time the phagocytes alone had been unable to reduce the numbers of pneumococci in the lesions.

Opsonins allow the phagocytes to use not only non-specific but also specific recognition for particle uptake. This is termed *immune phagocytosis*, and is mediated by virtue of the affinity of the phagocyte membrane for the Fc regions of certain immunoglobulins especially IgG1 and IgG3. Many types of immune complex, both in the form of antibody-coated cells or particles and in the form of immune precipitates, are readily phagocytosed in this manner. Immune phagocytosis may happen in two ways. Firstly, opsonizing antibody may initially become attached to the antigenic particle by its Fab combining sites. On subsequent contact of the particle with the phagocyte the antibody links them by Fc binding to the phagocyte, thus facilitating ingestion. Secondly, *cytophilic* immunoglobulin of the subtypes mentioned above may become bound in the first instance to the surface of the macrophage or neutrophil by its Fc fragment. On later contact with a particle bearing the appropriate surface antigen, the Fab combining sites of the cytophilic antibody bind to it, thus allowing phagocytosis. For example, macrophages with cytophilic antibody on their surface take up *Listeria* more avidly than those without.

As well as antibody, activated complement also has opsonizing activity, which has been shown using complement-fixing antibody and antigen. For this the important step is splitting of C3, at which point C3b becomes bound to the particle and enhances its affinity for the surfaces of phagocytic cells. These cells—neutrophils and macrophages—have sites on their surfaces which bind C3b. Other non-immunoglobulin, non-complement opsonic factors have been reported in serum but not identified.

Intracellular Digestion and Bactericidal Activity

Following ingestion, the phagosome or pinosome is moved through the cytoplasm by the action of contractile proteins to the region of the Golgi apparatus. This is the region of the cell where a large number of hydrolytic enzymes with low pH optima are synthesized. These acid hydrolases are packaged into small vesicles (primary lysosomes) in the Golgi region. The membranes of the primary lysosomes fuse with the newly-entered phagosome to form a "phagolysosome" (Fig. 3). The lysosomal hydrolases are then released into the phagosomes and are able to attack its contents without damaging the

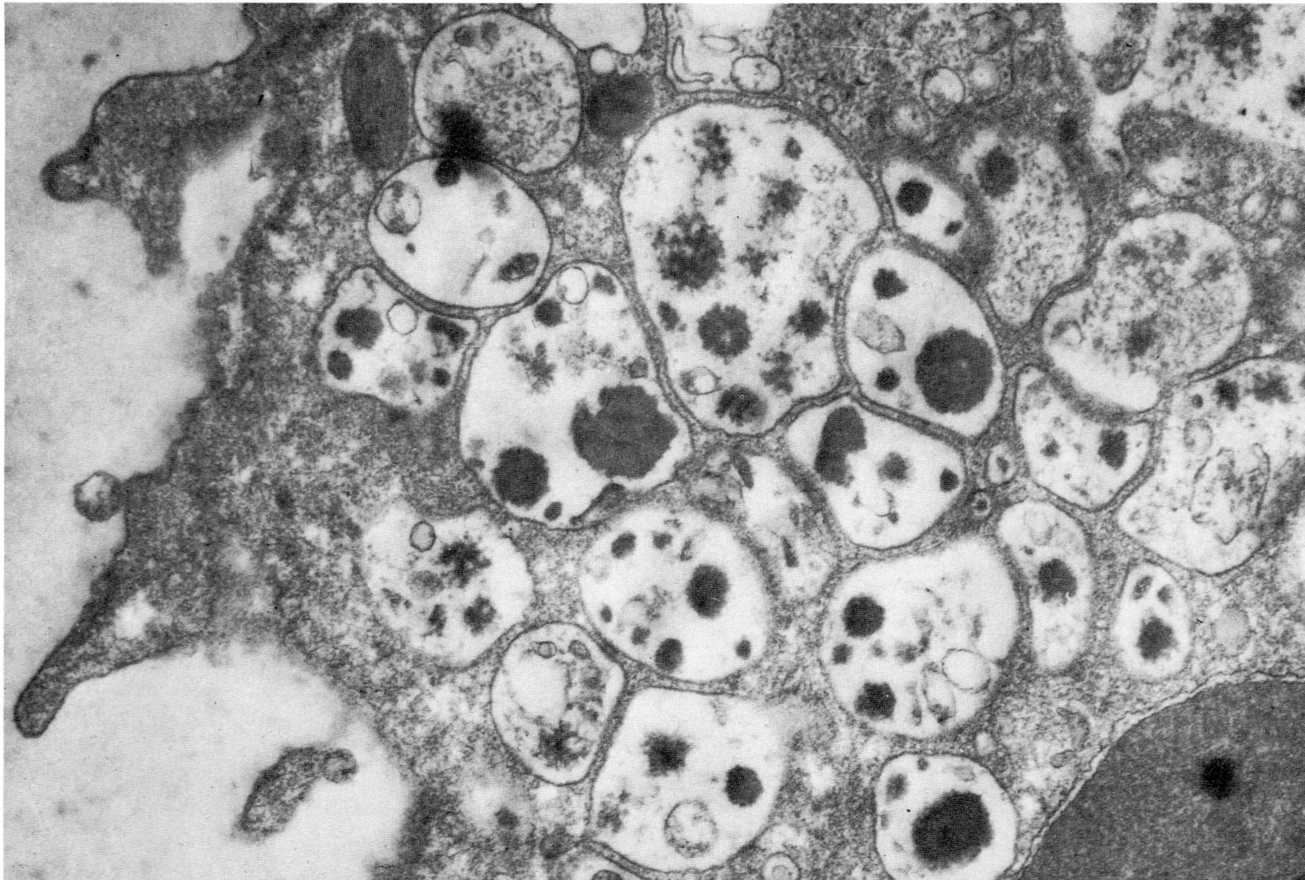

Fig. 3. Neutrophil leucocyte (bovine) containing numerous phagosomes with ingested casein. The blood leucocytes were added to milk *in vitro*. Note lack of granules (lysosomes) in the cell cytoplasm. These have fused with the ingested phagosomes. × 31,400. Photograph by courtesy of Dr B. Reiter, National Institute for Research in Dairying, Shinfield, Berks.

cytoplasm of the phagocyte itself. Numerous hydrolases have been shown to be associated with lysosomes including proteases, nucleases, glycosidases, phosphatases, lipases and others. Pinocytosed serum albumin can be shown to be digested rapidly to its constituent amino acids within pinosomes following fusion with lysosomes. Pinosomes or phagosomes which have fused with lysosomes and contain hydrolases are still functional. These are termed secondary lysosomes. In macrophages, they may play a part in further digestion if phagocytosis or pinocytosis occur again, by fusion with the new ingested vacuole and release of hydrolases into it. The terminology primary and secondary lysosome should not be confused with the terms primary and secondary granule used of neutrophils. The primary or "azurophil" granule is a granule which develops at the promyelocyte stage and which contains acid hydrolases and is therefore a lysosome. The secondary or "specific" granule develops at the myelocyte stage and contains hydrolases with a higher pH optimum, e.g. alkaline phosphatase or lysozyme.

The properties of phagocytosis and intracellular digestion which probably developed as a means of nutrition have become specialized in the phagocytes as a means of defence. Bacteria and other microorganisms taken into phagosomes are exposed to a full battery of hydrolases, so that *in vitro* it can be shown that practically the whole population of a test sample of staphylococci or *Escherichia coli* taken up by neutrophil leucocytes are rendered non-viable within 30 minutes or so of uptake. This bactericidal assay is frequently used as a clinical leucocyte function test. The mechanism of bacterial killing has been well studied in neutrophil leucocytes and it has been shown that, to kill catalase-positive organisms such as *Staphylococcus aureus*, the cell requires hydrogen peroxide produced by oxidation of glucose through the hexose monophosphate shunt, and a myeloperoxidase present in primary granules. The action of myeloperoxidase on H_2O_2 within phagosomes causes an incompletely understood halogenation reaction which may result in formation of a compound lethal for the ingested bacteria. This bactericidal metabolic pathway has been particularly closely studied because it is defective in children with *chronic granulomatous disease*, a syndrome characterized by repeated bacterial infections, chronic suppurating lymphadenitis, granulomatous pulmonary lesions and chronic skin lesions. The neutrophils of these children are deficient in their capacity to kill catalase-positive organisms like *Staph. aureus* or *E. coli*. The defect in these neutrophils can also be detected in the laboratory by their failure to reduce the dye nitroblue tetrazolium (NBT). NBT in the oxidized form is a yellow dye which is soluble (with some coaxing) in aqueous solutions and is taken up by neutrophils only in the course of phagocytosis. When stimulated by the addition of phagocytosable material, normal neutrophils take up the dye and reduce it to an insoluble form forming bluish-purple intracellular formazan crystals. The neutrophils of patients with chronic granulomatous disease fail to perform this reduction.

Neutrophils of these patients kill catalase-negative bacteria such as streptococci quite efficiently. Moreover, the myeloperoxidase system is poorly represented in macrophages yet these cells also kill bacteria efficiently. This suggests that there may be a number of other bactericidal pathways available to phagocytes to kill the large number of different organisms with which they come into contact, but as yet we know little about them.

Exocytosis

Phagocytosis stimulates intracellular fusion of lysosomes with the phagosome. In other situations the lysosomes may move to the periphery of the cell and fuse with the plasma membrane, discharging their contents into the extracellular medium. Such exocytosis can be induced in phagocytic cells, both neutrophils and macrophages, by a number of extracellular agents such as chemotactic factors or material such as immune complexes which come into contact with the cell surface under circumstances where the phagocyte is unable to ingest them. It is possible to detect significant digestion of extracellular protein by hydrolases after release from neutrophils. These released enzymes may have some extracellular bactericidal effect although, through dilution, this is likely to be less efficient than intracellular bacteriolysis. Released enzymes have been incriminated in tissue damage in sites where immune complexes are present, as in the glomeruli in glomerulonephritis or in the joints in rheumatoid arthritis. It is likely that, in migrating out of blood vessels, leucocytes are enabled to penetrate the basement membrane, which may otherwise form an impermeable barrier, by releasing hydrolases which attack the macromolecular constituents of the basement membrane thus allowing the leucocyte to pass through the hole it has itself made.

Exocytosis of enzymes from phagocytes may happen not only by the mechanism described above, but also when lysosome–phagosome fusion occurs *before* complete ingestion of the particle, so that enzyme escapes from the incompletely closed-off vacuole.

Chronic Inflammation and Granuloma Formation

Many organisms, of which *Mycobacterium tuberculosis*, *Brucella* spp. and *Bordetella pertussis* are well-studied examples, are relatively resistant to hydrolase action and therefore capable of surviving and of dividing inside phagocytic cells. Such bacteria are likely to survive the phagocyte which ingests them; indeed they may kill it and thus be passed from cell to cell. These bacteria are eventually taken up by macrophages and their continued presence induces formation of a macrophage granuloma, probably, in the first instance, by chemotactic attraction of macrophages by products released from the bacteria or from damaged host cells, and later by the release of substances which induce mitosis and protein synthesis in the macrophages which have arrived in the lesion. After a week or two these macrophages become much more efficient at killing such bacteria than their precursors were. These are called "angry" macrophages or "activated" macrophages (Fig. 4) although the word "activated" has often been used rather loosely in ambiguous contexts without saying exactly which function has been activated and this has led to some confusion. Following experimental administration of *Bordetella pertussis* and also probably in clinical tuberculosis, there is present what is termed a "high turnover" granuloma (Ryan and Spector, 1970) with rapid recruitment of macrophages and frequent mitoses in those present in the lesion. An equilibrium between host and parasite may ensue in which killing and multiplication of the bacteria are evenly balanced. In high-turnover granulomata, macrophages infiltrating the lesion are usually accompanied by lymphocytes. Lymphokines released from the latter on contact with antigen may prevent macrophages from leaving the lesion and may activate metabolic and synthetic events in macrophages which are there. Organisms which induce formation of macrophage granulomata of this type also induce a high degree of cell-mediated hypersensitivity. It may be that close contact of macrophages with lymphocytes allows activation of the latter by contact with macrophage-borne antigen. This raises the question of how a cell which is normally very efficient in degrading antigenic material presented to it can retain intact antigen for sufficient time for it to make contact with a lymphocyte. It has been suggested that there may be a specialized form of macrophage which takes up antigen without degrading it. Another suggestion is that sometimes phagocytosis is not followed by lysosomal fusion so that the intracellular material is not digested and may possibly be exocytosed later, or that particles may get into the cell without being enclosed in a phagosome. Live tubercle bacilli inside macrophage phagosomes are able to inhibit the fusion of lysosomes with phagosomes and thus prevent their own destruction.

The importance of macrophage granulomata of the high-turnover type is not restricted to bacterial infections. A similar sequence of events may occur during tumour rejection and probably also in many clinical situations where macrophages are prominent in the tissue reaction. There is much current

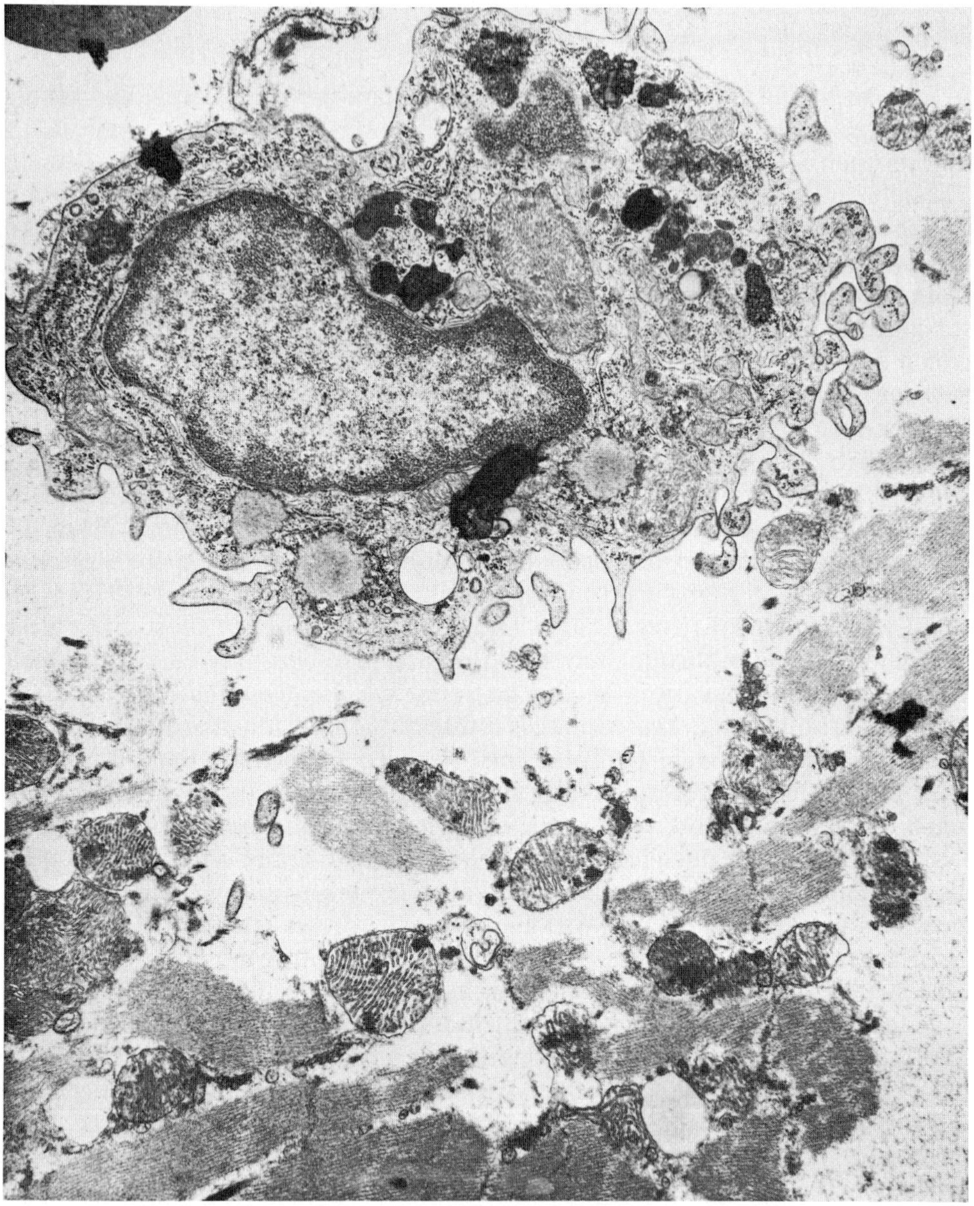

Fig. 4. Macrophage (upper) in a site of damaged cardiac muscle during rejection of an experimental heart transplant in a rat. The macrophage membrane is convoluted with numerous pseudopod-like processes and the cell contains ingested myocardial mitochondria and fragments of cardiac muscle. There is also rough endoplasmic reticulum. This is probably an "angry" macrophage associated with a cell-mediated immune response against the transplanted tissue. ×16,000. Osmium tetroxide fixation. Stain: uranyl acetate and lead citrate. From Wilkinson (1974).

interest in the cytotoxic properties of "angry" macrophages against tumour cells, the stimulation of such properties by use of bacteria such as BCG or the anaerobic coryneforms (including *Corynebacterium parvum*) as therapeutic agents, and the possibilities of macrophage interactions with T-cells in tumour rejection.

All this is in contrast with the appearance of "low-turnover" granulomata, described after experimental injection of carageenan, and probably similar to what happens following introduction of inert foreign bodies such as tattoo dyes. The recruitment of macrophages is much slower and the macrophages in the lesion which are long-lived cells show little evidence of increased protein synthesis or cell division, although there may be some formation of giant cells. Lymphocyte infiltration is not marked and specific immune reactions are not prominent. Such lesions may remain static for months or years.

Clearance Functions of Fixed Macrophages

The efficient removal of bacteria from the bloodstream by Kupffer cells in the liver has already been mentioned. These hepatic phagocytes form the main site of clearance of particles from both the systemic and portal circulations. If a large dose of particulate material is given it is possible to saturate the phagocytic capacity of the Kupffer cells temporarily. The same is true of any population of mononuclear phagocytes and the phenomenon is known as "reticulo–endothelial blockade". If hepatic phagocytes are blockaded and a subsequent dose of particles is given into the circulation, the particles which bypass the liver phagocytes are taken up by phagocytes in the spleen. Hepatic phagocytes are not in close contact with large numbers of lymphocytes, so that clearance of antigenic material in the liver is not normally followed by an immune response to the antigenic particles. However, splenic macrophages are contiguous with many lymphocytes and uptake of antigenic particles in the spleen is frequently followed by an immune response. In man, defects of Kupffer cell clearance may be found in cirrhotics in whom the blood is shunted away from Kupffer cells. These patients are, therefore, more likely to mount immune responses against circulating particulate antigens than normal persons. One of the major sources of antigen which is cleared normally by Kupffer cells is the gut. Probably food antigens and intestinal bacteria are normally cleared without inducing immune responses, but impairment of hepatic clearance may be associated with immunization against intestinal antigens.

MAST CELL FUNCTION

In reviewing the functions of the cells with which this chapter is concerned, one finds that mast cell function does not easily fit in with the rest. Mast cells are not phagocytes or cells which are known to kill invading microorganisms. Nevertheless, as I shall discuss later on, their best-studied function, exocytosis of granules, is closely related at the molecular level to such functions as chemotaxis and phagocytosis and to exocytosis in phagocytes. Mast cells are widely distributed in connective tissue, often close to blood vessels. They may easily be obtained in good quantity from the peritoneal cavity of the rat. Good places for histological study of mast cells are the tongue of the mouse or rat or the mesentery of the guinea pig. In man, they are abundant in serosal linings. They are found in increased numbers in the intestinal submucosa in parasitic infestations, in lesions of immediate hypersensitivity and often in chronic inflammatory granulomata. As mentioned earlier, mast cells and blood basophils are similar in both appearance and function.

Mast cells are immediately recognizable by their abundant heavy cytoplasmic granules. These stain particularly well with basic dyes such as toluidine blue. Their granules contain heparin, histamine, and serotonin, although there is doubt about the presence of the latter in human mast cells. It has long been known that mast cells could degranulate and that histamine was present in the tissues after degranulation. It is only fairly recently that it has been realized that, as well as releasing histamine on lysis of the cell, mast cells could release their granules by a precisely controlled mechanism of exocytosis. This has been demonstrated following contact of the cell membrane with certain activating agents such as the drug 48/80. Once the granules have been released, histamine leaves them to reach the tissues by ion-exchange across the granule membrane with sodium in the surrounding tissues. This histamine release is of interest to immunologists because it can be activated by IgE. The Fc portion of IgE antibody has an affinity for the mast cell membrane and IgE can easily be demonstrated bound by its Fc fragment on the mast cell surface. On binding to divalent or multivalent antigen these surface IgE molecules form a cluster by cross-linking with one another, which is believed to lead to a membrane perturbation which initiates exocytosis and histamine release. Degranulation is also accompanied by release of SRS-A (slow reacting substance of anaphylaxis) and an eosinophil chemotactic factor. A platelet activating factor has recently been described which is released from mast cells on degranulation and which causes platelet aggregation. The pharmacological effects of these mediators are primarily responsible for the lesions of classical immediate hypersensitivity. It is possible that mast-cell released factors play an important role in the inflammatory response to intestinal parasites although this role is still controversial.

EOSINOPHIL FUNCTION

The release of eosinophil chemotactic factors in immediate hypersensitivity, the presence of eosinophils in the lesions of immediate hypersensitivity and the blood eosinophilia common in allergic states raise the obvious question of what these cells are doing in these lesions. There is at present no satisfactory answer to this question. Eosinophils are phagocytic cells whose lysosomes, the prominent eosinophil granules, contain hydrolases, albeit a different pattern of hydrolases from neutrophils. These granules also contain large quantities of cationic peptides whose function is still not known. It has been suggested that eosinophils are specialized repair cells which enter immediate hypersensitivity lesions once they are established and are specially adapted to phagocytose mast cell granules and other products of this type of lesion. It has also been suggested that eosinophils release products which neutralize the vasoactive mediators in such lesions. For example, an arylsulphatase present in eosinophil granules can be shown to neutralize SRS-A. These are interesting possibilities which require further clarification. Eosinophils are also present in many other types of lesion. For instance, they are often prominent in chronic inflammatory granulomata possibly playing a role in cell-mediated responses as suggested earlier. Eosinophils migrate towards chemotactic factors such as C5a to which neutrophils and monocytes also migrate, so they may play an unknown role in many types of inflammation.

BIOCHEMICAL EVENTS IN CELLS WHICH MEDIATE NON-SPECIFIC IMMUNITY

Metabolic Events

It has become clear over the last decade or so that many of the functions discussed in this chapter, chemotaxis, phagocytosis, lysosome-phagosome fusion and exocytosis whether of mast cell granules or of lysosomes from phagocytic cells, require the expenditure by the cell of considerable energy which is mainly derived from the dephosphorylation of ATP formed by the metabolism of glucose. The cells are normally in a resting state using little energy until called upon to perform one or several of the above-mentioned functions. When this happens they show what has been called a metabolic burst, a term usually prefixed by the adjective "dramatic" by those authors who have studied it. Their consumption of oxygen and utilization of glucose increase sharply. The glucose may be derived from cytoplasmic glycogen granules which are abundant in neutrophils. Much of the energy is derived from anaerobic glycolysis and during the metabolic burst lactate accumulates in the cell. Neutrophils contain only scanty mitochondria and their capacity to derive ATP from oxidative phosphorylation may be limited. Macrophages may have a greater capacity to use oxidative sources of energy, but it seems that in them, too, anaerobic glycolysis is the major energy source during the metabolic burst. It has been suggested that the functions of phagocytic cells are also controlled by intracellular levels of cyclic AMP and cyclic GMP, since these functions are claimed to be facilitated by low intracellular cyclic AMP levels or by high cyclic GMP levels, and conversely, to be depressed by high intracellular cyclic AMP levels or by low cyclic GMP levels.

Contractile Proteins

The two major proteins, actin and myosin, which interact with one another during the contraction of muscle are now known to occur, not only in muscle, but also in many other cells including neutrophil leucocytes, mononuclear phagocytes and mast cells. In these cells actin is arranged within the cytoplasm in the form of *microfilaments* composed of long fine strands, about 5 to 8 nm wide, of helically polymerized actin which become "decorated" at regular intervals with heavy meromyosin when this is added *in vitro*. This decoration of the actin strand gives rise to the "arrowhead" appearance of microfilaments described by electron microscopists. On activation, cytoplasmic actin and myosin are believed to slide along on one another, as happens in a muscle fibre so that the apparent result is a contraction of the microfilament. If the microfilament is tethered at both ends, for instance to the plasma membrane or to the membranes of intracellular structures, this contraction will lead to a change in shape of the cell or part of the cell. Myosin is an ATPase and the conversion of ATP to ADP is a necessary step in the contraction which is also dependent on the local Ca^{++} concentration as discussed below. Actin in the cell cytoplasm is in equilibrium between a soluble form and the polymerized microfilamentous form, so that there is an equilibrium between assembly and disassembly of microfilaments which allows their rapid formation or dissolution as required in appropriate sites in the cell. It is believed that the detailed changes in shape which occur during phagocytosis, during the movement of the cell in chemotaxis, and during the movement of intracellular organelles in exocytosis, mast cell degranulation and lysosome-phagosome fusion, are all mediated by contraction of microfilaments and that, if the microfilaments are paralysed, these functions are blocked. This is a compelling idea but the evidence for it is still rather weak, being based partly on extrapolation from electron microscope appearances, and partly on inhibition of these functions by a drug, cytochalasin B, whose action is not truly microfilament-specific. However, the idea seems so attractive that better evidence may be expected soon.

There is another system of filamentous processes widely distributed in tissue cells, the *microtubule* system. This consists of an intracytoplasmic network of hollow cylinders which appear coarser in the microscope (outer diameter about 20 to 25 nm) than the microfilaments. It is based on the protein tubulin, which, like actin, is in equilibrium between a soluble and a tubular polymerized state, so that microtubules, like microfilaments, are in equilibrium between assembly and disassembly. Microtubules have been studied chiefly in the cilia and flagella of simple invertebrates and little is known of the molecular biology of microtubule function in leucocytes. They are known to form the mitotic spindle and it is believed that they are important in a number of cell functions because they form a rigid cytoskeleton, a sort of intracytoplasmic scaffolding which gives a cell the right sort of shape to perform a given function. For instance, as mentioned earlier, locomoting neutrophils and macrophages take on an oriented polarized shape with a defined front and back when they begin to move. Probably when this happens, the microtubules become oriented in the cell's long axis. If the microtubules are depolymerized using colchicine or vinblastine or a number of other anti-tubulin drugs, the cells still migrate vigorously but their shape is ill-defined and they may take on bizarre forms. This incoordination of movement destroys the cell's ability to detect chemotactic gradients, although they still show strong chemokinesis (see the definitions of these words above). To take another example, when normal phagocytes take in phagosomes, the phagosomes are normally moved in an orderly manner towards the Golgi region. Cells without microtubules still phagocytose well but the phagosomes move within the cytoplasm in a haphazard manner. Lysosome-phagosome fusion still occurs, so this is presumably a microfilament-mediated function. Microfilaments thus appear to operate cell movements, and microtubules to coordinate the movements.

In contracting muscle there is a critical requirement for divalent cations. The cytoplasmic Ca^{++} concentration is normally low (10^{-8}M to 10^{-7}M). When the muscle is activated by a nerve impulse, depolarization of the membrane occurs and this allows an influx of Ca^{++}, raising the cytoplasmic concentration of Ca^{++} to 10^{-6}M to 10^{-5}M and allowing a contraction. This Ca^{++} probably comes not from outside the cell, but from the sarcoplasmic reticulum, an intracytoplasmic vesicular network containing high concentrations of bound calcium. Since the membrane of the sarcoplasmic reticulum is in direct contact with the plasma membrane, it itself becomes depolarized when the plasma membrane is depolarized and releases its bound calcium into the cytoplasm. After contraction, and in order for the muscle to relax, it is required that the cytoplasmic Ca^{++} be removed rapidly and this Ca^{++} is taken back into the sarcoplasmic reticulum by an ATP-driven cation pump. This mechanism in muscle is described here because it is probable that the initiation of contractile events in phagocytes is very similar to that in muscle, although in phagocytes it has not, as yet, been intensively studied. It is known that cation fluxes are important for initiating these events but the site of intracellular storage of divalent cations has not been established. Also, the way in which the leucocyte membrane is activated is clearly different from a nerve impulse.

This account suggests that there are many analogies between phagocytes or mast cells at work and muscles at work. The body is able to use similar molecular mechanisms to serve very different functions in different cells.

Control and Recognition

The metabolic and contractile events described above are activated when certain molecules outside the cell make contact with the cell membrane. Chemotactic factors activate locomotion, phagocytosable particles activate the ingestion process and membrane-bound immunoglobulin interacting with antigen activates several functions in different cells. How do these extracellular molecules pass their message on to activate events inside the cell? The answer is not known with any certainty yet, but there is much interest in the idea that leucocytes, like nerve and muscle, are excitable cells whose membranes are influenced by appropriate signals from outside and that the transmission of the signal involves a transient increase in membrane permeability allowing cation fluxes as described above. If such a cation flux occurs locally at a particular site in the cell where the activating agent has made contact with the cell membrane, local contractile events will follow whose detailed pattern will differ according to the type of stimulus received. Thus contact with a particle leads to enclosure of the particle by extension of pseudopods, contact with a chemotactic factor leads to the assumption of an oriented, locomotor morphology and so on. How this is achieved in detail is not understood.

This brings us back to the problem of recognition mentioned at the beginning of this chapter. Why for instance are capsulated bacteria resistant to phagocytosis whereas the same bacteria without capsules are phagocytosed readily? Why do certain proteins evoke a chemotactic response whereas closely related proteins do not? The answer probably lies in the way these bacteria or proteins interact with the cell membrane. It may be that those agents which can bind to the membrane in such a way as to increase its permeability to ions and therefore initiate contractile events will be "recognized" by the phagocyte, while those which bind in a different way or fail to bind will not. Since membranes are composed of a fluid lipid bilayer with protein molecules floating in the lipid and able to move laterally, it is possible that permeability changes might occur either if the bilayer is disturbed directly by molecules which are able to penetrate it or if proteins cluster to allow formation of hydrophilic "pores" through the hydrophobic lipid. There is some evidence that chemotactic agents or the surface components of phagocytosable particles are able to penetrate directly into the hydrophobic interior of the lipid bilayer of the cell membrane perturbing the arrangement of water- and ion-excluding hydrophobic groups there and increasing the membrane's permeability. It is the energy of the hydrophobic interactions within the bilayer which maintains the barrier segregating the inside of the cell from the outside world, thus preserving the cell's integrity. To penetrate into the bilayer, the activating substance would itself have to possess hydrophobic sites whose thermodynamic properties would favour integration into a non-polar environment such as the interior of a lipid bilayer. Thus the relative hydrophobicity of substances in the extracellular medium may be important in enabling them to "excite" leucocytes. If this is true, the capsulated bacterium with its hydrophilic polysaccharide coat is not phagocytosed because its outer molecular layer has little or no affinity for hydrophobic areas in the cell membrane, whereas, when the capsule is removed, more hydrophobic groups are exposed which allow a chance of an interaction between the bacterium and the phagocyte leading to phagocytosis. I have suggested elsewhere (Wilkinson, 1974), that chemotactic factors act in a similar way.

Activation of phagocyte functions following membrane changes associated with protein clustering is another possibility. Immune phagocytosis and mast cell degranulation are examples of functions activated following clustering of opsonizing or cytophilic immunoglobulin cross-linked by antigen on the cell surface. However, to form pores in the membrane permeable to ions, the clustered proteins would themselves have to penetrate through the bilayer as integral membrane proteins do, but as cytophilic immunoglobulin does not. I personally favour the idea that activation of these cell functions follows a conformational change in the Fc fragment induced by cross-linking antigen, which increases the hydrophobic character of the Fc fragment and allows it to penetrate the bilayer. In this view membrane activation mediated by cytophilic immunoglobulin is not essentially different from non-immune activation. However the evidence at present is compatible with several hypotheses.

This concept of "recognition" in non-specific immunity is quite different from recognition based on the highly stereospecific interaction between complementary macromolecules with which immunologists are familiar. Accordingly, a completely different concept is required to explain the capacity of leucocytes to respond to the multitude of apparently completely dissimilar factors which have been described as activators of their various functions.

A BRIEF ACCOUNT OF SOME METHODS FOR PURIFYING THE CELLS DESCRIBED IN THIS CHAPTER

Human Blood Granulocytes and Monocytes

The red cells from heparinized venous blood can be sedimented by addition of dextran (e.g. 1 part of 6% dextran 110,000 mol. wt. to 9 parts of blood). After about an hour, the leucocyte-rich supernatant plasma is removed. This is layered on top of a mixture of Ficoll® and Triosil® (Sp. G. 1·078) in a centrifuge tube and spun at about 500 ***g*** for 30 minutes. Granulocytes and residual red cells are present in the button at the bottom of the tube, monocytes, lymphocytes and platelets in a layer at the interface. Residual red cells can be lysed by washing with 0·85% NH_4Cl or by brief exposure to distilled water or low molarity buffer at any stage. If it is required to obtain monocytes free of lymphocytes, an additional step separating the cells by virtue of the greater adhesiveness of monocytes than of lymphocytes, e.g. to nylon wool or to glass, must be used. However, it must be said that it is a matter of faith rather than of established fact that such methods produce pure populations of either cell type. If the Ficoll-triosil interfacial monocyte-lymphocyte layer is washed once or twice and centrifuged at × 500 ***g***, it can be freed of most of the platelets. These remain in the supernatant whereas nucleated cells spin to the bottom of the tube. The above procedure can be done in reverse, i.e. centrifugation of whole blood on Ficoll-triosil followed by addition of dextran to the mixed red cell and granulocyte layer.

Note that in all tests of leucocyte function, balanced salt solutions containing divalent cations and glucose are required. There is not a requirement for added protein in short-term experiments. Note also that the more elaborate the procedures used to purify a given cell population, the less viable the population will turn out to be. It is often best to compromise in order to obtain a cell population of good functional quality.

Eosinophils

These are difficult to purify. They can be obtained in workable quantity from the blood of persons with eosinophilia, or from the peritoneal cavity of the guinea-pig following repeated injections of antigen-antibody complexes or of whole human serum (Litt, 1961).

Peritoneal Exudate Neutrophils and Macrophages

Following injection of casein, paraffin oil or glycogen into the peritoneal cavity of the guinea pig or rabbit, large quantities of neutrophils in purity of greater than 90 per cent can be obtained between 5 and 18 hours later. Between 3 and 5 days after injection the predominant cell is the peritoneal macrophage, but many lymphocytes are also present. Macrophages can be obtained from the peritoneal cavities of normal mice without prior stimulation.

Alveolar Macrophages

These can be obtained from various species by transtracheal lavage of the lungs. Much higher quantities of these cells are obtained from the lungs of animals 10 days after administration of mycobacteria (BCG) than from those of normal animals (Myrvik *et al.*, 1961). Chickens are a good source of alveolar macrophages.

Hepatic Macrophages

These have been obtained by disaggregation of hepatic cells from one another by treatment with trypsin and EDTA and separation of the macrophages from hepatocytes on an albumin density gradient (Roser, 1968). The cells thus obtained after enzyme treatment may not be completely normal functionally.

Mast Cells

Probably the best source of free mast cells is the peritoneal cavity of the normal rat. No pre-treatment of the animal is required.

REFERENCES

Aschoff, L. (1924). Das reticuloendotheliale system. *Ergeb. Inn. Med.* **26**, 1.

Basten, A. and Beeson, P. B. (1970). Mechanism of eosinophilia. II. Role of the lymphocytes. *J. Exp. Med.* **131**, 1288.

Boyden, S. V. (1962). The chemotactic effect of mixtures of antibody and antigen on polymorphonuclear leucocytes. *J. Exp. Med.* **115**, 453.

Furth, R. van, Cohn, Z. A., Hirsch, J. G., Humphrey, J. H., Spector, W. G. and Langevoort, H. L. (1972). The mononuclear phagocyte system: a new classification of macrophages, monocytes and their precursor cells. *Bull. Wld Hlth Org.* **46**, 845–852.

Florey, Lord (1970). "General Pathology", 4th edition, Lloyd-Luke, London.

Litt, M. (1961). Studies in experimental eosinophilia III. The induction of peritoneal eosinophilia by the passive transfer of serum antibody. *J. Immunol.* **87**, 522.

McCutcheon, M. (1946). Chemotaxis in leukocytes. *Physiol. Rev.* **26**, 319.

Metchnikoff, E. (1893). "Lectures on the Comparative Pathology of Inflammation." Kegan Paul, London.

Myrvik, Q. N., Leake, E. S. and Fariss, B. (1961). Studies on pulmonary alveolar macrophages from the normal rabbit. A technique to produce them in a high state of purity. *J. Immunol.* **86**, 128.

Roser, B. (1968). The distribution of intravenously injected Kupffer cells in the mouse. *J. Reticuloendothelial Soc.* **5**, 455.

Ryan, G. B. and Spector, W. G. (1970). Macrophage turnover in inflamed connective tissue. *Proc. Roy. Soc. London*, B. **175**, 269.

Wilkinson, P. C. (1974). Surface and cell membrane activities of leucocyte chemotactic factors. *Nature* **251**, 58.

Zigmond, S. H. and Hirsch, J. G. (1973). Leukocyte locomotion and chemotaxis: New methods for evaluation and demonstration of cell derived chemotactic factor. *J. Exp. Med.* **137**, 387.

OTHER USEFUL SOURCES

Macrophages

Furth, R. van (ed.) (1970). "Mononuclear Phagocytes", Blackwell, Oxford. A report of a conference in Leiden. The proceedings of the second conference (same editor and publisher) are in press.

Gordon, S. and Cohn, Z. A. (1973). The macrophage. *Int. Rev. Cytol.* **36**, 171.

Nelson, D. S. (ed.) (1975). "Immunobiology of the Macrophage." Academic Press, New York and London.

Stuart, A. E. (1971). "The Reticuloendothelial system." Livingstone, Edinburgh.

Kupffer cells

Bradfield, J. W. B. (1974). Control of spillover: The importance of Kupffer cell function in clinical medicine. *Lancet* **ii**, 883.

Mast cells

Austen, K. F. and Becker, E. L. (eds.) (1971). "Biochemistry of the Acute Allergic Reactions." Blackwell, Oxford. There are several papers in this symposium report dealing with mast cells and some papers on other leucocytes.

Phagocytosis

Stossel, T. P. (1975). Phagocytosis: Recognition and ingestion. Seminars Hematol. **12**, 83.

Stossel, T. P. (1974). Phagocytosis. *New Eng. J. Med.* **290**, 717, 774 and 833. This three-part review covers similar ground to the above, but the final section is on clinical defects.

Chemotaxis

Sorkin, E. (ed.) (1974). "Chemotaxis: Its Biology and Biochemistry." Karger, Basel.

Wilkinson, P. C. (1974). "Chemotaxis and Inflammation." Churchill-Livingstone, Edinburgh.

Microbicidal actions

Elsbach, P. (1973). On the interaction between phagocytes and microorganisms. *New Eng. J. Med.* **289**, 846.

Karnovsky, M. L. (1974). The biochemical basis of the functions of polymorphonuclear leukocytes and macrophages. *In* "Progress in Immunology II", Vol. 4. (Eds. L. Brent and E. J. Holborow), p. 83. North Holland Publishing Co., Amsterdam and Oxford.

Klebanoff, S. J. (1971). Intraleukocytic microbicidal defects. *Ann. Rev. Med.* **22**, 39.

9

Lymphokines

M. A. BRAY and J. MORLEY

THE MEDIATOR CONCEPT IN DELAYED HYPERSENSITIVITY

The delayed hypersensitivity reaction is an immune response that has proved difficult to define. Zinsser, in 1925, was the first to appreciate the distinction between the delayed skin reaction to bacterial allergy and more immediate responses due to antibody. However, enlargement of the delayed hypersensitivity (cellular immunity) class of reactions to include other phenomena such as contact sensitivity to chemical antigens, the homograft reaction and reaction to virus-induced tumours was achieved only gradually over the next 40 years (see *Brit. Med. Bull.*, 1967). A reaction of delayed hypersensitivity (cellular immunity) would then have been distinguished from other immune responses by its transfer to a non-sensitized individual by live lymphoid cells from a sensitized donor; by a skin reaction of delayed onset and by the occurrence of hapten/carrier, rather than hapten, specificity. However, allergic phenomena exist whose classification cannot be achieved by these criteria. These include the reactivity conferred by the use of transfer factor preparations in man and the Jones-Mote reaction featured both by laboratory animals and man, which, whilst possessing the above characteristics of the delayed hypersensitivity response, exhibits, in addition, other distinctive features (especially a pronounced basophil infiltration) separating it from the delayed hypersensitivity reaction (Dvorak and Dvorak, 1974). These anomalies pose a challenge to the designation of delayed hypersensitivity (cellular immunity) reactions as expressions of T-cell activation and imply that the criteria characterizing delayed hypersensitivity responses are too loosely defined. These difficulties of definition have been compounded by the problems of quantitative evaluation of local or systemic delayed reactions and the absence, until quite recently, of chemically defined antigens.

The passive transfer experiments of Landsteiner and Chase indicated that the lymphocyte was likely to be a principal agent of the reaction of cellular immunity and, by analogy with the release from mast cells of stored vaso-active amines capable of mimicking a reaginic reaction, it was proposed that the lymphocyte might release *preformed* material capable of mimicking the delayed hypersensitivity reaction. This concept led to the investigation of the inflammatory potential of lymphocyte components by Willoughby and co-workers (see Pick and Turk, 1972). An emphasis on the microvascular actions of the material derived from disrupted lymphocytes (termed lymph node permeability factor or LNPF) retarded its evaluation as a mediator of cellular immunity; but now it seems unlikely that LNPF plays a major role in determining the inflammatory reactions of delayed hypersensitivity. Although guinea-pig LNPF has certain properties of relevance to the delayed hypersensitivity skin reaction, the soluble products generated following *in vitro* interaction of sensitized lymphocytes with specific antigen induce a much wider range of cellular responses (e.g. lymphocyte mitogenicity, monocyte chemotaxis and macrophage activation) that correspond closely to *in vivo* manifestations of delayed hypersensitivity (cellular immunity) (Bloom, 1971; David and David, 1972).

In vitro investigation of cultured lymphoid cells as indicators of cellular immunity stems from Rich's observation that small portions of spleen placed in culture medium failed to exhibit an outgrowth of cells in the presence of old tuberculin if the spleen fragments were derived from donor animals with positive skin reactions to old tuberculin, whilst spleen fragments from non-sensitized animals were unaffected by old tuberculin in the culture medium (Rich and Lewis, 1932). This *in vitro* technique was modified by George and Vaughan (1962) to permit the use of inflammatory cell populations derived from the guinea-pig peritoneal cavity, packed into capillary tubes and allowed to migrate *in vitro* as a fan on the floor of a culture chamber.

David and co-workers utilized this later technique to demonstrate firstly, that the phenomenon of antigen-induced cell migration inhibition is not only associated with cellular immunity but additionally exhibits the hapten/carrier specificity of the delayed hypersensitivity response rather than the hapten specific characteristics of the antibody-mediated hypersensitivity reaction; secondly, that the response is dependent upon the presence of a proportion of live sensitized *lymphoid* cells in the predominantly macrophage-rich cell exudate: thirdly, that the response is inhibited by the presence of protein synthesis inhibitors (David and David, 1972). This work progressed to the experimental demonstration by David (1966), and independently by Bloom and Bennett (1966) that such cell populations following contact with antigen can produce in the culture medium material capable of inhibiting the *in vitro* migration of peritoneal exudate cells from *unsensitized* animals (Fig. 1a).

DEFINITION OF LYMPHOKINES

Once the capacity of lymphoid cells to produce this biological activity had been demonstrated, it became necessary to characterize the material causing cell migration inhibition and to distinguish it from other agents which might have been responsible for this phenomenon. The association of this *in vitro* response with delayed hypersensitivity (cellular immunity) as well as its hapten/carrier specificity, implied that this phenomenon was not due to antibody. It was evident that the addition of supplementary antigen could enhance the responses to certain lymphokine preparations and indeed in some situations it has been shown that antigen addition may be a prerequisite for the *in vitro* manifestations of cell migration inhibition. However, such dependence appears to involve a restricted range of antigens and a more usual observation is that the biological activity of these materials is in no way dependent upon the presence of antigen. When bovine gamma globulin is used as an antigen it is possible to resolve this point as well as the question of possible antibody contributions to these *in vitro* responses by the simple expedient of precipitating both antigen and antibody from the active culture medium by addition of ammonium sulphate up to 50% saturation. Such a procedure does not exclude the possible contribution of small quantities of antigen or antibody, but it would seem unlikely that these are involved as the reintroduction of supplementary antigen or antibody has little or no effect on the extent of biological activity exhibited by these solutions. Differentiation from complement has received little attention but the generation of substantial levels of macrophage migration inhibitory activity in serum-free medium or in heat-inactivated sera make identity of lymphokines with complement components unlikely. The absence of antigen specificity as well as the non-dialysable nature of the material causing macrophage migration inhibition (and other lymphokine activities) serves to differentiate lymphokines from transfer factor preparations whose *in vitro* properties one might otherwise associate with such products of activated lymphocytes. Additionally, the capacity of transfer factor injections to confer delayed hypersensitivity on unsensitized individuals differentiates it from these soluble materials.

Once it was established that lymphocyte interaction with antigen results

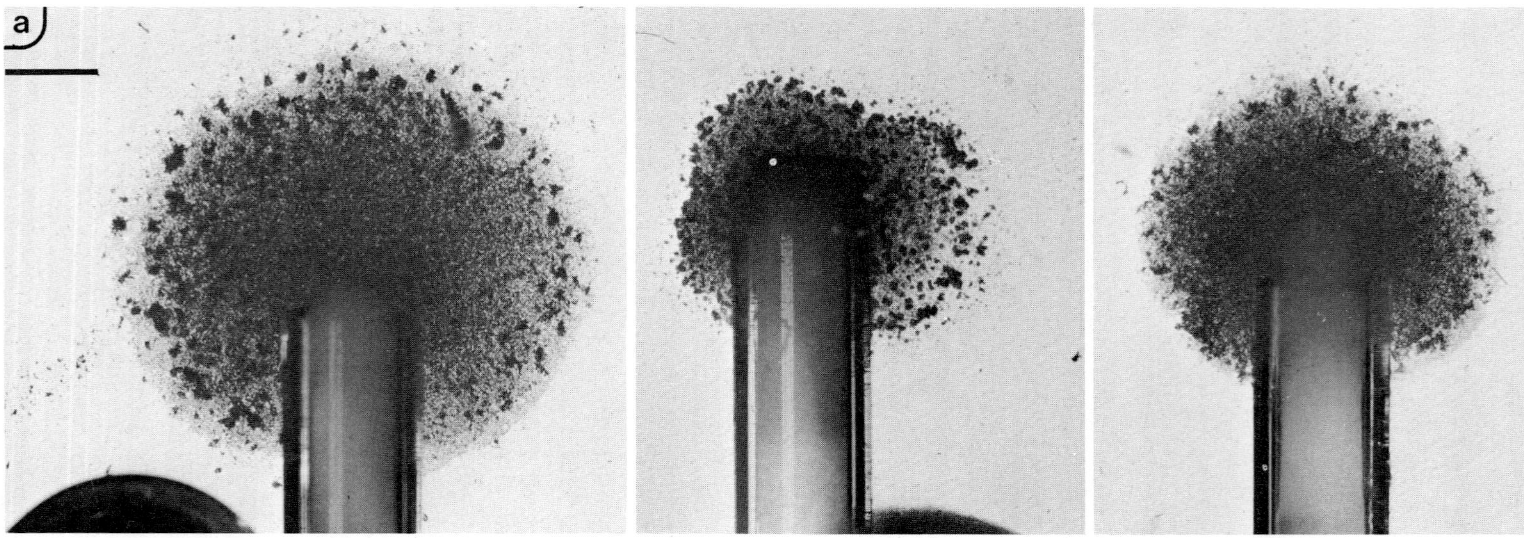
a

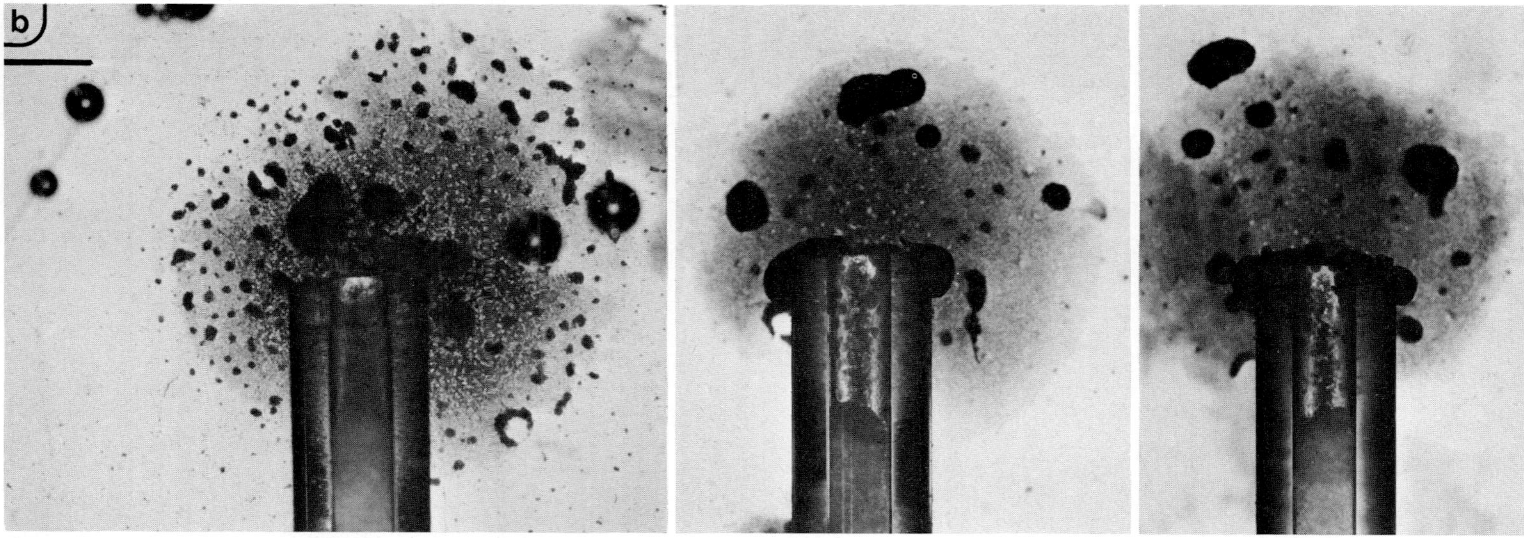

Fig. 1. Cell migration inhibition. (a) Migration of guinea-pig peritoneal exudate cells from normal animals (left); from sensitized animals in the presence of antigen (1·0 μg/ml PPD) (centre); and from normal animals in the presence of lymphokine (400 μg/ml BGG induced lymphokine) (right). (b) Migration of human peripheral blood leucocytes from a normal subject without antigen (left); from a tuberculin sensitive subject with antigen (5 μg/ml freeze-dried sonicate of *Mycobacterium tuberculosis*) (centre) and from a normal subject in the presence of lymphokine (500 μg/ml *M. tuberculosis* induced lymphokine) (right). 1·0 mm.

in formation of a material with biological activities distinct from those generated in other immunological systems, a term was needed to describe this material. Bloom and Bennett ascribed the activity they observed to a factor present in the culture supernatants, which they called migration inhibitory factor (MIF) (Bloom and Bennett, 1966). Following the demonstration of a succession of other activities in such culture fluids (for example mitogenic, chemotactic, cytotoxic and inflammatory), each was referred to by a name relevant to the activity in question (Table 1). This proved unwieldy as the number of factors is limited only by the number of test systems and it is likely that the number of biological activities ascribed to these materials will considerably exceed the actual number of active agents. The number of factors

TABLE 1
Some activities of lymphokines

Cell type affected	Action	Species
In vitro		
Macrophage	Migration inhibition	Guinea-pig
	Aggregation	Guinea-pig
	Chemotaxis	Guinea-pig
	Electrophoretic mobility	Guinea-pig
	Morphological changes	Guinea-pig
	Biochemical changes	Guinea-pig
	Chemotaxis	Rabbit
Lymphocyte	Mitogenesis	Guinea-pig
	Mitogenesis	Human
	Chemotaxis (mononuclear)	Human
Polymorphs	Migration inhibition (leucocytes)	Human
	Chemotaxis (neutrophil)	Guinea-pig
	Chemotaxis (eosinophil)	Guinea-pig
Other cells:		
HeLa cells, Mouse L-cells, Fibroblasts	Lymphotoxin	Guinea-pig, mouse, rat, rabbit, cat; Human
HeLa cells	Cloning inhibition	Human
HeLa cells	Proliferation inhibition	Human
Various cells	Interferon	Human
In vivo		
Macrophage	Disappearance from the peritoneal cavity	Guinea-pig
Vascular endothelium	Increased vascular permeability	Guinea-pig
Skin	Skin reactive	Guinea-pig
Lymph node	Lymph node activating (germinal centres)	Guinea-pig
	Lymph node activating (paracortex)	Guinea-pig

described had risen into double figures when, in 1969, Dumonde and his colleagues proposed *lymphokines* as a generic term to encompass these biologically active materials generated by lymphocytes in response to antigen or mitogen stimulation (Dumonde *et al.*, 1969). Lymphokines were consequently defined as "soluble non-antibody products of lymphocyte activation of specific antigen which produce increased vascular permeability following intradermal injection; which increase tritiated thymidine incorporation by cultured lymphocytes; and which inhibit macrophage migration *in vitro*. In the guinea-pig lymphokines can be distinguished from classical immunoglobulins by their solubility at 40% saturated ammonium sulphate and by their behaviour on gel filtration chromatography" (Morley *et al.*, 1973). This definition, though long overdue, could nonetheless be considered to be inadequate, for it was quite evident that the association of these several properties was based on the prejudiced notion that the various activities are regular components of lymphokine preparations although evidence justifying such a view was, for the most part, anecdotal.

LYMPHOKINE HETEROGENEITY

Once it had been established that more than one biological property could be exhibited by lymphokine preparations, attempts were made to separate such activities by biochemical techniques. Notwithstanding the imprecision of some of the tests of lymphokine function, it soon proved possible to differentiate between selected activities. Thus, by techniques such as gel filtration, caesium chloride gradients and susceptibility to enzymes, MIF could be distinguished from lymphotoxin, and both of these could be separated from the material chemotactic for macrophages (David, 1973) (Table 2). The problem of distinguishing those biological activities referred to in the above definition of lymphokines proved less amenable to a biochemical solution and the Kennedy Institute group (Bray *et al.*, 1976) adopted the use of repeated, multiple point, parallel line bioassay and by this means were able to dissociate the mitogenic, vascular permeability and migration inhibitory activities in guinea-pig lymphokine preparations (Fig. 2). This approach clearly establishes the heterogeneity of guinea pig lymphokine preparations and this analysis has been extended to include chemotactic activity, which appears to be associated with the inflammatory component of lymphokine. Such heterogeneity of lymphokines is consistent with observations that generation of particular lymphokine activities can be modified

TABLE 2

Physio-chemical properties reported for some lymphokines

Property	Lymphokine activity	Species
Molecular weight estimate (Sephadex G100)		
50–67,000	Migration inhibitory	Guinea-pig
25,000	Migration inhibitory	Human
50,000	Chemotactic	Guinea-pig
30–80,000	Mitogenic	Guinea-pig
80–90,000	Cytotoxic	Human
35–55,000	Cytotoxic	Guinea-pig
Electrophoretic mobility		
Pre-albumin	Migration inhibitory	Guinea-pig
Albumin	Migration inhibitory	Human
Albumin	Mononuclear chemotactic	Guinea-pig
Albumin	Mitogenic	Guinea-pig
Albumin	Cytotoxic	Mouse
β- and γ-Globulin	Cytotoxic	Human
Heat stability (56–60°C)		
Labile	Interferon	Human
Stable	Migration inhibitory	Guinea-pig
Stable	Migration inhibitory	Human
Stable	Chemotactic	Guinea-pig
Stable	Mitogenic	Guinea-pig
Stable	Mitogenic	Human
Stable	Cytotoxic	Mouse
Stable	Cytotoxic	Guinea-pig
Stable	Cytotoxic	Human
Sensitivity to Neuraminidase		
Sensitive	Migration inhibitory	Guinea-pig
Sensitive	Macrophage activating	Guinea-pig
Resistant	Migration inhibitory	Human
Resistant	Chemotactic	Guinea-pig
Resistant	Cytotoxic	Guinea-pig
Sensitivity to Trypsin		
Sensitive	Migration inhibitory	Guinea-pig
Sensitive	Migration inhibitory	Human
Sensitive	Interferon	Human
Resistant	Cytotoxic	Mouse
Resistant	Cytotoxic	Human
Sensitive	Cytotoxic	Guinea-pig

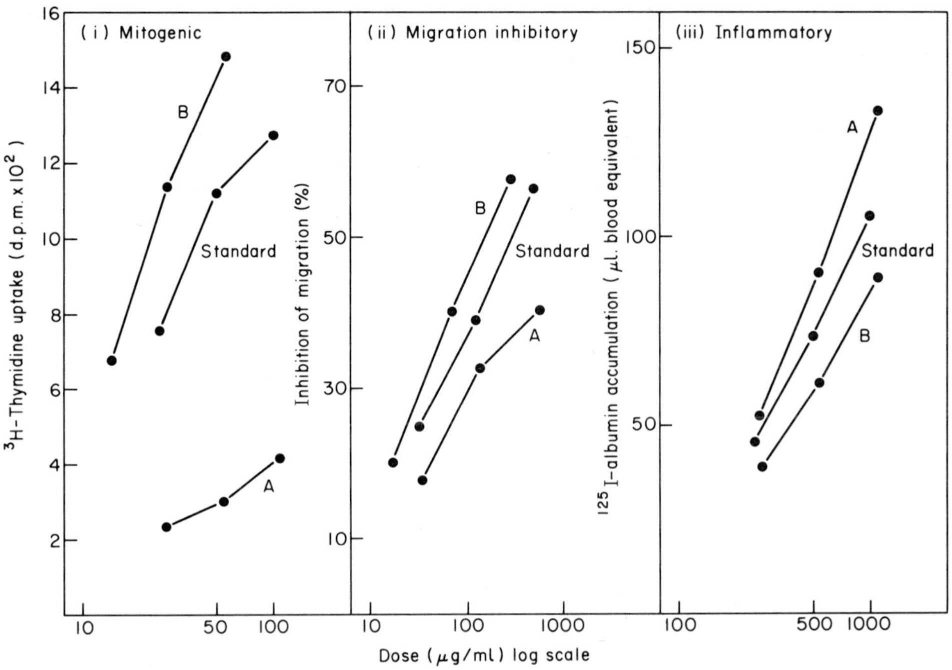

Fig. 2. Lymphokine heterogeneity. Two unknown lymphokine preparations (A and B) assessed with reference to a lymphokine standard using lymphocyte transformation (i), macrophage migration inhibition (ii); and increased vascular permeability (iii). Preparation A has little mitogenic activity, less than the standard for migration inhibition, but substantial inflammatory activity. Preparation B, on the other hand, has substantial mitogenic activity, a little more migration inhibitory activity, but less inflammatory activity than the standard. Both the standard preparation and lymphokines A and B were generated using identical preparative procedures.

independently of other activities. Thus, in animals exhibiting Jones-Mote reactivity, there is a mitogenic response of sensitized lymphocytes that is not paralleled in tests of macrophage migration inhibition. Also, in individuals treated with transfer factor, clinical improvement may be accompanied by altered leucocyte migration in response to antigenic stimulation in the absence of altered mitogenic activity. In the case of guinea-pig lymphokine production, it has been shown that E-type prostaglandins are able to inhibit production of mitogenic and macrophage migration inhibitory lymphokines whilst at the same time stimulating production of material producing increased vascular permeability (Bray *et al.*, 1975). These results may reflect the existence of separate lymphocyte subpopulations responsible for the production of particular lymphokine activities and such a system could provide the basis for considerable flexibility in the expression of an allergic response and, by implication, in pathogenic processes involving cellular hypersensitivity. Lymphokine heterogeneity is becoming increasingly evident (Table 2) and it is apparent that equating one activity with another is a practice liable to result in unnecessary disputes. This is particularly relevant to the clinical application of lymphokine measurement, where there is interest in an *in vivo* parameter which may only be assessed indirectly by recourse to the corresponding *in vitro* action. For example, the chemotactic action of lymphokines *in vitro* is generally regarded as indicating that lymphokines determine chemotaxis *in vivo*. It remains to be established that lymphokines alone will suffice to subserve this function as it is clear that single injections of lymphokines of established *in vitro* potency fail to cause mononuclear cell accumulation in the guinea pig.

MEASUREMENT OF LYMPHOKINE ACTIONS

Lymphokine activity is measured mainly by use of *in vitro* culture techniques (Bloom and Glade, 1971). A wide range of techniques are employed and for a given assay system (e.g. cell migration inhibition), methodological details show considerable variation between laboratories. The idiosyncrasies of various laboratories engaged in lymphokine studies have hampered progress in this field by limiting the extent to which it is possible to compare or correlate results from different groups. Use of response units (e.g. that amount of material necessary to cause a reduction in cell migration of a specified area in mm^2 or a reduction of 25%) is impracticable for there is a general reluctance of workers to modify their own techniques to conform to a common test system so that it would be exceedingly difficult to secure agreement on the optimal method of measurement in a particular assay system. On the basis of many precedents, the mechanism for resolving such a difficulty would be to utilize a standard lymphokine preparation (a fixed weight of which would constitute one unit of activity) whose properties and potency would be acceptable to the principal active laboratories in this field.

Despite the obvious need for reference material, it remains the practice of individual laboratories to either generate small quantities of lymphokine preparations for use as internal laboratory standard or to make all their comparisons within a single experiment. This latter practice is commonplace in studies using experimental animals where, for instance, one is comparing the effect of different treatments on a pool of reactive cells. In studies on patients, it is more usual to wish to compare the reactivity of a series of patients (who necessarily are investigated over a period of time, ranging from weeks to months) or to investigate the reactivity of an individual patient during the course of treatment. In view of the considerable daily variation in basal reactivity (e.g. the area of leucocyte migration or the level of ^{3}H-thymidine incorporation in untreated leucocyte populations) the use of a standard preparation in this sort of study would be of considerable advantage.

Provision of a guinea-pig standard in adequate quantities would necessitate sacrifice of very large numbers of donor animals and poses many technical difficulties. Moreover, as the major interest in lymphokine measurement lies in its application to man, it would seem more logical to utilize human cells for lymphokine standard preparations. It is of considerable interest therefore, that human continuous cell lines are capable of generating substantial levels of certain lymphokine activities (Papageorgiou *et al.*, 1973). Since such cell lines are, for other reasons, cultured on a major scale (e.g. in 100 litre batches), this would seem a most promising future source of reference material. However, it is necessary at present for laboratories to generate their own preparations and it is therefore appropriate to describe methods for preparation of human and guinea pig lymphokines.

Preparation of Lymphokine Reference Material

The method described below is meant only as a guide to general technique and many laboratories employ minor variations.

Lymphokines of animal origin may be prepared by *in vitro* culture of lymphoid cells from sterile inflammatory peritoneal cell exudates, or from teased lymph nodes. Cells from sensitized animals are gathered, either by washing out the peritoneal cavity with cold, sterile Hank's balanced salt solution three days after intraperitoneal injection of starch or oil, or by teasing lymph node tissue into culture dishes containing Eagle's minimal essential medium (MEM). After the cells have been removed from the animal, they are washed, counted and their viability is assessed by vital dye exclusion (eosin-Y or trypan blue). Cells are centrifuged at 400 ***g*** for 10 min and resuspended at concentrations from $0{\cdot}2$–$1{\cdot}0 \times 10^{7}$ viable cells/ml in Eagle's MEM containing appropriate serum (e.g. 5% heat-inactivated foetal calf serum, or normal guinea pig serum for guinea pig cell culture). Cell culture concentrations depend on culture conditions, viability and the sensitivity to the inducing antigen. Serum is not essential and can be substituted by carbowax or omitted, although in practice serum is usually included to improve culture viability. After resuspension, cells are incubated in sterile culture vessels with specific antigen, or mitogen, for 24 hr at 37°C in an atmosphere of 5% CO_2 in air. Dose levels of antigen or mitogen employed are somewhat arbitrary but the antigen dose is generally related to the antigen dose used in sensitization.

After culture, the supernatant is removed and ammonium sulphate added (to 40% saturation) in order to precipitate large molecular weight materials such as inducing antigen, antibody and immune complexes. This precipitate is removed and further ammonium sulphate added to give 90% saturation. The resulting precipitate containing the bulk of lymphokine activity is redissolved in a minimum volume of water and extensively dialysed (24 hr) to remove salts, first against running tap water and subsequently, for a further 24 hr, against cold 0·02 M volatile buffer so as to permit lyophilization, being finally stored in sealed containers at −20°C.

Guinea-pig lymphokine preparations prepared and stored in the above manner are stable for periods in excess of two years, in terms of their inflammatory, mitogenic and macrophage migration inhibitory properties.

Comparable preparative procedures have not been outlined for human lymphokine preparations, for, whilst it is possible to generate lymphokines from human lymphoid cells, it is less easy to secure large numbers of human lymphocytes. It is, however, possible to utilize this type of procedure for human lymphokine production and, the most readily available cell type is the peripheral blood lymphocyte, sedimented in 0·6% dextran; though, where available, other lymphoid cell sources (e.g. lymph nodes, or cells from thoracic duct drainage) could be employed.

Measurement of Lymphokine Activity

Some examples of technique for the assay of lymphokine activity are outlined below. These protocols serve as guides rather than obligatory procedures and alternative assay techniques have been described in considerable detail elsewhere (e.g. Bloom and Glade, 1971; Morley *et al.*, 1973). The test systems described here refer primarily to the guinea-pig, with, where possible, reference to the corresponding test for human lymphokine.

Cell Migration Inhibition

The capillary tube migration inhibition assay is the most widely characterized of the *in vitro* assays and, although becoming less popular, still provides the best correlation with *in vivo* reactivity.

Macrophage Migration Inhibition

Peritoneal exudate cells from non-sensitized donor animals are induced by intraperitoneal injection of 20 ml sterile light mineral oil or 2% soluble starch solution. After 3–4 days (oil) or 2–3 days (starch) the cells are removed, washed in Eagle's MEM and counted. Cells are resuspended at a concentration of approximately 4×10^7 viable cells/ml in cold (4°C) Eagle's MEM containing 10% heat-inactivated foetal calf serum, or 15% heat-inactivated normal guinea-pig serum. The cell suspension is used to fill 100 μl haematocrit tubes which are then sealed at one end with a wax plug and centrifuged at 400 ***g*** for 5 min in order to pack the cells against the plug. Tubes are cut at the cell/fluid interface and fixed by inert silicone grease into sterile 0·5 ml culture chambers, commonly in a prepacked sterile plastic plate of 12 chambers. Each chamber is promptly filled with serum-supplemented Eagle's MEM and sealed by a sterile coverslip, which is held in place by inert silicone grease placed on the upper surface of the chamber wall. Test materials are made up in serum-supplemented Eagle's MEM prior to the experiments and kept at room temperature. Lymphokine solutions are freshly prepared as storage of solutions at 4°C or −20°C can result in a reduction of potency. Cultures are incubated for up to 40 hr at 37°C when the cells migrating out of the capillary tubes form a fan on the floor of the chamber (Fig. 1a). This emigration can be measured by projecting the image of the fan onto paper using a microscope with a "camera lucida" attachment. The perimeter of the fan is recorded and the migration area is measured, either by means of a planimeter or by cutting out and weighing the recorded image. The response to lymphokine treatment is often expressed as a migration index (MI) derived as follows:

$$\mathrm{MI} = \frac{\text{(area of migration in presence of lymphokine)}}{\text{(area of migration in absence of lymphokine)}}$$

Multiplication of this ratio by 100 gives the migration area in the test chamber as a percentage of the response of untreated cells and this is most generally adopted because of the ease of assimilation of percentage interconversion (e.g. 75% response = 25% inhibition).

Leucocyte Migration Inhibition

Measurement of macrophage migration inhibition in man is not practicable. However, a comparable technique employing peripheral blood leucocytes has been widely adopted (Fig. 1b). Twenty to 25 ml of peripheral blood is sedimented in dextran (0·6% final concentration). The leucocyte-rich suspension is removed and the cells resuspended to approximately 1×10^8 viable leucocytes/ml in Eagle's MEM containing 10% heat-inactivated foetal calf serum or autologous human serum. Capillary tubes of 10 μl capacity are employed with an incubation period of 18–24 hr, as the difference between lymphokine-treated and untreated cultures is maximal at this time. It should be noted that by 40 hr the difference may no longer be evident in this test system.

Other Cell Migration Techniques

These have been described with the object of simplifying the execution or measurement of this phenomenon, but have been less widely used (Morley, 1974). Two techniques merit consideration, namely, the agarose plate technique of Clausen and the agarose drop method, introduced by Harrington and Stasny. In the former technique, the cell suspension is placed in a series of wells containing test material in an agarose plate. In the latter method, the cells are suspended in a drop of agarose which is incubated in a chamber containing test material in a culture fluid. Both methods yield regular migration areas (i.e. circular responses) so simplifying measurement of the response (e.g. permitting diameter measurement). These techniques are also advantageous in that they generally require less cells than the capillary tube migration test.

Lymphocyte Transformation (Lymphocyte Mitogenicity)

The technique of assessing the blastogenic activity of specific antigens and lymphokines via the uptake of radiolabelled thymidine is widely employed as both an experimental tool in animals and, because of the use of semi-automatic culture harvesting methods, as a clinical screen for lymphokine activity and lymphocyte function in man.

Regional lymph nodes are excised from animals treated with Freund's incomplete adjuvant and teased in Eagle's MEM. An increased cell yield can be achieved by passing a brei of cells and tissue through a wide mesh wire filter (80 gauge). After washing and counting, cells are resuspended to a concentration of 2×10^6 viable cells/ml in Eagle's MEM supplemented with 5% heat-inactivated pooled normal guinea-pig serum. The cell suspension is distributed in 1 ml volumes to sterile glass or plastic culture tubes, to which a further 1 ml of Eagle's MEM and serum, containing test material, is added. The cultures are incubated in an atmosphere of 5% CO_2 in air at 37°C for 24–48 hr, after which 1·0 μCi of tritiated thymidine in 10 μl of saline is added to each culture. Cells are incubated for a further 18–24 hr and then separated from the culture medium by centrifugation. This test measures uptake of tritiated thymidine by lymphocytes, a response parameter that shows a dose-related increase to lymphokine treatment. The cell population is washed in cold phosphate buffered saline; cells are lysed and the soluble protein is precipitated using 5% trichloroacetic acid. The resulting precipitate is washed in methanol to remove water, solubilized with hyamine hydroxide (10% w/v in methanol) at 56°C for 30 min and washed into scintillation counting vials with 10 ml toluene-phosphor scintillation fluid. Tritiated thymidine content is measured by means of an automatic beta-scintillation counter, the response being expressed as quench corrected disintegrations/min.

Human peripheral blood leucocytes can be utilized either following sedimentation and cell separation or as whole blood cultures. The whole blood technique is relatively simple and uses small volumes of blood, so lending itself to clinical applications. In this procedure, 0·1 ml of whole blood is added to 0·9 ml of Eagle's MEM with or without lymphokine, so that 10 ml of blood will suffice for up to 100 observations. The incubation time for human cell systems is usually 5–6 days and erythrocytes need to be lysed with 3% acetic acid before harvesting.

A microculture technique, using serological assay plates as culture chambers, has been described and uses smaller numbers of cells (Hartzman *et al.*, 1972). The post-culture cell separation and preparation for counting has been subject to some degree of automation whereby cells are collected on filter pads and subjected to serial washing without intermediate handling. Such filters are then placed directly into scinter, so avoiding the solubilization step.

Chemotaxis

Lymphokines are chemotactic for both neutrophils and macrophages *in vitro*, and the methods used to demonstrate chemotaxis for these two cell types differ significantly.

Neutrophils are induced by peritoneal injection of starch, cells being removed from the peritoneal cavity after 4 hr, washed, counted, and resuspended at 1×10^6 viable cells/ml in Eagle's MEM with 5% pooled normal guinea pig serum. In the case of macrophages, the starch is allowed to remain in the peritoneal cavity for 2–3 days. The culture chambers consist of a polyethylene specimen tube into which fits a smaller open-ended tube with a millipore filter glued over the lower end (5 μm pore size for neutrophils and 8 μm for macrophages). One ml of medium, with or without lymphokine is placed in the outer chamber and 1 ml of cell suspension in the inner chamber (care should be taken that the millipore filter is wetted with the cell suspension in medium in the inner chamber before medium is placed in the outer chamber and also that the depth of medium is equal in the two chambers). After a 4 hr incubation period, the degree of migration of cells through the millipore filters is measured.

For neutrophils, the number of cells appearing on the outer surface of the filter is counted after the filters have been removed and stained with toluidine blue. Macrophage chemotaxis can be measured in the same way or more conveniently by counting the number of cells passing into the lower chamber using either a Coulter counter or by counting the cell total in a 10 μl droplet of the culture medium from the lower chamber. A recently described technique utilizes two millipore filters, cell migration being assessed by counting the numbers of cells on the lower filter after the incubation period. In our experience this is less convenient and less precise than direct counting of cells in the lower chamber.

Human mononuclear cell chemotaxis may be measured by the above method and this technique has also been used to demonstrate an eosinophil chemotactic factor which is dependent upon the presence of immune complexes.

Increased Vascular Permeability

Guinea-pig lymphokine preparations produce increased vascular permeability when injected into the skin of unsensitized animals. This can be measured by an isotopic technique which has revealed the existence of three phases of activity. The first phase is mepyramine sensitive and probably relates to basic protein present in the preparations.

The assay involves assessing increased vascular permeability by counting accumulation of iodine-labelled guinea-pig serum albumin (GPSA) in dermal lesions (guinea-pigs receive intravenous injections via the dorsal hind foot vein of mepyramine maleate (1·5 mg/kg) in order to remove the first phase of activity). At the time of the injection of mepyramine, animals also receive 1–2 μCi of ^{125}I-GPSA in 0·5 ml of Evans blue dye. Immediately after this injection, lymphokines are injected intradermally into dorsal skin sites, and after 4 hr animals are killed and skinned. Discs of skin wholly including the inflammatory lesion are excised and counted to give their ^{125}I-GPSA content. One millilitre of venous blood is also removed and responses are calculated as μl of whole blood equivalent. By using three animals/assay, it is possible to arrange the dose allocations in a Latin square so permitting analysis of variance. Although there can be significant differences between sites, a more important source of variation eliminated by this approach is inter-animal variation. The confidence limits of 3+3 or 2+2 assays using this technique can be relatively wide. However, in practice, the ranking of potency of different preparations remains constant and successive potency assessments usually show satisfactory agreement.

Other methods for assessing intradermal reactivity of lymphokine preparations include the classical skin test where induration and erythema are measured visually, and the visual assessment of Evans blue dye extravasation.

Lymphocyte Cytotoxicity

The techniques outlined above are amongst the most common assays for lymphokine activity in both animals and man. Another method often employed is the assessment of lymphocyte cytotoxicity, and this technique is of particular interest in the study of tumour immunology. A wide variety of methods have been employed to measure the activity of cytotoxic lymphokines (lymphotoxins), the response parameter of this assay being death of specific target cells in tissue culture. Possible target cells include lymphocytes, tumour cells, mouse L-cells, fibroblasts and other established cell lines. The response may be measured in terms either of cytotoxic or cytopathic effects being assessed by vital dye staining, counting of intact cells, inhibition of uptake of radiolabelled amino acids or thymidine, ^{51}Cr or ^{125}I-deoxyuridine release from labelled target cells, or by time-lapse cinematography.

Other Lymphokine Assays

Apart from the techniques described above, a wide variety of other *in vitro* assays are currently being employed to assess lymphokine activity; for example, the ability of lymphokines to affect macrophage functions may be tested by techniques such as macrophage aggregation (assessed visually in suspension culture), or by increased spreading on culture plates. Other manifestations of macrophage activity include phagocytosis, which can be measured by uptake of radioactive gold, or biochemical assays such as glucose oxidation, assessed by using ^{14}C-labelled glucose. Lymphokines are also active on continuous cell line preparations and inhibition of proliferation or cloning of HeLa cells has been described. A bone resorbing factor measured by increased decalcification of bone tissue by osteoclasts can be demonstrated in lymphokine preparations. The range of materials, the cell types affected, and representative references have been listed in Table 1.

Bioassay of Lymphokines

The various biological actions of lymphokines have, in most instances, been shown to be dose-related, and in certain test systems dose-response curves have been described with reasonable precision. In the cases of macrophage migration inhibition, lymphocyte transformation, chemotaxis and increased vascular permeability, dose-response data has been utilized in conventional analytical dilution bioassays of the type adopted for many other biologically active materials. The purpose of employing multi-point analytical dilution bioassay is to provide maximal precision for a given expenditure of effort and materials (Finney, 1964). However, in the laboratory or clinical situation, there may be greater interest in evaluating the activity of large numbers of samples. For instance, it may be desirable to ascertain the level of chemotactic or mitogenic activity produced by a fixed number of cells in response to standard stimulation using a minimal quantity of blood. This type of situation

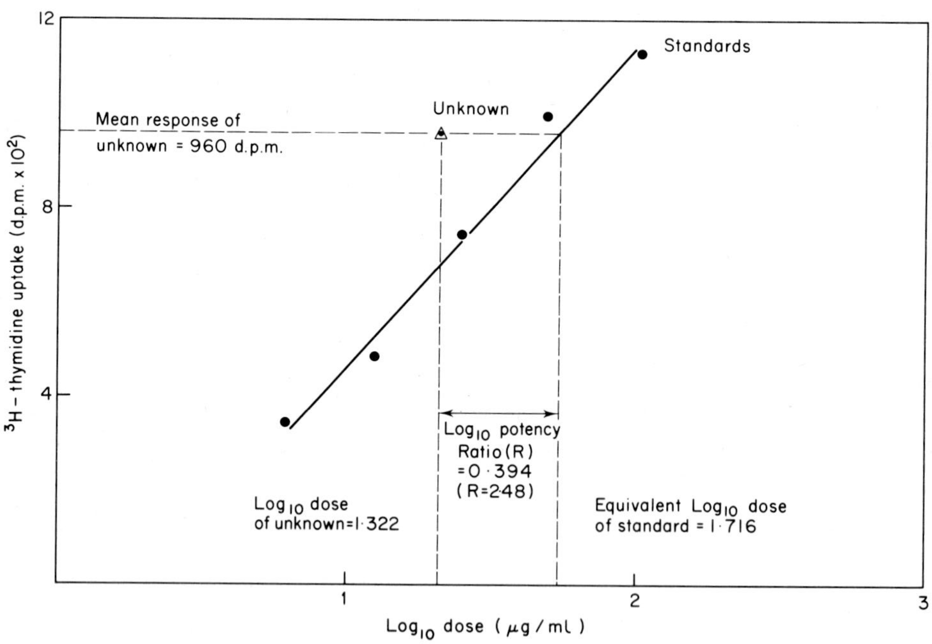

Fig. 3. Interpolation assay. Standard curve for a lymphokine standard assayed by lymphocyte transformation. The best fit straight line has been plotted and the mean response of an unknown lymphokine given at a dose of 21 µg/ml ($\log_{10}=1{\cdot}322$) is shown. The $\log_{10}$ potency ratio $=0{\cdot}394$ thus the potency ratio is 2·48 (i.e. for every 1 ml of unknown 2·48 ml of standard are needed to produce the same effect).

is illustrated in Fig. 3, which shows the interpolation assay of mitogenic lymphokine activity (see also Coloquhoun, 1971). It should be noted that such a procedure has inevitably less precision than the analytical dilution bioassay.

Many studies on lymphokine formation have generated idiosyncratic measuring systems with frequent recourse to the use of ratios to provide some form of normalization between individuals (for example, the use of the migration index) in order to accommodate the wide variations in reactivity between different individuals and, indeed, within the same subject from day to day. One problem in utilizing such ratios is that, with small numbers of replicates, the confidence limits can be very wide, yet such considerations are often overlooked or omitted. In practice, the error variance of an assay can be large (e.g. S of 10–20%) so that, for example, the migration inhibition index of 0·8, which is widely regarded as demonstrating significant inhibition, can require up to 10 replicates of both unknown and control in order to achieve a 95% level of significance. Thus, should ratios be preferred, it is instructive to consider the level of replication needed for the ratio to achieve significance in relation to the coefficient of variation of a particular experiment. This is illustrated by Table 3 which lists the upper confidence level for a migration index of 0·8 in experiments with standard deviations ranging from 0·01–0·2. Thus, if the standard deviation of an experiment is 0·1 then 4 replicates will suffice for a migration index of 0·8 (20% inhibition) to be significant at the 95% level. The form of the distribution of data is uncertain in many of these tests and this is of some consequence in determining the confidence limits of an observation. For normal distribution Fieller's theorem can be used to give confidence limits; for log-normally distributed data estimation is much simpler (Finney, 1964).

We would suggest that use of a reference preparation between experiments is preferable to use of, for example, the migration index, and that interpolation assays or analytical dilution bioassays be used so as to permit estimation of confidence limits. This would be particularly advantageous in a comparison of results from different laboratories.

LYMPHOKINE FUNCTIONS

It has been emphasized that the ability of lymphocytes to generate lymphokines is determined by the existence of delayed hypersensitivity in the donor animals *in vivo*. The assumption is made that, in the guinea-pig and man this lymphokine production is consequent upon T-cell activation, a conclusion

TABLE 3
Upper fiducial limits for M

S	2	3	4	5	6	7	8	9	10	11
0·01	0·840	0·821	0·816	0·813	0·812	0·811	0·810	0·809	0·809	0·808
0·02	0·881	0·842	0·832	0·827	0·824	0·821	0·820	0·818	0·817	0·816
0·03	0·924	0·864	0·848	0·840	0·836	0·832	0·830	0·828	0·826	0·825
0·04	0·969	0·886	0·865	0·854	0·848	0·843	0·840	0·837	0·835	0·833
0·05	1·017	0·908	0·882	0·868	0·860	0·854	0·850	0·846	0·843	0·841
0·06	1·067	0·932	0·899	0·883	0·872	0·865	0·860	0·856	0·852	0·850
0·07	1·119	0·955	0·916	0·897	0·885	0·877	0·871	0·865	0·861	0·858
0·08	1·175	0·980	0·934	0·912	0·898	0·888	0·881	0·875	0·870	0·867
0·09	1·235	1·005	0·952	0·927	0·911	0·900	0·892	0·885	0·880	0·875
0·10	1·298	1·030	0·971	0·942	0·924	0·911	0·902	0·895	0·889	0·884
0·11	1·366	1·057	0·990	0·957	0·937	0·923	0·913	0·905	0·898	0·893
0·12	1·440	1·084	1·009	0·973	0·951	0·935	0·924	0·915	0·908	0·902
0·13	1·519	1·112	1·028	0·989	0·964	0·948	0·935	0·925	0·917	0·911
0·14	1·605	1·141	1·048	1·005	0·978	0·960	0·947	0·935	0·927	0·920
0·15	1·699	1·171	1·069	1·022	0·992	0·972	0·958	0·946	0·936	0·929
0·16	1·803	1·201	1·090	1·038	1·007	0·985	0·969	0·956	0·946	0·938
0·17	1·918	1·233	1·111	1·055	1·021	0·998	0·981	0·967	0·956	0·948
0·18	2·047	1·266	1·133	1·073	1·036	1·011	0·993	0·978	0·966	0·957
0·19	2·192	1·300	1·156	1·090	1·051	1·024	1·005	0·989	0·976	0·967
0·20	2·357	1·336	1·179	1·108	1·066	1·037	1·017	1·000	0·987	0·976

Upper fiducial limits for a mean migration inhibition (M) of 0·8 (i.e. 20% inhibition) for standard deviation (S) values from 0·01 to 0·20 (i.e. 1–20%) with from 2–11 replicates. Values derived from the Behrens-Fisher analogue of Fieller's theorem (Finney, 1964, p. 32).

that is strengthened by the ability of plant mitogens such as phytohaemagglutinin (PHA) and concanavalin-A (Con-A) to mimic antigen activation of lymphocytes to produce lymphokine. However, in the mouse, where separation of T- and B-cells can be achieved, it has been demonstrated that activation of B-cell-rich populations by appropriate mitogens (e.g. pokeweed) yields similar mitogenic activity to that generated by T-cell activation (Mackler *et al.*, 1974). Nevertheless, it is reasonable to regard the process of lymphokine generation as reflecting primarily, a process of T-cell activation.

The impetus to develop *in vitro* indices of delayed hypersensitivity (cellular immunity) stems, in part, from the need for a convenient index of T-cell reactivity in conditions in which there is a likelihood that delayed hypersensitivity underlies pathological manifestations of the disease process. In such situations, there is the understandable tendency to relate *in vitro* phenomena to features of the delayed hypersensitivity reaction *in vivo*; thus, results of investigations of *in vitro* cellular immunity are frequently interpreted as accounting for features of cell dynamics *in vivo*. This is well illustrated by the *in vitro* effects of lymphokines on the macrophage where phenomena such as inhibition of cell migration, monocyte chemotaxis and macrophage activation are strongly suggestive of *in vivo* malfunctions of cellular immunity such as the accumulation and activation of monocytic cells in lesions of delayed hypersensitivity. Similarly, *in vivo* properties of lymphokines can be directly compared with the delayed hypersensitivity reaction, in terms of susceptibility to drug inhibition and the pattern of vascular changes where there is a similarity between lymphokine actions and the delayed hypersensitivity response.

This sort of evidence supports the view that lymphokines act as effectors of delayed hypersensitivity reactions, and the other component of the latter (i.e. cellular immunity) may also be subserved by release of lymphokine. The protective function of cellular immunity can be readily perceived but the significance of delayed hypersensitivity reactions is debatable, especially as it is clear that delayed hypersensitivity does not necessarily indicate protective immunity, and vice versa. The question therefore arises as to the nature and function of the system responsible for delayed hypersensitivity reactions.

In delayed hypersensitivity in the skin, there is a perivascular accumulation of mononuclear cells whose activities can result in tissue damage and necrosis if the reaction is of sufficient intensity. In other locations (for example, the joint) the lymphoid infiltrate can develop some degree of organization so that, in the rheumatoid joint, collections of lymphoid cells form aggregates which are suggestive of lymphoid follicles. Also, lymphokine production has been reported in the rheumatoid joint (Stastny *et al.*, 1973), and it is of particular interest to note that the intralymphatic injection of small quantities of lymphokine is able to effect a marked modification in the response of a lymph node to antigen presentation (including increased cellular proliferation in the germinal centres and paracortical distension due to increased cellular infiltration). Such evidence suggests that lymphokines are involved in the lymphocytic response to antigen, a view not inconsistent with observations establishing the ability of T-cells to modify B-cell activation (Raff, 1973). The potency of lymphokines in modifying accumulation of small lymphocytes from the circulation across the lymphatic endothelial venules is further circumstantial evidence that lymphokines are capable of modifying the reactivity to antigen. The existence of this phenomenon in the lymph node in reactions to small doses of antigen raises the possibility that the cellular accumulation of lymphocytes in response to extralymphatic accumulation of antigen, for example in the skin, represents an inappropriate attempt by mononuclear cells to collect and process antigen as if located in the lymph node. Should this interpretation of delayed hypersensitivity be valid, then it is possible to regard the lymphokines as agents of potential utility in the lymph node, which inadvertently cause adverse reactions in other loci, such as the skin or joint, simply as a consequence of their mislocation. Such a concept permits reconciliation of the adjuvant and potentially useful function of lymphokines in the lymph node with the adverse effects of lymphokine production in situations such as the delayed hypersensitivity response in the skin. At the systemic level, reactivity to antigen stimulates cellular immunity in a non-specific manner (Blanden *et al.*, 1969), being consistent with the non-specific action of macrophages provoked by lymphokine treatment. Evidence of increased circulating lymphokine levels in such responses is not extensive and the situation would seem less simple than previously envisaged since intravenous lymphokine can induce defective antigen reactivity in macrophages *in vitro* (Poulter and Turk, 1976) and systemic treatment with a starfish extract, which has similar action *in vitro* to MIF will depress, rather than enhance, cellular immune responses (Willenborg and Prendergast, 1974). This is clearly an area in need of further study.

The ability of lymphokines to cause monocyte accumulation *in vitro* and to activate non-sensitized lymphocytes implies that, once initiated, the cellular immune response will be amplified as a positive feedback system. There is thus apparently a need for mechanisms to limit the extent and duration of lymphocyte activity in reactions of cellular immunity. One regulatory system for which there is some evidence is the existence of a "suppressor"

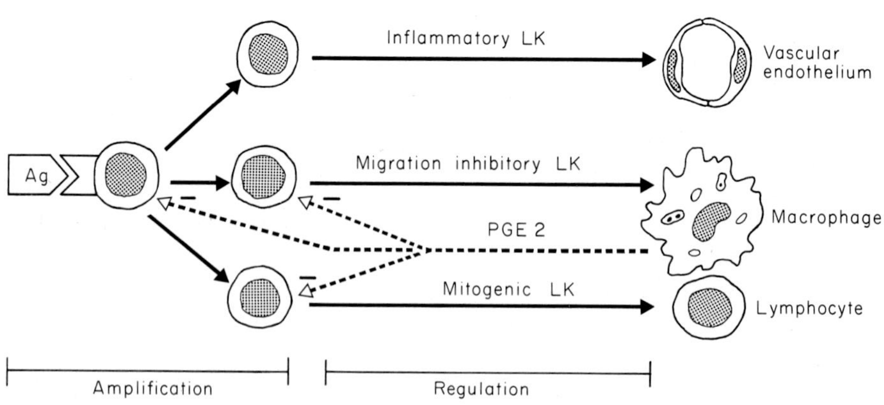

Fig. 4. Proposed negative feedback response to limit the extent and duration of cellular immune reactions.

T-cell which is capable of interfering with the optimal development of the antibody forming B-cells (Katz and Benacerraf, 1972). Our own work has indicated another control mechanism which involves the production of E-type prostaglandins by macrophages in response to lymphokines with consequent suppression by the prostaglandin of antigen-induced lymphocyte production of lymphokine (Bray *et al.*, 1975). Such a negative feedback system would serve to regulate the inflammatory reactions of delayed hypersensitivity (Fig. 4) and possibly the response of lymphoid tissue to antigen.

LYMPHOKINE MEASUREMENT IN MAN

The attraction of measurements of lymphokines or lymphokine actions in man is that, in principle, it provides an index of cellular immunity which does not necessitate exposure of the patient to antigenic stimulation. However, it must be acknowledged that the evidence in man (as opposed to the guinea-pig) for the existence of a correlation between delayed hypersensitivity, cellular immunity and *in vitro* lymphokine production remains insubstantial. Several population studies have been undertaken in which the *in vitro* reactivity has been correlated with *in vivo* responses, but longitudinal studies of individuals over periods during which there are marked changes in the *in vitro* cellular immune status have received little attention. This is a serious omission, for, as Poulter (1976) has recently demonstrated, the response in guinea-pigs to an infection (*Leishmania*) is accompanied by a period during which macrophages become unreactive in terms of *in vitro* cell migration inhibition to *Leishmania* antigen, or to preformed lymphokine prepared in response to an unrelated antigen. It is thus possible that in the analogous situation in man, strong cellular immunity may not be reflected in an *in vitro* test based on lymphokine production.

Nonetheless, measurement *in vitro* of lymphokine activities in response to antigenic stimulation of leucocytes has been undertaken in a wide variety of conditions (see Table 4). It has not been established in many cases that this type of measurement has any advantage over the use of skin tests. For instance, in the case of PPD reactivity, the relative insensitivity of *in vitro* tests in comparison with skin reactivity *in vivo* suggests that *in vitro* lymphokine tests will not easily supersede the simple, inexpensive and highly specific *in vivo* test. However, the advantage of *in vitro* tests in not subjecting the host to antigenic stimulation is a point of considerable importance when the host is man and the antigen is potentially hazardous (e.g. transplantation antigens,

TABLE 4

Some conditions associated with cellular immunity and/or lymphokine production

Condition
Viral infection
Tobacco mosaic virus
Vaccinia
Mumps
Pox viruses
Lymphocytic choriomeningitis virus
Bacterial infection
Mycobacteria
Staphylococcus
Listeria
Fungal infection
Parasitic infection
Leishmaniasis (cutaneous)
Chagas' disease
Schistosomiasis
Anergy
Sarcoidosis
Candidiasis
Hodgkin's disease
Contact sensitivity
Rheumatoid arthritis
Systemic lupus erythematosus
Multiple sclerosis
Glomerulonephritis
Cystic fibrosis
Encephalitis
Peripheral neuropathies—Guillain-Barré syndrome
Granuloma
Viral tumours
Tumour immunity
Transplantation immunity
Drug hypersensitivity

tumour antigens or pathogenic agents). There is also a further advantage of *in vitro* test systems in experimental investigation in which *in vivo* tests could be compromising (e.g. testing for cellular immunity in individuals undergoing transfer factor therapy). Attempts are being made with varying degrees of success to measure human lymphokine activity on more convenient target cells from individual patients. For example, leucocyte migration inhibition factor has been reported to inhibit guinea-pig macrophage migration and these cells have been used as indicator cells in cell migration studies, mixed with patients' cells. The use of established human cell lines as indicators has also been attempted with promising results. Thus, although the relationship of the *in vitro* tests to *in vivo* cellular immunity remains obscure there is, at least, hope that these tests will acquire some degree of standardization and reproducibility. Measurement of lymphokine production is a laboratory test of established value in certain areas of experimental medicine, but it is fair to state that, at present, its theoretical potential in the study of human disease remains unfulfilled.

ACKNOWLEDGEMENTS

The authors gratefully acknowledge the assistance of Mr K. Smith in the compilation of Table 3, and thank Dr R. A. Wolstencroft for helpful discussion.

REFERENCES

Blanden, R. V., Lefford, M. J. and Mackaness, G. B. (1969). The host response to Calmette: Guérin bacillus injection in mice. *J. Exp. Med.* **129**, 1079.

Bloom, B. R. (1971). *In vitro* studies of cell-mediated immunity. *Adv. Immunol.* **13**, 101.

Bloom, B. R. and Bennett, B. (1966). Mechanism of a reaction *in vitro* associated with delayed type hypersensitivity. *Science* **153**, 80.

Bloom, B. R. and Glade, P. R. (1971). "*In vitro* Methods in Cell-mediated Immunity." Academic Press, London and New York.

Bray, M. A., Gordon, D. and Morley, J. (1975). Regulation of lymphokine secretion by prostaglandins. *In* "Future Trends in Inflammation, II". (eds. G. P. Velo, J. D. Giroud and D. A. Willoughby). Piccin Medical Books, Italy.

Bray, M. A., Dumonde, D. C., Hanson, J., Morley, J. and Wolstencroft, R. A. (1976). Heterogeneity of guinea pig lymphokines revealed by parallel bioassay. *Clin. Exp. Immunol.* **23**, 333.

Colquhoun, D. (1971). "Lectures on Biostatistics." Clarendon Press, Oxford.

David, J. R. (1966). Delayed hypersensitivity *in vitro*; its mediation by cell-free substances formed by lymphoid cell-antigen interaction. *Proc. Nat. Acad. Sci. (Wash.)* **56**, 72.

David, J. R. (1973). Lymphocyte mediators and cellular hypersensitivity. *New Eng. J. Med.* **288**, 143.

David, J. R. and David, R. R. (1972). Cellular hypersensitivity and immunity. *Progr. Allergy* **16**, 300.

Delayed hypersensitivity. (1967). *Brit. Med. Bull.* **23**.

Dumonde, D. C., Wolstencroft, R. A., Panayi, G. S., Matthew, M., Morley, J. and Howson, W. T. (1969). Lymphokines. *Nature* **224**, 38.

Dvorak, H. F. and Dvorak, A. M. (1974). Cutaneous basophil hypersensitivity. *Progr. Immunol. II*, **3**, 171.

Finney, D. J. (1964). "Statistical Method in Biological Assay." Griffin and Company, London.

George, M. and Vaughan, J. H. (1962). *In vitro* cell migration as a model for delayed hypersensitivity. *Proc. Soc. Exp. Biol. Med.* **111**, 514.

Hartzman, R. J., Bach, M. L., Bach, F. H., Thurman, G. B. and Sell, K. W. (1972). Precipitation of radioactive labelled samples: a semi-automatic multi-sample processor. *Cell Immunol.* **4**, 182.

Katz, D. H. and Benacerraf, B. (1972). The regulatory influence of activated T-cells on B-cell responses to antigen. *Adv. Immunol.* **15**, 1.

Mackler, B. F., Altman, L. C., Rosenstreich, D. L. and Oppenheim, J. J. (1974). Induction of lymphokine production by EAC and of blastogenesis by soluble mitogens during human B-cell activation. *Nature* **249**, 834.

Morley, J. (1974). Cell migration inhibition: An appraisal. *Acta Allergologica* **29**, 185.

Morley, J., Wolstencroft, R. A. and Dumonde, D. C. (1973). The measurement of lymphokines. *In* "Handbook of Experimental Immunology" (ed. D. M. Weir), Chapter 28, 2nd edn. Blackwell, Edinburgh.

Papageorgiou, P. S., Henley, W. L. and Glade, P. R. (1973). Production and characterization of migration inhibitory factor(s) (MIF) of established lymphoid and non-lymphoid cell lines. *J. Immunol.* **108**, 494.

Pick, E. and Turk, J. L. (1972). The biological activities of soluble lymphocyte products. *Clin. Exp. Immunol.* **10**, 1.

Poulter, L. (1976). Ph.D. Thesis. University of London.

Poulter, L. and Turk, J. L. (1976). Changes in macrophages *in vivo* induced by desensitization. *Cell. Immunol.* In press.

Raff, M. C. (1973). T- and B-lymphocytes and immune responses. *Nature* **242**, 19.

Rich, A. R. and Lewis, M. R. (1932). Nature of allergy in tuberculosis as revealed by tissue culture studies. *Bull. Johns Hopk. Hosp.* **50**, 115.

Stastny, P., Rosenthal, M., Andreis, M. and Ziff, M. (1973). *Arthr. Rheum.* **16**, 572.

Willenborg, D. O. and Prendergast, R. A. (1974). The effect of sea star coelomocyte extract on cell-mediated resistance to *Listeria monocytogenes* in mice. *J. Exp. Med.* **139**, 820.

III

General Aspects of Immunological Disease

10

Mechanisms in Immunological Disease

A. M. DENMAN

An immune response accompanies many diseases in which significant tissue damage does not develop. Indeed it has in all its forms evolved primarily to protect the host from infection by pathogenic microorganisms and the current enthusiasm for invoking aberrant immune reactions to explain a variety of puzzling features of different diseases should not obscure this fundamental point. Moreover the immune system has been considered responsible for preventing the emergence or proliferation of malignant cells, although it may function primarily by limiting infection with oncogenic viruses. However, immune reactions directed at many environmental antigens are either of no obvious biological advantage to the host from the outset or else damage the tissues later as they develop. Adverse reactions to exogenous antigens include disorders such as atopic diseases of the skin and respiratory tract, dietary hypersensitivity and many forms of drug reaction. Immune responses to auto-antigens are known to be responsible for some diseases and have been implicated in the pathogenesis of many others.

Despite the neat way in which the various forms of immunological disease can be classified, it is evident from experimental models and still more from clinical practice, that several immune processes combine to induce tissue damage. Their relative contribution in different diseases is often a matter of individual interpretation. This point is well illustrated by the controversy which still surrounds the mechanism by which foreign tissues are rejected in the homograft reaction, the most obvious of immunological reactions. Although re-circulating small lymphocytes are beyond any doubt the cells which are initially sensitized, the subsequent contributions of cellular and humoral immunity in effecting graft rejection are still imprecisely defined. It is most logical to consider each mechanism in turn without assuming that only one is exclusively responsible for a particular form of hypersensitivity reaction. A six-fold classification is introduced in Chapter 1 (pp. 18–21) and forms the basis for discussion here (Table 1).

ANTIBODY MECHANISMS

Classically immediate hypersensitivity has been distinguished from delayed hypersensitivity by the time course after immunological challenge, by the histological appearances of the skin reaction and by the ability to transfer the reaction with serum but not with mononuclear cells. Such criteria have proved useful in analysing laboratory experiments but have been less valuable in clinical practice. The timing of reactions provoked by skin testing or by inhalation often fail to indicate the mechanisms which are operating. Biopsies of skin lesions, whether induced by spontaneous disease or by the injection of suspected antigens, can rarely be interpreted unquivocally, whilst the transfer of reactivity with serum to human recipients—i.e. the Praüsnitz-Küstner

TABLE 1
Summary of mechanisms of immunological damage

	Title	Triggering device	Mediators
ANTIBODY MECHANISMS	Reaginic	Reaginic antibody (IgE or possibly IgG_4)	Histamine, SRS-A,[a] ECF-A,[b] etc.
	Membrane reactive	Antibody (IgG, IgM or IgA) with specificity for membrane-bound antigen	Complement, polymorphs and their lysosomal enzymes
	Immune complex	Cell-free antigen–antibody complexes	Complement, polymorphs and their lysosomal enzymes
CELLULAR MECHANISMS	T-cell	T-lymphocytes	Lymphokines ± membrane effects
	K-cell	Other cytotoxic mononuclear cells plus membrane-fixed antibody	Soluble factors ± membrane effects
	Macrophage	Macrophages plus antibody, antigen–antibody complexes or other activating factors	Lysosomal enzymes ± membrane effects

[a] SRS-A = slow-reacting substance of anaphylaxis
[b] ECF-A = eosinophil chemotactic factor of anaphylaxis

reaction—is usually excluded by ethical considerations. A more satisfactory means of ascribing a disease to immediate hypersensitivity is to show that factors are operating which are known to characterize this type of reaction. The first three types of immunological damage are triggered by antibody and may be given the descriptive terms: reaginic, membrane-reactive and immune-complex (see Table 1).

Reaginic Mechanism

Acute hypersensitivity is characterized by the release of histamine and other pharmacological substances which produce a variable clinical picture depending upon the site and extent of their release. In its extreme form it presents as acute anaphylaxis. The antibody molecules which initiate this response are by tradition referred to collectively as "reagins" (Stanworth, 1971). These antibodies bind to tissue receptors through sites within their Fc region. IgE constitutes the major class of reaginic antibody but it seems likely that some IgG (e.g. subclass IgG_4) antibodies also contribute. The cells which possess receptors for reaginic antibodies are predominantly mast cells and basophils. The combining sites within the Fab region of these cell-bound antibody molecules are still able to react with antigen. This combination induces conformational changes in the cell membrane, thereby activating intracellular enzyme systems, in turn followed by the selective release of the mediators of acute hypersensitivity. The materials which are secreted are either pre-formed or synthesized in response to the cell's activation. These mediators account for the highly variable picture which hypersensitivity reactions present in clinical practice. In man, the respiratory and vascular systems bear the brunt of acute systemic reactions. There are considerable species differences in the relative importance of the numerous mediator substances and the particular target organs involved. Although histamine release is undoubtedly associated with clinically important reactions it is not the only mediator involved and may well not be the most critical. Bradykinin, slow-reacting substance (SRS-A), the eosinophil chemotactic factor of anaphylaxis (ECF-A) and possibly prostaglandins, contribute to the increased capillary permeability, platelet aggregation and perivascular aggregation of inflammatory cells which constitute acute hypersensitivity. Moreover, whilst it is convenient to regard this form of reaction as neatly circumscribed, its effects are often ramified through pathways which have traditionally been considered entirely separate. These include the activation of both the classical and alternative complement pathways and the initiation of intravascular coagulation. Furthermore, since the antibody response is probably never restricted to the production of IgE, immune complex formation with antibody of other classes is a common accompaniment.

There are practical difficulties in diagnosing acute hypersensitivity reactions of this nature. The history of an acute illness which produces vasomotor collapse and symptoms suggestive of anaphylaxis can be mimicked by other mechanisms which are in no way immunological.

Laboratory tests are of some assistance in establishing the mechanism of the disorder, particularly in its more persistent form. Radioimmunoassay will often permit the detection of raised serum IgE levels with specificity for the responsible antigen even in patients with negative skin tests (Higgins and Brostoff, 1975) and is the most precise method yet available.

An indirect means of implicating this form of immunological hypersensitivity in various disease states will undoubtedly be the ability of drugs with fairly precise pharmacological actions to suppress their clinical manifestation. Thus sodium cromoglycate has no effect on the events which lead to the combination of antigen and reaginic antibody on the surface of mast cells or basophils. Yet by preventing the release of mediators from such cells, this agent commonly suppresses the clinical manifestations of allergic rhinitis and bronchial asthma. There are also indications that it blocks hypersensitivity reactions in the gastro-intestinal tract to dietary antigens of which milk allergy is the best documented.

It must be emphasized that many forms of atopy, such as extrinsic asthma, are not simply the result of sensitization to a specific antigen but involve defects elsewhere in the pathway between entry of antigen and the reaginic antibody triggered release of inflammatory mediators (see Chapter 22). Another example is chronic urticaria, which has many of the features of acute hypersensitivity but is rarely accompanied by any demonstrable increase in serum reaginic antibody. The difficulties in attributing this complaint to any specific immunological mechanism are illustrated by the following case history:

A housewife aged 36 years presented with typical urticaria which characteristically became more florid towards evening and largely remitted in the morning. It responded partially to anti-histamine drugs. Skin biopsy revealed a pericapillary infiltration with mast cells and eosinophils. However, the serum IgE was not elevated and no specific abnormality was detected in the complement or any other immunological system. Circulating immune complexes were not detected.

An exclusion diet induced a rapid remission in her symptoms which could be reproducibly provoked by adding cheese to her diet. This sequence of events is common in chronic urticaria but the usual mechanisms of atopic reactions could not be firmly incriminated. This is not an uncommon example of a disease process in which no obvious immunological mechanism can be defined precisely.

Membrane-reactive Mechanism

Although immunopathological damage is only a minor feature of most microbial infections, the antibody response can cause tissue injury by a variety of mechanisms. The majority of these involve the activation of various mediators of which complement is the most important. Nevertheless, the direct interaction of antibody with tissue antigens can itself have injurious effects in which complement is not involved. This has been most evident in experimental systems. Thus rats which have been injected with antisera which react with the glomerular basement membrane, still sustain renal damage even when they have been decomplemented. The ability of microbial antigens and drugs to bind to cell membranes commonly provokes a response in which antibody reacts directly with antigen at these sites. However, it is uncertain to what extent this interaction can be damaging unless complement is fixed as a result. Antibodies which fix complement at sites of tissue binding initiate pathological processes which are considered below.

Immune Complex Disease

The antibody mechanism of tissue damage which has received greatest attention is the formation of circulating soluble complexes between antigen and antibody. There is a stage in the immune response to most antigens when such complexes are formed. Initially unbound antigen is found in the blood before the antibody response has become fully operative. When the antibody titre rises there is a brief phase during which antigen and antibody combine to form immune complexes. Thereafter antigen is rapidly cleared from the blood and is found only intermittently and in the presence of excess antibody. This is the pattern of events in most human infections. However there are conditions in which circulating immune complexes persist long enough to induce secondary events which lead to tissue damage. In general there are two sets of circumstances, sometimes interrelated, in which this may occur. In the first, the disease process is such that a continuous source of antigen is available so that antigen and antibody periodically circulate in combination. In the second, the character of the antibody response is such that the efficiency with which antigen is cleared from the blood is impaired. It is also apparent that immune complexes may be formed locally in the tissues or may be found in the circulation.

Sources of Persistent Antigen

Infections are the commonest cause of immune complex disease, since, in replicating, the responsible organism releases fresh antigen into the circulation. This may be a transitory phase if the infection is eliminated by a combination of host resistance and appropriate therapy. Persistent infections are liable to provide a constant source of immune complexes. These may be bacterial, parasitic or viral in nature. Thus subacute bacterial endocarditis is a disease in which continued bacterial infection of the heart valves is followed by a series of serological and inflammatory events in other tissues which may be hard to distinguish from those provoked by other causes. Indeed the immunopathological features of many diseases may be identical,

TABLE 2

Immune complex disease: principal causes in man

A. *Infections*	1. *bacterial*	sub-acute bacterial endocarditis; meningococcal infection
	2. *mycobacterial*	leprosy
	3. *protozoan*	malaria
	4. *viral*	dengue; hepatitis B
B. *Exogenous*	1. *dietary*	gluten sensitivity
	2. *occupational*	allergic alveolitis
	3. *drugs*	"serum sickness" (penicillin, sulphonamides) SLE syndrome; (procainamide; hydralazine; practolol)
C. *Auto-antigens*	1. *IgG*	rheumatoid disease
	2. *nucleic acids*	SLE
D. *Neoplastic*	1. *tumour antigens*	lymphoma; carcinoma
E. *Unknown*	1. *renal disease*	nephrotic syndrome
	2. *gastro-intestinal*	Crohn's disease; ulcerative colitis

This is not an exhaustive list but immune-complexes have been shown to contribute significantly to the disease picture in those instances which have been included.

irrespective of the aetiology, and may cause diagnostic difficulties as the following case report illustrates;

> A six-year-old boy presented with an intermittent fever and severe night sweats. Vasculitic lesions were noted on both feet and particularly over the great toes. At this stage the heart was not obviously abnormal and blood cultures were negative. Amongst other findings laboratory tests revealed greatly reduced levels of C3 and total haemolytic complement activity whilst immune complexes were detected by a variety of methods. The diagnosis of "immune complex disease" was clear and at this stage the findings seemed compatible with a "connective tissue disease". It was only after some time that *Moraxella kingii* was grown regularly in blood cultures and it became evident that the aortic valve was infected.

Tissue antigens can also provoke continuous immune complex disease. Thus in rheumatoid arthritis, circulating immune complexes formed between native IgG and either IgG or IgM rheumatoid factor probably account for the vasculitis which may complicate this disease. Tumour antigens complexed with antibody have been detected in the blood of patients with malignant disease and whilst leukaemias, lymphomas and neuroblastomas have been given most attention in this respect, many other neoplasms have been implicated.

Antigen can also be continuously absorbed from the environment thereby provoking the formation of immune complexes. Dietary antigens are one cause and immune complexes containing gluten have been detected in the diseased jejunal mucosa of patients with coeliac disease. Drugs are a potent source of haptens which, by combining with tissue proteins, can induce an antibody response and hence formation of immune complexes.

It is evident that virtually any encounter with an antigen is liable to induce immune complex formation. Indeed the more assiduously immune complexes have been sought in different disease states, the more commonly they have been detected. Furthermore, as no single laboratory technique can, as yet, detect all forms of immune complex, the frequency with which they can be found is largely dependent on the number of appropriate techniques the investigator is prepared to utilize.

Failure to Clear Soluble Complexes

The formation of immune complexes may become a process of pathological significance rather than an incidental finding if, for a variety of reasons, they are not readily cleared from the blood by the reticulo–endothelial system. In general there are three main factors which can predispose to the failure of elimination of complexed material:

(i) the nature and quantity of antigen,
(ii) the nature of the antibody response,
(iii) clearance by the reticulo–endothelial system.

(*i*) *The Nature and Quality of Antigen*

Complexes in which the antigen is predominantly monovalent or divalent will be poorly cleared from the circulation, particularly if they contain IgG subclasses for which monocytes and other reticulo–endothelial cells lack receptors. Lattice formation and hence clearance is limited if antigen is present in excess. Clearly some forms of antigen load such as those imposed by infections are particularly likely to provoke immune complex disease even in individuals without overt immune defects which might impair their ability to dispose of circulating complexes. Resistance to infectious disease is dependent on many host factors, some genetically determined, not all of which are linked to any obvious immunological function. Excessive production of antigen can in some infections, particularly by intracellular parasites, produce overwhelming amounts of soluble complexes. Nevertheless it must be conceded that other unexplained factors are probably operating since free antigen, antibody and soluble complexes can commonly be detected in the serum of patients without obvious ill-effects.

(*ii*) *The Nature of the Antibody Response*

It has long been recognized that the repeated injection of soluble antigens such as bovine serum albumin into rabbits is harmless in those animals which make antibody of sufficiently high affinity to eliminate antigen rapidly from the circulation. Rabbits which fail to clear antigen without a prolonged period in which soluble complexes circulate in the blood develop glomerulonephritis of variable severity. In mice, such susceptibility to immune complex disease has been attributed to the production of antibody of low affinity in certain inbred strains. These characteristics of the antibody response are probably under the control of immune response (Ir) genes whose immunopathological importance is summarized in a later section.

(iii) Clearance by the Reticulo–Endothelial System

The ways in which immune complexes are cleared from the circulation and catabolized are only partly understood. Whereas large complexes are readily phagocytosed by fixed or circulating cells, other mechanisms are involved in the clearance of smaller soluble complexes. Animal experiments indicate that the failure of such mechanisms potentiates the survival of complexes in the circulation. Human B-lymphocytes and cells of the monocyte–macrophage series bind immune complexes by their receptors for the Fc portion of the antibody molecule or for complement. Although it has not been formally demonstrated in man, it seems likely from experiments in other species that immune complexes are carried to the germinal centres of the lymph nodes and spleen by mononuclear cells and there degraded.

Disturbances of the complement system or of the pathways by which immune complexes are catabolized, are liable to prolong their period of circulation. Thus the complement components C1 to C3 enhance the neutralization of complexes between polyoma virus and antiviral antibody by agglutinating such complexes and thereby accelerating their phagocytosis (Oldstone *et al.*, 1974). The ability of complement to solubilize immune complexes (Miller and Nussenzweig, 1975) may well facilitate their clearance by phagocytic cells. Immune complex disease is associated with various forms of complement deficiency, whose number is likely to increase with improved methods of laboratory detection. This may take the form of deficient biosynthesis of a complement component, such as C2 deficiency in association with Henoch-Schönlein purpura (Epstein *et al.*, 1975). Furthermore, activation of the complement sequence leading to hypocomplementaemia has been proposed as the primary abnormality in some patients with mesangio–capillary glomerulonephritis (Peters and Lachmann, 1974). Abnormalities of this kind have two major consequences; firstly the ability to combat infection is impaired, thereby increasing susceptibility to immune complex disease, and secondly the period during which immune complexes circulate is prolonged.

Tissue Damage Induced by Immune Complexes

The mechanisms by which immune complexes induce tissue damage (Fig. 1) depends upon their site of production. The combination of antigen and antibody in the tissues produces local damage which is analogous, at least in its early stages, to a classical Arthus reaction. The predominant features of early lesions are the accumulation of polymorphonuclear leukocytes and the deposition of complement in sites of complex formation. Subsequently mononuclear cell infiltration becomes more prominent. The precise sequence of events can only be established if the lesions are examined at frequent intervals by a combination of techniques. This is obviously more practicable in animal models than in human disease. Thus, the transfer of auto-immune

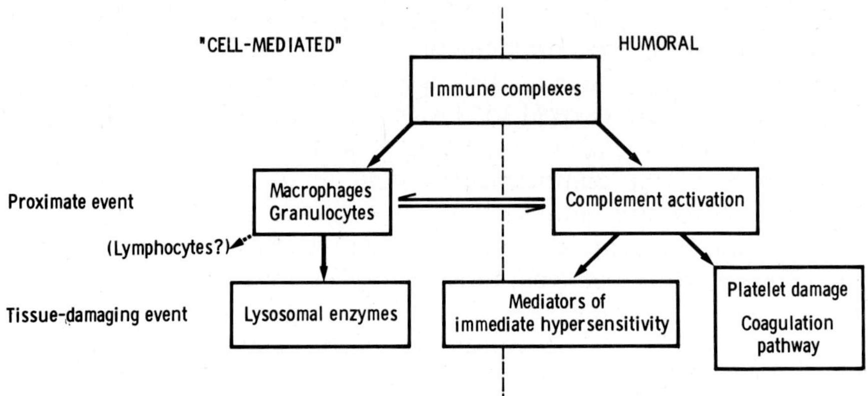

Fig. 1. Immune complexes and their immunopathological consequences. This is a grossly over-simplified representation of the *major* pathways only. The most important omissions are the control mechanisms which make most of these events the exception rather than the rule. The interaction of "cellular" and "humoral" factors is emphasized.

thyroiditis to normal rabbits and other species by the injection of serum containing thyroid auto-antibody has pointed strongly to the primary importance of antibody in the pathogenesis of this disease. Sequential studies of auto-immune thyroiditis (Clagett *et al.*, 1974) have clarified the sequence of events which leads to tissue damage at least in this experiment model. Circulating auto-antibody reacts with autologous thyroglobulin in the space between the basement membrane and the follicular cells. This interaction is marked by the deposition at this site of immunoglobulin and complement detectable by immunofluorescence, or visible as dense deposits by electron microscopy. In the early stages of the lesion polymorphonuclear granulocytes are prominent histologically and their influx in response to the deposition of immune complexes is probably accounted for by the complement binding. Later in the course of the disease, mononuclear cells accumulate in large numbers giving rise to the erroneous conclusion that these lesions are primarily cell mediated.

Sequential observations of this kind have, inevitably, been less frequently recorded in clinical medicine. Nevertheless opportunities have arisen for studying the series of immunopathological events provoked by defined causes of immune complex formation. Thus gluten has been administered to susceptible patients during remission thereby provoking the deposition of immune complexes and complement in the jejunal epithelium. Similarly improved techniques for examining the synovial membrane in the early stages of inflammatory arthritis have emphasized that immune complex deposition with infiltration by polymorphonuclear leucocytes is a prominent feature (Schumacher and Gall, 1974).

Blood vessels throughout the body are susceptible to damage initiated by circulating immune complexes but the kidneys are particularly vulnerable because the glomeruli allow the selective trapping and filtration of circulating material. This deposition can itself damage the blood vessel but the pathological consequences for the most part result from a variety of secondary events. Complement is both deposited and activated at sites of immune complex deposition. Polymorphonuclear leucocytes are attracted directly by the complexes and also by the chemotactic stimulus generated by complement activation. Immune complexes are ingested by these cells within vacuoles which merge with the lysosomes, thereby stimulating the selective secretion of lysosomal hydrolases which are toxic to a variety of tissue constituents (Page *et al.*, 1974) although the granulocyte itself remains viable. Moreover by the process of "reverse endocytosis" the granulocytes can secrete lysomal enzymes without the need for phagocytosing complexes. Reverse endocytosis is also stimulated by the generation of the complement component C5a following activation of either the classical or alternative complement pathways. Finally, the coagulation pathway can be activated in immune complex disease whilst histamine release may ensue as a result of the generation of anaphylotoxin during complement activation.

Some forms of complex attach preferentially to circulating red cells and fix complement. Such complexes tend to be of low molecular weight and, being easily detached from their binding sites on the membrane, readily reattach to other red cells. Complement, however, remains more firmly bound and all the red cells to which immune complexes have at some stage adhered, are prematurely removed from the circulation (Petz and Garretty, 1974). This is also seen in some auto-immune haemolytic anaemias (Fig. 2). Even morphological differences between various types of immune complex nephritis have been attributed to the selective distribution within the glomerulus of complexes with varying molecular weight and composition (Evans, 1974). For example, membranous glomerulonephritis seems likely to be produced by a combination of antigen and antibody which only reaches equivalence in the subepithelial zone. As a result little attraction of polymorphonuclear leucocytes leading to an inflammatory reaction would be expected.

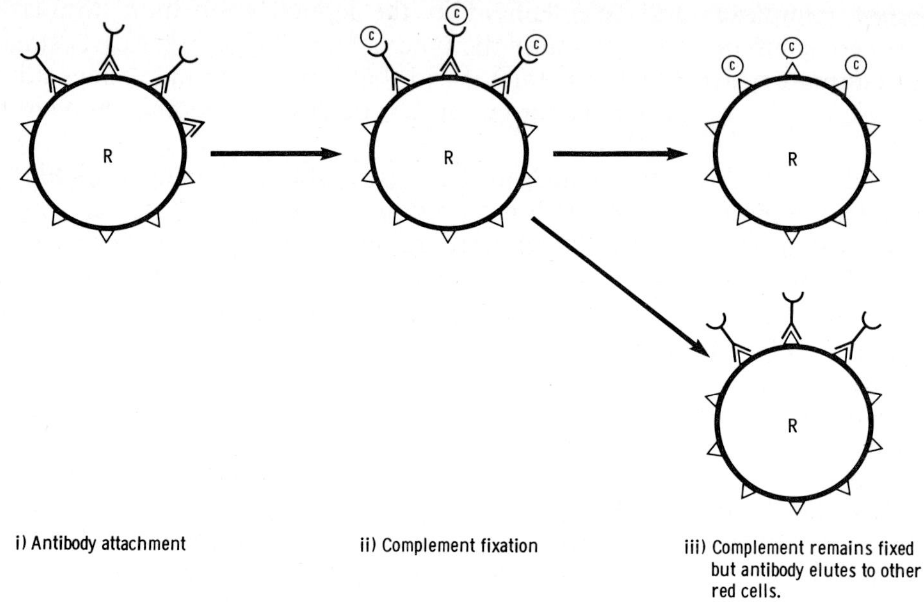

Fig. 2. Complement fixation by antibody to red cells. R = red cell; △ = red cell antigen; Ꭹ = red cell auto-antibody with Fc fragment; © = complement.

Local Antibody Synthesis

Antibody is synthesized in tissues which are the site of chronic immune reactions. In animal models such as auto-immune thyroiditis induced by immunization with heterologous thyroglobulin, local production of antibody to thyroglobulin can be demonstrated by a plaque technique. Similarly antibody to basic myelin is synthesized in the brains of animals with experimental allergic encephalomyelitis. Such experiments show that the antibody is not merely sequestered from the circulation but is secreted by lymphoid cells in the lesions. There is a clear advantage to the host in conveying cumbersome immunoglobulin macromolecules on the membranes of lymphocytes or macrophages which can readily penetrate intercellular spaces and even traverse the plasma membrane of other cells (Hall, 1969). There is little direct evidence that specific antibody is synthesized in comparable lesions in man although the direct demonstration of immunoglobulin synthesis in tissues such as rheumatoid synovial membrane and salivary glands affected by Sjögren's disease makes this highly probable. Indeed, in the former site the synthesis of rheumatoid factor has been specifically detected.

CELLULAR MECHANISMS

There are four principal grounds for believing that cell mediated immunity contributes significantly to tissue damage in human disease. Firstly, patients commonly give delayed hypersensitivity skin reactions to antigen which are related to the initiation of their disease. The best known example is the skin reaction to tuberculoprotein in patients with tuberculous infection. However this observation does not in itself prove that lymphocytes produce the tissue lesions which characterize tuberculous disease nor settles the time-honoured controversy about the contribution of hypersensitivity in this complaint. Secondly, lymphocytes often react *in vitro* to antigens related to disease in tests such as blast transformation or the release of radioisotopes from target cells bearing the relevant antigen. Positive results of this kind imply that the patient is sensitized to a particular antigen but again do not prove that the disease is cell-mediated. Thirdly, steroids and cytotoxic drugs have powerful therapeutic effects in many diseases in which the affected tissue is infiltrated by mononuclear cells. Such agents affect tissues in a variety of ways and are not sufficiently selective in their action even on the immune system to distinguish between the relative importance of different forms of immune responses. Finally, mononuclear cell infiltrations are a prominent histological feature in many tissues affected by immunological processes. However this can be misleading as firm conclusions cannot be drawn about the nature and function of the infiltrating cells. Techniques for isolating these cells and characterizing them either immediately or after short-term tissue culture give some indication of the relative numbers of lymphocytes and other mononuclear cells of various populations but again do not prove that a disease is cell mediated. Clearly the classical criterion for such a reaction, namely transfer of the disease by cells, cannot easily be tested with human material. The best hope of establishing the pathogenic importance of lymphocytes in inflammatory lesions is likely to be the development of suitable *in vitro* systems for examining the interaction between the responsible antigen and the infiltrating cells.

The mononuclear cells in chronic inflammatory lesions belong to heterogeneous populations with separate functions; these have to be fully evaluated before their pathological importance can be defined. The more this is achieved the less meaningful a rigid distinction between "immediate" and "delayed" hypersensitivity is likely to appear.

There is no doubt that under a variety of conditions lymphocytes can be shown to kill other cells *in vitro*. This has been demonstrated in numerous experiments in which lymphocytes sensitized to specific antigens destroy cells bearing those antigens. The antigenicity of such "target cells" can be related to the histocompatibility antigens they carry, their neoplastic nature, the antigens of viral or other infections or antigens specific to the organ or species of origin. This destruction can be monitored morphologically or by measuring the release of a suitable isotope such as radioactive chromium from the target cells. A major difficulty in the interpretation of the results is the propensity of lymphocytes to attack target cells such as fibroblasts with indiscriminate enthusiasm. This is particularly true of experiments in which the contact between lymphocytes and target cells is prolonged over a period of several days. In animal experiments this problem may not be insoluble because the appropriate controls can easily be devised. The specificity of interactions between human lymphocytes and cells such as fibroblast monolayers needs careful assessment.

The mechanisms of damage mediated by specifically sensitized T-lymphocytes (T-cell mechanism) and by non-sensitized mononuclear cells and macrophages (K-cell and macrophage mechanisms) must be clearly distinguished (Fig. 3). Specifically sensitized lymphocytes destroy only those target cells with antigenic determinants on their surface which are recognized by the effector cells. This mechanism of cell destruction does not depend on the release of antibody from the surface of cells of the lymphocyte series, contrasting with other situations in which cells carrying passive antibody can become cytotoxic, i.e. the K-cell and macrophage mechanisms.

T-cell Mechanism

The exact details of target cell killing by sensitized lymphocytes are still controversial. Most of the experimental evidence indicates that it results from a direct surface interaction between the effector and target cells (Ferluga and Allison, 1974). The first requirement, therefore, is for mobile lymphocytes which can make effective contact with the target cells. As a result of

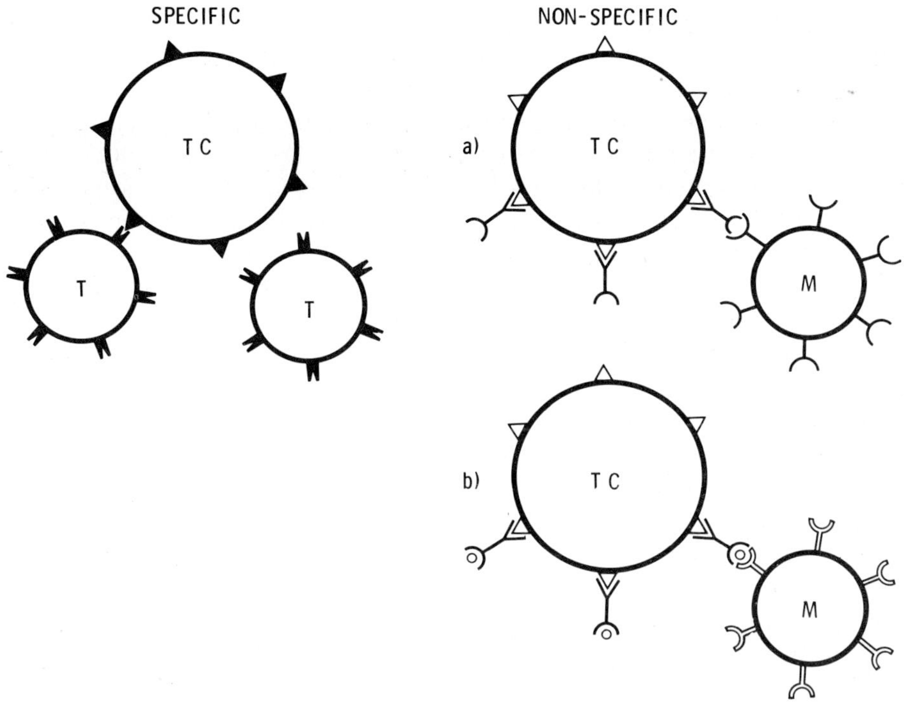

Fig. 3. Varieties of cytotoxicity mediated by mononuclear cells. Specific killing: ▲ — antigen on TC, the target cell; ▙ = specific receptor on T-lymphocyte (T). Non specific killing: (a) △ is a receptor on TC, the target cell, for specific antibody with an Fc portion ⋎. Receptors for the Fc portion of the antibody molecule ⋎ are present on mononuclear K-cells and macrophages (M). (b) the Fc portion of the molecule binds complement, O, for which receptors are also present on mononuclear cells and macrophages (M).

this apposition of membranes, damage to the target cell is initiated within minutes and will proceed even after the lymphocyte has disengaged and has moved away from the site of the reaction. Possibly the structure of the target cell membrane becomes altered in a way which renders it abnormally permeable to the leakage of intracellular ions and, possibly, also cytoplasmic proteins; thereafter osmotic processes complete the destruction of the cell. Nevertheless it must be stressed that the elucidation of this process is incomplete and of the greatest importance. It already seems unlikely that it can be accounted for by complement release or by the generation of lysolecithin, both of which have been adduced to explain the phenomenon.

Although theories based on the direct interaction between effector and target cells have been widely favoured by immunologists, the possibility remains that immune lymphocytes can release factors which diffuse through the tissues and damage cells at a distance. This notion is particularly appealing to clinicians because much of the evidence favouring it has been derived from observations in experimental pathology rather than *in vitro* reactions between cells. Moreover if this mechanism is accepted a pathogenetic role could still be attributed to sparse lymphocytic infiltrates in biopsies from diseased tissues whose destructive effects would be thereby greatly amplified. Such products are termed lymphotoxins and belong to that group of soluble factors or "lymphokines" which are released from activated lymphocytes (see Chapter 9). As an example, it has been claimed that factors released by the interaction of lymphocytes and antigen, produce demyelination in the central nervous system of guinea-pigs (Wisniewski and Bloom, 1975). It is also noteworthy that muscle fragments from patients with dermatomyositis or polymyositis stimulate the production of lymphotoxins by autologous lymphocytes which are toxic to muscle (Johnson *et al.*, 1972).

K-cell Mechanism

There are also *in vitro* systems in which mononuclear cells, which are not themselves specifically sensitized, are cytotoxic to target cells which have been sensitized with antibody (Fig. 3). Cytolysis of this kind results from interaction between the Fc portion of the sensitizing antibody and Fc receptors on the effector cells. The latter also possess receptors for complement which potentiate cytolysis by enhancing contact between the reacting cells (Perlmann *et al.*, 1975). The effector cells for this kind of reaction have proved rather difficult to characterize but they can be distinguished by morphological criteria and by their cell surface characteristics from most recognized populations of lymphocytes and macrophages. In particular, the cells in human peripheral blood which mediate what has been called "antibody dependent cytotoxicity" belong to a separate population with distinctive properties. Cytotoxic activity of this nature has been demonstrated in the pathogenesis of human immune disorders. For example, effector cells for this cytotoxic reaction contribute to the cellular infiltrate in auto-immune thyroiditis and in renal homografts undergoing rejection. Normal blood also contains cells which are cytotoxic for target cells which have been sensitized by coating them first with thyroglobulin and then with anti-thyroglobulin antibody obtained from the sera of patients with Hashimoto's thyroiditis (Calder *et al.*, 1973). Although cytotoxic reactions have mainly been demonstrated *in vitro*, the pathological features of many diseases are compatible with damage inflicted by this kind of process. Moreover the discovery of the K-cell type of damage which utilizes specific antibody resolves a major difficulty in understanding the significance of cellular infiltrates in chronic inflammatory lesions; this is the failure to demonstrate specific sensitization to tissue antigens in more than a small proportion of the cells which are attracted to sites of immunological damage whether in experimental models or in clinical material.

Macrophage Mechanism

Macrophages are prominent in many chronic inflammatory lesions. These cells have characteristic features by which they can be readily distinguished in tissue culture, such as their glass adherence, phagocytic powers and prominent lysosomes. In standard histological preparations these properties cannot be utilized for diagnostic purposes and thus their importance has been overlooked in many diseases. However, their contribution to chronic inflammatory lesions which have been experimentally induced is now fully accepted. The monocytes from which macrophages are derived reach sites of inflammation predominantly from the blood (Fig. 4). Here they differentiate into functional macrophages and can persist in this form for prolonged periods. Macrophages are stimulated to secrete lysosomal enzymes through a process of exocytosis by phagocytosing substances which they are unable to degrade and catabolize; these include many substances which are relevant to human disorders such as silica and asbestos particles, streptococcal cell walls and antigen–antibody complexes (Page *et al.*, 1974). The acid hydrolases that are produced by the lysosomes of macrophages have the same ability to attack numerous tissue components as those released by polymorphonuclear granulocytes. Moreover fixed macrophages also contribute to tissue damage in inflammatory lesions, the type A lining cells of the synovial membrane being a particular case in point. The importance of this kind of tissue damage lies in the link it provides between the specific immunological events which often initiate an inflammatory reaction and the nonspecific nature of later events which may prolong it indefinitely.

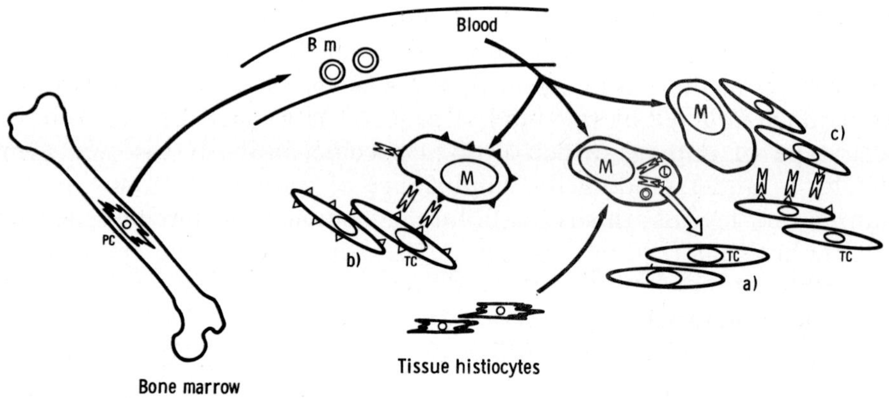

Fig. 4. Macrophages and immunopathology. Macrophage precursor cells (PC) are found predominantly in the bone marrow which gives rise to blood monocytes (Bm) which migrate to the lesion and there differentiate as macrophages (M). Tissue histiocytes also contribute to this pool. Three principal events ensue: (a) macrophages ingest immune complexes (≊◃) (or other irritants) which stimulate enzyme secretion by lysosomes (◎). These enzymes (⇒) are toxic to tissue components. (b) Macrophages become "armed" with antibody (≊) bound to their receptors (▲) and thereby react with antigens (△) on tissue cells (TC). (c) Macrophages separate target cells (TC) in the tissue planes and thereby allow access for antibody (≊) to react with surface antigen (△).

FAILURE OF CONTROL MECHANISMS

General Mechanisms

The mere demonstration of an immune response to an antigen does not imply that this will have pathological consequences. Thus antibody and specifically sensitized lymphocytes can be detected in individuals who show no signs of clinical hypersensitivity to the relevant antigen; the extent of the reaction is limited by homoeostatic mechanisms. Immune responses are subject to regulatory mechanisms which control both their intensity and duration. Elucidating the various ways in which different lymphoid cell populations collaborate in the induction of immune responses has also clarified the manner in which such responses are inhibited (Gershon, 1974) (Fig. 5). The details are still the subject of debate and certainly vary with different antigens. Nevertheless the triggering of B-lymphocytes to produce antibody depends upon the interaction of T-lymphocytes or their products with antigen, and specialized macrophages. Similarly, the most important feed-back pathway is that by which 7S antibody inhibits the production of both 19S and 7S antibody, the critical site being most probably the macrophage (Abrahams *et al.*, 1973). Cell-mediated immunity is also subject to homoeostatic control by circulating 7S antibody.

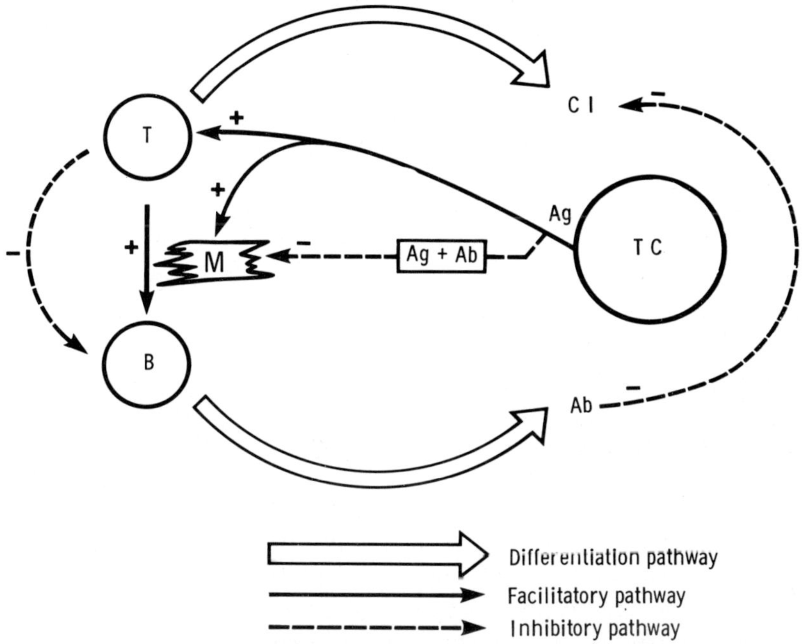

Fig. 5. Control mechanisms in immune responses. This is a simplified diagram of the principal facilitatory (+) and inhibitory (−) pathways. TC = target cell (e.g. infected host cell); Ag = antigen; T = T-lymphocytes; B = B-lymphocytes; M = Macrophages; CI = Cellular immunity; Ab = antibody; Ag + Ab = immune complexes.

Whilst the physiological role of antibody in regulating the immune response has been particularly stressed, a similar function is now attributed to subpopulations of T-lymphocytes. There are numerous experiments which indicate that such cells release factors which suppress the induction or amplification of immune responses involving both antibody production and cell-mediated immunity. The majority of these experiments involve the transfer of immune responses to animals by lymphoid cells and manoeuvres which interfere with such transfers. However a number of clinical observations suggest that the abrogation of control mechanisms by disease or therapy results in immune disorders. This can take the form of exaggerated reactions to infectious agents, drugs or simple skin tests to infectious agents, drugs, or sensitizing materials. It has also been suggested that prolonged hyper-immunization will induce a lymphoproliferative disease with auto-antibody production and cryoglobulinaemia by over-riding normal control mechanisms (Schultz and Yunis, 1975). This sequence of events has been observed frequently in experimental animals.

Immune Response (Ir) Genes

Variations in immune responsiveness could predispose different individuals to disease in a variety of ways which would be genetically determined. Hypersensitivity to drugs or a deficient response to microorganisms are obvious possibilities. In many species the immune response is controlled by genes which are closely related to the histocompatibility genes and have been termed Ir genes. These are inherited as autosomal dominants and their influence on immune response has for the most part been considered to operate through T-lymphocyte populations. Thus Ir genes determine the response to thymus dependent but not thymus independent antigens (see Chapter 2) with respect to both circulating antibody and delayed hypersensitivity. The lack of response to a particular antigen controlled by these genes is usually fairly specific; it is only detectable if they are challenged with relatively small quantities of antigen, being no longer apparent with larger doses. However, the inability to respond to a low dose of a particular thymus dependent antigen can still be overcome if the T-lymphocytes of the recipient are activated by other means at the time antigen is given (Fig. 6).

Such considerations are not entirely of academic interest since they indicate how patients may be provoked into undesirable reactions to antigens such as drugs and auto-antigens by intercurrent infections. Conversely they suggest means of increasing the immune response for therapeutic purposes.

It now seems likely that Ir genes function in ways which are more complex than simply determining the level of T-lymphocyte responsiveness to antigen. These include modifying the receptors for antigen on T-lymphocytes and inducing "acceptor" sites on T- and B-lymphocytes which are necessary for their interaction.

A number of associations between histocompatibility genes and human diseases have been clearly established (Möller, 1975). The majority of such studies have relied on specific anti-sera to HLA antigens but other markers on lymphocytes have been used which are detected by mixed lymphocyte reactions with selected panels of lymphocytes from other individuals and are termed LD (lymphocyte determined) antigens (see Chapter 29). The results of testing for LD antigens are more variable and extraneous factors such as drug treatment and intercurrent virus infection are more likely to interfere.

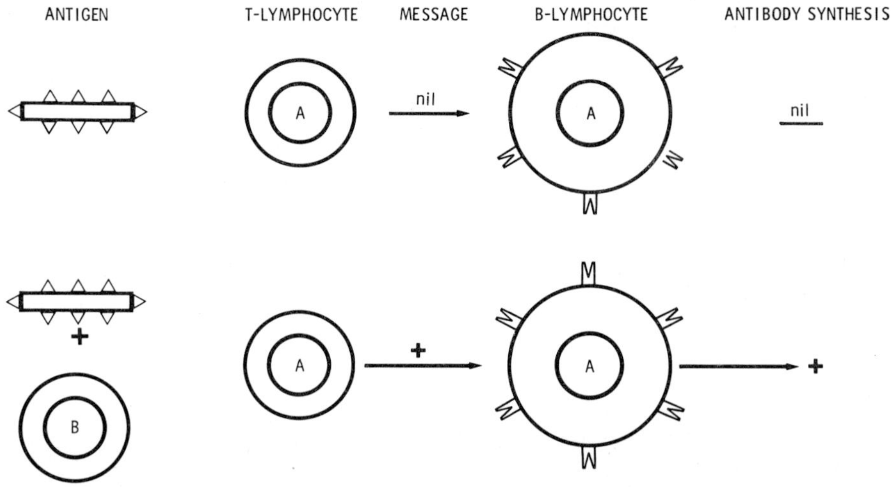

Fig. 6. The allogeneic effect. The T-lymphocytes of mouse strain A have no receptors for the determinant △ on the antigen, and are unable to trigger B-lymphocytes which possess the appropriate receptor M, into division and hence into antibody synthesis. Interaction with lymphocytes of strain B is followed by the proliferation of T lymphocytes of strain A with the production of a message which, together with antigen △, stimulates a specific antibody response. This effect may be exploitable in conditions of unresponsiveness to infectious diseases in man.

The increased frequency with which some HLA antigens occur in patients with a variety of chronic inflammatory and auto-immune diseases is particularly striking. Moreover, there is a preponderance of second locus HLA-B antigens over those of the first HLA-A locus in this connection (Table 3). An unexpectedly high occurrence of these alleles, either singly or in combination, has often been observed not only in the patients presenting with these diseases but also in their family members. The term "linkage disequilibrium" is used when two alleles, each occurring at two different loci, e.g. the HLA-A and HLA-B loci, appear together in individuals of a particular population more often that one would expect by chance. Such a phenomenon has been linked to disease proneness although in order to explain its occurrence one has to postulate that some biological advantage is conferred by the linked state or that the population is not fully out-bred.

TABLE 3

HL-A associations and disease

Disease	HLA type
Arthropathies	
ankylosing spondylitis	B27
Reiter's syndrome	
post-infective arthritis	
psoriatic arthritis	
juvenile rheumatoid arthritis	
associated with gastro-intestinal disorders	
Skin diseases	
psoriasis	A10
dermatitis herpetiformis	B8
Eye complaints	
uveitis	B27
Gastrointestinal disease	
coeliac disease	B8
chronic active hepatitis	B8
Central nervous system disorders	
multiple sclerosis	A3, B7, B18, D7a
Auto-immune disease	
insulin dependent diabetes mellitus	B8, B15, D8a
thyrotoxicosis	B8
Addison's disease	B8, D8a

Despite the strength of these HLA associations, particularly those with ankylosing spondylitis and related diseases, they do not prove that susceptibility to such disorders is determined by Ir genes or even by immunological mechanisms in general. Only in the arthritis which follows some bacterial infections are there firm grounds for attributing the influence of an HLA gene to the variabilities of host resistance to the responsible agent and even in this instance factors may be operating other than the obvious parameters of the immune response. Direct attempts to link HLA antigens with the patterns of response to specific antigens have so far had limited success. Family studies in ankylosing spondylitis and psoriasis make it extremely unlikely that possessing the B27 antigen is the only factor which determines susceptibility and other factors both genetic and environmental seem certain to be involved. Furthermore these antigens may predispose to disease through other mechanisms such as the distribution of virus receptors on human cells (Möller, 1975).

Nevertheless some evidence has been gathered which suggests that genetically determined patterns of immune response may govern susceptibility to some diseases. With respect to acute hypersensitivity, hay fever caused by ragweed pollen and IgE antibody production to its principal allergen, antigen E, are significantly associated with HLA haplotypes in successive generations of families with these complaints (Levine *et al.*, 1972). This feature of the immune response may only be revealed after challenge with antigens which have a relatively simple structure and may be obscured after immunization with complex ones.

The immune response to microorganisms largely determines the clinical course and is also genetically controlled. Thus the polyarthritis induced by *Yersinia enterocolitica*, *Salmonella* and *Shigella* infections has immunopathological features which are highly suggestive of immune complex disease and the genetically determined character of the antibody response may predispose to this complication by one of the mechanisms which has been discussed.

AUTO-IMMUNE DISEASE

Auto-immunity is that state where an immunological response is directed at the patient's own antigens. It is essential to distinguish between diseases which are directly mediated by auto-immunity and those in which autoantibodies can be demonstrated but whose pathological effects are unproven. Examples of true auto-immune diseases are thrombocytopenic purpura and haemolytic anaemia in which antibodies directed at platelets or red cells lead to their destruction in the peripheral blood or premature sequestration by the reticulo–endothelial system. In contrast, anti-nuclear antibodies occur in several connective tissue diseases without inflicting obvious tissue damage whilst antibodies reactive with thyroid antigens are detected in many patients, particularly in the elderly, who show no other signs of overt thyroid disease. It is uncertain whether auto-immunity results from the acquisition of new antigen(s) by tissues such as red cells and the thyroid or from a primary abnormality in the lymphocytes which mediate these reactions.

Initiation of Auto-immunity

The theory of auto-immunity (Fig. 7) which has dominated medical thinking since it was first propounded is Burnet's hypothesis of "forbidden clones". This proposes that lymphocytes which are immunologically responsive to a particular antigen belong to an individual clone of cells and that self-reactive clones are eliminated. Any cells with the capacity to respond to self-antigens are, it is proposed, eliminated in the thymus, or at other sites by cells derived from the thymus. This theory of clonal deletion has had to be modified in the light of recent findings.

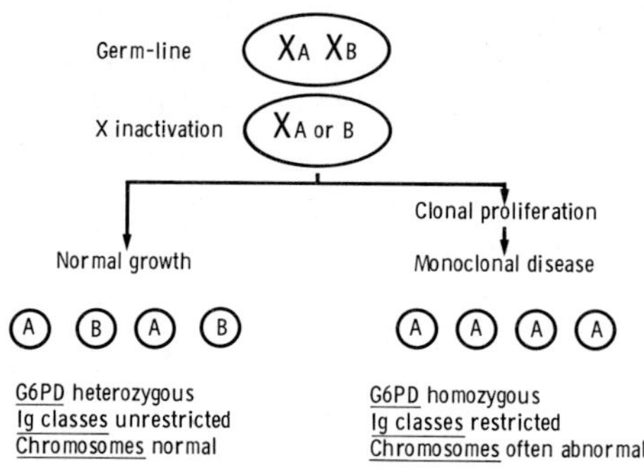

Fig. 7. Are autoreactive lymphocytes clonal? Three techniques have been used to show that Burkitt's lymphoma and other lymphoproliferative diseases are clonal. 1. Glucose-6-phosphate dehydrogenase (G6PD) markers: During X-inactivation one X-linked gene product is randomly inactivated, in this instance type A *or* B G6PD. Normal tissues are a mosaic of both types. Cells which are the progeny of a *single* cell are homozygous for G6PD. This technique is only applicable in black females, i.e. G6PD heterozygotes. 2. Ig classes: Surface Ig markers may be of limited heavy and light chain class but not *necessarily* so. 3. Chromosomal abnormalities: Clones often have a distinctive chromosomal marker (e.g. the Philadelphia chromosome in chronic myeloid leukaemia). The application of these techniques to the problems of auto-immunity is in its infancy.

B-lymphocytes with receptors for auto-antigens have been detected in the peripheral blood of normal subjects. Moreover, cells secreting auto-antibody are present in the lymphoid tissues of mice which do not in any way exhibit the signs of auto-immune disease. The validity of some of these experiments is still open to question since procedures for demonstrating the binding of auto-antigenic proteins such as thyroglobulins to human lymphocytes probably alter the structure and hence the immunogenicity of these proteins. If auto-reactive B-cells are normally present then an explanation has to be found for the loss of a controlling mechanism. The demonstration of co-operative interactions between T- and B-lymphocytes suggests that populations of T-lymphocytes may perform a regulatory function with respect to auto-reactive B-lymphocytes. A major advance would be to show that the lymphoid cells which produce auto-antibody are truly clonal in origin, that is the progeny of a single lymphoid cell which has escaped the control of T-lymphocytes; such a demonstration would strengthen the view that auto-immunity results from a primary defect in the lymphoid system. Techniques of the kind needed to test this possibility have been successful in demonstrating the clonal origin of several tumours including those originating from lymphoid cells such as Burkitt's lymphoma (Fialkow *et al.*, 1973a). They have not yet been applied to the analysis of human auto-immune disease but have provided strong evidence that clonal proliferation of lymphoid cells is a consistent feature in the spleens of NZB mice (Fialkow *et al.*, 1973b). Thus Damashek's suggestion that many auto-immune diseases are primary immuno-proliferative processes is amenable to experimental testing. The tendency of patients with lymphomas to develop auto-immune haemolytic anaemia is well recognized and, more recently, polyclonal hyper-gammaglobulinaemia with B-lymphocyte proliferation has been recorded in elderly patients with clinical features highly suggestive of graft-versus-host disease (Frizzera *et al.*, 1974).

Ablation of Control Mechanisms

If auto-immunity were proven to result from the uncontrolled proliferation of auto-reactive B-lymphocytes, the next step would be to show that this followed the failure of T-lymphocytes to suppress the process. To this end numerous reports have appeared concerning the distribution of lymphocyte subpopulations in auto-immune and connective tissue diseases, many of which purport to indicate a deficiency of "T-lymphocytes". However, there are difficulties in interpreting such results and in particular in deciding whether they indicate a primary deficiency of this nature. Immune function is commonly impaired as a non-specific consequence of persistent disease activity and abnormalities of lymphocyte transformation function *in vitro* or even of the immune responses *in vivo* cannot be assumed to be responsible for the onset of disease. Furthermore the selective sequestration of mono-nuclear cells within inflammatory tissues undoubtedly distorts the pattern of circulating cells observed in the peripheral blood. A resolution of this issue awaits the introduction of more specific assays of lymphocyte function and better screening of patient populations in the early stages of these disorders.

Altered Tissue Antigens

Another way of explaining the onset of auto-immune disease which does not mutually exclude theories invoking the regulation of B-lymphocytes is to attribute their pathogenesis to the stimulus provided by altered tissue antigens. This theory conforms with modern knowledge about the ability of simple, low molecular weight compounds to become antigenic after binding to carrier proteins. Thus the commonest causes of auto-immunity and, less frequently, auto-immune disease are drugs such as procainamide and methyl dopa. In addition the ability of virus infections, both transitory and persistent, to induce the formation of new antigens on cell surfaces is now well recognized. The frequent association of virus infection with auto-immune disease of variable duration suggests that viral modification of tissue antigens is an event of frequent clinical significance.

An eight-year-old boy presented with fever, muscle pains, lymphadenopathy, atypical mononuclear cells which exceeded 8,000 per cm and a rising titre of complement fixing antibody to cytomegalovirus which was initially 1/256. The Paul-Bunnell test was negative. The condition was diagnosed as uncomplicated cytomegalovirus infection. However over the next four weeks he developed a severe thrombocytopenia with the platelet count falling below 10,000 per cm and a strongly positive direct Coombs test. Steroid treatment was only partially successful and eventually splenectomy became necessary. An association with the initial cytomegalovirus infection seems inescapable.

The difficulty of this theory is to explain why only a small percentage of patients exposed to drugs or infections of this nature develop auto-immune disease. It has been postulated that drugs or viral antigens on cell surfaces are either closely related totographically to tissue antigens on host cells or else that the latter are modified as a result of this interaction. Cross-reaction with these altered antigens breaks tolerance in T-lymphocytes which thereby co-operate with and de-repress those B-lymphocytes which are potentially able to react with tissue antigens (Fig. 8). The variable susceptibility to auto-immune disease of people exposed to the same stimuli seems likely to depend on genetic factors for which the induction of auto-immune disease in animals can be cited as an appropriate analogy. The injection of thyroid or brain tissue from a foreign species in suitable form commonly induces auto-immune thyroiditis or encephalitis respectively in the recipient animal. The ease with which this can be accomplished varies with different strains of the same species and is genetically controlled. The precise level at which this control

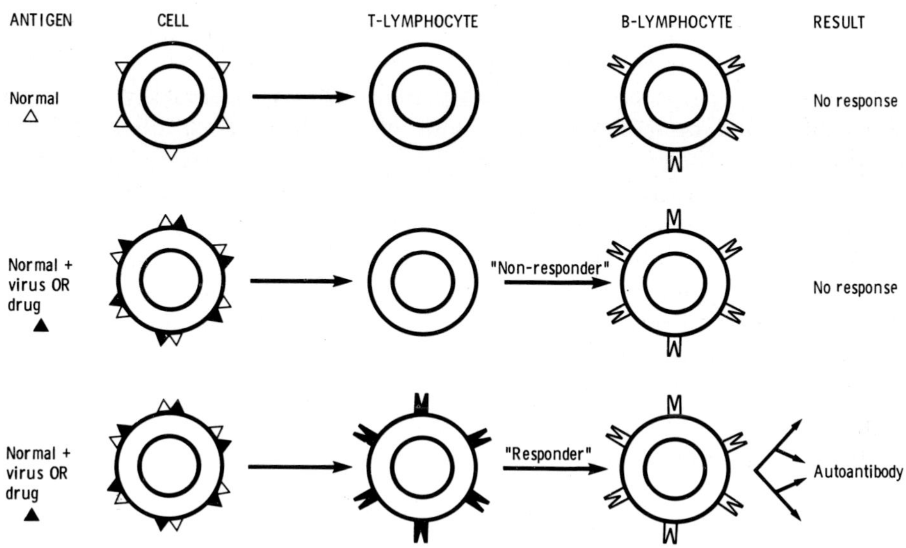

Fig. 8. Breaking of tolerance by exogenous agents. Normal cells do not induce an auto-antibody response by B-lymphocytes

operates is still debated but is likely to depend upon the speed with which homeostatic control can be restored and this in turn may prove to be related to T-lymphocyte function.

Mediators of the Auto-immune Response

The forms of immune response which are crucial to the development of human auto-immune disease have long been debated and the relative importance of circulating antibody and delayed hypersensitivity has been a particularly controversial issue. Much of the argument has centred on premises which, in retrospect, have been greatly over-simplified. Thus the mere observation that the diseased tissue is infiltrated by "mononuclear cells" in histological preparations does not constitute proof that the pathological changes result from "cell-mediated immunity" until the infiltrating cells have been characterized by other means. Claims that cell mediated immunity to auto-antigens have been detected in these diseases often rely on imperfect or inadequately controlled techniques, whose *in vivo* relevance remains to be established. Similarly the role of auto-antibody in these diseases has been over-simplified.

In different animal models there is evidence that auto-antibody may either initiate auto-immune disease or conversely can be shown to have a protective function. The heterogeneity of antibody classes involved could explain these discrepancies and the same caveat must be applied to human disease in which the presence of circulating auto-antibody is by no means synonymous with auto-immune disease. Theoretically auto-antibody could act synergistically with antibody dependent cytotoxic cells i.e. the K-cell mechanism (see above) to induce tissue damage (MacLennan, 1972) and direct evidence of this process has been obtained in auto-immune thyroiditis. On the other hand antibody complexed to auto-antigen might block tissue destruction by sensitized lymphocytes, a possibility suggested from studies of tumour immunology but which is as yet supported by few direct observations in human auto-immune disease. This issue will only be clarified after more data from human disease has been carefully and dispassionately analysed.

THE IMMUNOPATHOLOGY OF VIRUS INFECTIONS

The immunopathological consequences of virus infections (Fenner *et al.*, 1974) are complicated by two factors. Firstly viruses replicate in a variety of host cells whose distribution is determined mainly by the biological properties of individual strains, but to some extent also by the immune responses of the host at the time of infection. Moreover virus infection of host cells may take many different forms, some of which are particularly liable to result in persistent infection. A complete cycle of virus replication with the release of fresh virus particles is only one of several possible outcomes; many viruses become integrated in the cell with only partial expression of viral functions in the form of protein synthesis directed by viral nucleic acid. This produces a highly variable pattern of virus specific antigens which in turn stimulates an immune response by the host of varying form and intensity. Indeed, the cell may fail to express any readily detectable signs of virus infection unless it is reactivated by a physical or chemical stimulus or by some form of intercurrent stress whose precise nature is often hard to define. A pertinent example of the many forms infection by the same virus may take is provided by herpes simplex (Fig. 9).

The second factor which complicates the course of viral infections is the ability of many viruses to subvert host defences by interacting with the

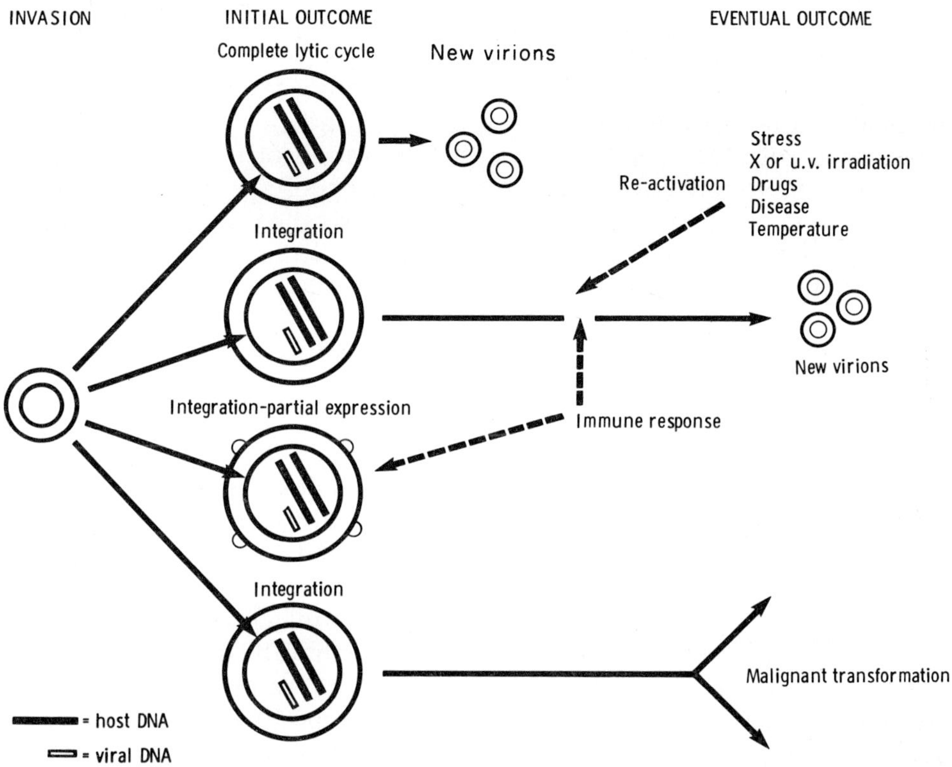

Fig. 9. Herpes simplex virus infection has several possible outcomes: 1. replication with death of the infected cell and the release of new infectious particles; 2. integration of viral DNA without the production of infectious particles, viral surface antigens or the death of the infected cell. There are many stimuli which can re-activate the virus but until then the cell does not provoke an immune response; 3. as in 2. but virus-coded antigens are expressed on the cell surface thereby provoking an immune response; 4. malignant transformation, an *in vitro* phenomenon whose clinical relevance is debatable.

different forms of immune response in a way which diminishes their effectiveness and encourages virus persistence.

Types of Immune Response in Virus Infections

The major problem in viral immunopathology is to determine the relative importance of tissue damage inflicted by viral cytopathic effects on the one hand and that resulting from the immune response by the host on the other. In a laboratory model of virus diseases such as lymphocytic choriomeningitis (LCM) virus infection it is relatively easy to attribute the characteristic acute encephalitis to T-lymphocyte cytotoxicity and the glomerulonephritis and other lesions of chronic infection to the deposition of immune complexes. Conversely the giant cell pneumonia seen in children with impaired cell-mediated immunity who contract measles is clearly the result of an abnormal pattern of virus infection in a compromised host. In most clinical infections the distinction cannot be readily made.

Acute Hypersensitivity

The majority of fleeting rashes in acute virus infections probably result from antibody reacting with widely disseminated viral antigen either expressed on the surface of the endothelial lining cells of blood vessels or encountered transiently in the blood. Occasionally the reaction is urticarial, as in the prodromal phase of acute infective hepatitis or of infectious mononucleosis. The infections are rarely of serious consequence and the morbidity is slight. However acute hypersensitivity may have more serious implications in respiratory infections of children and could account at least in part for the morbidity resulting from infections by agents such as reoviruses and respiratory syncytical virus.

Immune Complex Disease and Related Mechanisms

There are numerous examples of persistent virus infections in animals in which the agent circulates in combination with antibody. Although rising antibody titres in the blood enable the host to clear the blood of the major part of the circulating virus, residual virus commonly persists in the blood, usually bound to antibody in the form of infectious complexes. This sequence of events has been particularly well documented in mice infected with herpes simplex or lactic dehydrogenase viruses (Notkins, 1971). Antibody to the γ-globulin of the host enables the great part of this activity to be neutralized and provides an interesting analogy with rheumatoid factor. Virus probably continues to enter the blood from sites of replication in the tissues which are little affected by specific antibody. Indeed, it is a remarkable observation that cyclophosphamide treatment which ablates the antibody response to LCM virus in mice chronically infected with this virus has little effect on the amount of virus carried in the tissues (Hoffsten and Dixon, 1973). The amount of viral replication is itself controlled by independent genetic factors (Oldstone *et al.*, 1973).

The evidence suggests that infectious virus-antibody complexes incite tissue damage through the same mechanisms which have been considered in relation to the immunopathology of soluble complexes in general. Such mechanisms account for the glomerulonephritis and the perivascular aggregates of inflammatory cells of various type which are common features in these animal models.

Despite the tantalizing resemblance between many chronic inflammatory diseases of man and the immune complex disease induced by viruses in animals models (Table 4) there are relatively few of the former whose viral aetiology has been clearly established. Nevertheless there are already sufficient examples of viral diseases in man with immunopathological sequelae to show that these similarities are not wholly superficial. Thus the haemorrhagic shock syndrome which occurs principally during secondary dengue

TABLE 4

Principal virus diseases which induce immune complexes and are models of human disorders

Disease	Virus	Species
1. Glomerulonephritis	LCM, LDH, cytomegalovirus	mice
	oncornaviruses (oncogenic)	mice
	oncornavirus?	NZB × NZW mice
	Aleutian disease	mink
2. Haemolytic anaemia	oncornavirus?	NZB mice
	filtrable agent	African swine
	equine haemolytic anaemia agent	horses
3. Paraproteinaemia	Aleutian disease	mink
	oncornavirus?	mice
4. Endocrine diseases	possible filter-passing agent	chickens
5. Central nervous system		
a. neuropathy	Aleutian disease	mink
	oncornavirus?	mice
b. myasthenia	filter-passing agent	rodents
6. Tissue infiltrates	as in glomerulonephritis	
	arenaviruses (other than LCM)	mice

infections results from the formation of circulating antigen–antibody complexes in considerable amounts leading in turn to complement consumption, intravascular coagulation and the appearance of fibrin split products in the blood (Bokisch, 1974). The pathology of hepatitis B infection has been analysed in detail following the discovery of hepatitis-associated antigen and infectious (Dane) particles and this has allowed the relation between circulating antigen and antibody to be analysed by serological and ultrastructural techniques in a variety of patients with chronic hepatitis. Immune complexes

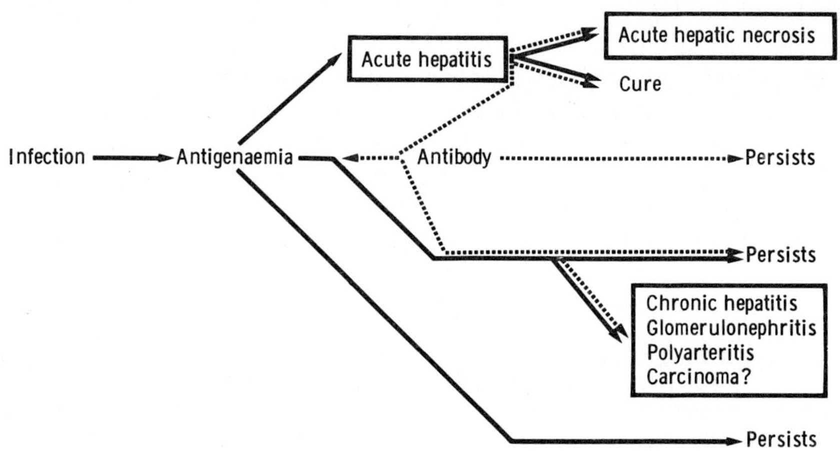

Fig. 10. Possible outcomes of infection with Hepatitis B (Australia antigen associated disease). Infection results in disease, as indicated in the squares, or with minor clinical disturbances. The outcome may be determined by immunological factors, i.e. T-lymphocyte cytotoxicity favouring liver necrosis and impaired control mechanisms favouring persistent complexes but these possibilities have not been clarified.

provoked by hepatitis-associated antigen have also been implicated in the pathogenesis of polyarteritis and glomerulonephritis, particularly in children. The exact mechanism of such diseases has not been fully clarified even in those patients in whom the viral antigens have been identified, and Australia antigen, antibody and complexes of the two have been detected in different patients but with highly variable immunopathological consequences (Fig. 10). Nor has a virus aetiology been established in the majority of chronic inflammatory disease of unknown aetiology in which circulating immune complexes have been detected in the blood or in tissue exudates.

Cellular Mechanism

The problem of distinguishing between the protective and destructive roles of the host response in virus infections is posed most acutely in relation to cell-mediated immunity. This is an issue of great therapeutic significance since the merits or hazards of prescribing immunosuppressive drugs in virus infections or their sequelae largely depend upon a correct interpretation of the salient immunological events. The outcome is hard to predict empirically as is well illustrated by the variable effect of anti-lymphocyte globulin in different infections, an agent which powerfully suppresses this form of immune response (Hirsch and Murphy, 1968). The answer may be unequivocal in experimental models such as LCM disease in mice where cytotoxic T-lymphocytes mediate cerebral damage by reacting with virus-coded antigens on the cell surface (Doherty and Zinkernagel, 1975). It is reasonable to suspect that encephalitis in man caused by other arenaviruses largely results from the destruction of infected cells by cytotoxic T-lymphocytes. Indeed the narrow limits to which cerebral swelling within the rigid confines of the skull can be tolerated probably accounts for the exceptionally deleterious effects of cell mediated immune reactions in the central nervous system. Indeed it must be emphasized that a T-cell mechanism is operative in the vast majority of virus infections of man and is responsible in large measure for the rashes which are characteristic of the common virus infections of childhood (Allison, 1967). In most such infections this reaction limits virus spread and replication and helps to protect the patient against re infection. Moreover patients with defective cell-mediated immunity but normal antibody production are abnormally vulnerable to infection by certain viruses, notably herpes simplex, varicella zoster, cytomegalovirus and measles. Thus children with congenital thymus deficiency are liable to develop progressive vaccinia after simple vaccination whilst patients receiving cytotoxic drugs or with lymphoproliferative disorders complicated by impaired cellular immunity are highly susceptible to varicella zoster infections.

Thus the detection of a mononuclear cell infiltrate within virus-infected tissues does not imply that this reaction must invariably be damaging to the infected cells. Indeed lymphocytes do not necessarily fulfill their protective function by destroying virus-infected cells but can block the replication of certain viruses in host cells which are susceptible to infection (Rouse and Babink, 1975). The protective function of mononuclear cell populations in virus infections is now better recognized (Fig. 11). The factors which lead to prolonged tissue destruction may only operate in a minority of patients and seem likely to depend on a genetically determined response by cytotoxic

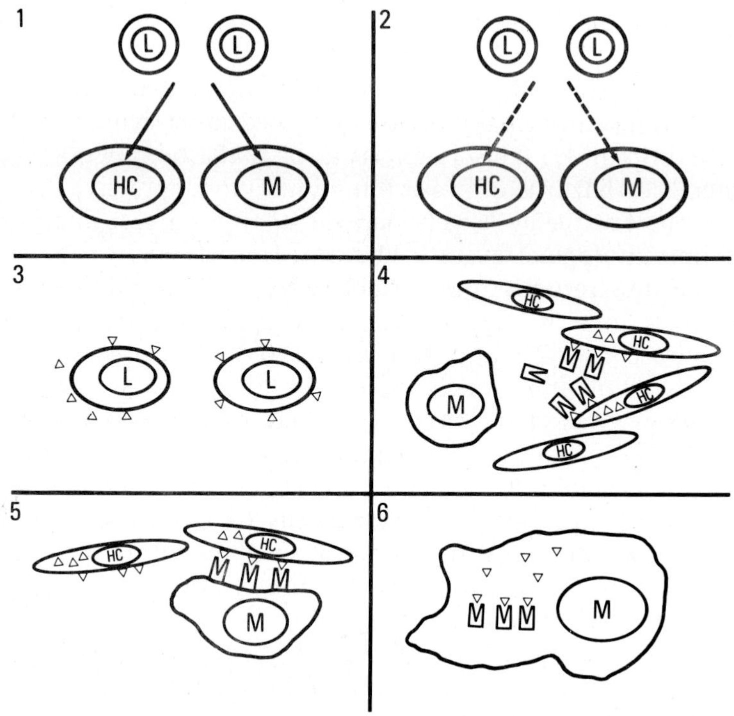

Fig. 11. Protective function of mononuclear cells in virus infections. The different functions are illustrated as follows: 1. lymphocytes confer virus-*specific* immunity on susceptible host cells or macrophages; 2. lymphocytes confer *non-specific* immunity on susceptible host cells or macrophages, not all of which is mediated by conventional interferon; 3. lymphocytes inactivate some viruses; 4. macrophages facilitate penetration by antibody molecules; 5. macrophages are "armed" with specific antibody; 6. macrophages are "activated" to destroy virus ingested in free form or bound to antibody. The relative importance of each defence mechanism varies with different virus infections. L = lymphocyte; HC = host cell; M = macrophage; △ = virus intracellular or budding from cell membrane; M = antibody; M = infectious complex.

T-lymphocytes which is excessively prolonged or is provoked by virus antigens to which the majority of those infected are not responsive.

Interference with Control Mechanisms

There are examples of virus infections in animals which increase the immune response to some antigens or interfere with the induction of tolerance to others (Fenner *et al.*, 1974). Similar instances have not been recorded in clinical practice but the almost invariable and transitory occurrence of skin rashes in patients with infectious mononucleosis given ampicillin raises the possibility that many virus infections act as adjuvants in increasing the immune response to exogenous antigens such as drugs (Fig. 12).

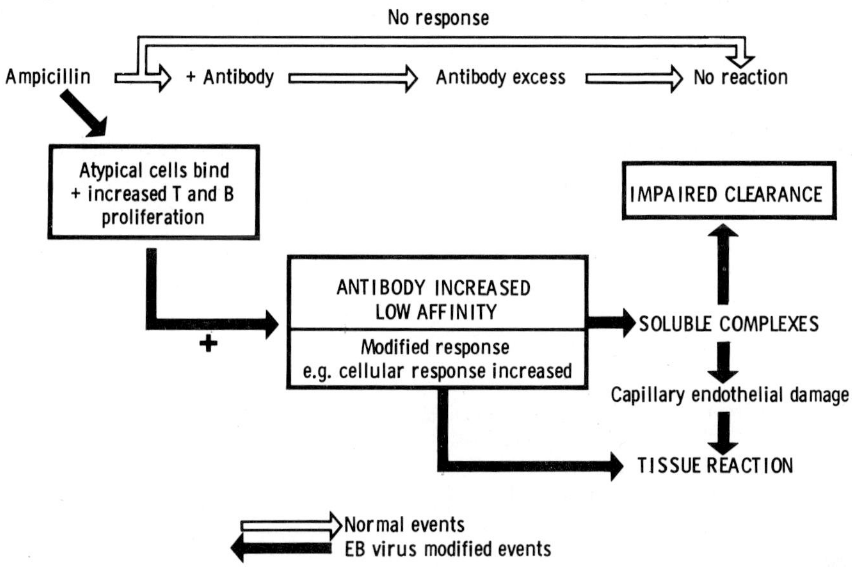

Fig. 12. Ampicillin rash in infectious mononucleosis—possible mechanisms. Penicillin and related drugs usually induce a specific antibody response but rashes occur in not more than 10% of treated patients. The events which may lead to a near 100% incidence of rashes in patients with infectious mononucleosis are illustrated in the figure. Those in boxes are *central* within the lymphoid tissues; the unboxed are *peripheral*.

Auto-immunity and Virus Infections

The theoretical attractions of attributing a viral aetiology to many human auto-immune diseases have been indicated but as yet the direct evidence for this view is fragmentary. Indeed in most animal models of persistent virus infection the arguments which were once used to ascribe chronic inflammatory lesions to auto-immunity have been replaced by those based on a more straightforward response to disseminated viral antigens. This issue is likely to be resolved by the introduction of more sensitive techniques. Important information may be uncovered by a more systematic search for evidence of specific virus infections in the acute early stages of connective tissue diseases. In chronic established disease the interpretation of anti-viral antibody titres, for example, is complicated by other factors, particularly a non-specific increase in serum γ-globulin.

Mechanisms for Evading the Host Response

Viruses can elude or subvert the host immune response in a variety of ways (Table 5).

TABLE 5
Possible mechanisms for virus persistence

Mechanism	Examples	Comments
I. Immunological		
A. Tolerance	impossible to demonstrate experimentally	not entirely excluded in all vertically-transmitted infections
B. non-responsiveness	slow infections of the CNS	genetic variation possible with some antigens on other viruses
C. Immune deficiency		
i. congenital	rubella	the effect of intra-uterine infection may be underestimated e.g. paramyxoviruses
ii. acquired	immunosuppression is common in virus infections	specific deficiency could persist in susceptible patients
D. Blocking (enhancing) antibody	sub-acute sclerosing panencephalitis; cytomegalovirus infection; loss of virus-specific surface antigen	not excluded in other infections; but *in vitro* demonstration only
II. Biological		
A. Direct cell-to-cell spread	myxoviruses; paramyxoviruses	may assist spread of other viruses by inducing cell fusion
B. Virus integration in host cells	demonstrated in numerous virus-host cell systems	
C. Defective virus infection	measles	likely to have important clinical implications

Immunological Unresponsiveness

In animal experiments it has proved impossible to induce tolerance to viruses by the same manoeuvre which will achieve this with other antigens, namely neonatal administration. Even murine oncornaviruses, which are vertically transmitted from the parent mice still excite an antibody response in the next generation. Despite such observations, the possibility remains that viruses which are acquired congenitally in man could damage the immune system with a variable degree of selectivity thereby inducing non-responsiveness to the invading virus and hence persistent infection. The widespread damage inflicted on the immune system by congenital rubella can ablate the antibody response to this virus (Ribon and Wasserman, 1974). There is also a special problem with regard to virus infections of the central nervous system since some viruses such as the agents responsible for kuru and Jakob Creutzfeld disease excite no detectable form of immune response. Two possible explanations can be envisaged; the central nervous system may be a site where replicating viruses are poorly immunogenic because of the relatively meagre circulation to this site of small lymphocytes which normally initiate the immune response. Alternatively the infecting agents may be "virioids" which are composed of a short sequence of nucleotides and fail to stimulate any immune response because they lack a protein coat.

Immunodeficiency

There is relatively little information about the genetic control of the immune response to viral antigens. Anti-viral antibody responses which are measured *in vitro* often have little relation to those which limit viral dissemination *in vivo*. With respect to tests for "cell-mediated immunity", a reduced responsiveness to some paramyxoviruses has been reported in patients with systemic lupus erythematosus and multiple sclerosis. However it is not clear whether such abnormalities precede the onset of disease and are truly genetic in nature or whether they result from the selective deletion of responding cells by virus. The reproducibility of these findings is still in question. The production of interferon by mononuclear cells has also been shown to be defective in some lymphoproliferative diseases.

An immunodeficient state can follow virus infections. Many viruses replicate in mononuclear cells of the central lymphoid tissues and the peripheral blood and can be demonstrated in circulating lymphocytes. Measles is an important example of such a virus (Osunkoya *et al.*, 1974) and is especially prone to replicate in the lymphocytes of patients suffering from malnutrition or other infections. It has been postulated that some viruses first stimulate the proliferation of lymphocytes in an immunologically specific response to that virus; these cells thereby become selectively vulnerable sites for replication of the same virus. This hypothetical sequence of events is quite plausible since EB (Epstein-Barr) virus, once acquired, remains permanently integrated in B-lymphocytes (Fig. 13). Indeed in some families, who are abnormally susceptible to EB virus for unknown reasons, the infection of lymphoid cells is progressive and terminates in hypogammaglobulinaemia (Provisor *et al.*, 1975). It seems probably that viruses which become integrated in lymphoid cells during the initial infection can be later reactivated if proliferation of these cells is stimulated by an appropriate immunological stimulus.

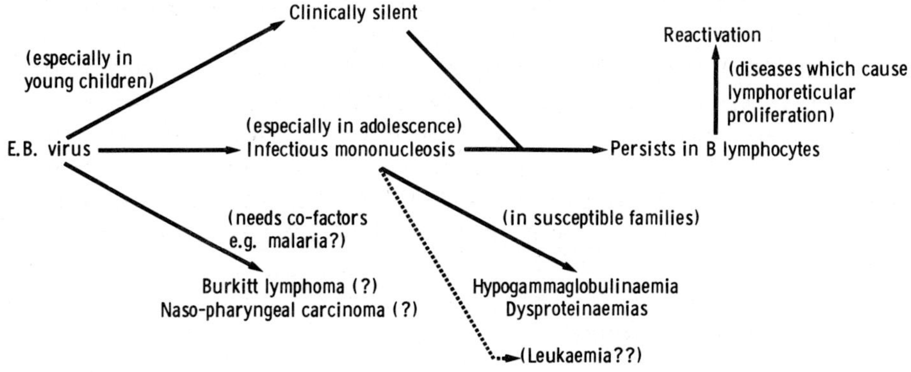

Fig. 13. The variable clinical expression of EB (Epstein-Barr) virus infection.

Chronic graft-versus-host disease provokes oncornavirus replication in this way and the activation of latent viruses such as cytomegalovirus in renal transplant patients is probably due as much to continuous immune stimulation by the graft as it is to treatment with cytotoxic drugs.

Enhancement of Virus Infections

Antibody whether free or complexed with antigen can block T-cell, K-cell and macrophage mechanisms of immunological damage. This paradoxical effect of antibody is probably a feature of antibody molecules appearing at a particular phase in immunization. The most important mechanism appears to be the blocking of receptor sites on the effector cells by complexes. This blocking effect, referred to as "enhancement" has been extensively investigated in tumour immunology and may prove apposite to problems of viral persistence. Enhancing complexes have been described in the cerebro-spinal fluid of patients with subacute sclerosing panencephalitis, a disease attributed to persistent infection by measles virus and in the plasma of patients with persistent cytomegalovirus infections. Furthermore, antibody can react with chronically infected host cells in a way which causes them to shed virus—specific antigens thereby preventing their destruction by sensitized lymphocytes with receptors for these antigens.

Direct Cell to Cell Spread of Viruses

Virus can spread directly to contiguous cells and thereby be inaccessible to neutralizing antibody or cellular defence mechanisms which operate in the extracellular space. The importance of this method of spread is emphasized by the so far rather disappointing therapeutic response to regimes which logically should have corrected those purely immunological defects to which the persistence of virus has been ascribed.

Subacute sclerosing panencephalitis (SSPE) is an example of a virus disease which has been treated by various immunotherapeutic manoeuvres. There have been many attempts to reverse the immune defects which have been considered to account for the persistent infection by measles virus. Thus the allegedly impaired cell-mediated responses to this agent has been treated by non-specific adjuvants or by transfer factor extracted from the leukocytes of donors who are demonstrably immune to measles virus. Similarly "blocking factors" in the plasma and cerebrospinal fluid which are postulated to prevent the destruction of measles-infected cells by cytotoxic lymphocytes have been removed by exchange transfusion of both these fluids. However, none of these measures have been convincingly effective and it seems likely that the measles strain responsible for the disease, which has many atypical features, is able to elude the immune response by spreading to neighbouring cells in the central nervous system (Fig. 14).

Latent Virus

The ability of many viruses to become integrated in host cells and undergo periodic cycles of activation and replication underlies the difficulty in eliminating such agents from the tissues. Thus the host response to herpes simplex

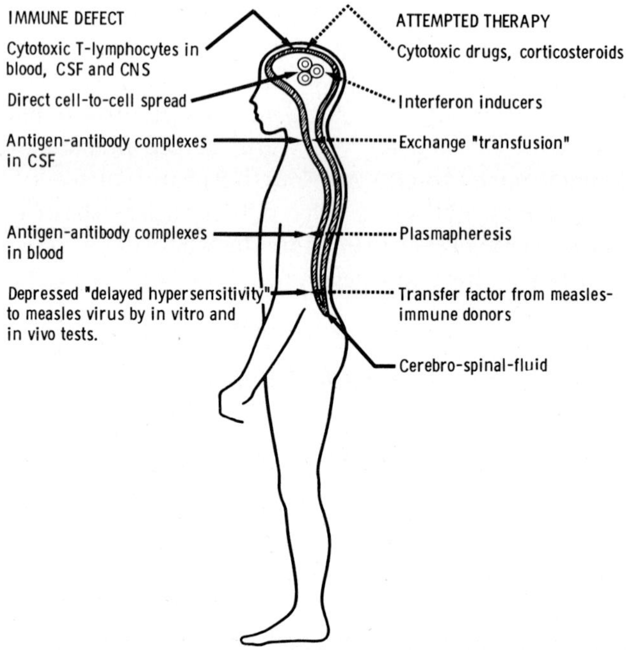

Fig. 14. Immunotherapy attempted in sub-acute sclerosing panencephalitis. This illustrates the practical application of the knowledge about the mechanism of virus persistence. It will be apparent that imperfect theory has given rise to conflicting therapy.

and varicella zoster infections probably acts primarily to limit the dissemination of these viruses during phases of activation.

Defective Virus Particles

Defective virus particles contain normal viral structural protein and a part of the viral genome but they interfere with the replication of the same virus in complete, non-defective form. This interference is not mediated by interferon. Host defence mechanisms are efficient at combating the spread of fully infectious virions and readily recognize cells which express the full complement of virus coded antigens. On the other hand it is likely that they are far less effective in eliminating cells which harbour defective virus. Moreover the stimulus to the immune response is liable to be incomplete if lymphoid cells do not come into contact with the complete virion. The defective measles virus of sub-acute sclerosing panencephalitis is an example of an agent whose persistence may be due in part to the incomplete expression of host immunity (Huang and Baltimore, 1970). These observations have therapeutic implications.

REFERENCES

Abrahams, S., Phillips, R. A. and Miller, R. G. (1973). Inhibition of the immune response by 7S antibody. *J. Exp. Med.* **137**, 870.

Allison, A. C. (1967). Cell-mediated immune responses to virus infections and virus-induced tumours. *Brit. Med. Bull.* **23**, 60.

Bokisch, V. A. (1974). The role of complement in haemorrhage shock syndrome (Dengue). *In* "Progress in Immunology" (eds. L. Brent and E. J. Holborow), p. 151. North-Holland Publishing Co., Amsterdam and Oxford.

Calder, E. A., McLeman, D. and Irvine, W. J. (1973). Lymphocyte cytotoxicity induced by preincubation with serum from patients with Hashimoto thyroiditis. *Clin. Exp. Immunol.* **15**, 467.

Clagett, J. A., Wilson, C. B. and Weigle, W. O. (1974). Interstitial immune complex thyroiditis in mice. The role of autoantibody to thyroglobulin. *J. Exp. Med.* **140**, 1439.

Doherty, P. C. and Zinkernagel, J. (1975). A biological role for the major histocompatibility antigens. *Lancet* **1**, 1406.

Epstein, L. P., Alper, C. A., Bloch, K. J., Herrin, J. T., Rosen, F. S., David, J. R. and Colten, H. R. (1975). Biosynthetic defect in monocytes from human beings with genetic deficiency of the second component of complement. *New Eng. J. Med.* **292**, 1169.

Evans, D. J. (1974). Pathogenesis of membranous glomerulonephritis. *Lancet* **1**, 1143.

Fenner, F., McAuslan, B. R., Mims, C. A., Sambrook, J. and White, D. O. (1974). *In* "The Biology of Animal Viruses", 2nd Edition, pp. 338–478. Academic Press, New York and London.

Ferluga, J. and Allison, A. C. (1974). Observations on the mechanism by which T-lymphocytes exert cytotoxic effects. *Nature (Lond.)* **250**, 673.

Fialkow, P. J., Klein, G., Klein, G., Clifford, P. and Singh, S. (1973a). Immunoglobulin and glucose-6-phosphate dehydrogenase as markers of cellular origin in Burkitt lymphoma. *J. Exp. Med.* **138**, 89.

Fialkow, P. J., Paton, G. R. and East, J. (1973b). Chromosomal abnormalities in spleens of New Zealand Black mice, a strain characterized by auto-immunity and malignancy. *Proc. Nat. Acad. Sci. (U.S.A.)* **70**, 1094.

Frizzera, G., Moran, E. M. and Rappaport, H. (1974). Angio-immunoblastic lymphadenopathy with dysproteinaemia. *Lancet* **1**, 1070.

Gershon, R. K. (1974). The control of immune responses. *In* "Contemporary topics in immunobiology" (eds. M. Cooper and N. Warner), p. 1. Plenum Press, New York.

Hall, J. G. (1969). Effector mechanisms in immunity. *Lancet* **1**, 25.

Hirsch, M. S. and Murphy, F. A. (1968). Effects of anti-lymphoid sera on viral infections. *Lancet* **2**, 37.

Hoffsten, P. E. and Dixon, F. J. (1973). Effect of immunosuppression on chronic LCM infection of mice. *J. Exp. Med.* **138**, 887.

Huang, A. S. and Baltimore, D. (1970). Defective viral particles and viral disease processes. *Nature (Lond.)* **226**, 325.

Huggins, K. J. and Brostoff, J. (1975). Local production of specific IgE antibodies in allergic rhinitis patients with negative skin tests. *Lancet* **2**, 148.

Johnson, R. L., Fink, C. W. and Ziff, M. (1972). Lymphotoxin formation by lymphocytes and muscle in polymyositis. *J. Clin. Invest.* **51**, 2435.

Levine, B. B., Stember, R. H. and Fotino, M. (1972). Ragweed hay fever: genetic control and linkage to HL-A haplotypes. *Science* **178**, 1201.

MacLennan, I. C. M. (1972). Antibody in the induction and inhibition of cytotoxicity. *Transplant. Rev.* **13**, 67.

Miller, G. W. and Nussenzweig, V. (1975). A new complement function: solubilization of antigen-antibody aggregates. *Proc. Nat. Acad. Sci. (U.S.A.)* **72**, 418.

Moller, G. (Ed.) (1975). HL-A antigens and disease. *Transplant. Rev.* **27**, 1.

Notkins, A. L. (1971). Infectious virus-antibody complexes: interaction with anti-immunoglobulins, complement and rheumatoid factor. *J. Exp. Med.* **134**, (suppl. 41).

Oldstone, M. B. A., Dixon, F. J., Mitchell, G. F. and McDevitt, H. O. (1973). Histocompatibility-linked genetic control of disease susceptibility to murine lymphocytic choriomeningitis virus infection. *J. Exp. Med.* **137**, 1201.

Oldstone, M. B. A., Cooper, N. R. and Larson, D. L. (1974). Formation and biologic role of polyoma virus-antibody complexes. A critical role for complement. *J. Exp. Med.* **140**, 549.

Osunkoya, B. O., Adeleye, G. I., Adejumo, T. A. and Salimonu, L. S. (1974). Studies on leucocyte cultures in measles II. detection of measles virus antigen in human leucocytes by immunofluorescence. *Arch. Gesamte Virusforsch.* **44**, 323.

Page, R. C., Davies, P. and Allison, A. C. (1974). Pathogenesis of the chronic inflammatory lesion induced by Group A streptococcal cell walls. *Lab. Invest.* **30**, 568.

Perlmann, P., Perlmann, H. and Müller Eberhard, H. J. (1975). Cytolytic lymphocytic cells with complement receptor in human blood. *J. Exp. Med.* **141**, 287.

Peters, D. K. and Lachmann, P. J. (1974). Immunity deficiency in pathogenesis of glomerulonephritis. *Lancet* **1**, 58.

Petz, L. D. and Garratty, G. (1974). Complement in immunohaematology. *In* "Progress in Clinical Immunology" (ed. R. S. Schwartz), p. 175. Grune and Stratton, New York, San Francisco and London.

Provisor, A. J., Iacuone, J. J., Chilcote, R. R., Neiburger, R. G., Crussi, F. G. and Baehner, R. L. (1975). Acquired agammaglobulinaemia after a life-threatening illness with clinical and laboratory features of infectious mononucleosis in three related male children. *New Eng. J. Med.* **293**, 62.

Ribon, A. and Wasserman, E. (1974). Immunodeficiency with congenital rubella. *Ann. Allergy* **32**, 35.

Rouse, B. T. and Babiuk, L. A. (1975). Host defence mechanisms against bovine rhinotracheitis virus II. inhibition of viral plaque formation by immune peripheral blood lymphocytes. *Cell Immunol.* **17**, 43.

Schultz, R. S. and Yunis, A. A. (1975). Immunoblastic lymphadenopathy with mixed cryoglobulinaemia. *New Eng. J. Med.* **292**, 8.

Schumacher, H. R. and Gall, E. P. (1974). Arthritis in acute hepatitis and chronic active hepatitis. *Am. J. Med.* **57**, 655.

Stanworth, D. R. (1971). Immunoglobulin E (reagin) and allergy. *Nature (Lond.)* **233**, 310.

Wisniewski, H. M. and Bloom, B. R. (1975). Primary demyelination as a non-specific consequence of a cell-mediated immune reaction. *J. Exp. Med.* **141**, 346.

11

Auto-immunity and Multi-system Disease: Systemic Lupus Erythematosus, Vasculitis and Progressive Systemic Sclerosis

J. V. JONES

When antigen enters the body, it may stimulate antibody production. Circulating antigen combines with free antibody to produce antigen–antibody complexes (see Chapter 10) which under normal conditions are rapidly eliminated. In certain circumstances complexes of antigen and antibody may persist in the circulation and eventually become deposited in tissues, where they then initiate inflammatory responses. A similar outcome may result from auto-immune responses against components of cells or tissues which have become antigenic within their own environment, thus providing a continual supply of antigen which both stimulates auto-antibody production and combines with the antibody produced to form soluble immune complexes. This mechanism of immune complex deposition in tissues is involved in diseases as varied as post-streptococcal glomerulonephritis, systemic lupus erythematosus, polyarteritis nodosa and many drug reactions. Little is known at present about the factors which favour formation of immune complexes of this type or which control the site of their deposition.

Von Pirquet and Schick (1905) described the condition of serum sickness which followed the injection of horse serum in man. Injections of serum from immunized horses were used extensively and with some success for the prophylaxis and treatment of infections such as diphtheria. Eight to twelve days after the first injection an urticarial rash developed in some subjects, which spread rapidly from the injection site to cover the whole body. This was accompanied by pyrexia, joint pains, generalized lymphadenopathy and proteinuria. An initial leucocytosis was often followed by a transient leucopenia. Von Pirquet and Schick showed that as serum sickness developed, antibodies to horse serum proteins appeared in the circulation, and they suggested that the antibodies were responsible for the disease. It was later found that features of serum sickness could be reproduced in animals by immunization with other protein antigens.

ANIMAL MODELS

Some consist of experiments in which animals are either injected with non-living antigens or receive cells transferred from animals that have been immunized. In other models, animals are studied in the course of natural or induced infections of various types.

Immunization with Non-living Agents

Claude Bernard is reported to have been the first to establish that the intravenous injection of heterologous serum in experimental animals could lead to proteinuria. Others have since shown that this is associated with a glomerulonephritis. Masugi found that the morphological changes produced in the kidneys of immunized animals when antigens were injected directly into the renal artery were similar to those found in polyarteritis nodosa. Rich and Gregory (1943) found that rabbits injected intravenously with horse serum developed an acute disseminated vasculitis. Over the next twenty-five years the detailed immunological mechanisms which lead to glomerulonephritis and vasculitis in serum sickness were studied in depth.

Animals (usually rabbits, rats or mice) are given either a single intravenous injection of an antigen, usually a protein such as human serum albumin (HSA) or bovine serum albumin (BSA), or, alternatively, a series of daily injections. Between eight and fourteen days after the injection of antigen, antibody begins to appear in the serum in increasing quantities and at this stage antigen–antibody complexes are formed which are taken up by phagocytic cells of the reticulo–endothelial system. During this phase the animals develop changes comparable to those of serum sickness, with inflammatory lesions in glomeruli (glomerulonephritis) and in the small vessels throughout the body (vasculitis). In the "one-shot" animal model, recovery is usually complete within a month. By giving a course of daily injections of antigen, a more prolonged disease (chronic serum sickness) can be established over several months. The distribution and severity of the inflammation is correlated with the size of the immune complexes produced and immunofluorescent techniques have demonstrated the deposition of immune complexes and complement in glomeruli and blood vessels elsewhere in the body. Free complexes may occur in the circulation and can be detected by a number of techniques. Components of the complement system may be depleted and fragments such as C3d may then appear. Free complexes are found in the circulation at a stage when renal and vascular damage is at its height (Dixon *et al.*, 1958). Similar methods have shown that circulating immune complexes are present in active or acute phases of systemic lupus erythematosus and polyarteritis nodosa.

The production of immune complex disease in animals has provided a most valuable tool for probing the mechanisms of immunologically mediated disease in man and this aspect has been reviewed by several authors (Cochrane and Koffler, 1973; Germuth and Rodriguez, 1973).

A different picture is seen when animals are immunized with suspensions of tissue in adjuvant. It is possible, for instance, to produce polymyositis by immunizing guinea-pigs with a homogenate of rabbit muscle, and the disease can be transferred from immunized to unimmunized animals by suspensions of sensitized lymphocytes (see Chapter 24).

It is also possible to produce an erosive arthritis in rats by injections of Freund's complete adjuvant alone. This disease can be transferred to syngeneic rats with lymphocytes. The relation of this condition to rheumatoid arthritis in man is far from clear.

Immunological Disturbances Associated with Infection

There are a number of virus-induced animal diseases which bear a striking resemblance to human disease. Although none of the human diseases under consideration in this section has been proved to be of viral origin, viral models in animals have one feature that gives them special interest and importance. Animal models produced by immunization with non-living agents are almost entirely self-limiting. "One-shot" serum sickness is not progressive, and chronic serum sickness persists in active form only as long as antigen injections are repeated. To this extent, these are defective models for human diseases such as systemic lupus erythematosus and polyarteritis nodosa, which often progress steadily unless modified by treatment. Virus-induced animal models, on the other hand, are often progressive and fatal, and are in this respect relevant to human disease.

Chronic Infection with Lymphocytic Choriomeningitis (LCM) Virus

The infection of mice with LCM virus provided one of the earliest models for a chronic viral disease whose features were determined by the immunological responsiveness of the host. Certain strains of mice carry the virus chronically and show no overt evidence of disease. If foetal mice are infected with a low dose of virus they remain apparently free of disease and were long regarded as immunologically inert (tolerant). One of the most important developments in the understanding of chronic virus disease was the finding by Oldstone and Dixon (1967) that neonatally infected mice are not, in fact, immunologically tolerant, but are chronic carriers of the LCM virus. By immunofluorescent study of the kidneys of carrier mice, they showed that deposition of mouse immunoglobulin, complement and virus antigen was associated with a persistent glomerulonephritis. By treating a homogenate of kidney with an acid buffer, which dissociates antigen–antibody complexes, they were able to elute antibody, which gave a positive complement-fixation reaction with LCM virus. They concluded that neonatally infected mice produced antibody which was inadequate to eliminate the virus, but which combined with virus to produce immune complexes, giving rise to a typical immune complex glomerulonephritis.

Aleutian Disease of Mink

This is a virus-induced disease of mink (Porter and Larsen, 1974). It is characterized by a generalized plasmacytosis and glomerulonephritis and there is a marked vasculitis affecting muscular arteries in the heart, liver, gastrointestinal tract, brain and kidneys. It is produced by a virus which has been well characterized and the disease can be transmitted to unaffected animals by cell-free extracts. Immunofluorescent studies demonstrate that mink immunoglobulin, complement and viral antigen are present in the vascular lesions and immune complexes are present in the serum. The disease can be suppressed completely by treatment with cyclophosphamide. All strains of mink are susceptible, but animals of the Aleutian genotype are more severely affected than others. This model has important similarities to systemic lupus erythematosus and polyarteritis nodosa.

NZB/W Mice

The inbred strain of mice known as New Zealand Black (NZB) were shown by Bielschowsky *et al.* (1959) to develop a spontaneous haemolytic anaemia. Breeding with the New Zealand White (NZW) gives a hybrid (NZB/W) which is especially prone to a rapidly progressive and fatal immune-complex glomerulonephritis, associated with an auto-immune haemolytic anaemia, and antibodies to deoxyribonucleic acid (DNA). Breeding experiments have shown that the genetic background is important in determining the age of onset and severity of the disease. It has also been found that NZB and NZB/W mice carry the Gross (G) leukaemia virus, and that much of the immunoglobulin lodged in the glomeruli consists of antibody to this virus. NZW and NZB/W hybrids are also unusual in their ability to produce large amounts of antibody when immunized with DNA. It seems likely that the NZB mouse harbours a virus against which the NZW mouse mounts an excessive, but ineffectual, response. The NZB/W hybrid, afflicted with a chronic antigen load and an overresponsive immune mechanism, dies of immune-complex disease. The striking feature of these animals is the close resemblance between the pathology of the lesions they develop and the changes found in systemic lupus erythematosus in humans.

A disease closely resembling SLE has also been found in dogs. The agent producing it appears to be transmissible. Immune complex diseases in animals illustrate the mechanism of glomerulonephritis and vasculitis in man. They cannot tell us what the trigger is in human disease, but some likely possibilities are discussed below.

SYSTEMIC LUPUS ERYTHEMATOSUS

The term "lupus" (Latin—a wolf) was first used to describe ulcerating, erosive skin lesions in the thirteenth century. Lupus erythematosus was originally confused with lupus vulgaris but later on the former was distinguished from the latter and subdivided into the localized cutaneous *discoid* form (DLE) and the systemic disorder in which the rash was associated with fever and generalized symptoms (SLE). The description of the LE-cell phenomenon by

Hargeaves *et al.* (1948) was an important landmark, since it enabled the disease to be defined more clearly. It was soon recognized that the LE-cell phenomenon was associated with antibodies against nucleoproteins and the fluorescent anti-nuclear factor (ANF) test (Holborow *et al.*, 1957) soon became the standard test for SLE. The measurement of antibodies to DNA by the Farr assay (Hughes *et al.*, 1971) has provided an even more specific test.

Clinical Outline

Systemic lupus erythematosus (SLE) is a progressive, generalized disease, normally accompanied by anti-nuclear antibodies (ANA) and a positive test for DNA binding. The American Rheumatism Association has attempted to establish diagnostic criteria (Cohen *et al.*, 1971), and lists 14 manifestations, suggesting that four or more of them, occurring simultaneously or serially, are necessary and sufficient for the diagnosis of SLE. Although these criteria make a useful framework for diagnosis, they fail to take account of several recent immunopathological findings. Most would now consider that the presence of ANA, an increased DNA binding in the serum, a characteristic renal biopsy, and typical findings on immunofluorescent study of a biopsy of light-exposed skin, are of diagnostic importance, and should be added to the list.

Estimates of the prevalence of SLE vary widely from 36 per million in Norway to 480 per million in Minnesota. In all centres the number of cases diagnosed has risen sharply in the last two decades. Much of the difference is likely to be due to increased awareness of the disease and to the increased sensitivity of diagnostic methods.

The clinical picture of SLE is highly variable. Dubois (1974, p. 237) lists no less than 64 clinical signs and symptoms, and comments that SLE has now replaced syphilis as "the great imitator". The commonest manifestations include fever, weight loss, joint pain, pericarditis, pleurisy, skin lesions (including butterfly rash, alopecia, and purpura), disturbances of the central nervous system, renal damage, hepatomegaly and lymphadenopathy. Approximately 10% of patients with SLE are first seen with discoid skin lesions. The skin lesions of the systemic disease, which appear first in areas of skin exposed to light, often show marked photosensitivity. On investigation, anaemia and leucocytopenia are common, with thrombocytopenia occurring in about 10% of cases. LE cells, anti-nuclear antibodies, and DNA-binding are considered under "immunological features".

The prognosis of SLE appears to have improved progressively over the past 20 years. Dubois in an analysis of a personal series of 249 fatal cases found that the median survival, which was less than two years before 1950, had increased, by 1973, to 8·5 years (Dubois, 1974). When non-fatal cases were included in the analysis, 57% were still alive 10 years after diagnosis.

Pathology

One of the characteristic features of SLE is the deposition of fibrinoid in the walls of small blood vessels. Fibrinoid is a homogeneous, acellular material, often showing a pattern of fibrils. It is eosinophilic, and stains with periodic acid Schiff (PAS). It is not unique to SLE, and occurs in polyarteritis nodosa, rheumatoid nodules and other forms of inflammatory vascular disease. Histochemical and immunochemical studies suggest that fibrinoid is a complex deposit including nucleoproteins, proteoglycans, fibrin and fibrinogen, immunoglobulins and complement. It seems likely that the deposition of immune complexes in vessel walls is one event that initiates the formation of fibrinoid. In contrast to the intense cellular infiltration and widespread necrosis associated with polyarteritis nodosa, SLE is usually accompanied by fibroblast proliferation, with some plasma cell and lymphocyte infiltration. Some workers have claimed that the presence of haematoxylin-stained bodies (round or oval, amorphous structures, of about the size of a cell-nucleus) in affected tissues is characteristic of SLE. Others have cast doubts on their specificity, and on their existence (Dubois, 1974). Granulomas have been reported in a number of tissues in SLE but they are not a specific feature and may also be associated with rheumatoid nodules.

The lesions described above may be found in any of the tissues or organs of the body in SLE, though there are some features characteristic of individual sites. The renal lesions are described in detail below (p. 345). In the spleen, there is often perisplenitis, with follicular hyperplasia, and perivascular fibrosis which, in its extreme form, produces "onion-skin" lesions. There may be generalized lymphadenopathy, with foci of necrosis and haematoxylin-stained bodies, proliferation of the sinus endothelium and follicular hyperplasia. Proliferative changes in the thymus have been reported with an increase in Hassall's corpuscles.

The extent to which the liver is involved in SLE has been the subject of considerable discussion. The group of cases originally characterized as "lupoid hepatitis" are now regarded as having chronic active hepatitis, and show one or two of the less specific laboratory features of SLE. Severe liver disease does not usually occur in patients with classical SLE, although minor histological changes may be seen on biopsy.

Despite the frequency of mental and neurological symptoms in the clinical presentation of SLE, pathological changes in the central nervous system are usually not striking. Proliferation of the vascular endothelium is found, but true vasculitis is rare. However, complexes of DNA with antibody and complement have been demonstrated in the choroid plexus in fatal cases of SLE.

Immunological Features

There are very few clinical and pathological features of SLE which cannot be demonstrated to be due to the presence of immune complexes in the circulation, or to their deposition in tissues. The fact that immunopathological mechanisms have been so clearly defined, now makes it necessary to consider the aetiology of the disease at a deeper level. The crucial question is to define the agents which stimulate the production of anti-nucleoprotein antibodies and immune complexes, and to clarify the relation between external agents and genetic factors in the aetiology of the disease.

The Antigens Involved

The LE cell phenomenon was first described by Hargraves *et al.* (1948), who demonstrated that when bone marrow from patients with SLE was incubated, free nuclear material appeared, which, when phagocytosed by polymorphonuclear neutrophils, gave rise to a cell of very characteristic appearance. It was subsequently found that the same type of cell was generated when defibrinated blood from patients with SLE was incubated *in vitro* (Fig. 1). It was later shown that the production of LE cells is dependent on serum factors, which were eventually characterized as antibodies to nucleoproteins and nucleic acids. Holborow *et al.* (1957) and Friou (1957) showed that these antibodies could be demonstrated by immunofluorescence.

Various patterns of staining have been described in the immunofluorescent test for anti-nuclear antibodies (ANA). Serum from lupus patients is allowed to react with sections of fresh tissue containing nucleated cells. The substrate cells do not need to be human: calf thymus and rat liver are often used. The sections are then stained with a fluorescent antibody to human immunoglobulin. The ANA may attach to the cells in a homogeneous pattern, staining

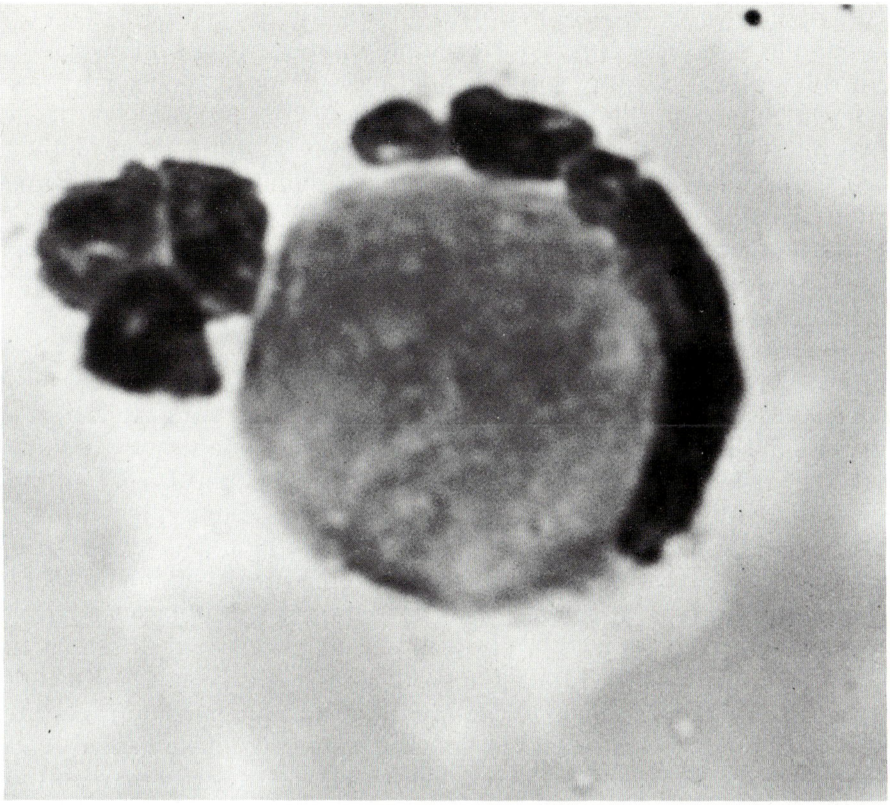

Fig. 1. LE cell. A polymorphonuclear leucocyte is shown, with a massive inclusion of degenerated nuclear material, partly surrounded by a stretched and deformed nucleus. ($\times$ 8,250) (Photomicrograph kindly provided by Dr I. Fraser.)

the whole nucleus diffusely. In the "peripheral" or "ring" staining, antibody outlines the nuclear membrane, while in the "speckled" pattern, it is deposited in granules over the nucleus. Occasionally, only the nucleoli are stained. It is claimed (Rothfield and Stollar, 1967) that the peripheral pattern of staining is produced by antibodies to native (double-stranded, ds) DNA, while the homogeneous staining corresponds to antibodies against DNA-histone complexes. Antibodies giving the speckled pattern include some reacting with complexes of RNA and protein.

Attempts to correlate the pattern of nuclear staining with the type and activity of disease have been inconclusive. However, patients with systemic sclerosis most commonly show anti-nucleolar antibody, while mixed connective tissue disease (p. 368) is most commonly associated with speckled staining, and with antibodies to extractable nuclear antigen (ENA).

With the advent of more sophisticated techniques it has become possible to define the nuclear antigens involved. This is clearly one of the most fundamental questions in the immunopathology of SLE, and has recently been reviewed by Stollar (1973). At least four kinds of antibody have been recognized in SLE:

i. antibodies reacting only with denatured (single-stranded) DNA;
ii. those reacting with both native (double-stranded) and denatured (single-stranded) DNA, but preferentially with the latter;
iii. those reacting equally with both forms, and
iv. those reacting preferentially with native DNA.

Using the sensitive Farr binding assay, it has been found that most sera from cases of SLE contain a mixture of all four types of antibody but that the fourth type is least common. An important general point is that antibodies specific for individual DNA bases will react preferentially with single-stranded DNA, on which DNA bases are exposed. In native, double-stranded DNA, the exposed determinants are related to the sugar-phosphate backbone of the molecule. It is of interest that antibodies to double-stranded DNA have been found to be most helpful in the diagnosis and management of classical SLE, while in the lupus-like syndromes associated with drug administration (p. 355) antibodies are principally directed against single-stranded DNA. Antibodies to histones and non-histone nucleoproteins and to RNA are also described in SLE but correlate less well with activity than antibodies to DNA.

DNA antibodies are usually of IgG class, though IgM antibodies have been described. They are detectable in between 80% and 100% of patients with active SLE, and in 40% or less of those with inactive disease. Changes in the level of DNA binding reflect the activity of the disease and are a useful guide to determining the degree of treatment required. A few patients with discoid lupus erythematosus have raised levels of antibodies to DNA, and this may be of prognostic significance.

Recently, a number of alternatives to the Farr method have been developed for the quantitation of antibodies to DNA. Picazo and Tan (1975) described a method in which nitrocellulose membrane filters were used to separate bound from unbound DNA. Aarden *et al.* (1975) described a hæmoflagellate, *Crithidia luciliae*, whose kinetoplast contains only double-stranded DNA. This is used as the basis of an immunofluorescent test for antibodies to native DNA which is only slightly less sensitive than the Farr assay. The same workers showed that the use of millipore filtration to separate bound and unbound

DNA gave higher values than the conventional assay. Further studies w... required to determine which of the tests for DNA antibodies is of greatest clinical value, and what type of DNA should be used in the test.

The Role of Anti-nuclear Antibodies

When antibodies to nucleoproteins were first demonstrated in SLE, it was considered that they might be directly toxic to cells but although the transfusion of anti-nuclear antibodies into normal subjects or experimental animals can lead to the transient appearance of the LE cell phenomenon, it does not produce the clinical or histopathological features of SLE.

Beck *et al.* (1966) reported studies on three infants born to mothers with SLE, who were exposed during gestation to placentally transmitted anti-nuclear antibodies. The infants were found to have ANA at the same level as the mothers, and antibodies persisted for up to ten weeks after delivery, declining slowly with a half-life similar to that of tetanus antitoxin. Despite the high levels of ANA, the infants remained free of clinical evidence of SLE. When immunofluorescence was applied to the kidneys of patients with SLE, it was shown that the glomeruli contained deposits of immunoglobulin, complement, and DNA. Immunoglobulin eluted from the kidneys of patients with SLE has antibody activity against a range of nucleic acid and nucleoprotein antigens. Moreover, on electron microscopy, the glomeruli of patients with SLE show changes which closely resemble those of animals with immune complex glomerulonephritis induced by injections of foreign protein antigens. These include extensive deposits of electron-dense material in the mesangium and in the sub-endothelial and sub-epithelial zones (Figs. 2a, 2b).

Immunofluorescent studies of the skin lesions in both discoid and systemic LE show that immunoglobulins and complement are deposited at the epidermal–dermal junction. In discoid lupus, these deposits are usually seen only in clinically affected skin, but in SLE, unaffected skin may also be positive (see Chapter 23).

Cormane and van Joost (1973) carried out auto-transplantation experiments, in which small areas of affected and unaffected skin were exchanged between different parts of the body in patients with discoid and systemic lupus erythematosus. They found that when affected skin from a patient with discoid LE was grafted to an unaffected area on the same patient, the skin was rejected like an allograft. Normal skin transplanted to an affected area was not rejected, and no rejection was seen after any form of transplantation in

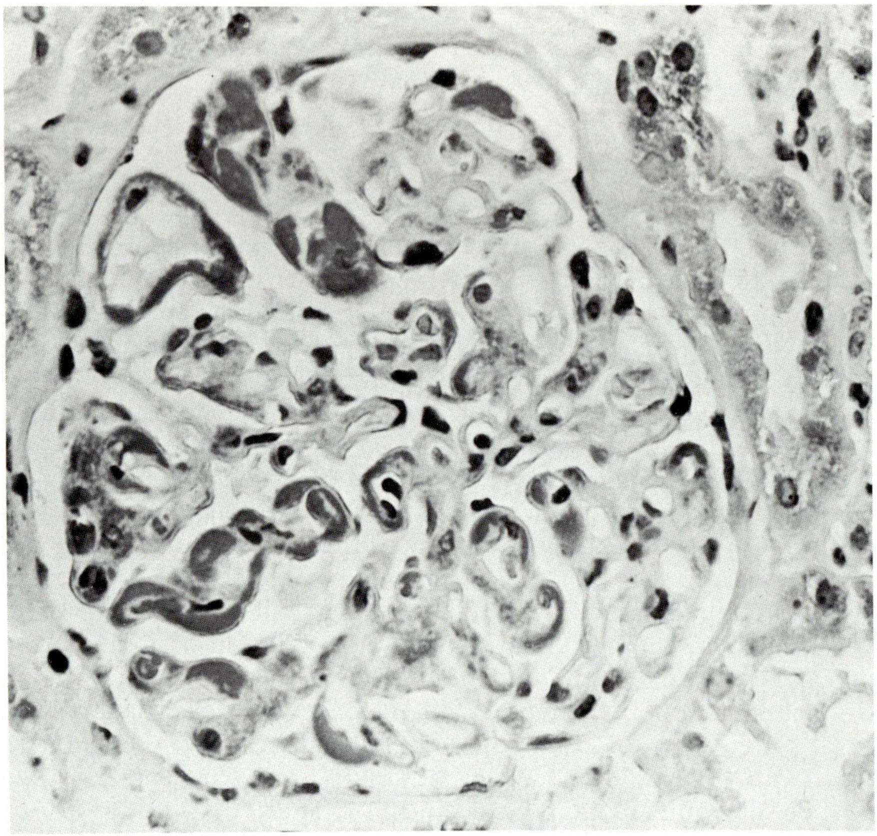

Fig. 2(a). Lupus nephritis. Glomerulus from a patient with systemic lupus erythematosus and early renal failure. Note the severe basement membrane thickening (wire-loop lesion) with many areas of intramembranous fibrinoid material. (Martius Scarlet Blue ×1,200.)

patients with SLE. This interesting work requires confirmation but it appears to suggest that new antigens appear in areas of skin affected with discoid LE but that the immune response to these antigens is blocked until the skin is transferred to a normal site. Since it is known that immune complexes can block the response to foreign antigens, it is attractive to speculate that the immunoglobulins and complement found in the epidermal–dermal region form a barrier, protecting antigens which appear locally.

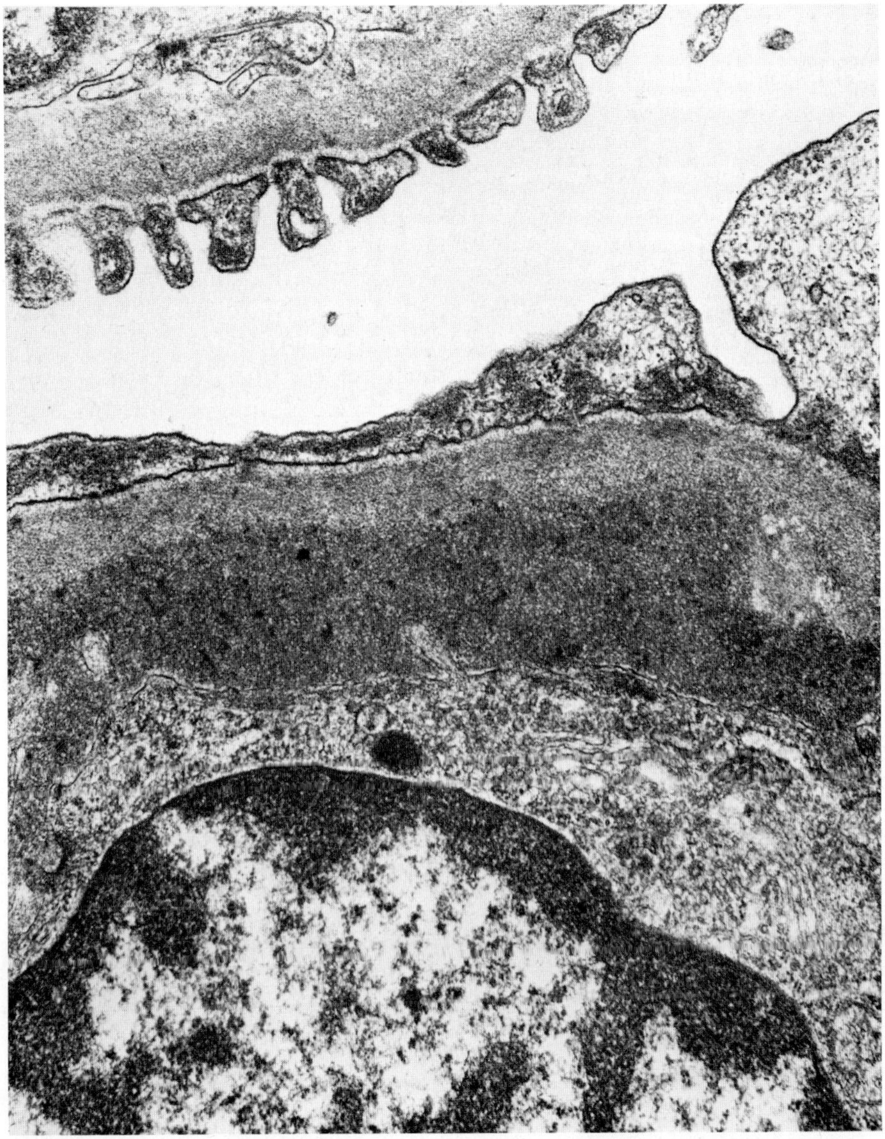

Fig. 2(b). Electron micrograph (×13,500) of renal biopsy tissue of a patient with SLE. Two basement membranes are shown with the intervening urinary space. The upper basement membrane is normal, with typical epithelial foot processes. The lower basement membrane is thickened, due to massive sub-endothelial electron-dense deposit. (Photomicrographs kindly provided by Dr C. R. Tribe.)

Circulating Complexes

Hypocomplementaemia may be found when antigen–antibody complex formation occurs within the vascular compartment. In the active phase of SLE, circulating levels of most of the complement components are reduced. The fact that the early components (C1, C4 and C2) are reduced in active SLE suggests that C3 is activated through the classical pathway. Further evidence for the presence of circulating immune complexes has been obtained by *in vitro* studies. It has been found that C1q, and monoclonal rheumatoid factors, both of which precipitate with immune complexes, give a positive reaction with sera from some cases of SLE (Agnello *et al.*, 1971).

Cryoglobulins are often a marker of circulating immune complexes and are frequently found in SLE. Some workers have claimed to find DNA in the cryoprecipitates (Barnett *et al.*, 1970), although others have been unable to confirm this.

Other Antibodies

While antibodies to nuclear antigens have attracted most attention, a wide range of other antibodies are found in SLE and may be of clinical importance. Antibodies to erythrocyte antigens are found in about 65% of patients with SLE, and are usually warm-acting antibodies of the IgG class. The specificity of the antigens with which they react has not yet been determined. Dacie and Worlledge (1969) found that among 210 patients with warm-antibody autoimmune haemolytic anaemia, 8% had SLE. Significant haemolysis is frequently present at the time of diagnosis of SLE.

Cytotoxic antibodies to leucocytes have been detected in 90% of patients with SLE. Of great interest are reports that sera from patients with SLE may contain antibodies specific for an antigen on human T-lymphocytes (Lies *et al.*, 1973). Antibodies to platelets have also been detected in SLE and may lead to significant thrombocytopenia. There is a degree of overlap between SLE and idiopathic thrombocytopenic purpura (ITP), and a number of patients presenting with apparently typical ITP may later develop SLE. This is said to be particularly common after splenectomy.

A false positive Wasserman reaction (WR) for syphilis is present in 20% of patients with inactive SLE, and 40% of cases of active disease. The antigen used in the Wasserman reaction is a phospholipid (cardiolipin) extracted from sheep heart. Other, more specific, tests for syphilis are negative.

Circulating anticoagulants are also common in SLE, particularly among the group with a false-positive WR. The anticoagulant appears to interfere with the interaction of the prothrombin activator with prothrombin and there is some evidence that it reacts with the phospholipid component of the activator complex. Since the Wasserman antigen is also a phospholipid, the association with a false-positive WR reaction is of particular interest. Patients with a circulating anticoagulant are especially likely to have thrombocytopenia, and since platelet membranes provide the phospholipid necessary for the intrinsic system of prothrombin activation, the three phenomena may be linked by an antibody to phospholipid.

Antibodies to thyroglobulin have been reported in 20% of patients with SLE, though only 1% have clinical evidence of thyroiditis. Antibodies to striated muscle and to mitochondria have occasionally been reported.

Cell mediated Responses

A few reports suggest that patients with SLE show cellular immunity to nuclear antigens. Freedman *et al.* (1960) injected a suspension of autologous or homologous leucocytes intradermally in 20 patients with SLE, and found a positive delayed skin response in 16, which was maximal at 24 hours. Such a reaction could, at least in part, be due to an Arthus reaction, particularly if there were a slow breakdown of the injected cells, liberating nuclear antigens which would then react with circulating antibodies. However, similar results have been demonstrated with various preparations of nuclear antigens, including double and single-stranded DNA and more recently *in vitro* studies have provided evidence for cellular immunity to DNA, both from positive lymphocyte transformation tests and from the liberation of macrophage inhibitory factor by lymphocytes.

The Immunological Status of Patients with SLE

It has been suggested that patients with SLE may suffer from an underlying instability of the immune mechanism. In a study of antibody production, Lee *et al.* (1971) found no abnormality in the primary or secondary response to monomeric flagellin derived from *Salmonella adelaide* in sixteen cases of SLE. Abe and Homma (1971) also described normal primary and secondary responses to tetanus toxoid, but, in common with other workers, found a significant depression in the ability to produce a cellular immune response to dinitrochlorobenzene, and to PPD. The basis for this reduction in cellular immunity is not clear: it may be associated with some form of antigenic competition with the antigens responsible for SLE, or it may be a consequence of the antibodies to human T-lymphocytes recently described in this condition.

Aetiological Factors in SLE

Antibodies to nuclear antigens are a striking feature of SLE, and many of the pathological features of the disease can be attributed to the deposition in tissues of these antibodies, complexed to antigen and complement. It is still not known why these antibodies arise and why their presence is perpetuated in established lupus. A number of possible factors will be discussed in this section, but it is clear that the mere presence of antibody itself is not sufficient to cause disease. Animals have been extensively immunized with cell nuclei, nucleoprotein, nucleic acids and histones, and it has been possible to produce high titres of antibody to DNA and to histones without any convincing evidence of a lupus syndrome. Moreover, the experimental transmission of anti-nuclear antibodies to volunteers by repeated transfusion, or to infants by transplacental passage, fails to reproduce the clinical features of SLE. Another factor or factors must be implicated in the initiation of antibody production, and in maintaining it at a high level. Infectious agents, and genetic factors are two possibilities in which there is currently much interest. The development of a lupus-like syndrome following drug administration may also have important implications. Finally there are increasing reports of the development of lupus syndromes in association with congenital abnormalities of the complement system.

Ultrastructural Studies

Ultrastructural studies of tissues in SLE have revealed three types of structure which may be related to viruses: (i) tubulo-reticular inclusions, (ii) material resembling C-type viruses and (iii) organized deposits on basement membranes.

Györkey *et al.* (1972) demonstrated arrays of filamentous structures in the endothelial cells of vessels in the skin and kidney of patients with SLE, and suggested that they resembled "unenveloped nucleocapsids of paramyxo- or related viruses". There is some doubt about whether these tubulo-reticular inclusions are specific for SLE, since others have reported them in Goodpasture's syndrome, and in the myocardium in Coxsackie B infection. Careful cytochemical studies have shown that these structures behave quite differently from Newcastle disease virus, a typical paramyxovirus, and that they are not digested by nucleases. They are more likely to consist of a phospholipid-protein complex than a nucleoprotein. Goodman *et al.* (1973) reported similar structures in the lymphocytes of patients with discoid and systemic LE and others have shown that the number of circulating lymphocytes containing tubulo–reticular structures correlates to some extent with disease activity.

The RNA viruses of the leukovirus genus are divided into subgenera A, B, C and D. The first two contain viruses known to cause tumours and leukaemia in cats and mice. The second two subgenera include visna (sheep) and the foamy agents of cats, cattle and primates. Viruses of subgenera A and C have been observed on electron microscopy to form structures termed "C-type particles". The characteristic feature of C-type particles is that no fully-developed, intracytoplasmic virus is distinguishable. Viral material only becomes visible immediately below the cytoplasmic membrane, from which it gains an envelope before its release.

Structures with some resemblance to degenerated C-type particles have been observed in the glomerular capillary walls of patients with SLE. The process of budding from plasma membranes has never been observed in human material, however, and the characterization of fuzzy round blobs in kidney biopsies seems at present to be more a matter of vivid imagination than of critical scientific analysis.

Among the most striking ultrastructural features of human SLE are the "thumb-print" deposits occasionally found lying beneath the glomerular basement membrane (Fig. 3). These organized deposits are extracellular, and show parallel dark lines enclosing a tubular space. Transverse striations can sometimes be seen, suggesting a helical configuration. Similar deposits are said to occur in the lupus-like syndrome of NZB/W mice. They bear no relation to any known viral structures, and may represent organized DNA or antibody molecules. Somewhat similar bodies have been described in the plasma and in the glomeruli of a patient with familial deficiency of lecithin-cholesterol acyl transferase (LCAT), and in that condition they are thought to represent layers of phospholipid membranes.

Infection and Transmissible Agents

There have been a large number of studies on the levels of specific anti-viral antibodies in patients with SLE. In general they are inconclusive. High levels

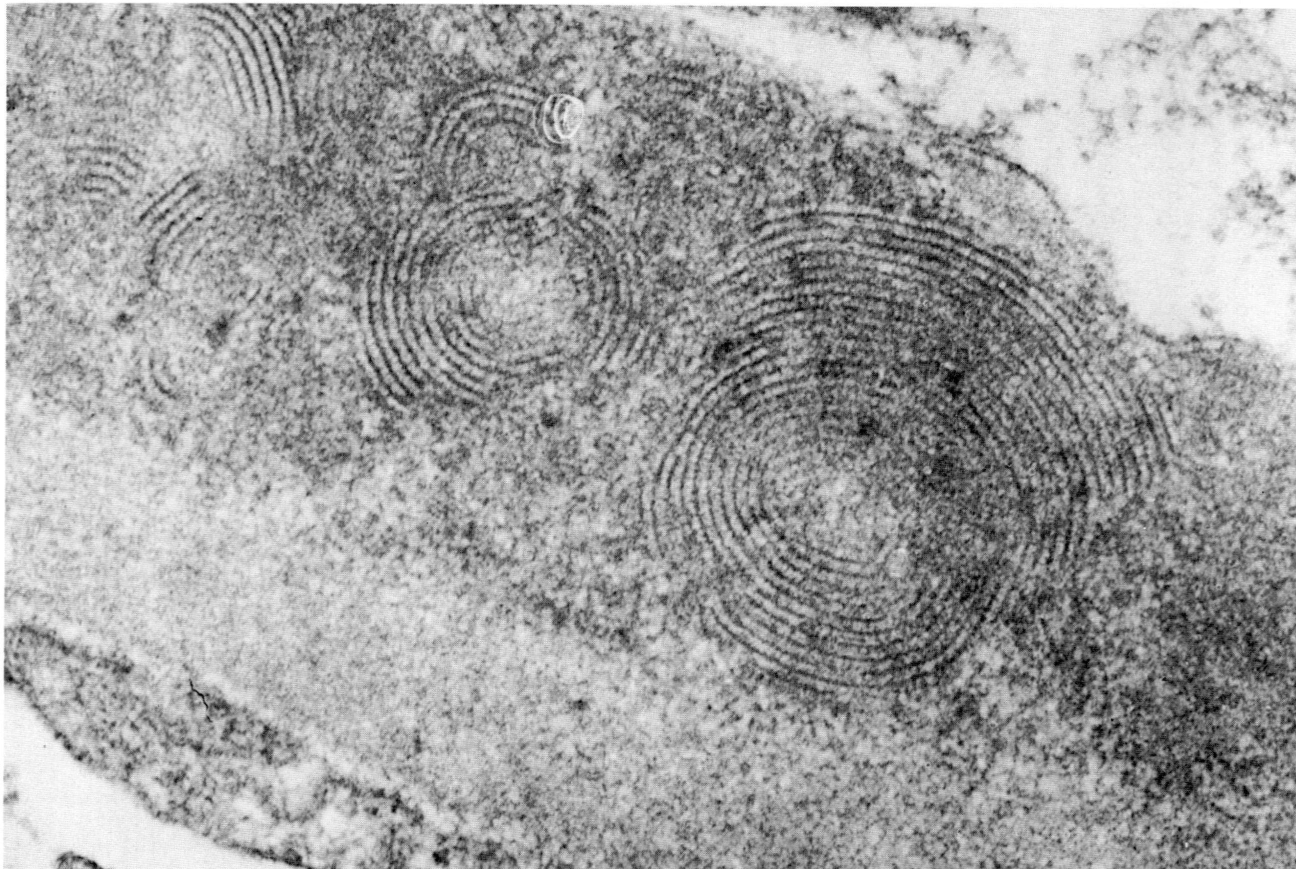

Fig. 3. Lupus nephritis. Thumb-print deposits lying beneath the glomerular basement membrane in a case of SLE. (× 24,400) (Photomicrograph kindly provided by Dr C. R. Tribe.)

of measles antibody are present in some patients with SLE but this is by no means specific, and it has been suggested that high levels of viral antibody in SLE correlate with the raised levels of gamma-globulin, and are part of a non-specific immunological hyperreactivity. Titres of antibody to Epstein–Barr virus (EBV) have been reported by some workers to be high and by others to be normal. Similar conflicting reports have appeared on the frequency with which hepatitis-B antigen (HBAg) and the corresponding antibody can be detected in patients with SLE.

There is increasing interest in the possibility that the virus associated with SLE may be a C-type RNA virus. These viruses are thought to operate by means of an RNA-dependent DNA polymerase, whose first product is a DNA:RNA hybrid. For this reason, Talal and Gallo (1972) examined sera for antibodies to a polydeoxythymidylio-polyribo-adenylic (dT.rA) hybrid, and found them in 14% of patients with SLE. They were only detectable, however, in the presence of antibodies to DNA and RNA, and their cross-reactivity made it difficult to draw firm conclusions.

Attempts have been made to detect C-type virus in the tissues of patients with SLE by biochemical means. Experiments to establish homology between RNA of C-type viruses and DNA from SLE have been unconvincing. However, a more promising and sensitive method is to look for typical virus antigens, by the method of competitive radioimmunoassay. An antiserum to purified viral protein is allowed to react with radioactively labelled preparations of the protein antigens under standard conditions, and a homogenate of the tissue under study is tested for its ability to block the reaction. Using this technique, Strand and August (1974) have reported the presence of C-type core protein in the spleen of a patient with SLE. These findings provide valuable evidence for the presence of C-type viruses in human tissues but they are far from establishing that such viruses are a *cause* of SLE.

Very extensive attempts to propagate a transmissible agent by culturing SLE tissue, and to transmit a pathogenic factor to experimental animals, have so far been unsuccessful. Lewis *et al.* (1973) were able to show that the serological abnormalities of canine lupus could be transmitted from an affected animal to newborn dogs, mice and rats by a cell-free filtrate from homogenized spleen cells. The activity of the transmissible agent could be enhanced by serial passage in mice and some of the mice treated with the filtrate developed lymphoid tumours, which were found to contain numerous viral particles, both of A-type and of C-type. Some of the RNA tumour viruses are known to be defective, requiring cells infected with a second virus strain in order to reproduce. These experiments suggest that a canine lupus virus exists which is capable of activating RNA tumour viruses when administered to mice.

Although the transplacental passage of anti-nuclear antibody may have little effect on the foetus (p. 345) there are reports of abnormalities in children born to mothers with SLE which are compatible with the existence of a transmissible agent. Individual cases have been described in which infants develop either discoid or mild systemic LE shortly after birth, which usually clears spontaneously (Dubois, 1974, p. 384). There is also a report of an infant with discoid LE whose mother developed SLE 11 months later.

Familial and Genetic Factors

Many have shown familial aggregations of cases of SLE. Such aggregations have been reported both for discoid and for systemic LE, and two of the most impressive studies are those of Leonhardt (1967) from Sweden, and Larsen (1972) from Norway. Both have shown that, in the families of probands with SLE, there is not only a higher incidence of SLE and of anti-nuclear antibodies, but also a significant elevation of serum immunoglobulins. These abnormalities may point to a genetic predisposition to SLE, or to a transmissible agent of low infectivity, operating against a background of genetic susceptibility. Simple vertical transmission (from mother to offspring by transplacental infection) is certainly not the only explanation, since a number of father–daughter pairs have been recorded. A recent study has shown that both non-consanguineous and consanguineous relatives of patients with SLE have an abnormally high incidence of lymphocytotoxic antibody when compared to a control population (Dehoratius and Messner, 1975). A number of studies on the incidence of various blood group and HLA antigens have been made with various results. A recent study by Kissmeyer-Nielsen *et al.* (1975) failed to find any deviation from the normal distribution of HLA antigens among patients with SLE, and discusses some explanations of earlier, probably spurious, findings.

Thus most of the epidemiological data are equally compatible with the existence of a transmissible agent of low infectivity, perhaps requiring genetic or immunological factors for its expression.

Complement Deficiencies

A number of cases have been reported in which diseases resembling SLE have developed in subjects suffering from primary abnormalities of the complement system (Stroud, 1974). Deficiencies of C1r, C1s, C2 and the C1 esterase inhibitor have each been found to be associated with lupus-like conditions in certain individual cases. These complement disorders are described more fully in Chapter 7, but it is of interest that they are all disorders affecting the early part of the classical pathway which plays an important role in the opsonization and phagocytosis of microorganisms and which may be necessary for effective antibody production.

Drug-induced Lupus-syndromes

A lupus-like syndrome occurs in about 10% of patients treated with *hydrallazine* and anti-nuclear antibodies are found in the serum in 98% of cases. Most patients recover spontaneously when the drug is withdrawn. It has been found that most of the patients reacting to hydrallazine are "slow-acetylators", when acetyl transferase activity is determined from the rate of acetylation of a standard dose of sulphamethazine. Hahn *et al.* (1972) found that patients with active hydrallazine lupus had antibodies to hydrallazine, as well as antibodies to both native (double-stranded) and heat-denatured (single-stranded) DNA. Lymphocytes from these patients also showed brisk responses when stimulated *in vitro* with hydrallazine, and with both types of DNA. Longitudinal studies are reported in one patient who developed antibodies and cellular immunity to hydrallazine during her first exposure, which disappeared when the drug was withdrawn. Antibodies and cellular immunity to DNA, however, appeared only *after* withdrawal of the drug. When the drug was recommenced, symptoms developed, antibodies to hydrallazine reappeared, and antibodies to DNA became undetectable.

Procainamide is the commonest cause of drug-induced lupus in the USA. The incidence is related to the dose and duration of treatment, and most cases recover when the drug is withdrawn. When Dubois (1974, p. 393) reviewed a group of 22 patients treated with procainamide, he found antibodies to DNA in 36%. It is of interest that the antibodies in this condition are directed against single-stranded rather than double-stranded DNA. This suggests that the antibodies are directed against the purine and pyrimidine bases of DNA (which are exposed only in the single-stranded form). Blömgren *et al.* (1972) found antibodies both to DNA and to procainamide, and suggested that procainamide might complex with DNA to produce a potent immunogen. A possibility which does not appear to have been considered is that procainamide is antigenically cross-reactive with one of the pyrimidine bases. If procaine is protein-bound at or near the HCl group, the terminal aminated benzene ring has a configuration similar to cytosine. It would be of interest to know if the antibodies in procainamide lupus react preferentially with poly-C.

Chlorpromazine and other members of the *phenothiazine group* of drugs are also able to induce a lupus syndrome associated with antibodies to single-stranded DNA. It has been shown that chlorpromazine will bind to single-stranded and, more slowly, to double-stranded DNA *in vitro* when exposed to ultraviolet light. The phenothiazine ring is similar in dimensions to the phenoxazone ring, which is known to intercalate between adjacent guanine bases in DNA, and it is possible that these drugs interact with DNA in this way, rendering it more antigenic.

Many other drugs can produce lupus syndromes and one of the most recently reported is practolol. The mechanism in this and many other instances is obscure. Drug-induced lupus is less severe than spontaneous SLE and usually subsides when the drug is withdrawn. This is further evidence that anti-DNA antibodies cannot be held responsible for self-perpetuating disease. The antibodies produced are mainly against single-stranded DNA in contrast to SLE, in which antibodies also appear against double-stranded DNA, and against a variety of nucleoproteins. Some drugs may cross-react antigenically with DNA bases, while others may form immunogenic complexes with DNA, particularly on exposure to ultraviolet light.

It has been argued that drug-induced lupus is expressed only in individuals predisposed by a "lupus diathesis", but this seems unlikely, in view of the variable frequency of lupus induced by various drugs, and the clinical and epidemiological differences between drug-induced lupus and SLE.

Therapeutic Aspects

The milder cases of SLE, with joint manifestations alone, may respond for a time to treatment with salicylates. When the disease becomes more aggressive, with widespread skin involvement, pleuritis, pericarditis, and haematological involvement, treatment with corticosteroids is urgently required. Forty to 60 mg of prednisone or its equivalent may be needed daily, initially, and the response is usually dramatic. When the initial symptoms and signs have subsided, long-term management with smaller doses of steroids is required to prevent or delay the development of permanent damage, particularly to the kidneys. A sufficient dose of steroids will be required to suppress symptoms, and return the ESR or plasma viscosity to normal. Repeated serological studies are required and, ideally, treatment should be adjusted to maintain DNA binding and complement levels within the normal range. If the disease proves steroid resistant, or if the dose of steroids required for maintenance is so large as to produce complications, then cytotoxic drugs will be needed. Azathioprine may be given in doses up to 150 mg daily, and cyclophosphamide can be used in oral or intravenous regimes. Both of these drugs can, of course, produce severe, and potentially fatal bone marrow depression, and need to be controlled with regular haematological investigations.

If there is clinical evidence of renal disease, with proteinuria, haematuria, a rising blood urea, or falling creatinine clearance, a renal biopsy will be required to establish the degree of renal damage, and cytotoxic drugs may be essential, since renal function can deteriorate rapidly. There is still much disagreement over the best way to administer cytotoxic drugs (see Chapter 30), and further therapeutic studies are required. If the central nervous system is involved, the prognosis is particularly poor, and the response to treatment is likely to be disappointing. Patients with cerebral lupus may die without major disturbances of serum complement although the c.s.f. complement is usually depressed (Petz *et al.*, 1971). Chloroquine and hydroxychloroquine may be a useful adjunct to treatment in milder cases of SLE, but both may produce irreversible ocular changes, and should be administered according to a strict dosage schedule (Dubois, 1974) and under the supervision of an ophthalmic surgeon.

Dubois has reported that the prognosis of SLE has improved strikingly in the past 20 years, and much of this improvement must reflect a more rational approach to therapy, and recognition of the dangers of renal damage.

VASCULITIC DISORDERS

In 1866, Kussmaul and Maier described two cases of a fatal, rapidly progressive disease, characterized by the presence of numerous nodules along the course of small arteries, with fever, progressive weakness, and glomerulonephritis. Within the nodules they found inflammation and necrosis of the arterial wall, and they therefore termed the condition periarteritis nodosa. With the recognition that the inflammatory lesions were not only "periarterial" but might involve any of the layers of the arterial wall, the term "polyarteritis nodosa" was preferred by many workers. By 1950, it was clear that polyarteritis nodosa had features in common with a number of other inflammatory diseases of blood vessels, and Zeek (1952) suggested "necrotizing angiitis" as a generic term to include a wide group of diseases characterized by inflammation of the whole thickness of the walls of blood vessels, and associated with necrosis and fibrin deposition. Rich and Gregory (1943) showed that rabbits immunized with horse serum developed vascular lesions closely resembling those of polyarteritis nodosa and Zeek (1952) suggested that a group of cases having "hypersensitivity angiitis" (due to serum, sulphonamides, or other drugs) should be separated from the other forms of vasculitis, and from polyarteritis nodosa. However, continuing study has suggested that many other types of vasculitis, including polyarteritis nodosa, are associated with hypersensitivity, and this classification now seems unstable.

Alarcon-Segovia and Brown (1964) suggested that it is helpful to visualize a spectrum of diseases associated with vasculitis, with a group of conditions characterized by a necrotizing vasculitis at one end, and a group of predominantly granulomatous conditions at the other. In between lie conditions such as Wegener's granulomatosis, in which there are varying combinations of vasculitis and granulomatous change (Fig. 4). This concept provides a useful and flexible framework for classification of the vasculitic disorders.

In general, it is preferable to use the term "*necrotizing vasculitis*" to describe the whole range of non-suppurative inflammatory diseases of blood vessels, distinguishing various subgroups, such as polyarteritis nodosa, within this broader definition. There is now increasing evidence that most of the diseases in this group are associated with some form of hypersensitivity. A number of cases have been reported in which a syndrome resembling polyarteritis nodosa has followed the administration of certain drugs.

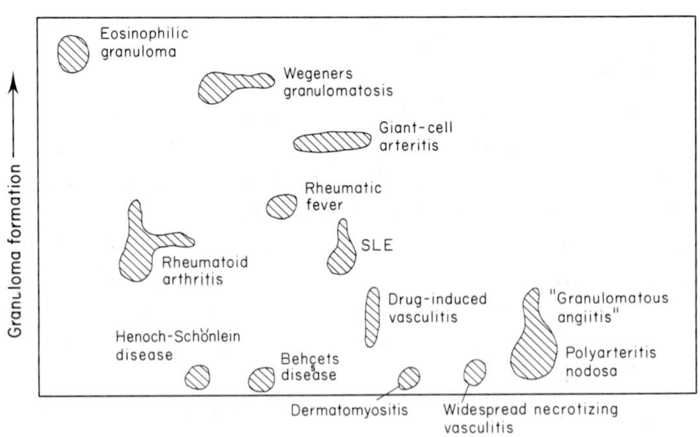

Fig. 4. The vasculitic disorders can be classified according to the relative proportions of vasculitis and granuloma formation, which are here indicated on an arbitrary scale (modified after Alarcon-Segovia and Brown).

Because there is controversy over whether these cases should be considered as having polyarteritis nodosa, they are discussed separately as examples of "drug-induced vasculitis" (p. 363). The distinction between polyarteritis nodosa and allergic vasculitis is still arbitrary but as more aetiological factors are identified and the immunological mechanisms become more completely understood, it should be possible to classify these conditions more logically.

POLYARTERITIS NODOSA

The incidence of the disease is unknown. In the Registrar General's statistical review of England and Wales for 1973, 227 deaths were ascribed to "polyarteritis nodosa and allied conditions", giving a death rate of 5 per million in men, and 4 per million in women. The value of this information is diminished by the surprising fact that this heading also includes deaths from systemic lupus erythematosus.

Clinical Features

Rose and Spencer (1957) and Frohnert and Sheps (1967) have documented the clinical symptoms and signs. Most patients have fever and weight loss, and more than half have joint symptoms: 60% have skin involvement, with a petechial rash, or more rarely, ischaemic ulcers. Nodules occurred in 20% of Frohnert and Sheps' series. Mononeuritis multiplex was the commonest neurological complication, and in the respiratory system, bronchitis, pneumonia and asthma were prominent features. Rose and Spencer (1957) suggested that the group with pulmonary involvement had more eosinophilia and a worse prognosis than the non-pulmonary group, but this was not supported by Frohnert and Sheps' (1967) finding that hypertension and renal involvement were the only recognizable factors affecting prognosis. Renal biopsy studies show arteritis or glomerulonephritis in 70% of cases and some 45% of patients die of renal disease (Rose and Spencer, 1957). Abdominal pain is a common presenting symptom, and arteritis involving the coronary system may produce angina or myocardial infarction. Myalgia is present in about 30% of cases. In general, the clinical course of patients with polyarteritis nodosa is one of progressive deterioration and death.

Pathological Features

Polyarteritis nodosa is characterized by focal inflammatory lesions affecting arterioles and, to a lesser extent, small or medium-sized arteries. There is necrosis, perhaps beginning in the media, but spreading to involve the intima and adventitia, and accompanied by the deposition of fibrinoid material. Dense leucocytic infiltration of the vessel wall occurs, with neutrophils, eosinophils and mononuclear cells (Fig. 5). The vasculitis process may proceed to healing, or may end in arterial occlusion and infarction. Giant cells and granuloma-formation are rarely seen. Most tissues and organs can be affected e.g. the gastrointestinal tract, kidneys, pancreas, gall-bladder, testes, heart, lungs, muscles and peripheral nerves. Renal involvement is common, with arteritis lesions and infarcts. The glomeruli may show fibrinoid necrosis with cellular proliferation leading to glomerular scarring.

The only investigation which is diagnostically convincing in this disease is a positive tissue biopsy and there has been much debate regarding the most suitable site. If skin is affected, the chances of a positive biopsy are high. Muscle biopsy is positive in only a third of cases but a positive biopsy is more likely if the muscle is clinically involved. Renal, testicular and rectal biopsies are often helpful and if the diagnosis is strongly suspected, it may be necessary to take biopsies from a number of sites. Recently, it has been claimed that the appearance of multiple small aneurysms on renal arteriography may be an important pointer to the diagnosis.

The lack of any serological test of diagnostic value helps to explain why this condition has been so much less studied than systemic lupus erythematosus. The diagnosis may be suggested by a mild anaemia, raised serum viscosity or ESR, leucocytosis and eosinophilia. The lungs may show patchy infiltrates, or pleural effusions, and cardiomegaly may be accompanied by ECG evidence of pericarditis or myocardial ischaemia. Immunoglobulin levels may be high. Complement changes are discussed below.

Immunological Features

Rich and Gregory (1943) emphasized the histopathological similarity between the lesions of polyarteritis nodosa and those of serum sickness, and established that animals immunized with a foreign protein develop a disease which is clinically and histologically similar to polyarteritis nodosa. Several workers, including Paronetto and Strauss (1962) showed that immunoglobulins were deposited in the walls of affected arteries in various organs and

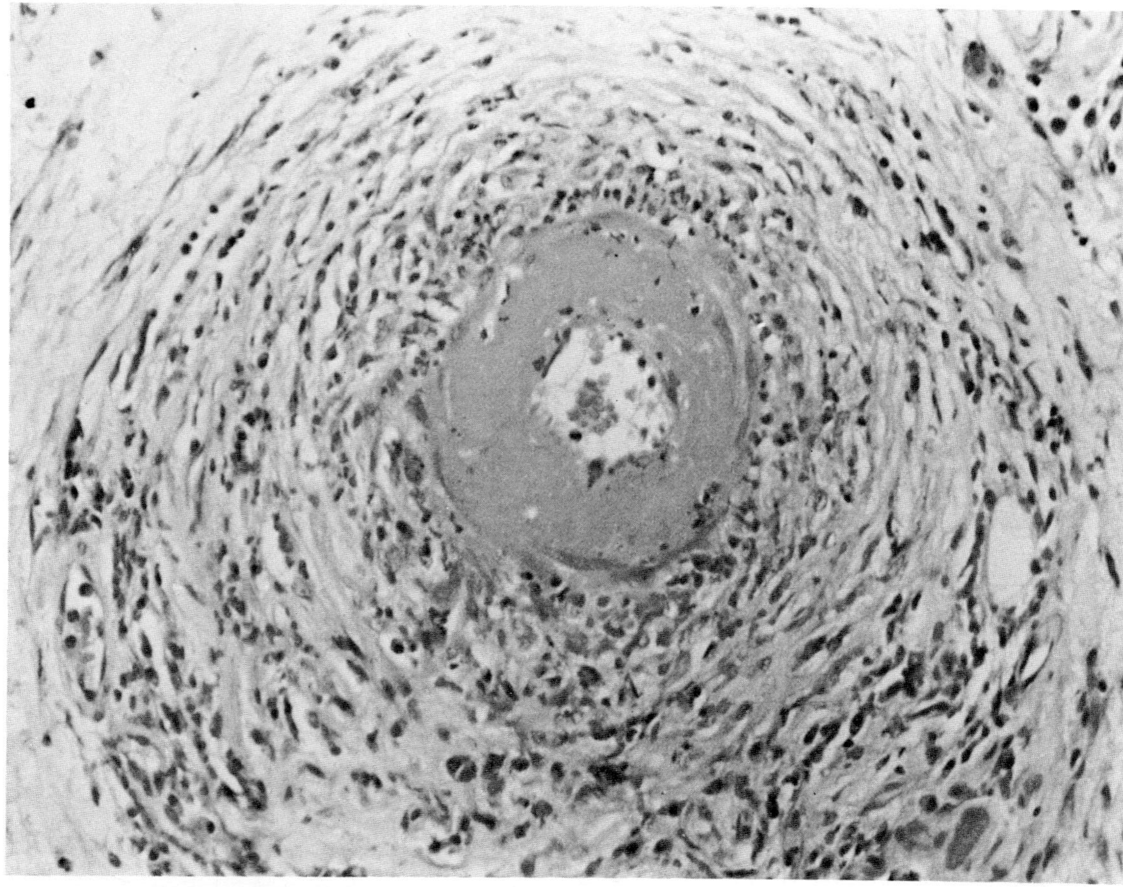

Fig. 5. Acute necrotizing vasculitis. Small submucosal artery in the rectum of a patient with rheumatoid arthritis and clinical signs suggestive of polyarteritis nodosa. Note the fibrinoid necrosis of the intima and infiltration of all coats by acute inflammatory cells. (Haematoxylin and eosin $\times 315$) (Photomicrograph kindly provided by Dr C. R. Tribe.)

Lachmann *et al.* (1962) demonstrated complement deposition in renal arteries and in the glomerular tufts.

Little progress was made until 1970 when Gocke *et al.* reported 4 out of 11 cases of polyarteritis nodosa in whom there was evidence of circulating Australia antigen (hepatitis B antigen). In all four cases circulating immune complexes were demonstrated by ultracentrifugation and precipitation with C1q. In one case, immunofluorescent studies showed that hepatitis B antigen, IgM, and complement were deposited in the skin lesions. Trepo *et al.* (1974) investigated 55 cases of polyarteritis nodosa from Lyons. In 30 they detected hepatitis B surface antigen (HBs Ag), and in 13 they found the corresponding antibody (anti HBs Ag). Five cases had both antigen and antibody. Antibody to the HB core antigen was found in 35 cases, indicating active viral replication. Cases with the most active vasculitis had both antigen and antibody, and in two patients, clinical remission was followed by the disappearance of HBs Ag, and the appearance of low levels of antibody.

This interesting development has provided a much needed stimulus to studies of the immunopathology of polyarteritis nodosa. Many patients are known to carry hepatitis B antigen for years without developing arteritis, and there are also symptomless carriers of HBs antigen–antibody complexes. There is also a strong impression that the incidence of HBs Ag in polyarteritis nodosa is less in Britain and Holland than in the USA and France.

Therapeutic Aspects

There is a strong clinical impression that corticosteroid drugs are life-saving in polyarteritis nodosa, although there is disappointingly little objective evidence of this. The Medical Research Council (Collagen Diseases and Hypersensitivity Panel, 1957, 1960) attempted to match a group of cortisone-treated cases with a retrospective control group, but because of the limitations of this type of study, were unable to draw any firm conclusions. After three years, 13 out of 21 cases in the treated group were alive. It is clear from these and other studies that the presence or absence of hypertension or renal involvement have an important correlation with the prognosis.

Frohnert and Sheps (1967) found a five-year survival of 13% for untreated cases, compared with 48% in a group of 110 treated with ACTH or corticosteroids. It is now generally assumed that corticosteroids should be given in doses sufficient to control symptoms, and if possible, to return the ESR to normal. The therapeutic question of current interest is which, if any, cytotoxic drugs should be used in addition to corticosteroids. Individual case reports have appeared, describing excellent responses to azathioprine or cyclophosphamide, but a large-scale, controlled trial of the effectiveness of these drugs is urgently needed. In practice, some patients will probably be controlled on moderate doses of corticosteroids. Those with an aggressive, life-threatening disease are likely to need larger doses, and in these the long term complications of corticosteroid therapy can be reduced by the judicious use of azathioprine or cyclophosphamide. In those who show evidence of disease progression, with increasing neuropathy or deteriorating renal function despite corticosteroids, cytotoxic drugs should be used promptly. It is reasonable to hope that a wider application of tests for circulating immune complexes in polyarteritis nodosa may give information on disease activity which will be of value in controlling treatment.

VASCULITIS ASSOCIATED WITH DRUGS

The first group of drugs to be suspected of producing vasculitis were the sulphonamides, and Black-Shaffer (1945) pointed out that the arterial lesions, of which the most striking feature was a widespread fibrinoid necrosis, were very similar both to those induced in animals by immunization with protein antigens (experimental serum sickness), and to those found in polyarteritis nodosa. He argued that sulphonamide hypersensitivity should be regarded as an immunologically determined disease having affinities with serum sickness and polyarteritis nodosa.

Other reports have extended the list of drugs which can produce vasculitis, without adding to our understanding of the mechanism involved. Among the agents for which claims have been made, often on rather slender evidence, are several antibiotics, including chloramphenicol, erythromycin, griseofulvin, penicillin, streptomycin and tetracycline; barbiturates, promazines, and hydantoins: hypotensive drugs including hydrallazine and guanethidine; thiazide diuretics; corticosteroids; gold, mercury, bismuth, and organic arsenicals; phenylbutazone; iodides and uracil compounds; quinine and quinidine derivatives; aspirin and phenacetin. Epsilon-aminocaproic acid, glibenclamide, pentazocine, and dynamite have been added to the list in the past few years, and exposure to weed-killers, insecticides and petroleum products has also been incriminated. Vasculitis occurring in drug addicts is likely to be associated with hepatitis B antigen.

There have been very few attempts to investigate the immunopathological aspects of drug-induced vasculitis. Björnberg and Gisslen (1965), who reported necrotizing vasculitis following thiazide administration, described one woman to whom a challenge dose of hydrochlorothiazide was given after her skin lesions had recovered. A severe recurrence of cutaneous vasculitis appeared on the next day. Later, she was given a test dose of the related drug, chlorthalidone. The result was even more dramatic, with a relapse of the skin lesions and frank haematuria, which persisted for over six months. Copeman (1970) reports the results of immunofluorescent studies on skin biopsies from a group of patients with "cutaneous angiitis" but it is not clear which patients were considered to have drug hypersensitivity. McDuffie (1970) has reported low levels of total haemolytic complement in one patient with a necrotizing vasculitis possibly due to chlorothiazide but few other immunological studies have been reported in drug-induced vasculitis.

CUTANEOUS VASCULITIS

This group of disorders is discussed more fully in Chapter 23. Although antibody and complement deposition may be detected in the skin and soluble complexes may be detectable in the circulation, these are not consistent findings and often do not correlate with each other.

Jones *et al.* (1975) have studied a case of necrotizing vasculitis in which IgG and complement were found in the skin lesions, particularly at the epidermal/dermal junction. Tests for circulating immune complexes were negative, but autologous serum produced lesions very similar to the spontaneous eruption both in histological appearance and on immunofluorescence. Fractionation of the serum suggested that the activity was closely associated with IgG, but had a molecular weight rather higher than that of normal IgG. It seems likely that this active component was a small immune complex.

GRANULOMATOUS VASCULITIS

Some vasculitic disorders are associated with the formation of granulomata, either in the walls of blood vessels, or in adjacent extravascular sites. As already mentioned, Alarcon-Segovia and Brown (1964) suggest that it is helpful to visualize a spectrum of related diseases (Fig. 4). At one end, in polyarteritis nodosa, and in the arteritis associated with rheumatoid arthritis and with dermatomyositis, there is a severe necrotizing vasculitis, with little or no evidence of granuloma formation. At the other end, in conditions such as eosinophilic granuloma and lethal mid-line granuloma, there is much granuloma formation, and little evidence of vasculitis. Conditions such as rheumatic fever and Wegener's granulomatosis occupy intermediate positions, with varying proportions of both components. This concept is a helpful one, but should not be considered as more than a descriptive convenience. Several diseases in this group are sufficiently characteristic to be considered individually, and in a few instances, there are features suggesting an immunopathological process.

Wegener's Granulomatosis

This is a condition in which necrotizing granulomata of the respiratory tract are associated with a generalized necrotizing vasculitis affecting particularly the lungs, spleen and kidneys. The kidneys often show a focal glomerulitis, in addition to their vascular changes. Immunofluorescent studies of renal biopsies in this condition have shown granular deposits of immunoglobulin and complement in glomeruli, suggesting the deposition of immune complexes and Horn *et al.* (1974) found sub-epithelial electron dense deposits in the glomeruli. There have been no detailed immunopathological reports of the vasculitic lesions in Wegener's granulomatosis, and limited studies of circulating complement components in this condition have been normal (Jones and Cumming, 1975).

Giant Cell Arteritis and Polymyalgia Rheumatica

This group of conditions lies towards the granulomatous end of the spectrum of vasculitic diseases. Characterized histologically by focal necrotizing arteritis in larger arteries, a typical feature is the development of granulomatous lesions, with foreign-body giant cells, in the media and intima of the vessels. The clinical presentation depends on the location of the vessels involved initially. The superficial temporal arteries, and less commonly, the ophthalmic and vertebral arteries, may be the main site of attack in the elderly, producing headache and arterial tenderness, often proceeding to blindness, and brain stem strokes. The histological features of Takayasu's disease (pulseless disease, aortic arch aortitis) are similar. Many patients with giant-cell arteritis also have symptoms and signs of generalized disease: fever, malaise and weight loss are common, and the ESR is raised, often to very high levels.

Polymyalgia rheumatica is also a disease of elderly patients, in which localized or generalized muscle pain and tenderness is associated with similar evidence of systemic involvement, and also typically, with a very high ESR. About 50% of patients also show changes of giant-cell arteritis on arterial biopsy. There has been one report in which immunoglobulins were detected in the media of affected arteries but little other immunological investigation appears to have been done. One case is reported to have been due to a hypersensitivity to indomethacin and one to sulphonamides. Giant cell arteritis responds dramatically to corticosteroids but direct evidence for the involvement of immunological mechanisms is almost completely lacking.

PROGRESSIVE SYSTEMIC SCLEROSIS

Progressive systemic sclerosis (PSS) is a condition characterized by inflammation, fibrosis and degenerative changes in the dermis, with thinning of the epidermis, and widespread involvement of other systems, including the heart, lungs, gastrointestinal tract, and kidney. It may be associated with vasculitis, myositis, kerato-conjunctivitis sicca (Sjøgren's syndrome) and the presence of anti-nuclear antibody. Similar skin changes are found in localized patches in morphoea, and in more extensive areas of skin in generalized scleroderma without systemic involvement.

The main clinical and histopathological features of PSS often begin in the fingers and hands, where the skin becomes progressively more tight, smooth and inelastic, with a striking increase in collagen in the dermis, and thinning of the epidermis. These changes may be preceded by Raynaud's phenomenon in the fingers. Fleischmajer *et al.* (1972), found that fat in the subcutaneous tissues was replaced by hyalinized connective tissue, containing masses of irregular collagen fibrils. Panniculitis was a striking feature in the deeper layers. Dysphagia, accompanied by collagen deposition in the lower two-thirds of the oesophagus, with mucosal ulceration, is the commonest gastro-intestinal feature, though small and large bowel involvement may occur, leading to malabsorption, and to the formation of wide-mouthed diverticula in the colon. The lungs commonly show diffuse interstitial and alveolar fibrosis. Renal involvement may take the form of changes in the afferent arterioles, and glomerular damage is sometimes seen (Fig. 6).

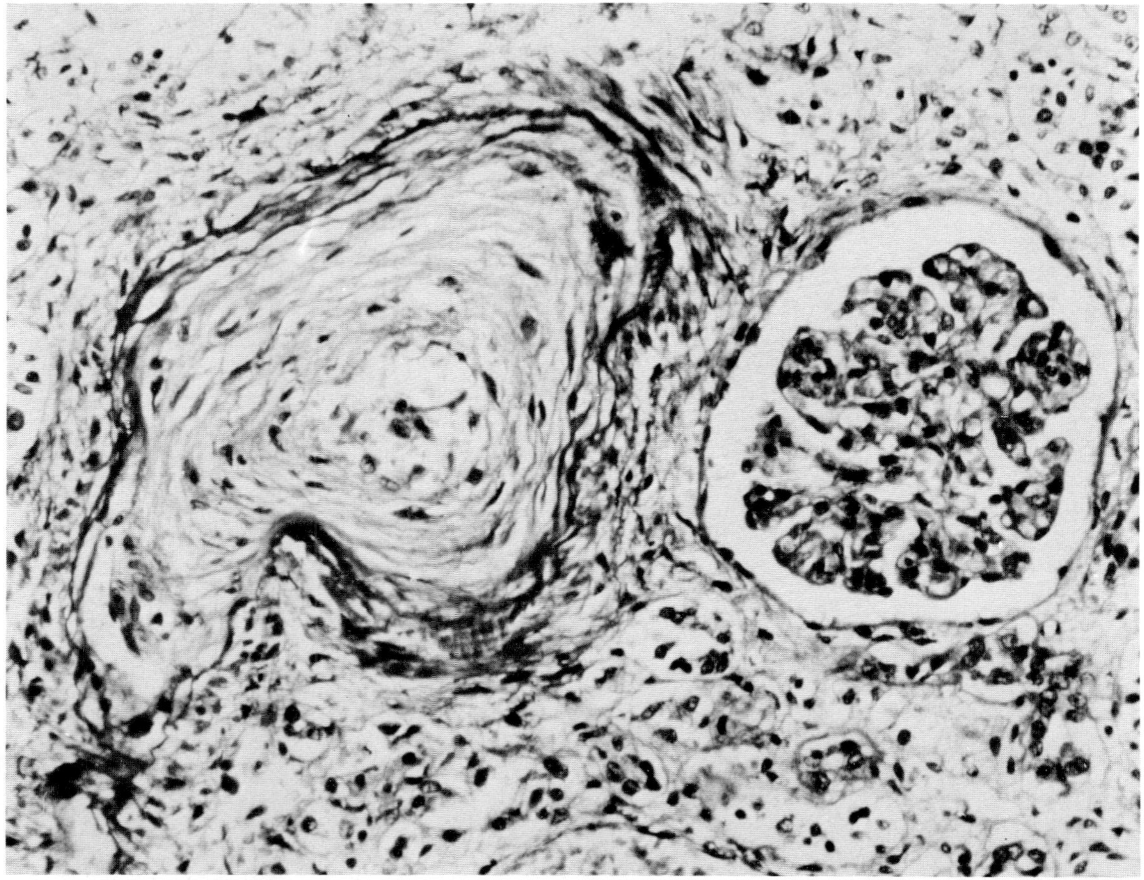

Fig. 6. Scleroderma kidney. Glomerulus and adjacent interlobular artery in the kidney of a patient with systemic sclerosis who died in renal failure with malignant hypertension. Note the severe narrowing of the artery by loose mucinous intimal thickening with only slight elastic reduplication. (Verhoeff elastic ×875) (Photomicrograph kindly provided by Dr C. R. Tribe.)

Immunological Features

LE cells and anti-nuclear antibodies are often found in PSS but the speckled, and the nucleolar pattern of immunofluorescent staining are more common in PSS than in SLE. Anti-nuclear antibodies occur more frequently in PSS than in localized scleroderma. Recently the presence of RNA antibodies has been found to be a characteristic feature of this condition (Alarcon-Segovia *et al.*, 1975).

There have been no convincing experimental models for scleroderma, though Stastny *et al.* (1963) found that by injecting allogeneic lymphocytes in rats, they could produce skin changes which had some histological resemblance to scleroderma, and to SLE. Jablonska *et al.* (1970) found immunoglobulin and complement deposited at the epidermal–dermal junction in those areas of sclerodermatous skin which showed telangiectasia, but not in indurated skin without vascular changes. There is some evidence that immunoglobulin, complement and fibrin are occasionally found in the glomeruli of patients with PSS, but the changes are less consistent and less dramatic than those seen in SLE.

Winkelstein *et al.* (1972) evaluated reactivity to delayed hypersensitivity antigens in 24 patients with PSS, and found them all to be normal. The response to PHA was also normal. Direct studies using white cells from patients with PSS, showed an inhibition of leucocyte migration with a range of antigens. More directly, Currie *et al.* (1971) found that lymphocytes from patients with PSS could be stimulated *in vitro* by exposure to collagen. Those from patients who had myositis as well as PSS were also stimulated by a homogenate of muscle. PSS lymphocytes were also found to be cytotoxic to fibroblasts in tissue culture.

There are many examples of overlap with other immunologically determined diseases. One subgroup is the "mixed connective tissue disease" described by Sharp *et al.* (1972) in which clinical features of SLE, polymyositis and PSS are combined, and antibodies are detectable to an "extractable nuclear antigen", presumably RNA. Parker (1973) has confirmed that this group of patients has antibodies to ribonucleoprotein. Hanson *et al.* (1974) found raised levels of immunoglobulins in children with PSS, and described a case in which scleroderma developed in a child following an episode of infective mononucleosis, accompanied by a rise in antibody titres suggesting active infection with EB virus.

REFERENCES

Aarden, L. A., Lakmaker Fieke., de Groot Els R., Swaak, A. J. G. and Feltkamp, T. E. W. (1975). *Scand. J. Rheumat.* Suppl. **11**, 12–19.

Abe, T. J. and Homma, M. (1971). Immunological reactivity in patients with systemic lupus erythematosus. *Acta Rheum. Scand.* **17**, 35.

Agnello, V., Koffler, D., Eisenberg, J. W., Winchester, R. J. and Kunkel, H. G. (1971). C1q precipitins in the sera of patients with systemic lupus erythematosus and other hypo-complementemic states: Characterization of high and low molecular weight types. *J. Exp. Med.* **134**, 228s.

Alarcon-Segovia, D. and Brown, A. L. (1964). Classification and etiologic aspects of necrotizing angiitides: an analytic approach to a confused subject, with a critical review of the evidence for hypersensitivity in polyarteritis nodosa. *Proc. Mayo Clin.* **39**, 205.

Alarcon-Segovia, D., Fishbein, E., Garcia-Ortigoza, E. and Estrada-Pana, S. (1975). Uracil – specific anti-R.N.A. antibodies in scleroderma. *Lancet* **i**, 363.

Barnett, E. V., Bluestone, R., Cracchiolo, A., III, Goldberg, L. S., Kantor, G. L., and McIntosh, R. M. (1970). Cryoglobulinemia and disease. *Ann. Intern. Med.* **73**, 95.

Beck, J. S., Oakley, C. L., and Rowell, N. R. (1966). Transplacental passage of anti-nuclear antibody. *Arch. Derm.* **93**, 656.

Bielschowsky, M., Hellyer, B. J. and Howie, J. B. (1959). Spontaneous haemolytic anaemia in mice of the NZB/BL strain. *Proc. Univ. Otago Med. School* **37**, 9.

Björnberg, A. and Gisslen, H. (1965). Thiazides: A cause of necrotizing vasculitis? *Lancet* **ii**, 982.

Black-Shaffer, B. (1945). Pathology of anaphylaxis due to sulfonamide drugs. *Arch. Path.* **89**, 301.

Blomgren, S. E., Condemi, J. J. and Vaughan, J. H. (1972). Procainamide-induced lupus erythematosus. Clinical and laboratory observations. *Am. J. Med.* **52**, 338.

Cochrane, C. G. and Koffler, D. (1973). Immune complex disease in experimental animals and man. *Adv. Immunol.* **16**, 185.

Cohen, A. S., Reynolds, W. E., Franklin, E. C., Kulka, J. P., Ropes, M. W., Shulman, L. E. and Wallace, S. L. (1971). Preliminary criteria for the classification of systemic lupus erythematosus. *Bull. Rheum. Dis.* **21**, 643.

Collagen Diseases and Hypersensitivity Panel (1957). Treatment of polyarteritis nodosa with cortisone: Results – after one year. Report to the Medical Research Council. *Brit. Med. J.* **1**, 608.

Collagen Diseases and Hypersensitivity Panel (1960). Treatment of polyarteritis nodosa with cortisone: Results – after three years. Report to the Medical Research Council. *Brit. Med. J.* **1**, 1399.

Copeman, P. W. M. (1970). Investigations into the pathogenesis of acute cutaneous angiitis. *Brit. J. Derm.* **82** (Suppl. 5) 51.

Cormane, R. H. and Joost, T. van. (1973). Lupus erythematosus: Immunologic studies of the skin. *In* "Immunopathology of the Skin. Labelled antibody studies". (Eds. E. H. Beutner, T. P. Chorzelski, S. F. Bean and R. E. Jordon), p. 92. Dowden, Hutchinson and Roos, Inc., Pennsylvania U.S.A.

Currie, S., Saunders, M. and Knowles, M. (1971). Immunological aspects of systemic sclerosis: *in vitro* activity of lymphocytes from patients with the disorder. *Brit. J. Derm.* **84**, 400.

Dacie, J. V. and Worlledge, S. M. (1969). Auto-allergic blood diseases. *In* "Clinical Aspects of Immunology" (eds. P. G. H. Gell and R. R. A. Coombs), p. 804. Blackwell Scientific Publications, Oxford.

Dehoratius, R. J. and Messner, R. P. (1975). Family studies of lymphocytotoxic antibodies in systemic lupus erythematosus. *In* "The Immunological Basis of Connective Tissue Disorders" (ed. L. G. Silvestri), North Holland Publishing Co., Amsterdam and Oxford.

Dixon, F. J., Vazquez, J. J., Weigle, W. O. and Cochrane, C. G. (1958). Pathogenesis of serum sickness. *Arch. Path.* **65**, 18.

Dubois, E. L. (1974). "Lupus Erythematosus". Second Edition. University of Southern California Press, Los Angeles.

Fleischmajer, R., Damiano, V. and Nedwich, A. (1972). Alteration of subcutaneous tissue in systemic scleroderma. *Arch. Derm.* **105**, 59.

Friedman, E. A., Bardawil, W. A., Merrill, J. P. and Hanau, C. (1960). "Delayed" cutaneous hypersensitivity to leukocytes in disseminated lupus erythematosus. *New Engl. J. Med.* **262**, 486.

Friou, G. J. (1957). Clinical application of lupus serum – nucleoprotein reaction using fluorescent antibody technique. *J. Clin. Invest.* **36**, 890.

Frohnert, P. P. and Sheps, S. G. (1967). Long-term follow-up study of periarteritis nodosa. *Am. J. Med.* **43**, 8.

Germuth, F. G. and Rodriguez, E. (1973). "Immunopathology of the Renal Glomerulus". Little, Brown and Co., Boston.

Gocke, D. J., Hsu, K., Morgan, C., Bombardierei, S., Lockshin, M. and Christian, C. L. (1970). Association between polyarteritis and Australia antigen. *Lancet* **ii**, 1149.

Goodman, J. R., Sylvester, R. A., Talal, N. and Tuffanelli, D. L. (1973). Virus-like structures in lymphocytes of patients with systemic and discoid lupus erythematosus. *Ann. Intern. Med.* **79**, 396.

Gyorkey, F., Sinkovics, J. G., Min, K. W. and Gyorkey, P. (1972). A morphologic study on the occurrence and distribution of structures resembling viral nucleocapsids in collagen disease. *Am. J. Med.* **53**, 148.

Hahn, B. H., Sharp, C. G., Irvin, W. S., Kantor, O. S., Gardner, C. A., Bagby, M. K., Perry, H. M. and Osterland, C. K. (1972). Immune responses to hydralazine and nuclear antigens in hydralazine-induced lupus erythematosus. *Ann. Intern. Med.* **76**, 365.

Hanson, V., Kornreich, H. K. and Drexler, E. (1974). Some immunologic considerations in focal scleroderma and progressive systemic sclerosis in children. *Pediatric Res.* **8**, 806.

Hargraves, M. M., Richmond, H. and Morton, R. (1948). Presentation of two bone marrow elements: the "tart" cell and the "LE" cell. *Proc. Mayo Clin.* **23**, 25.

Holborow, E. J., Weir, D. M. and Johnson, G. D. (1957). A serum factor in lupus erythematosus with affinity for tissue nuclei. *Brit. Med. J.* **ii**, 732.

Horn, R. G., Fauci, A. S., Rosenthal, A. S. and Wolff, S. M. (1974). Renal biopsy pathology in Wegener's granulomatosis. *Am. J. Path.* **74**, 423.

Hughes, G. R. V., Cohen, S. A. and Christian, C. L. (1971). Anti-DNA activity in SLE. A diagnostic and therapeutic guide. *Ann. Rheum. Dis.* **30**, 259.

Jablonska, S., Chorzelski, T. and Maciejowska, E. (1970). The scope and limitations of the immunofluorescence method in the diagnosis of lupus erythematosus. *Brit. J. Derm.* **83**, 242.

Jones, J. V., Cumming, R. H., Asplin, C. M., Harman, R. R. M. and Tribe, C. R. (1975). Necrotizing vasculitis; a circulating immune complex producing inflammatory skin lesions. *Brit. J. Derm.* **94**, 123.

Jones, J. V. and Cumming, R. H. (1975). Unpublished observations.

Kissmeyer-Nielsen, F., Kjerbye, K. E., Andersen, E. and Halberg, P. (1975). HLA antigens in systemic lupus erythematosus. *Transplant. Rev.* **22**, 164.

Kussmaul, A. and Maier, R. (1866). Uber eine bisher nicht beschriebene eigenthumliche Arterienerkrankung (Periarteritis nodosa), die mit morbus Brightii and rapid fortschreitender allgemeiner Muskellahmung einhergeht. *Dtsch. Arch. Klin. Med.* **1**, 484.

Lachmann, P. J., Müller-Eberhard, H. J., Kunkel, H. G. and Paronetto, F. (1962). The localization of *in vivo* bound complement in tissue sections. *J. Exp. Med.* **115**, 63.
Larsen, R. A. (1972). I. A proband material from central eastern Norway in family studies in systemic lupus erythematosus (SLE). *Acta. Med. Scand.* (Suppl.) **543**, 11.
Lee, A. K. Y., Mackay, I. R., Rowley, M. J. and Yap, C. Y. (1971). Measurement of antibody-producing capacity to flagellin in man. IV. Studies in autoimmune disease, allergy and azathioprine treatment. *Clin. Exp. Immunol.* **9**, 507.
Leonhardt, E. T. G. (1967). Family studies in systemic lupus erythematosus. *Clin. Exp. Immunol.* (Suppl.) **2**, 643.
Lewis, R. M., Andre-Schwartz, J., Harris, G. S., Hirsch, M. S., Black, P. H. and Schwartz, R. S. (1973). Canine systemic lupus erythematosus. Transmission of serologic abnormalities by cell-free filtrates. *J. Clin. Invest.* **52**, 1893.
Lies, R. B., Messner, R. P. and Williams, R. C. Jr. (1973). Relative T-cell specificity of lymphocytotoxins from patients with SLE. *Arthr. Rheum.* **16**, 369.
McDuffie, F. C. (1970). Serum complement levels in cutaneous diseases. *Brit. J. Derm.* **82**, (Supp. 5) 20.
Oldstone, M. B. A. and Dixon, F. J. (1967). Lymphocytic choriomeningitis. Production of antibody by "tolerant" infected mice. *Science* **158**, 1193.
Parker, M. D. (1973). Ribonucleoprotein antibodies: frequency and clinical significance in systemic lupus erythematosus, scleroderma, and mixed connective tissue disease. *J. Lab. Clin. Med.* **82**, 669.
Paronetto, F. and Strauss, L. (1962). Immunocytochemical observations in periarteritis nodosa. *Ann. Intern. Med.* **56**, 289.
Petz, L. D., Sharp, G. C. and Cooper, N. R. (1971). Serum and cerebral spinal fluid complement and serum auto-antibodies in systemic lupus erythematosus. *Medicine* **50**, 259.
Picazo, J. J. and Tan, E. M. (1975). Specificities of antibodies to native DNA. *Scand. J. Rheum.* Suppl. **11**, 35.
Pirquet, C. F. von and Schick, B. (1905). "Die Serumkrankheit", Deuticke, Leipzig and Vienna.
Porter, D. D. and Larsen, A. E. (1974). Aleutian Disease of Mink *In* "Slow Virus Diseases" (Progress in Medical Virology 18) (ed. J. Hotchin) p. 32, Karger, Basel.
Rich, A. R. and Gregory, J. E. (1943). The experimental demonstration that periarteritis nodosa is a manifestation of hypersensitivity. *Bull. Johns Hopk. Hosp.* **72**, 65.
Rose, G. A. and Spencer, H. (1957). Polyarteritis nodosa. *Quart. J. Med.* **26**, 43.
Rothfield, N. F. and Stollar, B. D. (1967). The relation of immunoglobulin class, pattern of anti-nuclear antibody, and complement-fixing antibodies to DNA in sera from patients with systemic lupus erythematosus. *J. Clin. Invest.* **46**, 1785.
Sharp, G. C., Irvin, W. S., Tan, E. M., Gould, R. G. and Holman, H. R. (1972). Mixed connective tissue disease. An apparently distinct rheumatic disease syndrome associated with a specific antibody to an extractable nuclear antigen (ENA). *Am. J. Med.* **52**, 148.
Stastny, P., Stembridge, V. A. and Ziff, M. (1963). Homologous disease in the adult rat, a model for autoimmune disease. I. General features and cutaneous lesions. *J. Exp. Med.* **118**, 635.
Stollar, B. D. (1973). Nucleic acid antigens. *In* "The Antigens" (ed. M. Sela) Vol. 1, p. 2. Academic Press, New York and London.
Strand, M. and August, J. T. (1974). Type-C RNA virus gene expression in human tissue. *J. Virol.* **14**, 1584.
Stroud, R. M. (1974). Genetic abnormalities of the complement system of man associated with disease. *Transplant. Proc.* **6**, 59
Talal, N. and Gallo, R. C. (1972). Antibodies to DNA:RNA hybrid in systemic lupus erythematosus measured by a cellulose ester filter radioimmunoassay. *Nature* (*New Biol.*) **240**, 240.

Trepo, C. G., Zuckerman, A. J., Bird, R. C. and Prince, A. M. (1974). The role of circulating hepatitis B antigen/antibody immune complexes in the pathogenesis of vascular and hepatic manifestations in polyarteritis nodosa. *J. Clin. Path.* **27**, 863.
Winkelstein, A., Rodnan, G. P. and Heilman, J. D. (1972). Cellular immunity in progressive systemic sclerosis (Scleroderma). *Ann. Rheum. Dis.* **31**, 126.
Zeek, P. M. (1952). Periarteritis nodosa: a critical review. *Am. J. Clin. Path.* **22**, 777.

12

Auto-immune Disease of the Endocrine Glands and Stomach

DUNCAN ADAMS

Even by 1900, understanding of immunology was surprisingly detailed. In his classical studies on the lysis of red blood corpuscles by antisera, Paul Ehrlich learned that antibodies had myriad specificities and could direct the powerful complement system on to a specific type of red cell, causing it to be ripped open with release of its haemoglobin. Ehrlich established that animals do not normally make antibodies against their own tissues, and coined the term "horror autotoxicus". He realized, however, that breakdown of the "horror autotoxicus" mechanism might occur and postulated that possible failure of the internal regulation of immune processes might be the explanation of many disease phenomena. My colleague, Walter Griesbach, recounted that in his medical student days in Germany before the First World War, the search for auto-immunity as a basis of disease was very fashionable. After the war, a generation of immunologists emerged who misquoted Ehrlich's "horror autotoxicus" principle as proof that auto-immunity could not occur and evidence for its occurrence was disregarded except for Dameshek and Schwartz's report in 1938 that auto-antibodies occur in haemolytic anaemia. However, it was a discovery in the thyroid field which finally produced a long overdue revolution in thinking.

There is a type of goitre in which the thyroid is extensively infiltrated with lymphocytes and plasma cells (Hashimoto, 1912). Patients with this disorder tend to have increased levels of gamma-globulin in their plasma. The features of Hashimoto's disease suggested an immunological pathogenetic mechanism to Doniach and Roitt (1957), who looked for thyroid auto-antibodies in sera from these patients, using a precipitin reaction. The findings were spectacular. Antibodies against human thyroglobulin were demonstrable in 80% of the cases of Hashimoto's disease, in 20% of cases of myxoedema and not at all in over 200 patients with other conditions. It appeared that auto-antibodies against thyroglobulin not only existed, but that they played a pathogenetic role in Hashimoto's disease and that myxoedema was the end result of the process.

Meanwhile, in studies on the specific antigenicity of organs, Witebsky *et al.* (1957) observed that rabbits immunized against thyroid extracts mixed with Freund's adjuvant not only developed antibodies against thyroglobulin, but also showed changes in their thyroid glands resembling those seen in Hashimoto's thyroiditis in man. They furthermore confirmed the presence of anti-thyroglobulin auto-antibodies in patients with Hashimoto's thyroiditis.

FUNDAMENTAL CONCEPTS

The Functional Requirements

It seems obvious that the immune system has evolved for defence of the host against pathogenic microbial parasites and tenable that it acts against malignant neoplasms. It also seems obvious that there will have been evolutionary pressures against any tendency of the immune system to react harmfully against the host. Nevertheless the requirement to be able to produce specific clones to react selectively with any one of thousands of potential pathogenic microbial invaders without producing clones reactive with host tissues is evidently too stringent. Some people are unable to defend themselves against a particular infection and others make clones which cause disease. Similarly if failure of immune surveillance in some people is a significant cause of malignant tumours, an incidence of auto-immune disease may be the price the population has to pay to avoid a greater incidence of malignancy.

The functions of the immune system fall into two categories, selection and execution.

Selection

This is mediated by the specific reactivities of antibody molecules. Plasma cells and B-lymphocytes produce antibody molecules, and there is evidence that immunoglobulin-like molecules form receptors on T-cells (Marchalonis, 1975).

It is possible that there is another selection system based on the presence of non-antibody molecules on the surface of T-lymphocytes, but this is not established. The product of the immune response (Ir) genes (Benacerraf and McDevitt, 1972) could conceivably be a non-antibody specificity-determining molecule related to cell-to-cell interaction, possibly concerned with prevention of malignancy. At present, there is little evidence for the existence of a second selection system. If it can be ruled out, it seems very likely that the Ir genes are V-genes, i.e. structural genes for polypeptide chains which form antibody combining sites (paratopes). This possibility is discussed below.

Execution

Unless an antibody reacts with a metabolically sensitive site on a cell (as thyroid-stimulating antibodies react with the receptor site for thyrotrophic hormone) simple combination with antigen may have little effect. Consequently, a variety of non-specific executive systems exist. One is the complement system which lyses cells to which it is directed by specific antibody. The reaction between antibody and antigen causes a structural alteration to cascade through the antibody molecule from the paratope (Jerne's term for the antibody's specific combining style) to the complement-reactive site which changes from an inactive to an active configuration. Other executive mechanisms include opsonisation, the facilitation of phagocytosis; specific antibody-mediated cytolysis by K (killer) cells; release of lymphokines from antigen-stimulated T-cells (these substances affecting cell movement and possibly mitosis and cytolysis); release of pharmacologically-active substances such as histamine from mast cells by antibodies of the IgE class on contact with their specific antigen.

Selection of Pre-formed Antibodies

It was first thought that antibodies achieve specificity by being folded around the antigen molecule, the "antigen-template" theory. Burnet challenged this, suggesting an enzyme induction process. Jerne then produced the original idea that antibodies are pre-formed and selected by antigen, the natural selection theory of antibody formation (Jerne, 1955). Burnet saw that antibodies must come from cells, and that the cells must exist as clones, and put forward the clonal selection theory of antibody formation (Burnet, 1959).

With today's detailed understanding of the mechanism by which the genetic code (in the form of specific sequences in DNA of adenine, guanine, thymine and cytosine) dictates the amino acid sequences which determine the three-dimensional structure of proteins, the selection of pre-formed molecules is seen to be the only antibody-forming process for which cell machinery exists.

Experience with bacterial cultures and understanding of the key role played by genetic mutation in enabling colonies to adapt and survive gave Burnet insight into the behaviour of populations of bacterial cells which applied also to populations of cells in the human body, and revealed the immunological importance of the clone and the role of somatic mutation.

The Immunological Clone

If a potato is divided into portions and planted, the resulting group of genetically-identical plants is known in horticulture as a clone. Burnet adopted this term to describe a hypothetical group of immunocytes, all making identical antibody molecules. Evidence from the study of plasma cell tumours first indicated that a single immunocyte makes antibody of a single specificity and there is general acceptance that each immunocyte is not unique, but is a member of a group of cells of identical specificity, the immunological clone. Burnet also introduced the expressive term, forbidden clone, to describe the self-reactive clones, not present in normal people, which occur in inherited auto-immune disease.

Somatic Mutation

Each time a cell divides its DNA must be replicated, with a small but finite chance of a copying error. These errors provide the phenotypic variety needed for evolution of a species by natural selection. Familiarity with the phenomenon of mutation in germ cells has for long been so widespread amongst biologists that it is surprising that the occurrence of the same process in dividing somatic cells should have been previously overlooked. As Burnet points out, to convince oneself of the reality of somatic mutation, one need only look at the back of the hand of an old person and observe the variety of localized skin abnormalities. In the immunity system, somatic mutation in immunocytes appears to play an important role in helping to provide the enormous diversity of clones needed for adequate immune defence. Somatic mutation also seems to play an integral role in inherited auto-immune disease, leading to both the initial appearance of the forbidden clones and to their subsequent diversification.

Although it is convenient to speak of somatic mutation, it is possible that an equivalent process of genetic alteration in dividing somatic cells, such as crossing-over of portions of chromosomes, is responsible for part or all of the somatically occurring variation observed.

The Generation of Immune Diversity

The enormous diversity of reactivity of the immunity system poses a question. How is this diversity achieved? With the discovery of the molecular structure of the immunoglobulin molecule and the knowledge that antibody specificity depends on the amino acid sequence of a light chain variable region and a heavy chain variable region, each coded for by V-genes on separate chromosomes, the genetic basis was apparent. Edelman (1971) pointed out that as heavy and light chain V-genes appeared to be able to associate at random, a hypothetical number, p of light chain V-genes, together with q heavy chain V-genes would result in $p \times q$ clones. These "primordial" clones probably undergo further diversification by somatic mutations occurring in the V-genes. These mutations may well affect the hypervariable regions especially, and initially they may occur largely in the thymus. The final complement of reactivity would be $p \times q \times$ (the somatic mutation factor).

Somatic mutation can occur only in immunocytes which are dividing, which implies that antigenic stimulation plays a role in the generation of immune diversity (Cunningham, 1974).

The Structure of Antibodies

The elucidation of the structure of antibody molecules and the discovery of the controlling structural genes (see Chapter 4), have added a fascinating new page to biology. An immunoglobulin molecule is composed of four polypeptide chains, two identical light chains each of about 200 amino acids and two identical heavy chains each of about 400 amino acids, the chains being joined together by disulphide bonds. Study of the amino acid sequences of immunoglobulin chains has revealed a repetitive pattern which indicates that the molecules have evolved from a basic unit of about a hundred amino acids, the immunoglobulin "domain": this evolution being achieved by duplication of the original structural gene. In immunoglobulin chains, the domain at the N-terminal end of the polypeptide shows great variety of amino acid sequence (see Chapter 4) forming a "variable" region, the remaining domains being relatively invariable and forming a "constant" region.

The Paratope

Jerne introduced this term for that part of the immunoglobulin molecule which combines with the antigen. The variable regions of adjacent light and heavy chains combine to form the paratope, the specificity being determined by the amino acid sequences of the two chains. Each basic immunoglobulin molecule has two identical paratopes, each paratope being, in three dimensional structure, a cleft.

Hypervariable Regions

Particularly striking is the finding that each variable region of an immunoglobulin polypeptide chain has in turn three hypervariable regions, involving a few amino acids around positions 28, 55 and 99, numbered from the N-terminus. In the variable regions, sulphur-containing amino acids occur at intervals, enabling parts of the polypeptide chains to be pulled together by intrachain disulphide bridges. In this way, the three hypervariable regions of each V-region polypeptide chain come together, a total of six hypervariable regions contributing the specificity of the paratope.

If somatic mutation contributes to antibody variability, it is of interest to know whether it involves particularly the hypervariable regions and whether a special mechanism, such as prevention of action of DNA repair enzymes, favours its occurrence.

Structural Genes for Immunoglobulin Chains; V-genes and C-genes

Studying rheumatoid factor in the blood of patients with rheumatoid arthritis, Grubb (1956) discovered that normal people make antibodies against other peoples' antibodies. These reactions never occur between two paratopes, simply because a cleft cannot fit another cleft. However, antibodies are large molecules and have their own antigenic determinants (epitopes), both on the parts formed by the constant regions of the polypeptide chains and on the parts formed by the variable regions. Some constant region epitopes show allotypic variation, i.e. each person shows one or another of a limited number of alternative epitopes, called allotypes. These are markers of immunoglobulin constant region structural genes, and the distribution of the relevant genes can be determined by family studies. At present the data are best explained by postulating the existence of at least three linkage groups (probably on separate chromosomes), two for light chains (kappa and lambda) and one for heavy chains. Each linkage group probably contains a large set of genes for the variable region, the V-genes, closely linked to the genes for the constant regions, the C-genes. In man there are thought to be ten C-genes for the heavy chains, two for lambda light chains and only one for kappa light chains (see Chapter 4).

Antibodies against Specific Antibodies

The epitopes occurring on the variable domains of immunoglobulin molecules are known as idiotypes and antibodies reacting with them are known as anti-idiotype antibodies. Such antibodies could be of great biological significance, since a complement-fixing clone against the idiotype of another clone would conceivably delete it by cytolysis. Such a mechanism would be particularly effective against T-cells which secrete little or no antibody, whereas B-cells, with copious antibody secretion, might be protected by a muffling reaction between the idiotype of secreted antibodies and the paratope of the reactive clone. Since the specificity of an idiotype is determined by the amino acid sequences of the chains forming a variable domain it will have a relationship to the specificity of the paratope. This implies a possible evolutionary mechanism by which antibodies of undesirable specificity may be deleted by anti-idiotype immune reactions, in accord with the general concept of "immune networks" proposed by Jerne (1973). If specific complement-fixing antibodies against the idiotypes of pathogenetic auto-antibodies could be developed artificially they might supply a great therapeutic need in auto-immune disease, namely a means of selective destruction of forbidden clones.

Immune response (Ir) Genes

In animals, studies of the inheritance of the immune response to certain unusual antigens, artificially made by forming polymers of single amino acids and adding other amino acids, have revealed the existence of genes which affect the magnitude of specific immune responses (Benacerraf and McDevitt, 1972). The effect of these genes is transmitted as a dominant trait, which excludes the possibility that they code for antigens which affect immune responses by clonal deletion in foetal life. Ir genes are linked to the genes controlling synthesis of the major histocompatibility antigens. It has been postulated that the Ir gene product is the receptor for antigen on the T-lymphocytes. If the T-cell receptor were variable region in nature (Marchalonis, 1975) then Ir genes could be V-genes presumably forming a linkage group distinct from the established kappa, lambda and heavy chain groups, but possibly combining with V-genes from one of these groups to code for the two chains forming the complete receptor. The linkage of a group of V-genes with the major histocompatibility genes could possibly be a device for avoiding auto-immune reactions, as will be discussed in the next section. This would explain the association of certain histocompatibility types with certain diseases of probable auto-immune nature (McDevitt and Bodmer, 1974).

Tolerance Mechanisms

Antigen–Antibody Gene Linkage?

As mothers and fathers have histocompatibility antigens which can provoke immune reactions in each other, normal immunological tolerance does not at first sight seem to be explicable on the basis of inheritance of sets of antigens and antibodies which are non-reactive with each other. However, since we know that the specificity of an immunological clone is determined by two separate V-genes and that the genes of the major histocompatibility loci are closely linked to the Ir genes, then if the latter are V-genes, as postulated above, antigen–antibody genetic linkage could exist, and could contribute to defence against auto-immunity in various ways. For example, each histocompatibility gene might be linked to an Ir gene which combines with a universal V-gene on another translocon (see p. 422) to code for specificity against an anti-idiotype antibody reactive with the product of the histocompatibility gene in question. Alternatively, Ir genes and histocompatibility genes could be arranged in compatible non-reactive pairs, a form of whole animal allelic exclusion (see p. 419) allowing only a paternal or a maternal pair at each double locus. With such an arrangement F_1 animals of two inbred strains would lack some of the parental antigens and would react against grafts from animals of the parental strains. This is generally thought not to occur, but some studies suggest the contrary (Lotzova and Cudkowicz, 1972), and the possibility of antigen–antibody gene linkage for defence against auto-immunity remains open.

Clonal Deletion in Foetal Life

In cattle, it is not uncommon for twins to share a single placenta and so to have a common vascular system during foetal life. Owen (1945) observed that in dizygotic twins, this enabled red cells of incompatible type to survive indefinitely in a host which would normally be expected to eliminate them by an immune response. On the basis of this finding, Burnet and Fenner (1949) developed the theory that during foetal life clones of immature immunocytes are deleted by contact with their specific antigen, instead of being stimulated as in post-natal life. This theory offered an explanation for the normal absence of immunological reaction against the host and appeared to receive strong confirmation when Billingham *et al.* (1953) demonstrated the induction of an artificial tolerance by injecting foetal mice with a mixture of spleen, kidney and testis cells from adult mice of a foreign strain. Some of the treated mice, on becoming adult, tolerated skin grafts from the foreign strain animals.

Studying this classical experiment in the light of the advances of the last twenty years, one wonders whether the animals which became tolerant did so because some of the injected foreign spleen cells developed into clones of immunocytes which protected the foreign tissue from attack by mounting cytotoxic or muffling immune reactions with idiotypic determinants on the host clones reactive with the foreign tissue. A similar reaction by host immunocytes against idiotypic determinants on graft clones may have protected the host from immunological attack by the graft. There is evidence that tetraparental mice, made by fusion of embryos of two histo-incompatible strains, have activated self-reactive clones, but that these are made harmless by "serum blocking factors" (Wegmann *et al.*, 1971). If the serum blocking factors were anti-idiotype antibodies, the absence of effective anti-idiotype clones in most instances would account for the extremely low incidence of success in attempts to make tetraparental animals between histoincompatible strains. In the light of this, the absence of self-reactivity in F_1 animals can hardly be ascribed to clonal deletion in foetal life. Some genetic mechanism, such as linkage between histocompatibility antigens and a group of V-genes, with whole animal allelic exclusion, is indicated.

Clonal Inhibition

It has been shown that immune paralysis can be induced in adult animals by prolonged treatment with both very high and very low dosage of antigen (Mitchison, 1968). As the effect is often only partial, producing a submaximal immune response, it might be better if the term "tolerance" were not used for this phenomenon, to prevent confusion with natural, absolute tolerance (e.g. the inability of nonthyrotoxic people to make thyroid-stimulating auto-antibodies) which is probably based on an absence of the specific clones.

Immune reactions against the idiotypic determinants of specific clones, as already mentioned, could play an important role in inhibition of certain immune responses.

Tolerance Mechanisms in Relationship to Auto-immunity

It is not possible to cure the inherited auto-immune diseases of laboratory animals by induction of immune paralysis. We have tried the high dose method in NZB × NZW mice, injecting renal homogenate containing both nucleoprotein and renal cellular antigens, with complete lack of success (Adams and Adams, 1972). Further studies are required, for success in inducing paralysis would have implications for therapy of human auto-immune conditions.

It has been postulated that inherited auto-immune disease is caused by a premature loss of suppressor T-cells which normally delete or inhibit the forbidden clones (Allison *et al.*, 1971). Impressive evidence favouring this theory came from studies in A/Jax mice, which develop auto-antibodies against nucleoproteins. Injection of thymus cells from syngeneic, young, pre-autoimmune animals caused a striking reduction in the auto-antibody titre (Teague and Friou, 1969), but as thymus cells are mostly nuclear material, antibody neutralization or immune paralysis could have occurred rather than a specific cellular effect. Experimental injection of nucleoprotein or dead thymus cells would settle this. Evidence against the suppressor T-cell theory is the failure of repeated thymus cell injections from syngeneic, young, pre-autoimmune animals to inhibit the auto-immunity of NZB and NZB × NZW mice (Croft, 1974). Genetic considerations provide further contrary evidence. The NZB × NZW hybrid mouse (see Chapter 11) has an auto-immune condition (lupus nephritis) absent from the inbred parents, yet would be expected to possess all the genes of the parental strains. Therefore, NZB × NZW mice should possess all T-cell reactivities of the parents, unless certain clones were deleted by early contact with specific antigen, and it is difficult to envisage how suppressor T-cells could provide a defence against auto-immunity if they were subject to deletion in this way. The genetic abnormality causing lupus nephritis in the NZB × NZW mice appears to be a positive one, the possession of something the parental strains lack. This favours the concept, discussed below, that the auto-immune disease is based on V-gene specificity.

It has been shown that normal people have circulating B-lymphocytes which bind thyroglobulin (Roberts *et al.*, 1973; Bankhurst *et al.*, 1973) from which it has been deduced that they are capable of mounting an immune response to thyroglobulin but fail to do so because of T-cell suppression or lack of T-cell cooperation. Nevertheless, the striking lack of immune response to thyroglobulin which normal people show when their thyroid glands are severely damaged by viral thyroiditis argues against the concept that thyroglobulin-reactive B-cells are present in normal people. To establish the significance of the "binding" reaction, it is necessary to demonstrate that the binding cells are indeed capable of mounting an immune response to thyroglobulin.

As inherited auto-immune disease is not present at birth and appears to arise by somatic mutation in immunocytes, it is quite possible that there is no defect of pre-natal tolerance mechanisms in people destined to develop auto-immunity. There may be no post-natal defence against forbidden clones. This point will be taken up again later.

Auto-immune Reactions

Distinction from Allergic Reactions

Auto-immunity is readily distinguishable from allergic reactions such as asthma, hayfever and eczema. In allergic reactions the antibody specificity is not directed against host antigens, the presence of foreign antigen is necessary, mediation by histamine-like agents is required and there is no irreparable damage to parenchymatous tissues. In auto-immune reactions the antibody specificity is directed against host antigens, the presence of foreign antigen is not obligatory and host tissue destruction occurs if the auto-antibodies are of a class capable of activating cytotoxic effector mechanisms such as the complement system and K-cells.

Altered Host Antigens

Virus infections, neoplasia and the occurrence of somatic mutations in structural genes all cause new or altered antigens to appear on the surface of cells, or on extracellular structures, inviting attack by the immune system. Such reactions play an integral role in what we regard as normal manifestations of virus infection and probably of ageing also.

Forbidden Clones

The fundamental characteristic of these is that they react with normal, unaltered host antigens. The reaction may or may not be pathogenic depending on the specificity (e.g. reaction with a hormone receptor site) and the class (e.g. complement-fixing) of the auto-antibodies. Forbidden clones occur as a genetically-determined abnormality, and become more common with advancing age.

THE RELATIONSHIP OF TISSUE DAMAGE AND INFECTION TO AUTO-IMMUNITY

When cells are infected by viruses, new antigens foreign to the host may appear on the surface of the cells. If the immune system of the host has clones responsive to the new antigens, which is usual, an immune attack will be mounted with eventual destruction of the infected cells. Thus, part of the cell destruction caused by a virus infection is mediated by reactions of the host immunity system to foreign antigens. In inherited auto-immune diseases, however, the situation is different.

The Fundamental Defect in Inherited Auto-immune Disease

The auto-antibodies of inherited auto-immune disease invariably react with the antigens of normal people, indicating that in these diseases the abnormality does not lie in altered antigens but in the capacity of the immune system to respond to certain unaltered host antigens.

The Effect of Thyroid Damage in Thyrotoxicosis

When auto-antibodies to thyroglobulin were discovered in thyroid disease, the anatomical isolation of this protein, inside the thyroid acini, gave rise to the idea that its auto-antigenicity is a consequence of its sequestration from the immunity system. This might prevent it from imposing tolerance by deletion of reactive clones of immature immunocytes during foetal life (Burnet, 1959). This idea was challenged by Irvine (1964), who observed that thyroid damage inflicted by ^{131}I treatment for thyrotoxicosis, causes an increase in the titre of pre-existing anti-thyroglobulin and thyroid cell auto-antibodies, as expected from the increased antigenic stimulation arising from the tissue damage. However, if one of these auto-antibodies was not present before the ^{131}I treatment, even repeated treatments sometimes failed to elicit its presence. From this Irvine concluded that some thyrotoxic people lack the capacity to respond to one or other of the auto-antigens. The abnormality in thyroid auto-immunity would thus be ability to respond to certain thyroid antigens, which Irvine described as an inherited defect of immunological tolerance. In support of this concept is the fact that thyroglobulin is not sequestered but is constantly present in blood and tissue fluid (Roitt and Torrigiani, 1967).

The Response in Viral Thyroiditis

Epidemics of viral thyroiditis are rare, but are readily detected as affected patients present with recently-developed goitres which have the unusual features of being painful and tender. In severe cases the patient is very ill with fever and tachycardia, and needle biopsy of the thyroid may produce only fluid with necrotic cell remnants. The release of thyroid hormones into the blood, due to the cellular damage, causes transient thyrotoxicosis and thyroglobulin may reach high levels in the blood and tissues.

Seeing such an epidemic in the 1960s, involving fourteen patients, I waited expectantly for the appearance of high titres of thyroid auto-antibodies, and my thinking was profoundly stimulated when none appeared. In Canada, Volpé *et al.* (1967) made a similar observation and furthermore noted that in patients who had pre-existing thyroid auto-immunity, this was increased by the viral infection.

These observations imply that the majority of people cannot mount an immunological response against their own thyroid antigens, no matter how great the antigenic stimulus. Certain abnormal individuals have the capacity to respond, and from the known genetic basis of thyroid auto-immune disease (Bartels, 1941) it is clear that the abnormality is inherited. In modern terms it can be stated that the fundamental defect in thyroid auto-immune disease is the genetically-determined possession of forbidden clones reactive with certain antigens. There is evidence that other inherited auto-immune diseases have a similar basis.

No Defect of Immunological Tolerance?

It does not necessarily follow that inherited auto-immune disease is based on a defect of immunological tolerance. Auto-immunity is not present at birth, but first appears some time later, suggesting that somatic mutation in what might be called "pre-forbidden clones" is an essential step. If this is so, it is unnecessary to postulate that people who develop auto-immune disease have a defect of tolerance mechanisms. There may be no mechanisms for maintaining tolerance in post-natal life. This is discussed further below.

Apparent Lack of Antigenicity of Intact Tissue

It is probable that all immunological clones (except possibly those reactive with histocompatibility antigens) remain in an inactive state until stimulated by specific antigen and the forbidden clones of auto-immune disease seem to be no exception. Furthermore, the stimulating effect of cell damage on auto-immunity implies either that auto-antigens on the surface of undamaged cells are not capable of stimulating the corresponding forbidden clones, or that the forbidden clones come into existence through antigenic stimulation of "pre-forbidden" clones, in accord with the concept of antigen-mediated diversity (Cunningham, 1974).

Irvine's (1964) evidence that radiation damage to the thyroid stimulates thyroid auto-immunity has been amply confirmed and there is also evidence that tissue damage inflicted by surgery, ischaemia and trauma provokes or aggravates auto-immunity of the heart and eye in predisposed people (Adams, 1969). As already mentioned, tissue damage inflicted by virus infection has a similar effect, but there is an additional mechanism by which microbial infection can provoke auto-immunity.

Stimulation of Forbidden Clones by Cross-reactive Microbial Antigens

Reactions between antigens and apparently unrelated antibodies, ascribable to chance, occur not infrequently, e.g. the Wasserman reaction performed with ox heart as antigen in place of *Treponema pallidum*, the Weil-Felix reaction, and the widespread occurrence of the Forssman antigen, similar to that occurring on sheep red blood cells. Such chance serological reactions are called "heterophile". Their occurrence indicates that similar antigens are widely distributed in the cells and tissues of different and unrelated species of animals and microorganisms. This means that an invading microorganism can be expected sometimes to have antigens in common with its host. Usually, when this happens, the host immune system does not react to the host antigen, eliminating the microorganism by reacting with their foreign antigens. However, if the host possesses a forbidden clone reactive with a host antigen present on the microorganism, the clones will be stimulated and auto-immunity will ensue.

Rheumatic Fever and Post-streptococcal Glomerulonephritis

Attacks of rheumatic fever often follow infection by group A β-haemolytic streptococci (see Chapter 16). The timing fits well with the concept that the infection triggers an auto-immune attack on the heart and this is supported by Kaplan's (1969) demonstration that immunoglobulin and complement are bound to heart muscle cells in cases of fatal rheumatic carditis. Kaplan has also demonstrated the nature of the triggering mechanism by showing that the human myocardium and group A β-haemolytic streptococci of some types have an antigen in common and that auto-antibodies to this antigen occur in patients with rheumatic fever.

It seems, therefore, that streptococcal antigens, cross-reactive with the human myocardium and heart valves, provoke an auto-immune attack in people predisposed to rheumatic fever. What is the nature of the predisposition? There is evidence that this has a genetic basis (Glynn and Holborow, 1961). I have suggested that the susceptibility lies in the possession of the requisite forbidden clones (Adams, 1969), which in turn could be due to the possession of the requisite V-genes and their development by somatic mutation.

Kaplan's work, combined with Burnet's theory provides an attractive, rational and detailed explanation of the pathogenesis of rheumatic fever. Furthermore, it suggests a possible method of prophylaxis for members of susceptible families, namely, immunization of infants with streptococcal vaccines before the forbidden clones have had time to develop, or, later, with streptococcal vaccines free of the cross-reactive antigens (Adams, 1969). This type of prophylaxis should be applicable to any auto-immune disease triggered by infection by a microorganism which possesses antigens cross-reactive with host antigens.

In contrast to rheumatic fever, glomerulonephritis follows infection by certain "nephritogenic" strains of streptococci only, especially group A, type 12. Clinically indistinguishable immune complex glomerulonephritis occurs in various other disorders and these conditions are discussed more fully in Chapter 17.

Other Diseases in which Infection Appears to Trigger Auto-immunity

It seems likely that disorders based on the activity of forbidden clones need an antigenic trigger provided by slight damage to the relevant tissue, as by infection with a virus. Infections with viruses are common and often sub-clinical, and almost all tissues in the body seem to be subject to at least minor attack.

Post-infective and Post-vaccinial Encephalomyelitis

Encephalomyelitis, frequently fatal, occurs very occasionally one to two weeks after the onset of smallpox, measles, rubella, mumps, varicella infections or after immunization against smallpox or rabies. The time of onset fits well with the concept that forbidden clones to neural tissue are triggered by the infection or by immunization and the low incidence, e.g. 0·1% following measles infection (Miller *et al.*, 1956), suggests that this highly detrimental disorder is due to germ line gene mutations which carry a heavy survival disadvantage and are thus seldom propagated. These mutations could be in the V-genes. The trigger mechanism might be trivial but antigenically effective damage to neural tissue, or the occurrence of cross-reactive antigens on the viruses. Encephalitis is extremely rare after measles immunization suggesting that the attenuated virus fails to cause neural damage or that it has lost antigens cross-reactive with neural antigens which occur on the wild-type virus. It would be of interest to look for such cross-reactive antigens.

Thyrotoxicosis

A mild epidemic of this disorder occurred in Denmark in 1941–1945 (Meulengracht, 1949). A possible mechanism was infection by a virus causing subclinical thyroid damage and so provoking thyrotoxicosis in people with latent thyroid-stimulating antibody clones. I have observed apparently non-random case presentation and exacerbation, which could be ascribed to a similar mechanism. In this as in other suspected auto-immune conditions onset during recovery from an infection suggests the infective triggering of forbidden clones (Adams, 1969).

THYROID AUTO-IMMUNE DISEASE

Thyrotoxicosis

Working in a region of endemic goitre, due to deficiency of iodine, H. S. Plummer (1928) discovered that there are two types of thyrotoxicosis. One, associated with nodules in the thyroid gland, tends to occur about ten years after development of a non-toxic goitre, is usually of only moderate severity and is not associated with eye signs. Histological signs of thyroid activity tend to be confined to the nodules. Plummer believed the condition to be due to an adenomatous change in thyroid tissue resulting in development of intrinsically active nodules. This view was confirmed by subsequent studies with radioactive iodine and recently by demonstration that blood thyrotrophin levels are below normal and that thyroid-stimulating antibodies do not occur in the condition (Adams *et al.*, 1975). Plummer's name for the condition, toxic adenoma, remains most appropriate.

The other type of thyrotoxicosis, by far the more common of the two in regions where iodine is not deficient, has been variously known as Graves' disease, von Basedow's disease or diffuse toxic goitre. The cause of the thyroid hyperactivity was for long a complete mystery. With the discovery of pituitary thyrotrophin, which stimulates the thyroid gland, the question arose whether the condition is due to excessive secretion of this hormone. Seeking an answer to this question, Purves and I developed a bioassay for thyrotrophin, based on measurement of thyroid hormone secretion in baby guinea-pigs.

Long-acting Thyroid Stimulator (LATS)

The bioassay involved injecting the guinea-pigs with ^{131}I iodide which was taken up by their thyroid glands, labelling the iodine-containing thyroid hormones, thyroxine and triiodothyronine. The animals were treated with non-radioactive thyroid hormone in dosage sufficient to suppress the secretion of thyrotrophin from the pituitary, this in turn causing cessation of thyroid secretion. After two days, the original radioactive iodide had been cleared from the blood leaving the animals with low levels of blood radioactivity but with large amounts of radioactivity in their thyroid glands in the form of labelled thyroid hormone. Injection of thyrotrophin caused secretion of labelled thyroid hormone into the blood where it increased the level of radioactivity. The increase in blood radioactivity following an injection of thyrotrophin proved to be a satisfactory index of the amount of thyrotrophin injected.

Preparations of thyrotrophin obtained from pituitary glands, or from the blood of patients with myxoedema, were found to produce a maximum increase in blood ^{131}I level about three hours after injection. In contrast, a serum sample from a thyrotoxic patient elicited a much more prolonged effect, with a maximum guinea-pig blood ^{131}I level about 16 hours after the injection (Fig. 1). The material responsible for this prolonged stimulation of the guinea-pig thyroid was eventually given the temporary, non-committal name of *long-acting thyroid stimulator* (LATS) (Adams, 1965) and its existence in a proportion of thyrotoxic patients was confirmed and understanding of its origin extended by McKenzie (1965) and Munro (1971). A particularly important contribution was McKenzie's assay which remains the key method.

The Chemical Nature of LATS

Fractionation of the proteins in LATS sera with 27% ethanol in the cold and with Sephadex G-200 showed that the activity was in the immunoglobulin fraction. Convincing evidence that LATS is an immunoglobulin molecule, and not some other compound associated with the immunoglobulins, was ob-

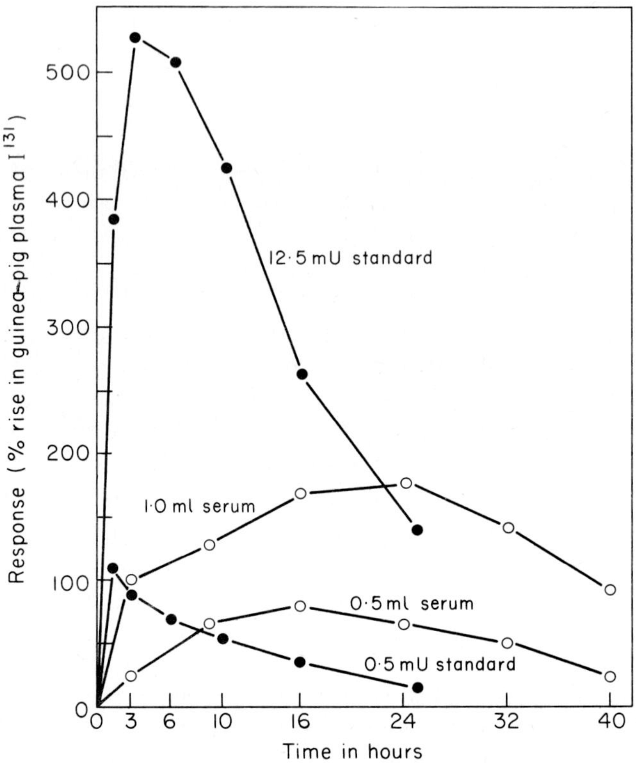

Fig. 1. The time course of the responses to two doses of thyrotrophin (U.S.P. Standard) and two doses of LATS (serum from a patient with thyrotoxicosis and exophthalmos), bioassayed in the guinea-pig. The prolonged nature of the LATS response is apparent. (From Adams, 1958 by kind permission of the Editor.)

tained by Smith *et al.* (1969) who split LATS-containing immunoglobulins into light and heavy polypeptide chains, with loss of thyroid-stimulating activity, then recombined the chains to recover the activity.

The Auto-antibody Nature of LATS

The immunoglobulin nature of LATS, together with its thyroid-stimulating action, establishes it as a thyroid-stimulating auto-antibody, as first claimed by Kriss *et al.* (1964) who demonstrated that LATS activity was reduced after incubation *in vitro* with thyroid gland homogenates. This was to be expected if the antigen to which LATS is directed is in thyroid tissue and the thyroid-stimulating property is a function of the molecule's paratope.

LATS as the Cause of Thyrotoxicosis

A causative role for LATS in thyrotoxicosis seemed highly probable after it was shown that blood thyrotrophin levels in untreated thyrotoxic people were below normal (Adams *et al.*, 1969). The negative feed-back action of the raised thyroid hormone levels in thyrotoxicosis would be expected to inhibit thyrotrophin secretion from the pituitary if an agent other than thyrotrophin itself were responsible for the thyroid overactivity. However, against a causative role for LATS were the anomalies that (a) many of the most severe cases of thyrotoxicosis did not show it, and (b) the levels of LATS in patients' blood did not correlate adequately with the degree of activity of the patients' thyroid glands (Chopra *et al.*, 1970).

LATS-Protector, Another Thyroid Auto-antibody

Following the demonstration that LATS activity could be neutralized by incubation *in vitro* with thyroid gland homogenates, we noticed that LATS sera from various patients showed variable resistance to neutralization with a thyroid gland preparation (Adams and Kennedy, 1967), and showed that this resistance is due to the presence of another immunoglobulin which competes with LATS for reaction with its receptor in the thyroid extract (Table 1). To demonstrate the reaction it is necessary to use minimal amounts of thyroid extract as an excess obscures the phenomenon by reacting completely with both immunoglobulins. The newly discovered immunoglobulin was given the temporary name LATS-protector, since it protects LATS from neutralization. It appeared to be a blocking antibody and occurred only in people with thyrotoxicosis, where its incidence, surprisingly, was found to be higher than that of LATS.

At this point a crucial contribution was made by Professor Deborah Doniach, who suggested that the LATS protector phenomenon might be based on species specificity. Noting that the thyroid extracts used in the studies were of human origin, she suggested that LATS protector was a specifically-human thyroid auto-antibody which did not cross-react with mouse thyroid. This was tested by using mouse thyroid extracts for neutralizing the LATS in the LATS protector reaction. The protector effect was

TABLE 1
The LATS-protector phenomenon

Materials assayed, dose/mouse made up to 500 μl with saline or euthyroid serum	No. of mice	Mean 17-hour response[a]
LATS serum W, 25μl in euthyroid serum	7	1677
		P↔0·001
LATS + human thyroid V, 25 μl in euthyroid serum	7	82
		P↔0·001
LATS + human thyroid + LATS-P serum B, 450 μl	7	692
LATS + LATS-P serum B, 450 μl	7	1402
LATS-P serum B, 450 μl	7	105
		n.s.
Euthyroid serum, 450 μl	7	74

Injection of LATS into prepared mice causes thyroid stimulation, manifest by an increase in the mouse blood radioiodine level. Prior incubation of the LATS with a human thyroid preparation causes loss of the thyroid-stimulating activity because the LATS has reacted with thyrotrophin receptors in the thyroid preparation. This neutralizing reaction is blocked if LATS-protector is added to the thyroid preparation before addition of the LATS. Thus, LATS-protector "protects" LATS from neutralization by thyroid preparations. LATS-protector does not block the action of LATS in the mouse and does not itself stimulate the mouse thyroid.

[a]The response is the percentage increase in the mouse blood ^{125}I level 17 hr after intravenous injection of the test material.

invariably absent, confirming Doniach's suggestion and opening up the possibly that, in man, LATS-protector is a thyroid stimulator (Adams and Kennedy, 1971).

Evidence that LATS-Protector Stimulates the Human Thyroid

A study of the incidence of LATS protector in fifty consecutive cases of diffuse toxic goitre (cases of toxic adenoma were excluded) is shown in Table 2. In 60% of the cases, LATS protector occurred alone and in a further 30% it

TABLE 2

The incidence of LATS and LATS-protector and their relationship to other features in 50 consecutive cases of untreated diffuse toxic goitre

	Patients showing:		
	LATS and LATS-P	LATS-P only	No LATS or LATS-P
Number of patients	15	30	5
Number with eye signs	10	11	1
Sex ratio, female : male	12:3	25:5	4:1
	Mean values and range		
Age in years	45 (20–65)	45 (19–72)	51 (40–70)
Thyroid ^{131}I uptake rate factor (k_1)	14·6 (3·0–25)	11·1 (1·8–36)	2·3 (0·7–3·7)
Thyroid size on scan, cm^2	23 (14–40)	22 (9–58)	34 (22–38)
Serum thyroxine, μg/100 ml	18·7 (11·6–23)	19·2 (10–26·6)	13·5 (11·2–17·6)
T_3 resin uptake, % standard	155 (100–192)	139 (93–197)	110 (105–113)
Free thyroxine index	29 (13–44)	27 (10–41)	15 (13–20)
LATS, % increase in mouse blood ^{125}I[a]	99·8 (24–407)	—	—
LATS-P, % protection[a]	all positive	32 (3·9–73)	—

[a]Lower values obtained by testing immunoglobulin concentrates and dividing result by concentration factor corrected for recovery (10 × 60% = 6).
From Adams *et al.* (1974a).

occurred together with LATS, making a total LATS-protector incidence of 90%. The five negative cases had only slight thyrotoxicosis, with an element of doubt in the diagnosis, as the dependable TRH (thyrotrophin-releasing hormone) test was not then available. The finding of LATS-protector in all but the mildest cases of thyrotoxicosis was in striking distinction to the findings with LATS and supported a causative role for LATS-protector. Further evidence was sought by testing whether there is a correlation between patients' LATS-protector levels and their thyroid gland activities as measured by thyroid ^{131}I uptake (Adams *et al.*, 1974a). The relationship is shown in Fig. 2.

Infusion of LATS Protector into Man

In four human volunteers a study was made of the effect of LATS-protector on thyroid activity (Adams *et al.*, 1974b). The subjects took a tracer dose of

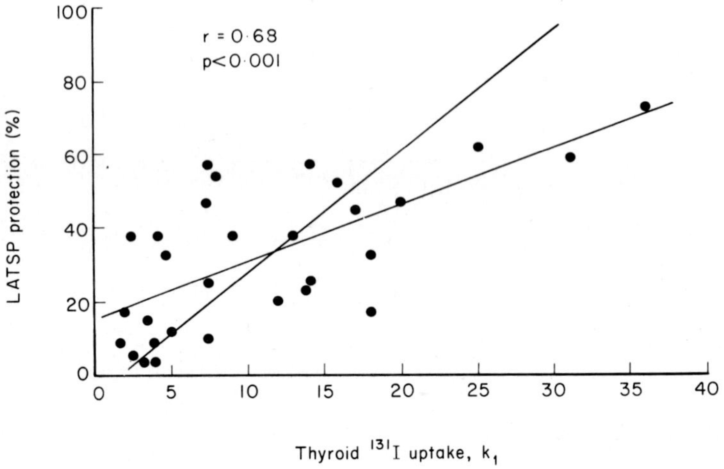

Fig. 2. The relationship between LATS-protector level and thyroid ^{131}I uptake in thirty patients with diffuse toxic goitre. There is a strong ($r = 0{\cdot}68$) and highly significant ($p < 0{\cdot}001$) correlation, despite the large error in the LATS-protector values, which were obtained by the division of one bioassay value by another. The existence of this correlation indicates that LATS-protector is the direct cause of the thyroid over-activity in auto-immune thyrotoxicosis. (From Adams *et al.*, 1974a, by kind permission of the Editor.)

^{125}I, followed by continuing treatment with thyroid hormone, and received infusions of plasma from thyrotoxic patients and control infusions from healthy people. The effects of thyroid secretion were monitored by measurements of blood ^{125}I levels, as in the McKenzie mouse bioassay. Plasma samples from three thyrotoxic patients, with high LATS-protector content but no demonstrable LATS, produced significant increases in the blood ^{125}I levels of the subjects, indicating that thyroid stimulation had occurred. Plasma samples from three normal people and one from a treated thyrotoxic patient with a low LATS-protector content had no effect. The result in one of the subjects is illustrated in Fig. 3. This study, providing direct evidence that LATS-protector has a stimulating action on the human thyroid, complements the indirect evidence that this auto-antibody is the cause of the thyroid hyperactivity occurring in auto-immune thyrotoxicosis.

Lack of Action of LATS in Man

It is possible to measure LATS and LATS-protector individually in a single serum sample. This was done in twenty untreated thyrotoxic patients who had both auto-antibodies and in whom thyroid activity had been measured by thyroid uptake of ^{131}I (Adams *et al.*, in press). In these patients the correlation between LATS-protector level and thyroid ^{131}I uptake was as close as that in thyrotoxic patients without LATS. If LATS had a thyroid-stimulating action in man, its presence in widely varying amounts would be expected to impair the correlation between LATS-protector and thyroid uptake. There was no correlation between thyroid uptake and the levels of LATS itself in these patients.

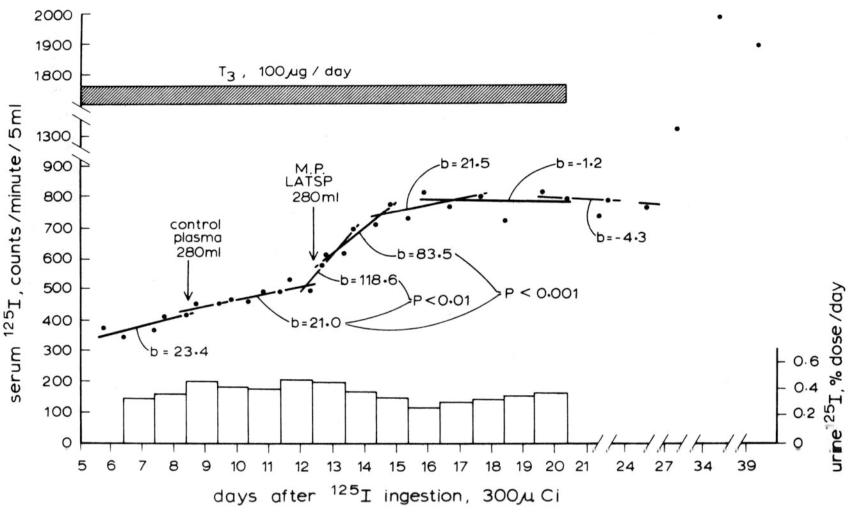

Fig. 3. The effect of infusing LATS-protector into a human volunteer. The serum ^{125}I level has risen significantly, indicating that thyroid stimulation has occurred with secretion of ^{125}I-labelled thyroid hormone into the blood. A control infusion of plasma from a normal person has had no effect. Taking the distribution space of infused immunoglobulin to be 5 litres, the LATS-protector level in the experimental subject would have been 1/18th of the level in the thyrotoxic patient who donated the LATS-protector plasma. (From Adams *et al.*, 1974b, by kind permission of the Editor.)

This indicates that LATS does not stimulate the human thyroid, and explains occasional anomalous observations where high LATS levels have been found in people without thyrotoxicosis. As LATS does not appear to occur in the absence of LATS-protector, the lack of activity of LATS is usually obscured. Very high levels of LATS probably have some effect in blocking the thyroid-stimulating action of LATS-protector.

Reaction of Thyroid-stimulation Antibodies with the Thyrotrophin Receptor

Although a neutralizing reaction between LATS and thyroid extracts incubated *in vitro* is readily demonstrable, it proved difficult to show a similar reaction with thyrotrophin. However, using highly purified thyrotrophin, labelled with ^{125}I, Manley *et al.* (1974a) and Mehdi and Nussey (1975) demonstrated binding to thyroid cell membrane protein and inhibition of binding by unlabelled thyrotrophin (Fig. 4). This reaction provides a hormone receptor assay for thyrotrophin.

LATS inhibits binding of labelled thyrotrophin (Fig. 5) indicating that it reacts with the thyroid cell receptor for thyrotrophin (Manley *et al.*, 1974b).

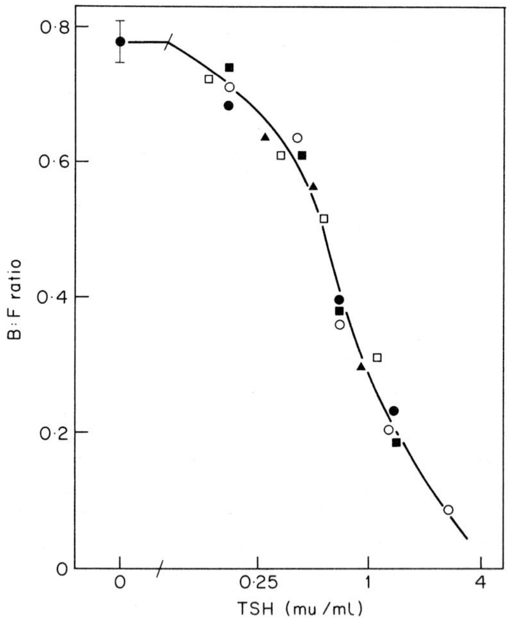

Fig. 4. The binding of highly-purified, ^{125}I-labelled thyrotrophin to thyroid cell receptors, *in vitro*, and its inhibition by unlabelled thyrotrophin (TSH). The effect is shown by the change in the ratio of bound to free (B : F) labelled thyrotrophin, which decreased progressively as the concentration of unlabelled thyrotrophin was increased. The reaction provides a hormone receptor assay for thyrotrophin. Similar effects were obtained with thyrotrophin preparations of widely varying purity (various symbols) indicating the specificity of the reaction and the lack of interference by other proteins. (From Manley *et al.*, 1974a, by kind permission of the Editor and Authors.)

This reaction explains the thyroid-stimulating action. Binding to the thyrotrophin receptor is believed to cause a molecular change to cascade through the molecule, producing a structural change at a distant site which becomes an active enzyme catalysing the conversion of adenosine triphosphate (ATP) to cyclic adenosine monophosphate (c-AMP), with activation of the cell.

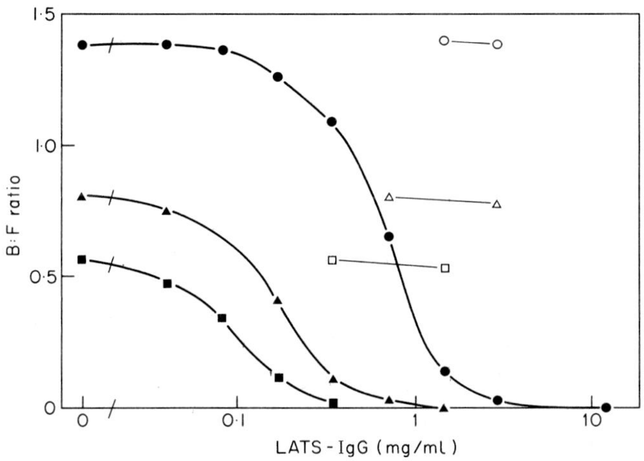

Fig. 5. Demonstration that LATS competes with thyrotrophin for reaction with the thyrotrophin receptor on the thyroid cell. The effect is shown by the change in the ratio of bound to free (B:F) ^{125}I-labelled thyrotrophin, which decreased progressively as the concentration of LATS immunoglobulin was increased (solid symbols). The reaction provides a hormone receptor assay for LATS. The three curves show the effect with varying concentrations of the receptor. Immunoglobulin from normal people had no effect (open symbols). (From Manley *et al.*, 1974b, by kind permission of the Editor and Authors.)

The species specificity differences between LATS and LATS-protector show that the human thyroid cell's thyrotrophin receptor is structurally different from that in mice, guinea-pigs and monkeys.

Smith and Hall (1974) have applied the receptor assay to clinical use, using human thyroid receptors. This assay would be expected to measure both LATS and LATS-protector, so the expected correlation with patients' thyroid activity would be lower than in the LATS-protector assay as performed in the mouse. In a first series of patients, thyrotrophin-displacing activity was found in the immunoglobulins of the great majority of a group of thyrotoxic patients (Fig. 6). This test may be expected to be developed for routine clinical use.

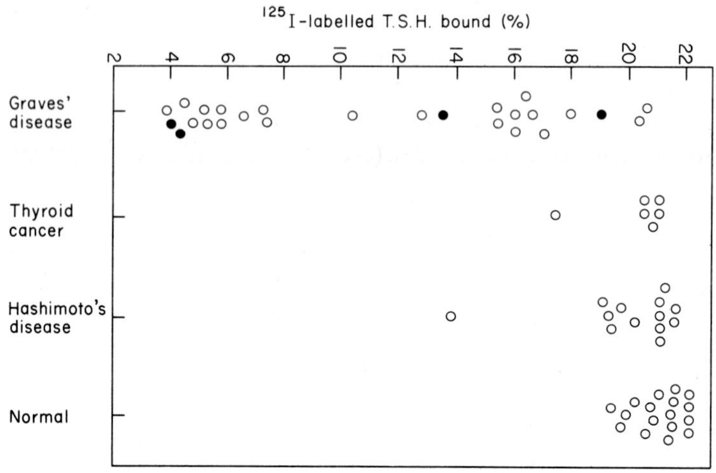

Fig. 6. Clinical application of a thyrotrophin receptor assay for thyroid-stimulating antibodies. The receptors are from human thyroid tissue and are therefore reactive with the human thyroid stimulator (HTS) as well as LATS (mouse thyroid stimulator, MTS). Activity was demonstrable in 88% of a group of patients with Graves' disease including both treated cases (open circles) and untreated cases (closed circles). One of 13 cases of Hashimoto's disease showed activity but there was none in a group of normal people. (From Smith and Hall, 1974, by kind permission of the Editor and Authors.)

Rationalization of Terminology of Thyroid-stimulating Antibodies

Table 3 summarizes the reactions of the thyroid-stimulating antibodies and shows the agreed new terminology Adams *et al.*, 1975). The term long-acting thyroid stimulator (LATS) is replaced by thyroid-stimulating antibody (TSAb); antibodies which have stimulatory activity in the McKenzie mouse bioassay are called mouse thyroid stimulator (MTS); and antibodies stimulating the human thyroid are called human thyroid stimulator (HTS). The dichotomy of the antibodies into HTS and MTS molecules seems very distinct, but it is possible that variants with partial or double reactivities occur. Antibodies reactive in the human receptor assay, which would include both HTS and MTS, could appropriately be designated human reactive (HR) TSAb.

Auto-immune Thyroiditis and Myxoedema

Witebsky and his group (1957) introduced the sensitive tanned red cell haemagglutination technique of Boyden for measuring antibodies to thyro-

TABLE 3

Properties and terminology of thyroid-stimulating antibodies

Old name	Reaction with				New name
	Mouse thyroid		Human thyroid		
	Binding	Stimulating	Binding	Stimulating	
LATS	+	+	+	−	Mouse thyroid stimulator (MTS)
	Neutralized by mouse thyroid extract	Active in mouse bioassay	Neutralized by human thyroid extract	Not active in man	
LATS-protector	−	−	+	+	Human thyroid stimulator (HTS)
	No neutralization with mouse thyroid extract	Not active in mouse bioassay	Neutralized by human thyroid extract, "protecting" LATS	Causes thyrotoxicosis	

From Adams *et al.* (in press).

globulin. This revealed that anti-thyroglobulin was present not only in patients with Hashimoto's thyroiditis and myxoedema, but also in a large proportion of patients with thyrotoxicosis and in a few percent of normal people. This finding caused general disappointment because it was not compatible with a causal role for anti-thyroglobulin in thyroiditis and its presumed end result, myxoedema. Recent work has provided further evidence that anti-thyroglobulin is a non-pathogenic auto-antibody. Plasma thyrotrophin levels can rise several hundred fold above normal, if necessary, to increase thyroid activity to protect the host from hypothyroidism. Because of this protective mechanism goitre (thyroid enlargement) is common and hypothyroidism is rare. Minor reductions in thyroid efficiency are compensated for unobtrusively by a slight rise in plasma thyrotrophin level. It follows that a normal plasma thyrotrophin level is a very sensitive index of a healthy thyroid gland. As to the biological effect of anti-thyroglobulin, a group of people having this auto-antibody alone were found to have a normal level of plasma thyrotrophin (Evered *et al.*, 1974). This suggests that anti-thyroglobulin does not damage the thyroid gland.

Mechanisms of Thyroid Damage

Trotter *et al.* (1957) found that many patients with thyroid disease and occasional normal people have complement-fixing auto-antibodies against thyroid gland tissue. These are quite distinct from anti-thyroglobulin, since they react with the microsomal fraction of thyroid cells (Roitt and Doniach, 1960). Microsomal fractions contain the cell membranes, including the surface membranes and their protein molecules, so these were auto-antibodies reacting with antigens which might be expected to have surface expression on thyroid cells. The anti-microsomal antibodies are demonstrable by immunofluorescence (Holborow *et al.*, 1959). As these auto-antibodies activate the powerful cytolytic complement system, they are a likely cause of thyroid cell damage and Buchanan *et al.* (1962) have shown that their presence correlates well with histological evidence of thyroiditis. In a relatively small series of patients with thyroid auto-antibodies, Evered *et al.* (1974) found that high serum TSH levels, indicative of reduced thyroid efficiency, were invariably associated with the presence of antimicrosomal auto-antibodies. Thyroid cells with auto-antibody on their surface are also likely to become targets for the killer (K) mononuclear cells discovered by Perlmann *et al.* (1972). T-lymphocytes, of the same specificity as the auto-antibodies, may also have a cytotoxic action against thyroid cells.

There are thus several mechanisms mediating cell damage in auto-immune thyroiditis, and in each the abnormal specificity may be generated by a forbidden clone reactive with thyroid cell surface epitopes.

Exophthalmos

Patients with auto-immune thyrotoxicosis quite frequently show changes in the orbit which are given the generic name of exophthalmos. Occasional patients without thyrotoxicosis also show exophthalmos, but these patients frequently (and possibly always) have some degree of auto-immune thyroiditis which can compensate for the action of low levels of HTS by reducing thyroid efficiency. If it could be demonstrated that exophthalmos may occur in the absence of HTS and thyroiditis it would be of significance in indicating that an independent forbidden clone, as opposed to an HTS mutant, is responsible.

The features of exophthalmos can be divided into four groups, as follows.

i. *Retraction of the upper eyelids.* This causes stare and lid lag and is apparently due to the overactivity of the sympathetic nervous system which is such a feature of thyrotoxicosis. It usually disappears as the patient is made euthyroid by treatment, indicating that it is mediated by the high thyroid hormone levels.

ii. *Conjunctival inflammation.* This includes a sense of "grittiness", epiphora, distension of the vessels (injection) and chemosis (conjunctival oedema). The exact cause is not known, but chemosis in particular responds well to treatment with adrenal steroids in low dosage.

iii. *Proptosis and peri-globular swelling.* Rundle (1964), measured orbital contents at post-mortem in exophthalmic patients and controls, and found that the former had an increased amount of fat in the orbit. Sometimes this seems to be entirely behind the globe, pushing it forwards, in other patients the fat seems to protrude around the globe causing fullness in the upper and lower eyelids with little protrusion of the globe. As fat cells possess a receptor for thyrotrophin, it is tempting to think that an HTS somatic mutant is responsible for the increase in bulk of the fatty tissue. Severe cases of proptosis occurring in the absence of MTS indicate that MTS itself is not the causative agent. Mahieu and Winand (1972) have evidence for the existence of orbital-reacting clones in patients with exophthalmos.

iv. *Myopathy of the extra-ocular muscles.* This causes strabismus in some patients, so-called ophthalmoplegia. Many patients with severe proptosis lack ophthalmoplegia, which might mean that it is caused by separate forbidden clones which affect the muscles specifically. The suggestion that the muscle damage is mediated by thyroglobulin/anti-thyroglobulin immune complexes (Konishi *et al.*, 1974) requires, for confirmation, the consistent demonstration of anti-thyroglobulin complexes in patients with ophthalmoplegia.

The production of exophthalmos in fish by injections of pituitary extracts may have no relationship to human exophthalmos. Fish kept in fresh water battle against the tendency of their osmotic pressure to draw in water and produce oedema, which causes protrusion of their eyes. It would be salutary if "exophthalmos-producing substance (EPS)" assayed in fish were renamed "fish oedema producing substance".

Exophthalmos in occasional patients with Cushing's syndrome seems likely to be due to the same or similar forbidden clones as those which cause exophthalmos in thyrotoxicosis. However, the spectacular potency of Cushing's serum in producing fish exophthalmos (Der Kinderen, 1967) is more likely to be due to a salt-retaining action of adrenal steroids.

Pre-tibial Myxoedema

Also called thyrotoxic dermopathy, this is a lumpy, subcutaneous thickening which occurs over the shins of some patients with exophthalmos. In severe cases it may involve most of the lower leg, ankle and foot. The condition can be well controlled by topical application of adrenal steroids. It seems likely that is is caused by forbidden clones which are similar to, or identical with, those that cause increase in bulk of the orbital contents.

Neonatal Thyrotoxicosis

Babies of mothers suffering from thyrotoxicosis sometimes show a transient form of thyrotoxicosis which disappears in a few weeks, if the baby survives. Where the mother shows MTS, auto-antibody is demonstrable in the affected baby (McKenzie, 1964) and similar findings have been made with HTS, (Munro, personal communication). The phenomenon is due to the transfer of maternal IgG across the placenta. Transplacental thyroid damage has not been observed, which implies that auto-immune tissue injury requires the presence of cells of forbidden clones.

Forbidden Clones in Thyroid Auto-immune Disease

In the present state of knowledge, Burnet's hypothesis that auto-immune disease is caused by the occurrence of forbidden clones of immunocytes reactive with host epitopes provides the only rational explanation of the variety of phenomena seen in thyroid auto-immune disease. Four main types of clone appear to occur, namely,

i. thyroid-stimulating, producing HTS and MTS;
ii. thyroid-damaging, e.g. those producing complement-fixing anti-microsomal thyroid auto-antibodies;
iii. exophthalmos-producing. Not yet established, possibly somatic mutants of TSAb.
iv. non-pathogenic, e.g. clones producing anti-thyroglobulin.

The specificities of the first three types of clone may be related, since they all react with epitopes on the surface of thyroid cells or cells which may have similarities, i.e. orbital fat cells with a receptor for thyrotrophin. Whether or not anti-thyroglobulin has any similarity of specificity with the other three types of forbidden clone is a question of great interest; is there one V-gene in common?

Evidence that Mouse Thyroid Stimulator (MTS) is a Somatic Mutant of Human Thyroid Stimulator (HTS)

Amongst the thyroid auto-antibodies, the two thyroid stimulators are alone in showing a relationship to each other. The mouse thyroid stimulator (MTS) does not seem to occur in the absence of the human thyroid stimulator (HTS), but the latter commonly occurs in the absence of MTS. This suggests that MTS is a somatic mutant of HTS. Only HTS causes stimulation of the human thyroid cell, but both auto-antibodies react with the thyrotrophin receptor, which suggests that the paratopes are quite similar, but that the fit between MTS and the receptor is not quite good enough to trigger the molecular cascade needed to change the adenyl cyclase site into its active configuration. The difference between HTS and MTS could be the result of a single point somatic mutation in one of the V-genes, presumably an alteration of a base in a sequence coding for one of the hypervariable regions which form the paratope.

Remission and Relapse in Auto-immune Thyrotoxicosis

When thyrotoxic patients are treated with anti-thyroid drugs, and after a year or so the treatment is stopped, about half the patients remain well for a variable period, a phenomenon known as remission. Presumably the HTS has fallen to a subpathogenic level, but this has not yet been demonstrated. Frequently the thyrotoxicosis subsequently recurs, the so-called relapse.

From current knowledge it seems likely that the HTS clone remains latent until it is stimulated, perhaps by thyroid cell damage, e.g. from a minor virus infection which might be subclinical. Thyrotrophin receptor from the damaged thyroid cell presumably provides the antigenic stimulus which re-activates the HTS clone. It may be necessary for the receptor particle to pass via a lymphatic and be taken to a lymph node. If, in addition to the thyroid-stimulating clone, a thyroid-damaging clone is present, the process could become self-perpetuating and then remission would not occur. If, however, no thyroid-damaging clones are present, then once the thyroid damage by virus ceases, HTS production would decline, giving a remission. If this concept is correct it should be possible to demonstrate a dissociation between the presence of thyroid microsomal antibody and the occurrence of remission.

AUTO-IMMUNE DISEASE OF THE OTHER ENDOCRINE GLANDS AND THE STOMACH

There is evidence indicating that the other endocrine glands and the gastric mucosa are affected by disorders which are based on auto-immunity (Doniach, 1975) (Table 4). Furthermore, these conditions show a genetic association. Gastric auto-immunity is described in detail in Chapter 18; here it is considered in the light of its similarities to thyroid auto-immunity and its association with auto-immunity in the endocrine glands.

Gastric Auto-immunity

Embryologically, the thyroid is derived from the fore gut, and cells of the gastric mucosa are similar to thyroid cells in having the capacity to concentrate iodide. The parietal cells in the mucosa lining the body and fundus of the stomach secrete the intrinsic factor which combines with vitamin B_{12} (the extrinsic factor) to allow its absorption from the small gut and so to constitute

TABLE 4

The variety of auto-antibodies so far discovered in auto-immune diseases of the endocrine glands and the gastric mucosa

Organ	Auto-antibodies against				
	Cells (microsomes)			Secretory product (protein)	
	Detected by Immunofluro-escence	Destructive, complement-fixing	Stimulating, e.g. v. THS receptor	Complement-fixing	
				No	Yes
Thyroid	+	+	TSAb: HTS MTS	Thyroglobulin	
Gastric mucosa parietal cells	+	+		Intrinsic factor	
Adrenal cortex	+	+	?		
Parathyroid	+	+	?		
Pancreatic islets	+	+	β cell-stimulating		Insulin
Testes, Leydig cells	+	+			
Ovaries, granulosa cells	+	+			
Anterior pituitary	+		?		

The question marks indicate the possibility that certain other auto-antibodies exist.

the haemopoietic factor recognized by W. B. Castle as necessary for the normal maturation of erythrocytes.

In pernicious anaemia there is insufficient intrinsic factor for adequate B_{12} absorption. The commonest cause of this condition appears to be an auto-immune attack on the gastric mucosa which shows atrophy of the epithelial cells and infiltration with lymphocytes and plasma cells. There is reduced or absent acid formation and the stomach condition is appropriately known as chronic atrophic gastritis.

The first gastric auto-antibodies found were discovered by Taylor (1959) and independently by Schwartz (1960) in the sera of patients with pernicious anaemia. These antibodies were directed against the intrinsic factor, blocking its combination with B_{12}. It now appears that there is also a second type of anti-intrinsic factor auto-antibody, reacting with a different part of the molecule (Roitt *et al.*, 1965). Neither of these auto-antibodies is complement-fixing.

Auto-antibodies against the gastric parietal cells also occur (Irvine *et al.*, 1962; Markson and Moore, 1962). They are found in pernicious anaemia and in atrophic gastritis, they fix complement and react with a microsomal component of the parietal cell (Taylor *et al.*, 1962). They may well play a pathogenetic role in the epithelial cell destruction of atrophic gastritis.

The genetic association between gastric and thyroid auto-immunity is shown by a significantly high coincidence of auto-immune disease of the two organs (Tudhope and Wilson, 1960) and by a significantly high occurrence of thyroid auto-antibodies in patients with gastric auto-immune disease and vice versa. However, the anti-thyroid and anti-gastric auto-antibodies are immunologically entirely distinct, showing no cross-reaction. A possible explanation for the association is offered below.

There is a striking similarity between thyroid and gastric auto-immunity in that the anti-cellular auto-antibodies of both organs are complement-fixing and directed against a microsomal component of the cells which probably has surface expression; in both instances there are also auto-antibodies against the secretory products of the cells, thyroglobulin and intrinsic factor. Furthermore, neither of these anti-secretory product auto-antibodies are complement-fixing (Table 4).

Adrenal Auto-immunity

Hot on the heels of the discovery of thyroid auto-immunity came the finding of complement-fixing auto-antibodies against cells of the adrenal cortex in patients with idiopathic Addison's disease (Anderson *et al.*, 1957). The indirect immunofluorescence technique revealed that about 60% of patients with Addison's disease show auto-antibodies against adrenal tissue. Most commonly these are specific for adrenal only but occasional patients show additional auto-antibodies which also react with other steroid-producing cells, namely the granulosa cells of the ovary, the Leydig cells of the testis and trophoblast cells of the placenta (Anderson *et al.*, 1968; Doniach, 1975).

The analogy with auto-immune destructive disease of the thyroid and stomach is close; the adrenal histology shows loss of parenchymal cells and infiltration with lymphocytes and plasma cells. Again the auto-antibodies react with a microsomal component. It is highly probable that idiopathic Addison's disease is caused by an auto-immune adrenalitis.

Cushing's syndrome, when due to bilateral adrenal hyperplasia, is at present believed to be invariably mediated by excessive secretion of corticotrophin from the pituitary. However, raised levels of this hormone are not demonstrable in all cases and destructive irradiation of the pituitary with radioactive yttrium is unsuccessful in about a third of the cases. It seems possible that an adrenal-stimulating auto-antibody, analogous to the thyroid-stimulating auto-antibodies may occur in some cases. A recent finding is the existence of auto-antibodies against pituitary cells, which were found in a group of patients with auto-immune adrenalitis (Doniach, 1975), and raise the very interesting possibility that in Cushing's syndrome there may be auto-antibodies which cause hyperactivity of the adrenal cortex by stimulating the corticotrophic cells of the anterior pituitary.

Auto-immune adrenalitis shows a strong association with thyroid and gastric auto-immunity, hypoparathyroidism and diabetes mellitus (Irvine, 1974).

Juvenile and Maturity-onset Diabetes

Diabetic patients can be divided into two groups according to age of onset and this corresponds roughly to a division based on whether or not the patient needs insulin treatment. This in turn suggests two separate pathogenic mechanisms, but there is evidence suggesting that at least the majority of the maturity-onset, non-insulin-dependent patients have a mild form of the condition which causes severe diabetes. Thus,

i. juvenile and maturity-onset probands show a heavy incidence of the alternative condition in their families (Pilgrim and Adams, unpublished);

ii. the treatments for maturity-onset diabetes, namely diet and oral hypoglycaemic agents, reduce the requirement for insulin or enhance its production;
iii. in both types of diabetes there is loss of the first peak of the biphasic rise in blood insulin level which normally follows intravenous glucose administration (Donnelly and Turtle, 1974).

When glucose is administered via the gut, the plasma insulin level rises much higher than when the intravenous route is used (McIntyre *et al.*, 1965), owing to the action of hormones from the gut mucosa (secretin, gastrin, pancreozymin) which stimulate insulin secretion. It has been suggested that in many persons with maturity-onset diabetes there is a loss of effectiveness of one or more of the gut hormones, perhaps due to failure of production following mucosal atrophy (Beavan *et al.*, 1974). Such atrophy could be based on auto-immune destruction as in pernicious anaemia, but it also seems possible that anti-beta cell membrane auto-antibodies could prevent the action of these hormones.

Evidence for a Possible Auto-immune Basis in Diabetes Mellitus

This is four-fold:

i. *Association with auto-immune disease.* Diabetes co-exists with thyroid, gastric and adrenal auto-immune disease significantly more often than expected. About 14% of patients with Addison's disease have diabetes, which is six times higher than in the general population. In addition, diabetic subjects show an increased incidence of thyroid, gastric and adrenal auto-antibodies.

ii. *Histology of the islets.* Many early cases of diabetes show insulitis, consisting of lymphocytic infiltration of the islets with cellular degeneration and sometimes fibrosis (Gepts, 1965). Recently, studying post-mortem material, Doniach (1974) found that cases of untreated juvenile diabetes showed a gross reduction in the number of islets and beta-cells, atrophic changes in surviving islets and increased interacinar fibrosis. Treated cases showed the same changes to a greater degree. Maturity onset cases also showed a reduction in the number of islets. In contrast to the histology seen in auto-immune thyroiditis and gastritis, diabetic islets seldom show plasma cells.

iii. *Occurrence of islet-cell auto-antibodies.* These were discovered by Bottazzo *et al.* (1974) in thirteen cases with destructive auto-immune disease of various endocrine organs, including ten cases with diabetes. The auto-antibodies were detected by the indirect fluorescence technique and are complement-fixing. Similar auto-antibodies have been found in five cases of diabetes with Addison's disease (MacCuish *et al.*, 1974). In striking contrast are the findings of Lendrum *et al.* (1975) who looked for anti-islet cell auto-antibodies, again using immunofluorescence in children with diabetes of recent origin. Of 105 diabetic children, 51 showed islet cell auto-antibodies and none had anti-adrenal auto-antibodies.

The finding of these anti-islet cell auto-antibodies is significant. Experience with thyroid and gastric auto-immunity teaches that a spectrum of related auto-antibodies exists and also that immunofluorescence has limited sensitivity. For example, it cannot detect the thyroid-stimulating auto-antibodies which cause thyrotoxicosis by reacting with the thyrotrophin receptor on the thyroid cell. Therefore, now that islet cell auto-antibodies have been demonstrated by an insensitive method, it becomes probable that a variety of auto-antibodies occurs in diabetes which may exert varying effects on the islet cells through reactions with their surface components. Such reactions could account for the apparent defects in diabetes in the beta cell receptors for glucose or hormones, postulated by Donelly and Turtle (1974).

The occurrence of transient neonatal hypoglycaemia, lasting a few weeks, in the babies of some diabetic mothers (Scott, 1966), analogous to neonatal thyrotoxicosis, was the first indication that beta cell-stimulating auto-antibodies may cross the placenta in the same way as thyroid-stimulating auto-antibodies. A further possible hint of such auto-antibodies is the occurrence of hypoglycaemia in some people who later become diabetic.

iv. *Auto-antibodies to insulin.* Recently evidence has been forthcoming for the existence of auto-antibodies against insulin (Hirata *et al.*, 1974).

High levels of insulin-precursor proteins in the urine of juvenile diabetics (Crossley and Elliott, 1973) may also be an indication of an islet-damaging process. The synalbumin insulin antagonist in the plasma of diabetics (Vallance-Owen and Lilley, 1961) might conceivably be a product of beta-cell damage with sufficient resemblance to insulin to exert a blocking action.

The Role of Virus Infection

A lack of clustering of cases and the variable course of diabetes mellitus favours an auto-immune basis rather than a simple virus infection of the islets, but as in other auto-immune conditions, cellular damage caused by virus infection might well initiate diabetes in subjects with genetic predisposition (i.e. possessing the requisite forbidden clones). A triggering effect of this sort could account for the observed seasonal variation in diabetes mellitus and the increased incidence of antibodies against Coxsackie B viruses in diabetes of recent origin (Gamble and Taylor, 1973). However, it remains quite possible that direct islet cell destruction by virus infection, without auto-immunity, may also cause diabetes. At present, with only sketchy evidence available, it is obviously desirable to keep all possibilities open, including viral destruction of the islets, islet failure due to inherited error of protein structure and islet failure due to auto-immune attack.

Parathyroid Auto-immunity

Blizzard (1969) discovered that many patients with idiopathic hypoparathyroidism have auto-antibodies against parathyroid cells. He found them in 38% of 74 patients with idiopathic hypoparathyroidism compared with 6% of control subjects. At least some of these auto-antibodies were complement-fixing. In the 74 cases, the incidence of Addison's disease was remarkably high at 24% and the incidence of thyroid disease and pernicious anaemia was also raised. Furthermore, in the patients without overt thyroid or gastric auto-immunity, the incidence of thyroid and gastric auto-antibodies was high at 15% and 12% respectively. There is thus good evidence that idiopathic hypoparathyroidism is based on auto-immunity and that the condition is genetically associated with adrenal, thyroid and gastric auto-immunity.

Hyperparathyroidism, which causes calcium and phosphate to be removed from the bones and deposited in the kidneys, (osteitis fibrosa cystica) is sometimes caused by a parathyroid gland tumour but in other cases there is diffuse hypertrophy of all four glands. The cause is unknown. Unlike the thyroid, the parathyroid has no known trophic hormone. However, as auto-antibodies against parathyroid cells are known to occur, it is possible that idiopathic hyperparathyroidism is caused by a parathyroid-stimulating auto-antibody.

Gonadal Auto-immunity

Auto-antibodies against ovarian cells have been demonstrated in Addison's disease (Anderson *et al.*, 1968) and in this condition 20% of young women show hypogonadism with ovarian fibrosis (Doniach, 1975). It is therefore possible that auto-immune destruction of the ovaries occurs, although not yet well established. I have seen hypogonadism, with enlarged ovaries in a mother and daughter, which perhaps suggests auto-immunity rather than enzyme deficiency, since the latter is always a recessive condition. Auto-antibodies to the Leydig cells of the testis have been demonstrated in Addison's disease (Doniach, 1975).

In man, post-mumps orchitis may be an auto-immune disorder, as it occurs at the time of expected full immune response to the virus, and the virus is not demonstrable in the affected testes. The incidence is higher in men (20% of mumps cases) than in boys (1·5%). This difference in incidence has been ascribed to an effect of sexual maturation, but an alternative explanation is provided by the forbidden clone concept. As forbidden clones arise by somatic mutation in post-natal life, their incidence increases with age, and so forbidden clones reactive with testicular antigens would occur more commonly in men than in boys. The link with parotitis could be the occurrence of a cross-reactive tissue-specific antigen in the two glands, so that an antigenic stimulus from the damaged parotid activates a latent anti-testicular forbidden clone, if it is present. Alternatively, the mumps virus may carry a testicular antigen. Search for such cross-reactive antigens is indicated.

In a small minority of infertile men auto-antibodies against sperm exist and appear to cause the infertility (Rumke, 1969).

Pituitary Auto-immunity

Histological evidence of auto-immunity affecting the adenohypophysis was first reported by Goudie and Pinkerton (1962). In a second case, a woman who died after a hypopituitary coma, there was co-existent pernicious anaemia, hypoadrenocorticism and hypothyroidism (Hume and Roberts, 1967). At post-mortem examination the gastric mucosa, adrenals and thyroid all showed atrophy of the parenchyma. The thyroid and gastric mucosa showed lymphocytic infiltration indicative of auto-immune thyroiditis and auto-immune gastritis. The pars anterior of the pituitary was atrophied to one-quarter of normal size and showed loss of parenchyma, fibrosis, heavy lymphocytic infiltration, occasional plasma cells and no giant cells. Recently Bottazzo *et al.* (1975) have demonstrated the existence of auto-antibodies against prolactin-secreting anterior pituitary cells.

The discovery of pituitary auto-immunity promises advances in understanding of acromegaly and Cushing's syndrome as well as mono-hormonal pituitary failure and idiopathic general hypopituitarism. The presence of gastric and thyroid auto-immunity in Hume and Roberts' case above suggests that pituitary auto-immunity is genetically associated with the organ-specific disorders already discussed.

DIAGNOSIS AND TREATMENT

Current diagnostic methods and therapeutic practice for the disorders discussed above are outlined in Table 5. It is noteworthy that current treatments are almost entirely based on endocrinology. If a general method for selective destruction or inhibition of forbidden clones could be developed, prevention of tissue destruction or stimulation would become possible, making therapy much more effective.

ANIMAL MODELS OF AUTO-IMMUNE DISEASE

Ehrlich found that it was not possible to produce an auto-immune reaction by actively immunizing an ordinary laboratory animal against its own tissues, a finding which explains why auto-immune disease is not universal. However, by immunizing an animal (e.g. a duck) with a tissue extract from another species (e.g. a rabbit) and injecting the antiserum into the tissue donor (the rabbit), early investigators found that the immune system had the power to cause severe lesions, such as lysis of erythrocytes and destruction of the renal glomeruli (Masugi, 1934), if antibodies of the requisite specificity were present.

Freund's Adjuvant Auto-immunity

With the introduction by Freund of adjuvants to antigenicity (consisting of oil and dead mycobacteria) the situation changed (Freund *et al.*, 1953). When homologous tissue extracts were injected emulsified in Freund's adjuvants, a proportion of laboratory animals mounted a transient immune attack against the relevant tissue, e.g. testis and brain. Witebsky *et al.* (1957) used the method to induce thyroiditis in rats. Since then, a transient auto-immune inflammation with auto-antibodies and tissue destruction has been induced in many organs by this method. In outbred animals only a proportion show the auto-immune response but some inbred strains show universal responsiveness and in a study with many different inbred strains of mice Vladutiu and Rose (1971) found that ability to develop thyroiditis is linked to histocompatibility type. It is therefore likely that genetic predisposition is involved. The association with histocompatibility suggests that the genetic predisposition lies in the immune response genes (Benacerraf and McDevitt, 1972) which as argued above, may be a set of V-genes.

Freund's adjuvants stimulate lymphocyte division and thus favour mutation, creating new clones. There are distinct limits to the induction of auto-immunity by the use of active immunization with tissue extracts in Freund's adjuvants. For example, the induction of thyroid-stimulating auto-antibodies comparable with those occurring in thyrotoxicosis, has not been demonstrated. Antibodies releasing ^{131}I from thyroid glands have been elicited but this is probably a simple cell-damaging action. Stimulating antibodies would increase thyroid ^{131}I uptake.

Spontaneously Occurring Auto-immune Disease in Animals

Certain animals suffer from spontaneous auto-immune disease with a genetic basis, and are thus good models for human auto-immune disease. The animals most extensively studied are NZB mice and obese chickens.

Obese Chickens

In a colony of white Leghorn fowls it was discovered that occasional animals developed spontaneous hypothyroidism, with small stature, obesity, defective feathers and reduced fertility (Wick *et al*., 1974). These changes can be corrected by treatment with thyroid hormone. The thyroid glands are reduced in size, and are infiltrated by lymphoid cells and plasma cells with loss of follicles and formation of germinal centres. The picture is closely analogous to that seen in human auto-immune thyroiditis. There are circulating auto-antibodies to thyroglobulin. Unlike human anti-thyroglobulin antibodies these are complement-fixing and no antibodies against thyroid cells have been demonstrated.

The occurrence of this auto-immune disease in fowls provided the opportunity to test the role of the bursa of Fabricius, a prime source of B-lymphocytes. It was found that surgical bursectomy on the day of hatching caused a marked reduction in the incidence and severity of the auto-immunity in 7-week-old animals of the obese strain. On the other hand, neonatal thymectomy had no retarding effect on the auto-immunity and may have enhanced it slightly. The development of adjuvant thyroiditis in ordinary chickens is impaired by prior thymectomy. This suggests that the obese chicken's forbidden clones develop in the bursa and that in ordinary chickens the

TABLE 5

Diagnosis and treatment of diseases of the endocrine glands and stomach which have an established or possible auto-immune basis

Disease	Main symptoms and signs	Diagnostic tests	Treatment
1. Thyrotoxicosis	Tiredness, nervousness, heat intolerance, weight loss, tachycardia, tremor, light periods, goitre	*Routine*: Blood T_4[a], T_3 resin uptake, T_3[a], TSAb.[1,2] Thyroid ^{131}I uptake 4 h, ^{99m}Tc scan *Doubtful case*: TRH test,[3] suppression with T_3 (4-hr thyroid ^{131}I uptake, T_3 100 μg/day for 7 days, count residual thyroid ^{131}I, repeat 4-hr ^{131}I uptake)	Carbimazole 10–80 mg/day or ^{131}I 3–25 m Ci or subtotal thyroidectomy
2. Exophthalmos	Proptosis, lid lag, conjunctival grittiness, epiphora, chemosis, diplopia	Ensure that there is adequate lid coverage of cornea. *Blood*: TSAb,[1,2] antithyroglobulin, antithyroid microsomes	Prednisone 5–20 mg/day. Best used early, in low dosage. Up to 5 mg b.d. is fairly safe for long periods. Tarsorrhaphy S.O.S. Avoid thyroid damage
3. Thyroiditis	Goitre, not tender	*Blood*: T_4[a], T_3 resin uptake, T_3[a], TSH[a], TSAb,[1,2] anti-thyroglobulin, anti-thyroid microsomes	Thyroxine 0·2–0·3 mg/day
4. Myxoedema	Tiredness, slowness, cold intolerance, weight gain, constipation, heavy periods, deep voice	*Routine*: Blood T_4[a], T_3 resin uptake, T_3[a], TSH, anti-thyroglobulin, anti-thyroid microsomes, cholesterol. E.C.G. Thyroid ^{131}I uptake, ^{99m}Tc scan *Doubtful case*: Therapeutic trial	Thyroxine 0·2–0·3 mg/day
5. Hypoparathyroidism (idiopathic)	Tetany, emotional lability, muscular weakness, numb phalanges, stridor, epilepsy, cataract, candidiasis, Trousseau's sign, Chvostek's sign	*Blood*: Ca, PO_4, CO_2, pH proteins, para-thormone[a], anti-parathyroid cell[b], E.C.G.	Calcium lactate 0·3 g × 16/day. Use calciferol also only if necessary (danger of nephrolithiasis) 25,000–100,000 v/day. Monitor by blood Ca level, aiming at 2·25 mmol/l

6. Hyperparathyroidism (hyperplasia)	Tiredness, polydipsia, polyuria, anorexia, nausea, constipation, hypotonicity, pathologic fracture	*Blood*: Ca, PO_4, CO_2, pH parathormone[a], anti-parathyroid cell[b]. E.C.G. X-ray: bones, kidneys. Slit lamp for band keratopathy	Surgery with frozen section biopsy, excision of 7/8 of all parathyroid tissue
7. Addison's disease (ncn-tubercular)	Tiredness, weight loss, anorexia, vomiting, hypotension, pigmentation	*Blood*: Na, K, Cl, CO_2, pH, cortisol, ATCH[a], anti-adrenal cell[b]. Synacthen test (I.M. ACTH, measure change in plasma cortisol in 30 minutes). X-ray: small heart	Cortisol 20 mg mane, 10 mg nocte. Fludrocortisone 0·1 mg/day. Increase dosage with infection or stress
8. Cushing's syndrome	Tiredness, central obesity, striae, muscle atrophy, hypertension, hirsutism, light periods	*Blood*: Na, K, Cl, CO_2, pH, differential white blood cell count. Glucose tolerance test. Plasma cortisol and ACTH[a] at 8·30 am and 4·30 pm for 3 days *Urine*: 17–OH corticosteroids, mg/g creatinine. 2 days control. 2 days on dexamethasone 5 μg/kg body weight aid (normal, <1 mg/g). 2 days on dexamethasone, 2 mg qid (no effect, adrenal tumour). *Urine*: 17-keto-steroids concurrently. X-ray sella turcica, IVP *S.O.S.*: Adrenal vein catheterization for left and right-sided plasma cortisols. Scan after giving radioactive cholesterol. Adrenal arteriograms. Computerized axial tomography of adrenals	1. Tumour of adrenal or pituitary; excision 2. Plasma ACTH measurable; 4,500r to pituitary, or 10,000r by cyclotron, or ^{90}Y implantation, or trans-sphenoidal partial or complete hypophysectomy using dissecting microscope 3. Plasma ACTH not measurable; total adrenalectomy and replacement therapy

continued

TABLE 5—continued

Disease	Main symptoms and signs	Diagnostic tests	Treatment
9. Diabetes Mellitus	Tiredness, weight loss, polyuria, polydipsia, polyphagia, skin infections, pruritus vulvae, coma	Glucose tolerance test. Blood insulin[a]. Check lens, retina, kidney function, nervous system, cardiovascular system	Diet (increase proportion of protein and fat and distribute calories throughout day in frequent small meals. Correct obesity) Sulfonylureas, Biguanides, Insulins
10. Panhypopituitarism in adults	Tiredness, anorexia, weight loss, hypotension, hypothermia, hypoglycaemia, loss of body hair, genital atrophy, amenorrhoea, diabetes insipidis, coma	Give insulin, TRH and GnRH simultaneously,[4] monitor blood glucose, T_4[a], T_3[a], cortisol, GH[a], TSH[a], LH[a], FSH[a]. Check optic fields, fundi. X-ray for sella size, pneumoencephalography, carotid angiography, SOS. Karyotype	Remove tumour SOS. T_4 0·05 mg initially, rising to 0·2–0·3 mg/day. Cortisone 5–15 mg b.d. Fludrocortisone 0·1 mg/day SOS. Women: oestradiol valerate 1 mg/day for 3 out of 4 weeks. Men: See "Testicular failure" below
11. Pituitary dwarfism	Small statue, reduced bone age	*Blood*: GH[a] before and 60 min after neutralized arginine hydrochloride 0·5 mg/kg body weight infused over 30 min. Exclude pituitary or suprasella tumour. Karyotype	Human growth hormone, 20–45 mg/month.[5]
12. Acromegaly	Headache, visual impairment, prognathism, soft tissue growth, enlarged sella, bone thickening	*Blood*: GH[a]. Check suppression 90 min after 75 g glucose orally. (GH is not always elevated, which could indicate the occurrence of autoantibodies with GH activity)	Remove tumour SOS. Partial or complete hypophysectomy with microdissection, or external irradiation of pituitary, or ^{90}Y implantation

13. Gigantism	Excessive height	As for acromegaly	As for acromegaly
14. Ovarian failure	Amenorrhoea, loss of secondary sexual characteristics, possible virilization from androgenic precursors of ovarian hormones	Maturation index of vaginal epithelium. Bioassay of urinary FSH. Blood LH[a] and FSH[a]. Exclude pituitary or ovarian tumour. Karyotype	Oestrogen–progesterone combination cyclically as with contraceptive pills. If not well tolerated use oestradiol valerate 2 mg b.d. plus medroxyprogesterone acetate 5 mg b.d. For best tolerance halve dosage in 1st week post-period
15. Testicular failure	Loss of drive, potency, libido, reduced secondary sexual characteristics	Karyotype, sperm count, urinary FSH (bioassay), blood LH[a] and FSH[a]. Testicular biopsy. Exclude pituitary tumour	Testosterone ester depot injections, e.g. "Sustanon 100", 1 ml. i.m./2 weeks, supplemented by testosterone 10 mg/day sublingually towards the end of the 2 weeks
16. Stomach autoimmunity Achlorhydria and pernicious anaemia	Indigestion, tiredness, possibly subacute combined degeneration with paresthesiae, ataxia, spastic weakness of legs, psychosis	Gastric analysis. Blood and marrow cell counts. Blood B_{12} level, antiparietal cell.[b] Check nervous system	Fruit juice with meals, 150 ml, for achlorhydria. For anaemia-hydroxocobalamin, 1,000 μg i.m. stat., replenish stores, then 1,000 μg i.m./2 months for maintenance

[a]Radioimmunoassay.
[b]Immunofluorescence sandwich technique.

thymus plays a role in providing the pre-forbidden clones required for adjuvant thyroiditis.

A colony of obese chickens has been obtained by selective breeding of the originally rare birds, but the mode of inheritance has not been determined. It would be of great interest to know whether it is compatible with the action of two dominant genes, as in human thyroid auto-immunity.

The NZB Mice and Their Hybrids

The general features of these mouse strains are described in the previous chapter.

A claim that the auto-immune haemolytic anaemia in NZB mice is caused by virus infection (Mellors and Huang, 1967) has not been confirmed and strong evidence against this concept is provided by the beneficial effect of treatment with ACTH and betamethazone (Howie, 1968), which would be expected to aggravate a virus infection. Treatment with cyclosphosphamide is very beneficial in the NZB/NZW mice (Russell and Hicks, 1968), presumably by inhibiting the development or activity of forbidden clones, but severe immunosuppression induced by gamma radiation (Adams and Adams, 1972) or azathioprine (Casey, 1968) causes a high incidence of malignant tumours, mostly lymphomas, suggesting that oncogence viruses are present. Such viruses, and the tumours they may induce, seem to have nothing to do with the auto-immunity (Adams and Adams, 1972).

To test the possibility that forbidden clones causing auto-immunity in NZB and NZB × NZW mice develop because of a loss of suppressor T-cells, NZB and NZB × NZW mice were given repeated injections of lymphoid cells including thymus cells from young, pre-autoimmune, syngeneic animals, but there was no beneficial effect (Croft, 1974).

The possibility that the forbidden clones develop as a result of unusual mutations permitted by a defective DNA repair enzyme system was tested by exposing NZB, NZB × NZW and outbred animals to continuous irradiation from radium at a low dosage equivalent to about 200 times the normal background (Croft *et al.*, 1975). The NZB × NZW mice showed no effect. The NZB and outbred mice died a little earlier than un-irradiated controls but there was no detectable effect on the auto-immunity, which could have been expected to show a spectacular acceleration if based on the absence of effective DNA repair.

The negative results of these experiments are compatible with the hypothesis that auto-immunity in the NZB and NZB × NZW mice is due to a positive, not a negative genetic effect, in accord with the predominantly dominant mode of inheritance. This is discussed further below.

THE NATURE OF THE GENETIC BASIS OF INHERITED AUTO-IMMUNE DISEASE; WHICH GENES?

The evidence that human and animal auto-immune diseases have a genetic basis leads to the question: which genes cause the disorder? Genes code for polypeptide chains and three general types are known, namely structural genes, regulator genes and DNA repair enzyme genes. All genes are codominant in that they code for their polypeptide chain regardless of the nature of their allele on the homologous chromosome, but characteristics (including diseases) determined by genes may be dominant or recessive. Conditions based on an enzyme deficiency are recessive because both alleles must be defective for the relevant polypeptide chain to be absent. On the other hand, antibody specifications would be inherited in dominant fashion as each allele of a pair of homologous V-genes will contribute its polypeptide chain to an antibody specificity, regardless of the nature of its homologous partner.

Understanding of genetic mechanisms is still incomplete. In trying to interpret genetic phenomena one needs to be conscious of the probable existence of undiscovered additional special devices. Two recently-discovered examples are X-chromosome exclusion and allelic exclusion.

X-chromosome exclusion. In each somatic cell of a female animal, only one of the two X-chromosomes is transcribed, the exclusion being random so that both chromosomes are equally expressed in the animal.

Allelic exclusion. In immunoglobulin-producing cells which are heterozygous for the structural genes for constant regions of heavy chains, each cell uses only one of these alleles, the choice being random, so that in the whole animal both alleles are expressed in co-dominant fashion. The phenomenon is known as allelic exclusion and appears to be part of the mechanism whereby a single immunocyte makes only a single type of antibody molecule.

As antibody specificity depends on two V-genes, one for a light chain and one for a heavy chain, the inheritance of antibody specificity will show features normally associated with recessiveness, such as a greater frequency in the sibs of a proband than in the parents.

The Mode of Inheritance of Thyroid Auto-immune Disease

For many years the pattern of inheritance of thyroid auto-immune disease has been puzzling. Bartels (1941), tentatively concluded that the mode of inheritance is recessive because of increased frequency in sisters of probands compared with mothers. However, he found instances where the condition occurred in three successive generations, a feature which had caused other investigators to conclude that the manner of inheritance is dominant with incomplete penetrance.

A hypothesis that the condition depends upon the presence of two co-dominant genes at separate loci would go far to explain the observed pattern, and would be consistent with the concept that the basis of thyroid auto-immunity lies in the V-genes. There is evidence that other auto-immune disorders have a similar pattern of inheritance.

Inheritance of Auto-immunity in the NZB Mouse and its Hybrids

Erythrocyte Auto-antibodies

Measuring auto-antibodies against red cells in F_1 and F_2 hybrids between NZB and NZC strains of mice, Bielschowsky and Bielschowsky (1964) concluded that the mode of inheritance was autosomal dominant although other studies have given less clear results (Ghaffar and Playfair, 1971). When NZB mice are mated with the C3H strain, there is a long delay in the appearance of erythrocyte auto-antibodies in the F_1 mice, and also an interesting difference between the sexes, the antibodies appearing about six months later in the males than the females (Holmes and Burnet, 1964). In NZB × NZW hybrids the females develop erythrocyte auto-antibodies about six months earlier than the males (Burnet and Holmes, 1965). These sex differences prompted Burnet to postulate that some of the genes involved must be on the X-chromosome.

The V-gene theory offers an explanation of these sex differences. On the assumption that one of the two V-genes contributing to the erythrocyte auto-antibodies of the NZB mice is not expressed in the hybrid, the late-appearing auto-antibody may result from the repeated somatic mutation of a clone in which the second V-gene has been contributed from the X-chromosome. As each cell in the female has two X-chromosomes compared to only one in the male, it seems possible that the female may have twice as many immunocytes as the male in clones coded for by a V-gene from an X-chromosome, so that with twice as many cells at risk, the necessary somatic mutations would occur sooner. A similar "gene dosage" effect expressed through the number of immunocytes at risk for somatic mutation could conceivably cause homo- or heterozygosity at expressed V-gene loci to influence the time of appearance of the forbidden clones. This would explain observations on back-cross animals (Holmes and Burnet, 1964), where one-quarter behave like homozygous animals of the parental strain and one-quarter like F_1 animals in accord with a two dominant gene hypothesis; the remaining half, which would be homozygous at one of the two loci, develop auto-antibodies rather sooner than the F_1 animals.

Lupus Nephritis

Braverman (1968) found that the renal disease of the New Zealand (NZ) mouse strains was transmitted independently of anti-nuclear and anti-erythrocyte auto-antibodies. This might be because the presence of additional cytotoxic clones is necessary to make nuclear material available for reaction with anti-nuclear auto-antibodies for development of immune complex glomerulonephritis.

The occurrence of auto-immune renal disease in hybrids of the NZB and NZW strains is a revealing genetic clue. As the parental strains lack the condition, its occurrence must depend on the action of at least two co-dominant genes at different loci. This would be expected if the genes concerned were immunoglobulin V-genes.

Another most significant genetic feature is that hybrids of NZB mice with a second inbred strain, the NZY mice, also show a high incidence of lethal lupus nephritis (Howie and Helyer, 1968). The NZY strain is derived from the same random-bred colony as the NZB and NZW strains. It is most unlikely that the same rare genetic mutation could have occurred in both the NZW and the NZY strains. More probably, in the parental, random-bred colony there exist V-genes which are capable of combining with an unusual V-gene in the NZB mice to form clones capable of mutating to the forbidden clones which cause the lupus nephritis.

The V-gene Theory of Inherited Auto-immune Disease

It is thus possible that the genetic basis of inherited auto-immune disease lies in the specificity of genes coding for the variable portions of immunoglobulin chains, the V-genes. The invariable absence of auto-immunity at birth suggests that in people destined to develop auto-immune disease, as in normal people, forbidden clones are successfully avoided (as for example by antigen/V-gene linkage) or deleted in foetal life. Auto-immune disease occurs because in post-natal life forbidden clones arise by a process of somatic mutation occurring in the V-genes. There is evidence that this process is largely restricted to the hypervariable regions and the probable explanation of the occurrence of the thyroid-stimulating auto-antibody, MTS, as a sequential mutant of HTS, indicates that certain base sequences in V-genes arise only as sequential variants of other sequences. It is postulated that the specificities determined by certain V-gene combinations can be transformed into autoreactivities by relatively few somatic mutations, whereas other specificities require a prohibitively large number. The operation of an undiscovered mechanism of differential DNA repair (e.g. excluding hyper-variable regions, including the remainder of V-regions) might preclude certain base sequences from arising by the mutation of other sequences.

Postulated Arrangements of V-genes on the Chromosomes to Explain Various Features of Human Auto-immune Disease

A V-gene marker has been discovered in rabbits but not so far in man, so the distribution of the V-genes on the human chromosomes is largely unknown. Gally and Edelman (1972) have coined the useful term, "translocon", for a linked set of V-genes and C-genes. A variety of evidence, including that obtained by study of markers for constant region genes and from analogy with rabbits and mice, indicates the existence of at least four translocons in man (H, κ, λ and Ir). There may be others.

The relative organ restriction and the genetic association of the various human "organ specific" auto-immune diseases, together with the high female to male sex incidence of thyroid auto-immune disease and the dissociation between anti-nuclear auto-immunity and thyro-gastric auto-immunity (Doniach *et al.*, 1963) might all be explained on the basis of arrangement of the relevant V-genes on the chromosomes. It is assumed that two V-genes on separate chromosomes are necessary for each clonal specificity and that each clone is capable of conversion to a forbidden clone by somatic mutations. If thyroid, gastric, adrenal, parathyroid and pancreatic islet auto-immunity were based on one common V-gene together with five separate V-genes, the organ specificity and genetic association would be explained. If the common V-gene had an alternative allele which contributed to the specificity of anti-nuclear factor (ANF) it would explain the observed dissociation between ANF and thyro-gastric auto-immunity. If one of the V-genes for thyroid auto-immunity were on the X-chromosome it would cause a 2:1 female sex preponderance. This is less than the observed value of 4·5:1, but could be a factor contributing to the sex ratio. The 9:1 female:male sex ratio for systemic lupus erythematosus is explained by postulating involvement of several V-genes on the X-chromosome, including one for ANF and one for the cytotoxic auto-antibody (Lies *et al.*, 1973) which would be expected to make nucleoprotein accessible to ANF, and so enable pathogenic immune complexes to form. The existence of a V-gene group on the X-chromosome has not yet been demonstrated, so explanations invoking this feature are speculative. However, Burnet has suggested that some of the genes affecting the inheritance of auto-immunity in mice are on the X-chromosome (Burnet and Holmes, 1965), and Burch and Powell's studies suggest three X-linked genes are implicated in systemic lupus erythaematosus.

Inherited Auto-immunity as Balanced Genetic Polymorphism

The inherited auto-immune diseases are surprisingly common for wholly deleterious conditions. This suggests that there may be some associated advantage. People heterozygous for the sickle cell gene have increased resistance to infection by the malaria parasite, which explains why sickle cell anaemia is unexpectedly common in people living in malaria-infested areas (Allison, 1954). This genetic effect is called balanced polymorphism. Environmental selection against a genetically-determined defect causing reduced reproduction is balanced by an associated reproductive advantage. The sickle cell gene is severely disadvantageous in the homozygous state, but in a malarial environment is advantageous in the heterozygote.

If balanced polymorphism is maintaining the incidence of inherited human auto-immune disease, the associated advantage is presumably related to the value of maximal diversity of immune response for defence against infection and neoplasia, with minimization of the immune reactive blanks necessary for avoidance of auto-immunity. More specifically, certain V-genes may be advantageous except in combinations which carry a high risk of the development of auto-immune disease. The incidence of infectious and malignant diseases in patients with auto-immune diseases and their families is therefore of interest.

SUMMARY

The immune system has evolved for protection of the host against microbial parasites and malignant tumours. In essence it consists of cell-destroying and toxin-removing effector systems together with a selector system (the antibody molecules) which (i) discriminates between invaders and host constituents and (ii) directs the effector systems towards invading cells or molecules so that they are eliminated. The basic cell of the selector system is the lymphocyte. Each lymphocyte makes antibody of only a single specificity and groups of lymphocytes making the same antibody are described as clones. About one million clones are necessary for adequate immune defence and it is believed that this great diversity arises partly through the existence of considerable numbers of V-genes coding for the amino acid sequences of the polypeptide chains forming antibody combining sites, and partly due to copying errors occurring during DNA replication in dividing lymphocytes, a phenomenon known as somatic mutation.

A growing number of common diseases are being recognized as resulting from failure of the selector function of the immune system, so that the effector mechanisms are mis-directed on to host tissues, or hormone receptor sites are inappropriately activated. The name given to a disorder of this type is auto-immune disease and that affecting the thyroid gland is understood in greatest detail.

Thyroid auto-immune disease is based on a genetic abnormality which permits the development of forbidden clones of lymphocytes. These react with certain host antigens on the thyroid cell and on its secretion product, thyroglobulin. The auto-antibodies against thyroglobulin may be harmless, but other forbidden clones make the thyroid-stimulating antibodies which cause thyrotoxicosis by reacting with the thyroid cell's receptor for thyrotrophic hormone. A further set of forbidden clones make auto-antibodies which direct the complement system on to components of the thyroid cell membrane causing the thyroid cell destruction of auto-immune thyroiditis, which can progress to cause myxoedema.

Gastric auto-immune disease appears to cause atrophic gastritis and pernicious anaemia. There is a close parallel with the auto-immune disease of the embryologically related thyroid gland in that complement-fixing auto-antibodies against parietal cell membrane components occur and also auto-antibodies against the parietal cell's secretory product, intrinsic factor. Complement-fixing auto-antibodies against membrane components of parenchymal cells of the damaged tissue have been demonstrated in idiopathic Addison's disease of the adrenals and in idiopathic hypoparathyroidism. Auto-antibodies against cells of the ovaries, testes and anterior pituitary have been demonstrated in certain patients and may have pathogenetic roles in diseases involving these glands. In diabetes mellitus, discovery of a genetic association with thyroid-gastric-adrenal auto-immunity suggested involvement of auto-immunity and this has been confirmed by the demonstration of auto-antibodies against islet cells in cases of juvenile diabetes. The insulin deficiency of diabetes may be caused by an auto-immune attack on the islets.

Observation of the effects of tissue damage inflicted therapeutically (as in radioactive iodine treatment of thyrotoxicosis) or by virus infection, has provided insight into the pathogenesis of auto-immune disease. In patients with thyroid auto-immune disease, damage to the thyroid gland aggravates the auto-immunity, presumably by providing increased antigenic stimulation of the forbidden clones. In the great majority of ordinary people thyroid damage, no matter how severe, does not provoke an auto-immune reaction. The simplest explanation is that normal people lack the forbidden clones which, when stimulated, cause auto-immune disease. The established genetic basis of thyroid and other auto-immune diseases indicates that the presence of forbidden clones is genetically determined. Animal models of auto-immune disease, such as the NZB mouse with auto-immune haemolytic anaemia and the obese chicken with auto-immune hypothyroidism illustrate its genetic basis.

The genes responsible for auto-immune disease are not yet known, but a number of clues suggest that they are the structural genes for antibody combining sites, the V-genes. If this is so, it could explain, (i) the dominant mode of inheritance, (ii) the need for at least two appropriate genes, (iii) the highly restricted nature of auto-antibodies, including organ specificity, (iv) the genetic association of organ-specific auto-immune disorders, (v) the observed dissociation of thyroid-gastric and anti-nuclear auto-immunity, and (vi) the high female sex incidence of thyroid auto-immune disease. The absence of auto-immune disease at birth and in the first years of post-natal life suggests that the forbidden clones arise by somatic mutation in "pre-forbidden" clones, and if this is so there may be no defect of tolerance mechanisms in people who develop auto-immune disease.

Auto-immune disease is remarkably common for a genetically-determined disadvantageous condition. This may mean that genetic polymorphism is involved and that the disadvantage of auto-immune disease is balanced by the advantage to the population of having the widest possible diversity of immune reactivity for defence against infection and neoplasia.

REFERENCES

Adams, D. D. (1958). *J. Clin. Endocr. Metab.* **18**, 699.

Adams, D. D. (1965). Pathogenesis of the hyperthyroidism of Graves' disease. *Brit. Med. J.* **1**, 1015.

Adams, D. D. (1969). A theory of the pathogenesis of rheumatic fever, glomerulonephritis and other autoimmune diseases triggered by infection. *Clin. Exp. Immunol.* **5**, 105.

Adams, D. D. and Kennedy, T. H. (1967). Occurrence in thyrotoxicosis of a gammaglobulin which protects LATS from neutralisation by an extract of thyroid gland. *J. Clin. Endocr. Metab.* **27**, 173.

Adams, D. D. and Kennedy, T. H. (1971). Evidence to suggest that LATS protector stimulates the human thyroid gland. *J. Clin. Endocr. Metab.* **33**, 47.

Adams, D. D., Kennedy, T. H. and Purves, H. D. (1969). Comparison of the thyroid-stimulating hormone content of serum from thyrotoxic and euthyroid people. *J. Clin. Endocr. Metab.* **29**, 900.

Adams, D. D., Kennedy, T. H. and Stewart, R. D. H. (1974a). Correlation between long-acting thyroid stimulator protector level and thyroid ^{131}I uptake in thyrotoxicosis. *Brit. Med. J.* **2**, 199.

Adams, D. D., Fastier, F. N., Howie, J. B., Kennedy, T. H., Kilpatrick, J. A. and Stewart, R. D. H. (1974b). Stimulation of the human thyroid by infusions of plasma containing LATS protector. *J. Clin. Endocr. Metab.* **39**, 826.

Adams, D. D., Dirmikis, S., Doniach, D., El Kabir, D. J., Hall, R., Ibbertson, H. K., Irvine, W. J., Kendall-Taylor, P., Manley, S. W., Mehdi, S. Q., Munro, D. S., Purves, H. D., Smith, B. R. and Stewart, R. D. H. (1975a). Nomenclature of thyroid-stimulating antibodies. *Lancet* **1**, 1201.

Adams, D. D., Kennedy, T. H., Stewart, J., Utiger, R. D. and Vidor, G. (1975). Hyperthyroidism in Tasmania following iodine supplementation; measurements of thyroid-stimulating antibodies and TSH. *J. Clin. Endocr. Metab.* (in press).

Adams, D. D., Kennedy, T. H. and Stewart, J. (in press). *Aust. N.Z. J. Med.*

Adams, S. and Adams, D. D. (1972). Evidence that autoimmune renal disease and tumour formation in NZB/W mice are due to separate defects. *Clin. Exp. Immunol.* **11**, 565.

Allison, A. C. (1954). Protection afforded by sickle cell trait against subterian malarial infection. *Brit. Med. J.* **1**, 290.

Allison, A. C., Denman, A. M. and Barnes, R. D. (1971). Cooperating and controlling functions of thymus-derived lymphocytes in relation to autoimmunity. *Lancet* **2**, 135.

Anderson, J. R., Goudie, R. B., Gray, K. G. and Timbury, G. C. (1957). Autoantibodies in Addison's disease. *Lancet* **1**, 1123.

Anderson, J. R., Goudie, R. B., Gray, K. G. and Stuart-Smith, D. A. (1968). Immunological features of idiopathic Addison's disease: an antibody to cells producing steroid hormones. *Clin. Exp. Immunol.* **3**, 107.

Bankhurst, A. D., Torrigiani, G. and Allison, A. C. (1973). Lymphocytes binding human thyroglobulin in healthy people and its relevance to tolerance for autoantigens. *Lancet* **1**, 226.

Bartels, E. C. (1941). "Heredity in Graves' disease". Munksgaard, Copenhagen.

Benacerraf, B. and McDevitt, H. O. (1972). The histocompatibility-linked immune response genes. *Science* **175**, 273.

Beaven, D. W., Arcus, A. C., Bell, J. P. and Smith, J. R. (1974). Epidemiology of diabetes mellitus. *N.Z. Med. J.* **80**, 291.

Bielschowsky, M. and Bielschowsky, F. (1964). Observations on NZB/B1 mice. Differential fertility in reciprocal crosses and the transmission of the autoimmune haemolytic anaemia to NZB/B1 × NZC/B1 hybrids. *Aust. J. Exptl. Biol. Med. Sci.* **42**, 561.

Billingham, R. E., Brent, L. and Medawar, P. B. (1953). "Actively acquired tolerance" of foreign cells. *Nature* **172**, 603.

Blizzard, R. M. (1969). Idiopathic hypoparathyroidism: a probable autoimmune disease. *In* "Textbook of Immunopathology", (eds. P. A. Miescher and H. J. Muller-Eberhard), Vol. II, p. 669, Grune and Stratton, New York.

Botazzo, G. F., Florin-Christensen, A. and Doniach, D. (1974). Islet-cell antibodies in diabetes mellitus with autoimmune polyendocrine deficiencies. *Lancet* **2**, 1279.

Bottazzo, G. F., Pouplard, A., Florin-Christensen, A. and Doniach, D. (1975). Auto-antibodies to prolactin-secreting cells of human pituitary. *Lancet* **ii**, 97.

Braverman, I. M. (1968). Study of autoimmune disease in New Zealand mice. *J. Invest. Dermatol.* **50**, 483.

Buchanan, W. W., Koutras, D. A., Crooks, J., Alexander, W. D., Brass, W., Anderson, J. R., Goudie, R. B. and Gray, K. G. (1962). The chemical significance of the complement-fixing test in thyrotoxicosis. *J. Endocr.* **24**, 115.

Burch, P. R. J. and Powell, N. R. (1965). Systemic lupus erythematosus. *Am. J. Med.* **38**, 793.

Burnet, F. M. (1959). "The Clonal Selection Theory of Acquired Immunity." Cambridge University Press, Cambridge.

Burnet, F. M. and Fenner, F. (1949). "The Production of Antibodies." 2nd Edition. Macmillan, Melbourne.

Burnet, F. M. and Holmes, M. C. (1965). Genetic investigations of autoimmune disease in mice. *Nature* **207**, 368.

Casey, T. P. (1968). Azathioprine administration and the development of malignant lymphomas in NZB mice. *Clin. Exp. Immunol.* **3**, 305.

Chopra, I. J., Solomon, D. H., Johnson, D. E. and Chopra, U. (1970). Thyroid gland in Graves' disease: victim or culprit? *Metabolism* **19**, 760.

Croft, S. (1974). Studies on the pathogenesis of autoimmune disease in the NZB and NZB × NZW mice. Ph.D. thesis, Otago University, Dunedin.

Croft, S., Adams, D. D. and Purves, H. D. (1975). A study of the effect of low-dosage irradiation on NZB and NZB × NZW mice. *Clin. Exp. Immunol.* **20**, 549.

Crossley, J. R. and Elliott, R. B. (1973). High urinary insulin-precursor levels in juvenile diabetics. *Lancet* **1**, 1259.

Cunningham, A. J. (1974). The generation of antibody diversity. Its dependence on antigenic stimulation. *Contemp. Top. Mol. Immunol.* **3**, 1.

Dameshek, W. and Schwartz, S. O. (1938). Haemolysins as cause of clinical and experimental haemolytic anaemias, with particular reference to nature of spherocytosis and increased fragility. *Amer. J. Med. Sci.* **196**, 769.

Der Kinderen, P. J. (1967). EPS, LATS and exophthalmos. *In* "Thyrotoxicosis", (ed. W. J. Irvine), p. 221. Livingstone, Edinburgh.

Dixon, F. J. (1971). Glomerulonephritis and immunopathology. *In* "Immunobiology", (eds. R. A. Good and D. W. Fisher), p. 167. Sinauer Associates, Stamford.

Doniach, D. (1975). Autoimmunity in endocrine disease. *In* "Medicine" Vol. 6, 2nd series, Immunological Disorders (ed. J. Holborow), p. 277. Medical Education (International) Ltd., London.

Doniach, D. and Roitt, I. M. (1957). Autoimmunity in Hashimoto's disease and its implications. *J. Clin. Endocr. Metab.* **17**, 1293.

Doniach, D., Roitt, I. M. and Taylor, K. B. (1963). Autoimmune phenomena in pernicious anaemia. Serological overlap with thyroiditis, thyrotoxicosis and systemic lupus erythematosus. *Brit. Med. J.* **1**, 1374.

Doniach, I. (1974). Pathology of the islets of Langerhans in diabetes mellitus. *In* "Immunity and Autoimmunity in Diabetes Mellitus". (eds. P. A. Bastenie and W. Gepts), p. 175. Excerpta Medica, Amsterdam.

Donnelly, P. E. and Turtle, J. R. (1974). Diabetes mellitus – a membrane receptor defect. *Aust. N.Z. J. Med.* **4**, 228.

Edelman, G. M. (1971). Antibody structure and molecular immunology. *Ann. N.Y. Acad. Sci.* **190**, 5.

Evered, D., Dingle, P. R., Roberts, D. F. and Stephenson, J. (1974). A long-term follow-up of patients with autoimmune thyroid disease. *In* "Proceedings of the Fifth Asia and Oceania Congress of Endocrinology" (ed. G. K. Rastogi), Vol. II, p. 83. Endocrine Society of India, Chandigarh.

Freund, J., Lipton, M. M. and Thompson, G. E. (1953). Aspermatogenesis in the guinea pig induced by testicular tissue and adjuvants. *J. Exp. Med.* **97**, 711.

Gally, J. A. and Edelman, G. M. (1972). The genetic control of immunoglobulin synthesis. *Ann. Rev. Genetics* **6**, 1.

Gamble, D. R. and Taylor, K. W. (1973). Coxsackie B virus and diabetes. *Brit. Med. J.* **1**, 289.

Gepts, W. (1965). Pathologic anatomy of the pancreas in juvenile diabetes mellitus. *Diabetes* **14**, 619.

Ghaffar, A. and Playfair, J. H. L. (1971). The genetic basis of autoimmunity in NZB mice studied by progeny-testing. *Clin. Exp. Immunol.* **8**, 479.

Glynn, L. E. and Holborow, E. J. (1961). Relation between blood groups, secretor status and susceptibility to rheumatic fever. *Arthr. Rheum.* **4**, 203.

Goudie, R. B. and Pinkerton, P. H. (1962). Anterior hypophysitis and Hashimoto's disease in a young woman. *J. Path. Bact.* **83**, 584.

Grubb, R. (1956). Agglutination of erythrocytes coated with "incomplete" anti-Rh by certain rheumatoid arthritic sera and some other sera. The existence of human serum groups. *Acta Path. Microbiol. Scand.* **39**, 195.

Hashimoto, H. (1912). Zur Kenntnis der lymphomatosen Veranderung der Schilddruse (Struma lymphomatosa). *Langenbecks Arch. Klin. Chir.* **97**, 219.

Hirata, Y., Tominaga, M., Ito, J.-I. and Noguchi, A. (1974). Spontaneous hypoglycemia with insulin auto-immunity in Graves' disease. *Ann. Int. Med.* **81**, 214.

Holborow, E. J., Brown, P. C., Roitt, I. M. and Doniach, D. (1959). Cytoplasmic localization of "complement-fixing" auto-antigen in human thyroid epithelium. *Brit. J. Exp. Path.* **40**, 583.

Holmes, M. C. and Burnet, F. M. (1964). The inheritance of auto-immune disease in mice: a study of hybrids of the strains NZB and C3H. *Heredity* **19**, 419.

Howie, J. B. (1968). Autoimmune disease in mice. *In* "Textbook of Immunopathology" (eds. P. A. Miescher and H. J. Muller-Eberhard), Vol. I, p. 179. Grune and Stratton, London and New York.

Howie, J. B. and Helyer, B. J. (1968). The immunology and pathology of NZB mice. *Advan. Immunol.* **9**, 215.

Hume, R. and Roberts, G. H. (1967). Hypophysitis and hypopituitarism: report of a case. *Brit. Med. J.* **1**, 548.

Irvine, W. J. (1964). Thyroid autoimmunity as a disorder of immunological tolerance. *Quart. J. Exp. Physiol.* **49**, 324.

Irvine, W. J. (1974). Autoimmunity to thyroid, gastric mucosa and adrenal cortex. *In* "Immunity and Autoimmunity in Diabetes Mellitus" (eds. P. A. Bastenie and W. Gepts), p. 137. Excerpta Medica, Amsterdam.

Irvine, W. J., Davies, S. H., Delamore, J. W. and Williams, A. W. (1962). Immunological relationships between pernicious anaemia and thyroid disease. *Brit. Med. J.* **2**, 454.

Jerne, N. K. (1955). The natural selection theory of antibody formation. *Proc. Natn. Acad. Sci.* **41**, 849.

Jerne, N. K. (1971). The somatic generation of immune recognition. *Eur. J. Immunol.* **1**, 1.

Jerne, N. K. (1973). The immune system. *Scient. Amer.* **229**, 52.

Kaplan, M. H. (1969). Autoimmunity to heart. *In* "Textbook of Immunopathology" (eds. P. A. Miescher and H. J. Miller-Eberhard), p. 641. Grune and Stratton, New York and London.

Konishi, J., Herman, M. M. and Kriss, J. P. (1974). Binding of thyroglobulin and thyroglobulin-anti-thyroglobulin immune complex to extraocular muscle membrane. *Endocrinology*, **95**, 434.

Kriss, J. P., Pleshakov, V. and Chien, J. R. (1964). Isolation and identification of the long-acting thyroid stimulator and its relation to hyperthyroidism and circumscribed pretibial myxoedema. *J. Clin. Endocr. Metab.* **24**, 1005.

Lendrum, R., Walker, G. and Gamble, D. R. (1975). Islet-cell autoantibodies in juvenile diabetes mellitus of recent origin. *Lancet* **1**, 880.
Lies, R. B., Messner, R. P. and Williams, R. C. (1973). Relative T-cell specificity of lymphocytotoxins from patients with systemic lupus erythemetosus. *Anthr. Rheum.* **16**, 369.
Lotzova, E. and Cudkowicz, G. (1972). Hybrid resistance to parental WB/Re bone marrow grafts. *Transplantation* **12**, 130.
Mahieu, P. and Winand, R. (1972). Demonstration of delayed hypersensitivity to retrobulbar and thyroid tissues in human exophthalmos. *J. Clin. Endocr. Metab.* **34**, 1090.
Manley, S. W., Bourke, J. R. and Hawker, R. W. (1974a). The thyrotrophin receptor in guinea-pig thyroid: general properties. *J. Endocr.* **61**, 419.
Manley, S. W., Bourke, J. R. and Hawker, R. W. (1974b). The thyrotrophin receptor in guinea-pig thyroid homogenate: interaction with the long-acting thyroid stimulator. *J. Endocr.* **61**, 437.
Marchalonis, J. J. (1975). *In* "The Lymphocytes; Structure and Function" (ed. J. J. Marchalonis), Dekker, New York.
Markson, J. L. and Moore, J. M. (1962). Autoimmunity in pernicious anaemia and iron deficiency anaemia. *Lancet* **2**, 1240.
Masugi, M. (1934). Uber die experimentelle glomerulonephritis durch das spezifische antinieren serum. *Beitr. Path. Anat.* **92**, 429.
Mehdi, S. Q. and Nussey, S. S. (1975). A radio-ligand receptor assay for the long-acting thyroid stimulator. *Biochem. J.* **145**, 105.
Mellors, R. C. and Huang, C. Y. (1967). Immunopathology of NZB/B1 mice. VI. Virus separable from spleen and pathogenic for Swiss mice. *J. Exp. Med.* **126**, 53.
Meulengracht, E. (1949). Epidemiologic aspects of thyrotoxicosis. *Arch. Intern. Med.* **83**, 119.
Miller, H. G., Stanton, J. B. and Gibbons, J. L. (1956). Para-infectious encephalomyelitis and related syndromes. *Quart. J. Med.* **26**, 427.
Mitchison, N. A. (1968). The dosage requirements for immunological paralysis by soluble proteins. *Immunology*, **15**, 509.
Morris, B. (1968). The lymphatic system and the immune response. *Aust. J. Sci.* **31**, 13.
Munro, D. S. (1971). The long-acting thyroid stimulator. *Current Topics Exp. Endocr.* **1**, 175.
MacCuish, A. C., Barnes, E. W., Irvine, W. J. and Duncan, L. J. P. (1974). Antibodies to pancreatic islet cells in insulin-dependent diabetics with co-existent autoimmune disease. *Lancet* **2**, 1529.
McDevitt, H. O. and Bodmer, W. F. (1974). HL-A immune response genes and disease. *Lancet* **1**, 1269.
McIntyre, N., Holdsworth, C. D. and Turner, D. S. (1965). Intestinal factors in the control of insulin secretion. *J. Clin. Endocrinol. Metab.* **25**, 1317.
McKenzie, J. M. (1964). Neonatal Graves' disease. *J. Clin. Endocr. Metab.* **24**, 660.
McKenzie, J. M. (1965). Review: pathogenesis of Graves' disease: role of the long-acting thyroid stimulator. *J. Clin. Endocr. Metab.* **25**, 424.
Owen, R. D. (1945). Immunogenetic consequences of vascular anastomoses between bovine twins. *Science* **102**, 400.
Perlmann, P., Perlmann, H. and Wigzell, H. (1972). Lymphocyte mediated cytotoxicity *in vitro*. Induction and inhibition by humoral antibody and nature of effector cells. *Transpl. Rev.* **13**, 91.
Plummer, H. S. (1928). Function of thyroid gland containing adenomatous tissue. *Tr. A. Am. Physicians* **43**, 159.
Roberts, I. M., Whittingham, S. and Mackay, I. R. (1973). Tolerance to autoantigen-thyroglobulin. *Lancet* **2**, 936.

Roitt, I. M. and Doniach, D. (1960). Thyroid autoimmunity. *Brit. Med. Bull.* **16**, 152.
Roitt, I. M. and Torrigiani, G. (1967). Identification and estimation of undegraded thyroglobulin in human serum. *Endocrinology* **81**, 421.
Roitt, I. M., Doniach, D. and Shapland, C. (1965). Autoimmune phenomenon in relation to the gastric mucosa in human disease. *In* "Immunopathology". IVth International Symposium, (eds. P. Grabar and P. A. Miescher), p. 314. Schwabe, Basel.
Rumke, P. (1969). Antigenicity of spermatozoa and immunity to sperm. *In* "Textbook of Immunopathology" (eds. P. A. Miescher and H. J. Muller-Eberhard), Vol. II, p. 669. Grune and Stratton, New York.
Rundle, F. F. (1964). Eye signs of Graves' disease. *In* "The Thyroid Gland". Vol. 2, (eds. R. Pitt-Rivers and W. R. Trotter), p. 171. Butterworth, London.
Russell, P. J. and Hicks, J. D. (1968). Cyclophosphamide treatment of renal disease in (NZB × NZW) F_1 hybrid mice. *Lancet* **1**, 440.
Schwartz, M. (1960). Intrinsic factor antibody in serum from patients with pernicious anaemia. *Lancet* **2**, 1263.
Scott, J. S. (1966). Immunological diseases and pregnancy. *Brit. Med. J.* **1**, 1559.
Smith, B. R. and Hall, R. (1974). Thyroid-stimulating immunoglobulins in Graves' disease. *Lancet* **2**, 427.
Smith, B. R., Dorrington, K. J. and Munro, D. S. (1969). The thyroid-stimulating properties of long-acting thyroid stimulator and γ-globulin subunits. *Biochim. Biophys. Acta* **192**, 277.
Taylor, K. B. (1959). Inhibition of intrinsic factor by pernicious anaemia sera. *Lancet* **2**, 106.
Taylor, K. B., Roitt, I. M., Doniach, D., Couchman, K. G. and Shapland, C. (1962). Autoimmune phenomena in pernicious anaemia. 1. Gastric antibodies. *Brit. Med. J.* **2**, 1347.
Teague, P. O. and Friou, G. J. (1969). Antinuclear antibodies in mice. II. Transmission with spleen cells; inhibition or prevention with thymus or spleen cells. *Immunology* **17**, 665.
Trotter, W. R., Belyavin, G. and Waddams, A. (1957). Precipitating and complement-fixing antibodies in Hashimoto's disease. *Proc. Roy. Soc. Med.* **50**, 961.
Tudhope, G. R. and Wilson, G. M. (1960). Anaemia in hypothyroidism. *Quart. J. Med.* **29**, 513.
Vallance-Owen, J. and Lilley, M. D. (1961). An insulin antagonist associated with plasma insulin. *Lancet* **1**, 804.
Vladutiu, A. O. and Rose, N. E. (1971). Autoimmune murine thyroiditis. Relation to histocompatibility type. *Science* **174**, 1137.
Volpé, R., Row, V. V. and Ezrin, C. (1967). Circulating viral and thyroid antibodies in subacute thyroiditis. *J. Clin. Endocr. Metab.* **27**, 1275.
Wegman, T. G., Hellstrom, I. and Hellstrom, K. E. (1971). Immunological tolerance: "forbidden clones" allowed in tetraparental mice (serum blocking factor). *Proc. Natn. Acad. Sci. (U.S.A.)* **68**, 1644.
Wick, G., Sundick, R. S. and Albini, B. (1974). A review. The obese strain (OS) of chickens: an animal model with spontaneous autoimmune thyroiditis. *Clin. Immunol. Immunopath.* **3**, 272.
Witebsky, E., Rose, N. R., Terplan, K., and Pain, J. R. and Egan, R. W. (1957). Chronic thyroiditis and autoimmunization. *J. Am. Med. Assoc.* **164**, 1439.
Wrong, O. M. (1971). Glomerular disease. *In* "Textbook of Medicine" (eds. P. B. Beeson and W. McDermott), Vol. II, p. 1177. Saunders, London.

IV

Immunity and Infection

13

Infectious Diseases

W. PAGE FAULK and B. M. GREENWOOD

Infectious diseases are still the major health problem in many parts of the world. In most developing countries acute infections such as pneumonia, measles, malaria, gastroenteritis, typhoid and meningitis account for the majority of admissions to medical and paediatric wards. Chronic infections such as tuberculosis and leprosy are widespread and many apparently healthy people harbour at least one potentially harmful parasite (Humphrey, 1974). Much remains to be learnt about the immune response to infections; in many cases, vaccination is not yet possible or has been found to be only partially effective under field conditions.

Although diphtheria, typhoid and cholera have been largely eradicated from developed countries, venereal and respiratory tract infections still cause much ill-health. Increasing evidence that diseases such as systemic lupus erythematosus and multiple sclerosis are due to an unusual response to infection is a further stimulus to the study of the complicated sequence of events in the immune response to infections. We attempt in this chapter a balanced consideration of the immunology of infectious diseases in developed as well as in developing countries and aim to underscore the universality of immunological interpretations rather than to deal in depth with selected categories of disease.

CLINICAL ASPECTS OF THE IMMUNE RESPONSE TO INFECTIONS

Before consideration is given to the clinical immunology of a supposed infection, there should be good evidence that it exists; for instance, an inflamed joint may suggest infection, but it can also represent leukaemia, rheumatoid arthritis, or gout. Once the presence of infection is established, it is important to know whether or not it is primary or secondary. Congenital diseases such as cystic fibrosis, metabolic diseases such as diabetes mellitus, and acquired lesions such as hydronephrosis often present as infections, and long-term treatment in these circumstances should be adjusted to the underlying disease. The history and physical examination are often as important to a clinical immunologist as are sophisticated laboratory tests in establishing a diagnosis. Certain points in the history and physical diagnosis are especially useful, and will be reviewed before laboratory aspects are considered.

History

Immunological clues to the diagnosis of some infectious diseases can be obtained if a careful history is obtained from the patient or a well-informed member of the family. It is important to enquire about previous infections, vaccinations, and exposure to infectious diseases. Such information is often not spontaneously produced, but can be extremely helpful if obtained; for instance, in the evaluation of meningoencephalitis not associated with parotitis, a history of recent exposure to mumps may be significant since mumps meningoencephalitis can occur in the absence of parotitis. Enquiries should be made into a patient's habits (e.g. pica in a toddler suggests the possibility of several parasitic infections, especially visceral larva migrans), diet (e.g. fondness for rare pork may suggest the possibility of trichinosis), occupation (e.g. hepatitis in blood bank personnel, brucellosis in dairy farmers or hydatid disease in sheep farmers), and pets (e.g. ornithosis from parakeets or pigeons). Immunological tests are available for all these relatively uncommon diseases but are of no use to the clinician until such a disease is suspected. Queries concerning past and present medications should also be made because certain drugs such as corticosteroids, phenylbutazone, chloramphenicol and methimazole impair neutrophil bactericidal functions. A careful genetic history should be obtained when possible; this is important in a patient suspected of having an immunodeficiency disease.

Physicians in temperate areas should be prepared to consider tropical diseases in their differential diagnosis, and remember that vaccines against diseases such as cholera and typhoid offer only limited protection. In view of the ease with which great distances can be covered on business or holiday, it should be routine in a suspected infection to ask the patient "where have you been?" The answer has often resolved a diagnostic dilemma, for instance by suggesting the possibility of paratyphoid-B in a fever of unknown origin.

Such diseases can usually be rapidly diagnosed or ruled out by simple immunological or microbiological tests.

Useful immunological information concerning infections in neonates can be obtained from midwives, nurses, obstetricians and mothers. For instance, the time between rupture of the membranes and delivery, or the colour and odour of the amniotic fluid, may suggest intra-uterine infections. Pseudocysts in the placenta suggest congenital toxoplasmosis, and such an observation may be useful since congenital toxoplasmosis is sometimes not clinically evident until several months of age.

Physical Diagnosis

The physical diagnosis of infectious diseases is an art that cannot be adequately discussed in this chapter, but certain observations are relevant to clinical immunology. For instance, tetany in an infant might suggest several diagnoses, but is sometimes associated with a form of primary immunodeficiency caused by thymic aplasia (Di George syndrome) that results in a type of immune failure and life-threatening infections. Eczema in a young child may suggest a form of immunodeficiency, the Wiskott-Aldrich syndrome, often associated with increased susceptibility to infectious diseases. Cerebellar ataxia and/or conjunctival telangiectasia should suggest investigation for a combined defect of cellular and humoral immunity, since this combination has long been known to produce abnormal susceptibility to infectious diseases. *Candida albicans* infections occur in many debilitating diseases, but if repeated and extensive, it should be remembered that chronic mucocutaneous candidiasis is sometimes associated with a specific loss of cutaneous resistance to the fungus due to an absence of leukotactic mediators from sensitized lymphocytes. It is important to consider this possibility, because the disease can be treated with lymphocyte products. Certain types of dwarfism may also be associated with immunodeficiency and decreased resistance to infections.

Patients with some antibody deficiency syndromes often have hypoplastic tonsils, and the peripheral lymph nodes may or may not be grossly deficient. In lymphopenic forms of hypogammaglobulinaemia and in combined immunodeficiency diseases patients conspicuously lack lymphoid tissue and lymph nodes. Poor teeth are not uncommonly seen in primary immunodeficiency diseases. The clinical features associated with hypogammaglobulinaemia are varied, but complicating infection is the most common presenting symptom, and usually involves the lower respiratory tract. Such patients often have splenomegaly or hepatosplenomegaly, sometimes associated with lymphadenopathy, joint findings, and gastrointestinal symptoms such as sprue.

Children with acute infections sometimes appear to be more ill than would be expected from the duration of their illness or from the clinical course of the same infection in other children in the community. A surgical scar indicative of a previous splenectomy in such a child should suggest the possibility of a rapidly progressive and perhaps fatal outcome. Sudden, unexpected, and unexplained death during an acute infection in children who, months or years before, have had their spleens removed for any of a variety of causes has been reported (Erickson *et al.*, 1968), and indicates the importance of the spleen in the acute response to infectious disease. Splenectomized subjects have defective phagocytosis, perhaps in part due to the absence of a phagocytosis stimulating peptide, tuftsin, produced in the spleen (Constantopoulos *et al.*, 1973).

Hepatomegaly may be associated with a variety of malignant and metabolic disorders, but is also seen in certain acute (e.g., infectious hepatitis) and chronic (e.g., toxocariasis) infections. *Toxocara* infections, although sometimes thought of as an oddity, are not uncommon in Britain. Enucleations have been done following a mistaken diagnosis of eosinophilic granuloma when in fact retinal involvement in visceral larva migrans with *Toxocara canis* was the underlying disease.

NON-SPECIFIC IMMUNITY

Although an adequate immune response is one of the principal host defence mechanisms against infectious diseases, patients also have a number of protective mechanisms that do not necessarily depend on development of a specific immune response. Obvious examples are an intact integument, adequate endocrine responses, and so-called non-specific factors of resistance such as lysozyme, C-reactive protein, and the acute inflammatory response. These have been adequately reviewed (Braun and Ungar, 1973), and will not be discussed here. There are, however, other forms of non-specific immunity relevant to the clinical immunology of infectious diseases. For instance, the serum of some people who have not been previously exposed to an organism may contain antibodies, usually opsonins, that are capable of destroying small numbers of a potentially pathogenic invader. These are sometimes called natural antibodies and are probably formed as a result of infestation with commensal organisms possessing cross-reacting antigens. The possibility of enhancing this type of cross-reacting immunity has recently been investigated. It has been shown that the oral introduction of a harmless strain of *E. coli* can induce antibody formation to virulent *Haemophilus influenzae*, Type B, the cause of an increasing number of childhood cases of meningitis.

The complement system is described in Chapter 7, but it should be mentioned here that activation of this system plays an important part in protection from several infections. The classical complement pathway may be activated by antiten–antibody complexes during infections, or the alternative pathway by endotoxin-like compounds released by some invading organisms. Complement activation may also result from the action of proteolytic bacterial enzymes.

The complement break-down products C3a and C5a play an important role in promoting leukotaxis and phagocytosis. They attract phagocytes to sites of infection and increase local vascular permeability. C3 promotes phagocytosis by binding to antibodies on the surface of organisms and by interacting with C3 receptors on macrophages. Activation of the full complement sequence can also lead to bacterial lysis. Some components of antibody-activated complement can cause vasodilatation and the transudation of plasma containing more antibody and leukotactic factors, leading to more phagocytosis.

Phagocytic cells, discussed in Chapter 8, play an important role in the destruction of many pathogenic organisms, usually in co-operation with opsonizing antibodies and complement. For instance, polymorphonuclear neutrophils can ingest and kill many virulent encapsulated pneumococci after the bacteria have been coated with antibody against pneumococcal capsular polysaccharide. The spleen also plays an important role as a site where damaged organisms are trapped and destroyed. This appears to be particularly important in protection against pneumococcal infections and malaria.

Finally, there is a matrix of poorly understood non-specific host factors of resistance to infections such as age, sex, race, etc. Age seems to be particularly important; for example, different viruses tend to affect different age groups. Adenoviruses and enteroviruses affect children and adolescents, while parainfluenza viruses mainly affect young children and respiratory syncytial virus infection is usually seen in children under two years of age. By contrast, influenza and rhinoviruses attack all age groups equally.

THE IMMUNE RESPONSE TO INFECTIONS

Patients respond to most infections with a specific immune response aimed at neutralization of the invading organism or its products. Both cellular and humoral immune responses to microbial antigens can occur, and in many infections one or the other predominates. Thus patients with pneumococcal infections show a marked antibody response to the pneumococcus with little evidence of cell mediated immunity, while patients with tuberculosis produce a cell-mediated immune response and a less marked antibody response. The factors determining whether cellular or humoral immunity predominates in any infection are not fully understood. The chemical and physical nature of the antigens are important, as antigens with repeating subunits, such as pneumococcal polysaccharide, tend to be T-cell independent and are more likely to produce a predominantly humoral response. Host factors are also important in determining the type of immune response a patient will mount in response to an infection. Thus *Mycobacterium leprae* provokes a marked humoral immune response (lepromatous leprosy) in some patients and a predominantly cellular immune response (tuberculoid leprosy) in others.

The rate at which a patient can mount an immune response to an invading organism markedly affects the outcome of the infection. A non-immune person requires several days to mount an effective primary immune response. Thus, in untreated pneumococcal lobar pneumonia, resolution of the lesion usually does not occur until about the seventh day of the infection, i.e., the time required to mount a primary immune response as measured by the detection of circulating antibodies. Without antibiotics, the mortality during this period in a non-immune patient is high. In contrast, an immune patient, i.e., one who has been previously exposed to the same or a cross-reacting organism by means of either natural infection or by previous immunization, shows an accelerated or secondary immune response, and the morbidity is low.

Antigens

In viral infections, a relatively small number of antigens seem to be involved in provoking protective immunity; for example, in serum hepatitis protection depends upon immunity to the central core antigen and the surface coat antigen of the virus. Bacteria usually possess more antigens, but in some instances it has been shown that a single antigen is of overriding importance in producing protective immunity. Thus, it has been found that the capsular antigens of group A and group C meningococci play dominant roles in producing protective immunity to these infections, and this has led to the development of successful polysaccharide meningococcal vaccines. The situation is even more complicated in infection by large parasites such as schistosomes or trypanosomes which contain many antigens, some released as secretory products and others liberated on the death of the organism. Some success has been achieved in characterizing antigens of malaria parasites and trypanosomes immunochemically. This type of research is of central importance in the development of effective parasite vaccines.

Antibodies

Antibodies protect against infection in several ways. Neutralization of an exotoxin can be achieved by the binding of antibody to the biologically active site of the toxin, or by the binding of antibody to a part of the toxin distant from the active site thus producing conformational changes. Anti-toxic immunity effectively protects against diseases such as tetanus and botulism, the clinical features of which are almost entirely dependent upon the action of an exotoxin.

Opsonization of invading organisms is another important protective function of antibody, for it promotes uptake of organisms by phagocytic cells, leading to subsequent intracellular killing. Antibodies of subclasses IgG_1 and IgG_3 are cytophilic for macrophages and they, in addition to IgM, can also enhance phagocytosis via complement activation.

Antibody cannot reach intracellular parasites and is thus relatively ineffective in protection against many intracellular infections. However, antibody can play an important part in controlling or modulating infections by preventing spread to other cells. This type of protective immunity operates in malaria. Isotope incorporation experiments show that protective antibody cannot prevent the growth of merozoites already within erythrocytes, but that it can prevent the parasite from invading other cells.

Complement

The protective actions of antibody often involve the participation of complement. Blood complement promotes the phagocytosis of microorganisms through the formation of Ag–Ab–C complexes that bind to C3 receptors on the membranes of some phagocytic cells. Adherence of such complexes to red cells or platelets further favours phagocytosis by macrophages. The combination of antibody with surface antigens of some gram-negative bacteria such as *E. coli* leads to activation of complement and a lipolytic effect with sybsequent lysis.

Other complement components are activated by substances such as endotoxin through the alternative pathway which can operate independently of antibody. This introduces the possibility of complement fixation and the subsequent biological effects of complement components in the absence of complement-fixing antibodies. This is perhaps especially important in the gut, where IgA, which can fix complement by the alternative pathway, is the predominant immunoglobulin.

Secretory Immunity

Many, if not most, infectious disease vectors gain their portal of entry via mucosal surfaces such as those of the sino-pulmonary and gastrointestinal tracts. These surfaces are protected by secretory IgA (IgA–S) made by lymphoid cells in the lamina propria and serving as a main line of defence for mucosal epithelium. This immunoglobulin is a dimer of serum IgA linked by a joining or "J"-chain and one molecule of secretory piece (see Chapter 4). IgA and secretory piece are made by different cells, and IgA–S is secreted onto mucous membranes by virtue of its association with secretory-piece. It resists proteolysis and is thus uniquely suited to function in the gut. IgA–S is found in tears, colostrum, vaginal secretions, saliva, sino-pulmonary and gastrointestinal secretions, and accounts for most of the so-called copro-antibodies in stool (Tomasi and Grey, 1972).

Antibody activity can be shown in IgA–S, as for instance in virus neutralization tests following attentuated oral polio vaccine, or after influenza or common cold infections. Antibody in nasal secretions (e.g., to parainfluenza type 1) or in gut fluids (e.g., to polio) correlates better with protection than serum antibody does. Where antibody is present both in serum and in secretions, the serum antibody is usually IgG and the secretory or local antibody is IgA–S.

IgA–S interferes with bacterial attachment to mucosal epithelium as part of a general mechanism for antigen clearance (Williams and Gibbons, 1972). Persons lacking IgA–S often have repeated sino-pulmonary and gastro-intestinal infections, sprue-like syndromes, or milk allergies; however, some seemingly normal people lack secretory IgA. Patients with ataxia-telangiectasia often lack IgA–S, and not uncommonly suffer *Giardia lamblia* gut infestations and *Pneumocystis carinii* pulmonary infections. There is also some evidence that persons who lack IgA also lack IgE, but at present this is not conclusive.

Cell Mediated Immunity

Contact between antigens from an invading organism and antigen-reactive cells may initiate a number of cellular immune reactions which have important protective effects. Cell mediated protective responses usually take longer than antibody responses to become established, but their rate of development is accelerated by prior exposure to the same or a closely related antigen. This explains the successful use of BCG in preventing tuberculosis. Cell mediated immune reactions are of particular value in protection against infection by intracellular parasites not accessible to attack by antibody and thus play an important role in the development of immunity to tuberculosis, leprosy, leishmaniasis and many intracellular fungal and viral infections (W.H.O. Technical Report, 1973).

Cell mediated immune responses achieve destruction of a pathogen in at least two ways. Firstly, sensitized lymphocytes may cause direct destruction of organisms. The way in which this is achieved is not fully understood but close contact between the lymphocytes and the organism, or the infected host cell, is required. Death of the organism is often achieved at the expense of destruction of the host cell, and this process plays an important part in the immunopathology of many infectious diseases.

Secondly, contact between antigen and antigen-reactive lymphocytes may lead to the release of lymphokines. Lymphokines attract macrophages to a site of infection, increase their metabolic activity, and make them more "aggressive". Macrophages activated in this way do not necessarily show specificity towards the organism invoking the cell mediated immune response. For instance, macrophages activated by lymphokines as a result of contact between tubercle bacilli and T-lymphocytes specific for tubercle bacilli show enhanced phagocytosis of tubercle bacilli, but also show enhanced ability to ingest other organisms such as *Listeria monocytogenes* (Mackaness, 1971). This type of macrophage activation may be an important protective factor in populations exposed to repeated infections. Lymphokines also attract polymorphonuclear neutrophils to a site of infection. Interferon is produced on contact between antigen and antigen-reactive T-lymphocytes, and this may also have a protective action in viral infections. Although a great deal is now known about the nature and action of lymphokines *in vitro* (see Chapter 9), it has proved very difficult to assess their role in protection against infections *in vivo*.

It can be shown experimentally that cells may be destroyed as a result of the combined action of antibody and leukocytes. These leukocytes are distinct from the population of T-lymphocytes involved in direct cell mediated cytotoxicity, and are a special subgroup of leukocytes, known as K-cells. This type of antibody-mediated cytotoxicity may have an important role in protection against infection. It has been suggested that it may be involved in protection against hepatitis, but this has been little investigated.

IMMUNE DEFICIENCY

Most patients with infectious diseases were probably immunologically normal before their infections, but it is important to recognize that patients with immune deficiency have impaired resistance. Vaccination diminishes infections in normal people, but patients with some immunodeficiencies should not receive live vaccines, and respond poorly to killed ones. Ordinarily innocuous vaccination procedures, such as those for polio, smallpox, tuberculosis, etc. are contraindicated in primary and in some secondary or acquired immunological deficiency diseases.

The pathogens responsible for infectious diseases in patients with primary or secondary immunodeficiency fall into three major groups (Table 1). There are several general principles useful in evaluating an infection in a child also suspected of having an immunodeficiency (Good *et al.*, 1970). For instance, patients with agammaglobulinaemia are rarely ill during the first six months of life because they are protected by maternal antibody, but infants with lymphopenic agammaglobulinaemia start having infections during the early weeks of life. Infections in the agammaglobulinaemic group are usually caused by encapsulated pyogenic bacteria and present clinically as pneumonia, septicaemia, meningitis, skin infections, conjunctivitis, and sinopulmonary infections. Patients with agammaglobulinaemia are unusually susceptible to hepatitis virus and occasionally to *Pneumocystis carinii*. They are not unduly susceptible to recurrent viral or fungal infections or to infections with so-called low-grade pyogenic bacteria such as *Enterobacteriaceae*, *Klebsiella*, or *Serratia marcescens*, and develop normal immunity to chickenpox and measles.

TABLE 1

Pathogens that cause infections in patients with immunodeficiencies

Type of immunodeficiency	Pathogens usually responsible for infections in each immunodeficiency group	
Humoral immune responses	Pneumococci *Haemophilus influenzae* *Streptococcus* sp. *Meningococcus* sp.	*Pseudomonas aeruginosa* Hepatitis virus *Pneumocystis carinii*
Cellular immune responses	Measles Varicella Vaccinia Cytomegalic-inclusion-body virus	*Mycobacterium tuberculosis* *Candida albicans* *Histoplasma*
Disorders of phagocytosis	Staphylococci *Klebsiella* sp. *Aerobacter aerogenes* *Serratia marcescens*	*Candida albicans* *Aspergillus* *Nocardia*

Data have been assembled for patients suffering from immunodeficiency diseases and leukocyte bactericidal functional defects (Good *et al.*, 1970). Complement deficiencies have not been included, but it should be recalled that these patients also show increased susceptibility to bacterial infections.

Patients with defective cellular immune mechanisms are especially liable to virus infections such as chickenpox, measles, or cytomegalic inclusion disease, and also to tuberculosis, *Candida albicans*, and *Nocardia* infections. Children in the leukocyte bactericidal dysfunction group, especially those with chronic granulomatous disease, are susceptible to staphylococcal infections and infections with *Klebsiella*, *Aerobacter aerogenes*, and *Serratia marcescens* as well as with *Candida* and *Nocardia* infections (Good, 1975). The low-grade pyogenic bacteria responsible for infections in chronic granulomatous disease are all catalase positive, and it is thought that this is related to the biochemical lesion of the leukocytes, which are defective in hydrogen peroxide production.

The immunosuppressive effects of many parasitic and viral infections may also predispose to secondary bacterial infection. For instance, children with severe measles frequently develop bacterial pneumonia, persistent gastroenteritis, candidiasis and occasionally tuberculosis. Cell mediated immunity is impaired in patients with Hodgkin's disease, increasing their susceptibility to unusual infections such as cryptococcosis and their risk of developing generalized vaccinia following smallpox vaccination.

TABLE 2

Non-specific factors of resistance that are affected by alterations in the levels of particular nutrients

Non-specific factors	Relevant nutrient	Nutrient Status[a]
Anatomic barriers		
Mucosa, connective tissue	Protein	Deficiency
skin, secretions, etc.	Vitamin A	Deficiency
	Vitamin B_1, B_2, B_6, Niacin	Deficiency
	Vitamin C	Deficiency[b]
	Zinc	Deficiency[b]
Achlorhydria	B_{12}	Deficiency
Ventilatory capacity	D	Deficiency
	Calories, fat	Excess
Intestinal flora alterations	Protein-calorie	Deficiency
	Vitamin A	Deficiency
	Iron	Excess
Fever (endogenous pyrogens)	Protein–calorie	Deficiency—presumptive
Hormonal response		
Cortisone (stress)[c]	Protein–calorie	Deficiency
Cortisone[c]		
Thyroxin	Iodine	Deficiency
Interferon	Protein	Deficiency—presumptive
	Vitamin C	Deficiency[b]
Lysozyme	Protein	Deficiency—presumptive
	Vitamin A	Deficiency—presumptive
Properdin	Protein	Deficiency—presumptive
	Pantothenic acid	Deficiency
Metal binding proteins		
Transferrin and lactoferrin	Protein	Deficiency
Albumin	Protein	Deficiency
Ceruloplasm (↑ in infection)	Protein	Deficiency—presumptive
α_2 macroglobulin	Protein	Deficiency—presumptive

[a]Precedes infection—not a result of the infection.
[b]Relative deficiency—wound healing improves when normal levels supplemented.
[c]Occasionally in kwashiorkor, cortisone ↑
In infection and marasmus, cortisol ↑
This table was prepared by Dr Charlotte Neumann, Department of Paediatrics, UCLA School of Medicine.

Another type of secondary or acquired immunodeficiency is seen in patients with protein–calorie malnutrition. The predisposing role of malnutrition has been demonstrated in several different infections. Protein malnutrition appears to play a major role but other forms, for instance vitamin A deficiency, may also be clinically important. It now seems that malnutrition predisposes to infection mainly through its deleterious effect on the immune response; however, non-specific factors of resistance are also affected by the levels of particular nutrients (Table 2). Protein malnutrition affects nearly all components of the normal immune response including bactericidal killing by phagocytes, immunoglobulin and antibody production, and induction and expression of cell mediated immune responses. These defects in immunity are associated with atrophy of the thymus, lymphoid hypoplasia, loss of delayed hypersensitivity, and a decrease in the number of circulating T-cells and abnormal *in vitro* responses to phytohaemagglutinin and pokeweed mitogen. Some of the possible mechanisms underlying these changes in man have been reviewed (Faulk *et al.*, 1975).

Malnutrition can lead to severe infection but the reverse can also occur. Poor appetite, malabsorption, vomiting, negative nitrogen balance, and protein loss into the gut or other secretions can precipitate protein malnutrition in a patient with an infection who is either not eating or is on a marginally adequate diet. A vicious circle of malnutrition leading to infection and infection leading to malnutrition is then established, the net effect of which is to impair ability of the immune system to deal effectively with infections. The malnourished child with measles illustrates this (Fig. 1).

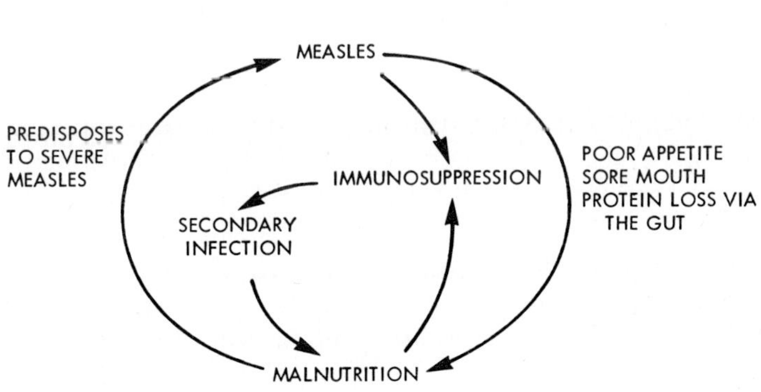

Fig. 1. Interaction of measles, malnutrition, and the immune response. The specific example of measles is used to demonstrate the general point that infection, malnutrition, and immunity can interact to the detriment of host defence mechanisms against many infectious diseases.

Many drugs impair immune function by causing marrow depression or by acting on the lymphoid system (see Chapter 30). Patients on prolonged treatment with immunosuppressive drugs, for example renal transplant recipients, are at high risk of developing severe infections, and these are one of the main hazards to life of patients surviving the early phase of potential graft rejection. Patients on immunosuppressive drugs are liable to develop unusual infections such as systemic herpes and invasive strongyloidiasis. As more powerful methods of modulating the immune response come into clinical use, iatrogenic infection is likely to become an increasing problem.

EVASION OF AND ESCAPE FROM HOST DEFENCE MECHANISMS

The immune response of the host ensures that many potential infections are aborted and that others are rapidly brought under control. However a number of microorganisms have evolved means of avoiding or counteracting specific and non-specific defence mechanisms (see Ciba Foundation Symposium No. 25, 1974). The following are among the most important.

Survival in a Protected Site

Intracellular parasites are protected from the harmful effects of serum antibody and can persist for prolonged periods in an immune host. Persistence may be favoured by the anatomical location of the organism; for instance, herpes simplex virus is frequently found in dorsal root ganglia, and cytomegalovirus can persist in the salivary gland. Viruses confined to mucosal surfaces, such as the common cold virus, are relatively protected from serum antibody, but are susceptible to secretory IgA. The localization of a virus has an important role in determining the duration of immunity that follows infection. For example, infections that confer life-long immunity, such as chickenpox or measles, have viraemic phases, long incubation periods and are not limited to mucosal surfaces. On the other hand, viral infections such as influenza and the common cold do not confer life-long immunity, partly because they have short incubation periods and are usually limited to mucosal surfaces. Some intracellular parasites, such as *Toxoplasma gondii* and the tubercle bacillus, can survive within phagocytic cells. This is thought to be due to their ability to resist fusion with acid protease-containing lysosomes in the cytoplasm of phagocytes.

Aggressins and Soluble Antigens

It has long been recognized that virulent strains of certain bacteria, such as the pneumococcus, can produce soluble factors called aggressins, and that these are able to block the protective action of antibody (Glynn, 1972). Some bacterial aggressins are soluble antigens, for instance the capsular polysaccharide of the pneumococcus, and these are able to neutralize opsonizing antibodies and thus prevent phagocytosis of the bacteria. Many larger parasites, such as *Plasmodia*, also release soluble anitigens into the circulation and these may block the immune response of the host. Bacteria can also produce other protective factors. Some staphylococci produce a mucopeptide that inhibits leukotaxis and certain strains of *E. coli* have an acid polysaccharide that inhibits agglutination, complement mediated lysis, and phagocytosis.

Antigenic Variation

Infection with influenza virus gives only limited protection against further infection, for the antigens of the virus can change to give a new variant which is no longer susceptible to protective antibody developed against the original strain. A gradual change in antigenic structure occurred in strains isolated between 1933 and 1946 and this culminated in the appearance of strain A1 that was responsible for a major epidemic. A more sudden change led to the appearance of strain A2 that was responsible for the pandemic of 1957.

Antigenic variation also occurs in malaria parasites and trypanosomes, making it difficult for the immune response to control infection by these parasites. Patients with African trypanosomiasis have antibody to trypanosome-derived antigens, but they are hardly ever able to overcome the infection and, untreated, nearly always die. The way in which antigenic variation allows a trypanosome to keep one stage ahead of the immune response of the host can be demonstrated in experimental trypanosome infections as shown in Fig. 2. The immune response to human malaria infections is more effective but repeated attacks of malaria are required to establish immunity, and continued exposure to the parasite is required if such immunity is not to be lost. Antigenic variation in malaria parasites perhaps accounts for this

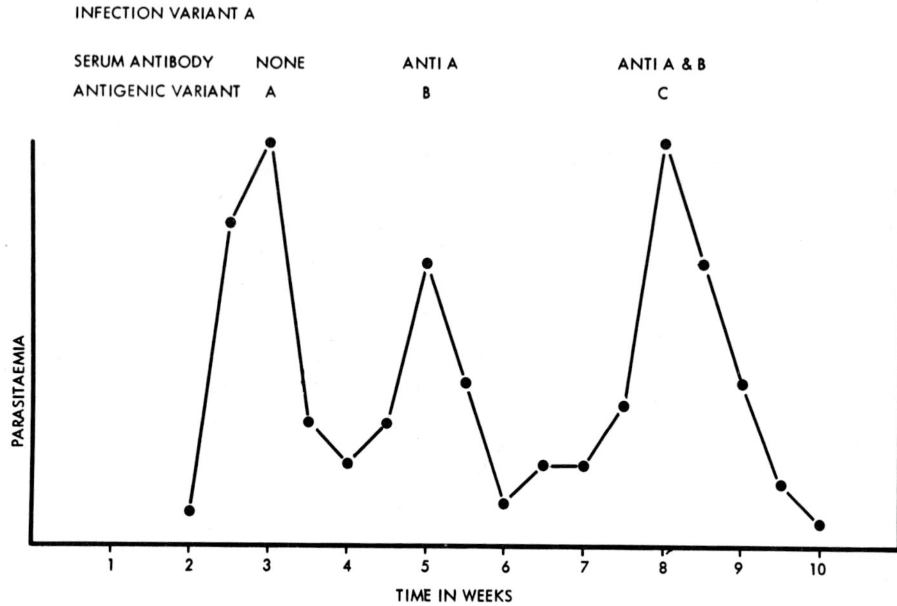

Fig. 2. Diagrammatic course of an experimental infection with *Trypanosoma rhodesiense*.

poor immune response. The mechanism of antigenic variation in trypanosomes and malaria parasites is not known, but "switching" on and off of controlling genes is thought to be more likely than true mutation. An antigenic change can probably be provoked by the formation of antibody to the initial variant and also perhaps by a rise in body temperature.

Antigenic Disguise

Many worms appear impervious to attempts of the host to destroy them, and adult schistosomes are frequently able to live out their natural life-span of up to 30 years unhindered within the portal vein. It has been shown that adult schistosomes are coated with substances that are closely related to blood group antigens of the host. This antigenic disguise appears to protect them from the immune response, because young and immature schistosomules, which do not possess this coat, can be successfully destroyed.

Immunosuppression

The occurrence of a generalized form of cellular or humoral immunosuppression has been demonstrated in viral, protozoal, and some mycoplasmal infections. It has not been clearly established in all cases that this aids the survival of the parasite in its host, but in several conditions such as lepromatous leprosy and chronic mucocutaneous candidiasis there is a specific suppression of immune responsiveness to antigens of the infecting organism which has serious consequences for the host.

In addition there is the group of slow virus infections such as kuru. It is not at present known how they evade or escape the host defence mechanisms, but they somehow manage to replicate and avoid inducing a measurable immune response.

IMMUNOPATHOLOGY OF INFECTIOUS DISEASES

There are now many clinical and experimental examples of damage resulting from the patient's immune response during an infectious disease (Notkins and Koprowski, 1973). The immunopathological mechanisms that between them account for most forms of immunologically mediated tissue injury are described in Chapter 10.

Reaginic Mechanisms

The clinical features are those of histamine release, either generalized anaphylaxis (peripheral circulatory collapse and severe bronchospasm) or local anaphylaxis (urticarial rashes, asthma, and diarrhoea). Helminth infections often provoke reaginic reactions, and the formation of large amounts of IgE is characteristic of many worm infestations. Collapse following rupture of a hydatid cyst during surgical removal is an example of a generalized anaphylactic reaction. Urticaria may occur in patients with various worm infections, and asthma may occur in patients with hookworm, ascaris, or strongyloides infections at the time of larval migrations through the lungs. Patients with pulmonary eosinophilia have high levels of serum IgE, and a reaginic reaction to microfilariae within the pulmonary circulation perhaps plays a part in the immunopathology of this disease. Destruction of a parasite by effective therapy may release large amounts of antigen and lead to development of a severe reaginic reaction. An example is the Mazzotti reaction of itching and iritis that may follow the start of diethylcarbamazine therapy for onchocerciasis.

The detailed role of infections in local anaphylactic reactions such as asthma and hay fever has yet to be determined, but there exists a considerable body of clinical literature suggesting that some forms of asthma and hay fever are related to antigens derived from bacteria, and vaccines are available commercially for use in these conditions. Reagins may also be involved in the pathophysiology of diarrhoea and sprue-like syndromes that result from gastrointestinal infections.

Tissue infiltration with eosinophils is a common finding in reaginic antibody reactions, and eosinophilia is a frequent accompaniment of infections giving rise to this type of antibody. The effect of eosinophilia remains uncertain but eosinophils can inactivate slow-reacting substance, suggesting that they may have a modulating effect on the severity of reaginic reactions.

Membrane-reactive Antibodies

Examples of membrane-reactive antibody mechanisms in the clinical immunology of infectious diseases are the Coombs' positive haemolytic anaemias due to anti-I auto-antibodies found in some *Mycoplasma pneumoniae* infections. Another type of cytotoxicity sometimes occurs in virus infections. Virus-infected cells expose certain antigens that are coded by the viral genome, and antibodies to either the virus or the virus-directed antigens are capable of cytotoxic reactions toward the cells that bear the virus, or virus-directed antigens. Such reactions generate immunopathological damage apart from the cytopathogenic effects of the virus itself (Allison *et al.*, 1972).

Antibodies in the blood directed toward microorganisms may invoke enhancement. The binding of enhancing antibodies to antigens on the surface of a microorganism tends to protect the organism from subsequent damage by sensitized lymphocytes.

It has also been suggested that certain antibodies and complement may have a stimulating as well as an enhancing or cytotoxic effect on certain cells, resulting in excessive metabolic activity. This may account for the proliferative effect of certain encephalitogenic viruses or for the destruction of normal liver cells that is seen in proliferative cirrhosis. This type of immunostimulation increases the rates of both cellular proliferation and the secretion of cell products in fibroblasts (Faulk and Temple, 1975).

Immune Complexes

Immune complexes have been shown to play a part in the immunopathology of many infectious diseases and some examples will now be considered.

Erythema nodosum leprosum is an immune complex type of reaction to antigens from leprosy bacilli present in high concentration in the affected areas of the skin. Also, the allergic complications of meningococcal disease are probably due to an immune complex reaction to meningococcal polysaccharide trapped in the skin and synovial tissues. The relationship between the clinical features and immunological findings in a patient with meningococcal disease developing allergic complications is shown in Fig. 3.

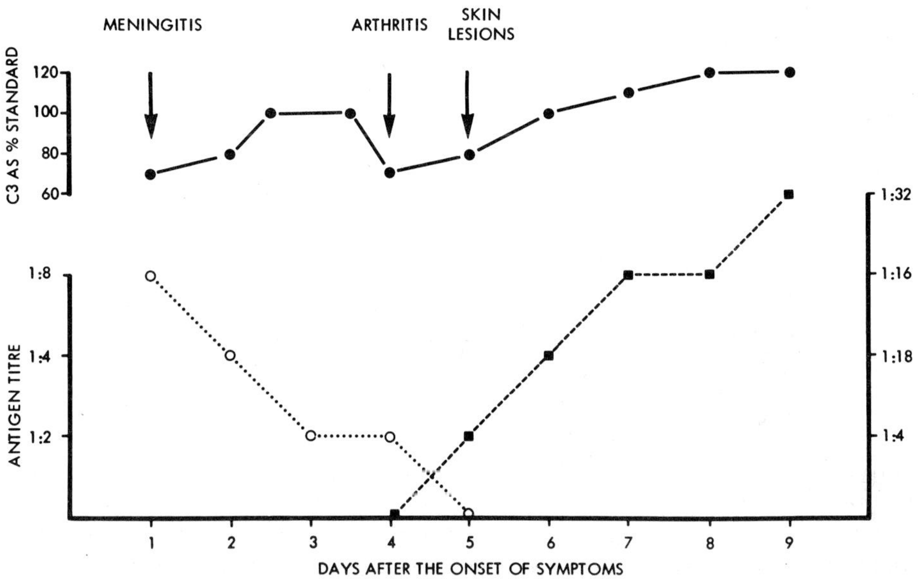

Fig. 3. Serological and clinical findings in a patient with meningococcal meningitis who developed allergic complications. These are seen in about 10% of patients with this infection.

An example of immune complex reaction to virus is seen in children who have received killed measles vaccine and subsequently develop local swelling and erythema when given live, attenuated vaccine. Children who have received such vaccine and who later sustain a natural measles infection sometimes experience more generalized and potentially dangerous disease with atypical skin lesions, pneumonia, oedema, and high fever. A similar phenomenon has been reported in respiratory syncytial virus (RSV) disease. This is seen with greater frequency and intensity in infants who have received transplacental antibody than in infants born of non-immune mothers. Also, natural disease with RSV is qualitatively and quantitatively more serious in infants who have received killed RSV vaccine than in unvaccinated controls. These examples show that high-titre circulating serum antibody may not always work to the advantage of the host.

Patients with serum sickness or immune complex disease have soluble immune complexes in their circulation that are eventually deposited in tissues, especially the kidneys, where they tend to provoke an inflammatory reaction. This mechanism is responsible for the nephritis of systemic lupus erythematosus, a disease possibly of viral origin. Such renal foci of inflammation occur during several infectious diseases including subacute bacterial endocarditis, some streptococcal infections, serum hepatitis, infectious mononucleosis, syphilis, typhoid, schistosomiasis and malaria. Glomerulonephritis following *P. malariae* infection is a major cause of childhood renal disease in tropical Africa (Adeniyi *et al.*, 1972). This form of immunopathology can be identified in renal biopsies as a "granular" pattern of immunoglobulins on the basement membrane by immunofluorescence, and as a "lumpy-bumpy" pattern in the electron microscope (see Chapter 17).

The formation of circulating immune complexes with consequent activation of the complement and kinin pathways is thought to play a role in the peripheral circulatory collapse and disseminated intravascular coagulation seen in haemorrhagic dengue fever. This syndrome is seen most frequently in patients who have been sensitized by previous exposure to a dengue virus of a different but related sero-group. Renal biopsies show the expected granular pattern of immunoglobulin staining by immunofluorescence, and complement break-down products are found in the sera. Similar events may account for the peripheral circulatory collapse sometimes seen in acute *P. falciparum* malaria.

Opportunities for immune complex formation occur in a wide variety of infections, and a great deal more needs to be known about the factors that influence its effects. In many instances only a small proportion of infected patients develop allergic complications, perhaps 10% in meningococcal meningitis (Fig. 3) and less than 1% in *P. malariae* infections. What determines this? Is the propensity to develop allergic complications related to the type of antibody, e.g. low affinity antibody? Are genetic factors involved? What determines whether the tissue damage produced is transitory, the common result in meningococcal infection, or persistent, as in most children with *P. malariae* nephritis? Answers to these questions may also help understanding of the pathogenesis of diseases such as systemic lupus erythematosus and rheumatoid arthritis where the nature of the initiating antigen or antigens is unknown.

Cellular Mechanisms

Contact between an infectious agent, or its products, and specifically sensitized T-lymphocytes may initiate reactions in which the organism is destroyed by the direct action of cytotoxic T-lymphocytes or by lymphokine activated macrophages. If the organism is an intracellular parasite its death is usually achieved at the cost of destruction of the host cell. Thus a cell mediated immune response to an infectious agent can play an important part in the pathogenesis of the tissue damage associated with that infection.

The granulomatous lesion of tuberculosis is an example. Patients with this disease usually develop a strong cell mediated immune reaction to products of the tubercle bacillus readily demonstrable by the tuberculin skin test. This strong cell mediated immune reaction can cause damage to host tissues. The characteristic caseating granulomatous lesion of pulmonary tuberculosis is probably produced by the combined toxic action of the tubercle bacillus itself and the immune response of the host. It is often difficult to detect tubercle bacilli in the pleural fluid of patients with tuberculous pleural effusions and an allergic reaction is thought to play an important part in the pathogenesis of this condition. Similar changes occur in the systemic mycoses.

Leprosy is another condition in which cellular mechanisms contribute to the clinical features of the disease. Patients with tuberculoid leprosy have strong cell mediated immunity to the leprosy bacillus and are eventually able to destroy it. However this is achieved only at the cost of extensive damage to the peripheral nerves. In contrast, patients with little cell mediated immunity to the organism (lepromatous leprosy) have less nerve damage but may succumb as a result of widespread and uncontrolled dissemination of the leprosy bacillus.

Lymphocytic infiltration of the brain is a prominent feature of many human viral encephalitides. In these infections it is probable that a cellular reaction to the virus contributes to destruction of host brain cells. In experimental viral encephalitides it has proved possible to diminish brain damage by depletion of T-lymphocytes by thymectomy or anti-lymphocyte serum.

Whilst there is no doubt that the immune response of the host contributes to the pathology of many infectious diseases, it is not always clear which mechanisms of immune tissue damage are involved, and it is likely that in many cases several are occurring together. In some infections immunological changes are found which do not fit into any of the recognized categories of immune tissue damaging mechanisms. Examples are the excessive immunoglobulin production in patients with African trypanosomiasis, the production of auto-antibodies by patients with parasitic infections, and the occurrence of immunosuppression in many viral infections. Malaria-induced immunosuppression has been implicated in the pathogenesis of Burkitt's lymphoma, and virally induced immunosuppression may play a role in the production of other tumours.

Extensive knowledge of immunopathology has not always led to clear understanding of pathogenesis. For example, the pathogenesis of rheumatic fever remains essentially unknown, despite the demonstration of heart antibodies and of serological cross-reactions between streptococcal and heart antigens and the significance of anti-measles antibodies in subacute sclerosing panencephalitis is similarly in doubt.

IMMUNODIAGNOSIS IN INFECTIOUS DISEASES

Laboratory Tests

Immunoglobulin Quantitation

Quantitative Ig determinations have particular relevance to the problems of intrauterine and neonatal infections (Alford *et al.*, 1975). The foetus and neonate are protected from many infections by maternal IgG acquired by trans-placental passage, but foetal and/or neonatal IgM may be made in response to an infection, and the measurement of IgM in the baby is thus a reasonable indication of whether or not infection has occurred. Children with congenital rubella have elevated IgM (and IgA) in the cord blood, and maintain elevated IgM levels in their blood for several months or years. Elevated cord blood IgM values are found as a consequence of other intra-uterine infections including cytomegalic inclusion disease, toxoplasmosis, and syphilis. A laboratory report of elevated cord IgM may thus confirm the general clinical impression of an intra-uterine infection, and the clinician is then faced with the need for specific antibody identification in order to establish a definitive diagnosis.

Diagnosis of the advanced stage of sleeping sickness can often be made by the detection of trypanosomes in the cerebrospinal fluid (CSF), but in some patients trypanosomes cannot be found. Detection of a markedly raised CSF IgM level in these patients is a valuable diagnostic aid since very large amounts of IgM are found within the central nervous system in the advanced stage of the disease.

Complement Determinations

Changes in total serum complement, measured by haemolytic assay, and in levels of individual complement components occur in many infections but are of limited value in diagnosis. Low levels of total haemolytic complement and of individual components, especially C3, are seen in many infectious diseases including post-streptococcal glomerulonephritis, bacterial endocarditis, gram-negative septicaemia, meningococcal septicaemia, malaria, trypanosomiasis and serum hepatitis. Conversely in typhoid fever and streptococcal skin infections serum complement levels are raised. In infections associated with the release of endotoxin, such as *E. coli* and meningococcal septicaemia, alternative pathway complement components are depressed more markedly than C1 and C4. Conversely when complement activation is due to immune complex formation, for example in malaria, C1 and C4 levels are markedly depressed.

Formation of immune complexes may lead to activation of the classical pathway of complement fixation, and organisms producing endotoxin, such as *E. coli* and the meningococcus, can activate the complement system by means of the alternative pathway (see Chapter 7).

There is a characteristic fluctuation in the serum levels of C3 in patients with acute viral hepatitis, and reductions in blood levels of practically all of the complement components except C4 have been reported in children with protein–calorie malnutrition.

Complement components are sometimes identifiable by immunofluorescence along with immunoglobulins and *P. malariae* antigen in renal biopsies from patients with malarial nephrosis. Similar findings have been reported in post-streptococcal glomerulonephritis, the renal lesion in dengue haemorrhagic fever, and in schistosomiasis. This indicates that components of complement participate in the pathogenesis of some of the nephropathies of infectious disease.

Antibody Measurements

Caution should be exercised in the assessment of antibody tests for infection. The significance of a raised antibody titre must be considered in the light of the rest of the clinical picture. For instance, a raised titre of brucella antibody in a suburban housewife with an unexplained fever would be a stronger indication of the presence of active brucellosis than the detection of a similar titre in the serum of a dairy worker. Similar caution and common sense is needed in the interpretation of results for the so-called febrile agglutinins in the evaluation of a fever of unknown origin. In these instances the history and physical examination are of central importance.

The diagnostic efficiency of antibody determinations can be increased in two ways. Detection of an increased antibody titre in convalescent serum compared with serum taken during the acute phase of the infection is strong evidence for the presence of an active infection. Examples of this are virus neutralization and haemagglutination procedures for anti-rhinovirus antibodies in sera from patients with common cold infections and immunized baboons as shown in Table 3. A retrospective diagnosis made in this way is of value in providing epidemiological data and in providing a definitive diagnosis, but is of little help to the clinician in deciding the clinical management of the patient during the acute phase of his illness. Determination of antibody class can also help to differentiate between active and previous infection, the

TABLE 3

Virus neutralizing and haemagglutinating titres in acute and convalescent paired sera in natural and induced active immunity to common cold viruses

Patient	Rhino-virus isolated	Virus neutralizing titre			Haemagglutinating titre	
		Acute	Convalescent	TCD_{50} in test	Acute	Convalescent
1	RV 14	4	32	1250	2	4
2	RV 14	4	8	500	2	2
3	RV 14	4	16	10	4	8
4	RV 14	4	6	100	2	2
5	RV 17	4	4	250	8	128
6	RV 17	8	128	50	32	128
Baboon 1	RV 14	2	25,600	100	2	1,056
Baboon 2	RV 17	2	3,200	100	2	512

The viruses used to coat the test erythrocytes for HA were isolated from nasopharyngeal swabs, and viral coating of the red cells was done with chromic chloride. The first baboon was immunized with RV 14 and the second with RV 17. TCD is tissue culture dose. Data taken from Faulk *et al.* (1971).

presence of a high titre of IgM antibody usually indicating a primary immune response and thus suggesting an active infection.

This approach has proved particularly valuable in the management of mothers who develop a rubella-like rash or who are exposed to rubella infection during pregnancy. Because of the high risk of congenital malformations following intra-uterine rubella infection, especially early in gestation, many mothers contracting rubella infection during pregnancy will wish to have an abortion. Definitive diagnosis of rubella infection is therefore essential. If no anti-rubella antibodies are found in the serum of the mother it is unlikely that she has been infected and this becomes almost certain if a second test repeated two weeks later is also negative. Detection of a raised antibody level indicates rubella infection but cannot differentiate between an active and a previous infection. If it can be shown by mercaptoethanol reduction, immunofluorescence, or gel filtration on agarose that most of the maternal anti-rubella antibody belongs to the IgM class it is likely that active infection is present, especially if there is a rising titre, and abortion may be indicated.

Many different immunological systems have been used to detect antibodies. Some of these are unique to the disease in question, such as the dye test of Sabin and Feldman for toxoplasmosis, but most tests involve standard immunological procedures such as precipitation in agar (e.g. in malaria as shown in Fig. 4), haemagglutination of antigen coated cells, agglutination of antigen-linked particles, agglutination of bacteria, or complement fixation. Immunofluorescence is particularly useful (Faulk and Hijmans, 1972) in that antibody identification can be made on intact organisms (e.g. trypanosomes), intracellular parasites (e.g. plasmodium-infected, fixed cells), or microbiological antigens coupled to carrier particles (e.g. membrane coupled viruses) as demonstrated in Fig. 5. Other tests employ biological assays such as the neutralization of viruses and bacterial toxins. Enzyme linked immunosorbent techniques are a promising new way for measuring antibodies to infectious agents that may be especially valuable in screening large numbers of sera collected during epidemiological surveys. Immediate type hypersensitivity skin tests can be used to detect the presence of reaginic antibodies.

For most infections antibody can be satisfactorily assayed by several of these systems. The type of test most frequently used in any infection is often a reflection of tradition rather than of intrinsic merit. It should however be mentioned that different immunoglobulins have different biological properties, and that different immunodiagnostic procedures are often designed to test for these specialized properties. For instance, some antibodies haemag-

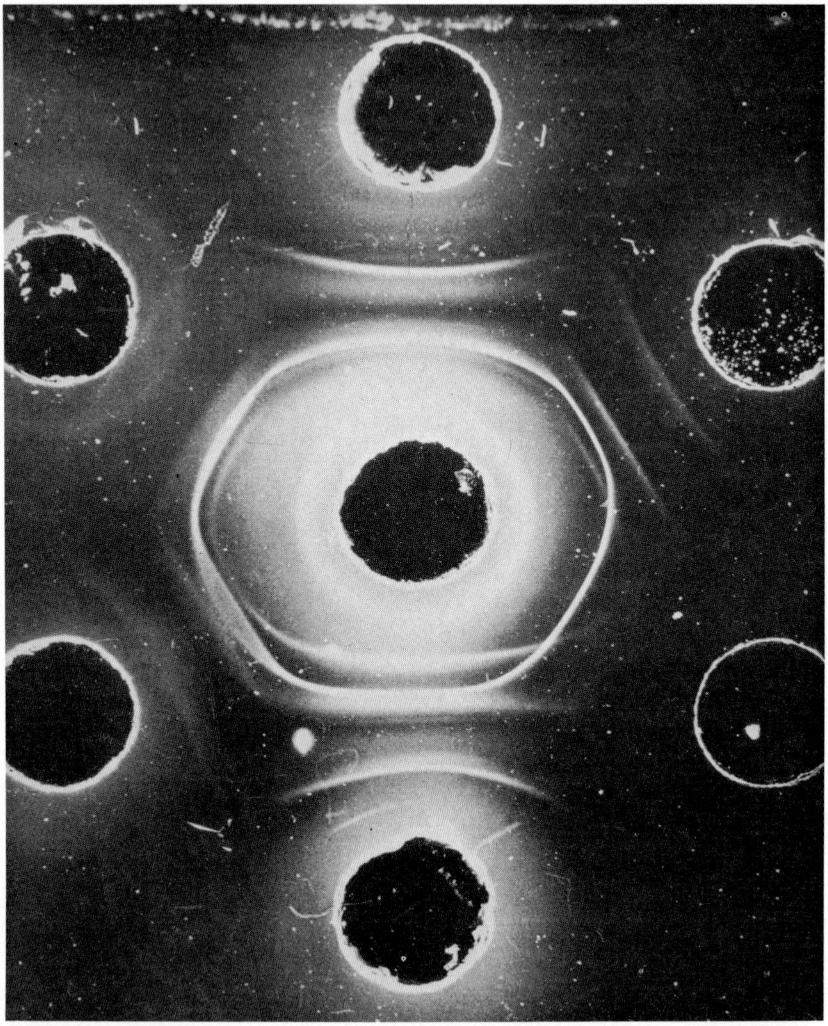

Fig. 4. Ouchterlony precipitation reactions in agar gel of human anti-plasmodial antibodies with plasmodial antigens. Sera from six patients with malaria in outside wells. *P. falciparum* antigens prepared from infected human placentae in centre well. Note that some antibodies show a continuous precipitation line of identity, while others are unique to individual patients.

glutinate very efficiently but are difficult to measure by complement fixation or by immunofluorescence.

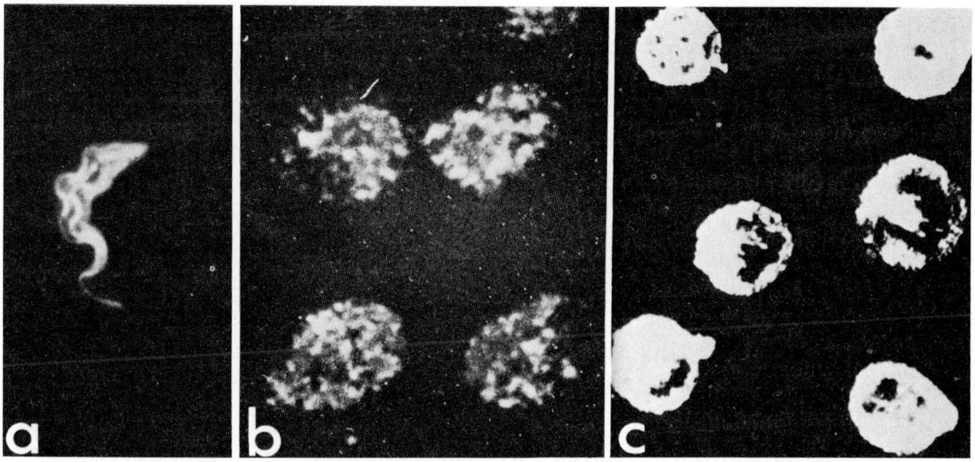

Fig. 5. Several different antigen preparations for immunofluorescence used in the immunodiagnosis of infectious diseases. Intact trypanosomes (a), intracellular malaria parasites (b), and membrane-coupled rhinoviruses (c) are examples of microorganisms that can be used as substrate for rapid diagnosis by immunofluorescence.

Most serological tests depend upon detection of antibody formed to an antigenic component or product of the invading organism. However, in some tests the antigen employed is derived from another source unrelated to the causative organism. Examples of these specifically reacting irrelevant antibodies are the antibody to beef heart detected in the Wasserman reaction, the antibodies agglutinating certain strains of Proteus bacteria formed in rickettsial infections, the anti-I cold agglutinins found in mycoplasma infections, the heterophile antibodies of infectious mononucleosis, and anti-T antibodies responsible for the panagglutination phenomenon sometimes seen in serious clostridial infections. These antibodies are usually found only in association with specific infections. Another group of specifically-reacting irrelevant antibodies occurs in a wide variety of infectious diseases, and their diagnostic usefulness is thereby diminished. Examples are rheumatoid factors and other antiglobulins, antinuclear antibodies, and cryoglobulins. Some infections give rise to other specific auto-antibodies such as the anti-smooth muscle antibodies often found in viral hepatitis and infectious mononucleosis.

Detection of Antigen

Detection of a component of an infective agent in a biological fluid is an accurate method of immunodiagnosis, for, unlike tests involving measurement of antibody, it indicates the presence of active or recent infection. The demonstration of polysaccharide antigens in the CSF of patients with pyogenic meningitis by means of a capillary tube precipitation assay was formerly used as a diagnostic test. Little interest was shown in immunodiagnosis by antigen detection until the discovery that the presence of Australia antigen in the serum was an accurate marker of infection by the serum hepatitis virus. Microbial antigen detection is now used to diagnose serum hepatitis, arborvirus infections, pneumococcal pneumonia, variola, cryptococcal meningitis and pyogenic meningitis. The success of this technique in establishing a diagnosis in patients with pyogenic meningitis is due partly to the fact that, unlike conventional bacteriology, the result is not influenced by prior administration of antibiotics.

Many antigens released during bacterial and viral infections are negatively charged and can be detected by counter-current immunoelectrophoresis, and this technique has been widely used for detecting microbial antigens. This and other methods including radioimmunoassay have been used for detecting Australia antigen.

Skin Tests

Skin tests are widely used in the immunodiagnosis of infectious diseases. Any of the clinical hypersensitivity reactions discussed above can be elicited in skin tests. For instance, the injection of pneumococcal polysaccharide antigen can give immune complex reactions in patients convalescent from pneumonia, and complement-independent enhancing antibodies may block the skin manifestations of delayed hypersensitivity. The type of reaction can often be determined by observation of the time-lag involved. Reaginic reactions usually occur within 10–20 minutes (e.g. the Casoni test for hydatid disease). Arthrus or immune complex reactions in 4–8 hours, and cellular reactions in 48–72 hours. Skin test procedures used in some infectious diseases are listed in Tables 4 and 5.

The tuberculin reaction is the best known and most widely studied form of delayed hypersensitivity and is a clinically acceptable measure of cell-mediated immunity. It is absent in children with T-cell deficiencies, and may also be lacking in conditions such as sarcoidosis, viral infections, certain

TABLE 4
Immediate type skin tests for infectious diseases

Disease or organism	Comments
Aspergillosis	(a) Patient may show immediate reaction only or a dual reaction consisting of an immediate reaction followed by an Arthus reaction (b) Positive in some patients with asthma due to aspergillosis
Hydatid disease (Casoni test)	(a) False positives common (b) Can cross-react with *Taenia saginata* and *Schistosoma mansoni* (c) May show a delayed type reaction
Filariasis Paragonomiasis	(a) Wide cross-reactions between different worm infections
Trichinosis	(a) Many false-positive and false-negative reactions (b) May show a delayed type reaction in 24–48 hr of 10–30 mm induration
Visceral larva migrans	(a) Test may remain positive for years after infection (b) Antigens of some Toxocara and Ascaris species may cross-react

forms of cancer, and in malnutrition. The role of malnutrition is particularly important. Many chronic infections such as tuberculosis lead to severe protein malnutrition and a resulting loss of delayed hypersensitivity reactions. This is the probable explanation for a recent finding in West Africa that 67% of the patients with proven pulmonary tuberculosis are tuberculin negative.

The tuberculin reaction is a useful diagnostic tool for tuberculosis, and many physicians feel that the conversion of a negative test to a positive reaction is adequate justification for anti-tuberculosis therapy except, of course, where BCG vaccination has been given.

Tests of Lymphocyte Function

A number of tests of T-cell function have been applied to patients with infectious diseases but at present these have been of more value in assessing pathological mechanisms that as an aid to diagnosis. One of the most commonly used techniques to measure T-cell numbers is the *in vitro* formation of spontaneous rosettes with sheep erythrocytes (see Chapter 3). The number of rosette forming cells is depressed in some chronic infections, such as lepromatous leprosy, and it is interesting that in this disease the number of B-cells is normal or elevated. The response to PHA is probably one of the

TABLE 5
Skin test antigens used for assessing delayed hypersensitivity in infectious diseases

Disease or organism	Name of antigen or test	Time of reaction, hr[a,b]
Blastomycosis	blastomycin	24–48
Brucellosis	brucellin	24–48
Candidiasis	candidin	24
Cat scratch	(footnote [e])	48
Coccidioidomycosis	coccidioidin	24–48
Histoplasmosis[c]	histoplasmin	24–48
Leishmaniasis	Montenegro test	24–48
Leprosy	lepromin (Mitsuda)	48 (Fernandez reaction) 4–5 weeks (Mitsuda reaction)
Lymphogranuloma venereum	Frei test	24
Mycobacteria		
M. tuberculosis	purified protein derivative (PPD)[d]	24–48
Atypical mycobacteria	PPD–A, PPD–B PPD–G, PPD–Y	24–48
Mumps	mumps antigen	24
Syphilis	luetin	24–48
Toxoplasmosis	toxoplasmin	24
Trichophyton mentagraphytes	trichophyton	24–48

[a] Evaluation of the skin test site should be made at 10–20 min and 2–6 hr, since strong immediate hypersensitivity reactions may interfere with interpretation of the delayed response.

[b] The absence of skin test reactivity in patients with minimal or histologically diagnosed disease (e.g., coccidioidomycosis, lepromatous leprosy, brucellosis, disseminated tuberculosis) is of prognostic value. However, skin tests may be negative in patients with active disseminated disease (e.g., coccidioidomycosis, lepromatous leprosy, brucellosis, miliary tuberculosis, leishmaniasis), probably indicating defective cell-mediated immunity at the stage of the illness. Malnourished patients may also have negative skin tests.

[c] Blood for serological analysis must be drawn before the skin test is applied.

[d] Tween-stabilized PPD should be used; alternatively, if test is performed with material that needs to be reconstituted it must be used within 30–60 min.

[e] Made from heat treated suspension of infected lymph nodes or pus.

most widely used *in vitro* metabolic tests for T-cells. Responses to PHA are depressed in several infections, including measles, congenital rubella, primary syphilis, and leprosy. It is also depressed in malnutrition. The PHA response is usually normal in tuberculoid leprosy but depressed in lepromatous leprosy.

T-cell activity may be measured by the response to specific microbiological or cell-membrane antigens based on incorporation of radiolabelled thymidine. This technique has been used with bacterial, viral and parasitic antigens, and also with cell-membrane-associated viral antigens. The complexity of tests of this type has precluded their widespread use as a diagnostic tool. However, recent simplifications of techniques such as lymphocyte transformation may allow their wider use in the future. Some success has already been achieved in determining the presence of subclinical leprosy infection (Godal and Negassi, 1973).

Tests for Phagocytic Function

These are discussed in Chapter 8.

THE ROLE OF IMMUNODIAGNOSIS

The clinical immunologist can help in the diagnosis and management of infectious diseases in several ways. He may be able to establish a diagnosis in a patient presenting a difficult clinical problem, such as a prolonged fever of uncertain origin; he may be able to determine the prevalence of a specific infection within a community, or he may be able to explain why a particular patient has succumbed to an infection, perhaps with a usually non-pathogenic organism.

One of the most important services to the community that he offers is in public health and preventive medicine. Immunological tests can indicate the prevalence of an infectious disease within a community. Although most tests will be unable to differentiate between active and past infection, information derived in this way may be of considerable value in planning public health measures. A few examples of the way in which immunodiagnosis may guide preventive health measures follow.

Skin testing of a community with PPD gives an indication of the prevalence of tuberculosis in that community, and analysis of the age related prevalence rate will indicate at which age infection is occurring. This information helps to establish the importance of tuberculosis as a cause of ill-health in the community, the need for a preventive service, and the age at which BCG vaccination should be given. Immunodiagnosis has also been used successfully at the community level in assessing the effectiveness of control campaigns against infectious diseases, e.g. a fall in serum IgM and anti-malarial antibody levels has been shown to follow successful malaria control.

Immunodiagnosis also has an important role to play in screening selected groups in the community who are particularly at risk of developing an infectious disease or who, if infected, are a hazard to others. Screening of pregnant mothers for syphilis has almost abolished congenital syphilis in many countries. More recently the introduction of screening of blood donors for Australia antigen has helped to reduce the incidence of post-transfusion hepatitis. Selective screening has proved of value in controlling rubella infections. Neonates with congenital rubella tend to shed infectious virus for several weeks or months and are a hazard to any pregnant members of the female attendant staff. This danger can be circumvented by screening nurses for anti-rubella antibodies and either immunizing those who are found to be non-immune or prohibiting non-immune nurses from working in the newborn nursery.

IMMUNOTHERAPY OF INFECTIOUS DISEASES

Before the discovery of antibiotics, serum therapy was the only effective form of treatment for several important human infections such as pneumococcal pneumonia and cerebrospinal fever. The major successes of antibiotics led to the abandonment of serum therapy, but during the past few years increasing attention has again been directed to the possibility of treating some infectious diseases by modulating the immune response of the host.

Blood Transfusion

It has long been a clinical impression that patients with a variety of infections benefit from transfusions of fresh blood. This beneficial effect could be due to passive transfer of antibody, lymphocytes or phagocytic cells, or to an effect on the nutritional state of the patient. Today the tendency is to use individual blood components rather than whole blood in the immunotherapy of infectious diseases. For instance, intravenous infusion of leukocytes from normal donors have been successfully used in the treatment of leprosy patients, and transfusions of fresh plasma to Wiscott–Aldrich patients improves their ability to resist infection.

Serum Therapy

Specific antisera are still used in the treatment of tetanus, botulism, generalized vaccinia and gas-gangrene, although, antisera are often ineffective in the treatment of tetanus and botulism if the toxins have fixed to tissues by the time the antisera are given. Serum has been used recently with apparent success in the treatment of Lassa fever, a viral disease with high mortality for which no other effective form of treatment is known.

Antiserum for immunotherapy is obtained by immunization of animals or human volunteers, or by collection of serum from a patient who has recovered from the infection. Horse antiserum, sometimes used in the treatment of tetanus, may lead to severe anaphylaxis or serum-sickness reactions such as glomerulonephritis. The likelihood of a severe anaphylactic reaction can be reduced by administration of a small subcutaneous test dose before giving the full dose intravenously. If it is essential to give the full dose to positive skin reactors it should be given very slowly with steroid cover. Recently human hyperimmune anti-tetanus serum carrying much less risk of anaphylaxis has become available. Antibody may be given either as whole serum or as purified gamma-globulin. Use of whole serum increases the risk of anaphylaxis but ensures the administration of IgA and IgM antibody which may be present in only small and variable amounts in commercial preparations of gamma-globulin.

In rabies the incubation period is particularly long, theoretically giving enough time for a full course of vaccination following exposure, but the World Health Organization recommends that antiserum be given together with vaccine to patients bitten by a proven rabid animal since there is evidence that the protective effect of giving both is greater than that of vaccine alone. The simultaneous administration of rabies antiserum does not appear to prevent the development of effective active immunity.

Lymphocytes and Transfer Factor

Serum or gamma-globulin therapy is likely to be of little value in the treatment of infections controlled by cell-mediated protective immune reactions. Attempts have therefore been made to influence the outcome in this group of infections by administration of lymphocytes or lymphocyte-derived transfer factor. This form of immunotherapy ought to be particularly successful in the treatment of patients with a defect in cell mediated immunity to the causative organism. A beneficial response to lymphocytes or transfer factor has been reported in several infectious diseases including leprosy, chronic mucocutaneous candidiasis, coccidioidomycosis, generalized vaccinia and hepatitis, but the evidence so far is anecdotal.

Polymorphonuclear Leucocytes

The development of continuous-flow blood cell separators has allowed the preparation of infusions rich in polymorphonuclear leucocytes, and these have been used with success in the treatment of neutropenic patients with infections.

Interferon Inducers

Most bacterial infections respond to antibiotic therapy, but this is of course not so for viruses. Viral replication is inhibited *in vivo* by interferon which de-represses cells and allows them to make an inhibitory protein which associates with cell ribosomes to attract viral mRNA and prevent translation from the polysome thus blocking virus synthesis. This has given rise to the concept of using interferon inducers to control virus infections. Interferon can be induced by double-stranded RNA of viral, bacterial, fungal or synthetic origin, while single-stranded RNA or DNA, or double-stranded DNA are without effect. If these inducers prove to be clinically effective, they may find their best use in diseases in which the multiplicity of antigenic types exceeds the number which could be put into a vaccine, as with the common cold virus.

Immunosuppression

The immune response of the host to an infection may play an important part in producing the clinical features of the disease, and the patient may be helped by treatment aimed at reducing the intensity of the immune response. The use of corticosteroids in the treatment of an acute lepra reaction or in the treatment of acute iritis provoked by treatment of onchocercasis with diethylcarbamazine are examples of such beneficial use of immunosuppression.

IMMUNOPROPHYLAXIS OF INFECTIOUS DISEASES

Immunoprophylaxis is one of the most useful contributions of immunology to clinical medicine. Effective vaccines are now available for the prevention of many infections, but there are still important problems to be solved. Prophylaxis is generally considered in terms of passive and active immunity (Table 6).

TABLE 6
Mechanisms of resistance to infections

Type		Examples
a) Non-specific immunity		Phagocytosis, lysozyme, interferon
b) Specifically acquired immunity:		
Passive	Natural	Maternally derived IgG in baby
	Induced	Protection by homolous or heterologous antibody or gamma globulin
Active	Natural	Exposure to infection
	Induced	Immunization with toxoid, or with killed or attenuated organisms

Passive Immunoprophylaxis

The placental transfer of antibody from mother to foctus provides a natural form of passive protection for neonates for about six months. An induced form of passive protection by antibody is clinically useful in the prevention of several infectious diseases (Table 7). Passive transfer of antibody can achieve only short-lasting immunity, but has proved especially valuable in subjects particularly at risk of infection. For instance, gamma globulin injections are useful in the prevention of bacterial infections in hypogammaglobulinaemia, but are not generally beneficial in other types of primary immunodeficiency states. Patients receiving corticosteroids should be given gamma-globulin if they are exposed to chickenpox, and measles may be prevented or modified if gamma-globulin is given within a few days of exposure. The same is true for polio, but less satisfactory results are obtained with rubella and varicella. The prophylactic administration of gamma-globulin is also of protective value in subjects entering an area of endemic disease to which they have had no or minimal exposure, such as hepatitis. Experience with Peace Corps volunteers has shown that protection from infective hepatitis can be successfully maintained by three-monthly injections of gamma-globulin. Physicians who give gamma-globulin to patients should be aware that they are also immunizing the patients to incompatible immunoglobulin allotypes.

TABLE 7

Conditions in which passive immunoprophylaxis is effective

Condition	Source of antiserum	Indications	Comments
Botulism	Horse	Suspected poisoning	Toxin rapidly bound to tissues. A trivalent antitoxin to types A, B and E now available.
Diphtheria	Horse	Close contact with active case	Given with toxoid
Gas-gangrene	Horse	Patient with a high risk of infection	Most toxin fixed rapidly to the tissues. Polyvalent antitoxin is of doubtful value
Measles	Human	Exposed children with an immune defect	Should be given as soon as possible after exposure
Rabies	Horse	Bites by a rabid animal	Given with vaccine.
Rubella	Human	Exposed pregnant woman	Should be given as soon as possible after exposure
Smallpox	Human	Close contact	
Tetanus	Horse or human	Patient with dirty wounds	Penicillin plus toxoid are an alternative prophylactic

Commercial gamma-globulin solutions contain 12·5–16·5% protein, and most of this is IgG, with small and variable amounts of IgA and IgM (Miller, 1971). Gamma-globulin injections have been recommended for the control of upper respiratory tract infections, but defences against these are dependent on local tissue immunity of mucosal surfaces, and the low amount of IgA (and unknown amounts of IgA–S) in commercial gamma-globulin speak against this as a useful therapeutic measure; and this conclusion is confirmed by clinical experience. Gamma-globulin injections have also been recommended for premature infants and newborns with transient hypogammaglobulinaemia because these babies are at risk of coliform infections, defences against which are dependent on IgM and complement for opsonization and phagocytosis. However, the small amount of IgM (and negligible amounts of complement) in commercial preparation of gamma-globulin do not support the use of gamma-globulin injections in these circumstances.

Active Immunoprophylaxis

Stimulation of active immunity by immunization is a much more satisfactory method of immunoprophylaxis than injectable gamma-globulin therapy, but has the disadvantage that days or weeks must elapse after immunization before effective immunity becomes established. Once achieved however, active immunity is likely to be long-lasting.

Two main types of vaccine are employed, those using killed organisms and those employing attenuated live strains (Edsall, 1975); the latter generally give more effective immunity. The vaccines that are used most frequently in clinical medicine are shown in Table 8. The immunization schedule should conform to the pattern of disease that prevails in the community and should not be determined only according to administrative dogma. Thus, BCG vaccination at secondary school entry may be entirely satisfactory in a temperate country where tuberculosis is rare, but this would be inappropriate in a developing country where most children have suffered a primary infection by their teens. In this situation, BCG will be most effective if given at or shortly after birth. Vaccines may be given by injection or by mouth, and the route of administration is important in determining the efficiency and type of immunity produced. For prevention of gut infections the vaccine must induce local mucosal immunity in the gastrointestinal tract, and this is much more likely to be achieved by an oral vaccine than by a parenteral injection.

Several vaccines occasionally produce serious side effects thus raising ethical problems over their use in a community where the infection in question is uncommon. A situation may be reached, as has occurred in the case of smallpox in the U.K., where more people suffer adverse effects from the vaccine than from the disease, thus creating strong pressures for its abandonment. This will be possible if, as now seems likely, smallpox is soon successfully eradicated in man, for there is no known animal reservoir. In other words, the vaccination schedule adopted in any community requires repeated reassessment in the light of changes in the prevalence of the disease in question throughout the world.

Problems in Immunoprophylaxis

Although progress has been made in the prevention of infectious diseases by immunoprophylaxis, several major problems remain unsolved. No effective vaccines are yet available for many important human infections, especially

TABLE 8

Vaccines used to promote active immunity in man[a]

Vaccine	Status	Vaccine	Status
Adenovirus	L, kf	Pertussis	K, KF, l
Anthrax	KF	Plague	L, K, kf
Botulism	KF	Polio	L, K
Brucella	L, k	Pneumococcus	KF
Chagas' Disease	k	Parainfluenza	k
Cholera	K, kf, l	Pseudomonas	kf
Coccidioidomycosis	k	Q Fever	k
Coli diarrhoea	l, kf	Rabies	L, K, kf
Cytomegalovirus	l	RSV	l, (k)
Dengue	l	Rhinoviruses	k
Diphtheria	KF	RMSF	K
Equine Encephalitis	L	Rubella	L
Gonococal	kf	Russian S. S. Encephalitis	K, l
Hepatitis	kf	Schistosomiasis	K, l
Influenza	KF, l	Shigellosis	L, (k)
Infectious Mononucleosis	kf	Smallpox	L, (k)
Japanese Encephalitis	K, l	Staphylococcus	kf
Leishmaniasis	k	Streptococcus	kf
Leprosy	l	Syphilis	k
Leptospirosis	K	Tetanus	KF
Malaria	k	Trachoma	k
Measles	L	Trypanosomiasis	k
Meningococcus A, C	KF	Tuberculosis	L, kf
Meningococcus B	kf	Tularaemia	L
Mumps	L	Typhoid Fever	K, l
Mycoplasma	l, (k)	Typhus Fever	K, L
Paratyphoid Fever	k	Yellow Fever	L

Key: L = live, K = killed, F = fractionated
Capital letters = usefulness established
Small letters = still in experimental stage
Parentheses = tried but results unsatisfactory

[a]This table has been produced by Professor G. Edsall, Department Microbiology, London School of Hygiene and Tropical Medicine (taken from manuscript to be published). We add the following contra-indications: a) live vaccine should not be given to subjects with leukaemia, lymphoma, primary or acquired immunodeficiency diseases, patients receiving immunosuppressive therapy, or women during the first trimester of pregnancy; b) smallpox vaccination should not be done in subjects with eczema; and c) whooping cough vaccine should not be given to children with a history of convulsions or to children with neurological diseases.

those caused by protozoa and helminths. There have, however, been recent reports of encouraging steps towards the development of an effective malaria vaccine (*British Medical Journal*, 1974).

The difficulties involved in vaccinating a child living in a village many miles from a main road have often resulted in the misuse of labile vaccines that have deteriorated as a consequence of adverse environmental conditions. Difficulties of this kind have led to the apparent failure of measles vaccination campaigns in several countries. This also contributed to the failure of a meningococcal-A vaccine trial in Africa. Further work on the production of more stable vaccines for the prevention of common infections is urgently needed. Stability might be achieved through the development of synthetic vaccines.

Vaccines against infections in which mucosal immunity plays an important part must be able to induce secretory IgA antibody formation. This has been achieved successfully in poliomyelitis by introducing the antigen directly to the mucosal surface, but this has not been so successful with cholera. Present cholera vaccines, which are injected subcutaneously, are relatively ineffective, perhaps because they do not produce local gut immunity. Investigations are currently underway to develop effective oral cholera and typhoid vaccines.

Finally, in some experimental systems the presence or absence of adjuvant, and the type of adjuvant, is of central importance in determining whether immunization will result in cellular or humoral immunity. Since some diseases in man are characterized by cellular immunity (e.g. tuberculosis, measles) and others by humoral immunity (e.g. pneumococcal pneumonia, tetanus) it is of practical value to match each vaccine with an adjuvant appropriate to the type of immunity that is most effective against the disease in question. This seems to be a real possibility in so far as some adjuvants are thought to mobilize T-cells in animals, and such may eventually prove to be the case in man.

REFERENCES

Adeniyi, A., Akingkugbe, O. O., Andres, G. A., Bassily, S., Brunner, T., Edington, G. M., Faulk, W. Page, Goodman, H. C., Hendrikse, R. G., Houba, V., Kibukamusoke, J. W., Milgrom, F., Ogunlesi, T. O., Oyediran, A. B. O. O., Soothill, J. F. and Soyannwo, M. A. O. (1972). Immunopathology of nephritis in Africa. *Clin. Exp. Immunol.* **12**, 291.

Alford, C. A. Jr., Stagno, S. and Reynolds, D. W. (1975). Diagnosis of chronic perinatal infections. *Am. J. Dis. Child.* **129**, 455.

Allison, A. C., Beveridge, W. I. and Cockburn, W. C. (1972). Virus-associated immunopathology: Animal models and implications for human disease (parts 1 and 2). *Bull. W.H.O.* **47**, 257 and 265.

Braun, W. and Ungar, J. (1973). "Non-Specific Factors Influencing Host Resistance". S. Karger, Basel, Munchen, Paris, London.

Ciba Foundation Symposium 25 (1974). Parasites in the Immunised Host: Mechanisms of Survival, (eds. R. Porter and J. Knight) Associated Scientific Publishers, Amsterdam.

Constantopoulos, A., Najjar, V. A., Wish, J. B., Necheles, T. H. and Stolbach, L. L. (1973). Defective phagocytosis due to tuftsin deficiency in splenectomized subjects. *Am. J. Dis. Child.* **125**, 663.

Edsall, G. (1975). *In* "Clinical Aspects of Immunology" 3rd edition, (eds. P. G. H. Gell, R. R. A. Coombs and P. J. Lachmann), p. 1601. Blackwell Scientific Publications, Oxford, London, Edinburgh, Melbourne.

Erickson, W. D., Burgert, E. D. and Lynn, H. B. (1968). The hazard of infection following splenectomy in children. *Am. J. Dis. Child.* **116**, 1.

Faulk, W. Page, Vyas, G. N., Phillips, C. A., Fudenberg, H. H. and Chism, K. (1971). Passive haemagglutination test for anti-rhinovirus antibodies. *Nature, New Biol.* **231**, 101.

Faulk, W. Page and Hijmans, W. (1972). Recent developments in immunofluorescence. *Progr. Allergy* **16**, 9.

Faulk, W. Page and Temple, Anne (1975). Fibroblast immunobiology. *In* "Regulation of Growth and Differentiated Function in Eukaryote Cells", (ed. G. P. Talwar), Raven Press, New York. In press.

Faulk, W. Page, Mata, L. J. and Edsall, G. (1975). Effects of malnutrition on the immune response in humans: A review. *Trop. Dis. Bull.* **72**, 89.

Godal, T. and Negassi, K. (1973). Subclinical infection in leprosy. *Brit. Med. J.* **3**, 557.

Good, R. A. (1975). *In* "Immunodeficiency in Man and Animals", (eds. D. Bergsma, R. A. Good and J. Finstad) Birth Defects: Original Article Series, Vol. XI. No. 1, p. 66. Sinaver Associates, Inc., Sunderland, Mass.

Good, R. A., Finstad, J. and Gatti, R. A. (1970). *In* "Infectious Agents and Host Reactions", (ed. S. Mudd) p. 76. W.B. Saunders Company, Philadelphia, London, Toronto.

Glynn, A. A. (1972). *In* "Microbial Pathogenicity in Man and Animals", (eds. H. Smith and J. H. Pearce), p. 75. Cambridge University Press, Cambridge.

Humphrey, J. H. (1974). The practical and potential contribution of immunology to the problems of developing countries. *J. Trop. Med. Hyg.* **77**, 282.

Leading article (1974). Malaria vaccines on the horizon. *Brit. Med. J.* **1**, 231.

Mackaness, G. B. (1971). Delayed hypersensitivity and the mechanism of cellular resistance to infections. *In* "Progress in Immunology", (ed. B. Amos), p. 413, Academic Press, New York and London.

Miller, M. E. (1971). *In* "Immunobiology", (eds. R. A. Good and D. W. Fisher), p. 280. Sinaver Associates, Inc. Stanford, Connecticut.

Notkins, A. C. and Koprowski, H. (1973). How the immune response to a virus can cause disease. *Scient. Amer.* **228**, 22.

Tomasi, T. B. and Grey, H. M. (1972). Structure and function of immunoglobulin A. *Progr. Allergy* **16**, 81.

Williams, R. C. and Gibbons, R. J. (1972). Inhibition of bacterial adherence by secretory immunoglobulin A: A mechanism of antigen disposal. *Science* **177**, 697.

World Health Organization (1973). Cell-Mediated Immunity and Resistance to Infection. Technical Report Series No. 519.

14

Immunodeficiency

A. D. B. WEBSTER

Many believe that various deficiencies in the immune system account for most of the immunopathology seen in human disease. The formation of soluble immune complexes may follow the production of low affinity antibody, systemic lupus erythematosus may be caused by a failure to deal with a particular virus and allergy by a failure to "neutralize" potential antigens. In this chapter I shall discuss only conditions where a demonstrable immune defect leads to recurrent and often life-threatening infections.

The success of gammaglobulin replacement therapy has provided the clinical immunologist with an incentive to screen all patients with recurrent infections for defects in antibody production. Many such patients can be diagnosed with ease but others may have subtle, and as yet poorly understood, defects. The penalties for missing the diagnosis may be high and it is not uncommon for patients to be referred for diagnosis when they have already developed irreversible lung damage due to chronic infection. It is also important to realize that primary antibody deficiency can occur at any age and is not, as was initially thought, predominantly confined to paediatric practice. Antibody deficiency may also occur as a secondary phenomenon in a number of diseases, particularly the lymphoid malignancies. Greater awareness of such problems may improve the prognosis in such patients.

The clinical significance of defects in cell mediated immunity (CMI) are still poorly understood. Isolated primary defects in CMI are exceptionally rare and only occur in infants and children. Unfortunately, studies on such children have not clarified the role of CMI in host defence. Secondary CMI defects are associated with a variety of infections and chronic inflammatory disorders but do not appear to have much clinical significance.

The physician should always bear in mind the possibility of a neutrophil polymorph or complement defect in patients, particularly children, who present with recurrent infections. Such defects are rare but some are amenable to treatment.

The various tests of immune function which are appropriate for an immune deficiency referral laboratory are enumerated below and form the basis for a classification of immune deficiency disorders that is still far from satisfactory.

DIAGNOSIS OF DEFECTS IN ANTIBODY PRODUCTION

Serum Immunoglobulin Concentrations

A severe defect in antibody production usually leads to hypogammaglobulinaemia. Most of these patients have a low concentration of total serum globulin and can be diagnosed by the simple technique of quantitative serum protein electrophoresis. However, this will not detect those with isolated immunoglobulin class defects or with border line levels of one or more classes. It is, therefore, necessary to screen all patients with suspected immunodeficiency by measuring the serum concentrations of the three main classes of immunoglobulin, IgG, IgA and IgM. This is easily performed by standard Mancini immunodiffusion techniques. Automated nephelometric methods have recently become popular but are only suitable for measuring IgG and IgA. There is some controversy at present as to how immunoglobulin concentrations should be expressed (see Chapter 4). There is no doubt that, for accuracy, they should be expressed in International Units/ml but many tend to prefer results converted to mg/100 ml. This problem has arisen because different laboratories have failed to agree on an absolute weight for the International Unit. Measurement of serum IgE and IgD concentrations may be of interest but are not diagnostically useful in this context.

Patients who are clearly hypogammaglobulinaemic need no further investigations except to exclude the presence of hypercatabolism or increased loss of gammaglobulin from the kidneys or gut. In practice, the great majority of patients with severe panhypogammaglobulinaemia have a primary defect in immunoglobulin production. In the absence of nephrosis, a sensible policy is to treat such patients with regular gamma-globulin injections. Further investigations are then indicated if adequate levels of serum IgG are not maintained. It should be remembered that patients with primary hypogammaglobulinaemia may also develop a protein losing enteropathy. This possibility can be tested by injecting I^{125} labelled IgG intravenously and measuring the half life. There are no direct methods for detecting loss of IgG from the gut but the associated albumin loss can be assessed by ^{51}Cr labelled albumin clearance in the stools.

Tests for Functional Antibody

Patients with recurrent infections and normal serum immunoglobulin levels should be screened for IgG subclass defects and further tests performed to clarify whether they can make functional antibody. A defect should be suspected if the serum level of IgG or IgM is bordering on the lower limit of normal in the face of recurrent infections. Useful screening tests in this situation are measurements of serum "natural" antibodies such as isohaemagglutinins and *E. coli* antibodies. The presence of serum isohaemaggluttinins indicates ability to produce functional IgM antibody. However, the titre range of anti-A and anti-B antibodies in the normal population is wide and only total absence is significant. On the other hand, antibodies to *E. coli* bacteria commensal in the gut are present in a reasonably high titre in all healthy children and adults. These are easily measured by a standard haemagglutination technique, the antigen being a pooled polysaccharide preparation from six or more common commensal *E. coli* serotypes (Webster *et al.*, 1974). The antibodies again tend to be IgM and it is often not possible to obtain specific information about IgG antibody production from this test.

Test Immunization

The next step is to proceed with test immunization. There are theoretical advantages in choosing antigens to which the subject has not previously been sensitized (primary antigens), but this leads to ethical difficulties in choosing safe antigens for human use. One such antigen, phage ϕX174 gives high IgG and IgM responses and is now generally accepted as safe (Peacock *et al.*, 1973). This DNA virus replicates only in a specific serotype of *E. coli* and does not induce anti DNA antibodies in humans. Well over a thousand immunizations have now been performed with this agent and no complications have arisen. Other protein antigens which have been used as primary immunogens are keyhole limpet haemocyanin and the flagella antigen from *Salmonella adelaide* (flagellin). The former is difficult to purify and the latter may not be a true primary antigen. Animal work has shown that proteins induce an antibody response requiring T-lymphocyte help and such antigens are considered as thymus dependent. On the other hand, polysaccharide antigens are thought to be T-cell independent. There is, therefore, good reason for immunizing with both a polysaccharide and a protein antigen since some patients may show a discrepancy between the two responses. Polysaccharides produce prolonged antibody responses in humans, and usually no secondary response can be elicited after a further injection six to eight weeks later. This type of "tolerance" is similar to that found in animals and the mechanism is debated. Synthetic polysaccharides such as levans and dextrans have been used as immunogens in humans but this should be discouraged in view of the possibility of inducing sensitization to a preparation which is often used in clinical practice as a plasma substitute. Although purified bacterial polysaccharides are not yet commercially available in Britain for immunization purposes, they are probably the safest preparations to use and may even offer some benefit to patients.

Secretory Immunoglobulins

IgA is the predominant immunoglobulin in secretions although, in its absence, IgM and, to a lesser extent, IgG may compensate. Both IgA and IgM can bind secretory piece which probably renders the molecule less susceptible to enzyme degradation. It is exceptionally rare for patients with normal serum concentrations of IgA immunoglobulin not to produce adequate amounts of secretory IgA in their saliva, tears and small bowel juice. The converse occasionally occurs when local immunity is relatively spared in the presence of severe hypogammaglobulinaemia. Accurate quantitative measurements of secretory immunoglobulins are difficult to obtain. The main reasons for this are that salivary IgA concentrations vary with salivary gland secretion rate, and are influenced by periodontal inflammation. The degree of protein transudation from inflammatory areas can be assessed by relating the immunoglobulin concentration to that of albumin in the same sample. Other aspects, including the use of correct standards in the measurement of secretory IgA are fully discussed by Tomasi and Grey (1972). However, for most practical purposes measurements on whole saliva, by a simple sensitive Mancini technique, identifies patients with major defects.

It must be said that the routine measurement of salivary immunoglobulin is of limited practical value since discrepancies between serum and secretory immunoglobulin are rare. However, the finding of secretory IgM or IgA in some patients with panhypogammaglobulinaemia may influence decisions on the necessity or frequency of gammaglobulin therapy.

Measurement of local specific antibody production following local test immunization has not been widely studied. Intranasal immunization with antigens such as diphtheria toxoid or influenza vaccine followed by measurement of antibody in nasal washings is not a difficult procedure. Further research in this area may uncover defects in local immunity in some patients with recurrent upper and lower respiratory tract infections.

Measurement of Circulating B-lymphocytes

B-lymphocytes mature and, probably after dividing, finally differentiate into plasma cells. They are recognized by immunofluorescent demonstration of immunoglobulin on their surface (see Chapter 3). Measuring the number of circulating B-cells is of little practical value for diagnosis except that their total absence may help identify patients with sex-linked agammaglobulinaemia. Most other patients with primary hypogammaglobulinaemia have normal or low numbers of circulating B-lymphocytes.

DIAGNOSIS OF DEFECTS IN CELL MEDIATED IMMUNITY

The term cell mediated immunity embraces a number of *in vivo* and *in vitro* phenomena which are generally recognized to require T-lymphocytes although other cells such as macrophages are also involved.

In vivo Tests

Delayed Hypersensitivity Skin Reactions

Patients are presumed to be presensitized to skin test antigens such as *Candida albicans*, streptokinase/streptodornase and usually also to purified protein derivative (PPD) and mumps antigens. It follows that positive skin reactions to these agents only indicate a functionally intact efferent limb of the immune responses. It is clearly important to distinguish between Arthus reactions seen between 16 and 24 hours following intradermal injection and delayed hypersensitivity skin reactions which usually appear after 48 hours. However, this is not always easy since both types of reactions may merge into each other.

Contact sensitizing chemicals such as dinitrochlorobenzene (DNCB) or picryl chloride are useful for testing both the afferent and efferent limbs of the immune response. A simplified test can be performed by painting 0·1 ml of a 5% solution of DNCB in acetone on the skin, accompanied by a control dose of 0·1 ml of a 0·1% solution painted at a different site on the arm. The control dose should give no reaction. Following challenge 7–14 days later with a 0·1% solution, normal persons develop erythema at this site within 24–48 hours. A recent afferent limb defect is suggested by the not uncommon finding of a positive Mantoux or Candida skin test in the presence of a negative DNCB reaction.

Delayed hypersensitivity skin reactions should be interpreted with great caution since they may be influenced by many factors such as drugs and protein/calorie malnutrition. It is important to use three or four skin test antigens since a negative result to only one means little. Positive tests indicate intact cell mediated immunity but negative reactions should not be relied upon for diagnostic purposes. However, taken together with *in vitro* tests for CMI, they can provide a fairly accurate picture of the patient's immunocompetence.

Severe primary defects in cell mediated immunity occur predominantly in infants and here it is important to make the diagnosis early. Delayed hypersensitivity skin tests are not very helpful in neonates who have not previously been exposed to antigens such as PPD and Candida. Furthermore, the direct irritant action of DNCB on infants' skin causes difficulty in interpretation since control doses tend to produce positive reactions. In these circumstances one generally relies on the *in vitro* correlates of cell mediated immunity.

Skin Graft Rejection

This is rarely used now as a diagnostic test of intact cell mediated immunity and carries the theoretical danger in patients with severe thymic deficiencies of transferring lymphocytes which might cause a graft versus host reaction. It requires only a minor surgical procedure but the graft needs to be observed regularly over a number of weeks.

In vitro Correlates of Cell Mediated Immunity (Asherson, 1972)

Lymphocyte Transformation

Lymphocytes separated from peripheral blood may be induced to form blast cells and divide by various mitogens (e.g. phytohaemagglutinin (PHA), pokeweed mitogen (PWM)) and by allogeneic lymphocytes (mixed lymphocyte reaction, MLR). Lymphocytes from preimmunized individuals also transform with specific antigens such as *Candida albicans* and PPD. The response is measured by the incorporation of radiolabelled thymidine into cells undergoing DNA synthesis. In practice, only the PHA transformation test is diagnostically useful and takes about 72 hours to perform. A quicker method using the uptake of radiolabelled uridine into RNA can give results within 24 hours.

Although lymphocyte transformation to PHA also involves some B-lymphocytes, it is regarded in clinical practice as predominantly an indicator of T-lymphocyte function. Neonates with isolated thymus defects (Di George syndrome) and severe combined immunodeficiency usually have very low or absent *in vitro* responses to PHA stimulation.

Measurement of Circulating Numbers of T-lymphocytes

T-lymphocytes (thymus processed) are recognized by their spontaneous ability to bind sheep erythrocytes to form rosettes (E-rosettes). The test can be performed in a few hours and is the most useful rapid screening method for detecting patients with significant T-cell deficiencies such as thymic aplasia and severe combined immunodeficiency. However, the presence of a normal number of circulating T-lymphocytes does not necessarily indicate intact T-cell function and other *in vivo* and *in vitro* functional tests are necessary. It is important to express the results both as a percentage of circulating lymphocytes and also as an absolute number per given volume of blood.

Lymphocyte Cytotoxicity

This phenomenon is regarded as one aspect of cell mediated immunity and involves the killing by lymphocytes of target cells, with or without the addition of anti-target cell antibody. It is thought to play a prominent role in defence against tumours, and may be involved in auto-immune diseases such as thyroiditis. Defects in this system are exceptionally rare and the test has little application to the diagnosis of primary defects in cell mediated immunity. Abnormalities may occur during immunosuppressive or cytotoxic therapy and in some patients with lymphoid malignancies although it is not clear whether such a defect plays any part in the aetiology of recurrent infections.

Macrophage Inhibition Factor (MIF)

This test measures the release of factors by antigen from stimulated immune lymphocytes which inhibit the movement of human white cells or guinea-pig macrophages (see also Chapter 9). The test is not useful in the diagnosis of immunodeficiency but there is interest in discrepancies which occur between MIF and lymphocyte transformation tests in patients with a variety of disorders, particularly mucocutaneous candidiasis.

Lymph Node Biopsies

Lymph nodes rarely need to be removed for purely diagnostic purposes but may give useful additional information on the severity and nature of the immune defect. Furthermore, the histological interpretation of such nodes is often difficult although pathologists are now beginning to understand the anatomical complexity and heterogeneity of lymph node responses. This "art" of interpretation has been greatly influenced by recognition of the characteristic appearances associated with certain immunodeficiency disorders.

Inguinal lymph nodes are the most accessible but are often fibrotic in older patients. Furthermore, the removal of an unstimulated lymph node may provide little information. Stimulation can be achieved by intradermal injection of antigens such as pneumococcal polysaccharide or painting the skin with contact sensitizing agents (e.g. DNCB) in the draining area of the node. The thigh is a particularly convenient place and intradermal injection of 0·1 ml of methylene blue at the immunization site, prior to removing the node usually helps to identify the draining node both macroscopically and microscopically. The optimal interval between immunization and removal of the node is not well defined in humans. However, animal experiments show that nodes removed about 7 days after immunization with pneumococcal polysaccharide contain many cortical germinal centres and medullary plasma cells while those removed 5 days after sensitization with DNCB show marked hypertrophy of the paracortical regions (Fig. 1a).

Lymph nodes from patients with primary hypogammaglobulinaemia characteristically lack germinal centres and plasma cells while those with isolated thymic deficiencies show a shrunken and lymphocyte depleted paracortical region (Fig. 1b). Peripheral nodes from infants with severe combined immunodeficiency contain very few lymphocytes, leaving only the fibrous anlage and histiocytes (Fig. 1c). Some patients with hypogammaglobulin-

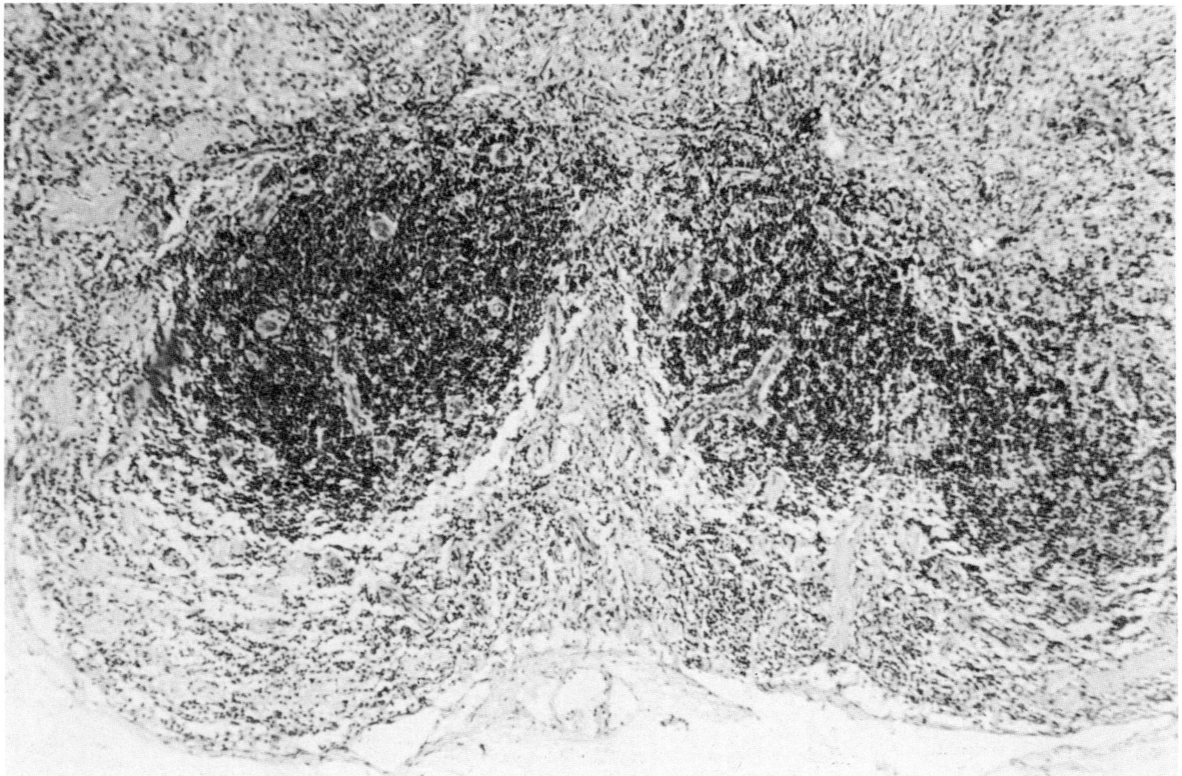

Fig. 1a. Normal lymph-node response five days after local stimulation with dinitrochlorobenzene. Note presence of cellular paracortical region. H and E ×112.

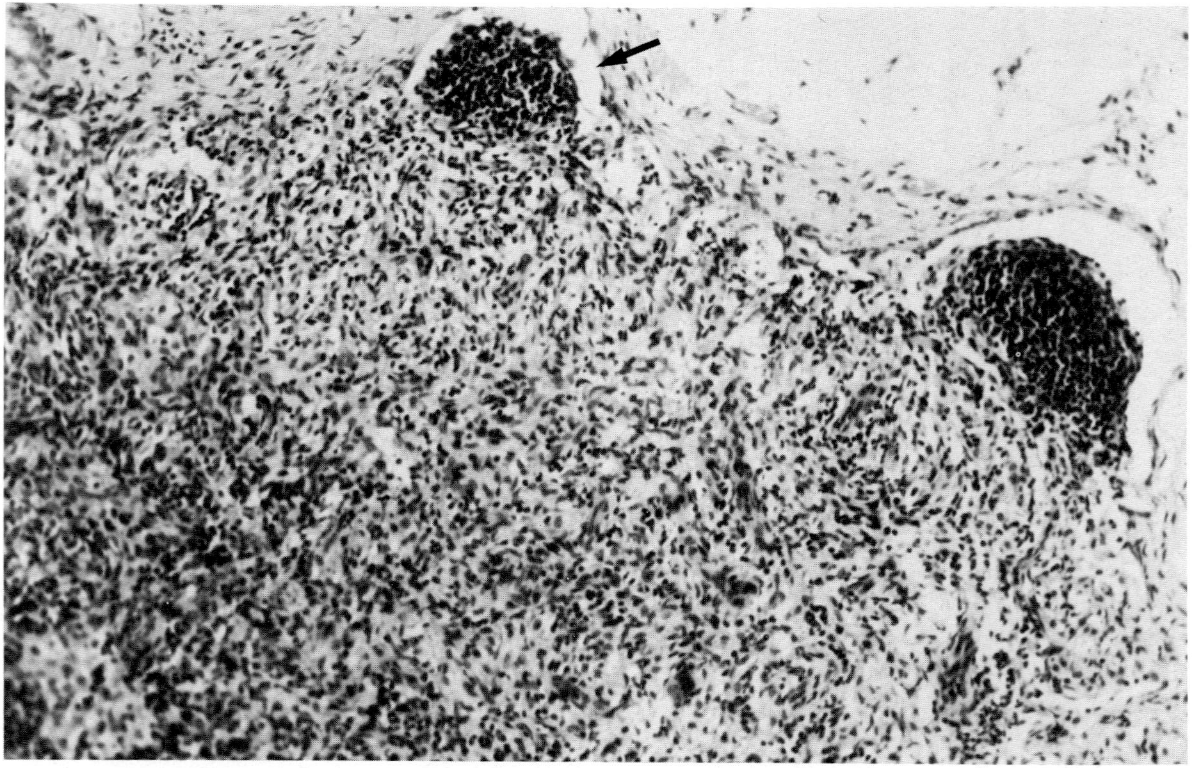

Fig. 1b. Inguinal lymph node removed from 3-month-old infant with thymic aplasia five days after local stimulation with dinitrochlorobenzene. Very few cells are present in the paracortical region, the node consisting predominantly of fibrous tissue and reticulum cells. There are some very small follicles just beneath the capsule (arrowed). No plasma cells were found in this biopsy despite normal serum immunoglobulin levels (H and E $\times 225$).

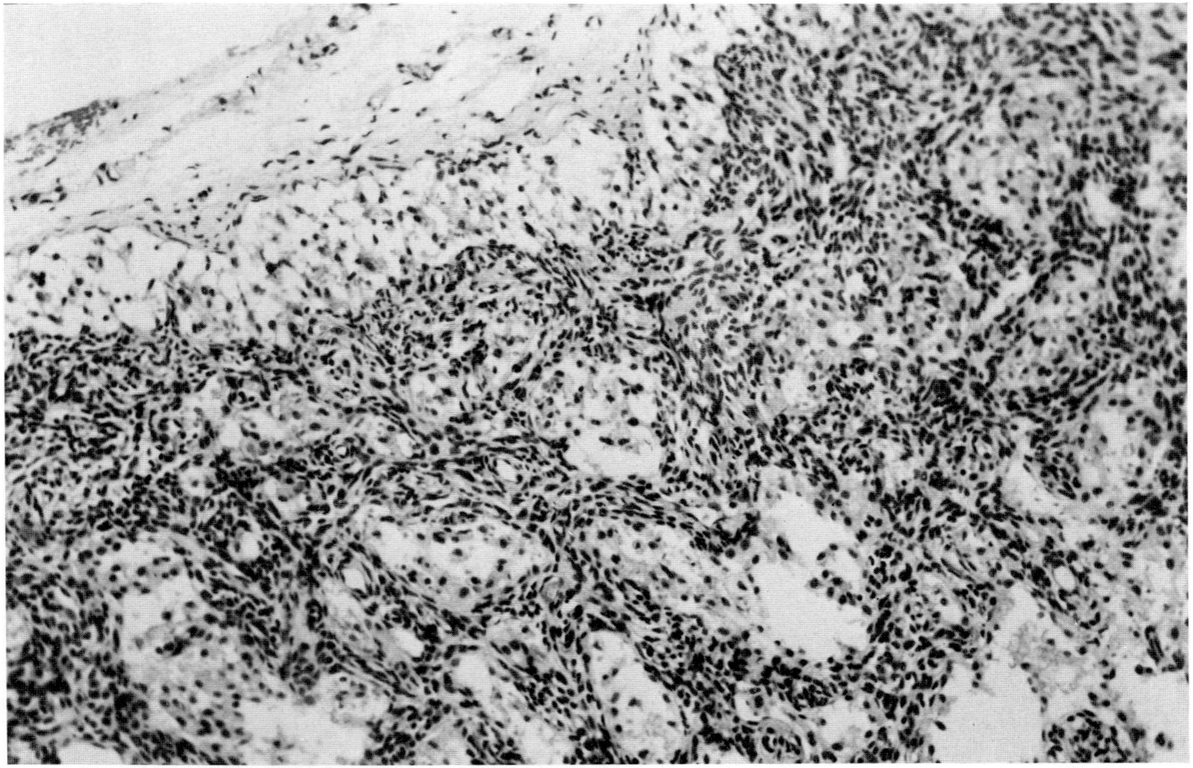

Fig. 1c. Inguinal lymph node from one-year-old infant with severe combined immunodeficiency removed five days after local stimulation with dinitrochlorobenzene. The node contains few lymphocytes, consisting predominantly of the fibrous anlage with some reticulum cells (H and E $\times 225$).

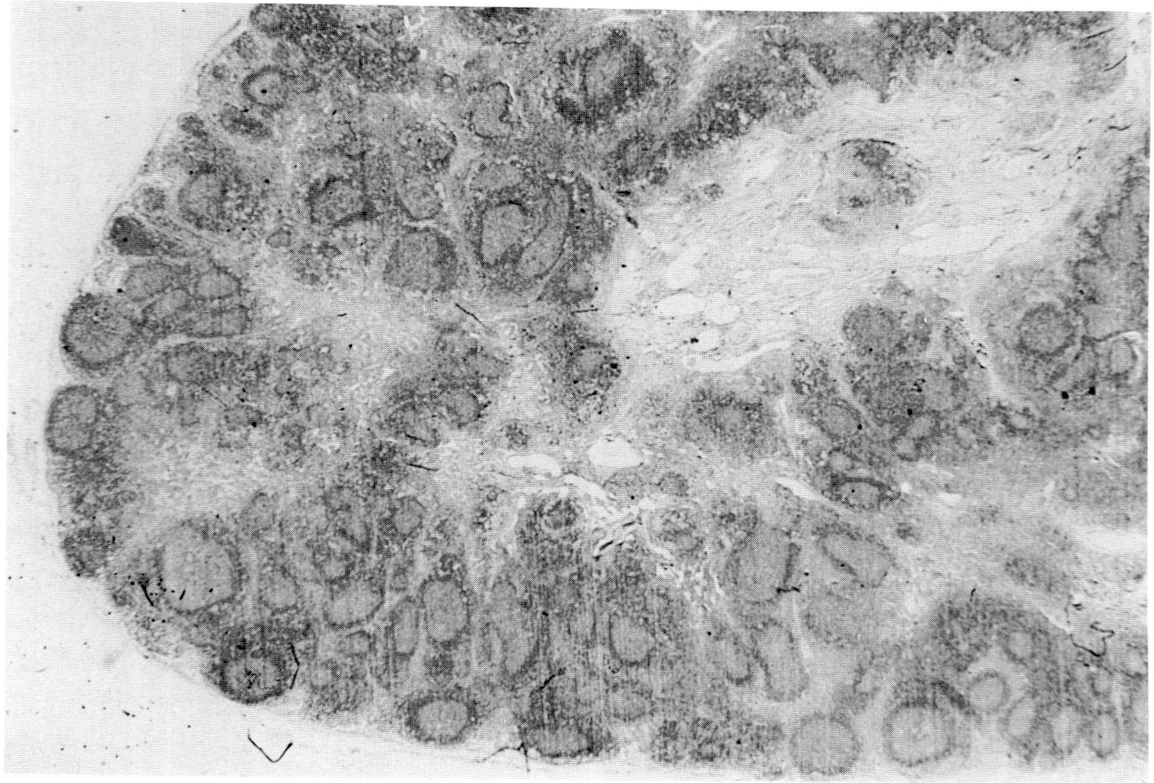

Fig. 1d. Axillary lymph node removed from 17-year-old boy with primary hypogammaglobulinaemia and a sarcoid-like granulomatous condition of the lungs and liver. Gross lymphadenopathy was also present and the nodes show germinal centre hyperplasia. No plasma cells could be identified in this biopsy (H and E $\times 60$).

aemia develop a generalized lymphadenopathy which histologically may show germinal centre hyperplasia (Fig. 1d). This appearance may identify a subgroup of patients where the block in antibody production occurs at a level different from that in the majority. The histology of nodes from some patients with hypogammaglobulinaemia may show a disordered structure and contain lymphoid cells of abnormal appearance. Such patients may be diagnosed incorrectly as suffering from a malignant lymphoma. If doubts remain about the diagnosis then a further lymph node should be examined and evidence of malignancy should be sought for in the gut. The lymphadenopathy in some of these patients disappears when they are given regular gammaglobulin injections.

PRIMARY IMMUNODEFICIENCY DISORDERS

The classification of primary immunodeficiency may be broadly subdivided into defects in antibody production, isolated thymic deficiencies and mixed deficiencies in both antibody production and cell mediated immunity (Table 1). Such divisions naturally tend to over-simplify since T- and B-lymphocyte collaboration is probably needed for most antibody responses.

Most patients with primary hypogammaglobulinaemia fall into the group called "common variable" immunodeficiency, a term coined by a World Health Organization committee (Fudenberg *et al.*, 1971). This does not mean that hypogammaglobulinaemia is common and the term is evidently intended to embrace in the future many other common immunopathological disorders such as immune complex disease and "allergic" phenomena.

DEFECTS IN ANTIBODY PRODUCTION

Transient Hypogammaglobulinaemia of Infancy

IgG immunoglobulin crosses the placenta and protects the infant for the first few months of life. The foetus and neonate is capable of mounting an IgM response and raised cord blood IgM concentrations usually indicate intrauterine infection. Production of IgG immunoglobulin is relatively depressed during the first year of life and IgA levels do not reach adult values until late childhood. However, there may be a delay in the ability of

TABLE 1
Classification of primary immunodeficiency

Defects in antibody production
Transient hypogammaglobulinaemia of infancy
Selective immunoglobulin deficiency IgA
IgG, M, E (very rare)
"Variable" hypogammaglobulinaemia
a) with normal or raised IgM
b) with defect in CMI
c) with thymoma
Sex linked hypogammaglobulinaemia
a) with absent B cells
b) with raised or normal IgM
Functional antibody defect with normal or raised serum immunoglobulins (dysgammaglobulinaemia)
Rubella syndrome with hypogammaglobulinaemia
Downs syndrome with functional antibody defect
Hypogammaglobulinaemia with neutropenia and exocrine pancreatic deficiency
Defects in cell mediated immunity
Thymus aplasia (or dysplasia)
Short limbed dwarfism
Familial lymphopenia
Mucocutaneous candidiasis
Mixed deficiencies in humoral and cell mediated immunity
Severe combined immunodeficiency
a) sex linked
b) autosomal recessive $\pm$ ADA deficiency
c) sporadic
Reticular dysgenesis
Ataxia telangiectasia
Wiskott–Aldrich syndrome

some infants, particularly those born prematurely, to produce IgG and IgM immunoglobulin. Some of these children suffer from recurrent infections between the age of three and twelve months and may benefit from regular gamma-globulin injections until their own production of immunoglobulin is adequate. This may take up to 2 years in some cases.

It is important to recognize patients in this group because early treatment can prevent morbidity. However, it should be remembered that the finding of panhypogammaglobulinaemia in the first year of life does not necessarily indicate a permanent defect. A reasonable policy is to give gammaglobulin injections and check the serum immunoglobulin levels about every four months. If panhypogammaglobulinaemia persists beyond 18 months then it is very likely that there is a permanent defect. Infants with transient hypogammaglobulinaemia have normal numbers of circulating B-lymphocytes and this distinguishes them from the sex-linked type of agammaglobulinaemia.

Selective Immunoglobulin Deficiencies

IgA Deficiency

It is estimated from screening blood donors that about one in seven hundred of normal healthy adults has total isolated IgA deficiency. IgA is absent in both the serum and secretions of these individuals and it is probable that those who remain healthy have compensated by secreting 7S IgM at mucosal surfaces. IgM also binds secretory piece and, although it is not as resistant to enzyme degradation as the dimer of IgA and secretory piece, it is probably functionally adequate. However, this is not the whole story since we have observed two such patients, who despite raised salivary IgM concentrations, have suffered from recurrent chest infections. The finding that lymphocytes from some patients with IgA deficiency and recurrent infections fail to release interferon after *in vitro* stimulation with mitogens may be relevant.

It is clear that many people with isolated IgA deficiency suffer from recurrent upper and lower respiratory tract infections. Affected children may present with asthma which appears to be triggered by bacterial bronchitis or they may only suffer from recurrent episodes of fever. Adults usually present with chronic bronchitis or recurrent attacks of acute bronchitis. Symptoms usually start in childhood or adolescence but can occur much later, suggesting an acquired defect. Amman and Hong (1971) in their excellent review of this condition, pointed out that about 40% of their cases had serum milk precipitins. This finding suggests a role for secretory IgA in preventing a systemic immune response to food antigens. Furthermore, there is some evidence of an increased incidence of atopic eczema in infants with low levels of serum IgA. The mechanism of these "allergies" is not known but a popular hypothesis is that IgA acts as a "blocking" antibody by reacting with potential antigens in the gut and rendering them non-immunogenic. Despite the possible link between allergic phenomena and IgA deficiency, serum IgE levels in these patients are not consistently raised.

A variety of disorders, many having a putative auto-immune basis, are associated with IgA deficiency. Amman and Hong (1971) suggest that IgA deficiency in apparently normal persons may not be such an innocuous defect as previously supposed since, if investigated and followed up, many will develop disorders such as Sjögren's syndrome, rheumatoid arthritis and thyroiditis. IgA deficiency is also associated with pernicious anaemia, particularly the familial type, and coeliac disease where plasma cells containing IgM, rather than IgA, are found in the jejunal infiltrate. Patients with A and B viral hepatitis also have an increased incidence of IgA deficiency. The cause and effect relationship is not yet settled but some patients are known to have had normal IgA levels prior to the hepatitis.

Family studies on patients with total isolated IgA deficiency usually show no evidence of inheritance. However, an autosomal recessive inheritance occurs in some patients with low, but not absent, serum IgA. The presence of total IgA deficiency is not linked to the Gm marker system. This means that a defect in the coding gene for IgA is unlikely since the regulating genes for the Gm types and IgA are closely linked. Furthermore, these patients have circulating B-lymphocytes with surface IgA which can be induced to synthesize and secrete IgA *in vitro*. There is a significantly increased incidence of abnormalities of chromosome 18, particularly partial deletions, in patients with low and absent IgA. However, it is unlikely that a major regulatory gene resides on this chromosome in view of the heterogeneity of these deletions. IgA deficiency occurs far more frequently than expected in near relatives of patients with variable hypogammaglobulinaemia suggesting a genetic link between the two types of immunodeficiency.

An important clinical aspect of this disorder is that more than half the patients have circulating serum antibodies to IgA. These antibodies are identified using a haemagglutination technique, the red cells being coated with IgA myeloma immunoglobulin. Vyas *et al.* (1969) have pointed out that some patients have antibodies against IgA myeloma proteins obtained from many different patients while others only react with the myeloma immunoglobulin from one particular patient. Those patients in the former category are particularly liable to reactions.

Subjects who are healthy need no specific treatment. However, there is some difference of opinion as to whether those with recurrent infections should receive regular replacement gammaglobulin injections. It has been said that injections of gammaglobulin, which contain about 5 mg/ml of IgA, are contraindicated in these patients because of the risk of anaphylactic reactions. This concern is based on the knowledge that some totally IgA deficient patients receiving blood transfusions have suffered severe reactions and a few have died. Screening for anti-IgA antibodies prior to gamma-globulin therapy may not be sufficient since, theoretically, patients may develop antibodies while receiving treatment. However, some patients with severe, but not necessarily total, IgA deficiency clearly benefit from regular gamma-globulin injections and we have treated three (one child and two adults) for more than a year with no complications and considerable reduction in frequency of chest infections. These patients presumably benefit from the passive diffusion of injected IgG onto mucosal surfaces since there is very little IgA in these preparations. Nevertheless, we have observed one patient with total IgA deficiency, Sjögren's syndrome and coeliac disease who developed a severe arthritis and immune complex glomerulonephritis after regular injections of gamma-globulin, both complications improving after the injections were discontinued.

It is clearly unwise to be dogmatic about treatment, and patients with infections should be considered for routine gamma-globulin injections. Nevertheless, the possibility of reactions should always be borne in mind and, if blood transfusions are required, washed red cells should be given. It is also essential that all patients be screened for anti-IgA antibodies and, if they are present, treatment with gamma-globulin may have to be withheld.

Isolated IgG Deficiency

This is a very rare defect and is said to be associated with an inability to neutralize bacterial toxins leading to formation of large necrotic lesions following infection. Although this fits in with the concept of IgG being particularly efficient at neutralizing toxins, it is hard to understand why patients with panhypogammaglobulinaemia do not develop such complications. We have observed only one case of isolated IgG deficiency, who suffered from "unremarkable" recurrent bronchitis but who also had an obscure liver disease with lymphocytic portal infiltration and gross hepatosplenomegaly. His chest condition improved considerably after regular gamma-globulin therapy.

Isolated Immunoglobulin Subclass Defects

Four subclasses of IgG (IgG 1–4) and two subclasses of IgA (IgA_1 and IgA_2) are known. The total serum IgG is made up of approximately 70% IgG_1, 20% IgG_2, 5% IgG_3 and 4% IgG_4. IgG subclass concentrations differ slightly in accordance with the genetic make up of their IgG as assessed by Gm typing. However, the relative concentrations of IgA_1 and IgA_2 are not associated with the Gm types; different genes presumably regulate this. The clinical significance of aberrations in IgA subclass concentrations is not yet apparent, but the possibility of IgG subclass defects must always be considered in patients with recurrent infections and normal levels of total IgG. One such patient has been described with isolated defects of IgG_2 and IgG_4 who benefited from regular gamma-globulin injections. Antibodies to most protein antigens (e.g. tetanus and diphtheria toxoids) are distributed in all IgG subclasses but polysaccharides, (e.g. dextran, pneumococcal polysaccharide) induce antibody only in the IgG_2 subclass. Patients with IgG_2 defects should thus be identifiable by their failure to produce an IgG response after immunization with polysaccharides. Disordered relative concentrations of IgG subclasses are seen in many patients with severe hypogammaglobulinaemia but are of no clinical importance.

Isolated IgM Deficiency

IgM antibody is thought to be important in protection against blood borne infections. This is supported by reports of meningococcal meningitis and generalized vaccinia in children with low levels of serum IgM. Total isolated deficiency of IgM is very rare and may be associated with recurrent infections. We have observed only two patients with this defect; one girl with pure red cell aplasia and a young woman with a familial chronic cholangitis. Both had recurrent chest infections which improved with regular gamma-globulin injections.

Isolated IgE and IgD Deficiencies

The normal serum IgE range is very wide and little is known about the interpretation of low levels. However, a few cases of apparently total IgE deficiency have been reported associated with recurrent infections while others are normal and healthy. The clinical significance of serum IgD is uncertain since many healthy persons have undetectable levels.

Familial Hypogammaglobulinaemia

There are some very rare families in which males and females have developed hypogammaglobulinaemia, suggesting an autosomal dominant or recessive mode of inheritance. However, a sex linked recessive inheritance can be clearly demonstrated in the great majority of cases.

Sex-linked Type

This condition only affects males, who develop recurrent infections, usually of the chest and ears, in the first two years of life. A rarer form is "sex-linked agammaglobulinaemia" where no serum immunoglobulin of any class is detectable by sensitive Mancini techniques. These children characteristically lack circulating B-cells and no plasma cells or germinal centres are found in the gut, bone marrow, spleen or lymph nodes. The tonsils and adenoids are absent, the latter being assessed by a lateral X-ray of the nasopharynx. Other affected children have low or normal numbers of circulating B-cells together with a low, normal or raised serum IgM. It is not clear whether this IgM represents functional antibody but it is rare for such children to have isohaemagglutinins or natural antibodies to *E. coli*. This pattern of immunoglobulin deficiency is similar to that seen in some infants with the rubella syndrome and the aetiology may be based on a foetal or infantile virus infection. The sex linked inheritance could then be explained by a genetically determined inability to deal with such a virus. On the other hand, sex linked agammaglobulinaemia is likely to be a defect in the gene coding for molecular assembly of immunoglobulins.

Both types of sex linked hypogammaglobulinaemia are associated with normal cell mediated immunity as assessed by delayed hypersensitivity skin tests, numbers of circulating T-cells and lymphocyte transformation to allogeneic and mitogenic stimuli. In contrast with other forms of panhypogammaglobulinaemia, splenomegaly and lymphopenia are rare. Eczema of the classical flexural type is common, but it usually becomes less troublesome after adolescence.

"Variable" Hypogammaglobulinaemia

This term embraces those who develop the disease in infancy or childhood or as adults, do not have affected relatives and who have low or normal numbers of circulating B-lymphocytes. Males and females are equally affected. A rough estimate, based on the findings of the Medical Research Council's working party (1971) suggests that the lifetime prevalence of this disorder lies between 5 and 10 per million of the population. However, with more widespread screening, this figure might be doubled. The pattern of the immunodeficiency varies but the majority of patients have unrecordable levels of serum IgA. Most patients have very low levels of serum IgG and IgM but, like some of the children with sex linked hypogammaglobulinaemia, a few have normal or raised levels of IgM. About 50% have splenomegaly which is often associated with a lymphopenia. 40% have defects in cell mediated immunity with negative delayed hypersensitivity skin reactions to common antigens and contact sensitizing agents together with depressed lymphocyte transformation to mitogens such as PHA and pokeweed mitogen. These abnormalities do not prejudice the short term prognosis of such patients but their long-term consequences have yet to be defined. Despite these *in vivo* and *in vitro* CMI defects, the relative percentage of circulating T-cells is normal although absolute numbers are diminished in those with lymphopenia. The cause of the lymphopenia is unknown and it is not usually associated with circulating lymphocytotoxins. Lymph nodes do not usually contain germinal centres and immunoglobulin containing lymphoid cells and plasma cells are also present. However, about 75% of patients do have such cells in the lamina propria of the gut, particularly the rectum. Nevertheless, the evidence to date shows that most fail to secrete significant quantities of immunoglobulin into the gut lumen.

Thymoma with Hypogammaglobulinaemia

About 2% of patients with primary hypogammaglobulinaemia have an associated thymoma. The tumour is usually benign and well encapsulated and the majority consist of spindle-shaped epithelial cells. Most patients have moderate or severe panhypogammaglobulinaemia but the cause and effect relationship with the tumour is not clear although its removal does not influence the hypogammaglobulinaemia. Nothing is gained, therefore, by routinely performing elaborate investigations to identify such tumours and a lateral chest X-ray is sufficient (Fig. 2). If necessary, further information on the tumour size can be gained from pneumomediastinography.

Patients with myasthenia gravis, another disorder associated with thymoma, often have deficient antibody responses to both protein and polysaccharide antigens, although frank hypogammaglobulinaemia is very rare. It is suggested that this is the primary defect which is in some way responsible for the development of the thymomata and myasthenia. Pure red cell aplasia is another condition associated with both thymoma and hypogammaglobulin-

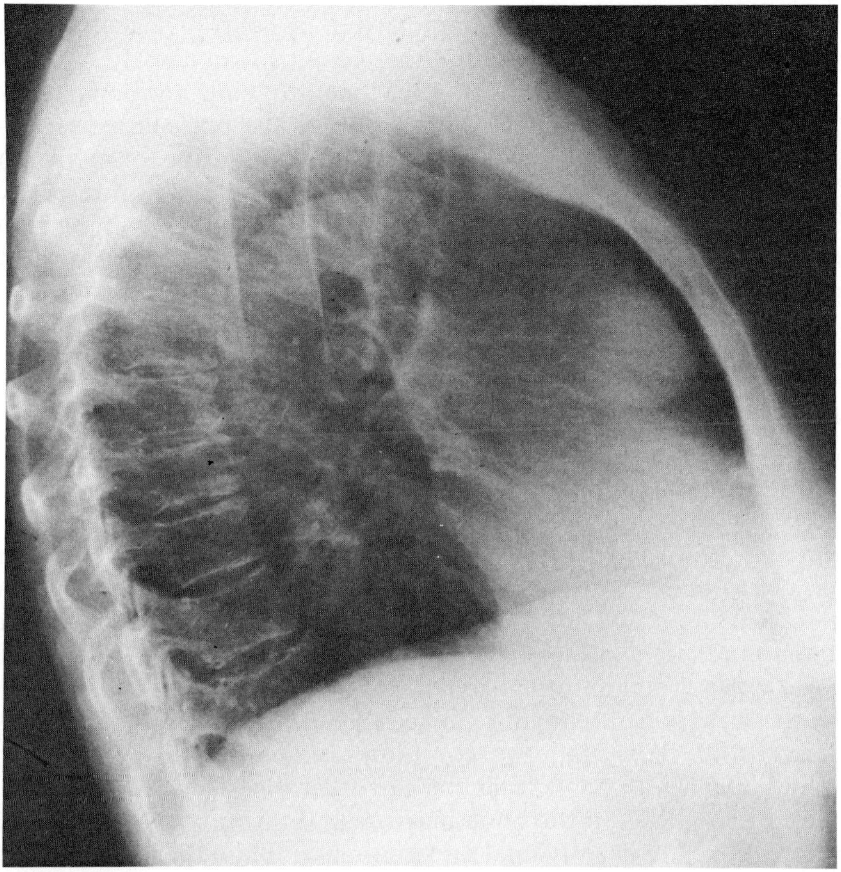

Fig. 2. Chest radiograph showing thymic mass in anterior mediastinum in a 63-year old woman with hypogammaglobulinaemia. The hypogammaglobulinaemia persisted after removal of the tumour.

aemia, although it is exceptional for all three conditions to occur in the same patient.

Severe watery diarrhoea, without steatorrhoea, occurs in some patients with thymoma and hypogammaglobulinaemia but usually disappears after removal of the tumour. It is possible that the tumour releases a factor which influences the lower bowel.

The Rubella Syndrome

A small proportion of infants with the rubella syndrome have a major antibody defect manifested by very low levels of serum IgG and IgA in infancy and childhood. The syndrome is characterized by neurological abnormalities, cataracts, deafness, cardiac defects and hepatosplenomegaly. Cord blood IgM concentrations are raised and IgM neutralizing antibody to rubella virus is present in high titres. However, despite the presence of serum antibody, virus can often be isolated from the throat and urine for many months. It is not clear what proportion of affected infants develop a permanent deficiency in IgG and IgA but recovery probably takes place in the majority. Permanent isolated IgA deficiency has been described in a few cases. However, it remains an open question whether the aetiology of childhood onset "variable" hypogammaglobulinaemia with raised or normal IgM levels is related to an infection with rubella or other similar virus.

Pancreatic Insufficiency, Neutropenia and Hypogammaglobulinaemia

Hudson and Aldor (1970) described a boy with exocrine pancreatic insufficiency, neutropenia, moderate hypogammaglobulinaemia and recurrent upper respiratory tract infections. Other members of the family also had immunoglobulin deficiencies. The condition resembled cystic fibrosis but the sweat test was normal and the malabsorption relatively easy to control with pancreatic extracts. Subsequent reported cases suggest an autosomal mode of inheritance and show that the condition is compatible with survival in relatively good health to at least the third decade. The neutropenia is due to myeloid hypoplasia in the bone marrow and thrombocytopenia may also occur. Infections are usually mild and gamma-globulin therapy is usually not indicated. The condition should be suspected in adults with pancreatic malabsorption, recurrent infections and neutropenia since a "forme fruste" of the syndrome probably exists.

Downs Syndrome

Recurrent bacterial infections of the upper and lower respiratory tract are common in this condition and there is also a high incidence of leukaemia. Despite a tendency to raised serum IgG levels, they have a significant defect in antibody production affecting both primary and secondary responses. There is also evidence that the physico-chemical nature of the immunoglobulin is abnormal. Lymphocyte transformation to PHA and numbers of circulating T-lymphocytes tend to become depressed in early adult life. The high incidence of leukaemia and auto-immune disease may be related to an inability to inactivate certain oncogenic viruses.

Gaucher's Disease

Children with this disorder accumulate large amounts of glycocerebroside in the reticulo–endothelial system. They tend to suffer from recurrent infections and about 70% have monoclonal or polyclonal increases in one or more immunoglobulin class. By analogy with the finding that long-chain fatty acids are mitogenic for circulating lymphocytes, it is possible that the glycocerebroside is mitogenic for B-lymphocytes, causing a consequent increase in immunoglobulin production.

Complications in Patients with Hypogammaglobulinaemia

Infections

Patients have difficulty in coping with bacteria and consequently most develop upper and lower respiratory tract infections, the commonest organism involved being *Haemophilus influenzae*. Middle ear sepsis is common in children and not infrequently leads to a permanent hearing defect. Osteomyelitis or septic arthritis may occur which characteristically have an insidious onset. The latter can sometimes be mistaken for rheumatoid or Still's disease with unfortunate consequences. Staphylococcal infections of the skin are surprisingly uncommon and are more characteristic of severe neutrophil polymorph defects (e.g. chronic granulomatous disease). Urinary tract infections are rare suggesting that defence mechanisms in this system is not primarily mediated by antibodies. However, three of our patients have developed dysuria, bladder pain and gross pyuria lasting for many weeks. No bacteria or viruses were isolated from the urine in two patients while mycoplasma was found in the third. All three patients recovered after 2–4 weeks therapy with oral tetracycline. This response suggests that a mycoplasma type organism was the causal factor in all cases. It is important to recognize this complication because such patients are usually treated with other ineffective antibiotics and remain in misery for months.

Amyloidosis has occurred in a few patients usually following chronic infection. It is interesting that immunoglobulin L-chain related proteins may be present in secondary amyloid fibrils in addition to amyloid A protein (Levin *et al.*, 1972).

Viruses

In general, patients tend to respond to virus infections normally and recover satisfactorily from measles and varicella infections. However, herpes zoster (shingles) is common and occurred in about 15% of patients in our series. There is also evidence of an increased incidence of paralytic poliomyelitis, some cases following systemic polio vaccination. In addition, some children immunized with oral polio vaccine have become long-term secretors of the virus. Hepatitis due to virus A or B is uncommon but a few patients have suffered recurrent acute episodes over a two to three year period.

A rare but usually fatal condition resembling dermatomyositis affects children with hypogammaglobulinaemia, particularly those with the sex linked type. Tense oedema in the subcutaneous tissues of the arms and legs, fever and malaise are associated with muscle rigidity and a violaceous skin rash. Affected children gradually deteriorate and usually die within about a year. In some cases the condition may be more a vasculitis than a true myositis since serum muscle enzyme levels (e.g. creatinine phosphokinase) are not always raised. The condition is very likely caused by viruses, particularly those of the enterovirus group, since several serotypes of ECHO virus have now been isolated from the cerebro-spinal fluid of a handful of such cases.

Such children are susceptible to a chronic brain disease which takes the form of an ultimately fatal encephalitis or meningitis. A number of different viruses have been isolated at post mortem from the brains of such patients and the histology is compatible with a virus infection (Dayan, 1971). We have managed a child with sex linked hypogammaglobulinaemia who suffered from a chronic meningoencephalitis with the simultaneous occurrence of "dermatomyositic" features. ECHO 11 virus was consistently isolated from the cerebro-spinal fluid and the child was treated with regular intravenous infusions of plasma containing anti-ECHO 11 antibody. The dermatomyositic features rapidly disappeared and the brain disease was probably modified since the child survived in relatively good health for almost 3 years (Fig. 3).

It is not clear why children with sex linked hypogammaglobulinaemia are particularly prone to this complication or why ECHO viruses should be involved. The fact that they characteristically have normal cell mediated immunity supports the conclusion from animal work that this system does not play a major role in protection against enteroviruses. Local production of antibody by lymphoid cells within the central nervous system probably plays an important part in recovery from viral encephalitis and meningitis in immunologically normal persons and these children almost certainly lack this capacity. It could be argued that, in order to protect such children against

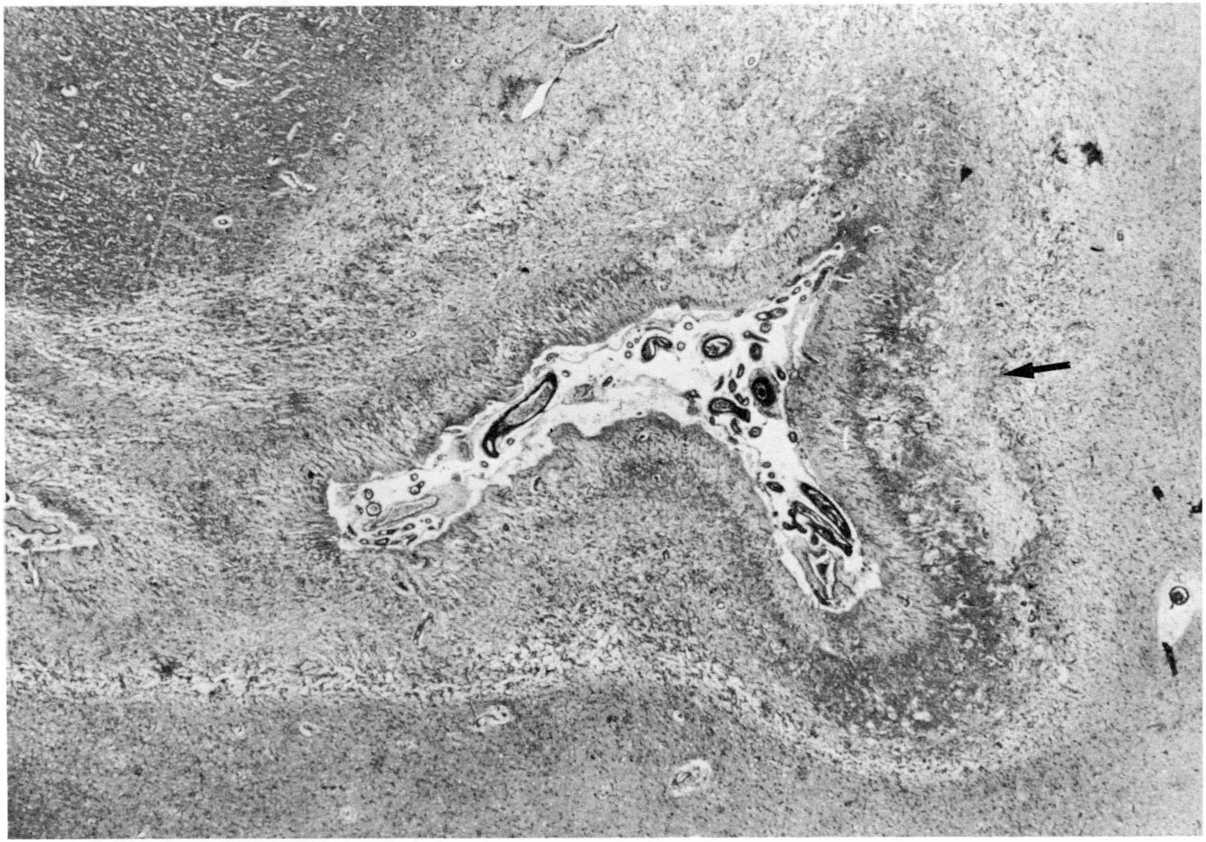

Fig. 3. Section of cerebral cortex from a boy of 11 years with sex linked hypogammaglobulinaemia showing a focus of neuronal loss and astrocyte proliferation (arrowed). Patient suffered with a chronic Echo 11 viral meningitis for two years (H and E ×23).

this complication, they should be given regular gamma-globulin containing antibody to all the common pathogenic viruses. However, the difficulty with enteroviruses is that the sero-types responsible for neurological disease in the general population vary from year to year and commercially available gamma-globulin rarely contains the relevant antibodies. The failure in our case to completely eliminate the brain disease with systemic injections of anti-ECHO antibody suggests that purified hyperimmune gamma-globulin should be injected intrathecally as early as possible. Experience with intrathecal gamma-globulin for neonatal tetanus in India has shown this to be a safe procedure.

Haemopoietic Disorders

Children with hypogammaglobulinaemia may present with a severe neutropenia which is usually associated with a chest infection or septicaemia. The aetiology is probably based on a depression of neutrophil precursor differentiation by high concentrations of circulating endotoxin which would normally be neutralized by antibody. It is important to be aware of this association because the neutropenia might be considered the primary defect. Neutrophil counts usually rapidly return to normal following antibiotic treatment but leucocyte transfusions may be necessary as a temporary measure. This complication does not occur once these children are receiving regular gamma-globulin injections.

Lymphopenia occurs in about 50% of patients with variable hypogammaglobulinaemia and may be related to the primary aetiology of the disease. Thrombocytopenia occurs in a minority of patients and, in our experience, is usually related to a drug sensitivity reaction or severe folate deficiency. However, four out of 30 patients in our series with adult onset hypogammaglobulinaemia developed an episode of thrombocytopenia in childhood or adolesence. This may have been caused by a virus-triggered auto-immune phenomenon and could be related to the subsequent development of the immunodeficiency. Haemolytic anaemia, sometimes associated with a positive Coomb's test, is rare and is again usually related to a drug sensitivity. Both the thrombocytopenia and anaemia tend to improve rapidly after withdrawal of the offending drug but platelet transfusions and steroids are indicated as a temporary measure in the more severe cases.

A mild hypochromic anaemia is common and is usually associated with a low serum iron. Total serum iron binding capacity is usually normal and we have found the estimation of bone marrow iron stores to be more helpful.

Some patients do have a true iron deficiency, often secondary to malabsorption, but others have adequate iron stores indicating a block in utilization. It is not always possible to pass this abnormality off as the "anaemia of infection" since some of the patients are in good general health.

Bone marrow depression causing anaemia, neutropenia and thrombocytopenia not uncommonly occurs when patients with unsuspected malabsorption are treated with prolonged courses of drugs containing trimethoprime (e.g. co-trimoxazole). This drug exacerbates the folate deficiency already present in these patients. Recovery is usually rapid after withdrawing the drug and giving oral folinic acid. Folate and vitamin B_{12} deficiency, secondary to malabsorption, may also lead to a megaloblastic anaemia.

Splenomegaly frequently occurs in patients with variable hypogammaglobulinaemia but the haematological sequelae of hypersplenism are rarely seen. However, there are some cases where a severe leucopenia, thrombocytopenia and haemolytic anaemia has necessitated splenectomy. Removal of the spleen in such patients usually improves the situation considerably and is not associated with an increased susceptibility to infections provided patients are given regular gamma-globulin therapy.

Arthritis

Infection should always be considered a possibility in patients with hypogammaglobulinaemia who develop a mono or polyarthritis. Septic arthritis tends to present insidiously and can be confused with rheumatoid or Still's disease. If, even after joint aspiration, doubts remain about the diagnosis then it is wise to give high doses of antibodies for up to six months. However, some children develop a truly aseptic monoarthritis which usually affects one knee. The joint fluid contains mostly lymphocytes and swelling may recur intermittently over many years. There is no specific treatment and the condition usually resolves spontaneously, without leaving any permanent damage, by adolescence. This type of arthritis may occur in patients already receiving gammaglobulin whereas septic arthritis is exceptional after commencement of such therapy.

About 5% of adults with variable hypogammaglobulinaemia suffer from a polyarthritis involving the large joints, particularly wrists and knees, associated with a tenosynovitis. The latter characteristically causes a carpal tunnel syndrome together with tendon sheath swelling on the dorsum of the hands and feet. The condition usually affects untreated patients and dramatically improves within a few weeks after commencing regular gamma-globulin injections. Joint erosions do not occur and the joint fluid contains mostly lymphoid cells. Rheumatoid factor is not present in the serum. The aetiology is unknown but presumably involves an agent or toxin which is neutralized by antibody in the gamma-globulin. This dramatic recovery after therapy prompted a trial of gamma-globulin in patients with classical rheumatoid arthritis which was unfortunately unsuccessful.

A few hypogammaglobulinaemic patients have developed apparent classical rheumatoid disease with joint erosions and subcutaneous nodules. There is a high incidence of auto-immune phenomena and immunodeficiency in the family members of some of these cases. Furthermore, there is an increased incidence of isolated IgA deficiency in rheumatoid arthritis.

Skin Disease

Eczema is particularly common in patients with sex linked hypogammaglobulinaemia but also occurs in a milder form in some children and adults with the "variable" type. Other skin conditions are rare. Psoriasis occurred in 2% and vitiligo in 3% of patients in our series.

Granulomata

Although the commonest lung pathology in these cases is bronchiectasis and fibrosis, patients occasionally develop a granulomatous condition with a reticulated lung pattern on chest radiography similar to sarcoidosis (Fig. 4). A few show positive Kveim tests and also have liver granulomata. Steroid therapy is generally ineffective and two patients with this complication in our series died young with cor pulmonale.

Allergies

About 10% of patients develop skin sensitivity reactions to antibiotics and other drugs. The mechanism of these reactions are not known but probably involves cell mediated immunity rather than a humoral mechanism. A similar number of patients develop anaphylactic reactions to gamma-globulin (see below). I have not seen a convincing case of asthma or allergic rhinitis in over 150 patients with primary hypogammaglobulinaemia.

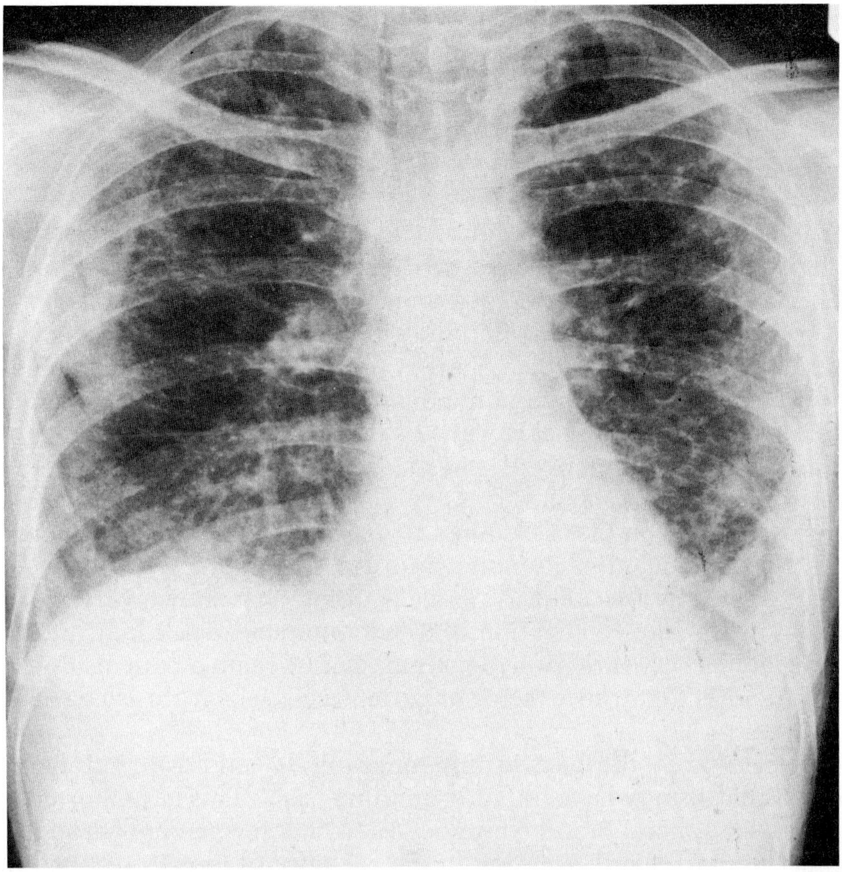

Fig. 4. Chest radiograph from 50-year-old woman with hypogammaglobulinaemia showing reticulated lung fields consistent with sarcoidosis.

Malignant Diseases

Kersey *et al.* (1973) highlighted the grossly raised incidence of lymphoreticular malignancies which account for about 10% of deaths in the Wiskott Aldrich syndrome and ataxia telangiectasia. They also showed a raised incidence of leukaemia and other solid tumours in sex-linked and variable hypogammaglobulinaemia. However, lymphadenopathy is not uncommon in these disorders and pathologists tend to diagnose lymphoreticular malignancy incorrectly when the lymph node architecture is abnormal. The experience in England over the past five years does not indicate an obvious association between malignancy of any type and sex-linked or variable hypogammaglobulinaemia.

Gastric Disorders

Between 40% and 60% of adults with hypogammaglobulinaemia have achlorhydria and many also have deficient intrinsic factor secretion which may ultimately lead to "pernicious anaemia" (PA) (Twomey *et al.*, 1970). However, the PA associated with hypogammaglobulinaemia differs in many respects from the classical form. This is probably because atrophic changes occur over the whole stomach in hypogammaglobulinaemic PA whereas the antrum is spared in the classical form. Gastrin secreting antral cells in the latter consequently remain functional and are released from the usual inhibitory influences of hydrochloric acid. This explanation is based on only a few careful histological studies on biopsies taken from different parts of the stomach in patients with hypogammaglobulinaemic PA and there is need for further investigation in this area. The available histology has shown varying degrees of atrophy, with intestinalization and a mononuclear cell infiltration. Not surprisingly, it is very rare for hypogammaglobulinaemia patients to have the serum antibodies to intrinsic factor or parietal cells which are usual in classical PA.

The aetiology of the gastric inflammation is unknown but there is a suggestion that it may have an auto-immune basis. This is supported by the finding that peripheral blood lymphocytes from a few patients produce MIF and undergo blast transformation in the presence of human or hog intrinsic factor. This parallels results in classical PA where about 70% of patients give positive responses to these tests. However, it is possible that these *in vitro* phenomena occur secondarily to gastric inflammation caused by chronic bacterial infection of the stomach mucosa.

Isolated IgA deficiency is also associated with the classical form of PA, particularly the familial variety. A further link between hypogammaglobulinaemia and pernicious anaemia is that vitiligo, which is also thought to have an auto-immune basis, occurs with increased frequency in both conditions.

Small Bowel Disorders

Mild malabsorption is very common and occurs intermittently in about 60% of adult patients with hypogammaglobulinaemia. Occasionally gross malabsorption occurs leading to a megaloblastic anaemia with a low red cell folate and vitamin B_{12}, osteomalacia and weight loss. This is often due to infection with the parasite *Giardia lamblia* which can be eliminated with a 10-day course of mepacrine or metronidazole. The diagnosis of giardiasis cannot always be confirmed by finding the characteristic cysts in the stools and small bowel biopsies or jejunal juice may have to be examined for the presence of *Giardia* trophozoites. Patients with hypogammaglobulinaemia are particularly prone to infection with *Giardia* which suggests that the normal defence mechanism against this parasite involves secretory antibody. However, some cases of severe malabsorption defy complete explanation and often remit spontaneously or following a course of antibiotics. Increased numbers of aerobic, and sometimes anaerobic, organisms are frequent in the jejunal juice of most of these patients but their concentration is often no greater than in other hypogammaglobulinaemic patients without malabsorption. It is debated whether such moderate increases in small bowel bacteria (less than 10^7/ml) could account for the malabsorption. Such bacteria might produce an irritant effect on the gut by producing deconjugated bile acids but C^{14} glycocholic acid breath tests are usually negative.

Jejunal biopsies in most cases of both mild or severe malabsorption are either normal or show partial villous atrophy (Fig. 5). Single biopsies are often normal when taken from patients with giardiasis but Ament *et al.* (1973) have demonstrated that mucosal abnormalities can nearly always be found if multiple biopsies are taken. Total villous atrophy with a cellular infiltrate is rare and is termed "hypogammaglobulinaemic sprue" because it may improve after antibiotic therapy. However, such a case in our series (Fig. 5) improved only after gluten withdrawal, demonstrating that coeliac disease may occur in the presence of profound hypogammaglobulinaemia. Unfortunately, this observation does not completely clarify the role of plasma cells in the mucosal lesions of coeliac disease since this patient, and most other patients with variable hypogammaglobulinaemia, have immunoglobulin containing cells in the lamina propria of the small and large bowel (Broom *et al.*, 1975).

A few cases of ulcerative jejuno-ileitis have been described with hypogammaglobulinaemia where there is gross oedema of the mucosa with polymorph leucocyte infiltration. This potentially lethal condition may respond to steroids and antibiotics. Crohn's disease has been described in a patient with hypogammaglobulinaemia but the association must be extremely rare.

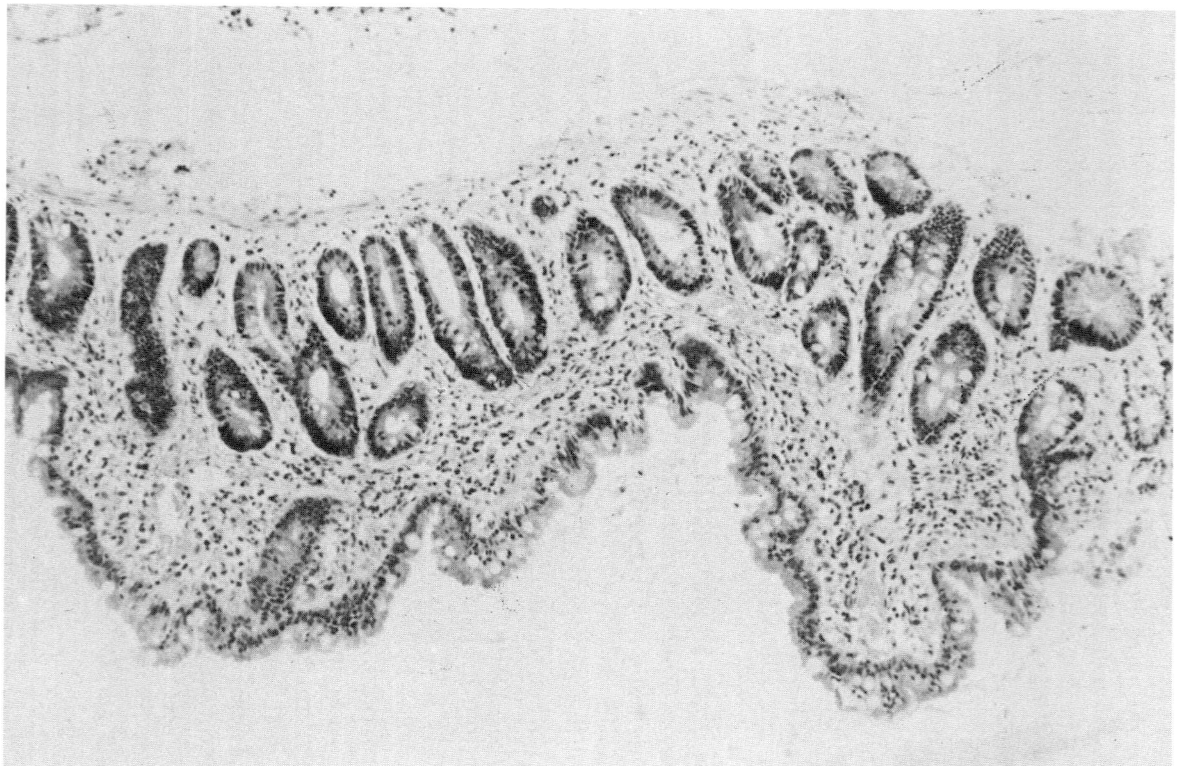

Fig. 5. Jejunal biopsy from 60-year-old man with hypogammaglobulinaemia showing severe villous atrophy and a mononuclear cell infiltrate. Patient was given a gluten free diet and biopsy appearances six months later were considerably improved (H and E ×135).

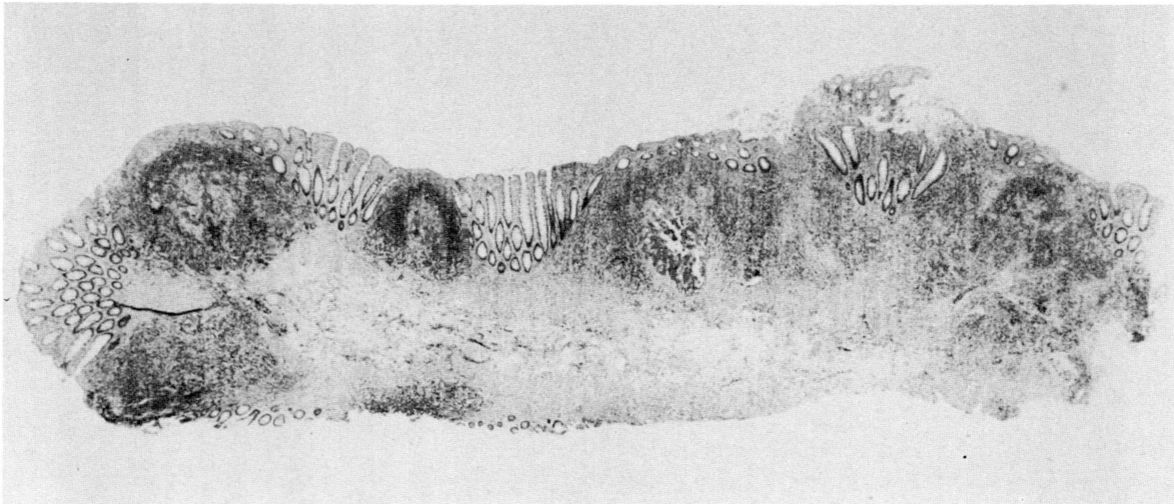

Fig. 6. Rectal biopsy showing extensive nodular lymphoid hyperplasia in a 43-year-old man with hypogammaglobulinaemia. Nodules were also demonstrated fibrescopically and by biopsy of the small bowel. The nodules are similar to the germinal centres of lymph nodes, having a peripheral tightly packed cuff of small lymphocytes and larger pale staining mononuclear cells in the centre (H and E $\times 23{\cdot}5$).

Nodular Lymphoid Hyperplasia (NLH)

This condition is virtually confined to adult patients with primary variable hypogammaglobulinaemia but is occasionally found in the colon or terminal ileum of immunologically "normal" children where it may cause gastro-intestinal bleeding or recurrent abdominal pain. I have also seen an immunologically normal adult with gross NLH of the small bowel which was discovered following a barium meal for abdominal pain. The condition has been described in isolated IgA deficiency but has not been reported in patients with the sex-linked form of agammaglobulinaemia.

The nodules consist of mononuclear cells, the whole structure bearing some similarity to the germinal centres of lymph nodes (Fig. 6). Our own investigations show that the cells within the nodules do not contain immunoglobulin. The nodules are usually small, being less than 3 mm in diameter, and may be seen at fibreoptic examination. They are usually confined to the small bowel but may occur in any part of the gastrointestinal tract. Patients who develop these nodules do not seem to form a subgroup within the spectrum of variable hypogammaglobulinaemia as assessed by the various *in vivo* and *in vitro* tests for humoral and cell mediated immunity. The aetiology of this condition remains a mystery but probably reflects an aberrant local immune response to bacteria or parasites in the gut.

The finding of NLH should cause no alarm since it is a benign disorder and causes symptoms only in exceptional circumstances when large nodules may cause obstruction. It is claimed that NLH may disappear after regular plasma therapy but regular gamma-globulin injections have no effect on the condition.

Large Bowel Disorders (Table 2)

Rectal mucosa taken from patients with hypogammaglobulinaemia frequently contains numerous crypt microabscesses although the macroscopic appearance is usually normal. Symptoms of proctocolitis are rare and ulcerative colitis has been described in only two cases. *Salmonella* and *Shigella* enterocolitis commonly affects such patients in the United States but is rare in Britain. Patients often become chronic *Salmonella* carriers after such an illness. Watery diarrhoea, without steatorrhoea, may rarely be due to the irritant effect of deconjugated bile acids produced by an overgrowth of bile splitting organisms. Oral cholestyramine, which binds bile salts, may alleviate symptoms. The diarrhoea associated with thymoma and hypogammaglobulinaemia is discussed above.

TABLE 2
Diagnosis and treatment of diarrhoea in patients with primary hypogammaglobulinaemia

Jejunal biopsy and analysis of gut flora		
normal mucosa	colistin syrup	If symptoms persist then trial of mepacrine is indicated for "missed" giardiasis
Villous atrophy +cellular infiltrate	Trial of gluten free diet, Colistin if this fails	
Severe mucosal oedema +polymorph infiltrate (v. rare)	Colistin + steroids	

Specific measures	
Giardiasis (look in jejunal juice if stool negative)	Mepacrine (100 mg tds for 10 days)
Bile acid deconjugation	Cholestyramine Colistin syrup (10 day course)
Dysentery (*Shigella* or *Salmonella*)	Antibiotics not indicated unless systemic infection occurs

Liver Disease

About 5% of patients with all types of hypogammaglobulinaemia have a variety of liver disorders. The most important is chronic cholangitis, which in most cases is probably due to an ascending bacterial infection of the biliary tree. The diagnosis can usually be confirmed by the ragged appearance of the extra and intrahepatic bile ducts on retrograde cholangiography. Once established, the condition is very difficult to reverse and, despite continuous antibiotics, patients either die with acute septicaemia or develop cirrhosis within two or three years.

Children may insidiously develop a gross hepatosplenomegaly where the histological abnormality is an intrahepatic portal infiltration with mononuclear cells. Cirrhosis usually develops over five to ten years. The aetiology is unknown but is probably chronic infection or an inability to neutralize

TABLE 3
Routine screening tests for complications in primary hypogammaglobulinaemia

Blood	Haemoglobin + film	(R)
	Differential blood count	
	Red cell folate	
Serum	Calcium	
	Aspartate transaminase	
	Alk. phosphatase	
	Bilirubin	
	Iron/iron binding capacity	
	Vitamin B12	
5-day faecal fat		
Pentagastrin stimulation test (+intrinsic factor measurement)		
Sputum, Urine	culture	(R)
Barium meal and follow through		
Sinus X-rays		
Chest X-ray (AP + lateral)		(R)
Lung function tests		(R)

(R) = Repeat routinely at annual intervals.

certain toxins from the gut. Table 3 shows the routine screening tests appropriate to investigation of complications in primary hypogammaglobulinaemia.

Treatment of Primary Hypogammaglobulinaemia

Antibiotics should be used freely and in high dosage for at least ten days when patients develop acute infections. It is usually wise to give patients supplies of antibiotics so that they can start treatment immediately symptoms are noticed. Long term prophylactic antibiotics should be avoided since these may encourage the growth of resistant organisms. However, some patients with advanced lung disease cannot do without continuous antibiotics.

Although co-trimoxazole is very effective chemotherapy for most acute chest infections, it should be used with caution since many patients have folate depletion secondary to malabsorption. Surgical drainage of middle ear or sinuses should be performed if necessary and lobectomy for isolated bronchiectatic areas may be very rewarding provided patients are already receiving regular replacement gamma-globulin. Steroids are not absolutely contra-indicated and may occasionally be appropriate for complications such as pulmonary granulomata, haemolytic anaemia and thrombocytopenia.

Gamma-globulin Replacement Therapy

All patients with recurrent infections and hypogammaglobulinaemia should be treated with regular intramuscular injections of gamma-globulin at a dose of 25–50 mg/kg body weight. There is also an argument in favour of giving gamma-globulin to those rare patients with severe hypogammaglobulinaemia who are not affected by recurrent infections in order to protect them from the possibility of a sudden potentially lethal complication such as meningitis. Patients should initially receive a loading course of five daily injections at a dose of 50 mg/kg body weight. Most patients then require weekly injections but a few with mild symptoms manage with fortnightly treatment. The amount injectable at any one time is limited because the material cannot be made more concentrated than about 150 mg/ml without becoming too viscous.

In Britain, the gamma-globulin used for intramuscular injections is made by alcohol fractionation of blood plasma and contains the following approximate concentrations of immunoglobulin: IgG 150 mg/ml, IgA 5 mg/ml, IgM 1 mg/ml, IgE 850 U/ml. The preparations contain aggregated gamma-globulin which can be eliminated by centrifugation but tends to reform on standing. Gamma-globulin contains antibodies to a wide variety of bacteria and viruses and has a half life of approximately 14 days in hypogammaglobulinaemic subjects. However, it should be remembered that specific antibody to an organism which was currently causing infection may be used up very quickly.

The type of gamma-globulin mentioned above cannot be administered intravenously without causing severe anaphylactic reactions probably because of the presence of aggregates. The formation of aggregates can be prevented by removing the Fc fragment by acid treatment. Such preparations have been used mainly in America but still give a high incidence of reactions, and the half life is much shorter than that of gamma-globulin used for intramuscular injection. Since much higher concentrations of serum immunoglobulin can be obtained with intravenous injection this form of therapy is nevertheless likely to become more popular in Britain once a safer preparation is available. Purified IgA immunoglobulin is now commercially available with a view to improving immunity at mucosal surfaces but it is too early to comment on its usefulness.

Provided the serum IgG level is kept above 200 mg/100 ml in patients with severe hypogammaglobulinaemia, infections are controlled unless there is already structural lung damage. Failure to maintain this level may indicate a co-existent protein losing enteropathy. This can be assessed by injecting appropriate radiolabelled immunoglobulin or, perhaps more conveniently, by measuring the half life of a specific antibody in the injected gamma-globulin which is not absorbed out by common pathogens (e.g. diphtheria antitoxin).

Plasma therapy is useful in acute infection since it supplies large amounts of all types of immunoglobulins. It is particularly indicated in septicaemia where IgM immunoglobulin is especially effective. Long-term use of plasma infusions carries a risk of antigen A hepatitis whereas purified gamma-globulin preparations for intramuscular or intravenous use do not transmit hepatitis virus. Acute reactions occur within minutes of injection in about 10% of patients receiving intramuscular gamma-globulin and in a much higher proportion receiving intravenous therapy. This takes the form of collapse, pain and tightness in the chest, breathlessness and rigors. Spontaneous recovery is the rule but the patients may be lethargic and pyrexial for many hours afterwards. Antihistamines, hydrocortisone and adrenaline may be needed for severe cases.

The reactions are unusual in that they are unpredictable. Skin tests with gamma-globulin a few days after the attack are usually negative and patients have no further trouble when they have their next injection a week later. However, it is customary to give graded doses under medical supervision at the subsequent injection. The mechanism of these reactions is not clear but there is evidence that aggregated gamma-globulin releases histamine *in vitro* from the circulating basophils of patients who have recently had reactions. The mediator for this may be an IgE antibody although serum levels of IgE are not raised in comparison with other patients without reactions. Serum antibodies to aggregated gamma-globulin giving a positive latex rheumatoid factor test were found in one patient with a reaction but may have been irrelevant. Antibodies to IgA have been implicated in a few other patients.

We have not yet had to abandon therapy in any patient giving repeated reactions. My impression is that twice weekly injection of gamma-globulin is useful in "tolerizing" patients. Intermittent fresh frozen plasma infusions, together with regular intramuscular gamma-globulin prevented reactions in one patient. In difficult cases, it is worth centrifuging the gamma-globulin preparation at 10,000 ***g*** for 60 min to remove aggregates immediately prior to the injection, as this has prevented reactions.

Aetiology of Primary Hypogammaglobulinaemia

A reasonable hypothesis for the aetiology of primary hypogammaglobulinaemia is that there is a major defect in the gene responsible for coding immunoglobulin. Such may hold for the rare disorder of sex-linked agammaglobulinaemia, but since patients with other types of hypogammaglobulinaemia have circulating B-lymphocytes, which by definition have immunoglobulin on their surface, this is no longer tenable. Nevertheless, most patients' B-cells cannot be induced to produce intracytoplasmic immunoglobulin when stimulated *in vitro* with pokeweed mitogen (PWM). This defect is not present in total isolated IgA deficiency where the cells with IgA on their surface can produce intracytoplasmic IgA on stimulation with PWM. Stimulated lymph nodes from patients with hypogammaglobulinaemia also do not contain plasma cells or lymphocytes with intracytoplasmic immunoglobulin, but lymphoid cells in the lamina propria of the gut of such patients do, although the immunoglobulin concentrations in the gut juices tend to be very low. This apparent functional dichotomy between circulating lymphocytes and those in the gut has yet to be explained.

Two appealing hypotheses have been put forward to explain these findings. Firstly, suppressor T-lymphocytes have been shown to depress both humoral and cell mediated immune responses in mice. Waldman *et al.* (1974) have demonstrated that lymphocytes from patients with variable panhypogammaglobulinaemia depress *in vitro* immunoglobulin production from normal lymphocytes when mixed together in the presence of PWM. However, the interpretation of this experiment is not straightforward since we have shown that depression of immunoglobulin production occurs in mixtures with lymphocytes from some normal donors but not others.

The second view compares the disease with the phenomenon of allotypic suppression in mice where an immunoglobulin allotype is permanently suppressed by neonatal injection of anti-allotype serum. This suppression can be transferred by "suppressor" T-lymphocytes, a finding which links together both hypotheses. However, the "whys and wherefores" of such a phenomenon occurring are hard to imagine.

Alternatively, the defect may lie in a congenitally determined enzyme deficiency leading to a defect of clonal expansion of lymphocytes or an inability to secrete immunoglobulin from the lymphoid cell. The latter suggestion is supported by a recent finding in some patients of a defect in attachment to the immunoglobulin molecule of certain sugars necessary for the secretory phase.

ISOLATED DEFECTS IN CELL MEDIATED IMMUNITY

Thymic Deficiency

Isolated severe defects in cell mediated immunity are very rare and probably only associated with congenital partial or complete absence of the thymus. The classical form (Di George syndrome) follows an intra-uterine "accident" at about 3 weeks gestation causing failure of formation of the third and fourth pharangeal arches. This leads to absence of the thymus and parathyroid glands with consequent neonatal hypoparathyroidism causing tetany and convulsions. Infants may also have skeletal abnormalities of the head such as hyperteliorism, shortened lip philtrum, low set notched ear pinnae and nasal clefts. Abnormalities of the large vessels in the thorax may occur, particularly Fallot's tetralogy and right sided aorta. Some affected infants suffer from repeated bacterial and viral infections and die within the first few years of life. Others remain relatively well, and with time recover part of their CMI as judged by increasing numbers of circulating T-lymphocytes and return of PHA lymphocyte transformation responses to normal. In these patients there is presumably only a partial thymic deficiency. A few children are described who have apparently developed a defect in cell mediated immunity with infections after infancy. Some of these have benefited from a thymus graft and one hypothesis is that the disorder is due to premature thymic involution.

There is controversy over whether these patients are hypo- or hyper-responders with respect to antibody production following immunization with various antigens. This question is relevant to the basic understanding of immune responses since the absence of T-helper cells would theoretically depress antibody production, while absence of T-suppressor cells might cause enhancement. The facts are contradictory but the majority of investigations so far show that most patients are poor antibody producers (Lischner, 1972).

The diagnosis depends upon the demonstration of low or absent numbers of circulating T-lymphocytes together with absent delayed hypersensitivity skin reactions and paracortical lymphocyte depletion in lymph nodes. About a third of patients have lymphopenia. Transformation of peripheral blood lymphocyte by PHA and allogeneic lymphocytes (MLR) is usually grossly depressed but may be normal. The discrepancy between the absence of T-cells, as judged by currently available markers, and the ability to transform in a mixed lymphocyte reaction is also seen in thymic deficient "nude" mice. The interpretation is not yet settled but it is possible that T-cell precursors, as yet uninfluenced by the thymus, are capable of reacting. Such cells have been identified in the bone marrow of patients with thymic aplasia and acquire the ability to rosette with sheep red cells after incubation with suitable thymic extracts.

The *in vitro* tests can sometimes be difficult to reconcile with the clinical events as is illustrated by our own case of partial thymic aplasia. This infant presented with fits due to hypoparathyroidism a few days after birth. Investigation showed a normal lymphocyte count with 6% of circulating T-lymphocytes (normal 55–75%) and 40% of B-lymphocytes (normal 15–22%). Contact sensitivity to dinitrochlorobenzene could not be induced. A lymph node biopsy taken five days after local stimulation with picryl chloride showed the characteristic abnormalities (see Fig. 1b). Serum immunoglobulins were normal for his age and by one year he had developed a normal level of natural antibodies to *E. coli*. However, immunization with diphtheria toxoid and pneumococcal polysaccharide failed to produce antibody responses. Lymphocyte transformation to PHA and allogeneic cells gave low normal responses. Despite these apparent severe defects, this baby has reached the age of 15 months without a day's illness. This suggests that the tests we use to assess CMI may bear little relation to clinical events. In addition, it casts doubts on the assumption that responses to polysaccharides in humans are thymus independent.

Treatment

Patients who suffer from infections and failure to thrive should be given a 13 to 16 week foetal thymus graft as soon as possible. There are now a number of reports of successful grafts which have provided some important clues to thymic function. Lymphocyte transformation responses to PHA have returned to normal within a few days of thymus grafting and there is evidence that the transformed cells are of recipient and not donor origin. Furthermore, successful reconstitution of T-cell function has been achieved by thymus grafts enclosed in millipore chambers. This strongly suggests that the grafted thymus is releasing a soluble substance which influences the patient's own precursor T-lymphocytes. Although it is unusual for thymus cells to initiate a graft versus host reaction, it is reasonable to recommend that future thymus grafts be enclosed in a millipore chamber. The surgical procedure involved is relatively minor, the millipore chamber being placed within the rectus sheath.

Ware *et al.* (1975) have isolated a factor from pig thymus which, injected into patients with thymic deficiency, restores T-lymphocyte function. This type of therapy is likely to supersede thymus grafting in the near future.

Documentation of Cases

In view of the puzzling heterogeneity of this condition, particularly in respect of antibody responses, it is very important that cases are investigated in as much detail as time allows. If the patient should come to autopsy, then particular attention should be paid to examining central and peripheral lymph nodes. A very careful search should also be made for the thymus by block sectioning the mediastinum, neck and pharynx in order to exclude the presence of a small undescended remnant of thymic tissue.

Cartilage Hair Hypoplasia

A syndrome characterized by dwarfism and thin sparse hair was first noticed in studies on the Old Amish sect in North America. Children have disproportionately short limbs similar to that seen in achondroplasia although this condition is inherited as an autosomal recessive. The skeletal abnormalities are due to metaphyseal dysostosis and other associated abnormalities include neutropenia, malabsorption, Hirschsprung's disease and recurrent infections. They are particularly susceptible to very severe varicella infection, and this is explained by a defect in cell mediated immunity characterized by absence of delayed hypersensitivity, depression of *in vitro* lymphocyte transformation to PHA and prolonged skin graft rejection. Serum immunoglobulin concentrations are normal or raised and specific antibody production is intact.

Chronic Mucocutaneous Candidiasis

This condition occurs in infants and children who develop oral and vaginal thrush together with lesions on the skin. Infection beneath the nails causes the fingers to have a characteristic "drumstick" appearance. A few patients develop grossly disfiguring lesions involving large areas of the body, particularly the head and neck. The precise aetiology is unknown, but the disease is probably caused by a primary defect in cell mediated immunity associated with other generalized metabolic or endocrine abnormalities.

Most patients have negative delayed hypersensitivity skin tests to *Candida* but *in vitro* lymphocyte transformation responses vary. Some have a generalized depression of lymphocyte transformation to all stimuli while others only show a specific inability to transform with *candida*. Patients also differ in the ability of their lymphocytes to produce MIF in the presence of *candida*.

Treatment

The disease is largely responsible for the recent renewal of interest in the therapeutic uses of transfer factor, which was first described by H. S. Lawrence in 1955. There are now many reports of patients whose skin lesions have disappeared within weeks following transfer factor injections. Delayed hypersensitivity skin tests to *Candida* and other *in vitro* lymphocyte tests for cell mediated immunity have also reverted to normal. However, the exact role of transfer factor remains debatable, especially as most patients have received additional therapy with antifungal agents such as amphotericin B. In addition patients often have associated endocrine abnormalities, particularly hypoparathyroidism, which should be treated simultaneously. It is also claimed that correcting the iron deficiency common in these patients may itself improve the skin lesions.

A double blind therapeutic trial of transfer factor is badly needed but is unlikely because of the rarity of the disease and because physicians feel bound to use multiple therapy as soon as possible to prevent further disfigurement. However, in the less severe cases, careful dissection of the response to individual treatments may help clarify the situation.

SYNDROMES ASSOCIATED WITH DEFECTS IN ANTIBODY PRODUCTION AND CELL MEDIATED IMMUNITY

Severe Combined Immune Deficiency of Infancy (SCID)

This disease nearly always leads to death within the first two years of life unless immunological reconstitution is successful. Infants usually present within the first two months of life with failure to thrive, oral thrush and recurrent upper and lower respiratory tract infections. Intractable diarrhoea, sometimes with steatorrhoea, is common and is usually not accounted for by known pathogenic bacteria or viruses. Jejunal biopsies in some patients have shown the presence of large submucosal vacuolated macrophages similar to those seen in Whipple's disease. Many infants die undiagnosed and it is suggested that the disease may account for as much as 10% of extra-neonatal infant mortality. A frequent cause of death is opportunistic infection with the protozoan *Pneumocystis carinii*, which causes an insidious pneumonia leading to gradual anoxia. The disease covers a spectrum, the most severe form having a gross defect in CMI and agammaglobulinaemia. Other affected infants, who tend to survive for two to three years, have a severe CMI defect but normal or grossly raised levels of serum immunoglobulins. Despite this, they fail to make functional antibody following immunization.

Diagnosis

Apart from the usually obvious clinical clues to the diagnosis, tests for cell mediated immunity are always grossly depressed or absent. There is a profound depression in numbers of circulating T-lymphocytes. Circulating B-cells may be absent in cases with agammaglobulinaemia but in others their number may be markedly expanded. Lymphopenia and eosinophilia are common, the latter possibly being due to a mild chronic graft versus host reaction (GVH) caused by maternal lymphocytes which have crossed the placenta. Delayed hypersensitivity skin reactions are absent and lymphocyte transformation by PHA is grossly depressed or absent. Peripheral lymph nodes contain very few lymphocytes, leaving only the fibrous anlage and histiocytic cells (Fig. 1c). In patients with normal or raised levels of immunoglobulins, mediastinal lymph nodes may become heavily infiltrated with plasma cells. The thymus is usually present but shrunken, containing few lymphocytes and no Hassall's corpuscles. The absence of Hassall's corpuscles indicates a failure of thymic maturation whereas lymphocyte depletion can occur secondarily to a chronic illness.

There are two other clinical entities recently described which should now be included under SCID. Cederbaum *et al.* (1975) have drawn attention to the difficulty in distinguishing SCID from Letterer-Siwe disease (LSD). Features of both conditions include hepatosplenomegaly, macular skin rash, failure to thrive and eosinophilia. The aetiology of LSD is based on widespread organ infiltration with apparently normal histiocytes and, in its true form, is not particularly associated with infections. The importance of differentiating the two diseases is that steroids and cytotoxic agents are used (with poor success) in LSD, but are absolutely contra-indicated in SCID. The reason why such histiocytic proliferation occurs in some cases of SCID is not clear but it may represent a GVH reaction initiated by maternal cells.

Purtulo *et al.* (1975) have recently described a kindred in whom six male children died of a lymphoproliferative disorder associated with a defect in CMI and hyper- or hypo-gammaglobulinaemia. These children developed infectious mononucleosis before or during the terminal events of their illness. The disease appears to be sex linked and might be considered a variant of SCID with apparent susceptibility to infection and malignant transformation by EB virus. SCID also occurs in the rapidly fatal condition of reticular dysgenesis, where there is a failure of all types of bone marrow stem cell to differentiate.

Genetics

SCID may occur spontaneously or show a sex-linked recessive or autosomal recessive mode of inheritance. This accounts for the male predominance in the disease. A considerable advance in understanding of the disorder has come from the finding that many infants with the autosomal form of the disease also have a deficiency of adenosine deaminase (ADA) (Pickering *et al.*, 1974). This enzyme is important in purine metabolism and catalyses the conversion of adenosine to inosine. However, although there are some theoretical possibilities, the link between ADA deficiency and the immune defect is unknown. More recently, deficiency of purine nucleoside phosphorylase has been described in a 5-year-old girl with infections and a defect in CMI. This enzyme catalyses conversion of inosine to hypoxanthine, which is only one metabolic step beyond the reaction involving ADA. ADA deficiency can be conveniently recognized by measuring the concentration of the enzyme in red cells, and tissue enzyme levels are also low. Mothers who are heterozygote carriers are immunologically normal but have low levels of red cell ADA. Although still in the research phase, prenatal diagnosis is possible by measuring the enzyme level in cells obtained by amniocentesis. This development should lessen the fear of further pregnancy in mothers who have already had an infant with SCID since they can be given the option of early therapeutic abortion.

Treatment

The only specific "cure" available is a bone marrow graft but unless the donor is an identical sibling, a GVH reaction usually occurs. Such reactions are clinically recognized by hepatosplenomegaly, lymphadenopathy, skin rash and spontaneous bleeding due to thrombocytopenia. Graft lymphocytes eventually destroy other haemopoietic stem cells leading to severe neutropenia, anaemia and death. Reactions can be modified with immunosuppresive drugs such as cyclophosphamide, steroids, azathioprine and antilymphocyte globulin (ALG) and a number of children have survived through such an episode to become successfully reconstituted. Mild GVH reactions may be self-limiting. Attempts to modify the grafted bone marrow cells by eliminating the lymphocytes causing the GVH reactions have proved unsuccessful. The use of foetal liver tissue containing lymphocytic stem cells has also led to fatal GVH reactions and carries no advantage.

All near relatives, particularly siblings, should be HLA typed. In the search for a suitable donor, lymphocytes from suitably matched individuals should be tested in a "two way" mixed lymphocyte reaction with the recipient's lymphocytes. Perfect HLA matches are unlikely to be found but success can be achieved using donors with minor HLA differences which may give rise only to mild self-limiting GVH reactions. The availability of suitable donors in the UK will be increased when tests are completed on the large number of volunteer potential donors currently being processed at the Westminster Hospital in London. Donating bone marrow involves multiple sternal and iliac crest aspirations under general anaesthesia. About 10^9 marrow cells are transferred to the receipient by intravenous injection.

An unexpected finding has occurred in patients with SCID and ADA deficiency who have been successfully reconstituted (Parkman *et al.*, 1975). Despite re-population by donor lymphocytes, the recipient's red cells do not show chimaerism and remain ADA deficient. This presumably means that ADA deficiency offers some survival advantage for red cells.

An alternative method of treatment for SCID is to graft a foetal thymus, thereby correcting the CMI defect, and then treat the remaining hypogammaglobulinaemia with regular injections of gamma-globulin. There have been a number of recent successes with this method and it is probably safer than risking a lethal GVH reaction following incompatible bone marrow graft. In view of one report of a GVH reaction following a thymus graft, it is advisable to graft the thymus within a millipore chamber. However, in most cases, the treatment of choice remains a bone marrow graft since, despite gamma-globulin treatment, a severe defect in antibody production often leads to chronic ill health.

Supporting Treatment Prior to Transplantation

A great deal of publicity has recently been given to the plight of infants and children with SCID who have been delivered by sterile techniques and then kept in sterile "cages" until a suitable bone marrow donor is available. Such patients can theoretically be kept alive indefinitely but the emotional and social problems involved are enormous. Long term maintenance in sterile environments should be discouraged but short term isolation in suitable sterile cabinets following a bacterial decontamination regime can be useful. However, a limited time of a few months should be allotted to the period of isolation at the outset. If an appropriate HLA matched donor is unavailable, then a foetal thymus transplant should be performed in the hope that the defect in cell mediated immunity can be reversed.

Pneumocystis carinii pneumonia is so common in this condition that it is worth giving prophylactic oral sulphadiazine up to the time of the transplant. Once established, *pneumocystis carinii* pneumonia is usually lethal, but intravenous pentamidine isethionate and intramuscular sulphadiazine are the drugs of choice.

Wiskott-Aldrich Syndrome

This sex-linked recessive condition only affects males and is characterized by thrombocytopenia, eczema and immunodeficiency (Cooper *et al.*, 1968). Bruising and recurrent epistaxis usually occur in early infancy. The eczema, which particularly affects the scalp and ears, is often superinfected by constant scratching. Most patients suffer from recurrent sinopulmonary and middle ear bacterial infections and some are susceptible to chronic virus infections. One patient in our clinic developed chronic anal warts which were resistant to treatment while another suffered from a recurrent Guillain–Barré syndrome. Auto-immune haemolytic anaemia occurs in a few patients. The severity of the condition varies and there seems to be a "forme fruste" of the syndrome which is mild and compatible with a normal life span.

About 60% of patients have low serum IgM levels while the serum IgE is high in 40%. The former is associated with an inability to produce antibodies to polysaccharides. Antibody responses to protein antigens are also significantly depressed in many patients. This may be related to an increased catabolism of IgG, IgA and IgM which is not accounted for by gastrointestinal or urinary protein loss. Serum isohaemagglutinins and "natural" *E. coli* antibodies are usually absent. The raised IgE levels may be related to the high incidence of drug sensitivity reactions in these patients. About 10% of patients develop leukaemia or other lymphoreticular neoplasms in childhood or adolescence but, the most frequent cause of death is an intracerebral or other haemorrhage. Splenomegaly occurs in most patients and is probably related to the constant sequestration of platelets which have a short half life. The platelets are also small in size and are functionally abnormal *in vitro* since they fail to aggregate with ADP and do not adhere to collagen. Heterozygote female carriers may also show such platelet abnormalities.

Cell mediated immunity, as judged by depression of delayed hypersensitivity and lymphocyte transformation to mitogens, is often impaired. Lymph nodes may be normal but, as the disease progresses, usually show loss of lymphocytes in the paracortical regions. The thymus is often small and atrophic at autopsy but contains Hassall's corpuscles. The number of circulating T-lymphocytes may be depressed and there is often an associated lymphopenia. The general impression is of a gradual deterioration in CMI with time, which suggests that the defects are secondary.

Treatment

The only definitive treatment is a bone marrow graft which will correct both the platelet defect and the immune defect. Thymus grafts have been implanted in a few patients in order to correct the CMI defect but these have been unsuccessful. More recently, there has been considerable enthusiasm for regular injections of transfer factor. Some patients seem to have benefited after such treatment with improvement in the eczema, general health and bruising. Delayed hypersensitivity skin tests may revert to normal and MIF tests may become positive. Circulating numbers of T-lymphocytes may increase but *in vitro* lymphocyte responses to mitogens and antigens remain depressed. This, together with the findings by Spitler *et al.* (1972) that only patients with a deficiency of monocyte receptors for IgG tend to respond, clouds the whole phenomenon in mystery and a double blind trial is urgently needed. The thrombocytopenia and bleeding is often exacerbated by infections which should be energetically treated with antibiotics. Steroids can be helpful in acute thrombocytopenic crises but should be avoided in the long term. Splenectomy improves the platelet half-life but has lost favour because of the high incidence of post-operative fatal pneumococcal septicaemia. However, it may be possible to prevent this complication with regular gamma-globulin replacement therapy. Gamma-globulin injections may also help prevent recurrent sinopulmonary infections and may also give protection against potentially oncogenic viruses which are presumably responsible for the high incidence of lymphoid tumours. Papovavirus, which shows some antigenic cross-reactions with the mouse oncogenic virus SV40, has been isolated from the reticulum cell sarcoma and urine of a patient with this syndrome. However, this patient had a high level of anti-papovavirus antibody at least a year before tumour detection.

Ataxia Telangiectasia

This multisystem disease is characterized by oculocutaneous telangiectasia, cerebellar ataxia, immunodeficiency and an autosomal recessive mode of inheritance (McFarlin *et al.*, 1972). Some patients have vitiligo with "cafe au lait" patches, hypoplastic ovaries, glucose intolerance and a tendency to develop progeric changes in early life. The ataxia becomes obvious when the child starts to walk and is progressive. Patients usually die in the second decade due to chronic infective lung disease although about 10% die of a lymphoreticular malignancy. There is a mild "forme fruste" of the disease which is consistent with survival to the fifth or sixth decade.

Most patients have some abnormalities of the immune system. About 70% have IgA and/or IgE deficiency and a few have severe panhypogammaglobulinaemia. Circulating lymphocytes from most patients show depressed *in vitro* lymphocyte transformation to mitogens and antigens and about a third have negative delayed hypersensitivity skin reactions. There is a general correlation between the severity of the CMI or immunoglobulin defect and the frequency of recurrent infections. The thymus is usually depleted of lymphocytes at autopsy and often does not contain any Hassall's corpuscles, a finding which suggests a primary thymic defect. Lymph nodes are usually depleted of lymphocytes but contain germinal centres. There is marked loss of Purkinje cells in the cerebellar cortex with demyelination of cerebellar tracts and posterior columns of the spinal cord.

Chromosome studies on lymphocytes have shown an increased number of "breaks" which may bear some relation to the high incidence of malignancy. A clone of circulating lymphocytes, identified by an abnormal chromosome pattern, has been shown in one patient to gradually expand over a number of years although this may not necessarily be related to lymphoid malignancy. Nucleomegalic cells, similar to those seen in progressive multifocal leuko-encephalopathy, have been found in the brain and other organs at autopsy. This may indicate the presence of a "slow" virus infection.

Treatment

No treatment of the neurological defect is available. Attempts to modify the immune defect by transfer factor and thymus grafts have not proved successful. Correction of the humoral immune defect with regular injections of gamma-globulin may be beneficial although it should be remembered that some patients have circulating IgA antibodies which might cause reactions.

Table 4 summarizes the complications seen in primary immunodeficiency, and Table 5 summarizes available lines of treatment.

TABLE 4
Complications affecting patients with primary immunodeficiency

Hypogammaglobulinaemia		
Lung disease	bronchiectasis	cor pulmonale
	fibrosis	cor pulmonale
	granuloma (rare)	cor pulmonale
Meningitis		
Ear and sinus infections		
Malabsorption	giardiasis	
	bacterial overgrowth	
	"coeliac" disease (rare)	
Nodular lymphoid hyperplasia		
Achlorhydria ± intrinsic factor deficiency		
Lymphadenopathy	"reactive"	
	germinal centre hyperplasia	
	lymphoid malignancy	
Arthritis	septic	
	aseptic + tenosynovitis	
Anaemia	iron deficient	
	deficiency of	Vit B12
		Folate (trimethoprim induced)
Inflammatory liver disease		
Thymoma *Ureaplasma* cystitis		

Herpes zoster
Lymphoid malignancy
Eczema

"Slow" virus — dermatomyositis / encephalitis } mainly in children

IgA deficiency

Recurrent chest infections
Sinusitis
Autoimmune disease — Sjögren's syndrome / rheumatoid arthritis / thyroiditis
Tendency to "atopy"
Malabsorption
Nodular lymphoid hyperplasia } rare
Pernicious anaemia

Thymus deficiency — Severe Combined Immunodeficiency (SCID)

Recurrent upper and lower respiratory tract bacterial infections
Lethal virus infections (measles, varicella, smallpox)
Moniliasis

Pneumocystis pneumonia
Diarrhoea ± malabsorption
Lymphoid malignancy

SECONDARY IMMUNODEFICIENCY (Table 6)

Immunodeficiency is being demonstrated in an ever increasing number of diseases but the cause and effect relationship in many is far from clear. The immune defect associated with some diseases seems to be largely of academic interest, having no apparent clinical significance. However, a greater understanding of such defects may help unravel the aetiology of the primary disease. In other cases, the immunodeficiency leads to recurrent infections which are sometimes dismissed by the clinician as being a conse-

TABLE 5
Treatment of primary immunodeficiency

Hypogammaglobulinaemia (including some cases of IgA deficiency)	Gamma-globulin i.m. (i.v. gamma-globulin, fresh frozen plasma)
	(N.B. Caution with blood transfusions and gamma-globulin in total IgA deficiency)
Isolated thymic deficiency	Thymus graft (millipore chamber) or Thymosin
Wiskott–Aldrich syndrome	Transfer factor Bone marrow graft Gamma-globulin
Mucocutaneous candidiasis	Transfer factor + amphotericin B Correct any endocrine or iron deficiency
Severe combined immunodeficiency	Bone marrow graft (thymus graft – millipore chamber + gamma-globulin) Prophylactic sulphadiazine for *Pn. carinii* Irradiated blood transfusions

quence of the patient's "general debility". Greater awareness of the existence of such defects should enable us to improve the management of such patients.

The Leukaemias

Over half of patients with chronic lymphatic leukaemia develop hypogammaglobulinaemia and consequently suffer from recurrent infections. In view of the relatively prolonged course of this disease, it is very important that all patients are screened for such a defect and, if necessary, given regular injections of gamma-globulin. However, measuring serum concentrations of immunoglobulin may not be sufficient since many patients have a severe defect in specific antibody production well before they develop hypogammaglobulinaemia. Measurement of serum isohaemagglutinins and *E. coli* antibody may be helpful in this context. Hypogammaglobulinaemia tends to progress with the severity of the primary disease and may be exacerbated if cytotoxic therapy is given. Some patients develop defects in cell mediated immunity but it is not clear whether this is of clinical significance.

Other varieties of lymphoid and myeloid leukaemias may be associated with humoral or cell mediated immune deficiency although the severity of the primary disease usually overshadows these aspects. Nevertheless, with improvement in the overall remission rate it is possible that gamma-globulin

TABLE 6
Secondary immunodeficiency

Disorders associated with recurrent infections	Recurrent infections not of major clinical significance
Chronic lymphatic Leukaemia Myeloma } (H) Hodgkin's disease (C)	Lymphoid and myeloid diseases Other paraproteinaemias (H) Other lymphoid and myeloid malignancies (C)
Protein calorie malnutrition (C+H)	Metabolic Uraemia Diabetes Hypothyroidism Iron Vit. C } deficiency Cyanocobalamin II deficiency } (C)
Malaria Trypanosomiasis } (H)	Infections Measles Infectious mononucleosis Tuberculosis Syphilis Leprosy Viral hepatitis } (C)
	Chronic inflammatory disorders Rheumatoid arthritis Sjögren's syndrome Biliary cirrhosis } (C)
	Granulomata Sarcoidosis Whipple's disease Crohn's disease Wegeners granulomatosis } (C)
Nephrosis Protein losing enteropathy Burns } (H)	Protein losing and hypercatabolic states Dystrophia myotonica
	Other conditions Ageing Malignancy Pregnancy } (C)

(C) = Predominantly affects cell mediated immunity.
(H) = Predominantly affects antibody production.

injections may be useful in patients with acute leukaemias when their immunocompetence is being additionally compromised by cytotoxic agents.

Protein Losing and Hypercatabolic States

Infections, particularly pneumococcal pneumonia, may occur in patients with the nephrotic syndrome, where there is considerable loss of gamma-globulin in the urine. The serum IgG, being a smaller molecule than IgM, tends to be predominantly affected because of its greater loss by diffusion through the damaged renal glomeruli. Replacement therapy with injections of gamma-globulin may be useful but it is very difficult to maintain an adequate level in the face of such rapid loss. In acute infections, it is better to give large quantities of fresh frozen plasma intravenously.

Protein-losing enteropathy with associated hypogammaglobulinaemia may occur secondarily to other gastrointestinal disorders (e.g. hypertrophic gastritis, Crohn's disease). Intestinal lymphangiectasia is a rare non-hereditary cause in children which is diagnosed by the finding of dilated mucosal lymphatics on small bowel biopsy. Apart from hypogammaglobulinaemia, patients may have lymphopenia and subcutaneous lymphangiomas with peripheral oedema. Fortunately the condition usually improves spontaneously before adolescence.

Extensive third degree burns lead to enormous protein loss through the skin. Some of the recent plasma substitutes used in such cases contain very little gamma-globulin and one should ensure that serum immunoglobulin levels are maintained with fresh frozen plasma.

Very little is known about the mechanism controlling metabolism of immunoglobulins. A primary hypercatabolic state, as opposed to loss from the gut or kidneys, is very rare. The diagnosis depends upon a decreased half life of injected I^{125} labelled immunoglobulin in the face of a failure to demonstrate albumin loss from the kidneys or gut (Waldman and Strober, 1969). This occurs in dystrophia myotonica where there is often a moderate decrease in serum IgG concentration. However, it is rare for such patients to suffer from recurrent infections although some have grossly inadequate specific antibody responses.

Myeloma and Paraproteinaemias

Most patients with myeloma have a significant defect in ability to produce specific antibody and many have low levels of the "normal" immunoglobulins outside the M-component. Serum concentrations of IgA and IgM are predominantly affected but may rise to normal levels during remissions induced by chemotherapy. Septicaemia and pneumonia, particularly pneumococcal, are common complications in patients with myeloma but attempts to prevent these with regular gamma-globulin injections have proved disappointing. However, now that the prognosis is improved by the use of more efficient therapeutic regimes, it might be appropriate to review the effect of temporary gamma-globulin injections until remission is induced. Other paraproteinaemias such as Waldenström's macroglobulinaemia may also be associated with infections and a defect in humoral immunity.

Solid Lymphoid Tumours

It is well known that the advanced stages of Hodgkin's disease are associated with a variety of infections, particularly herpes zoster and unusual opportunistic protozoal and fungal infections. Humoral immunity remains intact until the terminal stages but there is a significant defect in cell mediated immunity early in the disease which increases with time. Patients in stage 1 often have depressed delayed hypersensitivity skin reactions, poor lymphocyte transformation to PHA and show prolonged survival of skin grafts. Longmire *et al.* (1974) found that spleen cells from patients with Hodgkin's disease spontaneously produced large amounts of immunoglobulin *in vitro* when compared with cells from normal spleens. Furthermore, an IgG fraction of this immunoglobulin had a high binding affinity for the patient's own lymphocytes. This suggests an immune reaction in patients with Hodgkin's disease directed against antigenic structures on autologous lymphocytes. Such structures may turn out to be closely related to an aetiological virus.

Other solid lymphoid tumours (e.g. lymphosarcomas) may also be associated with defects in cell mediated and humoral immunity, particularly when there is widespread infiltration of the bone marrow, lymph nodes and spleen.

Drugs

The most important drugs causing immunodeficiency are those used for treatment of chronic inflammatory disorders and malignancy. Only antilymphocyte globulin (ALG) has a specific immunosuppressive effect and most of the other chemotherapeutic agents affect the metabolism and/or mitosis of most bone marrow and circulating blood cells. Fatal infections, due to overdosage and prolonged treatment, used to be common following administration of drugs such as prednisolone, azathioprine and cyclophosphamide. However, recent regimes employ short courses of intermittent high dose therapy and serious infections are now uncommon. Nevertheless, the occasional fatal infection still occurs and we need more information about the effect of these drugs on polymorphs and lymphocytes.

Renal transplant recipients often need to be on long-term immunosuppressive therapy and these patients are particularly prone to the development of opportunistic infections such as *Pneumocystis carinii* pneumonia and generalized cytomegalovirus infections. It is not clear how one can improve this situation since the very reason for therapy is to depress the immune response. Furthermore, such patients are prone to development of tumours particularly of the brain and lymphoid system. Although patients receiving immunosuppressive drugs other than to suppress graft rejection have a marginally increased susceptibility to tumours, a chronic graft versus host reaction induced by immunosuppression may be the relevant inducing factor in most of these malignancies.

The synthetic immunosuppressive drugs currently available for human use have optimal actions at different stages of the immune response (Makinodan *et al.*, 1970). All of them significantly depress both cell mediated and humoral immunity except the alkylating agent, busulphan, which has only a very weak immunosuppressive action. Many of these drugs act by preventing the lymphocyte division required for generation of an immune response. Steroids have a marked anti-inflammatory action, thereby preventing the expression of cell mediated immunity but studies in human volunteers show that they also induce a lymphopenia and depression of PHA induced lymphocyte transformation when injected intravenously.

There is increasing evidence that some drugs used in the treatment of infections are also immunosuppressive. The combination of trimethoprim and sulphamethoxazole can have a marked depressive effect on *in vitro* lymphocyte transformation to PHA. The mechanism of this action is not known and its clinical significance not yet investigated. Inidazole, an antihelminthic used in the treatment of schistosomiasis, causes depression of delayed hypersensitivity skin reactions and *in vitro* lymphocyte transformation. Rifampicin, now used extensively in the treatment of tuberculosis, causes humoral and cell mediated immune depression in animals. Tests in man suggest that CMI is not significantly affected but there is a depression of IgG production after test immunization with Phage ϕX174. The finding of light chains in the urine of some patients taking rifampicin also suggests disordered immunoglobulin production.

The relevance of these immunosuppressive side effects to the treatment of infections is not understood but it is possible that depression of certain aspects of cell mediated immunity might aid in the elimination of certain organisms. This is analogous to the additional use of steroids in patients with resistant pulmonary tuberculosis, the rationale for which is prevention of inflammation and fibrosis which tends to impede adequate tissue penetration of anti-tuberculous drugs.

Anaesthetic agents such as halothane slow the movement of lymphocytes *in vitro*, consequently causing depression of lymphocyte transformation to PHA. This may be an important factor in post-operative infections. Irradiation therapy for carcinoma of the breast leads to a moderate decrease in the number of circulating T-lymphocytes but is probably of no clinical significance. Phenobarbitone and hydantoins may depress both cell mediated and humoral immunity. The former is known to depress *in vitro* lymphocyte transformation while long term treatment with hydantoins in children is associated with a significant decrease in serum IgA immunoglobulin concentrations. However, epileptic patients on these two drugs do not seem to suffer clinical effects.

Infections

Many acute infections are associated with a transient defect in cell mediated immunity. Tuberculosis and syphilis are examples of chronic infections where a defect in cell mediated immunity may be partly due to serum inhibiting factors which can be demonstrated by their ability to depress lymphocyte transformation *in vitro*. This can be diagnostically important in severe tuberculosis when the Mantoux test is negative. However, *in vitro* lymphocyte transformation to PPD may be positive in the presence of heterologous normal serum but negative with autologous serum. The nature of such inhibiting serum factors is not known but α_2 macroglobulin has been shown to inhibit lymphocyte transformation.

The various types of leprosy are good examples of how the patient's immunocompetence affects the course of the disease. Patients who are able to mount an adequate cell mediated immune response limit the infection in the tuberculoid form. However, deficient CMI leads to widespread dissemination in the lepromatous variety. The reason for this heterogeneity in response is not known but it probably depends on a number of factors such as genetic susceptibility and degrees of secondary immunodeficiency caused by parasitic infections and malnutrition. Transfer factor, obtained from patients with the tuberculoid form, can be used to convert patients with lepromatous leprosy but the advantages of this manoeuvre are not yet clearly defined.

Severe secondary infections are common in patients suffering from malaria and trypanosomiasis. The former is associated with defects in antibody production and the presence of serum auto-antibodies. CMI defects occur in Gambian trypanosomiasis and light chains are also often found in the urine suggesting abnormal immunoglobulin synthesis. Hypergammaglobulinaemia occurs in most of these parasitic infections, the IgM level being particularly high. It is suggested that parasitic antigens may have a non-specific mitogenic action on B-lymphocytes stimulating them to produce large quantities of IgM immunoglobulin. Such an inappropriate response might prejudice specific antibody production to other infective agents. If this hypothesis is correct, regular gamma-globulin injections or plasma infusions should decrease the incidence of secondary infections in patients with these diseases.

Von Pirquet was the first to describe the cutaneous anergy which occurs to tuberculin during measles infection. Recently this virus has been shown to inhibit lymphocyte transformation to PPD *in vitro*. However, this may not be the entire explanation since high levels of serum cortisol, present during such infections, may also depress CMI. A number of viruses are known to infect lymphocytes (e.g. herpes viruses) and to replicate in transformed lymphoblasts. This may severely compromise lymphocyte function and may, for example, be responsible for the high incidence of auto-antibodies in infectious mononucleosis.

A non-specific cutaneous anergy occurs in sub-acute sclerosing panencephalitis (SSPE) caused by the measles virus. The patients have high titres of circulating measles antibody and *in vitro* lymphocyte cytotoxicity for measles-infected fibroblasts is inhibited in the presence of autologous, but not heterologous, serum. The nature of this serum factor is unknown but it may be antigen–antibody complexes (Valdimarsson *et al.*, 1974). Transfer factor, obtained from measles-immune donors, seems to reverse the cutaneous anergy and lowers the serum measles antibody titre, but progression of the encephalitis seems to be unaffected in the short term.

Common infections may induce either a lymphocytosis (e.g. pertussis) or lymphopenia (e.g. influenza) the latter perhaps caused by circulating lymphocytotoxins. This may account for the common occurrence of secondary bacterial infection following upper respiratory tract infections although mechanical damage to the bronchial tree is probably of prime importance.

In addition, viruses may also affect the chemotactic properties of leucocyte polymorphs.

Virus infections may rarely cause a permanent defect in antibody production with hypogammaglobulinaemia. Rubella, cytomegalovirus and EB virus infections have all been implicated in a few cases and antigen B hepatitis virus may lead to IgG deficiency.

Metabolic Disorders

Uraemia, iron deficiency anaemia and diabetes mellitus are all associated with defects in cell mediated immunity as assessed by delayed hypersensitivity skin reactions and *in vitro* lymphocyte transformation. Uraemia, which has received special attention because of its importance in renal transplantation, is also associated with a clearly demonstrable defect of humoral immunity. Nevertheless, with good management it is unusual for patients with chronic uraemia to suffer recurrent infections. However, a minority of patients on chronic haemodialysis develop repeated infections, particularly sepsis in the area of the arteriovenous shunt, and it may be appropriate to treat these with regular gamma-globulin injections.

One case of severe infantile hypogammaglobulinaemia has been described in association with absence of the vitamin B12 transport protein, cyanocobalamin II. Large doses of parenteral vitamin B12 eventually reversed the immunodeficiency.

Severe protein–calorie malnutrition is usually associated with a depression in cell mediated immunity and there is a high incidence of fatal virus infections, particularly measles, among children with this condition. Such starvation may lead to low numbers of circulating T-lymphocytes with depressed *in vitro* lymphocyte transformation. Gross lymphatic depletion of lymph nodes is often seen at autopsy. It should be remembered that many chronically ill patients, particularly those with advanced malignancy, suffer from a degree of malnutrition which may influence results of tests for cell mediated immunity.

Chronic Inflammatory and Granulomatous Disorders

The majority of patients with active sarcoidosis are anergic, have a nonspecific depression of *in vitro* lymphocyte transformation and show depressed lymphocyte cytotoxicity against EB virus infected cell lines. There is hypergammaglobulinaemia and specific antibody responses are increased when compared to normal controls. Similar defects in CMI are seen in some patients with other chronic inflammatory disorders (e.g. Sjögren's syndrome, rheumatoid arthritis, Chrohn's and Whipple's diseases) and some of the *in vitro* abnormalities may be due to inhibitory serum factors. However, recurrent infections are not generally a problem in such patients, a finding which further suggests that CMI, as we understand it, is not of major importance in host defence.

Non-lymphoid Malignancy

Much effort has been devoted to assessing immunity in patients with early and advanced malignancy. Recent work clearly confirms that defects in cell mediated immunity, as assessed by delayed hypersensitivity skin reactions and *in vitro* lymphocyte transformation, occur in patients with many varieties of solid tumour (e.g. breast and gastric neoplasms). Furthermore, these defects do not necessarily increase in severity as the disease progresses. Non-specific immunopotentiation with multiple BCG injections and with the anti-helminthic, levamisole, have marginally improved the prognosis in patients with melanoma and bronchial carcinoma respectively. However, it remains an open question whether these immune defects bear any real relationship to aetiology in cancer.

Ageing

Burnet postulated that the increased incidence of auto-antibodies and malignancy in old age is due to an immunodeficiency state. However, attempts to define this deficiency have not provided conclusive evidence. Humans reaching old age have a moderately depressed number of circulating T-lymphocytes and their lymphocyte transformation by PHA is significantly depressed. Numbers of germinal centres in axillary lymph nodes decrease with age but the paracortical thymic dependent regions usually remain well populated with lymphocytes. Serum immunoglobulin concentrations do not fall and there is a tendency in extreme old age to raised serum IgG levels. Specific antibody production following immunization remains intact.

Most of the investigations into the ageing process have been carried out in mice. There is good correlation in some strains between thymic atrophy, depression of cell mediated immunity and age. As in humans, ageing is associated with development of auto-antibodies and auto-immune disease. Such defects in cell mediated immunity may reflect a "run down" in the number of thymocytes in accordance with Hayflick's finding of a limited capacity for doubling in a dividing somatic cell population. This may explain the shortened lifespan and auto-immune disease found in the NZB strain of mice which is related to the presence of a vertically transmitted virus. Intact immunocompetence in young animals seems to keep the virus in a latent state whereas viral replication is widespread in older animals. Longevity can be conferred in these older animals by syngeneic lymphocyte transfers from young mice.

Some propose that the degenerative processes of ageing are related to a gradual immune destruction caused by a loss of "self-tolerance". However, it is unlikely that one of the commonest hallmarks of ageing, atherosclerosis, could be related to a failure of immunocompetence. Amyloidosis, which is ubiquitous in ageing vertebrates, may reflect an immune disorder, but so far only primary amyloidosis has been related directly with immunoglobulin light chain structure.

Pregnancy

The potential graft versus host relationship between foetus and mother is interesting. Cell mediated immunity, as assessed by delayed hypersensitivity skin reactions and *in vitro* transformation to mitogens is depressed in pregnancy. This is partly due to circulating serum inhibitory factors, such as chorionic gonadotrophin, which inhibit lymphocyte transformation to PHA. The trophoblast barrier between the foetal and maternal circulation is, curiously, nonimmunogenic. Faulk *et al.* (1974) have eluted an IgG antibody from trophoblast basement membrane which inhibited lymphocyte transformation to allogeneic lymphocytes and mitogens. Other studies have shown that maternal and other heterologous lymphocytes are inhibited from transforming in a mixed lymphocyte reaction with lymphocytes from neonates. This suggests that a soluble product is released from foetal lymphocytes which has a non-specific inhibitory reaction on lymphocyte transformation.

There are, therefore, a number of mechanisms whereby cell mediated immunity is markedly depressed both systemically and locally at the placental barrier. The systemic effects may predispose to the rapid progression of some cancers in pregnancy.

Transfer Factor

Transfer factor (TF) is a dialysable low molecular weight material extracted from human peripheral blood white cells. The extraction procedure involves separating "buffy coat" white cells on a suitable gradient, breaking up the cells by freezing and thawing and then treating with deoxyribonuclease. It has been customary to dialyse this material against distilled water but recent evidence suggests that culture medium is preferable. The dialysate is then freeze dried, leaving lyophilized transfer factor which remains stable at room temperature for many years. For treatment the lyophilized TF is reconstituted and injected subcutaneously. Lawrence (1965) claimed that TF could transfer specific cell mediated immunity but this is still not completely accepted. Most of the early experiments on TF depended upon demonstrating that delayed hypersensitivity skin sensitivity to antigens such as PPD could be transferred to a negative individual after injection of TF from a positive donor. However, the objection remains that any skin testing prior to TF treatment may immunize the individual. Although appropriate skin test controls have been performed, there is the difficulty that a low level of immunity already exists to such control antigens. These problems encouraged the use of *in vitro* models where cells were incubated with TF and their blastogenic responses to various antigens subsequently tested. Such experiments in man and monkeys have so far failed to provide convincing evidence that TF transfers specific immunity.

Nevertheless, there is reasonably good evidence that TF induces non-specific immunopotentiation by enhancing delayed hypersensitivity skin reactions to a variety of antigens, including contact sensitizing agents. It can also enhance the production of MIF but has only weak activity in potentiating lymphocyte transformation to mitogens and antigens.

TF has now been used in a large number of patients with chronic inflammatory disorders such as rheumatoid arthritis, Behcet's disease and mucocutaneous candidiasis (Rocklin, 1975). Double blind trials in rheumatoid arthritis have shown no benefit. At an anecdotal level, dramatic effects have been claimed in many other diseases. The amount of TF needed to produce an effect varies. The material extracted from about 10^9 lymphocytes is generally adequate, but injections may have to be repeated at regular intervals. Whole blood transfusions have produced dramatic improvement in some patients with mucocutaneous candidiasis but it is not clear whether this is as efficient as giving concentrated TF. The side effects from therapy are virtually negligible and the material is non-immunogenic.

The time has clearly come for widespread double blind trials on TF therapy in patients referred to special centres for such treatment. Until results are known scepticism about its activity will continue.

Complement and Polymorph Defects

It is not within the scope of this chapter to deal in detail with defects of the complement system or those of neutrophil polymorphs (see Chapters 7 and 8). Such defects should always be considered in children with recurrent infections, particularly staphylococcal abscesses. Clq, Clr, C2 and C3 deficiencies, all inherited primary defects, are associated with recurrent infections and may be diagnosed by the presence of a low total CH_{50} serum complement titre. C2 deficiency is closely associated with systemic lupus erythematosus and other auto-immune phenomena. Clq deficiency, probably due to hypercatabolism, occurs in some patients with primary hypogammaglobulinaemia and severe combined immunodeficiency and may be corrected after bone marrow transplantation. Patients with sickle cell disease fail to utilize the alternative complement pathway for the fixation of C3 to bacterial cell walls which may explain why they are particularly susceptible to pneumococcal septicemia.

Screening tests for immunodeficiency should always include a neutrophil polymorph count to exclude neutropenia which may be congenital, cyclic or secondary to drugs or infection. A number of primary metabolic defects of neutrophil polymorphs have now been described, the best known being chronic granulomatous disease (CGD) where there is an inability of the patient's polymorphs to kill staphylococci and gram-negative organisms. The condition is diagnosed by the failure of the polymorphs to reduce the salt nitrotetrazolium to blue formazan (NBT test). Other abnormalities include defects in phagocytosis, chemotaxis and random motility. Serum inhibitory factors, still largely unidentified, may be responsible for some of these defects. Unfortunately, there is no single screening test that identifies all of these rare abnormalities and laboratories involved in screening for immunodeficiency have to maintain a large number of techniques to ensure that they are detected.

REFERENCES

Ament, M. E., Ochs, H. D. and Davis, S. D. (1973). Structure and function of the gastro-intestinal tract in primary immunodeficiency syndromes: a study of 39 patients. *Medicine* (Baltimore), **52**, 227.

Amman, A. J. and Hong, R. (1971). Selective IgA deficiency: presentation of 30 cases and a review of the literature. *Medicine* (Baltimore), **50**, 223.

Asherson, G. L. (1972). The development of lymphocyte function tests. *Brit. J. Hosp. Med.* **8**, 665.

Broom, B. C., de la Concha, E. G., Webster, A. D. B., Loewi, G. and Asherson, G. L. (1975). Dichotomy between immunoglobulin synthesis by cells in gut and blood of patients with hypogammaglobulinaemia. *Lancet* **ii**, 253.

Cederbaum, S. D., Niwayama, G., Stiehm, E. R., Neerhout, R. C., Amman, A. J. and Berman, W., Jr. (1974). Combined immunodeficiency presenting as the Letterer-Siwe syndrome. *J. Paediatrics* **85**, 466.

Cooper, M. D., Chase, H. P., Lowman, J. T., Krivit, W. and Good, R. A. (1968). Wiskott-Aldrich syndrome – an immunologic deficiency disease involving the afferent limb of immunity. *Amer. J. Med.* **44**, 499.

Dayan, A. D. (1971). Chronic encephalitis in children with severe immunodeficiency. *Acta Neuropath.* **19**, 234.

Faulk, W. P., Jeannet, M., Creighton, W. R. and Carbonara, A. (1974). Immunological studies of human placenta. *J. Clin. Invest.* **54**, 1011.

Fudenberg, H., Good, R. A., Goodman, H. C., Hitzig, W., Kunkel, H. G., Roitt, I. M., Rosen, F. S., Rowe, D. S., Seligmann, M. and Soothill, J. R. (1971). Primary immunodeficiencies – report of a World Health Organization committee. *Paediatrics* **47**, 927.

Hudson, E. and Aldor, T. (1970). Pancreatic insufficiency and neutropenia with associated immunoglobulin deficit. *Arch. Int. Med.* **125**, 314.

Kersey, J. H., Spector, B. D. and Good, R. A. (1973). Primary immunodeficiency diseases and cancer: the immunodeficiency-cancer registry. *Int. J. Cancer* **12**, 333.

Levin, M., Franklin, E. C., Frangione, B., *et al.* (1972). The amino acid sequence of the major non-immunoglobulin component of amyloid. *J. Clin. Invest.* **51**, 2773.

Lischner, H. W. (1972). Di George Syndrome(s). *New Eng. J. Med.* **81**, 1042.

Longmire, R. L., McMillan, R., Yelenosky, R., Armstrong, S., Lang, J. E. and Craddock, C. G. (1973). *In vitro* splenic IgG synthesis in Hodgkin's disease. *New Eng. J. Med.* **289**, 763.

Makinodan, T., Santos, G. W. and Quinn, R. P. (1970). Immunosuppressive drugs. *Pharm. Rev.* **22**, 189.

Medical Research Council (1970). Hypogammaglobulinaemia in the United Kingdom. Medical Research Council, SRS 310.

McFarlin, D. E., Strober, W. and Waldermann, T. A. (1972). Ataxia telangiectasia. *Medicine* **51**, 281.

Parkman, R., Gelfand, E. W., Rosen, F. S., Sanderson, A. and Hirschhorn, R. (1975). Combined immuno and adenosine deaminase deficiency. *New Eng. J. Med.* **292**, 714.

Peacock, D. B., Jones, J. V. and Gouch, M. (1973). The immune response to ΦX 174 in man. I. Primary and secondary antibody production in normal adults. *Clin. Exp. Immunol.* **13**, 497.

Pickering, R. J., Pollara, B. and Meuwissen, H. J. (1974). Workshop on severe combined immunological deficiency disease and adenosine deaminase deficiency. *Clin. Immunol. Immunopath.* **3**, 301.

Purtilo, P. T., Cassel, C., Yang, J. P. S., Harper, R., Stephenson, S. R., Landing, B. H. and Vawter, G. F. (1975). X linked recessive progressive combined variable immunodeficiency (Duncan's disease). *Lancet* **1**, 935.

Rocklin, R. E. (1975). Use of transfer factor in patients with depressed cellular immunity and chronic infection. *In* "Immunodeficiency in Man and Animals", (eds. D. Bergsman, R. A. Good, J. Finstad and N. W. Paul), Vol. XI, No. 1, p. 431. (Birth Defects: original article series.)

Spitler, L. E., Levin, A. S., Stites, D. P., Fudenberg, H. H., Pirofsky, B., August, C. S., Stiehm, E. R., Hitzig, W. H. and Gatti, R. A. (1972). The Wiskott-Aldrich syndrome. *J. Clin. Invest.* **51**, 3216.

Tomasi, T. B. and Grey, H. M. (1972). Structure and function of immunoglobulin A. *Progr. Allergy* **16**, 81.

Twomey, J. J., Jordan, P. H., Laughter, A. H., Meuwissen, H. J. and Good, R. A. (1970). The gastric disorder in immunoglobulin-deficiency patients. *Ann. Int. Med.* **72**, 499.

Valdimarsson, H., Agnarsdottir, G. and Lachmann, P. J. (1974). Cellular immunity in subacute sclerosing panencephalitis. *Proc. Roy. Soc. Med.* **67**, 1125.

Vyas, G. N., Holmdahl, L., Perkins, H. A. and Fudenberg, H. H. (1969). Serologic specificity of human anti IgA and its significance in transfusion. *Blood* **34**, 573.

Waldman, T. A., Broder, S., Blaese, R. M., Durm, M., Blackman, M. and Strober, W. (1974). Role of suppressor T cells in pathogenesis of common variable hypogammaglobulinaemia. *Lancet* **11**, 609.

Waldman, T. A. and Strober, W. (1969). Metabolism of immunoglobulins. *Progr. Allergy* **13**, 1.

Wara, D. W., Goldstein, A. L., Doyle, N. E. and Amman, A. J. (1975). Thymosin activity in patients with cellular immunodeficiency. *New Eng. J. Med.* **292**, 70.

Webster, A. D. B., Efter, T. and Asherson, G. L. (1974). *Escherichia coli* antibody: a screening test for immunodeficiency. *Brit. Med. J.* **3**, 16.

V

System Disorders

15

Rheumatoid and Sero-negative Arthritides

E. J. HOLBOROW and A. J. SWANNELL

RHEUMATOID ARTHRITIS

Rheumatoid arthritis affects not only the joints but also the haematological, reticulo-endothelial, cardiovascular, nervous and respiratory systems and is a systemic disorder perhaps better called rheumatoid disease. It most commonly presents as painful swollen peripheral joints. Classically, middle-aged women 40–60 years are affected but the disease also occurs in teenagers and the elderly. Women are affected more frequently than men (ratio 3:1), pregnancy producing a remission sometimes followed by an exacerbation after childbirth.

The most common complaint is of pain, swelling and stiffness of the metacarpo-phalangeal and wrist joints, often with pain under the ball of the foot indicating metatarso-phalangeal involvement. Later larger joints such as the ankles, knees and elbows may become affected leading to limitation of movement of individual joints, flexion contractures and severe mechanical deformities which cripple and restrict the patient.

Occasionally, rheumatoid arthritis may start as a mono-arthritis or as a pleural effusion. Such presentations, however, are not common and other causes of mono-arthritis and pleural effusion have to be excluded before a label of rheumatoid disease is attached. The initial presenting arthritis may wax and wane over a period of months, the patient being virtually pain-free for periods of weeks. This "palindromic" presentation may continue for months before it becomes obvious from X-rays and blood tests that the patient is suffering from rheumatoid arthritis.

Systemic Features

Apart from joint involvement, if the onset is severe there is often a low grade fever, general malaise and weight loss. The patient may be found to be anaemic and the sedimentation rate raised. Some other common systemic features of rheumatoid disease reflect the accompanying immunological disorders.

Lymphadenopathy

Early in the disease there is often enlargement of the axillary and epitrochlear lymph nodes which show prominent secondary germinal centres. The axillary lymph nodes may become so large that an underlying malignancy and reticulosis is suspected, especially if there is associated weight loss.

Nodules

Gradually, subcutaneous nodules may form over the olecranon process and pressure areas such as the fingers, Achilles tendon, sacrum, occiput and occasionally the ear. Single nodules vary in size from being just palpable to about the size of a small plum, and collections of nodules may occur which feel like a bag of peas. Always associated with positive tests for rheumatoid factor in the serum, nodules help to substantiate the diagnosis of rheumatoid arthritis and generally indicate a poor prognosis. Microscopy shows fibrinoid necrosis at the centre of the nodule surrounded by histiocytes arranged in a radial palisade. The central necrotic areas contain IgG and rheumatoid factor deposits and are evidently the seat of immune complex formation or deposition (Nowaslawski and Bryzosko, 1967). Nodules may ulcerate or become infected but usually come and go over months.

Vasculitis

When the disease has been present for some time small brown spots may be noticed around the nail bed (Fig. 1) or associated with nodules. These indicate small areas of endarteritis which have produced infarction due to underlying vasculitis. A more severe form can occur affecting mesenteric or limb vessels producing gangrene of the gut or limbs with serious consequences.

Patients with vasculitis usually have positive tests for rheumatoid factor and a worse prognosis generally. Recent work (see below) indicates that patients with vasculitis have circulating soluble immune complexes.

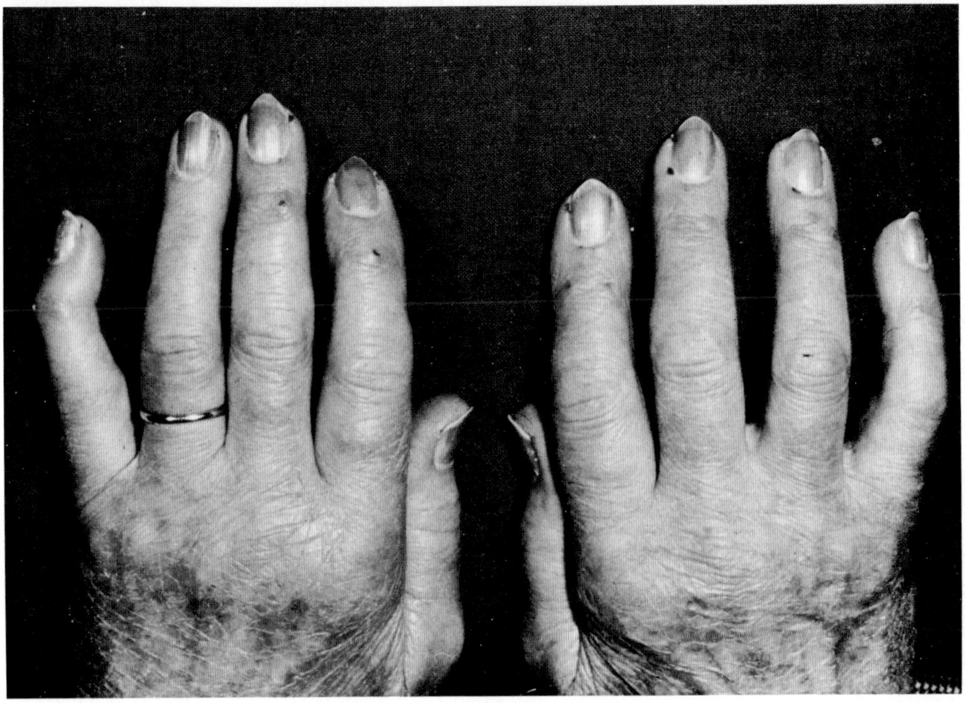

Fig. 1. Vasculitic nailfold infarcts in a patient with sero-positive rheumatoid arthritis.

Neuropathy

Many patients with arteritis and long-standing disease develop a peripheral neuropathy. This produces a severe burning pain, in the legs initially, and may lead to a "stocking and glove" distribution of anaesthesia. Associated motor involvement may produce foot or wrist drop. Independently of the sensorimotor peripheral neuropathy, isolated monoarthritis can occur producing median, lateral popliteal or ulnar nerve symptoms.

Chest Involvement

The lungs and pleura may be involved, and men with rheumatoid disease may present with pleural effusion followed some months later by the development of sero-positive rheumatoid arthritis. Rheumatoid nodules may develop within the lung substance producing diagnostic confusion on chest X-ray and sometimes necessitating biopsy. Diffuse interstitial pulmonary fibrosis is also seen, particularly in patients with long-standing disease and positive tests for rheumatoid factor. Clinically this produces progressive dyspnoea which can be extremely incapacitating. Caplan (1953) described a rheumatoid pneumonoconiosis in coal miners with a characteristic radiological appearance of rounded opacities later becoming confluent, resembling massive pulmonary fibrosis. This syndrome can also occur in miners without arthritis but with positive tests for rheumatoid factor and rheumatoid factor may also be present in patients with fibrosing alveolitis (Turner-Warwick and Haslam, 1971).

Immunological Features

A serological characteristic of rheumatoid disease is the presence of rheumatoid factors, a constellation of auto-antibodies reactive with antigenic determinants on IgG molecules. About a third of patients with classical or definite rheumatoid arthritis have raised levels of anti-nuclear antibodies.

Rheumatoid Factors (RFs)

Nature and Specificity

The sera of many rheumatoid patients agglutinate sheep or human erythrocytes sparingly coated with rabbit anti-erythrocyte antibody, often to high titre. This reaction is the basis of the Rose–Waaler test, the sheep cell agglutination test (SCAT) the human erythrocyte agglutination test (HEAT) and the differential agglutination test (DAT), all of which detect the antiglobulins of IgM class which are the classical rheumatoid factors. Human erythrocytes sensitized with appropriately selected human anti-erythrocyte antibodies, such as incomplete anti-D, also provide a useful indicator system. The essential feature of the reactant coating the red cells in such tests for rheumatoid factors is not that it is antibody but that it is IgG. Latex agglutination, utilizing polystyrene particles coated with human IgG, forms the basis of a convenient and simple slide agglutination test for rheumatoid factor.

The reactivity of rheumatoid sera with IgG has been exhaustively examined in order to settle three controversial questions, namely, is it due to the presence of antibodies? If so, are the antibodies in question auto-antibodies? And thirdly, if auto-antibodies, are these directed at, and perhaps engendered by, configurational changes taking place in antibody molecules as a result of interactions of the latter with antigen; or do they react directly with native IgG? Early in this controversy, Franklin *et al.* (1957) identified in the sera of some rheumatoid patients by ultracentrifugal analysis large protein complexes (22S) which proved to be dissociable into a 19S IgM fraction showing rheumatoid factor activity, and native 7S IgG. Subsequently the results of numerous investigations in which native, altered, autologous, homologous and heterologous gamma-globulins were used as reactants to analyse rheumatoid factor activity have all pointed to the conclusion that rheumatoid factors consist of a set of separate antibody specificities each reactive with part of a complex IgG determinant (Normansell, 1972), and that this explains the reactivity of rheumatoid sera with rabbit as well as with human and other species IgG. There is little doubt that these anti-IgG antibodies arise as auto-immune responses in rheumatoid disease. What imparts so striking an immunogenic property to autologous IgG in these patients is not clearly understood, but circular dichroism studies show that conformationally altered IgG molecules are present in rheumatoid serum (Johnson *et al.*, 1975).

Incidence and Diagnostic Specificity of Rheumatoid Factors

IgM Rheumatoid Factors

IgM antibodies are especially efficient as agglutinators in serological tests, such as those classically used to detect rheumatoid factor, which depend upon haemagglutination or particle agglutination, and, as noted above, such tests selectively detect rheumatoid factors of the multivalent IgM antibody class. As with many serum antibodies, the distribution of titres is a continuous variable within the population studied (Zutshi *et al.*, 1969), so that any level purporting to separate the sero-positive from the sero-negative is one arbitrarily chosen to include as many patients clinically acceptable as rheumatoid, and to exclude as many non-rheumatoid subjects as possible.

The agglutinating titres usually taken as positive are 1:16 or more in the DAT test, 1:20 or more in the latex test and 1:200 or more in the "FII test". In the latter, tannic acid treated sheep red cells coated with a fraction of human serum rich in gamma-globulin (FII) provide an especially sensitive indicator of rheumatoid factor activity. The frequency of positives according to this scale obtained in one survey of rheumatoid and other subjects is shown in Table 1. When a line dividing negatives from positives is drawn in this way, some patients with a variety of other diseases, and some normal people, still fall into the sero-positive group, while a minority of patients with undoubted rheumatoid disease appear persistently sero-negative.

TABLE 1

Anti-globulin antibodies (rheumatoid factors) in health and rheumatic disease

	Number	Age (range) (years)	DAT+ (%)	Latex +/++ (%)	FII titre	
					1/200 or more (%)	Mean tube titre[a]
Control subjects						
healthy	70	39 (17–80)	0	0	11	1·4
sick adults	71	40 (16–82)	0	4	16	1·2
chest disease (adults)	65	53 (16–76)	1·5	11	26	1·8
Degenerative joint disease	84	57 (33–76)	1·2	1·2	20	1·7
Rheumatoid arthritis						
classical/definite	435	53 (18–84)	42	75	87	7·4
probable/possible	69	50 (20–79)	5	30	50	3·8
Ankylosing spondylitis	65	38 (15–65)	0	1	31	2·1
Gout	52	56 (31–80)	2	6	21	1·8

Modified from Zutshi *et al.* (1969).
[a] tube 1 = 1/25, tube 2 = 1/50, tube 3 = 1/100 . . . tube 10 = 1/12,800.

Among non-rheumatic conditions in which RFs are present, sometimes at high titre, are some bacterial and viral infections (for example, sub-acute bacterial endocarditis, viral hepatitis, and infectious mononucleosis), some chronic infections and parasitic diseases (leprosy, tuberculosis, schistosomiasis, trypanosomiasis) some monoclonal paraproteinaemias, and as noted above, some fibrosing lung conditions. In such sero-positive non-rheumatoid conditions, reactions with human IgG are more frequent than with rabbit IgG, but in many cases both are present.

Only about 25% of sero-positive subjects in random population samples have clinical evidence of rheumatoid disease (Ball and Lawrence, 1961), and among non-rheumatoid subjects there is a tendency for the incidence of sero-positivity to be greater in older age groups. The subsequent incidence of rheumatoid disease in sero-positive subjects without previous polyarthritis is low.

While positive tests for anti-human and especially anti-rabbit IgG activity thus have diagnostic value, especially at high titres, the finding of anti-globulin activity of the IgM rheumatoid factor type is clearly not to be simply equated with a diagnosis of rheumatoid arthritis. Attempts to increase serological sensitivity have led merely to a decreased diagnostic significance of positive reactions. Furthermore, a proportion of sero-negative rheumatoid subjects remains sero-negative no matter how much the sensitivity of any given test for IgM RF is increased.

IgG Rheumatoid Factor

As distinct from the large (22S) complexes noted by Franklin *et al.* (1957), some rheumatoid sera on ultracentrifugation yield complexes of intermediate (9–17S) size, which are composed entirely of IgG molecules but which on dissociation nevertheless also display rheumatoid factor activity (Kunkel *et al.*, 1961). Free IgG rheumatoid factor activity is often present in rheumatoid sera, as immuno-absorbent techniques capable of selectively detecting and measuring anti-globulin activity by Ig class show, and IgG anti-globulin levels measured in this way are about the same in both sero-positive and sero-negative individuals. IgG anti-globulins are apparently also present in the sera of patients with some rheumatic conditions hitherto regarded as typically sero-negative namely, Still's disease, psoriatic arthropathy and ankylosing spondylitis. The methods of detecting serum IgG rheumatoid factor available hitherto are open to criticism on technical grounds, and more experience of results with modified techniques (for example, the plastic tube binding method of Hay *et al.* (1975)) is needed before the pattern of distribution of serum IgG rheumatoid factor in disease and in health, and the clinical value of its determination becomes clearly defined. There can be little doubt, however, of its implication in the pathogenesis of rheumatoid synovitis.

Biological and Immunopathogenetic Significance of RFs

Most subjects with serum anti-globulin activity of IgM rheumatoid factor type do not have rheumatoid arthritis. On the other hand sero-positivity, especially at high titre, is associated in rheumatoid disease with a more rapid progression of the arthritis, and with a poorer prognosis, as well as with systemic complications such as nodules, vasculitis, intractable skin ulcers, neuropathy and Felty's syndrome. If RFs play a pathogenetic role in the disease it might thus be expected that rheumatoid RFs differ in some respect other than titre from non-rheumatoid RFs.

The physiological role of anti-globulins is largely conjectural. Under experimental conditions human RF can assist neutralization of virus by antibody, and may protect against inflammatory responses by competing with complement for sites on the IgG molecule.

In its reaction with human IgG, IgM RF activates complement through its own complement attachment sites via the classical pathway (Zvaifler and Schur, 1968). Although evidence is still scanty on the point, non-rheumatoid RFs appear to be poor complement activators (Bianco *et al.*, 1974).

The ability of rheumatoid RF to fix complement is an important, perhaps crucial factor in the production of rheumatoid synovitis, for a striking difference between non-rheumatoid sero-positive individuals and rheumatoid subjects is that in the latter a principal site of production of RF is in the affected joints themselves. The cellularity of the inflamed rheumatoid synovial membrane is predominantly due to infiltration of lymphocytes and plasma cells, and immunofluorescent studies have repeatedly shown that many of the latter synthesize IgG or IgM in their cytoplasm (Fig. 2). In cryostat sections of synovial membranes from affected joints of sero-positive rheumatoid subjects especially, many of these IgM plasma cells display a cytoplasmic binding affinity for IgG which reflects precisely the specificity of the *in vitro* reactivity of IgM rheumatoid factors and shows the same complement fixing properties. Furthermore, as well as IgG and IgM plasma cells and plasma cells with RF activity, deposits of immunoglobulin, RF, and complement are regularly demonstrable in the interstitial connective tissue of the joint lining, in the walls of synovial blood vessels and as components of cytoplasmic inclusions in those synovial lining cells that have phagocytic properties (Brandt *et al.*, 1968).

Haemolytic complement activity in the sera of rheumatoid patients is often normal or somewhat raised, but in the synovial fluid of actively affected rheumatoid joints it is significantly lower than in non-rheumatoid joint fluids. This, with the fact that phagocytic cells in rheumatoid synovial effusions and in the synovial lining contain inclusions of IgG, IgM, complement components and RF in various combinations, strongly suggests that the rheumatoid synovial membrane is a site of extravascular immune complex disease, in which the complement-activating potential of anti-globulin: IgG interaction is one of the major immunopathogenetic mechanisms (Ziff, 1973).

A deficiency of this hypothesis has been its inadequacy as an explanation

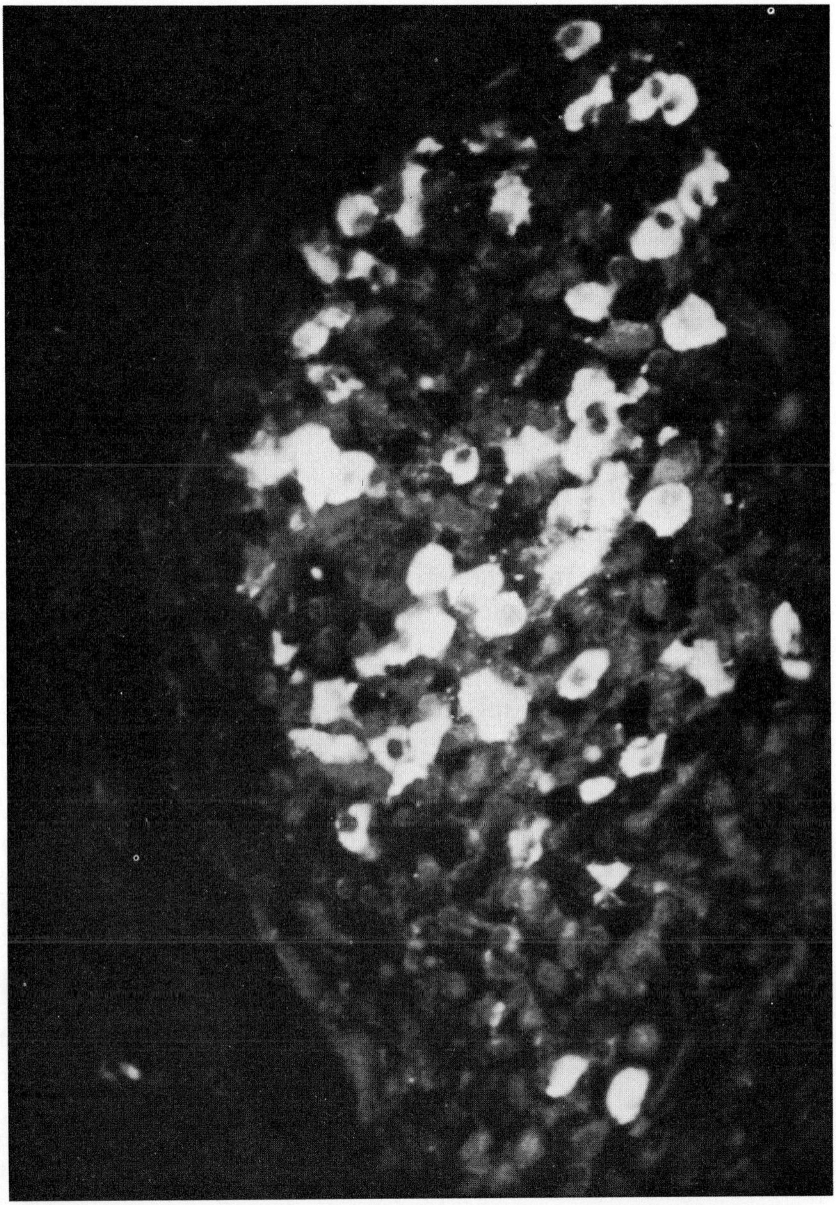

Fig. 2. Synovial membrane from a rheumatoid knee joint. Cryostat section of an area of mononuclear cell infiltration deep to the synovial lining cell layer, showing immunofluorescent staining of plasma cells with fluorochrome-labelled anti-human Ig antiserum. In consecutive sections stained with anti-IgM and IgG reagents, some plasma cells may be shown to be synthesizing IgM and others IgG, a few IgA. In some of these positive plasma cells the immunoglobulin synthesized, irrespective of class, is specific auto-antibody with anti-IgG activity, which contributes to immune complex formation in the joint.

of sero-negative rheumatoid arthritis. This objection was countered when it was shown that IgG rheumatoid factor is produced in the affected synovial membranes of sero-negative as well as of sero-positive rheumatoid patients. Complement binding in the synovial membranes of both, as demonstrated by immunofluorescence, is in fact identified more closely with IgG than with IgM deposits, and in the phagocytic synovial lining cells from sero-negative patients' joints, complement may be demonstrable in company with IgG alone (Kinsella *et al.*, 1970).

While complement depletion as measured by C4 and C2 levels, and the presence of conversion products, is usually more marked in joint fluids from sero-positive than from sero-negative patients, depletion of C4 only (a more sensitive indicator) is often demonstrable in fluids from the latter. High molecular weight IgG complexes have been found in rheumatoid synovial fluid as well as serum (Winchester *et al.*, 1970), and have also been eluted from rheumatoid synovial membranes (Munthe and Natvig, 1971). Whether from serum or from joint fluid these display an ability to fix complement via the classical pathway by binding Clq (Table 2). The results of allotype analysis of the IgG protein content of complexes derived from the joint show that it is of restricted type, and hence likely to have been synthesized in the joint rather than to have reached it from extra-articular sources. This conclusion has been strikingly confirmed by pepsin digestion experiments on rheumatoid synovial membrane sections, which show that the Fab fragments of the immunoglobulin product of many of the IgG plasma cells present in both sero-positive and sero-negative patients possess rheumatoid factor-like anti-IgG activity, but that this is blocked *in vivo* through complex formation with adjacent Fc portions of other intracellular IgG molecules

TABLE 2

^{125}I-Clq binding activity in rheumatoid serum and synovial fluid

	No. of samples	Bound ^{125}I-Clq %	
		serum	synovial fluid
Seropositive rheumatoid arthritis	19	56[a] ± 26	62 ± 16
Seronegative rheumatoid arthritis	20	35 ± 19	58 ± 15
Degenerative joint disease	12	20 ± 14	33 ± 12
Trauma	12	19 ± 6	35 ± 8
Other arthritis	9	17 ± 8	37 ± 7
Normal controls	48	15 ± 6	—

[a] Mean ± 1 SD.
Lambert *et al.* (1975).

which presumably have identical combining specificity (Munthe and Natvig, 1971). Thus the solely IgG intermediate complexes in rheumatoid serum, and also in rheumatoid joint fluids, appear to take origin as unique self-associating IgG RF molecules (Pope *et al.*, 1974) synthesized in rheumatoid synovial membrane plasma cells, and presumably also in lymph nodes and in lymphoid cell infiltrates which may occur elsewhere e.g. in the salivary glands in Sjögren's syndrome. It appears likely that the complement-binding sites of these complexes as they leave the parent plasma cell are potential triggers of the inflammatory sequence of complement activation. There is some evidence that, in addition, alternative pathway activation takes place in the rheumatoid joint (Gotze *et al.*, 1972). In rheumatoid subcutaneous nodules the presence of immunoglobulin and rheumatoid factor deposits argues that immune complex deposition plays a causative role here also (Nowaslawski and Bryzosko, 1967).

Anti-nuclear Antibodies

Nature and Specificity

Anti-nuclear antibodies were discovered as a result of Hargrave's observation of lupus erythematosus (LE) cell formation in bone marrow specimens from patients with systemic lupus erythematosus (SLE) and initial investigations into their nature and specificity were carried out in the context of SLE and lupus like conditions. The "LE cell factor" responsible for the phenomenon proved to be a complement-fixing IgG antibody against deoxyribonucleoprotein, and the precipitation, haemagglutination and complement-fixing reactions which established this fact also revealed that lupus sera may contain antibodies against other nuclear constituents including DNA, RNA-protein and other soluble non-nucleic acid constituents of nuclei, some of which have been partially characterized (Chapter 11).

The anti-nuclear antibodies characteristic of SLE are seldom present in rheumatoid arthritis sera, but the use of immunofluorescence as a method of screening sera for anti-nuclear reactivity revealed at an early stage that anti-nuclear antibodies (ANA) as a class have a much wider distribution, and are present in about a third of patients with classical or definite forms of rheumatoid arthritis (Ward *et al.*, 1964), the serum levels ranging from 25–1,600 U/ml. The highest levels of positivity are seen in patients with established rheumatoid disease, especially those with vasculitis, nodules, or infection, and in Felty's and in Sjögren's syndromes. Except for granulocyte specific ANA, discussed below, the specificity of the anti-nuclear antibodies detected by immunofluorescence in rheumatoid sera is not well characterized. Other methods of testing show that they are seldom directed at soluble deoxyribonucleoprotein, at Sm nuclear antigen or at ribonucleoprotein (RNP), although it is now reported that low levels of anti-DNA may be present in some rheumatoid sera (Notman *et al.*, 1975). In contrast to SLE the immunoglobulin class of rheumatoid ANA is preponderantly IgM (Holborow and Johnson, 1965), although it may be difficult to demonstrate this unequivocally since co-existing IgM RF can interact with IgG ANA, causing nuclei binding the latter to stain misleadingly for IgM.

Much ingenuity has been expended in attempts to relate different patterns of nuclear fluorescence—homogeneous, speckled, peripheral and others—to reactions with defined nuclear antigens. In tests where cryostat sections of rat or mouse liver provide the nuclear substrate, positive rheumatoid sera may give either homogeneous or speckled nuclear fluorescence, and indeed the pattern may change with increasing serum dilution. With substrates more carefully selected to permit interpretation of speckled staining as due to anti-Sm or anti-RNP antibody, rheumatoid sera do not give this pattern, but usually a homogeneous one. In our experience, the nuclear staining patterns under routine conditions of testing are diagnostically inconclusive.

Granulocyte Specific ANA

As well as ANA of anti-RNP specificity, patients with Felty's syndrome usually have a serum ANA with specificity for granulocyte nuclei. Felty's syndrome is the combination of neutropaenia and splenomegaly in a patient with rheumatoid arthritis. The lymp nodes are often enlarged and the patient may be anaemic. Clinically the neutropaenia predisposes to recurrent infections which may be fatal and the anaemia itself can produce symptoms.

Granulocyte-specific ANA (GS-ANA) is also present in the serum of about 75% of other rheumatoid patients and in 30% of SLE patients (Elling *et al.*, 1968). GS-ANA may sometimes be shown by immunofluorescence to have complement-fixing properties and when this feature is present it shows a strong association with neutropaenia in both Felty's syndrome and in rheumatoid arthritis (Wiik and Munthe, 1974), although a causal link is not proved.

Biological and Immunopathogenetic Significance of ANA in Rheumatoid Arthritis

The reason or reasons for the appearance of anti-nuclear antibodies in connective tissue disease are unknown. Popular hypotheses postulate impairment of T-cell control over B-cells programmed to produce ANAs, and antigenic stimuli arising directly or indirectly from viral infections, perhaps aided by the adjuvanticity of viral nucleic acids. At present evidence for such mechanisms in rheumatoid arthritis is even more scanty than in SLE.

The immunopathogenetic significance of ANAs in connective tissue disease has been most clearly established for anti-DNA antibodies participating in immune complex formation in SLE. In rheumatoid arthritis ANA has been regarded hitherto chiefly as a useful marker of cases likely to display complications such as vasculitis or neuropathy, and of complicated forms of the disease such as Sjögren's and Felty's syndromes, and particular antibody specificities for individual nuclear antigens have not been identified as clinically significant.

Despite this, there is good evidence that nuclear antigens, including native and denatured DNA, and soluble nucleoprotein, are often present in rheumatoid synovial fluid, as inclusions in phagocytic cells in rheumatoid synovial effusions and as deposits in rheumatoid synovial membranes (Cracchiolo *et al.*, 1971). Single-stranded DNA has been found in a majority of the cryoprecipitates which usually form in rheumatoid effusions on cooling, and complement fixing anti-nuclear antibodies of IgG and IgM classes and antiglobulin activity are also often present (Zvaifler, 1973). Eluates from rheumatoid synovial membrane may contain ANA, and the specific ANA activity in the joint fluid may in fact exceed that in the serum. There are thus grounds for postulating that the formation of immune complexes by anti-nuclear antibodies contributes to the immunopathology of rheumatoid joints, and these have been strengthened by the identification of GS-ANA as a component of such intra-articular complexes (Wiik, 1975a). More interesting is the parallel identification of GS-ANA as a component of circulating immune complexes in Felty's syndrome and in rheumatoid arthritis (Wiik, 1975b), since it points to a role for anti-nuclear antibodies other than anti-DNA in the formation of intravascular complexes which may be systemically damaging.

Circulating Immune Complexes

It has been known for two decades that protein complexes of different sizes from large (22S) to multiple intermediate (9–17S) may be present in rheumatoid sera as well as in rheumatoid joints, and that their presence is particularly associated with the severer forms of disease. Most attention has been paid to elucidating the role of such immune complexes in producing joint inflammation, but good evidence has also been forthcoming from immunofluorescent studies that systemic rheumatoid vascular lesions—such as occur in the skin and in the peripheral nerves, for example—are the result of deposition of circulating immune complexes apparently similar to those implicated in rheumatoid synovitis (Nowaslawski and Bryzosko, 1967; Conn *et al.*, 1972).

Whether extravascular (synovial) or intravascular (systemic) with regard to their site of formation, the complexes which have been most exhaustively investigated for their pathogenetic potential in rheumatoid disease are those resulting from the reactions of IgM and IgG rheumatoid factors. Recently, anti-nuclear antibodies—including the GS-ANA mentioned above—have been identified as significant contributors to immune complex formation in rheumatoid arthritis intravascularly as well as in the joint (Wiik, 1975a,b) and it may well be that other as yet unidentified antigens are implicated as participants in antigen–antibody reactions which produce soluble complexes circulating in rheumatoid blood.

With the demonstration of the pathogenic potential of such complexes, their detection in the blood of individual patients is becoming a matter of clinical interest to the rheumatologist looking for ways of bettering the management and treatment of patients. The multiplicity of tests for serum immune complexes now in use indicates the uncertainties of interpretation at the present stage of study of circulating immune complexes in rheumatoid disease, but progress in defining their place in management is likely to be rapid. The serum Clq binding activity is high in sero-positive rheumatoid subjects, and somewhat less, although still significantly raised in many sero-negative rheumatoid patients, in parallel with the joint fluid findings (Table 2). Sero-positive patients with severe progressive disease, who have had or are likely to have vasculitic complications, usually have soluble immune complexes in their sera in which IgM RF appears to be involved as a component. This appears to alter the behaviour of the complexes so that they enhance rather than (as in SLE) inhibit uptake by macrophages of labelled aggregates of human IgG *in vitro* (Onyewotu *et al.*, 1975). Preliminary studies in rheumatoid patients receiving penicillamine show that a decrease in IgM RF levels during therapy is frequently paralleled by a change from enhancing to inhibiting complexes (Mohammed *et al.*, 1976). Penicillamine does not, however, reduce anti-nuclear antibody titres, and may indeed induce ANA production, and sometimes anti-DNA antibody. It remains to be determined whether this effect of penicillamine explains the failure of some rheumatoid patients to improve on penicillamine therapy. At any rate, it appears that tests capable of detecting and measuring immune complexes in the blood and distinguishing their different biological properties are likely to be useful in identifying rheumatoid patients at risk of the more severe forms of systemic disease, and may provide a practical means of monitoring the effects of treatment.

Anti-collagen Antibodies

Humans have antibodies to denatured collagen (called anti-gelatin factors) in their sera (Maurer, 1954). Although there is agreement that normal sera react poorly with native as compared with denatured collagen, the serum factors responsible have not been identified in most cases. Beard *et al.* (1976) have found somewhat elevated titres of antibodies agglutinating fresh tanned sheep red cells coated with denatured collagen in several systemic rheumatic conditions, including rheumatoid arthritis, juvenile chronic polyarthritis and scleroderma. Steffen (1969) using an anti-globulin consumption test, has found antibodies to collagen in about 75% of patients with rheumatoid arthritis, Felty's syndrome, systemic lupus erythematosus, Sjögren's syndrome and scleroderma, while control sera were largely negative, and Michaeli and Fudenberg (1974a) have obtained similar results by haemagglutination. The distinction between anti-native and anti-denatured collagen antibodies is blurred by the fact that native and denatured collagen share some antigenic determinants. With regard to reactivity against native and denatured collagen, human auto-antibodies against the latter appear to be well authenticated, and to be present in raised titre in some systemic rheumatoid conditions and in some other chronic conditions, such as emphysema, associated with collagen breakdown (Michaeli and Fudenberg, 1974b). In addition to serum antibodies, Steffen has claimed that antibodies to collagen may be detected in the synovial fluid from rheumatoid joints by agglutination of collagen-coated red blood cells (Steffen, 1970). In view of the findings of Conochie *et al.* (1975) it is probable that the agglutinations obtained were not due to anti-collagen antibodies but to the presence of glycosaminoglycans. Non-covalent binding between collagen coated cells and various polyanions, especially chondroitin-4-sulphate, closely simulates immunological agglutination, and it seems likely that such substances are present in the synovial fluid of the rheumatoid joint.

With regard to reactivity against native and denatured collagen, therefore, human auto-antibodies against the latter are present in raised titre in some systemic rheumatic diseases and in other chronic conditions associated with collagen breakdown. The true incidence of anti-native collagen auto-antibodies in health and disease requires further investigation and bio-chemical characterization of anti-gelatin factors is also needed. Meanwhile it remains an open question whether anti-collagen antibodies contribute to the immunopathology of rheumatoid arthritis.

Serum Immunoglobulins

Serum immunoglobulin levels are of little diagnostic value in these conditions, but show some departures from normal (Table 3). The total Ig and the IgG levels are significantly if only moderately raised, especially in sero-positive patients. Several reports mention a more marked mean elevation of serum IgA in both sero-negative and sero-positive subjects; but in a few patients selective IgA deficiency has been found. Irrespective of rheumatoid factor titres, IgM levels are usually normal.

TABLE 3

Serum immunoglobulin levels in rheumatoid arthritis and Still's disease

	mg % (mean)			
	IgG	IgA	IgM	IgD
Control adults	1,100	270	125	n.d.
Rheumatoid arthritis	1,396	418	144	n.d.
Control children	1,123	199	73	4·4
Still's disease	1,464	341	91	2·9

Figures kindly supplied by A. Howard.

A minority of patients have a low molecular weight variant of serum IgM, termed 7S IgM, which reportedly has complement fixing properties superior to those of IgM RF. 7S IgM is found also in some normal people, and in other diseases, and probably has no special significance in rheumatoid arthritis, although one report associates its presence with rheumatoid vasculitis (Theofilopoulos *et al.*, 1974).

Cell Mediated Immunity

The ability to develop delayed hypersensitivity reactions to new antigens is somewhat impaired in sero-positive rheumatoid arthritis and in Sjögren's syndrome, but as in other instances of mild CMI defects in human disease this seems not to render patients unduly liable to infection. In contrast with this apparently general defect is the heightened responsiveness to human IgG of the leucocytes of these patients.

Leucocyte migration inhibition experiments show that rheumatoid blood lymphocytes are stimulated by aggregated human IgG (Brostoff and Roitt, 1975), and they produce macrophage inhibition factor on incubation with normal IgG (Sany *et al.*, 1975). Conversely, rheumatoid lymphocytes are specifically stimulated to mitosis by autologous rheumatoid factor (Astorga, 1975). There is evidence also that the responsiveness of rheumatoid lymphocytes to other forms of stimulation differs from normal. Rabbit antisera against rheumatoid lymphocytes have a weaker transforming effect on both RA and normal lymphocytes than antisera against normal human lymphocytes (Williams *et al.*, 1971). That the rheumatoid lymphocyte surface differs from normal was also suggested by the observation that in mixed lymphocyte culture (MLC) between cells from two rheumatoid subjects the response is weaker than that between cells from two normal subjects or between rheumatoid-normal combinations (Astorga and Williams, 1969). Impaired MLR reactions have been noted also between cell-pairs from ankylosing spondylitis and psoriatic arthritis patients and also from multiple sclerosis (Hedberg *et al.*, 1975).

In random one-way MLC reactions between rheumatoid patients and control subjects, Stastny (1976) has recently reported that low responses were given by the cells of 31 of 43 RA patients in cultures against 8 of the same RA patients' cells used as stimulators. The remaining 35 patients' cells used as stimulators yielded only normal MLC reactions, and used as responders did not produce low responses with non-RA lymphocytes. A few of the control subjects' cells, however, gave low responses to two RA stimulators.

To be taken into account in interpreting such results is the fact that in at least some patients with RA, many of the blood lymphocytes are coated with anti-lymphocyte antibodies (Winchester *et al.*, 1975) which might well interfere with the expression of lymphocyte recognition measured in the MLC. Alternatively, drug treatment might account for poor responsiveness. Stastny was able to exclude both these possibilities, and has produced an explanation which opens a new approach to enquiry into the genetics of RA. MLC stimulation is under genetic control regulated by a separate histocompatibility locus called HLA-D, at which several alleles governing major MLC or lymphocyte-defined (LD) determinants have been identified. Stastny's postulate is that the production of low MLC responses among RA patients is due to a sharing of LD determinants. If certain patients providing the stimulator cells are homozygous at the HLA-D locus, cells of other patients possessing the same LD determinants would be expected to produce very low MLC responses. Family studies of several RA patients whose cells are low MLC stimulators (Stastny, 1975), have shown that they are homozygous for identical or closely similar determinants, R and r, which characterize an allele designated HLA–DW4 (Bull W.H.O., 1975). The frequencies of R and r in rheumatoid patients, according to Stastny (1975), are shown in Table 4. The complexity of the genetics of the HLA region is such that associations observed between gene products and diseases have a number of possible interpretations, of which an effect due to the operation of immune response (Ir) genes (see Chapter 2) is a particularly attractive one, as yet unproved.

Rheumatoid synovial fluids exert a mitotogenic effect on autologous lymphocytes (Kinsella, 1973), and have the ability to inhibit macrophage migration without added antigen, but fluids from other inflammatory arthritides may have similar though lesser effects. Substances with similar lymphokine activity are produced by rheumatoid synovial cell cultures (Ziff, 1973).

These findings tell us little about which antigens or other stimuli induce lymphokine production by rheumatoid lymphocytes, but they evidently reflect the fact that T-cells are undergoing blast transformation in the rheumatoid synovial membrane, and presumably contributing in this way to the chronic local inflammation. The lymphocytes in some rheumatoid

TABLE 4
Frequency of the MLC determinants R and r in rheumatoid patients and controls

Population group	Number studied	Frequency of MLC determinants		
		R	r	R and/or r
		Percent positive		
Adult RA	44	51	21	72
Juvenile RA	38	26	6	32
Non-RA	54	7·4	3·7	11

From Stastny (1975).

synovial effusions are predominantly T-cells, and the fact that they nevertheless respond poorly to mitogens such as phytohaemagglutinin (Sheldon *et al.*, 1974) further argues that they are cells which have already undergone stimulation *in vivo*.

The numbers of T- and B-cells in the blood of rheumatoid patients are not significantly different from normal. The effects, if any, on the lymphocytes and the mononuclear cells in the blood of the circulating immune complexes now known to be often present in rheumatoid patients has not yet been studied.

Immunological Aspects of Treatment

Although immunological reactions are clearly involved in the pathogenesis of rheumatoid arthritis, most of the non-steroidal anti-inflammatory drugs commonly used in treatment in the early stages and in less severe cases have little detectable effect on the immune responses of the treated patient in the doses given. Most of them, including aspirin, inhibit mitogen-stimulated and antigen-stimulated lymphocyte transformation *in vitro* at appropriate dosage (Panush, 1975).

With progressive worsening of symptoms and the appearance of radiological evidence of erosive change in the affected joints it is often thought necessary to introduce chloroquine, gold, penicillamine, steroid or cytotoxic agents. Chloroquine reduces the titre of rheumatoid factor in the serum (Popert *et al.*, 1961) and has been shown to inhibit the response of cultured human lymphocytes to phytohaemagglutinin. Gold therapy reduces levels of acute phase proteins, and binds to albumin (Lawrence, 1961). At higher serum levels it binds to serum Ig, complement and rheumatoid factor (Lorber, 1971, 1972), which may explain its intracellular concentration in the rheumatoid joint in macrophages which have ingested immune complexes. Experimentally, gold interferes with phagocytosis (Jessop *et al.*, 1973), with migration of macrophages (Vernon-Roberts *et al.*, 1973) with lysosomal enzyme action (Freyberg, 1972) and inhibits complement activity (Schultz *et al.*, 1973).

Both gold and penicillamine therapy reduced the titre of serum rheumatoid factor, but there is little evidence that this plays any part in the therapeutic response (Huskisson *et al.*, 1974). The effect of penicillamine on circulating immune complexes in rheumatoid arthritis has been mentioned above.

The immunological effects of steroids, azathioprine and cyclophosphamide in rheumatoid disease are discussed in Chapter 30. These are drugs used in rheumatoid disease at least partly for their immunosuppressive properties. Recently, however, treatment with levamisole, a drug thought to produce an opposite, immunopotentiating effect has been reported to be beneficial in rheumatoid arthritis. Like penicillamine, levamisole is slow to take effect, and a prolonged course of therapy over months is required. Both drugs reduce the titre of rheumatoid factor, and stimulation of cell mediated immunity has been noted with both, as measured by increased delayed skin reactions to PPD and by inhibition of leucocyte migration by tuberculin as antigen. Huskisson *et al.* (1976) have suggested that penicillamine, as well as levamisole, may have an immunopotentiating effect in rheumatoid arthritis. If auto-immunity were a manifestation of immunodeficiency it would not be surprising if drugs stimulating immune responsiveness produced improvement in auto-immune disease. The relevance of this postulate to rheumatoid arthritis requires further investigation.

SJÖGREN'S SYNDROME

This is a syndrome consisting of dry eyes (keratoconjunctivitis sicca), dry mouth (xerostomia) and an underlying connective tissue disorder, usually rheumatoid arthritis. The lacrimal and salivary glands become infiltrated with lymphocytes and germinal centres may be present. The glands fail to produce their secretions, and this produces a gritty sensation in the eyes leading to conjunctivitis and corneal erosion. The dry mouth causes difficulty in swallowing and is often associated with bad teeth. Dryness may also affect the respiratory tract and the vagina and a renal tubular defect is also present which leads to a reduced capacity to produce an acid urine after an oral acid load.

Patients with Sjögren's syndrome are particularly liable to develop rashes after gold or penicillin (Bloch *et al.*, 1966). Their peripheral blood lymphocytes may show an increase in B-cell numbers and a depletion of T-cells (Talal *et al.*, 1974), and they have a high frequency of auto-antibodies.

Auto-antibodies

The incidence of rheumatoid factor is especially high (96–100% anti-human IgG, 72–74% anti-rabbit IgG) and there is a marked tendency to hypergammaglobulinaemia, especially in patients with the sicca syndrome but without rheumatoid arthritis (Bunim, 1965). Anti-nuclear antibodies are often present (56–80%), again with greater frequency in the latter group. Other auto-antibodies sometimes seen in Sjögren's syndrome are anti-smooth muscle (Feltkamp and van Rossum, 1968) low titre anti-thyro-globulin (Bloch and Bunim, 1963), and anti-reticulin (Rizzetto and Doniach, 1973).

The similarities between the changes in the salivary and lacrimal glands in Sjögren's syndrome and those in the thyroid gland in Hashimoto's disease prompted attempts to demonstrate serum antibodies specific for salivary and lacrimal tissue. More than half the patients tested have proved to have instead an antibody against the cytoplasm of salivary duct epithelium (Bertram and Hallberg, 1964), which is also found at lesser frequency in rheumatoid arthritis, SLE and myasthenia gravis (Feltkamp and van Rossum, 1968). The significance of this antibody is unknown.

Also related to the salivary gland is the recent finding in Sjögren's syndrome of an increase in salivary β_2 microglobulin concentrations, together with an increase in the serum levels, especially in cases with associated renal or lympho-proliferative complications (Michalski *et al.*, 1975). β_2 micro-globulin is a protein of molecular weight 11,800 daltons, with a striking homology of amino acid sequence with that of some homology regions of IgG. It is normally present on cell-surface membranes in close relation with the HLA transplantation antigens, and is in fact indistinguishable from a polypeptide component of the latter. Its presence on lymphocyte cell membranes presumably accounts for its presence in the saliva produced by the lymphocyte-laden salivary tissues in Sjögren's syndrome. Measurement of β_2 microglobulin serum levels may prove useful in identifying Sjögren's patients in whom renal disease or lymphoma is developing, and possibly more generally in assessing the effect of immunosuppressive drugs in reducing the lymphocyte mass or tumour.

ADULT SERO-NEGATIVE ARTHRITIS

Over the last ten years a group of sero-negative inflammatory arthritides occurring in adults has been split off from rheumatoid arthritis. It is suggested that certain of these inflammatory sero-negative arthritides have clinical similarities which encourage their common grouping (Wright and Reed, 1964; Moll *et al.*, 1974). There is evidence of genetic links between some conditions in this group which may prove to have immunological significance.

Ankylosing Spondylitis, Psoriatic Arthritis, Reiter's Disease, and the Intestinal Arthropathies

Ankylosing spondylitis is an erosive arthropathy with a strong hereditary character. It typically starts in the sacroiliac joints and later spreads to involve the spine with bony ankylosis. Presenting symptoms usually occur in the third decade and it is predominantly a male disease (sex incidence 5:1). The initial complaint is of low back pain, worse after resting and often passing down over the buttocks and backs of the legs. Over the following years the pain and stiffness may be felt higher up the spine associated with underlying pathological fibrosis and ossification of the apophyseal joints and annulus fibrosus. Eventually, the complete spine from occiput to sacrum may undergo bony fusion. Iritis occurs in 25% of patients with ankylosing spondylitis (Wilkinson and Bywaters, 1958) and can progress to glaucoma and blindness. A granulomatous aortitis also occurs (Ansell *et al.*, 1958).

Peripheral joints may also be involved, particularly the hips and knees, and some boys present with peripheral arthritis, only later developing the full picture of ankylosing spondylitis. Although the distribution of affected joints differs from that in rheumatoid arthritis, the histopathology of the joint tissues is similar.

Psoriatic arthritis is a sero-negative erosive inflammatory polyarthritis that affects people with psoriasis. It seems to differ from rheumatoid arthritis occurring with psoriasis in its epidemiology, pattern of joint involvement, radiology and serology (Wright, 1969). The arthritis may occur before, during or after the skin lesions of psoriasis and sometimes only the nails are affected, with characteristic pitting. Classically the terminal interphalangeal joints of the fingers and toes are involved. There may be considerable associated periostitis leading to swelling of the whole digit producing a sausage-like appearance, with obliteration of the normal "waist" between joints. If repeated attacks of arthritis occur, underlying bony resorption takes place, producing severe deformity of the digit which can then be pulled in and out like a concertina. Later, sacroiliitis may occur and in some instances spinal involvement indistinguishable from ankylosing spondylitis.

The arthritis of Reiter's disease is a sero-negative polyarthritis usually affecting the joints of the lower limb and sometimes the sacroiliac joints and spine. By definition the arthritis is associated with conjunctivitis and urethritis and commonly affects young men in their third decade. Of unknown cause, the arthritis is associated with non-gonococcal inflammation of the genital tract, dysentry or non-specific diarrhoea. Conjunctivitis occurs in a third of cases but only occasionally produces a purulent exudate. Iritis occurs in about 8% of first attacks but in chronic cases the incidence rises to 30–40% (Ford, 1963).

A sero-negative peripheral inflammatory synovitis also occurs in 10% of patients with ulcerative colitis. The arthritis is asymmetrical, affects large joints and disappears leaving no residua (Wright and Watkinson, 1965). A similar peripheral arthritis may occur in patients with Crohn's disease.

Another group of patients with ulcerative colitis or Crohn's disease develops sacroiliitis and ankylosing spondylitis, the final clinical picture resembling classical idiopathic ankylosing spondylitis. It is also known that among relatives of patients with ulcerative colitis there is an increased frequency of sacroiliitis and ankylosing spondylitis, and that in two rare diseases, Whipple's disease and Bechet's syndrome, there is also an increased prevalence of polyarthritis and sacroiliitis (Moll *et al.*, 1974).

Clinically it seems that this group of sero-negative arthritides overlap, with sacroiliitis as a common feature. In view of the strong association between each of these conditions and ankylosing spondylitis, Moll and his colleagues group them together as "the sero-negative spondarthritides", although spondyloarthritides might seem a preferable term.

Immunological Features

Although classically sero-negative for IgM rheumatoid factor, raised levels of IgG rheumatoid factor have been reported in both ankylosing spondylitis and psoriatic arthritis (Howell *et al.*, 1972).

In ankylosing spondylitis, moreover, cell mediated immunity to autologous IgG is present in a majority of patients, an immunological abnormality held in common with rheumatoid arthritis, and also present, though to a lesser extent, in Reiter's syndrome (Weisbart *et al.*, 1975); a differential point, however, is that cell mediated immunity to IgG is also likely to be found in the relatives of ankylosing spondylitis patients. The mixed lymphocyte reaction (MLR) is reduced in ankylosing spondylitis, and this appears to be largely associated with histocompatibility antigen type (Nikbin *et al.*, 1976). In the MLR, with mitomycin-treated pooled normal human lymphocytes as stimulating cells, lymphocytes from both ankylosing spondylitis patients and asymptomatic individuals (whether relatives or not) of HLA-B27 histocompatibility antigen type incorporate significantly less ^{3}H-thymidine than the lymphocytes of asymptomatic subjects without HLA-B27. This seems to indicate a defect of cell mediated immunity inherited with HLA-B27. The few ankylosing spondylitis patients who are not HLA-B27 also give diminished responses, so the presumed defect may also be heritable independently.

HLA-B27 and Arthritis

The histocompatibility antigen HLA-B27 was present in 96% of 75 patients with ankylosing spondylitis screened for histocompatibility type by Brewerton *et al.* (1973), and in only 7·4% of control subjects. HLA-B27 was present also in more than half the relatives of such patients. Although an individual with HLA-B27 is thus very much (300 times) more likely to develop ankylosing spondylitis than someone lacking it, only 5% of men and 0·6% of women with HLA-B27 in fact develop clinical disease. HLA-B27 is thus an important but clearly not the only susceptibility factor.

In patients with ulcerative colitis, psoriasis and Crohn's disease (conditions which, uncomplicated, themselves display genetic factors unrelated to HLA-B27) true spondylitis with or without other arthropathy is 30 times as likely to develop as in the rest of the population, and HLA-B27 is present in a high proportion (35–67%) of those so affected. This suggests a pattern of overlapping genetic factors linking these conditions and arthritis with the major histocompatibility complex.

HLA-B27 is present in an even higher proportion (70–90%) of patients with Reiter's disease following urethritis or *Shigella* dysentry, and with arthritis following *Yersinia* or *Salmonella* infection. There is thus a highly significant association between HLA-B27 and specific microorganisms in these examples of "reactive" arthritis in which the causative organism cannot be isolated from the joint.

The eye condition acute anterior uveitis is known to be associated with ankylosing spondylitis, Reiter's disease, ulcerative colitis, Crohn's disease, and more rarely with certain infections. It is rarely seen in psoriasis. Brewerton (1975) found that 58% of Caucasian patients attending an eye hospital with acute anterior uveitis were HLA-B27, which indicates a 20-fold increased susceptibility in those with this type, though only a 1% actual incidence. In patients with uveitis and one of the associated diseases mentioned the incidence of HLA-B27 was 90%.

Relevance to Immune Responsiveness

In inbred mouse and guinea-pig strains, the ability to produce a high antibody response to a chemically defined antigen such as a polypeptide is inherited, and a low response likewise. In hybrids the high response is dominant, and cross-breeding experiments show that the genes concerned, the immune response (Ir) genes, are closely linked to the major histocompatibility gene complex, in the mouse the H-2 system on chromosome 17. This localization of Ir genes to the H-2 region in mice suggested a search for associations between HLA antigen types and the incidence of certain diseases in man, especially diseases where abnormal immune responsiveness is suspected. The underlying assumptions in such a search are that specific immune response genes influence disease susceptibility, that human Ir genes are found in the major histocompatibility region (HLA, on chromosome 6, in man) and that Ir and HLA genes occur together not only in families but in the population manifesting the diseases in question. This type of non-random association of genes in populations is known as linkage disequilibrium, and its existence implies that the loci are more effective if they work together. The function of the histocompatibility system, however, is unknown.

The various degrees of association between HLA-B27 and arthritis, inflammatory bowel disease, infections and eye disease provide a thread linking the complex overlapping relationships noted clinically between these conditions. The less than one-to-one relationship, however, indicates that the associations are due to more or less closely linked susceptibility genes, and not directly to HLA itself. The facts so far known strongly imply that the susceptibility genes for ankylosing spondylitis are also involved in some other forms of seronegative arthritis, but direct evidence that they are in fact the immune response genes is still awaited.

Polyarthritis with Hypogammaglobulinaemia

A rare form of sero-negative polyarthritis occurs in adult onset hypogammaglobulinaemia, primarily affecting large joints and accompanied by tenosynovitis of the hands and feet. The condition resembles rheumatoid arthritis, but the joints show no erosions, and the joint effusions contain no polymorphs and have normal complement levels. Patients may present at rheumatology clinics and their hypogammaglobulinaemia becomes recognized because of their history of recurrent chest infections. The condition responds dramatically to gamma-globulin treatment (Webster *et al.*, 1976).

JUVENILE CHRONIC POLYARTHRITIS

Under this heading ("juvenile rheumatoid arthritis" in the USA) falls arthritis with onset before 16 years, involving four or more joints for a period of three months or more with pain, swelling and limitation of movement, in which the histopathology of the joint tissues is compatible with rheumatoid arthritis. Other causes of childhood joint disease, in particular rheumatic fever, virus infections, other systemic connective tissue disease (such as systemic lupus erythematosus, dermatomyositis and scleroderma) acute leukaemia and bone and joint infections have to be excluded.

Studies of the natural history of the disease show that juvenile chronic polyarthritis is heterogeneous. In a large series of patients followed for 15 years (Ansell *et al.*, 1974) about 10%, predominantly older girls, differed from the rest in being persistently sero-positive for IgM rheumatoid factor, rapidly developing joint erosions in the hands and feet, and often having elbow nodules. This subgroup closely resembles adult rheumatoid arthritis.

The large sero-negative group was further subdivisible. A small subgroup, constituting 12% of the cases and mostly boys, had ankylosing spondylitis with bilateral sacroiliitis and spinal limitation, or sacroiliitis of spondylitic type without spinal involvement. The remaining sero-negative subgroup included patients presenting with inflammatory polyarthritis, high fever, rash, lymphadenopathy and splenomegaly, as originally described by Still (1897).

Iridocyclitis involving the iris and ciliary body affects about 10% of children with sero-negative juvenile chronic polyarthritis. An acute type of brief duration occurs in patients with sacroiliac joint changes and ankylosing spondylitis, but this accounts for only about 10% of the iridocyclitis of Still's disease. Chronic iridocyclitis, characterized by an insidious onset, persistent ocular inflammation and residual scarring, band keratopathy and cataracts, occurs mostly in children with only few joints involved.

Anti-nuclear Antibodies in Iridocyclitis

Anti-nuclear antibodies detectable by immunofluorescence are present in 30% of children with chronic juvenile polyarthritis—predominantly females with pauci-articular onset of the disease. In patients with associated chronic iridocyclitis the incidence of ANA is much higher, at least 90% and perhaps more (Schaller *et al.*, 1974). The antibodies are predominantly of IgG class, and serum levels are 25 units/ml or more. No other auto-antibodies are reported. The appearance of ANA usually precedes rather than follows the iridocyclitis. Whether it has pathogenic significance is not known, but it provides a useful marker for identifying patients with Still's disease at risk for chronic iridocyclitis. Most patients with acute iridocyclitis are ANA-negative.

As well as non-organ specific ANA, granulocyte-specific ANA may be present in juvenile chronic polyarthritis, and was found in 20% of patients negative by routine ANA testing (Rosenberg *et al.*, 1975). Unlike the granulocyte-specific ANA of Felty's syndrome or rheumatoid arthritis, it has not been shown to fix complement.

IgG rheumatoid Factor

Raised IgG anti-globulin were initially reported in Still's disease by Torrigiani *et al.* (1969) and the presence of both IgG and IgA anti-globulins in juvenile chronic polyarthritis has been confirmed (Florin-Christensen *et al.*, 1974). Like IgM rheumatoid factors, their serum levels are affected by drug treatment.

HLA-typing

Patients developing ankylosing spondylitis or sacroiliitis of spondylitic type show the expected high incidence of HLA-B27 (Edmonds *et al.*, 1974) but the presence of this antigen is not always expressed as sacroiliitis in males with juvenile chronic polyarthritis. The incidence of HLA-B27 in patients with definite or probable juvenile chronic polyarthritis of less than five years duration is reported as 25% (Hall *et al.*, 1975), and shows a negative correlation with the presence of ANA. This is about three times the incidence of HLA-B27 expected in the population as a whole, but its relationship to the subsequent development of ankylosing spondylitis will be clarified only by long-term follow-up.

REFERENCES

Ansell, B. M., Bywaters, E. G. L. and Doniach, D. (1958). The aortic lesion of ankylosing spondylitis. *Brit. Heart J.* **20**, 507.

Ansell, B. M., Bywaters, E. G. L. and Wood, P. R. N. (1974). Is juvenile chronic polyarthritis (U.S. = JRA) more than one disease? *Abstr. VI Pan-American Cong. Rheumatic Diseases, Toronto*, Abstr. No. 144.

Astorga, G. P. (1975). Study of the effects of antigammaglobulin factors on lymphocytes from patients with rheumatoid arthritis. *In* "Immunological Aspects of Rheumatoid Arthritis" (Ed. J. Clot and J. Sany), p. 80. Karger, Basel.

Astorga, G. P. and Williams, R. C. (1969). Altered reactivity in mixed lymphocyte culture of lymphocytes from patients with rheumatoid arthritis. *Arth. Rheum.* **12**, 547.

Ball, J. and Lawrence, J. S. (1961). Epidemiology of the sheep cell agglutination test. *Ann. Rheum. Dis.* **20**, 235.

Beard, H. K., Faulk, W. P., Conochie, L. B. A. and Glynn, L. E. (1976). Some immunological aspects of collagen. *Progr. All.* **26** (in press).

Bertram, U. and Halberg, P. (1965). Organ antibodies in Sjögren's syndrome. *Acta Allerg. (Kbh)* **20**, 472.

Bianco, N. E., Dobkin, L. W. and Schur, P. H. (1974). Immunological properties of isolated IgG and IgM anti-gamma globulins (rheumatoid factors). *Clin. Exp. Immunol.* **17**, 91.

Bloch, K. J. and Bunim, J. J. (1963). Sjögren's syndrome and its relation to connective tissue disease. *J. Chron. Dis.* **16**, 915.

Bloch, K. J., Buchanan, W. W., Wohl, M. J. and Bunim, J. J. (1965). Sjögren's syndrome. A clinical, pathological and serological study of sixty-two cases. *Medicine (Baltimore)* **44**, 187.

Brandt, K. D., Cathcart, E. S. and Cohen, A. S. (1968). Studies of immune deposits in synovial membranes and corresponding synovial fluids. *J. Lab. Clin. Med.* **72**, 631.

Brewerton, D. A. (1975). HL-A 27 and acute anterior uveitis. *Ann. Rheum. Dis.* **34** Suppl. 33.

Brewerton, D. A., Caffrey, M., Hart, F. D., James, D. C. O., Nicholls, A. and Sturrock, R. D. (1973). Ankylosing spondylitis and HL-A27. *Lancet* **i**, 904.

Brostoff, J. and Roitt, I. M. (1975). Cellular reactions to mycoplasma and aggregated IgG in patients with rheumatoid arthritis. *In* "Immunological Aspects of Rheumatoid Arthritis" (Ed. J. Clot and J. Sany), p. 106, Karger, Basel.

Bulletin World Health Organization (1975). Nomenclature for factors of the HLA system. **52**.

Bunim, J. J. (1965). The frequent occurrence of hypergammaglobulinanaemia and multiple tissue antibodies in Sjögren's syndrome. *Ann. N.Y. Acad. Sci.* **124**, 852.

Caplan, A. (1953). Certain unusual radiological appearances in the chest of coalminers suffering from rheumatoid arthritis. *Thorax* **8**, 29.

Conn, D. L., McDuffie, F. C. and Dyck, P. J. (1972). Immunopathologic study of sural nerves in rheumatoid arthritis. *Arthr. Rheum.* **15**, 135.

Conochie, L. B., Scott, J. F. and Faulk, W. P. (1975). A passive agglutination method using collagen-coated tanned sheep erythrocytes to demonstrate collagen glysosamizoglycan interaction. *J. Immunol. Meth.* **7**, 393.

Cracchiolo, L. S., Goldberg, L. S., Barnett, E. V. and Bluestone, R. (1971). Studies of cryoprecipitates from synovial fluid of rheumatoid patients. *Immunology* **20**, 1067.

Edmonds, J., Morris, R. I., Metzger, A. L., Bluestone, R., Terasaki, P. I., Ansell, B. and Bywaters, E. G. L. (1974). Follow-up study of juvenile chronic polyarthritis with particular reference to histocompatibility antigen W27. *Ann. Rheum. Dis.* **33**, 289.

Elling, P., Graudal, H. and Faber, V. (1968). Granulocyte-specific antinuclear factors in serum and synovial fluid in rheumatoid arthritis. *Ann. Rheum. Dis.* **27**, 225.

Feltkamp, T. E. W. and Van Rossum, A. L. (1968). Antibodies to salivary duct cells and other autoantibodies in patients with Sjögren's syndrome and other idiopathic auto-immune diseases. *Clin. Exp. Immunol.* **3**, 1.

Florin-Christensen, A., Arana, R. M., Morteo, O. G., Roux, M. E. B. and Hubscher, O. (1974). IgG, IgA, IgM and IgD antiglobulins in juvenile rheumatoid arthritis. *Ann. Rheum. Dis.* **33**, 32.

Ford, D. K. (1963). The incidence of uveitis in Reiter's disease. *Brit. J. Vener. Dis.* **39**, 18.

Franklin, E. C., Holman, H. R., Muller-Eberhard, H. J. and Kunkel, H. G. (1957). An unusual protein component of high molecular weight in the serum of certain patients with rheumatoid arthritis. *J. Exp. Med.* **105**, 425.

Freyberg, R. J. (revised by Ziff, M. and Barren, J.) (1972). Gold therapy for rheumatoid arthritis. P. 455 in Arthritis and allied Conditions, 8th edition (Ed. J. L. Hollander and D. J. McCarty), Philadelphia.

Gotze, O., Zvaifler, N. J. and Muller-Eberhard, H. J. (1972). Evidence for complement activation by the C3 activator system in rheumatoid arthritis. *Arthr. Rheum.* **15**, 111.

Hall, M. A., Ansell, B. M., James, D. C. O. and Zylinski, P. (1975). HL-A antigens in juvenile chronic polyarthritis (Still's disease). *Ann. Rheum. Dis.* **34**, Suppl. 1, 36.

Hay, F. C., Nineham, L. and Roitt, I. M. (1975). Routine assay for detection of IgG and IgM antiglobulins in sero-negative and sero-positive rheumatoid arthritis. *Brit. Med. J.* **3**, 203.

Hedberg, H., Kallen, B., Löw, B. and Nilsson, O. (1975). Mixed leucocyte reaction (MLR) in arthritides. *Rheumatology* **6**, 90.

Holborow, E. J. and Johnson, G. D. (1965). The nature of antinuclear immunoglobulins. *Ann. N.Y. Acad. Sci.* **124**, 833.

Howell, F. A., Chamberlain, M. A., Perry, R. A., Torrigiani, G. and Roitt, I. M. (1972). IgG antiglobulin levels in patients with psoriatic arthropathy, ankylosing spondylitis and gout. *Ann. Rheum. Dis.* **31**, 129.

Huskisson, E. C., Gibson, T. J., Balme, H. W., Berry, H., Burry, H. C., Grahame, R., Hart, F. D., Henderson, D. R. F. and Wojtulewski, J. A. (1974). Trial comparing D-penicillamine and gold in rheumatic arthritis. Preliminary report. *Ann. Rheum. Dis.* **33**, 532.

Huskisson, E. C., Scott, J. Balme, H. W., Dieppe, P. A., Trapnell, J. and Willoughby, D. A. (1976). Immunostimulant therapy with levamisole for rheumatoid arthritis. *Lancet* **i**, 393.

Jessop, J. D., Vernon-Roberts, B. and Harris, J. (1973). Effects of gold salts and prednisolone on inflammatory cells. I. Phagocytic activity of macrophages and polymorphs in inflammatory exudates, studied by a skin window technique in rheumatoid and control patients. *Ann. Rheum. Dis.* **32**, 294.

Johnson, P. M., Watkins, J. and Holborow, E. J. (1975). Antiglobulin production to altered IgG in rheumatoid arthritis. *Lancet* **1**, 611.

Kinsella, T. D. (1973). Induction of autologous lymphocyte transformation by synovial fluids from patients with rheumatoid arthritis. *Clin. Exp. Immunol.* **14**, 187.

Kinsella, T. D., Baum, J. and Ziff, M. (1970). Studies of isolated synovial lining cells of rheumatoid and non-rheumatoid synovial membranes. *Arthr. Rheum.* **13**, 784.

Kunkel, H. G., Muller-Eberhard, H. J., Fudenberg, H. H. and Tomasi, T. B. (1961). Gamma globulin complexes in rheumatoid arthritis and certain other conditions. *J. Clin. Invest.* **40**, 117.

Lambert, P. H., Nydegger, U. E., Perrin, L. H., McCormick, J., Fehr, K. and Miescher, P. (1975). *In* "Immunological Aspects of Rheumatoid Arthritis", p. 52, Karger, Basel.

Lawrence, J. S. (1961). Studies with radioactive gold. *Ann. Rheum. Dis.* **20**, 341.

Lorber, A., Bovy, R. A. and Chang, C. C. (1971). Binding of gold to rheumatoid factor: Correlation with serum gold levels. *Arthr. Rheum.* **14**, 172.

Lorber, A., Bovy, R. A. and Chang, C. C. (1972). Relationship between serum gold content and distribution to serum immunoglobulins and complement. *Nature—New Biol.* **236**, 250.

Maurer, P. H. (1954). Antigenicity of oxypolygelatin and gelatin in man. *J. Exp. Med.* **100**, 497.

Michaeli, D. and Fudenberg, H. H. (1974a). The incidence and antigenic specificity of antibodies against denatured human collagen in rheumatoid arthritis. *Clin. Immunol. Immunopath.* **2**, 153.

Michaeli, D. and Fudenberg, H. H. (1974b). Antibodies to collagen in emphysema. *Clin. Immunol. Immunopathol.* **3**, 187.

Michalski, J. P., Daniels, T. E., Talal, N. and Grey, H. M. (1975). Beta$_2$ immunoglobulin and lymphocyte infiltration in Sjögren's syndrome. *New Engl. J. Med.* **293**, 1228.

Mohammed, I., Barraclough, D., Holborow, E. J. and Ansell, B. M. (1976). The effect of penicillamine therapy on circulating immune complexes in rheumatoid arthritis. *Ann. Rheum. Dis.* (in press).

Moll, J. M. H., Haslock, I., Macrae, I. F. and Wright, V. (1974). Associations between ankylosing spondylitis, psoriatic arthritis. Reiter's syndrome, the intestinal arthropathies and Bechet's syndrome. *Medicine* (*Baltimore*) **53**, 343.

Munthe, E. and Natvig, J. B. (1971). Characterization of IgG complexes in eluates from rheumatoid tissue. *Clin. Exp. Immunol.* **8**, 249.

Nikbin, B., Brewerton, D. A., James, D. C. O. and Hobbs, J. R. (1976). Diminished mixed lymphocyte reaction in ankylosing spondylitis, relatives and normal individuals all with HL-A27. *Ann. Rheum. Dis.* **35**, 37.

Normansell, D. E. (1972). Anti-globulin in rheumatoid sera. 111. The reactivity of anti-globulin rheumatoid factors with heterologous-globulin. *Immunochemistry* **9**, 725.

Notman, D. D., Kurata, N. and Tan, E. M. (1975). Profiles of antinuclear antibodies in systemic rheumatic diseases. *Ann. Intern. Med.* **83**, 464.

Nowaslawski, A. and Bryzosko, W. J. (1967). Immunopathology of rheumatoid arthritis. II. The rheumatoid nodule (the rheumatoid granuloma). *Path. Europ.* **2**, 302.

Onyewotu, I. I., Johnson, P. M., Johnson, G. D. and Holborow, E. J. (1975). Enhanced uptake by guinea pig macrophages of radio-iodinated human aggregated immunoglobulin G in the presence of sera from rheumatoid patients with cutaneous vasculitis. *Clin. Exp. Immunol.* **19**, 267.

Panush, R. S. (1975). Effects of certain antirheumatic drugs upon normal human peripheral blood lymphocytes. Inhibition of mitogen- and antigen-stimulated incorporation of tritiated thymidine. (Abstr.). *Arthr. Rheum.* **18**, 418.

Pope, R. M., Teller, D. C. and Mannik, M. (1974). The molecular basis of self-association of antibodies to IgG (rheumatoid factors) in rheumatoid arthritis. *Proc. Nat. Acad. Sci.* **71**, 517.

Popert, A. J., Meijers, K. A. E., Sharp, J. and Bier, F. (1961). Chloroquin diphosphate in rheumatoid arthritis. *Ann. Rheum. Dis.* **20**, 18.

Rizzetto, M., Doniach, D. (1973). Types of reticulin antibodies detected in human sera by immunofluorescence. *J. Clin. Path.* **26**, 841.

Rosenberg, J. N., Johnson, G. D., Holborow, E. J. and Bywaters, E. G. L. (1975). Eosinophil specific and other granulocyte-specific antinuclear antibodies in juvenile chronic polyarthritis and adult rheumatoid arthritis. *Ann. Rheum. Dis.* **34**, 350.

Sany, J., Mathieu, O., Clot, J., Mandin, J. and Serre, H. (1975). Production of MIF-like supernatants by rheumatoid arthritis lymphocytes stimulated by immunoglobulin G. *In* "Immunological Aspects of Rheumatoid Arthritis", p. 131 (Ed. J. Clot and J. Sany), Karger, Basel.

Schaller, J. G., Johnson, G. D., Holborow, E. J., Ansell, B. M. and Smiley, W. K. (1974). The association of antinuclear antibodies with the chronic iridocyclitis of juvenile rheumatoid arthritis (Still's disease). *Arthr. Rheum.* **17**, 409.

Schultz, D. R., Gottlieb, N. L. and Arnold, P. I. (1973). Effects of gold on functional activities of individual complement components. *Arth. Rheum.* **16**, 131.

Sheldon, P. J., Papamichail, M. and Holborow, E. J. (1974). Studies on synovial fluid lymphocytes in rheumatoid arthritis. *Ann. Rheum. Dis.* **33**, 509.

Stastny, P. (1975). MLC determinants associated with rheumatoid arthritis. *In* "Histocompatibility Testing 1975" (Ed. F. Kissmeyer-Nielsen), p. 797, Munksgaard, Copenhagen.

Stastny, P. (1976). Mixed lymphocyte cultures in rheumatoid arthritis. *J. Clin. Invest.* **57**, 1148.

Steffen, C. (1969). Tissue antibodies in rheumatoid arthritis and other connective tissue diseases. *Ann. Immunol.* **i**, 47.

Steffen, C. (1970). Consideration of pathogenesis of rheumatoid arthritis as collagen autoimmunity. *S. Immunoforsch.* **139**, 219.

Still, G. F. (1897). On a form of chronic joint disease in children. *Med. Chir. Trans.* **80**, 47.

Talal, N., Sylvester, R. A., Daniels, T. E., Greenspan, J. S. and Williams, R. C. (1974). T- and B-lymphocytes in peripheral blood and tissue lesions in Sjögren's syndrome. *J. Clin. Invest.* **53**, 180.

Theofilopoulos, A. N., Burtonboy, G., Lospalluto, J. J. and Ziff, M. (1974). IgG rheumatoid factor and low molecular weight IgM in association with vasculitis. *Arthr. Rheum.* **17**, 272.

Torrigiani, G., Ansell, B. M., Chown, E. E. A. and Roitt, I. M. (1969). Raised IgG antiglobulin factors in Still's disease. *Ann. Rheum. Dis.* **28**, 424.

Turner-Warwick, M. and Haslam, P. (1971). Antibodies in some chronic fibrosing lung diseases. 1. Non-organ-specific antibodies. *Clin. Allergy.* **1**, 83.

Vernon-Roberts, B., Jessop, J. D. and Doré, J. (1973). Effects of gold salts and prednisolone on inflammatory cells. II. Suppression of inflammation and phagocytosis in the rat. *Ann. Rheum. Dis.* **32**, 301.

Ward, D. J., Johnson, G. D. and Holborow, E. J. (1964). Antinuclear factor in rheumatoid arthritis. *Ann. Rheum. Dis.* **23**, 306.

Webster, A. D. B., Loewi, G., Dourmashkin, R. D., Golding, D. M., Ward, D. J. and Asherson, G. L. (1976). Polyarthritis in adults with hypogammaglobulinaemia and its rapid response to immunoglobulin treatment. *Brit. Med. J.* **1**, 1314.

Weisbart, R. A., Bluestone, R. and Goldberg, L. S. (1975). Cellular immunity to autologous IgG in rheumatoid arthritis and rheumatoid-like diseases. *Clin. Exp. Immunol.* **20**, 409.

Wilk, A. (1975a). Joint fluid immune complexes involving granulocyte specific antinuclear factors in rheumatoid arthritis. *Acta Path. Microbiol. Scand.* Sect. C. **83**, 365.

Wiik, A. (1975b). Circulating immune complexes involving granulocyte specific antinuclear factors in Felty's syndrome and rheumatoid arthritis. *Acta Path. Microbiol. Scand.* Sect. C. **83**, 354.

Wiik, A. and Munthe, E. (1974). Complement-fixing granulocyte-specific antinuclear factors in neutropenic cases of rheumatoid arthritis. *Immunology* **26**, 1127.

Wilkinson, M. and Bywaters, E. G. L. (1958). Clinical features and course of ankylosing spondylitis as seen in the follow-up of 222 hospital referred cases. *Ann. Rheum. Dis.* **17**, 209.

Williams, R. C., Emmons, J. D. and Astorga, G. P. (1971). Studies of antilymphocyte antigen produced against normal and rheumatoid arthritis lymphocytes. *Arthr. Rheum.* **14**, 697.

Winchester, R. J., Agnello, Y. and Kunkel, H. G. (1970). Gamma globulin complexes in synovial fluids of patients with rheumatoid arthritis. II. Partial characterization and relationship to lowered complement levels. *Clin. Exp. Immunol.* **6**, 689.

Winchester, R. J., Fu, S. M., Hoffman, T., Winfield, J. B. and Kunkel, H. G. (1975). Delineation of peripheral blood lymphocyte populations; analysis of some interfering factors. *In* "The Immunological Basis of Connective Tissue Disorders" (Ed. L. G. Silvestri), p. 209, North Holland Publishing Co., Amsterdam.

Wright, V. (1969). Psoriatic arthritis. *In* "Textbook of Rheumatic Diseases" (Ed. W. S. C. Copeman), p. 632, Edinburgh.

Wright, V. and Reed, W. B. (1964). The link between Reiter's syndrome and psoriatic arthritis. *Ann. Rheum. Dis.* **23**, 12.

Wright, V. and Watkinson, G. (1965). The arthritis of ulcerative colitis. *Brit. Med. J.* **2**, 670.

Ziff, M. (1973). Pathophysiology of rheumatoid arthritis. *Federation Proceedings* **32**, 131.

Zvaieler, N. J. (1973). Immunopathology of joint inflammation in rheumatoid arthritis. *Adv. Immunol.* **16**, 310.

Zvaifler, N. J. and Schur, P. (1968). Reactions of aggregated mercaptoethanol treated gamma globulin with rheumatoid factor—precipitin and complement fixation studies. *Arthr. Rheum.* **11**, 523.

Zutshi, D. W., Reading, C. A., Epstein, W. V., Ansell, B. M. and Holborow, E. J. (1969). FII haemaglutination test for serum antigammaglobulin factors in arthritides sero-positive and sero-negative by other tests. *Ann. Rheum. Dis.* **28**, 289.

16

Immunology of Heart Diseases

E. G. L. BYWATERS

This Chapter will deal with the immunological mechanisms involving the heart in such conditions as rheumatic fever, other connective tissue diseases and other myocardiopathies, including endomyocardial fibrosis and their experimental counterparts. An excellent earlier review of this field was published by Kaplan and Frengley (1969). This review will exclude consideration of graft rejection (except insofar as it throws light on, for instance, the development of cross-reacting antibodies). That is a specialized field of considerable current importance, well reviewed by Roberts and Lessof (1973).

The intrinsic antigens of the heart consist for the most part of myocardial fibres and their constituent proteins (Espinosa and Kaplan, 1970; Lin *et al.*, 1973). Antigenic components include sarcolemmal membrane and other cytoplasmic and nuclear components of non-specific character. We must consider also the connective tissue framework, including that of the valvular apparatus and the serosa of the pericardium as well as blood vessels. In addition, the heart may become the site of extrinsic antigen deposition and by virtue of its vascular system it may participate in general allergic reactions.

The myocardium has been the seat of fatal allergic reactions due to drugs such as penicillin, cincophen or sulfonamide (Langsjoen and Stinson, 1965) to phenindione (Kerwin, 1964) and to other drugs. Reactions to foreign serum are known occasionally to affect the heart. Viral, e.g. Coxsackie (Hirschman and Hammer, 1974) or vaccinial (Matthews and Griffiths, 1974) as well as Chagasic infection (Cossio, 1975), often involve both myo- and pericardial tissues in a reaction which is probably due as much if not more to immunological mechanisms as to direct cell damage (Woodruff and Woodruff, 1974). The long persistence of undegradable streptococcal cell wall mucopeptide antigen in the heart (Ohanian *et al.*, 1969) may give rise to rheumatic fever-like lesions in mice and rabbits and in the joints in rats (Yang *et al.*, 1970). The heart disease produced in experimental animals originally by repeated injections of streptococci (Murphy and Swift, 1949) and more recently by auto-heart antigen (Halbert *et al.*, 1973) resembles closely that of rheumatic fever (Murphy, 1960), the major cause of heart disease in developing countries such as Great Britain in the nineteenth century or Egypt in the 1960s (Abdin and Eissa, 1965).

POST-STREPTOCOCCAL CARDITIS

Rheumatic fever and the resultant rheumatic heart disease has been known since 1930 to be due to preceding Group A β-haemolytic streptococcal infection. The mechanism by which the streptococcus induces rheumatic fever in 0·3% or 3% of the infected population in sporadic and epidemic conditions respectively has been a major problem since that time. Rheumatic fever is not associated with any particular streptococcal type of the 60 or so far ascertained, differing here from post-streptococcal nephritis. Nor does it seem to be genetically determined by HLA antigens (Falk *et al.*, 1973) although the blood group polymorphism of rheumatic fever subjects shows an excess of both non-secretor and non-O individuals (Glynn and Holborow, 1969): the occurrence of multiple cases within a family is almost certainly associated with environmental conditions, particularly overcrowding and multiple infections by virulent, rapidly "passaged" streptococci. The virtual disappearance in the last 20 years of rheumatic fever and the mild, often M-deficient and non-typeable strains of streptococci characteristic of well-to-do societies are both due primarily to improvement in social conditions and a resultant decrease in virulence of Group A β-haemolytic streptococci. This organism is still with us but no longer rampant, except in poor societies.

The discovery by Kaplan of cross-reaction between antibody to Group A streptococci and heart-tissue antigens, using Coon's immunofluorescence staining technique, started a new era in our understanding of rheumatic fever. Auto-antibodies to heart antigen had previously been demonstrated by complement fixation and agglutination techniques: Kaplan and Suchy (1964) were able to demonstrate anti-streptococcal antibody reacting with subsarcolemmal myocardial antigen and vice versa. This appeared in 41% of acute rheumatic fever cases (Hess *et al.*, 1962). The streptococcal antigen was originally thought to be M protein but it is now thought to be usually a mucopeptide of the cell membrane. Antibodies against certain group A strains may show cross-reactivity with cells other than myocardial: synovial cells and astrocytes, fibroblasts, endothelial cells and epidermal cells (Kingston and

Glynn, 1971), perhaps accounting for the varying symptomatology of rheumatic fever. The cardiac antigen with which streptococcal antibody reacts appears now to be not the C-polysaccharide-like material incriminated by Goldstein *et al.* (1968) and Halpern *et al.*, (1967) but a plasmalogen (Kasp-Grochowska *et al.*, 1972, Kasp-Grochowska and Glynn, 1975), a membrane phospholipid and a new class of antigen extractable from human myocardium.

Such a heart reactive antibody appears in the serum not only in rheumatic fever but after heart damage from infarction (associated with Dressler's syndrome) and post-cardiotomy, even in cases of congenital and non-rheumatic heart disease (see below). It is found also after streptococcal sore throats without the complication of rheumatic fever. Is it therefore a *post hoc* phenomenon and not *propter hoc*? Zabriskie *et al.* (1971) have been able to identify two types of sarcolemmal antibody, one of which is absorbed out only by heart, the other by both heart and streptococcus. It is the latter antibody which in high titre is associated with streptococcal heart damage.

According to Zabriskie, what determines whether recurrences of rheumatic fever occur after streptococcal infection (presumably by a different M type) is the interval level of cross-reacting antibody. If this is raised and streptococcal infection occurs, another rheumatic fever episode will ensue. The rise in cross-reacting antibody seen in post-cardiotomy states is usually less and the antibody is different—being absorbed out by cardiac antigen but not by streptococcus. It is still unclear, however, how circulating auto-antibody at whatever titre can affect individual myocardial cells without some other damaging factor. Experiments on rats in fact indicate that some factor additional to streptococcal infection may be necessary e.g. isoproterenol (Gazenfeld *et al.*, 1966). Cellular immunity, shown to develop with streptococcal infection and to be transferable (Lawrence, 1960) may well be involved.

Delayed hypersensitivity to Group A haemolytic streptococci is known to be present in rheumatic fever, but its role is still not clear, chiefly because cellular immunity is difficult to quantify. However, Read *et al.* (1974) have recently shown, using peripheral blood leucocyte migration inhibition, that cellular immunity to streptococcal cell membrane is considerably increased in active rheumatic fever as compared with normals and in active rheumatic fever as compared with non-rheumatic acute streptococcal sore throats. This abnormal response appears to last for up to five years after the initial attack of rheumatic fever and it may well be that the lymphocytes seen in and around the acute lesion in the heart of rheumatic fever patients in the neighbourhood of damaged fibres and Aschoff nodes are cytotoxic.

Another approach (Dudding and Ayoub, 1968) demonstrated a long continued group A polysaccharide antibody rise only in those patients with continuing cardiac lesions but this was not confirmed by Zimmerman *et al.* (1971). Certainly some explanation is needed why some people with rheumatic fever get carditis and even residual valvular damage and some do not. We are still searching for the factors which render the myocardial fibre susceptible to the circulating auto-immune antibody and perhaps a separate mechanism determining the progressive fibrosis of valvular disease: the latter is seen also (Brigden *et al.*, 1960) in systemic lupus erythematosus, where fibroblast activation by immune complex deposits may be operative. However, both in SLE with and SLE without carditis, anti-heart antibodies may be found in about 60% of cases, staining both sarcolemmal and subsarcolemmal regions of human infant myocardial fibres (Das and Cassidy, 1973).

THE POST-INFARCTION SYNDROME

Dressler's (1956) recognition of a systemic upset following infarction (including fever, raised sedimentation rate, pleurisy and sometimes pericarditis), differed from and was greater than that expected from the small amount of necrotic tissue involved. The recognition of a similar syndrome following operations on the heart (Robinson and Brigden, 1963) has provided us with further information on the significance of heart auto-antibodies and has allowed serial prospective observation. Van der Geld (1964) using Steffen's anti-globulin consumption test and indirect immunofluorescence showed auto-antibody to human heart in about half the infarction cases, a proportion similar to that found by Heine *et al.* (1966) and Strausz and Dobias (1967). Several immunofluorescent staining patterns are seen—subsarcolemmal, endomysial, interfibrillary and striational. The reaction is maximal at two to four weeks and was associated with IgA and IgG containing cells in the heart, particularly near necrotic areas (Schenk, 1973) and with soluble complex formation and the appearance of inactivation products of C3 and C4 (Versey and Gabriel, 1974). Other auto-antibodies may also be present e.g. thyroid and gastric parietal cell antibodies (Lawrence and Wright, 1972).

THE POST-CARDIOTOMY SYNDROME

Similar observations have been made following cardiotomy not only in patients with rheumatic heart disease but also in congenital heart disease

(Ito *et al.*, 1968), where the syndrome occurred in 26 out of 86 consecutive long-term survivors mostly in the age group 5–15 years but not in those under one year of age (Engle *et al.*, 1974). It responded to prednisone and salicylate. Auto-antibody occurred in six out of these 26 cases (Robinson and Brigden, 1963) as shown by a haemagglutination technique and in five of these six the clinical syndrome developed later, e.g. at 7 weeks. The antibody appears first usually between 6–40 days and may last for months (Ehrenfeld *et al.*, 1961). It is absorbed out by heart muscle but not by streptococcal membrane, but apparently is not toxic to homologous heart cells *in vitro* (Gery *et al.*, 1960). Because the clinical syndrome is always associated with antibody the latter appears to be more than just a by-product. It obviously plays a much more important role in transplant rejection.

HEART REACTIVE ANTIBODY IN TRANSPLANTATION

This develops between the fourth and eleventh day preceding rejection and is depressed by treatment with steroid, immunosuppressive drugs and anti-lymphocytic serum. It reappears on stopping treatment (Ellis *et al.*, 1970). Indeed these authors have utilized the streptococcal cross-reacting antigen to aid transplantation. Tolerance to allografted heart was induced in mice by Group A streptococcal pre-treatment: both humoral and delayed hypersensitivity failed to develop (Ellis *et al.*, 1974).

OTHER CONDITIONS WITH IMMUNOLOGICAL INVOLVEMENT

Other heart conditions with associated immunological abnormalities include sub-acute bacterial endocarditis with multiple auto- and exo-antibodies (Bacon *et al.*, 1974), recurrent idiopathic pericarditis where 30% of symptomatic patients show circulating autoantibody (Robinson and Brigden, 1968) and other types of myocardial disease (Robinson *et al.*, 1970), including cardiomyopathy (Fowler, 1971), and particularly idiopathic hypertrophic sub-aortic stenosis (Das *et al.*, 1973). Endomycocardial fibrosis, common in the tropics and distinguishable from rheumatic heart disease (Parry and Abrahams, 1965), has also been shown to manifest heart antibodies and Van der Geld *et al.* (1966a,b) have shown not only fibrin and bound globulin near myofibrils in this condition, but also a cryoprecipitate of IgG and IgM in the serum, high circulating anti-heart antibody and auto-antibodies against gastric mucosa and thyroid. However, as Das *et al.* (1971) showed, specific fixation of antibody in myocardium can occur in cardiomyopathy in the absence of circulating heart reactive antibody. Familial cardiomyopathy also shows myocardial auto-antibody in 50% of those clinically affected and in 20% of unaffected relations compared with about 5% of controls (Klajman *et al.*, 1971).

Immunological advance has usually depended on biochemical expertise, especially in the preparation of pure antigens, and biochemical advances have begun recently to utilize the specificity of immunological reactions. Recent progress in characterization of muscle and cell membrane proteins can be expected to add considerably in the near future to our knowledge in this field, but, in the absence so far of intelligible genetic factors, there is still a need for imaginative clinical assessment, since environmental and historical factors may well play a considerable part in determining why only a fraction of those exposed to myocardial damage develop auto-antibodies and why an even smaller fraction get diseases therefrom. It seems likely, as in other fields, that auto-antibody may perform a scavenger function but that if persistent it may, if combined with some other factor—toxic damage, cellular hypersensitivity or cytotoxicity, produce symptoms of "auto-immune" or, perhaps better, "auto-aggressive" disease.

REFERENCES

Abdin, Z. H. and Elissa, A. (1965). Rheumatic fever and rheumatic heart disease in children below the age of five years in the tropics. *Ann. Rheum. Dis.* **24**, 389.

Bacon, P. A., Davidson, C. and Smith, B. (1974). Antibodies to candida and autoantibodies in sub-acute bacterial endocarditis. *Quart. J. Med.* **43**, 537.

Brigden, W., Bywaters, E. G. L., Lessof, M. H. and Ross, I. P. (1960). The heart in systemic lupus erythematosus. *Brit. Heart J.* **22**, 1.

Cossio, P. M. (1975). Chagasic cardiopathy: antibodies reacting with plasma membrane of striated muscle and endothelial cells. *Circulation* **50**, 1252.

Das, S. K. and Cassidy, J. T. (1973). Antiheart antibodies in patients with systemic lupus erythematosus. *Am. J. Med. Sci.* **265**, 275.

Das, S. K., Callen, J. P. and Dodson, V. N. (1971). Immunoglobulin binding in cardiomyopathic hearts. *Circulation* **44**, 612.

Das, S. K., Cassidy, J. T. and Petty, R. E. (1972). Antibodies against heart muscle and nuclear constituents in cardiomyopathy. *Am. Heart J.* **83**, 159.

Das, S. K., Cassidy, J. T., Dodson, V. N. and Willis, P. W. (1973). Antiheart antibody in idiopathic hypertrophic subaortic stenosis. *Brit. Heart J.* **35**, 965.

Dressler, W. (1956). A post-myocardial-infarction syndrome. Preliminary report of a complication resembling idiopathic, recurrent, benign pericarditis. *J. Am. Med. Ass.* **160**, 1379.

Dudding, B. A. and Ayoub, E. M. (1968). Persistence of streptococcal group A antibody in patients with rheumatic valvular disease. *J. Exp. Med.* **128**, 1081.

Ehrenfeld, E. N., Gery, I. and Davies, A. M. (1961). Specific antibodies in heart disease. *Lancet* **1**, 1138.

Ellis, R. J., Lillehei, C. W. and Zabriskie, J. B. (1970). Heart-reactive antibody in heart transplants. *J. Am. Med. Ass.* **211**, 1505.

Ellis, R. J., Zabriskie, J. B. and Ebert, P. A. (1974). Tolerance to myocardial tissue allografts by pretreatment with cross-reactive streptococcal membrane antigen. *Surgery* **76**, 142.

Engle, M. A., McCabe, J. C., Ebert, P. A. and Zabriskie, J. (1974). The postpericardiotomy syndrome and antiheart antibodies. *Circulation* **49**, 401.

Espinosa, E. and Kaplan, M. H. (1970). Antigenic analysis of human heart tissue. Antigens with restricted organ distribution in acid extracts of human myocardium. *J. Immunol.* **105**, 416.

Falk, J. A., Fleischman, J. L. and Zabriskie, J. B. (1973). A study of HL-A antigen phenotypes in rheumatic fever and rheumatic heart disease patients. *Tiss. Antigens* **3**, 173.

Fowler, N. O. (1971). Autoimmune heart disease. *Circulation* **44**, 159.

Gazenfeld, E., Rosemann, E., Davies, A. M. and Leufer, A. (1966). Isoproterenol induced myocardial lesions in the immunized and non-immunized rat. II. Histopathological lesions after specific immunization. *Immunology* **10**, 193.

Gery, I., Davies, A. M. and Ehrenfeld, E. N. (1960). Heart-specific autoantibodies. *Lancet* **1**, 471.

Glynn, L. E. and Holborow, E. J. (1969). Blood groups and their secretion in rheumatic fever. *In* "Rheumatology: an Annual Review", Vol. 2, p. 113, Karger, Basel.

Goldstein, I., Rebeyrotte, P., Parlebas, J. and Halpern, B. (1968). Isolation from heart valves of glycopeptides which share immunological properties with streptococcus haemolyticus group A polysaccharides. *Nature* **219**, 866.

Halbert, S. P., Lin, T.-M. and Smith, S. (1973). The cardiac auto-immune system. IX. Autoimmune myocarditis in rabbits immunized with rabbit heart. *Int. Arch Allergy* **44**, 783.

Heine, W. I., Friedman, H., Mandell, M. S. and Goldberg, H. (1966). Antibodies to cardiac tissue in acute ischemic heart disease. *Am. J. Cardiol.* **17**, 798.

Hess, E. V., Fink, C. W., Taranta, A. and Ziff, M. (1962). Circulating heart antibodies in rheumatic fever: a clinical study. *Arthr. Rheum.* **5**, 301.

Hirschman, S. Z. and Hammer, G. S. (1974). Review: Coxsackie virus myopericarditis. A microbiological and clinical review. *Am. J. Cardiol.* **34**, 224.

Ito, T., Engle, M. A. and Goldberg, H. P. (1958). Postpericardiotomy syndrome following surgery for nonrheumatic heart disease. *Circulation* **17**, 549.

Kaplan, M. H. and Frengley, J. D. (1969). Autoimmunity to the heart in cardiac disease. Current concepts of the relation of autoimmunity to rheumatic fever, postcardiotomy and postinfarction syndromes and cardiomyopathies. *Am. J. Cardiol.* **24**, 459.

Kaplan, M. H. and Suchy, M. L. (1964). Immunologic relation of streptococcal and tissue antigens. II. Cross-reaction of antisera to mammalian heart tissue with a cell wall constituent of certain strains of group A streptococci. *J. exp. Med.* **119**, 643.

Kasp-Grochowska, E., Kingston, D. and Glynn, L. E. (1972). Immunology of bovine heart valves. I. Cross-reaction with the C-polysaccharide of streptococcus pyogenes. *Ann. Rheum. Dis.* **31**, 282, 290.

Kerwin, A. J. (1964). Fatal myocarditis due to sensitivity to phenindione. *Can. Med. Ass. J.* **90**, 1418.

Kingston, D. and Glynn, L. E. (1971). A cross-reaction between Str. pyogenes and human fibroblasts, endothelial cells and astrocytes. *Immunology* **21**, 1003.

Klajman, A., Kamin-Belsky, N. and Feldman, S. (1971). Immunologic studies in familial cardiomyopathy. *Am. J. Cardiol.* **28**, 707.

Langsjoen, P. H. and Stinson, J. C. (1965). Acute fatal allergic myocarditis. *Dis. Chest* **48**, 440.

Lawrence, H. S. (1960). *In* "Cellular Aspects of Immunity" (Ed. G. E. W. Wolstenholme and M. O'Connor), p. 249, Churchill, London.
Lawrence, M. S. T. A. and Wright, R. (1972). Tamponade in Dressler's syndrome with immunological studies. *Brit. Med. J.* **1**, 665.
Lin, T.-M., Halbert, S. P. and Bruderer, R. (1973). The cardiac auto-immune system. VIII. Immunofluorescence patterns of cultured rat heart cells exposed to rabbit anti-rabbit heart autoantibodies. *Int. Arch. Allergy* **44**, 62.
Matthews, A. W. and Griffiths, I. D. (1974). Post-vaccinal pericarditis and myocarditis. *Brit. Heart J.* **36**, 1043.
Murphy, G. E. (1960). Nature of rheumatic heart disease with special reference to myocardial disease and heart failure, *Medicine* **39**, 289.
Murphy, G. E. and Swift, H. F. (1949). Induction of cardiac lesions, closely resembling those of rheumatic fever, in rabbits following repeated skin infections with group A streptococci. *J. Exp. Med.* **89**, 687.
Ohanian, S. H., Schwab, J. H. and Cromartie, W. J. (1969). Relation of rheumatic-like cardiac lesions of the mouse to localization of group A streptococcal cell walls. *J. Exp. Med.* **129**, 37.
Parry, E. H. O. and Abrahams, D. G. (1965). The natural history of endomyocardial fibrosis. *Quart. J. Med.* **34**, 383.
Read, S. E., Fischetti, V. A., Utermohlen, V., Falk, R. E. and Zabriskie, J. B. (1974). Cellular reactivity studies to streptococcal antigens. *J. clin. Invest.* **54**, 439.
Roberts, C. I. and Lessof, M. H. (1973). Immunological aspects of cardiovascular disorders. *In* "Progress in Cardiology", Vol. 2 (Ed. N. Yu and J. F. Goodwin), p. 31, Lea and Fibiger, Philadelphia.
Robinson, J. F. and Brigden, W. (1963). Immunological studies in the post-cardiotomy syndrome. *Brit. Med. J.* **2**, 706.
Robinson, J. and Brigden, W. (1968). Recurrent pericarditis. *Brit. Med. J.* **2**, 272.
Robinson, J. A., Grieble, H. G. and Anderson, T. O. (1970). The serological abnormalities of idiopathic myocardial disease. *Cardiovasc. Res.* **4**, 14.
Schenk, E. A. (1973). Immunopathologic studies in myocardial infarction. *Am. J. Path.* **70**, 50a.
Strausz, I. and Dobias, G. (1967). Autoantibodies reacting with heart muscle tissue in coronary heart disease. *J. Clin. Path.* **20**, 161.
Van der Geld, H. (1964). Anti-heart antibodies in the post-pericardiotomy and the post-myocardial infarction syndrome. *Lancet* **2**, 617.
Van der Geld, H., Somers, K. and Peetroom, F. (1966a). Endomyocardial fibrosis. *Lancet* **1**, 48.
Van der Geld, H., Peetcom, F., Somers, K. and Kanyerezi, B. R. (1966b). Immunohistological and serological studies in endomyocardial fibrosis. *Lancet* **2**, 1210.
Versey, J. M. B. and Gabriel, R. (1974). Soluble complex formation after myocardial infarction. *Lancet* **2**, 493.
Woodruff, J. F. and Woodruff, J. J. (1974). Involvement of T lymphocytes in the pathogenesis of coxsackie virus B_3 heart disease. *J. Immunol.* **113**, 1726.
Yang, C. H., Anderle, S. K. and Cromartie, W. J. (1970). Relation of experimental arthritis in rats to localization of group A streptococcal cell walls. *Fed. Proc.* **29**, Abstr. No. 238.
Zabriskie, J. B., Read, S. E. and Ellis, R. J. (1971). *In* "Progress in Immunology", Vol. 1 (Ed. B. Amos), pp. 212, Academic Press.
Zimmerman, R. A., Auernheimer, A. H. and Taranta, A. (1971). Precipitating antibody to group A streptococcal polysaccharide in humans. *J. Immunol.* **107**, 832.

17

Glomerulonephritis

J. S. CAMERON and D. GWYN WILLIAMS

Human glomerulonephritis is recognized to be a condition in which allergic mechanisms play a prime role, initiating or continuing the tissue damage associated with the disorder. Evidence for this is derived indirectly from the production of analogous diseases in experimental animals, and directly from the demonstration of the participation of antigen–antibody complexes and anti-basement membrane antibodies in human disease.

GLOMERULONEPHRITIS IN EXPERIMENTAL ANIMALS

The study of experimental glomerulonephritis has markedly increased our understanding of the pathogenesis and modes of glomerular damage. Two different mechanisms of experimental glomerulonephritis are recognized—one due to circulating immune complexes, and the other to antibodies directed against constituents of renal basement membrane.

Immune Complex Disease

There are two varieties of experimental immune complex nephritis.

Acute, or "One Shot" Serum Sickness

Injection of a single dose of foreign protein causes an illness characterized by glomerulonephritis, arthritis and arteritis. These inflammatory lesions occur when complexes of antibody and injected antigen are circulating in the animal, and in most instances are short-lived, subsiding after the elimination of the antigen.

Chronic

In this model, repeated injections of a foreign protein into an experimental animal lead to a prolonged state of circulating immune complexes which result in a chronic glomerulonephritis.

In both forms, immunofluorescent techniques have demonstrated complement, immunoglobulin and antigen deposited in granular fashion in the glomeruli.

The variety of antibody response to even a single antigen has been outlined in earlier chapters. The type of complex formed may be critical to the development of nephritis, and it is likely that a whole family of complexes may circulate in a single patient. Germuth and Rodriguez (1973) have produced evidence from bovine serum albumin-induced nephritis in rabbits that the size of complexes is critical in determining the site of deposition in the glomerulus; large complexes of a size greater than 10^6 daltons deposit preferentially in the mesangium, smaller complexes localizing to the glomerular capillary walls. However, it would be unwise to ignore the effects of possible events occurring after the deposition of complexes in the glomerulus in determining the final pattern. Most attention has been directed to complexes formed at equivalence or in moderate antigen excess, since these may best activate complement. The presence of free antibody as well as complexes may be of importance, since complexes formed in antibody excess are also capable of inducing an experimental nephritis of focal distribution. Moreover, complexes formed in antibody excess have a different phlogistic capacity in that they activate the coagulation system more effectively than complexes formed in antigen excess.

Anti-basement Membrane Disease

The glomerulonephritis following injection of heterologous anti-basement membrane antibody provides the other basic type of experimental glomerulonephritis. Characteristically, such antibody ("nephrotoxic" antibody) produces a disease of two phases. In the first 'heterologous' phase, the injected antibody fixes to the host's glomerular basement membrane (GBM) and produces a lesion with minor microscopical changes resulting in proteinuria.

The second phase is due to the host's production of antibody against the foreign immunoglobulin comprising the anti-GBM antibody, and is therefore called the autologous phase. The host's antibody fixes to the glomerular basement membrane and a proliferative nephritis follows. Immunofluorescence can demonstrate the fixation of both heterologous and autologous antibody on the GBM in their respective phases.

An important development in this field was the demonstration that the immunization of sheep with homologous or heterologous GBM, and of rabbits with GBM fragments extracted from their urine, results in the production of anti-GBM auto-antibodies with an associated nephritis.

Combination of Non-renal Antigen and Antibody in Renal Tissue

Anti-GBM nephritis is an example of antibody combining, within tissue, to an antigen. In this case the antigen is a specific one belonging to renal tissue and thus determines the localization of the disease. Before soluble complex formation and localization were described, deposition of antigen unrelated to the organ in tissue, with subsequent fixation of antibody, was postulated. This mechanism can induce renal disease and may play a part in some forms of nephritis. If aggregated protein is injected, it will be taken up by the mesangium of the kidney. If, subsequently, specific antibody is injected, this will fix to the antigen deposited in the mesangium and lead to a brisk nephritis. A nephritis model using heterologous aggregated IgG has been described in which this is the sequence of events.

HUMAN GLOMERULONEPHRITIS

It is now clear that human types of glomerulonephritis occur which are analogous to the experimental types described above. These are described in more detail later in this chapter, and it is sufficient here to list the evidence for these mechanisms operating in human disease.

Immune Complex Nephritis

Indirect evidence is provided by the immunofluorescent pattern of granular deposition of immunoglobulin and complement components, and the demonstration of circulating immune complexes in some forms of nephritis (e.g. systemic lupus). More convincing evidence is the elution of antigen, and antibody against it, from diseased glomeruli, with the demonstration that the antibody does not react directly with the GBM.

Anti-GBM Nephritis

Immunofluorescence again provides indirect evidence in that the characteristic linear pattern of immunoglobulin or globulin basement membrane can be demonstrated. Direct evidence lies in the demonstration of circulating anti-glomerular basement antibodies, their elution from the glomeruli, and the production of anti-GBM nephritis in primates by injecting the eluate.

THE MEDIATION OF GLOMERULAR INJURY

The glomerular damage in both types of nephritis is produced by inflammatory processes induced by complement, fibrinogen and polymorphs and other unidentified mechanisms. In human disease, the evidence for these mechanisms is circumstantial, e.g. demonstration of the relevant material in the diseased glomeruli by immunofluorescence and the presence of hypocomplementaemia and circulating and urinary fibrin degradation products (FDPs). In experimental nephritis more direct proof is the failure to induce nephritis in animals in which one of the mediators is blocked or depleted.

Complement

In animal nephritis a role for complement has been defined in only the heterologous phase of anti-GBM nephritis: in complement-depleted animals polymorph accumulation failed to occur. This was not the case in the autologous phase nor in "one-shot" serum sickness in rabbits, in which the arteritis is prevented, but not the glomerulitis. The relevant studies have not yet been performed in experimental chronic immune complex disease.

The complement system has been extensively studied in human glomerulonephritis, and abnormalities have been most frequently found in acute glomerulonephritis (AGN), systemic lupus (SLE) and the histologically-defined mesangiocapillary glomerulonephritis (MCGN) (Williams *et al.*, 1974).

Hypocomplementaemia

In AGN and SLE, there is reduction of C3 associated with low C1q and C4 levels indicating classical pathway activation. In MCGN the serum levels of the early classical pathway components are usually normal, and the reduced C3 is considered to be due to activation of complement via a bypass such as the alternative pathway.

Circulating C3 Breakdown Products

These have been demonstrated in the fresh plasma of patients with each type of nephritis, and indicate C3 breakdown *in vivo*.

C3 Splitting Activity

This was first demonstrated in the serum of patients with MCGN, and was given the name of C3 nephritic factor (C3NeF). It has been shown to break down C3 via the alternative pathway, which accords with the normal C1q, C4 and C2 levels found in most patients with hypocomplementaemic MCGN. C3 splitting activity has more recently been found in SLE and AGN; in the former the classical pathway of complement is activated, and also in most cases of the latter, although in a minority the alternative pathway only is activated.

The nature of the serum factors which can break down C3 *in vitro* is unknown. Those acting via the classical pathway are most likely to be immune complexes; C3NeF has been the object of differing reports, one group of workers (Vallota *et al.*, 1974) claiming it to be a separable protein demonstrable immunochemically in normal sera, while another group has failed to separate the C3NeF activity from IgG, suggesting that it is an immune complex (Thompson, 1972).

Hypercatabolism and Hyposynthesis of C3

Turnover studies using radioactive C3 in these diseases have shown that hypocomplementaemia is accompanied by hypercatabolism of C3 (Charlesworth *et al.*, 1974; Ruddy *et al.*, 1975). This is not the only factor contributing to the hypocomplementaemia, since C3 hypercatabolism may be accompanied by hyposynthesis of C3. The reason for this unusual relationship is unknown; it may be postulated that it is a protective mechanism, the reduced synthesis of C3 making less C3 available for the production of tissue damage.

Glomerular Deposition of Complement

Immunofluorescent studies have shown complement components in diseased glomeruli in many types of glomerulonephritis.

Complement abnormalities have also been found in other human nephritides, e.g. haemolytic–uraemic syndrome, shunt nephritis, and the nephritis accompanying subacute bacterial endocarditis, although they have received less detailed studies. These changes in complement, and our knowledge of the biological activities consequent on complement activation, make it reasonable to assume that complement contributes to the glomerular damage in human nephritis.

Fibrin

There is little doubt that fibrin deposition causes glomerular damage in experimental nephritis (Josso *et al.*, 1972). Defibrination has been shown to reduce both crescent formation and functional impairment in both anti-GBM (Naish *et al.*, 1972) and immune complex models (Thomson *et al.*, 1975). Nonetheless, in both models disease is still present, as manifest by the accumulation of polymorphs and the existence of proteinuria. Fibrin deposition cannot be regarded as essential to glomerular damage.

In human nephritis the finding of fibrin in glomeruli, with evidence that fibrin metabolism is altered—increased serum levels, catabolism and urinary excretion of fibrin and its breakdown products—indicate that there is intraglomerular fibrin deposition and fibrinolysis. On the other hand, fibrin excretion has been recorded in the absence of glomerular deposition which has led others to suggest that the excess urinary fibrin is simply a manifestation of the proteinuria accompanying glomerular damage. The experimental work discussed above, however, indicates that in some, but not necessarily all patients, fibrin is directly involved in causing glomerular damage.

How fibrin is involved is not clear, particularly in man. In animals such as the rabbit, with platelets showing immune adherence, local release of platelet factors produce coagulation. In man, whose platelets do not show immune adherence, coagulation may be initiated by polymorphs, complement activation, or activated Hageman factor. The situation is further confused by the failure to demonstrate factor VIII in the glomeruli of many cases of human nephritis, which raises the question whether fibrinogen is deposited in the glomerulus by the normal pathway of coagulation.

Polymorphonuclear Leucocytes

In both the heterologous and autologous phases of experimental anti-GBM nephritis, depletion of polymorphs lessens the severity of the nephritis, diminishes proteinuria and, in the autologous phase, decreases fibrin deposition and crescent formation (Henson, 1972; Naish *et al.*, 1975). Polymorph activity thus seems to precede fibrin formation. In human disease circumstantial evidence for the role of polymorphs is providing by their accumulation in glomeruli, and by recent work demonstrating lysosomal protease, presumed to originate from polymorphs, in the urine of patients with glomerulonephritis (Sanders *et al.*, 1976).

Platelets

In experimental models acute soluble complex injury is platelet-dependent and in many forms of human glomerulonephritis platelet turnover is markedly accelerated and platelet localization within the kidneys is increased (George *et al.*, 1975). Although platelets are inflammatory cells capable of participating in immunological events as well as in coagulation, it appears most likely that they play a role in secondary injury of glomeruli where endothelial damage has already occurred.

Other Mechanisms of Glomerular Damage

Experimental work has shown that glomerular damage independent of complement, fibrin and polymorphs occurs in disease produced by avian nephrotoxic antibody and the γ-2 fraction (non-complement fixing) of sheep nephrotoxic antibody. Further, anti-GBM nephritis in the guinea-pig is independent of polymorphs and complement not only when intact antibody fixes to the GBM but also when $F(ab)_2$ fragments of the antibody are used, excluding events requiring Fc piece (Simpson *et al.*, 1975). This mode of damage may be due to fixation of the antibody itself, or to involvement of mediators either unknown, or not yet incriminated (e.g. the kinin system).

Cell-mediated injury has been inferred in rats immunized with homologous kidney, their lymphocytes demonstrating blast transformation and MIF production on exposure to antigen. In humans, cell-mediated mechanisms do not seem to be very prominent although the production of migration inhibition factor (MIF) has been detected in some cases of proliferative glomerulonephritis and anti-GBM disease.

SOLUBLE COMPLEXES IN HUMAN NEPHRITIS

It is usual to suppose that the majority of patients suffering from glomerulonephritis have some form of immunological disorder leading to the formation, circulation and glomerular localization of phlogistic immune complexes. While there is a good deal of evidence to support this suggestion, it is well to remember that in the great majority of patients the evidence for direct involvement of immune complex deposition is lacking. It is possible that some forms of nephritis result from non-immunological events with or without later recruitment of immune mechanisms, but if this is the case we are ignorant of their nature.

The many possible events in the genesis of immune complex nephritis must also be considered. Table 1 lists some of the circumstances which may influence the formation, circulation and deposition of complexes; there are certainly others. There is a tendency to think in over-simple terms about the antigens involved. It is possible that more than one antigen–antibody system may participate in the formation of soluble complexes, each with a different potential for damaging the glomerulus. This may particularly be the case when the agent causing the nephritis is an infectious organism. In the spontaneous nephritis of the NZB/NZW mouse which so closely resembles human SLE (Chapter 11) there is good evidence that complexes formed against viral antigens are present in the kidney, as well as DNA/anti-DNA complexes. Multiple antigens are, of course, present in most of the infectious agents incriminated in human nephritis (see Table 2). The antigens hitherto identified in these organisms are usually those important in serotyping, and are probably not those involved in the genesis of nephritis.

The work of Germuth *et al.* (1973), Dixon (1968) and others working with experimental animals has shown that almost all the patterns of histological

TABLE 1

Known variables in the formation, deposition and damaging effect of antigen–antibody complexes

Antigen	type and number of antigen(s) quantity rate and timing of exposure persistence in circulation
Antibody	class subclass ? ratio of classes affinity/avidity
Complement	quantity biological activity

Glomerular localization of complexes	size of complex
	circulatory hydrodynamic events
	  local
	  systemic
	events affecting capillary permeability
	  ? cytotropic antibody

Removal of complexes from glomeruli	reticulo–endothelial system activity
	  systemic
	  local (mesangial)

Phlogistic activity of complexes	complement activation platelet activation coagulation

Inhibition of phlogistic damage	fibrinolysis
	  plasmin(ogen activator)
	  fibrinolysis inhibitors
	complement inhibitors
	removal of complement and IgG by proteolysis

damage seen in human proliferative glomerulonephritis may be reproduced in a single species with a single antigen, by varying the immunization schedule or the previous treatment of the animal. Presumably some or all of the events listed in Table 1 are involved. The number of histological reactions identifiable in the glomerulus is limited and it is likely that the grouping of patients with similar histological patterns has been overemphasized. There is also evidence that in man several of the antigens listed in Table 2 are capable of producing almost all the varieties of glomerular damage seen; for example, HB_s (Australia antigen), DNA and tumour antigens.

TABLE 2

Some antigens believed to be responsible for human glomerulonephritis

			Evidence[a]			Type of nephritis and comments
			Antigen	Antibody	Clinical + IgG or C3	
EXOGENOUS	Bacteria:	Streptococci	Yes	Yes	Yes	Acute, sometimes chronic
		Staphylococci	Yes	—	Yes	In association with SBE or infected shunts
		Pneumococci	Yes	—	Yes	Acute, single case studied
		Enterococci	—	—	Yes	In SBE
		S. typhi	—	—	Yes	Acute with nephritis
		M. leprae	—	—	Yes	May be common
	Viruses:	Measles	—	—	Yes	In sub-acute sclerosing panencephalitis
		Hepatitis B	Yes	—	Yes	Acute, chronic and arteritis Antigen identification in tissue doubtful
		Oncornavirus	Yes	—	Yes	In acute leukaemias
		Echo 9	—	—	Yes	Acute; also in animals
		EB	Yes	—	Yes	Single case
		Ascending polyneuritis agent	—	—	Yes	Circumstantial evidence only
	Rickettsiae:	Coxiella, etc.	—	—	Yes	Especially in SBE
	Parasites:	*P. malariae*	Yes	Yes	Yes	Chronic
		P. falciparum	—	—	Yes	Acute nephritis only
		S. haematobium	Yes	—	Yes	Epidemiological evidence only
		S. Mansoni	—		Yes	Epidemiological evidence only
		Toxoplasma	—	—	Yes	Single case
		Filariae	—	—	Yes	

	Treponemes *T. palliaum*	—	Yes	Yes	Secondary and congenital syphilis
	Drugs[b] Tridione	—	—	Yes	Membranous nephropathy. Mode of injury not established. ? complexes. ? tissue damage plus release of immunizing endogenous antigen
	Penicillamine	—	—	Yes	
	Gold	—	—	Yes	
	Mercury	—	—	Yes	
	? Heroin	—	—	Yes	May be due to contaminants, or infection
ENDOGENOUS	DNA	Yes	Yes	Yes	In SLE
	Tumour antigen(s)	Yes	Yes	Yes	A few well-studied patients
	Carcinoembryonic antigen	Yes	—	Yes	Single case
	Renal tubular brush border antigen	Yes	—	Yes	? only in Japan
	Thyroglobulin	Yes	—	Yes	A single case
	Ig	Yes	—	Yes	Mixed cryoglobulinaemias

[a] *Antigen*, antigen demonstrated in glomerular deposits. *Antibody*, specific antibody eluted from kidneys postmortem, or from biopsy. *Clinical + IgG or C3*, clinical evidence of association (e.g. healing of nephritis on removal of putative agent) plus granular or irregular deposits of IgG or C3 in the glomeruli.

[b] Also many others not listed which may lead to acute arteritis with accompanying glomerulonephritis.

Localization of complexes in the kidney has been extensively studied, and some factors important in the site of localization within the glomerulus have already been discussed. There are good morphological reasons why the kidney is involved so readily in soluble complex diseases, whereas to induce an arteritis or lesions in other organs may require the presence of prior inflammation. The kidney receives one-fifth of the cardiac output at high pressure straight from the aorta, and transmits this blood flow through short channels directly into the glomeruli at relatively high capillary pressure. The glomerular capillaries have a unique structure which allows them to act as filters. The principal modification is that the endothelium, instead of being a thick layer of cytoplasm, with opportunities for filtration only at the tight junctions between cells, is reduced to a thin fenestrated sheet barely detectable in an electron micrograph of a capillary cross-section. Molecules or complexes of molecular weights of up to 10^6 can pass this barrier and penetrate the basement membrane very readily. The main filtration barrier in glomerular capillaries lies at the extracapillary junction of the podocyte (found only in the kidney) and the membrane, and material at this site is relatively inaccessible to polymorphs. In soluble complex disease the kidney is thus involved as an "innocent bystander" in immunological events which are not related specifically to that organ. It is now known that in a variety of acute infections many individuals deposit soluble complexes in the kidney, leading to the transient proteinuria formerly called "febrile" proteinuria. It may even be a physiological role of the kidney to receive soluble complexes and remove them from the circulation, the abnormal event being the genesis of chronic irreversible disease as a result of this deposition.

The final event to be considered is the removal of complexes from the kidney. It could be argued from the previous paragraph that here is the most likely site of deficiency leading to chronic disease. We know almost nothing of the removal of deposited complexes from any site within the glomerulus. In particular, the mechanism by which extracapillary deposits are removed (for example in healing after acute post-streptococcal glomerulonephritis) is quite unknown. Although the mesangium is usually assumed to have a phagocytic function, deposits are rarely seen within the mesangial cell cytoplasm, but are detected between the cells. The evidence for phagocytosis is, in fact, poor, although the mesangium as a whole undoubtedly acts as a receptacle for foreign matter deposited in the glomeruli. How it removes this material from the glomeruli is unknown, but the macula densa has recently been suggested as a route of removal into the distal tubules and hence into the urine.

Antigens Believed to be Involved in Human Glomerulonephritis

Table 2 lists the antigens currently believed to be involved in human glomerulonephritis. At first sight the list appears impressive; but when one remembers that in many instances the evidence is extremely slender, and that even with well-established agents the number of cases studied is usually in single figures, some sense of perspective is restored. When it is realized further that in more than 95% of patients with presumed soluble complex nephritis no connection can be established with *any* of the agents listed, the size of the problem becomes apparent. We are usually investigating patients months or years after the onset of their disease, and it may be that by this time secondary events are of greater importance in determining the outcome, and may obscure the initiating events.

The complete proof that a putative antigen is involved in a soluble complex glomerulonephritis requires first that antibody be demonstrable in the glomeruli. Second, that elution of tissue or biopsy cryostat section with acid buffer (to dissociate the antibody–antigen complex) results in an eluate containing antibody which will refix onto the antigen *in vitro*. The antigen must also be demonstrable in the biopsy, preferably in the same distribution as the antibody, with or without prior elution of antibody. Finally, soluble complexes should be demonstrable in the circulation, and it should be possible to show that these contain the antigen found in the kidney. These are ideals rarely even approached in the clinical study of nephritis.

It is worth noting here the difficulty of detecting antigen in the glomeruli, even in an experimental situation where it is known to be present. This may result in part from the small quantities involved, or from the fact that the antigen is covered with IgG and associated complement. However, even when these reactants are eluted with acid buffer, potassium iodide or potassium thiocyanate, it may still be impossible to demonstrate antigen known to be present, even with powerful monospecific antisera. In the clinical situation the antibodies are often not monospecific, and crude eluates of kidney tissue often contain a variety of proteins. The failure to demonstrate an antigen is frustrating, but obviously does not imply absence of antigen nor denies it a role in the production of the nephritis.

In Table 2 the antigens detected in the glomeruli or for which specific antibody has been eluted from the glomeruli, are indicated. Only in the case of post-streptococcal nephritis, SLE, malaria, and one or two patients with tumours have both antigen and antibody been successfully demonstrated. For the great majority of agents listed, the evidence is circumstantial or coincidental only.

A glance at Table 2 shows that many of the factors listed are common infectious agents, and that many organisms are represented. By analogy with the spontaneous nephritides found in other animal species so far studied, it is likely that the many patients whose nephritis is not yet associated with any of the listed antigens have an unusual response to common pathogenic and commensal viruses. Several of the known agents in human nephritis are worth discussing in more detail.

The Nephritis of SLE

This has already been mentioned in Chapter 11. Here, evidence is very strong that complexes formed with native double-stranded DNA (ds-DNA) and deposited in the kidney are the cause of the renal manifestations. Even those patients with entirely normal urine and renal function commonly show evidence of immune complex deposition in their kidneys if renal biopsy is performed. Anti-DNA antibody may be of IgG, IgM or IgA class, although IgG predominates. There is some correlation between the amount of circulating anti ds-DNA and the progression of the disease, but the initial severity shows no correlation and even the relationship with activity is present only in some patients. The role of viruses in relation to immune complex disease is discussed in Chapter 10.

Nephritis in Association with Sub-acute Bacterial Endocarditis (SBE)

This has been recognized for many years (Gutman *et al.*, 1972) but the immunological nature of the lesions has only recently been emphasized (Boulton-Jones *et al.*, 1974). Nephritis is much more common in patients with a prolonged course and frequently with negative blood cultures. There is a particular association with staphylococcal and other less common organisms such as rickettsiae, rather than the commoner *Str. viridans* or *Str. faecalis*. The serum complement concentrations are sometimes low and resolution of the renal lesions may follow treatment of the valvular infection. The finding of focal and segmental glomerulonephritis is common, and it is possible that this results from the formation and deposition in the kidneys of insoluble complexes in antibody excess, the antigen being released from the infected valves into plasma containing a high titre of antibody. Removal of the infection usually arrests the progress of the disease.

The relationship between the nephritis of SBE and those cases of nephritis associated with infected jugulo-atrial shunts inserted for hydrocephalus is obvious. The organism (*Staph. albus*) is often that found in SBE and in one patient with a shunt and nephritis staphylococcal antigen was identified in the glomeruli after antibody elution. The serum complement is usually very low for long periods, and interestingly the histological pattern in the glomeruli is usually one of mesangiocapillary glomerulonephritis with subendothelial deposits (often associated in the idiopathic form with persistently low complement concentrations). Dramatic improvements from renal failure have been recorded when the infected shunt is removed.

Nephritis Associated with P. malariae

This has attracted much attention, partly because it may be a common cause of nephritis in the tropics. Other plasmodia (e.g. *P. falciparum*) may be associated with a transient nephritis and even a nephrotic syndrome, but only *P. malariae* seems to give rise to a progressive nephritis. Malarial antigen and malarial antibody have both been demonstrated in the glomeruli of affected patients, and there is good evidence of circulating complexes in many patients.

Post-streptococcal Nephritis

Although it has been studied for nearly 200 years, this is still a source of controversy. Streptococcal antigen has been demonstrated in the glomeruli of only a few patients, and antibody from convalescent patients will refix to glomeruli in the biopsies of the same patients. Although evidence has been produced for a single nephritogenic antigen common to all nephritogenic strains, there is undoubtedly some cross-reactivity between human basement membrane antigens and some streptococcal antigens. The role of post-streptococcal nephritis in the production of chronic disease is also controversial. In the United States the view is widely held that it is a common antecedent of chronic nephritis. Apart from the present rarity of streptococcal nephritis in the United Kingdom, most workers in Britain believe that while well-documented, this is an unusual event characterized by different histological appearances early in the course of the disease and probably resulting from an unusual host response to the infection.

Chronic Australia Antigenaemia

This is now firmly associated with various forms of proliferative nephritis, polyarteritis with nephritis, and membranous nephropathy. The demonstration of the antigen in tissue is still somewhat dubious, for technical reasons, but the clinical association is strong; especially since the antigen subtypes are unequally and consistently represented in patients with nephritis.

Syphilis

Nephritis and a nephrotic syndrome have been described in association with both congenital and secondary syphilis, and recently specific antibody has been eluted from the biopsy from such a patient. The condition responds well to elimination of the antigen(s) by treatment of the syphilis.

Malignant Disease

Patients with tumours, usually either carcinomata or Hodgkin's disease, may develop a nephrotic syndrome. The renal lesion may parallel remissions and relapses in what appears to be the primary condition, and in a few patients tumour-specific antibody and tumour antigens have been identified in the glomeruli; in one patient carcinoembryonic antigen was found in the glomerular deposits by indirect immunofluorescence.

Drug-associated Nephritis

Some cases occur as part of a generalized vasculitis in response to the drug. Others, particularly in association with tridione, penicillamine and gold, present with persistent proteinuria, nephrotic syndrome and membranous nephropathy in the renal biopsy. It is not clear whether the drug acts as a hapten itself, or whether it causes tissue damage with autoimmunization to tissue antigens released. The persistence after withdrawal in a few patients might suggest the latter, but gold at least may remain for many years in the proximal tubules in animals. Edgington *et al.* (1968) have shown that the nephritogenic antigens of experimental autologous immune complex nephritis are localized in the renal proximal tubular brush border. There is some evidence that this antigen may be involved in human nephritis.

Combination of Antigen and Antibody in the Kidney

Some forms of nephritis do not fit easily into the soluble complex theory of nephritis. One of these is that in which mesangial deposition of IgA is the sole or most prominent feature. It is possible that the IgA is the antigen, not the antibody deposited in this area; and that the IgG often found in association with it is deposited *in situ* after the IgA has localized. In systemic lupus erythematosus, there is evidence that DNA will fix to basement membranes. In SLE without clinical evidence of glomerulonephritis, a linear pattern of immunoglobulin deposition may be seen along the basement membrane which is lost in later phases with obvious nephritis. This may represent an early phase of the nephritis in which antibody combines, *in situ*, with DNA antigen deposited along the basement membrane.

Anti-Glomerular Basement Membrane Antibody Nephritis (Wilson and Dixon, 1973; Sissons *et al.*, 1974)

Perhaps the best understood animal model of glomerulonephritis is that induced by the injection of antibody specifically directed against glomerular basement membrane antigens as outlined above. The human analogue of this experimental model is thus of some importance, and again has been much studied. However, the striking fact is how rare anti-glomerular basement membrane (anti-GBM) antibody appears to be as a cause of human disease. Peters *et al.* (1974) noted only 11 instances in 400 biopsies, and in a survey of nephritis in south-east England only four cases were seen in over 500 patients.

To prove that anti-GBM antibody is involved in glomerulonephritis antibody eluted from kidney or renal biopsy specimens must refix to the GBM of kidney *in vitro*. This has been demonstrated in only a handful of instances. The presence of circulating anti-GBM antibody is suggestive, but in many patients there is no antibody demonstrable, presumably because it is completely fixed to the GBM of the kidneys. In such circumstances, circulating antibody may become detectable only after the kidneys have been removed. A number of different techniques have been used to show anti-GBM antibody: the simplest is indirect immunofluorescence, where the patient's serum is layered on a cryostat section of normal human kidney and fixation of human IgG to the GBM is shown by fluorescent anti-IgG. Much more sensitive, and quantitative, are radioimmunoassay and haemagglutination methods, but these are not yet generally available. The finding of the characteristic linear, continuous fixation of IgG along the basement membrane by immunofluorescence may be taken as evidence of anti-GBM nephritis. There are a number of pitfalls in this observation, however. First, careful study under oil immersion at high magnification is required to show that sometimes apparently linear deposits are, not in fact, finely granular (Fig. 7b). Second, non-specific linear fixation is seen along the basement membrane in a number of situations where this structure is diffusely abnormal; it has been noted in diabetic nephropathy, in patients with dense intramembranous deposits with mesangiocapillary glomerulonephritis and is regularly seen in sections of normal kidney which have been subjected to washing in saline or buffer. It is also seen occasionally in kidneys presumed to have lesions which are not immunological in origin, for example polycystic disease.

Clinical Characteristics and Definition of Human anti-GBM Disease

The principal character of human anti-GBM disease is an aggressive form of glomerulonephritis, associated with a rapid fall in the glomerular filtration rate with evidence of persisting glomerular disease, or even sudden onset of anuria. Histologically, there is usually extensive extracapillary proliferation (crescents) although milder changes may be seen in the initial stages, principally a focal and segmental glomerulonephritis confined to only a part of some glomeruli. Even at this stage, however, there is diffuse fixation of IgG to the basement membrane in the characteristic linear fashion (Fig. 7a), although other immunoglobulins are absent and complement usually discontinuous or absent. In a proportion of patients (impossible to state accurately at present, but probably no more than 50%, there are also disproportionate anaemia and lesions in the lungs. These consist of interstitial pulmonary haemorrhages showing as a diffuse pulmonary infiltrate on X-ray; this combination is usually given the name of Goodpasture's syndrome (lung purpura and nephritis). To avoid confusion the following terminology should be adopted (Wilson and Dixon, 1973):

i. *anti-GBM nephritis with Goodpasture's syndrome:* preferably, with demonstration of circulating anti-GBM antibody. A nephritis with (at least) linear immunofluorescent IgG in the kidney and lung lesions;
ii. *anti-GBM nephritis:* with *or without* lung lesions, circulating antibody is demonstrated, or linear immunofluorescent IgG seen (presumed anti-GBM nephritis).

The term Goodpasture's syndrome should not be applied to patients with anti-GBM nephritis without the characteristic lung lesions; nor should every patient with lung lesions and nephritis be assumed to have anti-GBM nephritis. Polyarteritis, and occasionally Henoch-Schönlein purpura, may present with this combination of features; and without proper study it may be impossible to say whether anti-GBM nephritis is present or not.

The Pulmonary Lesions

The origin of the pulmonary lesions and their relation to the renal disease is still obscure. A simple and attractive explanation is that the anti-GBM antibody cross-reacts sufficiently with pulmonary basement membrane to deposit within the lung and cause injury. In favour of this hypothesis is that in a few patients linear IgG may also be demonstrated in the lung, and *in vitro* some anti-GBM antibodies will fix to lung tissue. Further, in some patients removal of the kidneys may result in a dramatic and immediate improvement in the lung lesions. However, this has been reported in only about half the small number of patients submitted to nephrectomy for lung involvement. In view of the rise in anti-GBM antibody titres following nephrectomy it might be expected to worsen the pulmonary lesions. IgG is, however, only rarely noted fixed to the basement membranes in the lung. It may be that in some patients the lung is the primary site of the immune events, and the anti-GBM nephritis a secondary event. It has been suggested that there is an association between anti-GBM nephritis and inhalation of organic solvents, particularly petroleum products. The condition of Goodpasture's syndrome is commonest in young people who are perhaps more likely to be in contact with fuels than other members of the community.

Pulmonary lesions may precede the apparent onset of nephritis in some patients, or appear later in a patient in whom anti-GBM nephritis has already been noted. Either of these two manifestations may dominate the clinical picture, but it is important to re-emphasize that half the patients with demonstrated anti-GBM nephritis do not have lung lesions at all. Either the lung or the kidney lesion may result in death; the former from massive pulmonary haemorrhage and hypoxaemia, the latter from rapidly worsening uraemia. Before dialysis was available the great majority of patients with anti-GBM nephritis died of uraemia within a few months but occasional well-documented instances of spontaneous resolutions are recorded. After dialysis has been started the pulmonary lesions may be a problem and in some cases, as noted above, nephrectomy has been dramatically successful. Others die of pulmonary disease despite nephrectomy whilst maintained on dialysis.

The data on renal transplants in these patients is of exceptional interest, but no clear picture has emerged. With or without nephrectomy, anti-GBM antibody often disappears from the circulation within a few months. This disappearance may be accelerated by immunosuppressive treatment, although there is no proof of this. Even in the absence of detectable antibody before transplantation, however, the graft has sometimes been destroyed immediately by a similar extracapillary glomerulonephritis with linear fixation of IgG on the GBM. On the other hand, even in the presence of demonstrable antibody successful grafting has been carried out without, apparently, recrudescence of the nephritis in the kidney. In one interesting patient, transplantation before nephrectomy led to immediate recurrent disease and loss of the graft. After nephrectomy, a second graft was performed without trouble.

Anti-TBM Nephritis

Both experimental and human glomerulonephritis are not infrequently accompanied by disease of the tubules and tubular dysfunction. Deposition of Ig and C3 in the tubule is, however, rare. Although these findings are clear, lesions of the tubules received little attention from immunologists until recently (Andres and McCluskey, 1975), more attention having been given to obvious glomerular disease.

Experimentally, anti-tubular basement membrane (anti-TBM) nephritis may be induced by immunization of an animal with heterologous TBM. Characteristically, there follows linear deposition of Ig and C3 on the recipient's TBM with interstitial inflammation. Passive transfer of the disease may be achieved with the recipient's serum, and anti-TBM antibody may be eluted from the diseased kidney. In certain instances a cross-reaction of the anti-TBM antibody with GBM occurs, and indeed in anti-GBM nephritis in rabbits a proportion of cases produced by immunization with GBM develop tubular disease. The sharing of antigens by both tubular and glomerular basement membrane is thus demonstrated. Experimental anti-TBM nephritis has also been produced in allograft kidneys, and in a rat model in which immunization of one species (Norway Brown) with the kidney of another (Sprague–Dawley) produced anti-TBM antibodies, and also immune complex glomerular disease.

A different form of tubular lesion has been produced in rats and rabbits by injection of homologous kidney. Granular deposits of Ig and C3 are detectable on the TBM, but anti-TBM antibodies are not found. It is suggested that this condition is due to the demonstrable antibodies directed against cytoplasmic constituents of the tubular cells. More recently, the TBM has been shown to be the site of lesions with granular deposition of Ig and C3 in rabbits with chronic immune complex disease induced by a schedule of frequent high dose BSA injections.

In the human, anti-TBM disease with circulating anti-TBM antibodies has been found in anti-GBM disease, in association with immune complex glomerular disease, and also alone with evidence of tubular dysfunction without glomerular disease. Anti-TBM antibodies have also been demonstrated in patients bearing renal allografts; in the cases investigated, the antibodies were auto-antibodies. The only exception was one case in which the TBM of the allograft was involved but the patient's own TBM was spared. Linear deposition of Ig and C3 has been found in methicillin-associated interstitial nephritis; in this condition it is suggested that the hapten dimethoxyphenyl penicillyl is fixed in the TBM (and interstitium) with resultant antibody formation.

TBM involvement in human immune complex disease has been noted in SLE, occasionally in other forms of glomerulonephritis, and in allografts (Lehman *et al.*, 1975). There are granular deposits of IgG and C3, and in SLE DNA has been demonstrated by immunofluorescence in the deposits (Fig. 7i).

The deposition of C3 indicates the participation of complement in mediating damage in TBM disease; experimentally this has been confirmed by the failure of passive transfer of anti-TBM antibody-mediated disease to decomplemented animals. A role for polymorphs has also been demonstrated experimentally. In human disease, the question whether the anti-TBM antibodies are primary or arise secondarily to tubular damage remains unresolved.

Interstitial Nephritis

Interstitial nephritis is a common accompaniment of both glomerular immune complex and anti-GBM disease. The infiltrating cells are primarily lymphocytes and plasma cells, and it is commonly supposed that these cells indicate cell mediated forms of immunological damage. One of the most frequently identified associated factors in human interstitial disease is drug ingestion, e.g. methicillin, sulphonamides and rifampicin, presumably acting as haptens. Immunoglobulin and sometimes complement may be seen in the interstitium in such cases.

IMMUNE DEFICIENCY AS A CAUSE OF GLOMERULONEPHRITIS

The view that nephritis may result from a relative deficiency of some part of the immune response arises from observations of both experimental disease in animals, and of patients with glomerulonephritis.

In various species and strains of laboratory animals, chronic infection may be associated with immune complex disease. This appearance of immune complexes in situations where antigens are not eliminated promptly leads to the idea that the inability to eliminate the infection might be the primary event in the genesis of immune complex disease. One example of this is lymphocytic choriomeningitis in mice. This is caused by a chronic virus infection, which in some animals leads to an immune complex nephritis. Strains of mice differ greatly in their susceptibility to develop nephritis, and this has been related to their ability to produce high affinity antibody: nephritis-prone animals produce only antibody of low affinity, and also have poor macrophage function. In NZB/NZW mice (see Chapter 11) T-cell function is markedly deficient and despite the production of antibody against a variety of viruses the organisms persist and cause chronic infections. The viruses include the Gross leukaemia virus, and the Scripps leukaemia virus. Antibodies to the latter cross-react with the host's DNA and RNA.

A possible human counterpart of these situations of failure to eliminate antigen and nephritis may be seen in the association of both SLE and glomerulonephritis with deficiencies of various complement components, and of recurrent infections with C3 deficiency (reviewed by Peters and Williams, 1974). An intact complement system is required for rapid and effective immune elimination. The lack of complement does not, however, inhibit the antibody response so that when the host encounters an appropriate antigen, both antibody and antigen persist together in the circulation, and damaging immune complexes may arise.

Partial Lipodystrophy (PLD)

Recent observations on the association between hypocomplementaemia, mesangiocapillary glomerulonephritis, and the condition of partial lipodystrophy (PLD) (Peters *et al.*, 1973; Sissons *et al.*, 1975) have provided another instance of lack of complement associated with glomerulonephritis, in which the evidence suggests that hypocomplementaemia precedes the onset of nephritis. The basis for this suggestion is that PLD itself may be associated with circulating C3NeF (see Chapter 7 and p. 585) and a low serum C3 in the absence of nephritis. When PLD is associated with nephritis, in every instance so far recorded the PLD preceded the nephritis, usually by many years. Thus it is suggested that C3NeF, and the consequent low C3, is the primary abnormality in this form of hypocomplementaemic nephritis. Such a sequence would explain hitherto puzzling features of this disease, namely the continuation of the complement abnormalities in patients who have had a bilateral nephrectomy, and the lack of correlation between the course and severity of the disease on the one hand and the degree of hypocomplementaemia and the presence of C3NeF on the other. The presence of C1q and C4 in the diseased glomeruli, and the occasional low serum levels of these components of complement in a disease in which complement activation (by C3NeF) proceeds via the alternative pathway could be explained by activation through the classical pathway by immune complexes, although it must be admitted that direct proof of an immune complex aetiology for MCGN is lacking. Another possible mode of pathogenesis of the glomerular lesion in MCGN is that the complement activation by C3NeF alone leads to tissue damage; this is a particularly attractive explanation for the variety of MCGN with intramembranous deposits, where C3 is found in the basement membrane without IgG, and the C1q and C4 concentrations are normal. Attempts to induce glomerular disease experimentally by chronic activation of complement have, however, been unsuccessful.

Other Abnormalities

Other instances of specific immune deficiency preceding and predisposing to glomerulonephritis are as yet not described, although we have seen recently a young man with typical congenital hypogammaglobulinaemia who at the age of eleven developed an acute nephritis, confirmed histologically. The immune response is a complex interplay of several mechanisms, and it is not unreasonable to propose that defects in these, e.g. production of antibody of normal affinity, T-cell function, or macrophage function, will be demonstrated in association with glomerulonephritis.

THE HISTOLOGICAL APPEARANCES OF GLOMERULONEPHRITIS

This is a complex subject and the recent texts and illustrations of Heptinstall (1974) and Burkholder (1974) should be consulted for a full account. However, some general points concerning the morphology of renal disease are worth mentioning. First, it is likely that none of the groups into which glomerulonephritis is classically divided on morphological grounds arises from exposure to a single antigen, or possibly even by a single mechanism. Second, it follows that while a general description of prognosis is possible on the basis of morphology (Cameron, 1973), within each group there will be variation ranging from early renal failure to complete and permanent recovery. The important consideration is the proportion of patients within the histological group that follows each clinical course.

The first broad histological division is into patients with obvious evidence of structural damage and those without, despite the fact that they show proteinuria and sometimes a nephrotic syndrome. This latter group is usually referred to as having the "minimal change" lesion in the United Kingdom, and "lipoid nephrosis" in the United States. There is no direct evidence that this condition is immunologically determined, and much evidence that it is not a soluble complex disease. No deposits are usually visible upon electron microscopy and immunofluorescence is usually negative. However, some indirect evidence suggests that allergic responses may be involved: occasional patients are seen whose nephrotic syndrome is associated with specific antigens, and IgE levels in the group as a whole are greater than normal (Reeves *et al.*, 1975). A number of facts points to a possible disorder of T-cells (Shalhoub, 1974) but at the moment no theory of causation is adequate. The classical finding that this group, alone in nephritis, responds promptly to corticosteroid or cytotoxic agents with disappearance of proteinuria, may also be taken as evidence. It is extremely rare for patients with this condition to develop uraemia, although segmental or global glomerular lesions appear 5–15 years from onset with some frequency.

The remainder of patients with clinical evidence of glomerulonephritis show a variety of glomerular changes. In these, both existing glomerular structures may be modified and added features become evident. These principally relate to the appearance of material believed to represent immune complexes deposited within the glomeruli and the reactions to this deposition: evidence of inflammation, fibrin deposition, and scarring.

Deposition of Immunological Material

Evidence of immune deposits may, of course, be obtained by immunofluorescent techniques (see below) but detailed comparison shows that in virtually all patients with positive fluorescent findings, electron-dense material may be identified in the glomeruli. Such changes can be seen in the light microscope if 1 μm plastic-embedded sections are used with special stains. Again the correlation with immunofluorescence findings is very close.

Material believed to represent deposits may be seen within the mesangium (Fig. 5) or along the capillary walls (Figs 1–4, 6). In this latter site, the deposits may be between the subendothelial cell and the basement membrane (Fig. 1); extracapillary, lying on the outside of the basement membrane underneath the cytoplasm of the podocyte (epithelial cell) (Figs 2 and 3); or within the substance of the basement membrane itself (Fig. 4). It is often forgotten that the sites of deposits may be multiple (Fig. 6), and that if studied carefully, at least two sites and often three are involved, with one predominating to give the condition its "classical" character. In the nephritis of SLE it is usual to see obvious deposits at several sites.

The Cellular Reaction

The cells of the glomerulus may react to the presence of phlogistic material. Either mesangial, endothelial, or extracapillary cells may proliferate, or any two, or all three may be involved. The important divisions here are whether the lesions are confined to the mesangium (in which case the lesion has in general a relatively benign course); involve the capillary wall as well (which usually carries a poorer prognosis) or involve the epithelial cells with extracapillary proliferation (which usually carries a bad prognosis). Polymorphonuclear leucocytes are seen, often in association with deposits (Fig. 3) presumably attracted by complement-induced leucotaxis. Whether all other increase in cells represents division of cells *in situ* is not yet known. This is probably true for endothelial and epithelial cells, but the mesangium may receive circulating cells, possibly macrophages.

Other Added Features

The matrix of the mesangium is most frequently and consistently increased, and may extend round the capillary wall subendothelially (mesangial interposition). Areas of the glomerulus may show sclerosis, either diffusely or segmentally. Acute reactants in the inflammation process, such as fibrin, are rarely seen in conventional microscopy, although they are more frequently identifiable on immunofluorescent studies. Platelets are rarely seen except in

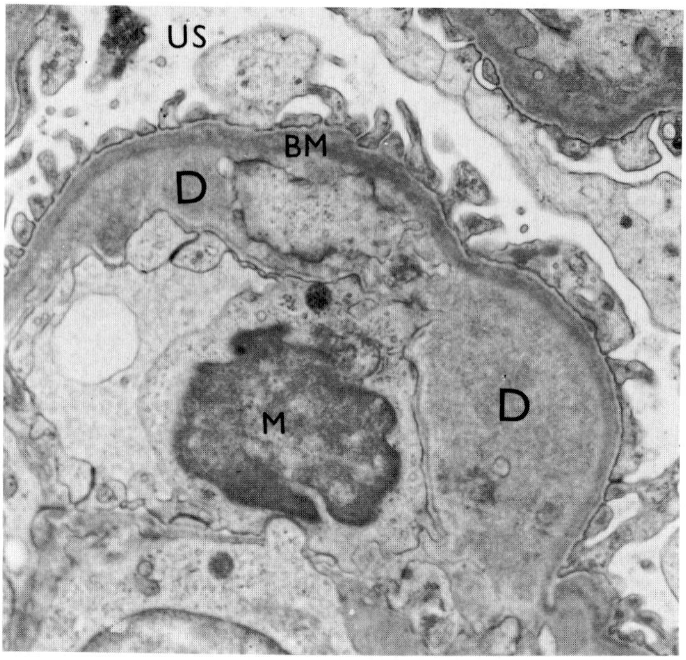

Fig. 1.

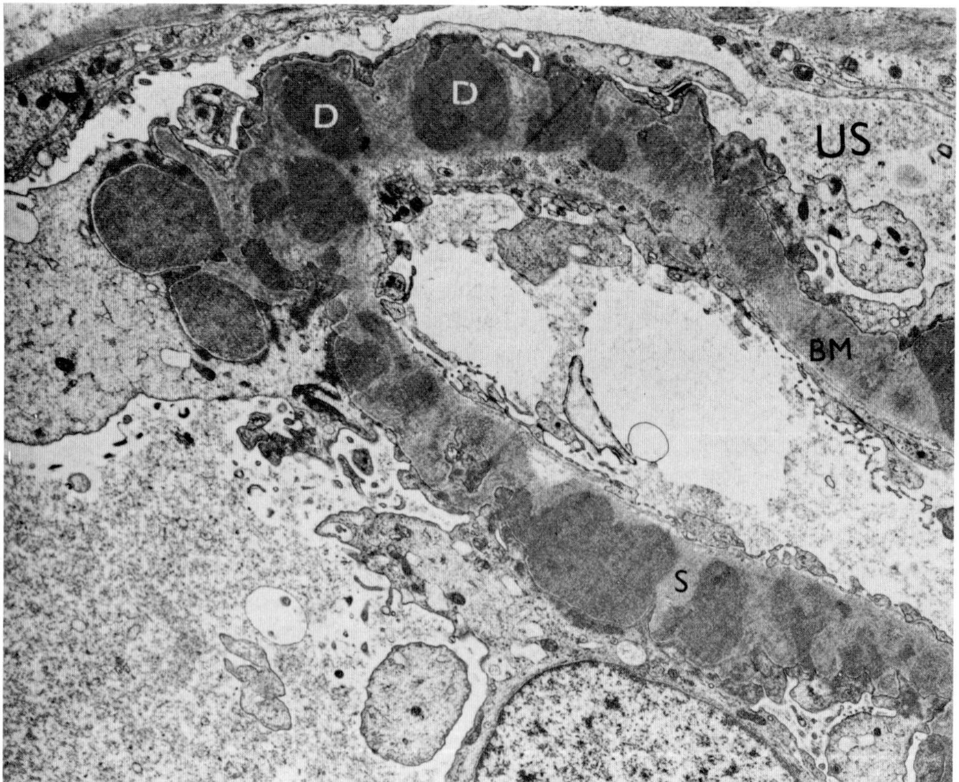

Fig. 2.

acute lesions, although their role in experimental nephritis seems well established. More often, at high power or on electron microscopy the capillary lumen is filled with an amorphous material whose origin is in doubt.

These diverse elements make up the pattern of deposits, proliferation and capillary wall alterations that constitutes the histological appearances of glomerulonephritis. The great majority of these are described under the one heading of "proliferative glomerulonephritis" encompassing all those conditions with obvious increase in glomerular cellularity. It is clear from the description above that this is a very heterogeneous group, and it has been extensively, enthusiastically (and repeatedly) subdivided. The important divisions from a clinical and morphological viewpoint may be summarized thus:

i. *acute exudative glomerulonephritis:* no scarring, cellularity prominent, polymorphs visible, mesangial and extracapillary deposits;
ii. *mesangial proliferative glomerulonephritis:* lesions confined to mesangium; deposits, proliferation, sclerosis;
iii. *mesangiocapillary (membranoproliferative) glomerulonephritis:* mesangial lesions as in (ii) but also mesangial interposition and capillary wall deposits, usually subendothelial but occasionally within the membrane;
iv. *extracapillary glomerulonephritis:* predominant lesions are extensive extracapillary proliferation to form crescents; but the glomerulus may be affected by any of (i)–(ii) in addition, or be relatively normal;

Fig. 1. In this figure, and in Figs 2–6, part of a single glomerulus is illustrated at high magnification to show the various intraglomerular sites of immune deposits. Material believed to be immune deposit is seen in a subendothelial site (D) between the basement membrane (BM) and the endothelial cells lining the capillary. In the centre of the glomerular lobule is the nucleus of a mesangial cell (M) and the urinary space (US) with foot processes of the podocyte (epithelial cell) are seen at the top and on the right. From a patient with mesangiocapillary glomerulonephritis and subendothelial deposits. Electron micrograph of araldite-embedded material, ×3900 (Dr D. R. Turner).

Fig. 2. Immune deposits in an extracapillary (subepithelial, extramembranous) site (D). A portion of a glomerular capillary loop is shown, with the urinary space (US) at the top and on the left. Multiple extracapillary deposits are seen, lying on the outer surface of the basement membrane (BM) which is considerably disorganized. Extensions of basement membrane-like material lie between the deposits, and because of their appearance on silver staining of paraffin-embedded material are called "spikes" (S). From a patient with membranous nephropathy and a nephrotic syndrome. Electron micrograph of araldite-embedded material, ×5,600 (Dr D. R. Turner).

v. *endocapillary glomerulonephritis:* may be occasional crescents but changes principally in mesangium and capillary wall. No exudative changes as in (i) but sclerosis present;

vi. *focal/segmental proliferative glomerulonephritis:* any of (i)–(v) affecting part of, or some glomeruli only.

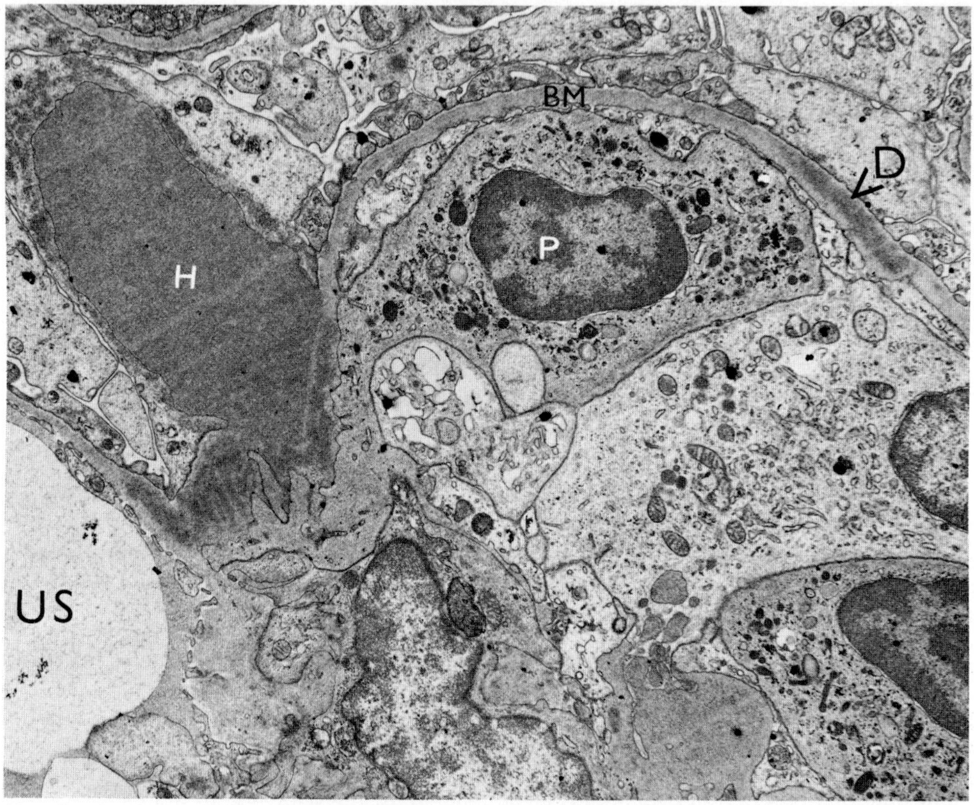

Fig. 3. A large, solitary extramembranous deposit (a "hump", H) lying beneath the cytoplasm of an epithelial cell (or podocyte) and outside the capillary basement membrane (BM). In contrast to the appearance in Fig. 2, the "hump" is longer than its base, is solitary, or at most infrequent, on the capillary wall, and is not flanked by "spikes". Within the capillary lumen, a polymorphonuclear leucocyte (P) may be seen, which has stripped the endothelial cell cytoplasm off the basement membrane and interposed its own cytoplasm against the membrane, allowing digestion of this structure by lysosomal enzymes. This attraction of a polymorph presumably occurs in response to complement-mediated chemotaxis from material in the "hump". A minor linear deposit (D) within the basement membrane itself may also be seen on the right of the figure. The urinary space (US) is at the lower left. From a patient with an acute nephritic illness and acute exudative glomerulonephritis on biopsy. Electron micrograph of araldite-embedded material, ×7,000 (Dr D. R. Turner).

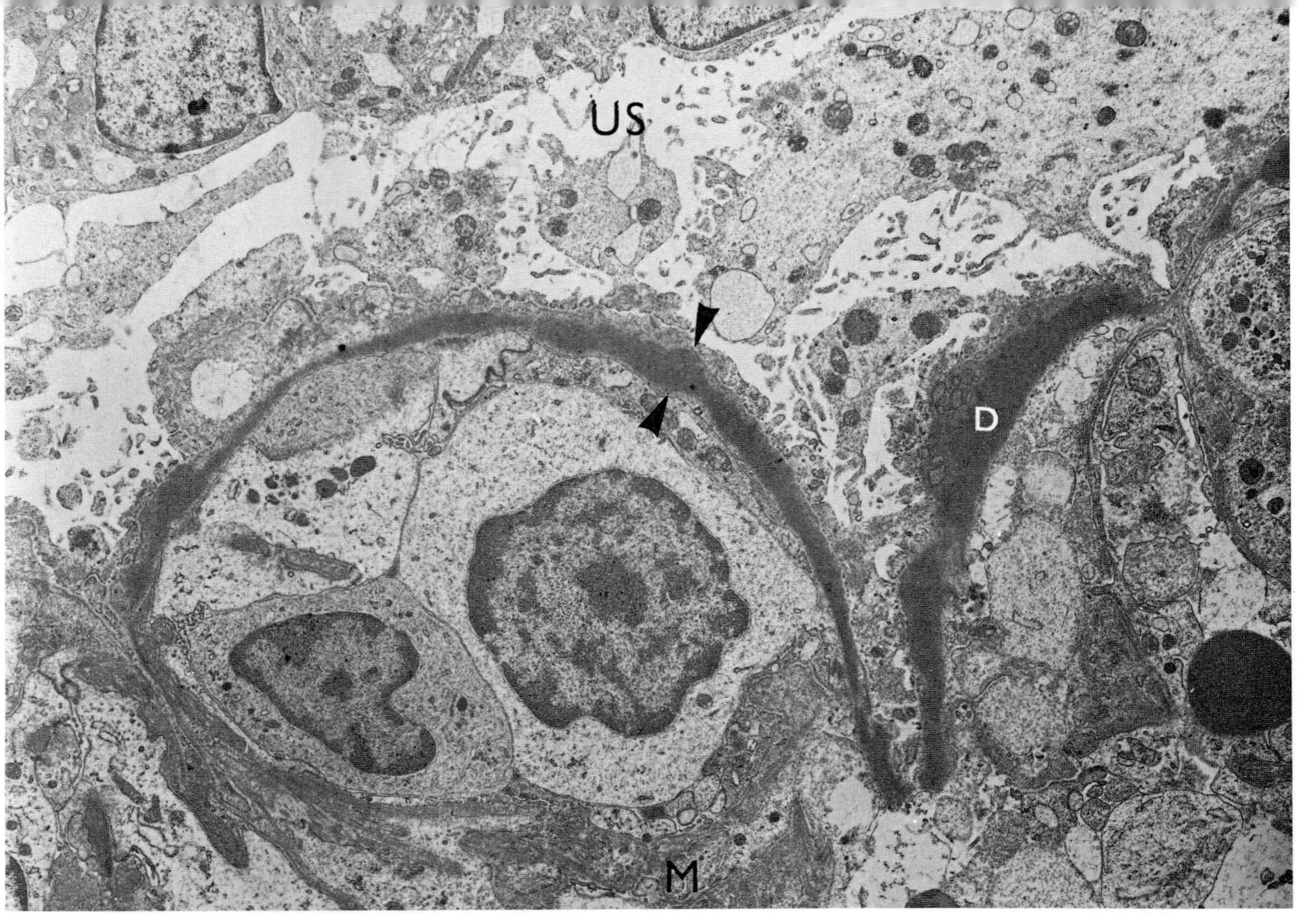

Fig. 4. An extensive, rather continuous, very electron-dense "deposit" (D) within the substance of the basement membrane itself. This is usually called "dense deposit disease" and it is not yet clear whether this represents deposition of immunological material or not. The mesangium (M) below, is expanded, hypocellular and also contains material believed to represent immune deposits. The urinary space (US) is at the top. From a patient with mesangiocapillary glomerulonephritis and a nephrotic syndrome. Electron micrograph of araldite-embedded material, $\times 4{,}700$ (Dr D. R. Turner).

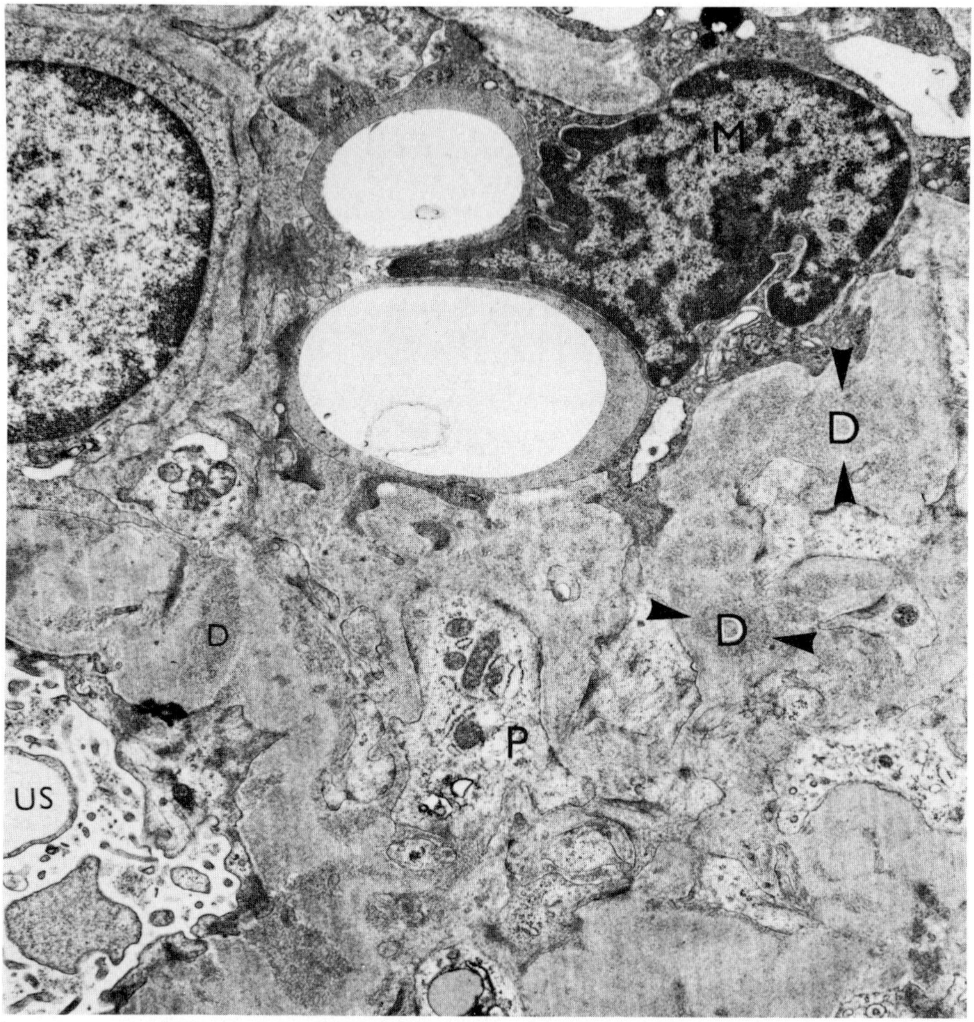

Fig. 5. Deposits within the mesangium (D and arrows). These are less electron-dense than deposits within or around the capillary wall (D, seen at lower left, next to the urinary space, US) and are often more difficult to detect and demonstrate. The mesangium, in addition to containing deposits, shows an excess of mesangial matrix. A mesangial cell nucleus (M) is seen at top right; the other material seen is mesangial cell cytoplasmic processes (P). The two lucent areas are probably artefacts. Electron micrograph of araldite-embedded material, $\times$ 5,600 (Dr D. R. Turner).

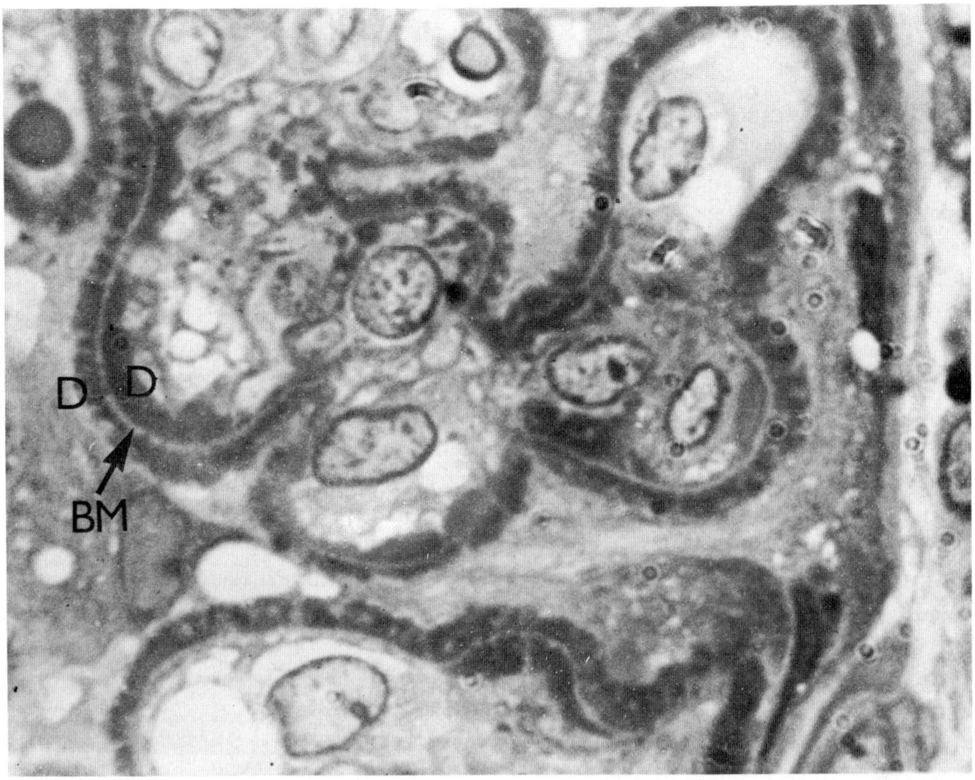

Fig. 6. Deposits at both subendothelial site and an extracapillary site in a glomerulus from a patient with systemic lupus erythematosus. Deposits were also present in the mesangium. Optical microscopy of araldite-embedded material cut at 1 μm, ×1,200 (Dr D. R. Turner). (This picture is taken from material from the same biopsy as depicted in Fig. 7f, which also shows the extensive deposits at multiple sites.)

Two other broad groups are usually referred to. The first, *membranous nephropathy* (or glomerulonephritis) is characterized by diffuse capillary wall thickening arising from exclusively extramembranous (subepithelial) deposits. The mesangium appears relatively normal, although close examination reveals some proliferation and sclerosis, but no deposits. The second, *segmental hyalinosis* or *focal glomerulosclerosis* is at present controversial. Some regard it as a variety of proliferative glomerulonephritis, with more obvious sclerosis than usual and a segmental distribution; others believe that the similar lesions seen in longstanding "minimal change" lesions suggest it is a variant of that condition with a poorer prognosis. Others feel it is a separate entity altogether, of unknown aetiology.

IMMUNOFLUORESCENT STUDIES IN GLOMERULONEPHRITIS

Renal biopsy enables fresh, snap-frozen material to be prepared for sectioning in a cryostat. Autopsy material may be processed similarly but is less satisfactory. Usually, direct immunofluorescent techniques employing monospecific antisera to immunoglobulins, complement components and fibrin(ogen) are used (Morel-Maroger *et al.*, 1972; Burkholder, 1974; Thoenes, 1976). The few antigens that can be identified are usually sought by indirect techniques. Most work has been done with FITC-conjugated antisera (Figs 7–11) although peroxidase-conjugated sera have some advantages, particularly permanence of the preparations (Fig. 12). The degree of ultrastructural localization which can be obtained is much higher (Fig. 13), especially if material embedded in plastic is used. As with optical and electron microscopy, various elements and appearances may be seen with labelled antibody techniques. These, together with other evidence, may be arranged into useful patterns. It must be admitted that we are far from being able to assemble this information in an entirely coherent fashion at present.

The basic patterns of localization are shown in Figs 7a–7h. Figure 7a shows the characteristic linear deposition (of Ig) along the basement membrane in a patient with anti-GBM nephritis and Goodpasture's syndrome. Before a deposit is classed as truly linear it must be examined under oil immersion to see that it is not, in fact, finely granular (Fig. 7b). Other kinds of deposition may be confined to the mesangium (Fig. 7c); may be purely peripheral within the capillary wall (Fig. 7d) or show a combination of peripheral and mesangial deposit round the capillary wall. At higher magnifications the site of deposition within the capillary wall may be determined, as in some patients with SLE nephritis who show both subendothelial and subepithelial deposits (Fig. 7f). Finally, immune reactants may be localized within the glomeruli in a segmental fashion in only part of the glomerulus (Fig. 7g). Deposition of fibrin may be irregular or segmental but one characteristic pattern is within extracapillary crescents (Fig. 7h) which may be the only site of fibrin visible.

The presence of immunoglobulins suggests an immunological origin for the glomerular disease. IgG is most frequently found, but there are histological appearances associated specifically with deposition of IgA and IgM, although this is less common. Subclasses of IgG may be studied if appropriate antisera are available, but as yet no clinical significance has been attached to the findings. IgD has also been studied, but seems to follow IgG deposition and to add little to the diagnosis. IgE is found in the glomeruli in a number of forms of nephritis, but again no particular significance has yet

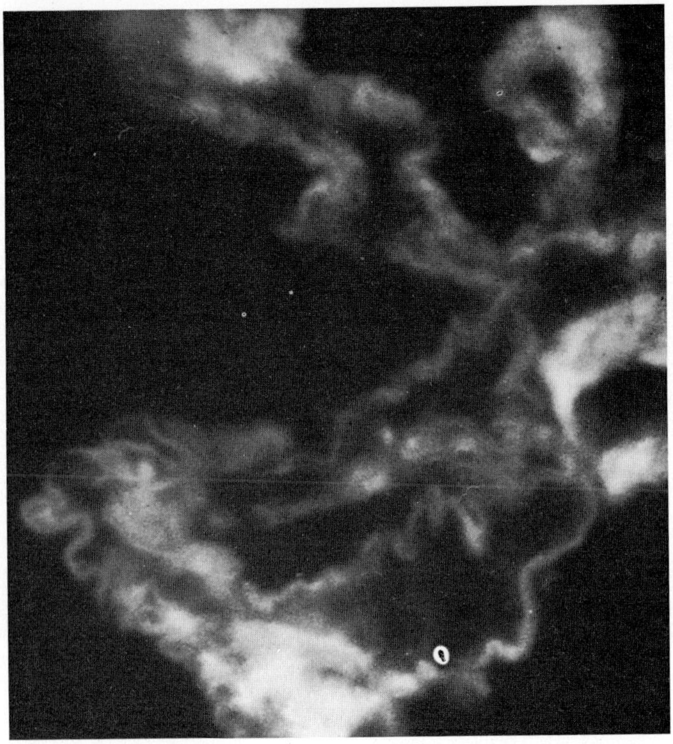

Fig. 7a.

Fig. 7. The basic patterns of glomerular deposition of immune reactants, as revealed by the use of specific fluoresceinated antisera. 7a shows the classical linear pattern of immunoglobulin G deposition seen in anti-GBM nephritis from a patient with Goodpasture's syndrome. This cannot be resolved into granules even when oil-immersion is used at high magnification, but 7b demonstrates that careful study may be necessary before the description of "linear" can be applied. This patient had obvious membranous nephropathy on electron microscopy, but the finely granular deposits of IgG within the glomerular basement membrane appear linear at this magnification, except at a few points on the capillary wall (arrows). In some patients, deposits are confined to the mesangium, as in 7c and presumably represent complexes which localize only at this site. In contrast, 7d shows a pattern of nearly pure peripheral deposition of immune reactants, again presumably representing complexes localizing exclusively at this site. In many patients, deposits may be seen throughout the glomerulus, at both a mesangial and a peripheral site, as in 7e. In patients with a peripheral pattern of deposits, examination under oil immersion may reveal that there are both subendothelial and subepithelial deposits, as in 7f; this is frequent in systemic lupus erythematosus. As well as deposition of immune reactants in a diffuse fashion within the glomerulus, in some lesions (principally but not exclusively affecting only part of the glomerulus on optical microscopy) a segmental distribution of immunoglobulin or complement may be seen (7g). Immune reactants are rarely seen in an extraglomerular site, with the exception of fibrin (7h) which is frequently seen in the epithelial cell proliferation forming "crescents" (C) round the glomerular tuft. Finally, both immunoglobulins and complement components may be found in the tubular basement membrane in some patients (7i), especially in lupus and mesangiocapillary glomerulonephritis. (Figures 7a–7h by courtesy of Dr S. Leibowitz; Figs 7b and 7i, Dr D. J. Evans.)

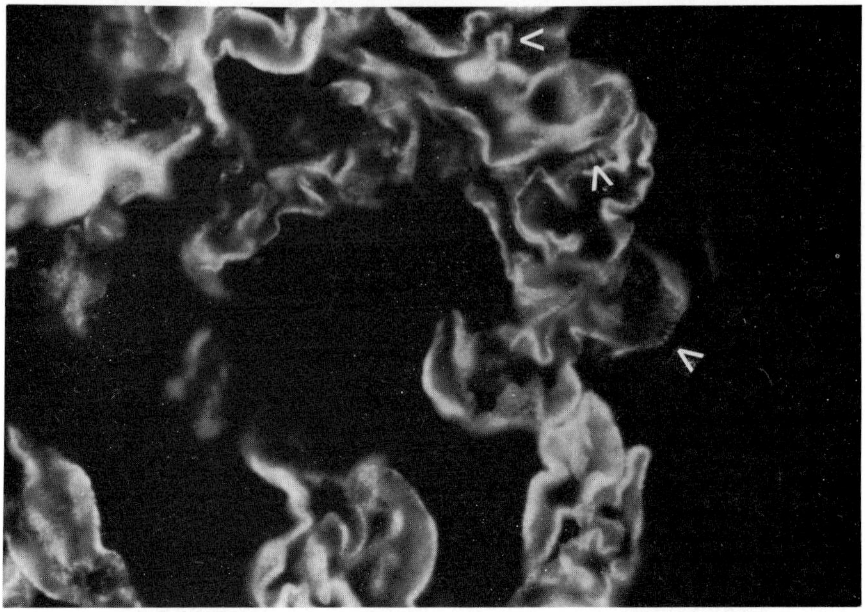

Fig. 7b.

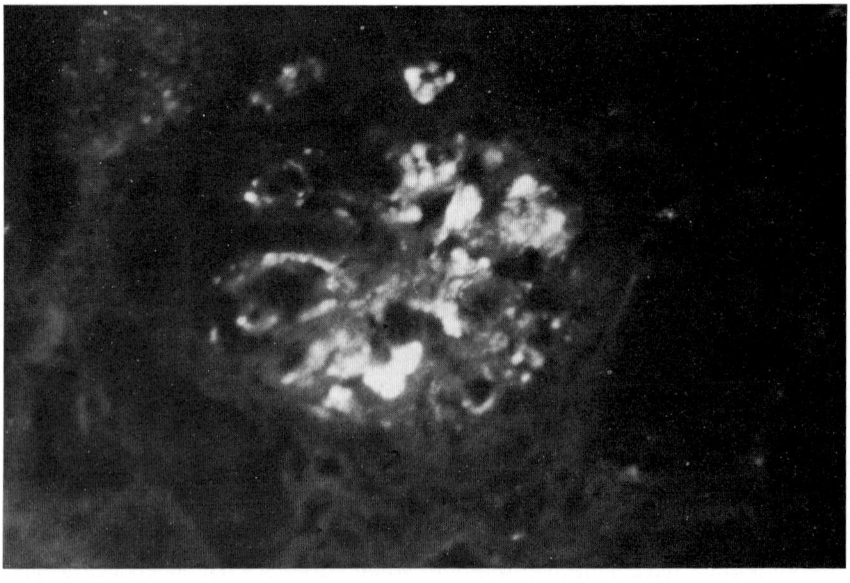

Fig. 7c.

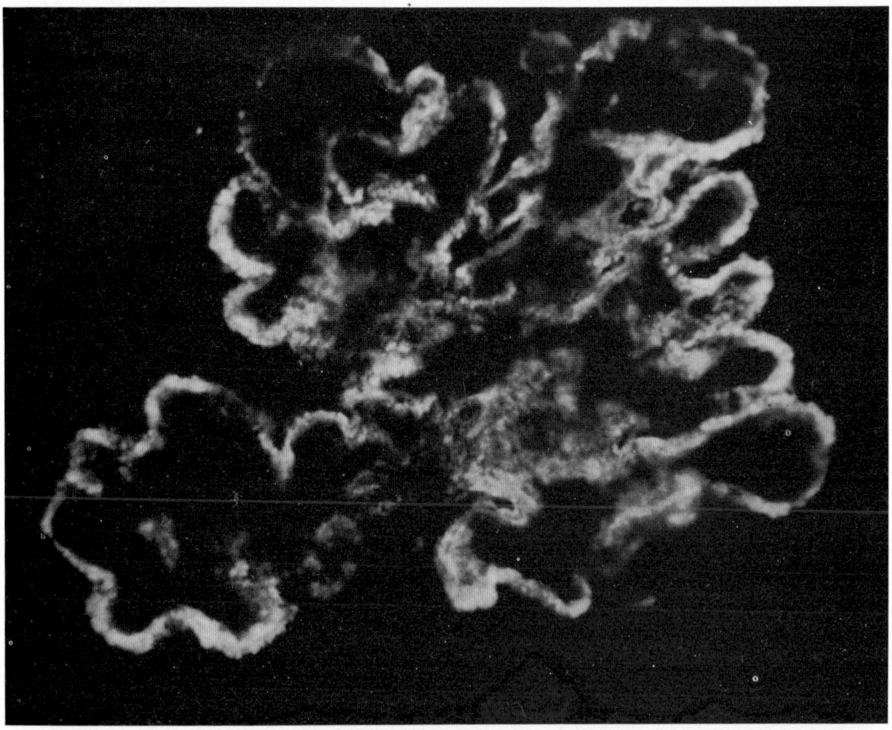

Fig. 7d.

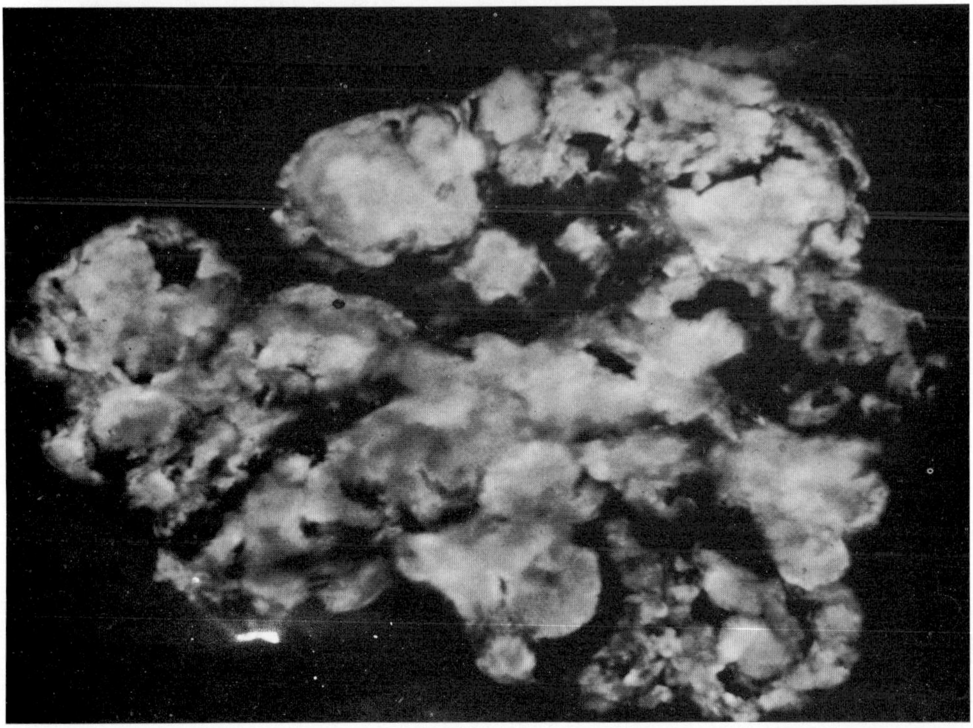

Fig. 7e.

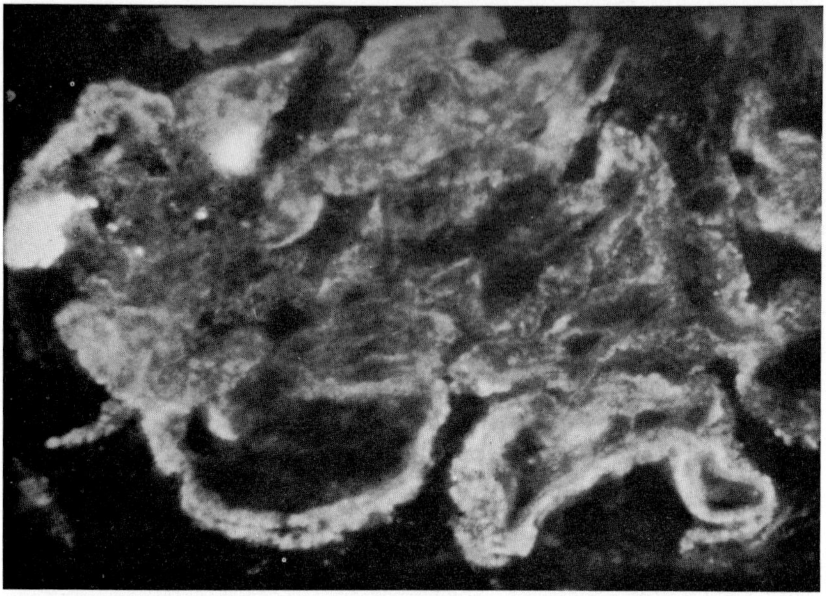

Fig. 7f.

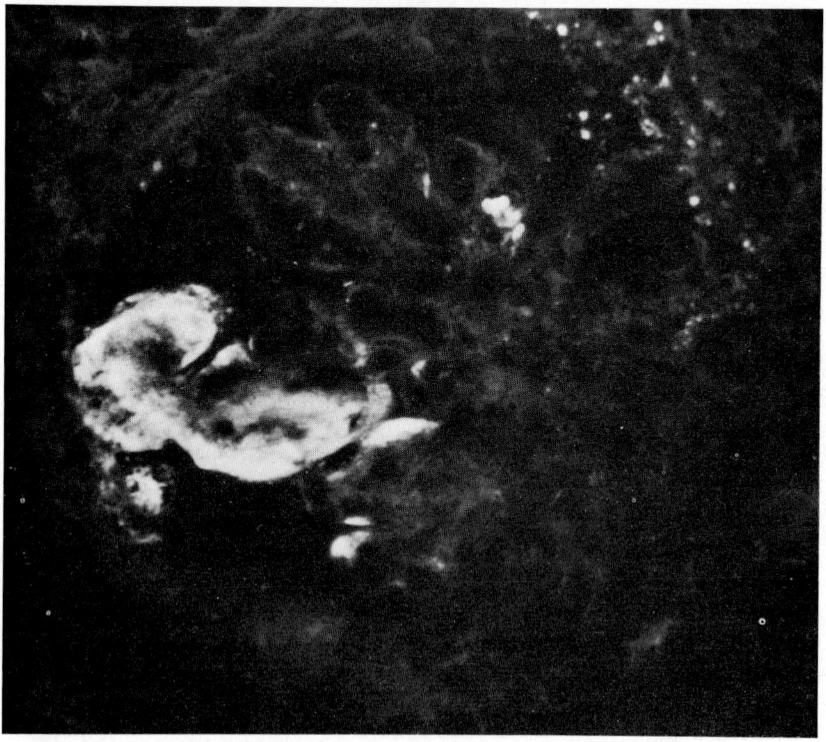

Fig. 7g.

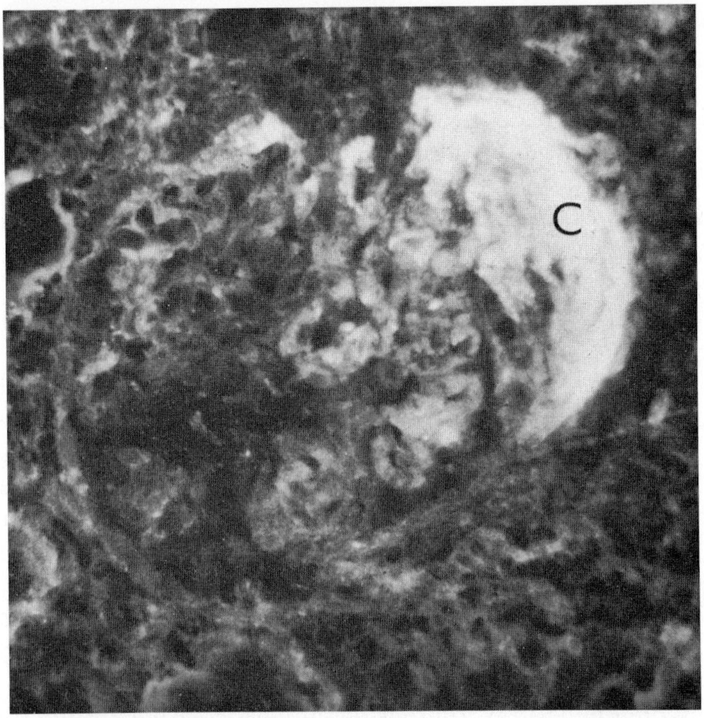

Fig. 7h.

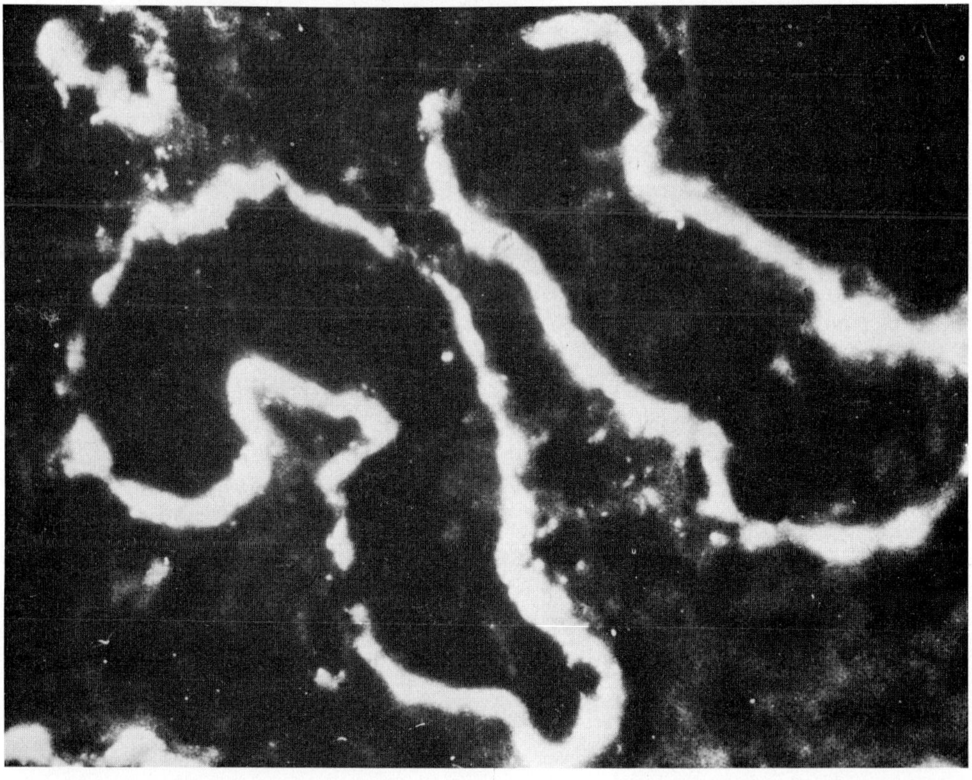
Fig. 7i.

been found for these observations; the early reports of IgE deposition alone in patients with "minimal change" lesions have not been confirmed.

Study of the glomerular deposition of complement components (Berger, 1974) may not only show the presence of complement within the glomerulus, but may also suggest whether the classical (C142) or alternative (properdin) pathway is the mode of activation. The obligatory examination is for C3, but it is worthwhile studying C1q and/or C4 to see whether classical pathway components are also present. Factor B has not been noted to fix to tissue, but if anti-sera are available properdin may be sought as an indicator of alternative pathway activation. The presence or absence of the distal components C5–9 does not seem to add greatly to the information gained by seeking the presence or absence of C3. Apart from fibrin, little attention has been paid to other coagulation factors. Factor VIII, however, is known to be absent in the prominent fibrin deposition within crescents, perhaps suggesting that the fibrin is deposited by mechanisms other than the classical coagulation cascade.

Figures 7–11 illustrate the immunofluorescent finding commonly associated with the different varieties of histology discussed above. Further detail will be found in the captions.

In minimal change lesions, there is usually no positive finding on immunofluorescent study, although flecks of C3 may be seen in the arterioles and in the glomerular tuft, where they may be accompanied by a small amount of IgM. These findings are probably non-specific.

In acute exudative glomerulonephritis bright deposits of IgG are usually seen, probably corresponding to the subepithelial deposits usually visible on electron microscopy. C3 is also present, is often stronger and persists longer than the IgG. Other immunoglobulins are usually absent (Fig. 8).

In mesangial proliferative glomerulonephritis deposits seen on immunofluorescent study are confined to the mesangium (Fig. 9). Usually this consists of IgG and C, but if the clinical setting is one of recurrent attacks of macroscopic haematuria then IgA may be found, alone or accompanied by C3 or IgG. IgA may also be seen in the mesangial or focal nephritis seen in Henoch-Schönlein purpura (HSP), in patients with SLE, and with cirrhosis and nephritis. It is not yet clear whether this is secretory IgA or not, or whether it is acting as antigen, antibody or both. Properdin is also present with the IgA, suggesting that the C3 often accompanying it has been activated via the alternative pathway.

In mesangiocapillary glomerulonephritis the findings depend upon the predominant site of the deposits in the capillary wall. In the commoner group with subendothelial deposits, peripheral IgG, occasionally accompanied by IgM is seen (Fig. 10). C3 is always present, and C1q and C4 usually found also, suggesting a predominant classical pathway activation of C3; however, properdin is also present. The mesangium is relatively spared and fibrin is usually absent. In the rarer group with continuous intramembranous deposits (Fig. 11) there may be nothing at all on immunofluorescent study, or C3 in isolation. This usually stains the basement membrane faintly but in contrast to the subendothelial variety the mesangium may be the site of large bright C3 deposits. Properdin may sometimes be found but immunoglobulins and classical complement components are always absent.

In predominantly extracapillary glomerulonephritis with crescents the striking finding is of fibrin within the crescents (Fig. 7h); often the glomeruli show no fluorescence, but depending upon the type of deposit seen there may be granular mesangial or peripheral Ig or C3. If the crescents occur in association with circulating anti-GBM nephritis, then the pattern of linear IgG is seen (Fig. 7a). This is often an isolated finding, and if C3 is also present then it is in an interrupted pattern along the basement membrane.

In focal and segmental glomerulonephritis the clinical setting of the nephritis may predict what is seen. Often this group of patients have a systemic vasculitis such as Henöch–Schonlein purpura, polyarteritis nodosa or systemic lupus. In the case of a focal nephritis with HSP, there is diffuse IgA in the mesangium of all glomeruli in a high proportion of patients. In polyarteritis, there may be no findings at all except some fibrin deposition. In SLE, usually all immunoglobulins and complement components are present, the pattern depending upon the variety of histology seen. In the milder and more focal forms, however, the immunofluorescent findings are usually diffuse with Ig and complement (C) components in the mesangium of all glomeruli. In contrast to the more severe forms of diffuse proliferative glomerulonephritis often seen in SLE, however, there are no deposits of Ig or C components in the capillary walls.

In membranous nephropathy the immunofluorescence is confined to the peripheral capillary walls. IgG and C3 are nearly always present, and IgM and IgA may be seen (Fig. 7d). Early complement components are almost always absent. Fibrin is rarely found.

In segmental sclerosis the lesions contain fibrin, IgM and C3 (Fig. 7g). Whether this is non-specific secondary fixation to a scarred area of glomerulus or represents immunological reactants mediating the injury is not clear. Immunofluorescence is very helpful in distinguishing this group of patients from those with old scarring segmental glomerulonephritis, since the latter usually show diffuse deposits in the mesangium on immunofluorescence.

In systemic lupus erythematosus almost any pattern or combination of immune deposits may be seen. The commonest, however, are confined to

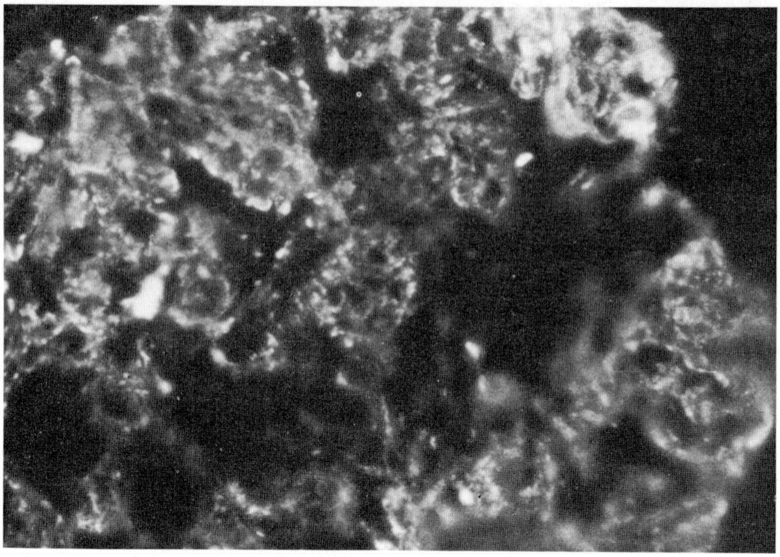

Fig. 8. C3 deposition in a patient with classical acute post-streptococcal glomerulonephritis. There is widespread deposition of C3 throughout the glomerulus, with large bright aggregates scattered around the periphery of the glomerular lobules; these correspond to the "humps" as shown in Fig. 3 (Dr S. Leibowitz).

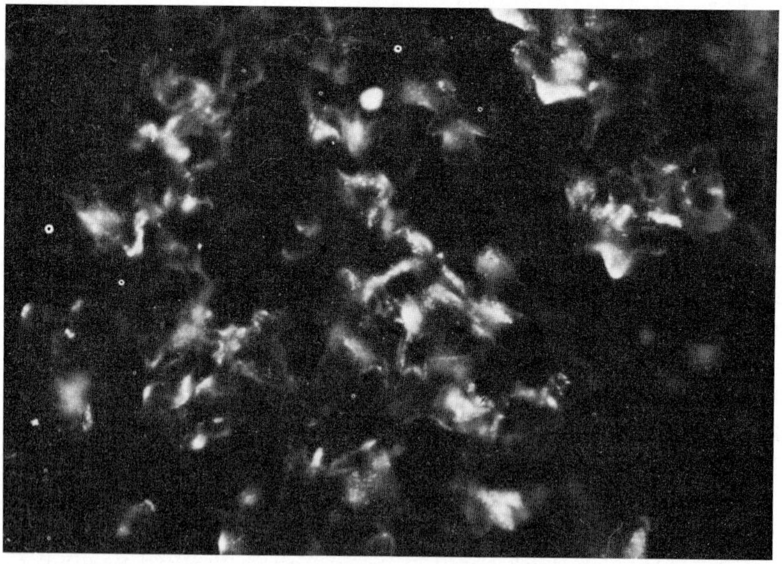

Fig. 9. Mesangial deposition of IgA in a patient with recurrent attacks of macroscopic haematuria. This may be accompanied by IgG, and less commonly C3 in the same distribution; but in many patients the IgA may be seen alone, or together with properdin (Dr S. Leibowitz).

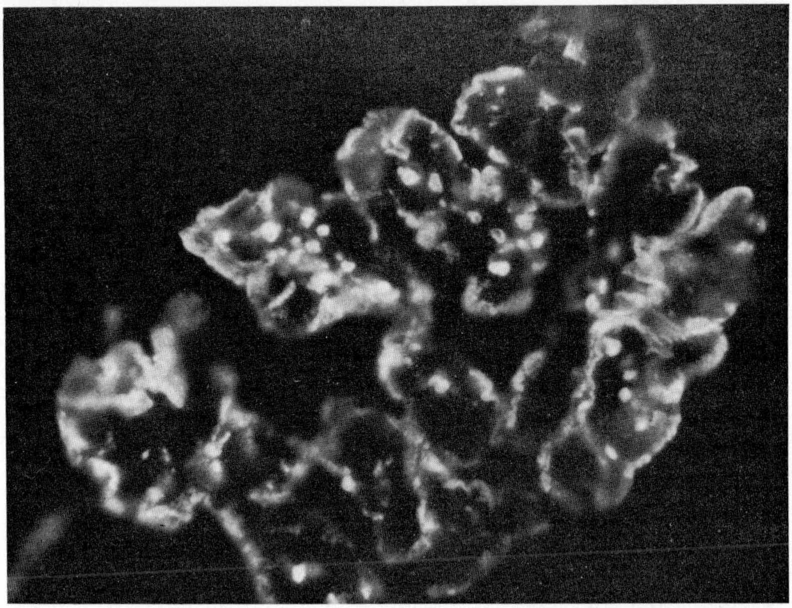

Fig. 10. Mesangiocapillary glomerulonephritis with subendothelial deposits. Antiserum against C3. There are extensive deposits of C3 around the periphery of the glomerular lobules, in an interrupted fashion. In general, the central mesangial region is devoid of fluorescence, but in the upper half of the glomerulus shown, deposits of C3 are also seen in the mesangium. The C3 is always accompanied by IgG and sometimes IgM; rarely, IgA may also be present. Early components of the classical pathway of C3 (C1q and C4) are usually present also (Dr D. J. Evans).

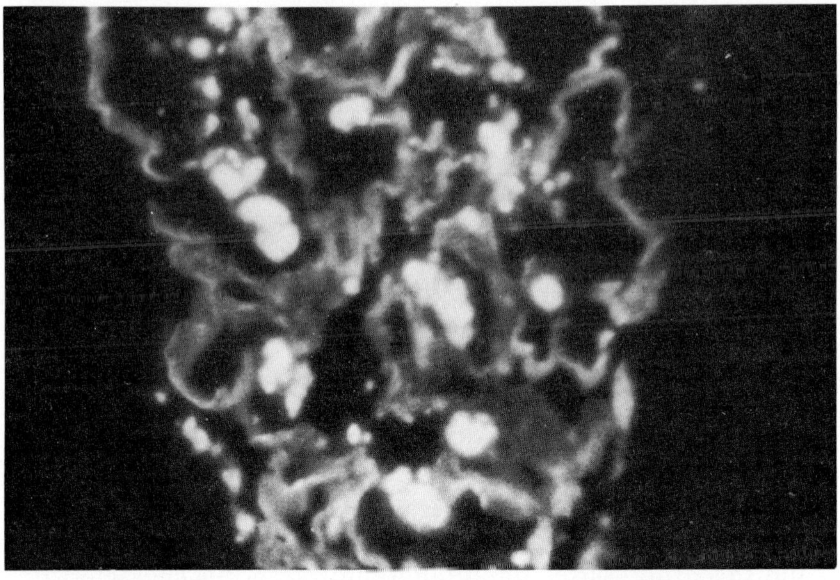

Fig. 11. Mesangiocapillary glomerulonephritis with continuous, intramembranous dense "deposits". In such specimens no immune reactants at all may be found in some patients, and the immune nature of the alterations in the basement membrane is in doubt. C3 is often found alone, as here, with prominent, bright coarse deposits within the mesangium. The peripheral capillary walls may show a linear deposition of C3 along the material in this site, but this is usually fainter than shown here, and probably represents non-specific fixation of C3 to altered basement membrane. Other C components and immunoglobulins are absent, although IgM may be noted in a minority (Dr D. J. Evans).

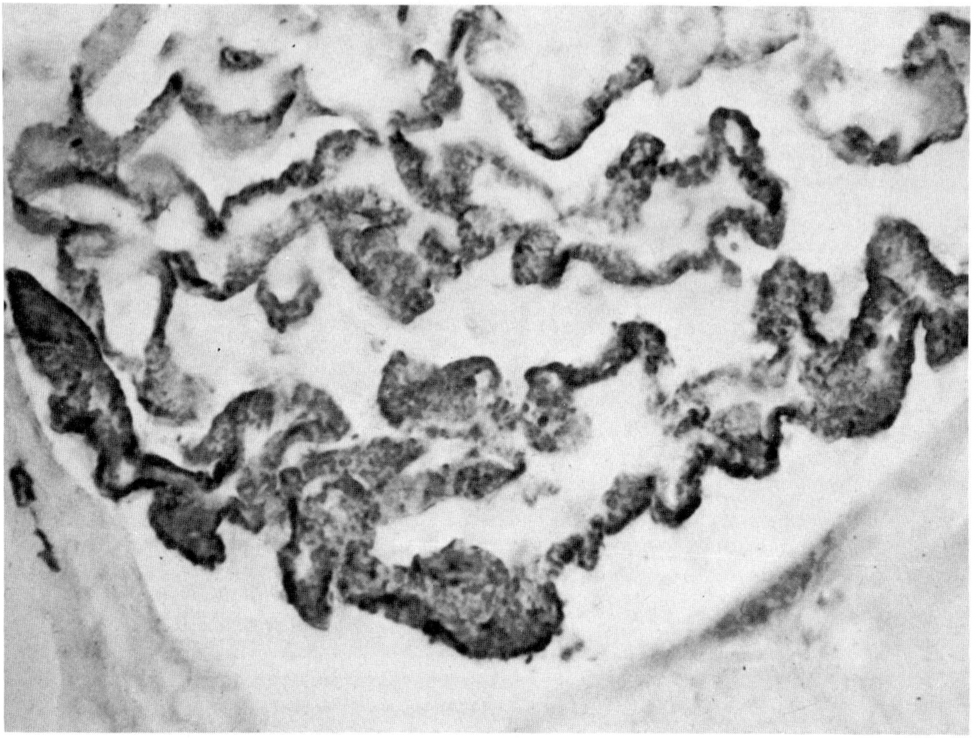

Fig. 12. Deposition of IgG in the peripheral capillary walls of a patient with membranous nephropathy, demonstrated by the use of monospecific antiserum conjugated with peroxidase. The snap-frozen tissue is prepared as for antisera conjugated with fluorescein, but after treatment with peroxidase-conjugated antiserum, the (brown) colour developed by the enzymatic activity of the peroxidase localizes the antigen. Resolution of the deposits into individual granules can be seen at centre right (Dr D. Wilson).

the mesangium, or both in the mesangium and around the capillary walls. Occasionally, a purely peripheral (membranous) pattern may be seen. In the capillary wall it is common to see extensive deposits at both a subendothelial and an extracapillary site (Figs 6 and 7f). Usually IgG and C3 are present, but in the majority of patients IgM, IgA, C1q and C4 will also be found, and this "full house" on immunofluorescence is characteristic of the nephritis of SLE. It is seen otherwise only in occasional patients with mesangiocapillary glomerulonephritis and subendothelial deposits.

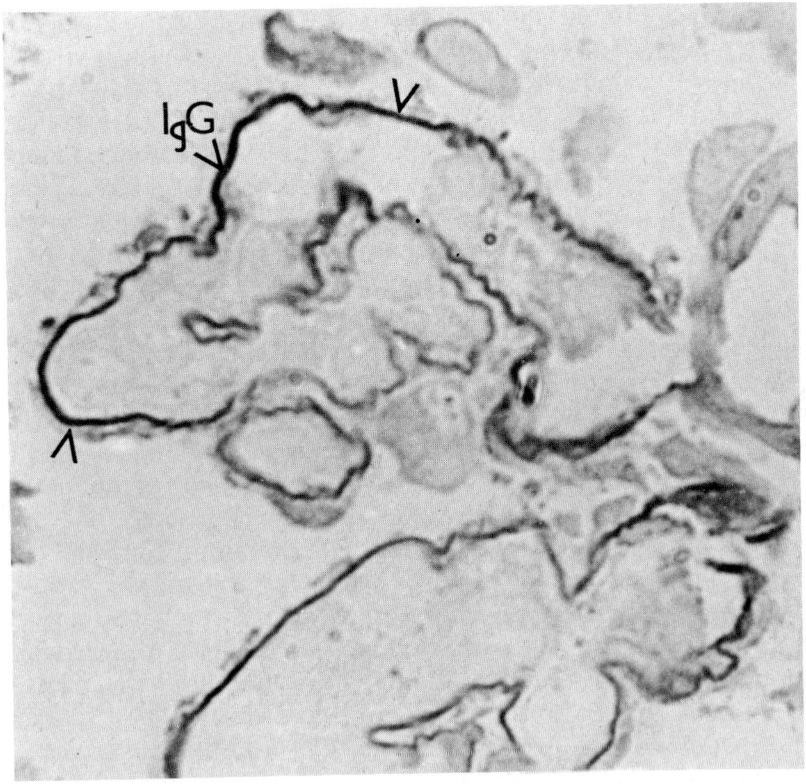

Fig. 13. A linear deposit of IgG in the peripheral capillary walls of a rabbit given specific anti-GBM antiserum (kindly donated by Dr D. K. Peters). Localization was with peroxidase-conjugated antiserum as in Fig. 12, but in this case the conjugate was layered onto a thick section of frozen tissue, which was subsequently mounted into araldite, cut at 1 μm thickness and viewed using optical microscopy (as here) or electron microscopy. Very precise localization of immune reactants is possible with this method, as can be seen. The deposited IgG is indicated by the arrows; no counterstain (Dr D. R. Turner).

IMMUNOLOGICAL TESTS IN THE CLINICAL MANAGEMENT OF PATIENTS WITH GLOMERULONEPHRITIS

Although there is a great variety of immunological tests available which may bear on the immunology of glomerulonephritis, only a handful of these are both clinically useful and widely available (Wilson and Dixon, 1974). The principal immunological technique of importance is immunofluorescent study of frozen biopsy material, discussed above.

Measurement of immunoglobulin levels is not useful in the management of individual patients with glomerulonephritis. Measurement of IgG concentrations depends more upon the amount and type of proteinuria present than upon the immunological status of the patient. In acute post-streptococcal glomerulonephritis, and in lupus, concentrations of IgG from 2,000 to more than 4,000 mg/dl may be found, and in mesangiocapillary glomerulonephritis IgG is disproportionately raised when proteinuria is accounted for, the rise being principally in IgG_3. In patients with IgA in the glomeruli, the plasma IgA levels may be as high as 1,000 mg/dl but this is not confined to patients with mesangial IgA, as has been suggested, nor is it frequent enough to be a useful clinical pointer. IgE levels are sometimes very elevated in patients with "minimal change" lesions and this should perhaps prompt a search for specific antigens.

Individual antibody titres are again of little use, except that a rising level of antistreptolysin O may suggest previous streptococcal infection. A single value however, is of small help especially in the age group 5–15 when acute post-streptococcal glomerulonephritis is most common. Carriage of HB_s is infrequent enough in England to make the search for antibody and antigen worthwhile in patients with nephritis, and the demonstration of a raised titre of anti-double stranded DNA antibody is of importance in the diagnosis of systemic lupus erythematosus. However, anti-DNA antibody titres do not correlate with biopsy findings, nor in our experience with the clinical progression of the disease (Cameron *et al.*, 1976), although Adler *et al.* (1975) claim that in patients with prolonged high titres the clinical course is unfavourable. If a particular agent is suspected of being the precipitant in a case of nephritis, it may be useful to determine the antibody to the particular bacterium, virus or parasite in question; but failure to demonstrate antibody may mean that all the antibody is complexed in the circulation, while demonstration of a high titre does not, of course, prove an association between agent and nephritis.

Few tests for detecting or concentrating soluble immune complexes (see Chapter 6) are yet in general use and it is unlikely that a single test will detect all the circulating complexes that may be relevant to glomerular disease. The ideal would be to detect the complex, identify its antigenic component, describe its physical properties (especially its size) and its biological activity (in particular its ability to activate complement and platelets). Antigen may be identified by immune electron microscopy if the antigen is an intact microorganism, or a recognizable part of one, or by immune diffusion. Suitable for the latter is the concentration of antigen and/antibody in cryoprecipitates from the serum of patients with glomerulonephritis.

Among the most useful groups of tests at present available are those based upon the analysis of serum complement. Although complement is probably involved in the glomerular injury of the majority of glomerulonephritides and can be demonstrated in the glomeruli in most cases, the serum complement concentration is normal in most. Turnover studies of individual complement components show that in some patients complement is being consumed at a more rapid rate than usual, but these studies are too complex for routine use.

Serum complement levels may be transiently depressed below normal in acute nephritis of various forms, particularly post-streptococcal nephritis, but usually returns to normal within eight weeks (Cameron *et al.*, 1973). In mesangiocapillary glomerulonephritis and lupus nephritis, however, the depression may persist, although fluctuations are the rule in the latter. The finding of a low serum complement, therefore, particularly if this finding persists, is a valuable aid to diagnosis.

A simple measure of complement is quantitation of C3 by radial immunodiffusion and this is the test most widely performed. However, it has two disadvantages: (1) in systemic lupus, C3 is relatively less depressed than C1q, C2 and C4, and may be normal when the latter show gross depression; (2) deficiencies of complement, which may predispose to nephritis (see p. 602) will not be detected unless they happen to affect C3. The total haemolytic complement assay lacks both these disadvantages, but requires fresh or freshly-frozen serum, which makes transport of samples to a distant laboratory a problem. In addition to screening total haemolytic complement and C3, it may be useful to know in patients with hypocomplementaemia, whether the C3 is being activated via the classical or the alternative pathway. Clues to this can be obtained by measuring the C4 concentration (immunochemically or by doing a functional "142" test (see Chapter 7) to see if the C142 components are also being consumed. Properdin levels may be measured to test the alternative pathway but as yet anti-properdin sera are in short supply. Measurement of the distal components C5–9 does not add to diagnostic precision.

The complement profiles in acute glomerulonephritis, mesangiocapillary glomerulonephritis and systemic lupus have been studied extensively (Williams *et al.*, 1974). In acute post-streptococcal glomerulonephritis, classical pathway activation is predominant but the alternative pathway is also involved. In mesangiocapillary glomerulonephritis with subendothelial deposits, the levels of C1q and C4 are frequently depressed, and both classical and alternative pathways seem involved. In patients showing intramembranous deposits, in contrast, C1q and C4 concentration are almost always normal, while properdin levels alone may be depressed and C3 concentrations are much more frequently abnormal. This, together with the immunofluorescent evidence already discussed suggests exclusive activation of C3 by the alternative pathway in this condition. In SLE, the principal activation of C3 is by the classical pathway, and C1 and C4 concentrations (in contrast with findings in the forms of nephritis just discussed) may be abnormal when C3 is within normal limits, and are more depressed than the C3 when this is low.

Numerous tests have been examined to see if they would provide an index of the "activity" of the glomerular disease and of its future course. The most recent of these is the measurement of fibrin degradation products (FDPs) in the urine, believed to result from intraglomerular fibrinolysis of fibrin deposited within the glomerular capillaries (Clarkson *et al.*, 1971). However, this has come under criticism (Hall *et al.*, 1975) and at the time of writing it appears most likely that a major contribution to urinary FDP is filtered fibrinogen and FDP, since correlation with histology and prognosis depends upon the quantity and type of proteinuria; measurements already known to correlate with severity of disease. Attempts to assess the excretion of complement breakdown products have also been made, but are at an early stage of evaluation. The red cell haemagglutination inhibition methods used in both these tests are time consuming but radioimmunoassay for individual FDP fragments is now possible.

THE TREATMENT OF GLOMERULONEPHRITIS

The recognition of the role of immunological phenomena in glomerulonephritis, suggested the use of immunosuppressants in treatment. Unfortunately, these have not proved to be effective in the majority of forms of glomerulonephritis. Evidence that they favourably alter the course of disease is found only in SLE (Chapters 11 and 30), in which their effectiveness may be due to their anti-inflammatory effect, and in the nephrotic syndrome associated with the minimal change lesion, which is notable for the lack of proof of its immunological pathogenesis. The concept that at least some glomerulonephritides are primarily immune deficiency diseases may explain this failure of immunosuppression.

The detailed studies of the last decade have indicated some other possible modes of treatment.

First, if an antigen is identifiable as responsible for an immune complex nephritis, its elimination should lead to improvement in the glomerular disease. Examples are (Table 2) the removal of infection in syphilis, SBE and jugulo-atrial shunt nephritis; the excision of a neoplasm; and the removal of immunogenic drugs such as penicillamine or gold. The marked reduction in the incidence of malarial nephropathy following eradication of the parasite in endemic areas is in contrast with the persistence of disease following apparent elimination of the parasite in infected individuals with nephritis. The identification of further antigens susceptible to removal will extend the possibilities.

A second approach arising out of immunological studies is the recent attempts to remove circulating anti-GBM antibodies, immune complexes and immune reactants from patients by plasmaphoresis. Early reports are encouraging, particularly in anti-GBM disease.

A third line of treatment has been to block mediators of glomerular damage. In human disease this has been widely attempted with heparin, warfarin and dicoumarol as anticoagulants. Convincing proof that these bring about improvement is lacking; it may be that they have been administered too late in the course of the disease. Animal work suggests that the dose of heparin employed in patients may be too low, and has also shown that arvin (ancrod) is more effective than heparin in preventing fibrin deposition and crescent formation. The use of arvin in human disease remains to be evaluated.

Fourthly, the correction of an underlying immunodeficiency disorder would be expected to result in alleviation of glomerular damage. Such therapy is still in its infancy and has yet been applied only to gross forms of immunodeficiency. It is likely that immune defects predisposing to glomerulonephritis will be more subtle in nature.

REFERENCES

Adler, M. K., Baumgarten, A., Hecht, B. and Siegel, N. J. (1975). Prognostic significance of DNA-binding capacity patterns in patients with lupus nephritis. *Ann. Rheum. Dis.* **34**, 444–450.

Andres, G. A. and McCluskey, R. T. (1975). Tubular and interstitial renal disease due to immunological mechanisms. *Kidney Int.* **7**, 271–289.

Berger, J., Noel, L. K. and Yaneva, H. (1974). Complement deposition in the kidney. *Adv. Nephrol.* **4**, 87–100.

Boulton-Jones, J. M., Sissons, J. G. P., Evans, D. J. and Peters, D. K. (1974). The renal disease of subacute infective endocarditis. *Brit. Med. J.* **2**, 11–14.

Burkholder, P. (1974). "An atlas of renal histopathology". Harper and Row, New York.

Cameron, J. S. (1976). The natural history of glomerulonephritis. *In* "Renal Disease" (Ed. D. A. K. Black), Blackwell, Oxford. 4th edition (in press).

Cameron, J. S., Vick, R. M., Ogg, C. S., Seymour, W. M., Chantler, C. and Turner, D. R. (1973). Plasma C3 and C4 in management of glomerulonephritis. *Brit. Med. J.* **3**, 668–672.

Cameron, J. S., Lessof, M. H., Ogg, C. S., Williams, B. D. and Williams, D. G. (1976). Disease activity in the nephritis of systemic lupus erythematosus in relation to serum complement concentrations, DNA binding capacity and precipitating anti-DNA antibody. *Clin. Exp. Immunol.* **25**, 418.

Charlesworth, J. A., Williams, D. G., Sherington, E., Lachmann, P. J. and Peters, D. K. (1974). Metabolic studies of the third component of complement and the glycine-rich beta glycoprotein in patients with hypocomplementaemia. *J. Clin. Invest.* **53**, 1578–1587.

Clarkson, A. R., Macdonald, M. K., Petrie, J. J. B., Cash, J. D. and Robson, J. S. (1971). Serum and urinary fibrin/fibrinogen degradation products in glomerulonephritis. *Brit. Med. J.* **3**, 447–451.

Cochrane, C. G. and Koffler, D. (1973). Immune complex disease in experimental animals and man. *Adv. Immunol.* **16**, 186–264.

Dixon, F. J. (1968). The pathogenesis of glomerulonephritis. *Am. J. Med.* **44**, 493–498.

George, C. R. P., Clark, W. F. and Cameron, J. S. (1975). The role of platelets in glomerulonephritis. *Adv. Nephrol.* **5**, 19–65.

Germuth, F. J. and Rodriguez, E. (1973). "The Immunopathology of the Renal Glomerulus". Little Brown and Co., Boston.

Gutman, R. A., Striker, G. E., Gilliland, B. C. and Cutler, R. E. (1972). The immune complex glomerulonephritis of bacterial endocarditis. *Medicine (Baltimore)* **51**, 1–25.

Hall, C. L., Pejhan, N., Terry, J. M. and Blainey, J. D. (1975). Urinary fibrin–fibrinogen degradation products in nephrotic syndrome. *Brit. Med. J.* **1**, 419–422.

Henson, P. M. (1972). Pathological mechanisms in neutrophil-mediated injury. *Am. J. Path.* **68**, 593–612.

Heptinstall, R. H. (1974). "Pathology of the Kidney" 2 vols, 2nd Ed. Churchill, London.

Edgington, T. S., Glassock, R. J., Dixon, F. J. (1968). Autologous immune complex nephritis induced with tubular antigen. *J. Exp. Med.* **127**, 555–571.

Josso, F., Cosson, A., Girot, R. and Gazeneger, C. (1974). Intravascular coagulation and nephropathies. *Adv. Nephrol.* **3**, 175–196.

Lehman, D. H., Wilson, C. B. and Dixon, F. J. (1975). Extraglomerular immunoglobulin deposits in human nephritis. *Am. J. Med.* **58**, 765–786.

Lockwood, C. M., Boulton-Jones, J. M., Lowentha, R. M., Simpson, I. J., Peters, D. K. and Wilson, C. B. (1975). Recovery from Goodpasture's syndrome after immunosuppressive treatment and plasmapheresis. *Brit. Med. J.* **2**, 252–254.

Morel-Maroger, L., Leathem, A. and Richet, G. (1972). Glomerular abnormalities in non-systemic diseases. *Am. J. Med.* **53**, 170–184.

Naish, P., Penn, G. B., Evans, D. J. and Peters, D. K. (1972). The effect of defibrination on nephrotoxic serum nephritis in rabbits. *Clin. Sci.* **42**, 643–644.

Peters, D. K., Williams, D. G., Charlesworth, J. A., Boulton-Jones, J. M., Sissons, D. G. P., Evans, D. J., Kourilsky, O. and Morel-Maroger, L. (1973). Mesangiocapillary glomerulonephritis, partial lipodystrophy and hypocomplementaemia. *Lancet* **2**, 535–538.

Peters, D. K. and Williams, D. G. (1974). Complement and mesangiocapillary glomerulonephritis. The role of complement deficiency in glomerulonephritis. *Nephrol.* **11**, 189–197.

Reeves, W. G., Cameron, J. S., Johansson, S. G. O., Ogg, C. S., Peters, D. K. and Weller, R. O. (1975). Seasonal nephrotic syndrome. Description and immunological findings. *Clin. All.* **5**, 121–137.

Ruddy, S., Carpenter, C. B., Chin, K. W., Knostman, J. N., Soter, N. A., Gotze, O., Muller-Eberhard, H. J. and Austen, K. F. Human complement metabolism: an analysis of 144 studies. *Medicine* (Baltimore) **54**, 165–178.

Saunders, E., Coles, G. A. and Davies, M. (1976). Role of lysosomal enzymes in the pathogenesis of human glomerulonephritis. *Kidney Int.* (in press).

Shalhoub, T. (1974). Pathogenesis of lipoid nephrosis: a disorder of T-cell function. *Lancet* **2**, 556–559.

Simpson, I. J., Amos, N., Evans, D. J., Thomson, N. M. and Peters, D. K. (1975). Guinea pig nephrotoxic nephritis. I. The role of complement and polymorphonuclear leucocytes and the effect of antibody subclass and fragments in the heterologous phase. *Clin. Exp. Immunol.* **19**, 499–511.

Sissons, J. G. P., Evans, D. J., Peters, D. K., Einsinger, A. J., Boulton-Jones, J. M., Simpson, I. J. and Macanovic, M. (1974). Glomerulonephritis associated with antibody to glomerular basement membrane. *Brit. Med. J.* **4**, 11–14.

Sissons, J. G. P., West, R. J., Fallows, J., Williams, D. G., Boucher, B. J., Amos, N. and Peters, D. K. (1976). The complement abnormalities of lipodystrophy. *New Eng. J. Med.* **294**, 461–465.

Symposium (1971). Proceedings of a conference on immune complexes and disease. *J. Exp. Med.* **134**, No. 3, Part 2.

Thompson, R. A. (1972). C3 inactivating factor in the serum of a patient with chronic hypocomplementaemic proliferative glomerulonephritis. *Immunology* **22**, 147–158.

Thomson, N. M., Simpson, I. J., Evans, D. J. and Peters, D. K. (1975). Deprivation with Ancrod in experimental chronic immune complex nephritis. *Clin. Exp. Immunol.* **20**, 527–535.

Theenes, G. H. (1976). The immunohistology of glomerunonephritis distinctive marks and variability. *Current Topics Pathol.* **61**, 61–106.

Vallota, E. H., Götze, O., Spiegelberg, H. L., Forristal, J., West, C. D. and Muller-Eberhard, H. J. (1974). A serum factor in chronic hypocomplementaemic nephritis distinct from immunoglobulins and activating the alternate pathway of complement. *J. Exp. Med.* **139**, 1249–1261.

Williams, D. G., Peters, D. K., Fallows, J., Petrie, A., Kourilsy, O., Morel-Maroger, L. and Cameron, J. S. (1974). Studies of serum complement in the hypocomplementemic nephritides. *Clin. Exp. Immunol.* **18**, 391–405.

Wilson, C. B. and Dixon, F. J. (1973). Antiglomerular-basement membrane antibody induced glomerulonephritis. *Kidney Int.* **3**, 74–89.

Wilson, C. B., Dixon, F. J. (1974). Diagnosis of immunopathologic renal disease. *Kidney Int.* **5**, 389–401.

18

Gastrointestinal Disease

O. EADE and R. WRIGHT

THE GUT-ASSOCIATED IMMUNE SYSTEM

The lymphoid tissue of the gastrointestinal tract plays an important role both in the immune defence of the body and in the pathogenesis of certain disorders. Intestinal colonization with bacteria, viruses and parasites provides a major stimulus to immunoglobulin production, and ingestion of dietary antigens induces antibody formation. Although immunoglobulin-producing and other lymphoid cells are sparse in the intestine before birth, they increase rapidly during the neonatal period. These cells are scattered throughout the lamina propria, and form aggregates in some areas, the Peyer's patches, which are particularly prominent in the distal small intestine. In addition, some lymphocytes are present in the epithelium, interposed between the enterocytes. Gowans and Knight (1964) demonstrated in rats that labelled large lymphocytes from the thoracic duct when injected into the femoral vein of a recipient animal, preferentially "home" to the lamina propria of the small intestine. Similar homing has been seen in subcutaneous implants of foetal gut in syngeneic animals, and is apparently due to an intrinsic property of the small intestine.

Some of the lymphoid cells of the gastrointestinal tract form part of the secretory immune system which transfers immunoglobulin locally into the gut. The majority of immunoglobulin synthesizing cells in the lamina propria contain IgA, and the predominant immunoglobulin in external secretions is secretory (11S) IgA. Only a small amount of secretory IgA is found in the serum. The molecule of secretory IgA is a dimer of 7S IgA, together with a glycoprotein, secretory piece. The immunoglobulin fraction of the secretory IgA molecule is released from the plasma cell, but secretory piece is probably synthesized within the enterocyte (see Chapter 4). An additional polypeptide J-chain is required for dimerization of IgA and formation of secretory IgA. The exact site of combination of IgA with secretory piece is unknown.

Shiner and Ballard (1973) suggest that locally produced IgA in the lamina propria passes through the epithelial basement membrane into the intercellular spaces, and thence into the upper third of the enterocyte, where it combines with secretory piece to form 11S IgA, and is transported across the microvilli into the lumen. The structure of the secretory IgA molecule probably protects it from proteolysis.

That the secretory immune system is important in defence against viral colonization of the gastrointestinal mucosa has been shown with polio-virus vaccine. Following parenteral administration of Salk vaccine a carrier state may persist after infection with the organism. This does not occur if the oral (Sabin) vaccine is given, implying that local immunity in the gut prevents the carrier state. Secretory IgA may also have important antibacterial properties. Opsonization promotes phagocytosis, and the finding that IgA can activate the alternative pathway of complement suggests that it promotes complement-mediated lysis of bacteria. Copro-antibodies provided better resistance to experimental cholera in guinea-pigs than circulating antibodies (Burrows, 1947), and human cholera stools contain a large amount of IgA.

The high incidence of dietary antibodies in selective IgA deficiency suggests that the secretory immune system also regulates absorption of dietary antigens. Predisposition to infestation with *Giardia lamblia* in selective IgA deficiency indicates that the secretory immune system plays a role in protection against this parasite. The main immunological response to helminthic infestation of the gut is the production of IgE antibodies. This is associated with infiltration of eosinophils and mast cells. The IgE system appears to be linked to T-lymphocytes since experimentally thymectomy with administration of antilymphocyte serum prevents worm expulsion in rats.

The precise function of the other lymphoid cells in the gastrointestinal tract, in particular intraepithelial lymphocytes and the Peyer's patch cells, is unknown. The latter are almost devoid of immunoglobulin-containing cells, and stimulation with a variety of antigens has failed to demonstrate specific antibody production in a Peyer's patch. Craig and Cebra (1971) suggest that Peyer's patch cells serve as precursors of IgA-producing cells.

Ultrastructurally the epithelial cells overlying the Peyer's patches are specialized into microfold cells (Owen and Jones, 1974). The formation of a latticework by processes from these cells allows lymphoid cells to approach the luminal surface of the epithelium closely. The microfold cells contain multiple vesicles, and it is possible that they transport antigenic material by pinocytosis. That ingested antigens may pass through the normal intestinal epithelium to allow oral immunization is well established (Walker *et al.*, 1973).

Immune deficiency Syndromes and the Gastrointestinal Tract

The importance of the integrity of the gut-associated immune system is reflected in the gastrointestinal manifestations of immune deficiency disorders, which is described in Chapter 14.

Malnutrition

The recurrent severe infections from which malnourished children suffer may be due to inadequate secretory antibody response locally. Chandra (1975) measured serum and nasopharyngeal IgA antibody levels in malnourished children and healthy controls after immunization with live attenuated measles or polio virus vaccine. Secretory IgA response in the malnourished children was impaired.

Alpha-chain Disease

This is one of the group of lymphoid cell dyscrasias collectively called heavy-chain disease. IgA heavy chains (alpha chains) in the serum are demonstrable as a broad band in the alpha-gamma region, and give an arc on immuno-electrophoresis with an anti-serum to IgA, but not with anti-light chain sera. Alpha-chain disease occurs predominantly in people of Mediterranean origin and is discussed more fully in Chapter 27.

PERNICIOUS ANAEMIA

Chronic, non-specific gastritis is probably due to a variety of causes, and can be separated histologically into chronic superficial gastritis, atrophic gastritis and gastric atrophy. In superficial gastritis, there is slight to severe infiltration of the mucosa with lymphocytes and plasma cells. In atrophic gastritis, the cellular infiltrate may be more pronounced and, in addition, there is atrophy of mucosal glands and intestinal metaplasia. In gastric atrophy, there is almost complete absence of gastric glands, and the cellular infiltrate is much less marked. Gastric atrophy may be the end result of the more acute inflammatory lesion. Biopsy of the gastric mucosa under direct vision with a flexible fibro-optic gastroscope has shown that the lesions may be patchy, and that a specimen from a single site may not be representative of the pathology of the stomach as a whole.

Chronic gastritis is probably due to a variety of causes, only some of which may have an immunological basis. Patients with chronic gastritis seldom have gastrointestinal symptoms, but may have impaired gastric secretion, including secretion of pepsin, hydrochloric acid and intrinsic factor (IF).

The clinical findings favouring a hypothesis that chronic atrophic gastritis with impaired IF secretion is due to an auto-immune process are summarized in Table 1. The association with other putative auto-immune disease is strongest for thyroid disease, including thyrotoxicosis and myxoedema. There is an increased incidence of pernicious anaemia (PA) in insulin-dependent (juvenile) diabetes and in idiopathic Addison's disease, and we have seen patients with both PA and auto-immune haemolytic anaemia. An interesting association is with immunodeficiency disorders, where the gastric mucosa is infiltrated with lymphocytes but devoid of plasma cells. In addition to the association in the patients themselves, there is a high incidence of auto-immune disorders in first degree relatives.

It is known that corticosteroid drugs facilitate the absorption of vitamin B_{12}, although the mechanism is not clear. Studies of the histology of the gastric mucosa in patients with PA given prednisolone suggest that the

TABLE 1
Clinical features suggesting auto-immunity in pernicious anaemia

1. Association with other auto-immune diseases,
    - Thyrotoxicosis
    - Myxoedema
    - Hashimoto's thyroiditis
    - Vitiligo
    - Juvenile diabetes mellitus
    - Auto-immune haemolytic anaemia
    - Late-onset immunodeficiency
2. Gastric lesion sometimes improved by corticosteroids and azathioprine
3. Vitamin B_{12} absorption improved by corticosteroids and azathioprine, (possibly because of regeneration of gastric parietal cells and increased intrinsic factor secretion)

improved IF secretion and Vitamin B_{12} absorption results from regeneration of gastric parietal cells. It has been claimed that azathioprine improves the gastric lesion, but further studies are required.

Immunological Features of Pernicious Anaemia and Gastritis

Two circulating auto-antibodies have been described in PA or latent pernicious anaemia (LPA); antibodies to intrinsic factor (IF) and to the gastric parietal cell cytoplasm (GPC) (Table 2).

TABLE 2
Auto-immune features in pernicious anaemia

1. Intrinsic factor antibodies (present in 50–70% of PA patients):
    - in serum, indicate PA or latent PA
    - in gastric juice, block B_{12} absorption
2. Gastric parietal cell antibody (present in 80–90% of PA patients):
    - in serum indicates gastric lesion

    Found in 20–30% of:
    - Relatives of PA patients
    - Thyroid disease
    - Addison's disease
    - Juvenile diabetes mellitus
    - Vitiligo

IF Antibodies in serum

Taylor (1959) showed that sera from patients with PA block absorption of Vitamin B_{12}, and that the inhibitory factor is a gammaglobulin. It has been characterized as an auto-antibody to IF. There are two types of antibody to IF, a blocking antibody (type 1), which links to IF at or near the site at which vitamin B_{12} binds, and thus prevents formation of B_{12}-IF complexes; and a binding antibody (type 2), which reacts with the B_{12}-IF complex at a site on the IF molecule remote from the combining site for B_{12}. In serum, blocking antibody occurs more commonly; binding antibody is usually found only when titres of blocking antibody are high and is rarely detected alone. The IF antibody seldom occurs in the absence of frank PA, and is invariably associated with histological evidence of severe gastritis. Even in the absence of frank anaemia, IF antibodies are usually associated with impairment of IF secretion, low serum vitamin B_{12} levels and achlorhydria, i.e. LPA. However, Rose *et al.* (1970) detected IF serum antibodies in 11 out of 23 patients with thyroid disease whose absorption of vitamin B_{12} was normal, and in whom acid and IF secretion in the gastric juice was unchanged for three to seven years without progression to frank PA. The type 2 antibody is more common in patients of blood group O. Both type 1 and type 2 IF antibodies in serum are usually of IgG class, and IgA antibody is rare.

Gastric parietal cell antibodies in serum

Irvine *et al.* (1962) detected complement-fixing antibody to homogenates of gastric mucosa in the sera of patients with PA. A more sensitive test is indirect immunofluorescence whereby the antibody may be shown to react with the cytoplasm of gastric parietal cells of a wide variety of animal species. The antigen is organ-specific, however, and although its distribution in the cell resembles that of the microsomal antigen in the thyroid, there is no serological cross-reactivity between the two.

By indirect immunofluorescence, GPC antibody is detected in the sera of over 80% of patients with PA, but lacks the high degree of diagnostic specificity for PA or LPA of IF antibodies (Doniach and Roitt, 1964). It is found in some apparently healthy people, particularly women over the age of 60. Allowing for this, there is an increased incidence of GPC antibodies in patients with thyroid disease, including myxoedema, thyrotoxicosis and Hashimoto's thyroiditis. There is also a high incidence in patients with idiopathic iron deficiency anaemia, particularly those who have associated mucosal and epithelial changes, such as post-cricoid webs. It is uncertain whether the mucosal changes seen in iron deficiency have an immunological basis, since they may respond to iron therapy. Patients with idiopathic adrenal insufficiency and young diabetics also have an increased incidence of GPC antibodies. This broader serological overlap confirms the less frequent clinical association between PA and the disorders mentioned previously.

GPC antibody in serum may be either IgG or IgA in class, although the latter is less common. Hoedemaker and Ito (1970) have localized the antigen to the microvillus of the parietal cell by electron microscopy. It appears to have both lipid and protein components, but has not been purified.

When GPC antibody is present, gastric biopsy almost invariably reveals evidence of gastritis (Fig. 1). The more severe the gastritis, the higher the frequency of the GPC antibody (Wright *et al.*, 1966). However, even severe

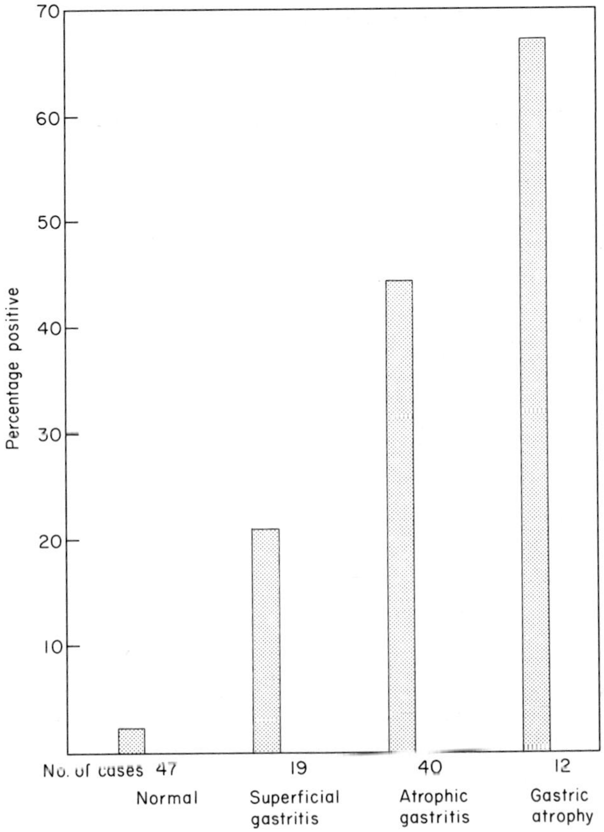

Fig. 1. Gastric parietal cell antibody in serum in relation to severity of gastritis (after Wright *et al.*, 1966).

atrophic gastritis and gastric atrophy can occur without detectable GPC antibodies in the serum. The presence of the antibody in atrophic gastritis is related to the disease in which the antibody occurs. This suggests that there may be more than one cause for the gastritis and that only certain cases are immunologically mediated. Strickland *et al.* (1971) have shown that patients with gastritis in whom the gastric antrum is spared usually have parietal cell antibodies and high serum gastrin levels, whereas antibodies are usually absent and gastrin levels low when there is antral involvement. It must be emphasized that the capacity of individuals to produce auto-antibodies, possibly genetically determined, may be the causal factor.

Auto-antibodies in Gastric Juice

Antibodies to both IF and GPC may also be present in the gastric juice of patients with PA or LPA (Fisher *et al.* (1966). Views on the predominant type of IF antibody and its immunoglobulin class however conflict. This is partly explained by technical problems created by complexing of IF and antibody in gastric juice. It is reported that there is a higher incidence of both types of IF antibody in gastric juice than in serum, and that they may be either IgG or IgA. In contrast, GPC antibodies are found in gastric juice less frequently than in serum, although they too may be of either class. It is thus unlikely that their presence is due to passive exudation from the serum, particularly as other antibodies present in serum, such as anti-thyroglobulin, are not detectable in gastric juice.

By combined immunofluorescent staining and radioautography, type 2 IgG IF antibodies have been demonstrated in plasma cells in the gastric mucosa, but cells producing IgA auto-antibody were not found, despite the presence of antibody activity in the IgA in serum and gastric juice. This suggests that the mechanism of production of auto-antibodies in the gastric mucosa may not be the same as that of antibody formation to ingested antigen, and that serum and gastric juice antibodies are produced at different sites in the gastric mucosa or draining lymph nodes (Taylor, 1972).

Despite the specific association of IF antibody with PA and LPA and the high correlation of GPC antibodies with the auto-immune type of gastritis, their role in the pathogenesis of the gastric lesions is still not clear.

The possibility that the GPC antibody is cytotoxic receives some support from animal experiments (see below), but the evidence in man is scanty. Low complement levels have been reported, and complement is fixed when parietal cell antibody is applied to gastric mucosa. There is also evidence from fluorescent studies that intrinsic factor antibodies fix complement in their reaction with parietal cells (Jacob and Glass, 1971).

Cell mediated Immunity

Lymphocyte transformation and leucocyte migration inhibition by a variety of gastric antigens has been reported in patients with PA. These studies have the major drawback that purified antigens have not been used and appropriate controls—that is, patients with gastritis but without evidence of PA—have usually not been included. Although cell mediated immunity has been demonstrated to a variety of antigens in gastric juice, including IF

(Chanarin and James, 1974), similar effects have been obtained with gastric mitochondria and microsomes, as well as with liver mitochondria, and with antigens in gastric juice which do not bind Vitamin B_{12}. Attempts to correlate evidence of cell mediated immunity with the presence of circulating antibody to IF or GPC have failed.

Animal Models of Gastritis

Attempts to produce in animals by immunological means gastritis similar to that seen in man have on the whole been unsuccessful. The parietal cell mass and the acid output in animals is reduced by repeated injections of human GPC antibody but gastritis does not develop. Immunization of animals with gastric homogenates is reported to produce a patchy gastritis and circulating GPC antibody (Krohn and Finlayson, 1973).

COELIAC DISEASE

Coeliac disease may present in childhood with steatorrhoea and failure to thrive. Some patients do not present until adult life, although often with a childhood history of bowel disturbance and poor growth. In other cases, the intestinal lesion may be entirely subclinical. The disease improves following exclusion of gluten from the diet, and recurs after re-challenge with gluten. Patients with gluten-sensitive enteropathy may respond to cortico-steroids despite continuing to take gluten in their diet.

The precise nature of the toxic component in gluten has not been identified. It resides in the alpha gliadin fraction of gluten and its *in vivo* instillation into the jejunum of patients with treated coeliac disease results in histological changes in the intestinal mucosa.

The Intestinal Lesion

In coeliac disease, the histological lesion is proximally situated in the small intestine. Varying degrees of villous atrophy occur with accompanying crypt cell hyperplasia, degenerative changes of the surface epithelium and dense infiltration of the lamina propria with lymphoid cells. The latter are predominantly plasma cells and the total number of lymphocytes in the lamina propria is reduced. However, the number of intra-epithelial lymphocytes is considerably increased.

Shiner (1973) has shown that in coeliac disease the earliest ultrastructural changes in the gut occur in the subepithelial connective tissue forming the basement membrane, and there is swelling of the endothelial cells of small blood vessels, oedema and infiltration with inflammatory cells including polymorphs.

The histological appearance has features of both an immune complex and a cell-mediated type of reaction.

Gluten-induced enteropathy, with an intestinal lesion identical in kind with that of untreated coeliac disease also occurs in dermatitis herpetiformis. In the latter, unlike coeliac disease, IgA deposits are present at the dermo-epidermal junction, a finding of diagnostic importance (see Chapter 23). The skin lesions respond to restriction of dietary gluten.

Other Lymphoid Tissue Changes

Splenic atrophy occurs in a high proportion of patients with adult coeliac disease, although this is not known to be a feature of the condition in childhood. In addition, small intestinal lymphoma may complicate both treated and untreated coeliac disease and it has been suggested that the malignant transformation may be related to lymphoreticular atrophy and impaired immune surveillance.

Associations with Other Conditions

Coeliac disease may be associated with fibrosing alveolitis and we have noted an association between coeliac disease and patients with extrinsic allergic alveolitis due to avian exposure. There is an increased incidence of carcinoma of the gastrointestinal tract, particularly of the oesophagus.

Familial Incidence

Coeliac disease has familial features, approximately 10% of first degree relatives being affected. Other evidence of a genetic factor is a preponderance of the histocompatibility antigens HLA-B1 and HLA-B8 and the possibility that an immune response gene is linked to the HLA loci in question has been suggested (Falchuk *et al.*, 1972).

Immunological Features (Table 3)

Antibodies

Antibodies to gluten may be demonstrated in the serum and intestinal juice of untreated coeliacs but antibodies to a variety of other dietary antigens also occur, indicating that they are secondary (Taylor *et al.*, 1964). The reticulin antibody described by Seah *et al.* (1971) occurs in 50–70% of untreated adults and 85% of children and is a useful screening marker for coeliac disease (Fig. 2). Anti-reticulin antibody is also found in 20–30% of patients with dermatitis herpetiformis, in about 25% of patients with Crohn's disease and in about 4% of apparently normal individuals. It disappears on a gluten-free diet and reappears after gluten-challenge (Alp and Wright, 1971). Reticulin antibody may be merely another example of an immune response to a dietary antigen, but the fact that the earliest lesion in coeliac disease after gluten challenge occurs at the basement membrane raises the possibility that it is also significant in pathogenesis. Evidence of cross-reactivity between reticulin and gluten is conflicting.

In coeliac disease, the serum IgA is often raised and the IgM lowered. This contrasts with the finding of a reduced proportion of IgA-containing plasma cells in the lamina propria, and increased numbers of IgM-containing cells. Unexplained also is the association between coeliac disease and selective

TABLE 3
Immunological features of coeliac disease

1. Serological abnormalities:
   - Antibodies to dietary proteins and reticulin
   - Increased IgA; decreased IgM
   - Selective IgA deficiency (rare)
   - Circulating immune complexes
2. Mucosal abnormalities:
   - Deterioration after gluten challenge suggestive of immune complex-type reaction
   - Infiltration with plasma cells and lymphocytes
   - Decreased IgA; increased IgM
3. Cell mediated reactions
   - Impaired lymphocyte PHA responsiveness
   - Impaired lymphocyte cytotoxicity
   - *In vitro* CMI to gluten fractions (lymphocyte transformation and MIF production)
4. Splenic and lymphoreticular atrophy
5. Lymphoma (rare)

IgA deficiency. The latter occurs in 1:700 of the general population but is seen in approximately 1:70 of patients with coeliac disease.

The humoral response to parenteral immunization in coeliac patients is deficient as compared with control subjects. Pettingale (1970) found reduced antitoxin production in coeliac patients following tetanus toxoid immunization, particularly after secondary immunization, and significantly lowered

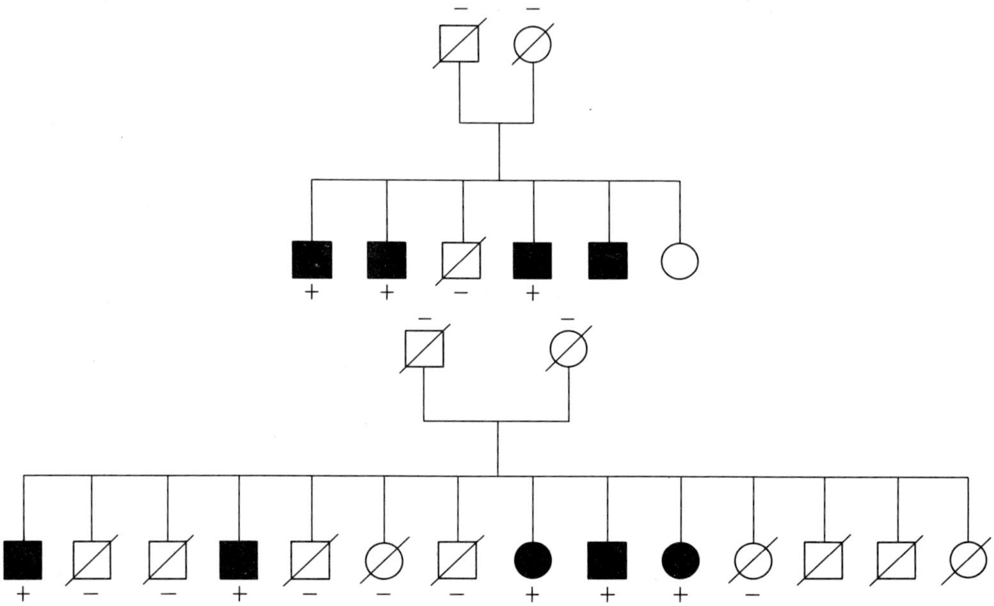

Fig. 2. Family trees illustrating the familial incidence of coeliac disease and value of reticulin antibody as a screening marker. (After Stevens *et al.*, 1975).
■ Male coeliac; ● female coeliac ◻̸ or ∅ male or female relative in whom a normal biopsy has been obtained □ or ○ male or female relative in whom no biopsy has been obtained. + or − above or below symbol indicates the presence or absence of reticulin antibody in serum. (No sign indicates reticulin antibody not tested for.)

IgM responses. Coeliac patients show low primary and secondary antibody responses to intravenous immunization with bacteriophage ΦX 174 and a defect in switching from IgM to IgG antibody production in the secondary response (Baker *et al.*, 1975). Enhancement of IgA antibody response was reported by MaWhinney (1973) in coeliac subjects, following a single dose of oral polio vaccine.

Role of Antibodies in Pathogenesis

The possibility that humoral factors play a part in the pathogenesis of coeliac disease has stimulated several studies. A precipitin reaction with the Clq component of complement given by the sera of a high proportion of adult coeliac patients (Doe *et al.*, 1973) suggests the presence of circulating immune complexes. The frequency of precipitin reactions is higher among untreated patients and this, together with the presence of immunoglobulin and complement on the basement membrane of the jejunal mucosa after gluten challenge *in vivo* favours an immune complex reaction. This interpretation is supported by the fall in the serum complement level and the development of circulating complement breakdown products in treated coeliacs following gluten challenge.

Organ cultures of jejunal biopsy fragments have been used to investigate the pathogenesis of coeliac disease. When cultures from untreated coeliacs are maintained for twenty-four hours they show histological and biochemical improvement of the mucosa. This is prevented by the addition of a gluten fraction to the culture fluid. Normal biopsies from treated coeliacs however, are unaffected by *in vitro* culture with gluten, so that it appears that prior contact with gluten *in vivo* is necessary for *in vitro* sensitivity to be demonstrated. However, in co-culture experiments, Falchuk *et al.*, (1975) have shown that a humoral factor released by jejunal biopsy fragments from an untreated coeliac patient appears to affect the normal jejunal mucosal tissue of a treated coeliac patient placed on the same grid. Approximately half the immunoglobulin produced by cultured coeliac jejunal biopsy tissue has anti-gliadin specificity, and it is possible that this is the humoral factor responsible for the co-culture results.

Cell mediated Reactions

Impaired PHA responsiveness of cultured lymphocytes from patients and their reduced cytotoxic properties toward target cells suggests a defect of cellular immunity. Lymphocyte transformation in response to gluten fractions has been shown (Holmes *et al.*, 1972) and there is evidence of MIF production by cultured jejunal biopsy fragments from coeliac patients in the presence of alpha gliadin. This was not seen in the absence of added antigen or with biopsies from normal controls (Ferguson *et al.*, 1975).

A lesion similar to that of coeliac disease occurs in allografts of small intestine in mice, suggesting that cellular immunity is involved in the pathogenesis of coeliac disease, and observations on the small intestinal mucosal lesion in rats infested with the worm *Nippostrongylus brasiliensis* lends support to this view. Thymectomized rats, though heavily infested with this parasite, do not develop the villous atrophy characteristic of non-thymectomized animals (Ferguson and Jarrett, 1975).

It is also possible that some of the immunological features of coeliac disease are secondary to the intestinal lesions and as yet there is no conclusive evidence that its pathogenesis is due to an immunological abnormality.

INFLAMMATORY BOWEL DISEASE

The Intestinal Lesions

Ulcerative colitis and Crohn's disease are chronic inflammatory disorders of the intestine with a tendency to remission and relapse. Their aetiology is unknown, but an infection or abnormal immunological response to an unidentified antigen are likely possibilities. Idiopathic ulcerative colitis is confined to the large intestine, and the lesion is mainly mucosal with polymorph, eosinophil, lymphocyte and plasma cell infiltration. Crohn's disease may affect any part of the gastrointestinal tract, though chiefly the ileum and colon. It produces thickening of the bowel wall with formation of lymphoid follicles and granulomas in the intestine itself and in the draining lymph nodes. Skip lesions (segmental areas of disease) are a characteristic feature.

Familial Incidence

Approximately 10% of patients with ulcerative colitis or Crohn's disease have affected relatives, and it is of interest that both conditions may occur in a family. One report has claimed an excess of histocompatibility gene HLA-B11, but this has been disputed. As one might expect, patients with inflammatory bowel disease who have ankylosing spondylitis show a strong association with HLA-B27. This does not appear to be the case in patients who have changes confined to the sacroiliac joints. An increased incidence of inflammatory bowel disease in Jews has been reported in several studies, and it appears to be extremely rare in natives of the developing countries.

Associations with Other Conditions

There is an increased incidence of atopy in ulcerative colitis, but the association of inflammatory bowel disease with auto-immune disorders is tenuous, although there have been case reports of association with chronic active hepatitis, systemic lupus erythematosus, pernicious anaemia, Hashimoto's disease and auto-immune haemolytic anaemia. Of special interest from an immunological point of view are the extra-intestinal manifestations such as arthritis, ankylosing spondylitis, uveitis, erythema nodosum and disorders of the liver including portal triaditis, chronic active hepatitis and sclerosing cholangitis. It is not clear whether these manifestations are true complications of the inflammatory bowel disease, possible independently mediated by immunological mechanisms, or whether they are part of a generalized disease, the brunt of which falls on the bowel. It is possible that both ulcerative colitis and Crohn's disease form a syndrome with various aetiologies.

Corticosteroid drugs and azathioprine may have a favourable effect on the clinical course, but it is not clear whether this occurs on the basis of an immunosuppressive or an anti-inflammatory action. A recent clinical trial has shown that Intal (sodium cromoglycate) significantly benefits patients with chronic proctitis. Intal is known to reduce degranulation of mast cells and modify anaphylactic reactions, and it is of particular interest that in this study the patients who responded to Intal were those with high circulating and tissue eosinophil counts (Heatley *et al.*, 1975).

Immunological Features

Circulating Antibodies and Immunoglobulins

Dietary allergy, particularly to milk, has been thought to be an important factor in the aetiology of ulcerative colitis, and a controlled clinical trial has shown that on a milk-free diet the relapse rate is reduced in about 20% of patients (Wright and Truelove, 1965). However, there is no evidence that this reflects a true allergic response in these subjects. High titre dietary antibodies and circulating and tissue eosinophilia are present in some patients but do not correlate with clinical response to a milk-free diet.

Circulating antibodies to colon were first detected in the serum of children with ulcerative colitis by Broberger and Perlmann (1959). They used as antigen a phenol–water extract of colonic tissue from stillborn infants, and found antibodies by a haemagglutination technique in 28 out of 30 children with ulcerative colitis and in only a small number of controls at low titre. Subsequently, with the immunofluorescent technique, they demonstrated that the colon antibody reacts with colonic epithelial cell cytoplasm. Using this technique, we and others have found colon antibodies much less frequently in adult patients with ulcerative colitis (Table 4). Unlike pernicious anaemia, ulcerative colitis and Crohn's disease have a very low incidence of other auto-antibodies, in line with the rarity of clinical association with auto-immune disease. The presence of circulating antibodies to colon cannot be correlated with any of the clinical features, and they often persist after colectomy.

TABLE 4
Auto-antibodies in ulcerative colitis and Crohn's disease

	Ulcerative colitis			Crohn's disease		
	No. of patients tested	Positive No.	Positive %	No. of patients tested	Positive No.	Positive %
Human colon	197	25	12·7	86	2	2·3
Rat colon	80	2	2·5	87	7	8·0
Smooth muscle antibody (SMA)	281	12	4·3	95	3	3·2
Mitochondrial antibody	280	3	1·1	94	0	0·0
Thyroid cytoplasmic antibody	281	9	3·2	95	0	0·0
Gastric parietal cell antibody	281	11	3·9	95	0	0·0
Anti-nuclear factor (ANF)	281	25	8·9	95	9	9·5
Thyroglobulin	269	29	10·8	98	17	17·3
Rheumatoid factor	222	14	6·3	95	10	10·5

After Perrett *et al.*, 1971.

The colon antigen is present in rat and human, and cross-reacts with the common enterobacterial antigen (the Kunin antigen), particularly of *E. coli* O14. It is probably a lipopolysaccharide and is related to blood group substance. The antigen is found in the colonic epithelial cells, in goblet cells in the small intestine and in proliferating bile-ducts, as well as in germ-free rat faeces, which presumably contain desquamated colonic epithelial cells. Because of the cross-reactivity of the colon antigen with common entero-bacterial antigens, Lagercrantz *et al.* (1966) have postulated that auto-immunization in ulcerative colitis arises from breaking of tolerance to such cross-reacting antigens. A possible abnormal response to normal endogenous bacteria is suggested by the work of Monteiro *et al.* (1971) who demonstrated by immunofluorescence antibodies in the colonic mucosa of patients with ulcerative colitis reacting against anaerobic organisms. These intramucosal antibodies were of the IgG class, but could not be demonstrated in serum.

Immune complex injury by endogenous bacteria is thus a possible mechanism of tissue injury in ulcerative colitis.

Reports of the immunoglobulin class of the antibodies produced by the infiltrating cells in ulcerative colitis are conflicting. Brandtzaeg *et al.* (1974) using alcohol-fixed tissue, and careful washing to remove extracellular immunoglobulins, found a striking increase in IgG cells, and a lesser increase in IgM cells. IgG cells were often present in the submucosa, where immunoglobulin-containing cells are rarely demonstrable in normal colon.

Serum immunoglobulins are usually normal in both ulcerative colitis and Crohn's disease, though some patients have elevated IgA and we have seen patients with inflammatory bowel disease who have hypogammaglobulinaemia and others with selective IgA deficiency.

Lymphocyte-mediated Cytotoxicity

Perlmann and Broberger (1963) studied the effect of colon antibodies on colonic epithelial cells in tissue culture and failed to find evidence of cytotoxicity, but demonstrated that lymphocytes from patients with ulcerative colitis have the property of specifically killing colon cells.

This work was extended by Watson (1969) and by Shorter *et al.* (1972), but the results are difficult to interpret. It appears that lymphocytes from both ulcerative colitis and Crohn's disease are cytotoxic for autologous and for allogeneic colonic epithelial cells *in vitro*. This cytotoxic effect disappears about ten days after colectomy, is blocked by preliminary incubation of the lymphocytes with lipopolysaccharide bacterial extracts, and can be induced in lymphocytes from healthy subjects by preliminary incubation with such lipopolysaccharide extracts. Patient's serum, particularly the IgM fraction, also induces normal lymphocytes to become cytotoxic for colonic epithelial cells. These results suggest that cell-bound antibody or immune complexes attached to the lymphocyte surface may be responsible.

A factor that makes interpretation of such experiments uncertain is the lack of appropriate controls for patients with idiopathic chronic inflammatory bowel disease. It would be of interest to examine lymphocytes from patients with chronic amoebic dysentery by similar techniques.

The evidence of sensitization to colon provided by the presence of circulating colon antibodies, is strengthened by Bendixen's (1967) report of inhibition of migration of blood leucocytes from patients with ulcerative colitis and Crohn's disease by sterile foetal human colon and ileal mucosa. Lymphocytes from patients with ulcerative colitis exposed to Kunin antigens or to a phenol-water extract of *E. coli* O119 B14 produce MIF, suggesting cell mediated immunity to these antigens also (Bull and Ignaczak, 1973).

It must be emphasized again that none of these immunological features has been shown to be specific to patients with ulcerative colitis, and all could be secondary phenomena.

Of greater interest is the possibility that immune mechanisms may be important in the pathogenesis of some of the extracolonic manifestations. Jewell and MacLennan (1973) demonstrated small immune complexes in the sera of patients with inflammatory bowel disease, by their ability to inhibit the lysis of sensitized target cells by non-immune lymphocytes. Sera from patients with ulcerative colitis and Crohn's disease producing much greater inhibition in this cytotoxic system than normal serum, and the circulating small immune complexes presumed to be demonstrated may be contributing to the pathogenesis of the extracolonic manifestations. However, immune complexes have not been demonstrated by direct means in the extracolonic tissues involved.

In view of the histological similarity between Crohn's disease and sarcoidosis several studies have examined hypersensitivity to Kveim antigen by skin tests and leucocyte migration inhibition. Results have been conflicting, largely because of differences in the batches of sarcoid spleen used as testing material. Despite reports suggesting that a proportion of patients with Crohn's disease show an abnormal response to sarcoid spleen antigen, the issue is still unsettled.

Similarly, there have been conflicting reports on reactivity to tuberculin, DNCB and fungal antigen in Crohn's disease. Although depression has been observed as compared with healthy controls, it is not clear whether this is a basic defect or whether it is merely due to a non-specific effect of severe illness.

GASTROINTESTINAL ALLERGY

Atopic hypersensitivity in the gastrointestinal tract may be manifest in infancy in the form of cow's milk allergy, and the more recently described soy protein allergy. Shiner *et al.* (1975) have demonstrated an increase in IgE-containing plasma cells in two infants with cow's milk allergy after challenge with cow's milk, in addition to local degranulation of mast cells. After a period the child outgrows the allergy to cow's milk and subsequent challenges with the antigen have no clinical effect.

The less well-defined condition of eosinophilic gastroenteropathy occurs among atopic individuals. There may be infiltration of the wall of the gastrointestinal tract with eosinophils to a variable extent. Infiltration can be quite dense, and in the small intestine there may be changes of villous atrophy which may extend through the muscle layers to the serosal surface. Typically, there is a history of gastrointestinal symptoms following ingestion of certain foods, although elimination diets are not always successful. Some cases respond to treatment with corticosteroids.

CONNECTIVE TISSUE DISORDERS AND THE GUT

Vasculitis of the mesenteric vessels may occur in rheumatoid arthritis, resulting in infarction of the bowel, perforation and peritonitis. In addition, longstanding rheumatoid disease may be associated with amyloidosis of the bowel.

The gastrointestinal tract may be affected by vasculitis in systemic lupus erythematosus. Malabsorption, with villous atrophy, has also been seen but the possibility of coexisting coeliac disease is not excluded.

Involvement of the alimentary tract in systemic sclerosis may extend from the mouth to the rectum. Early changes occur in the oesophagus, with atrophy of smooth muscle and submucosal sclerosis. Similarly, disorders of motility can affect both the small and large intestine with radiological evidence of dilation and pseudo-diverticulum formation. Abdominal pain, diarrhoea or constipation and frank malabsorption may supervene. As with other connective tissue disorders occlusion of mesenteric vessels may occur.

REFERENCES

Alp, M. H. and Wright, R. (1971). Autoantibodies to reticulin in patients with idiopathic steatorrhoea, coeliac disease and Crohn's disease and their relation to immunoglobulins and dietary antibodies. *Lancet* **ii**, 682.

Baker, P. G., Verrier Jones, J., Peacock, D. B. and Read, A. E. (1975). The immune response to ΦX174 in man. *Gut*, **16**, 538.

Bendixen, J. (1967). Specific inhibition of the *in vitro* migration of leucocytes in ulcerative colitis and Crohn's disease. *Scand. J. Gastroenterol.* **2**, 214.

Brandtzaeg, P., Baklein, K., Fausa, O. and Hoel, P. S. (1974). Immunohistochemical characterisation of local immunoglobulin formation in ulcerative colitis. *Gastroenterology* **66**, 1123.

Broberger, O. and Perlmann, P. (1959). Autoantibodies in human ulcerative colitis. *J. Exp. Med.* **110**, 657.

Bull, D. M. and Ignaczak, T. F. (1973). Enterobacterial common antigen-induced lymphocyte reactivity in inflammatory bowel disease. *Gastroenterology* **64**, 43.

Burrows, E. (1947). Studies on immunity to Asiatic cholera iv. Excretion of coproantibody in experimental enteric cholera in guinea pigs. *J. Infect. Dis.* **81**, 261.

Chanarin, I. and James, D. (1974). Humoral and cell-mediated intrinsic factor antibody in pernicious anaemia. *Lancet* **i**, 1078.

Chandra, R. K. (1975). Reduced secretory antibody response to live attenuated measles and polio virus vaccines in malnourished children. *Brit. Med. J.* **ii**, 583.

Craig, S. W. and Cebra, J. J. (1971). Peyer's patches; an enriched source of precursors for IgA-producing immunocytes in the rabbit. *J. Exp. Med.* **134**, 188.

Doe, W. F., Booth, C. C. and Brown, D. L. (1973). Evidence for complement binding immune complexes in adult coeliac disease, Crohn's disease and ulcerative colitis. *Lancet* **i**, 402.

Doniach, D. and Roitt, I. M. (1964). An evaluation of gastric and thyroid auto-immunity in relation to haematologic disorders. *Semin. Hemat.* **1**, 313.

Falchuk, Z. M., Rogentine, G. N. and Strober, W. (1972). Predominance of histocompatibility antigen HL-A8 in patients with gluten-sensitive enteropathy. *J. Clin. Invest.* **51**, 1602.

Falchuk, Z. M., Gebhard, R. L. and Strober, W. (1975). The pathogenesis of gluten-sensitive enteropathy (coeliac sprue): organ culture studies. *In* "Coeliac Disease". Proceedings of the Second International Coeliac Symposium (eds. W. Th, J. M. Hekkens and A. S. Peña), pp. 107–117. Medical and Technical Publishing Company Limited, Leiden, Holland.

Ferguson, A. and Jarrett, E. E. E. (1975). Hypersensitivity reactions in the small intestine; I. Thymus dependence of experimental partial villous atrophy. *Gut* **16**, 114.

Ferguson, A., MacDonald, T. T., McClure, J. P. and Holden, R. J. (1975). Cell-mediated immunity to gliadin within the small intestinal mucosa in coeliac disease. *Lancet* **i**, 895.

Fisher, J. M., Fees, C. and Taylor, K. B. (1966). Intrinsic factor antibodies in gastric juice of pernicious anaemia patients. *Lancet* **ii**, 88.

Gowans, J. L. and Knight, E. J. (1964). Recirculation of lymphocytes in the rat. *Proc. Roy. Soc. B*, 159, 257.

Heatley, R. V., Calcraft, B. J., Rhodes, J., Owen, R. and Evans, B. K. (1975). Disodium cromoglycate in the treatment of chronic proctitis. *Gut* **16**, 559.

Hoedemaker, P. J. and Ito, S. (1970). Ultrastructural localisation of gastric parietal cell antigen with peroxidase-coupled antibody. *Lab. Invest.* **22**, 184.

Holmes, G. K. T., Asquith, P. and Cooke, W. T. (1972). Cell-mediated mechanisms in adult coeliac disease. *Gut* **13**, 324.

Irvine, W. J., Davies, S. H., Delamore, I. W. and Williams, A. W. (1962). Immunological relationship between pernicious anaemia and thyroid disease. *Brit. Med. J.* **ii**, 454.

Jacob, E. and Glass, G. P. J. (1971). Localisation of intrinsic factor and complement fixing intrinsic factor antibody complex in the parietal cell of man. *Clin. Exp. Immunol.* **8**, 517.

Jewell, D. P. and MacLennen, I. C. (1973). Circulating immune complexes in inflammatory bowel disease. *Clin. Exp. Immunol.* **14**, 219.

Krohn, K. J. E. and Finlayson, M. D. C. (1973). Inter-relations of humoral and cellular immune responses in experimental canine gastritis. *Clin. Exp. Immunol.* **14**, 237.

Lagercrantz, R., Hammarström, S., Perlmann, P. and Gustafsson, B. E. (1966). Immunological studies in ulcerative colitis. III. Incidence of antibodies to colon–antigen in ulcerative colitis and other gastro-intestinal diseases. *Clin. Exp. Immunol.* **1**, 263.

MaWhinney, H. (1973). M.D. Thesis, Belfast.

Monteiro, E., Fossey, J., Shiner, M., Draser, B. and Allison, A. C. (1971). Antibacterial antibodies in rectal and colonic mucosa in ulcerative colitis. *Lancet* **i**, 249.

Owen, R. L. and Jones, A. L. (1974). Epithelial cell specialisation within human Peyer's patches: an ultrastructural study of intestinal lymphoid follicles. *Gastroenterology*, **66**, 189.

Perlmann, P. and Broberger, O. (1963). *In vitro* studies of ulcerative colitis. 2. Cytotoxic action of white blood cells from patients on human fetal colon cells. *J. Exp. Med.* 117, 717.

Pettingale, K. W. (1970). Immunoglobulin and specific antibody responses to antigenic stimulation in adult coeliac disease. *Clin. Sci.* **38**, 16.

Rose, M. S., Chanarin, I., Doniach, D. and Brostoff, J. (1970). Intrinsic factor antibodies in absence of pernicious anaemia. *Lancet* **ii**, 9.

Seah, P. P., Fry, L., Hoffbrand, A. V. and Holborow, E. J. (1971). Tissue antibodies in dermatitis herpetiformis and adult coeliac disease. *Lancet* **i**, 834.

Shiner, M. (1973). Ultrastructural changes suggestive of immune reactions in the jejunal mucosa of coeliac children following gluten challenge. *Gut* **14**, 1.

Shiner, M. and Ballard, J. (1973). Mucosal secretory IgA and secretory piece in adult coeliac disease. *Gut* **14**, 778.

Shiner, M., Ballard, J. and Smith, M. E. (1975). The small intestinal mucosa in cow's milk allergy. *Lancet* **i**, 136.

Shorter, R. J., Huizenga, K. A., Spencer, R. J., Aas, J. and Guy, B. S. (1972). Inflammatory bowel disease cytophilic antibody and the cytotoxicity of lymphocytes for colonic cells *in vitro*. *Am. J. Dig. Diseases* **16**, 673.

Strickland, R. G., Bhathal, P. S., Korman, M. G. and Hansky, J. (1971). Serum gastrin and the antral mucosa in atrophic gastritis. *Brit. Med. J.* **iv**, 451.

Taylor, K. B. (1959). Inhibition of intrinsic factor by pernicious anaemia sera. *Lancet* **ii**, 106.

Taylor, K. B., Truelove, S. C. and Wright, R. (1964). Serologic reactions to gluten and cow's milk proteins in gastrointestinal disease. *Gastroenterology* **46**, 99.

Taylor, K. B. (1972). Immune mechanisms and diseases of the gastrointestinal tract. "Recent Advances in Gastroenterology." (Eds. Badenock, J. and Brooke, B. N.), Churchill-Livingstone.

Walker, W. A., Isselbacher, K. J. and Bloch, H. A. (1973). Intestinal uptake of macromolecules. II. Effect of parenteral immunisation. *J. Immunol.* **221**.

Watson, D. W. (1969). Immune responses and the gut. *Gastroenterology* **56**, 944.

Wright, R. and Truelove, S. C. (1965). A controlled therapeutic trial of various diets in ulcerative colitis. *Brit. Med. J.* **ii**, 138.

Wright, R., Whitehead, R., Wangel, A. G., Salem, S. N. and Schiller, K. F. R. (1966). Autoantibodies and microscopic appearance of gastric mucosa. *Lancet* **i**, 618.

19

Liver Disease

O. EADE and R. WRIGHT

THE ROLE OF THE LIVER IN IMMUNOLOGICAL RESPONSES

The strategic interposition of the Kupffer cells of the liver between the gastrointestinal tract and antibody-forming cells elsewhere may regulate immune responses to antigenic stimuli arising from bacterial and viral colonization of the gut and ingestion of dietary antigens.

The Chase-Sultzberger phenomenon—that is, specific immunological unresponsiveness induced by oral administration of haptens—was first observed in guinea-pigs in which it was shown that feeding DNCB prevents subsequent development of delayed hypersensitivity to this hapten administered subcutaneously. Cantor and Dumont (1967) showed that the liver plays a central role in tolerance to orally administered haptens. Feeding of DNCB to adult dogs before subcutaneous injection of the hapten suppressed formation of specific circulating antibodies but this effect was abolished by prior porta-caval anastomosis when a normal antibody response was obtained. They suggested that the Kupffer cells of the liver sequester antigens rather than process them for antibody formation and that this results in immunological unresponsiveness to the antigen. Should Kupffer cells fail to sequester antigen absorbed from the gut either through functional impairment or because of shunting of portal blood, hypergammaglobulinaemia would result.

We have examined this possibility by comparing the immune response of rats to repeated injection of sheep red blood cells (SRBC) into the portal vein with that of rats injected via the inferior vena cava. The antibody response as measured by circulating haemagglutinins and haemolysins was reduced after portal vein injection as compared with inferior vena cava injection.

In addition, cell mediated immunity as determined by ear thickness twenty-four hours after intra-auricular injection of antigen was demonstrated in animals injected via the inferior vena cava but not in those injected by the portal vein. Studies of the organ distribution of labelled antigens support the concept that the Kupffer cells are capable of taking up and processing antigen without initiating antibody formation (Triger and Wright, 1973a).

Circumstantial evidence in man is the presence of high titre antibodies to two gut-associated bacteria, *E. coli* and *Bacteroides*, in patients with liver disease, especially chronic active hepatitis, whereas titres of antibodies to non-gut associated bacteria such as *Haemophilus influenzae B* are unremarkable. In addition, high-titre antibodies to dietary antigens such as gluten fraction III are significantly increased in cirrhosis (Triger *et al.*, 1972). Bjørneboe *et al.* (1972) have shown that *E. coli* antibody titres increase in patients with cirrhosis of the liver who have undergone porta-caval shunt. These findings have been reinforced experimentally by Keraan *et al.* (1974) who produced increased serum immunoglobulin levels and *E. coli* antibody titres in rats following porta-caval shunting.

Thomas *et al.* (1973) concluded that the nature of the antigen may be critical, since soluble antigen such as bovine serum albumin is not taken up by Kupffer cells but when preformed immune complexes are injected sequestration occurs. In cirrhotic rats there is impairment of the liver's ability to trap such immune complexes, as well as particulate antigens such as *Salmonella adelaide*.

We have found high titres of antibodies to measles, rubella and cytomegalovirus in chronic active hepatitis, but these cannot be explained in the same way and we think it likely that they may be due to release of antigen sequestered in the liver or to persistent viral infection. We have therefore suggested that a variety of non-specific factors may be important in the development of the hyperglobulinaemia in liver disease as well as a direct response to gut-associated bacteria or other infectious agents (Triger and Wright, 1973b). Products of liver tissue breakdown and bacterial endotoxin may also contribute by acting as adjuvants.

Failure of Kupffer cells to sequester antigen may have clinical consequences in cirrhosis, and probably accounts for the high incidence of gram-negative septicaemia. Liver macrophages may in addition play a role in the pathogenesis of liver disease by failing to terminate viral infection, by failing to sequester specific immune complexes or by participating in local cytotoxic immunological reactions by interaction with lymphocytes. In acute viral hepatitis in animals persistent viral replication occurs in Kupffer cells with spill-over and infection of the hepatocytes, or, after transient infection of the

Kupffer cells, replication may occur in the hepatocytes (Sabesin and Koff, 1974a,b). Impaired Kupffer cell function in man could be an intrinsic abnormality or result from blockade by competitive phagocytosis of autoantigens or exogenous antigens such as enterobacteria. Such impairment might produce acute or chronic liver injury.

ACUTE VIRAL HEPATITIS

Australia Antigen

The discovery of the Australia antigen (HB Ag) by Blumberg *et al.* (1965), and the recognition of its specific association with hepatitis B infections have been important steps towards understanding the immunopathology of acute viral hepatitis and the pathogenesis of certain chronic liver diseases.

The antigen, initially thought to be a new serum protein allotype, was detected by immunodiffusion against the serum of a haemophiliac patient who had had multiple blood transfusions. Subsequently, more sensitive techniques such as counter-immunoelectrophoresis, passive haemagglutination and radioimmunoassay have been used.

It was not clear at first whether the antigen was confined to hepatitis B infection, but Giles *et al.* (1969) at the Willowbrook State School in New York showed conclusively that the antigen was associated only with hepatitis B. They studied two human serum pools MS-1 and MS-2, the MS-1 pool from short incubation virus A infections, and the MS-2 pool from virus B infections. HB Ag was only found in the MS-2 serum pool and in the sera of children who had been inoculated with MS-2 serum. Serial studies showed that the antigen appeared in the serum before elevation of the transaminase, and that infection could also be transmitted by the oral route, although then the incubation period was longer.

There is a remarkable geographical variation in the frequency of positive tests for antigen in the sera of apparently healthy individuals, from 0·01% in North America and Western Europe to 20% in certain parts of Southeast Asia (Blumberg, 1972). The carrier state may be induced by inapparent inoculation or by insect vectors, scarification and tattooing. Chronic carriers are more likely to be male than female and often become so in early life. Carriers are usually symptom-free and their liver biopsy findings range from complete normality to chronic aggressive hepatitis with or without cirrhosis (see below).

Under the electron microscope, the antigen consists of small spherical forms 20 nm in diameter, long tubular forms and large particles which were first described by Dane *et al.* (1970) (Fig. 1). The Dane particle is 42–44 nm in diameter with a central hexagonal core, and a coat. The core (HBc Ag) is the virus and is immunologically distinct from the coat as well as from the small spherical and tubular forms, which are excess viral protein coat or surface material (HBs Ag), the Australia antigen itself. The core particles can be demonstrated in liver cell nuclei by electron microscopy and by immunofluorescence; the HBs Ag is added in the cytoplasm of the liver cells.

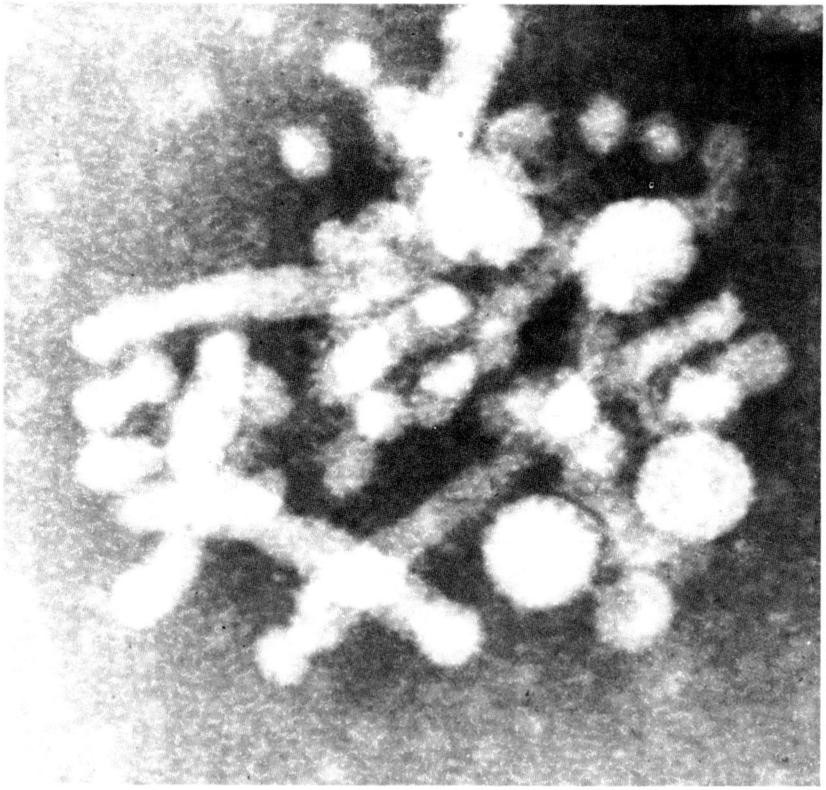

Fig. 1. Electron micrograph of hepatitis B antigen by negative staining (×300,000). Note the small tubular and Dane particles clumped by antibody—the Dane particle has an internal hexagonal core.

The hepatitis surface antigen is a beta-lipoprotein with a carbohydrate component. Nucleic acid cannot be demonstrated in purified small particles, and this, with their other biophysical characteristics, including low buoyant density for size, is evidence that the surface antigen is not the complete virus. It is resistant to heating at 56°C, to freezing and thawing, to treatment with Tween 80 and to moderate changes in pH. Loss of antigenic activity follows reduction of disulphide bonds, and digestion with faeces, intestinal homogenates and by certain bacteria.

There are antigenic differences in the hepatitis B surface antigen itself, and several subtypes have been defined (Le Bouvier, 1971; Bancroft *et al.*, 1972). There is a common antigenic determinant designated *a* and two other mutually exclusive determinants, *d* and *y*, all positive sera being either *ad* or *ay*. Two additional specificities, *w* and *r*, have also been described. The differential geographical distribution of these subtypes (Fig. 2) make them useful in epidemiological studies, but although subtypes may correlate with severity and type of liver disease in any given geographical location, there is no evidence that they directly determine virulence or the nature of the hepatic pathology.

Subtyping of HBs Ag-positive individuals can provide clues to the method of spread in a community. It has also provided information on the duration of the carrier state, e.g. subtyping of symptom-free blood donors in Toronto

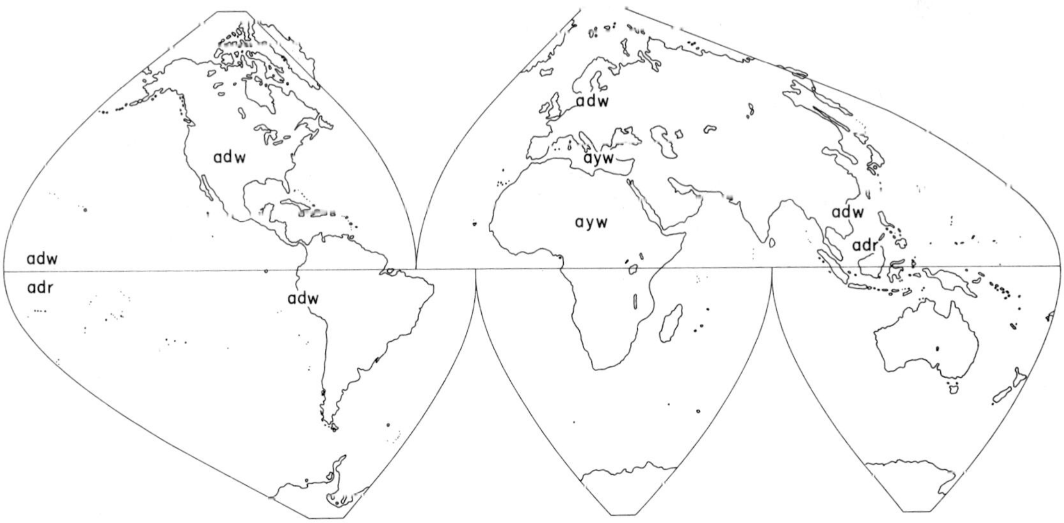

Fig. 2. Geographical distribution of HBs Ag subtypes (from Mazzur *et al.*, 1973).

showed that their subtype was determined by their country of birth rather than their country of domicile.

A different antigen–antibody system associated with HBs Ag-positive sera has recently been described by Magnius and Espmark (1972), and has been given the designation *e*. The *e* antigens and antibodies have been detected only in HBs Ag-positive sera and, according to one study from Copenhagen, the *e* antigen occurs most commonly in patients with chronic hepatitis. In acute hepatitis, its presence indicates a poor prognosis, progression to cirrhosis being common. The nature of the *e* antigen, whether virus or host derived, is still uncertain.

The core of the Dane particle (HBc Ag) is 27 nm in diameter, and can be clumped with anti-core antibody after removal of the outer coat (HBs Ag) by treatment with Tween 80. The core particles have a greater buoyant density than the HBs Ag, and have DNA polymerase activity. Double-stranded DNA has been isolated from these naked intranuclear particles, but it is not yet clear whether the DNA is double-stranded in the virion or whether a helper virus is necessary for replication.

Serial studies after infection with hepatitis B suggest the following sequence of events (Table 1): As early as two months after exposure, HBs Ag can be detected in the serum, followed by DNA polymerase activity (presumably at the height of viral replication) and the appearance of antibody to the HB core antigen (HBc Ag) just before or at the time of initial elevation of the serum transaminase. Later in the disease, usually five to six months after infection, antibody to the surface antigen (HBs Ag) appears. By immunodiffusion, antibody to HBs Ag is seldom detected after natural infection, but the more sensitive radioimmunoassay shows primary and secondary responses. Although anti-HBs Ag is protective, it is usually present only at low titre, and it is not known for how long it persists. There is evidence that a cell mediated immune response to HBs Ag also occurs early in the infection.

TABLE 1

Sequence of events after infection with Hepatitis B virus (after Krugman et al., *1974)*

Months after exposure	0	1	2		3	4	5	6	7	8
SGOT					+	+				
DNA polymerase				+						
HBs Ag		+	+	+	+					
Anti-HBc				+	+	+	+	+	+	
Anti-HBs							+	+	+	

Immunopathological Mechanisms in Acute Viral Hepatitis

Studies of the hepatitis B antigen have provided insight into possible immunopathological mechanisms involved in producing both the liver disease and the extrahepatic manifestations of acute viral hepatitis. Immune complexes of HBs Ag and antibody can be detected in serum by electron microscopy, and deposition of these immune complexes in extrahepatic tissues is responsible for the arthritis, polyarteritis and glomerulonephritis sometimes seen in hepatitis B infection. The HBs Ag and complement have been demonstrated by immunofluorescence in these tissues, and serum complement levels may be low.

The mechanism of the hepatic injury is, however, less clear cut. Initially it was thought that the severity of hepatic damage was correlated with the presence of immune complexes in serum, but there is no direct evidence of significant immune complex deposition in the parenchymal tissue in acute viral hepatitis. The HBs Ag, however, is readily detectable by immunofluorescence in the cytoplasm of the apparently normal hepatocytes of chronic carriers of the antigen. A cell-mediated immune response to the hepatitis B surface antigen may be responsible for eliminating the infection and a defect here might result in the carrier state, but it is not clear whether cell mediated immunity plays a role in tissue injury. Analogy with viral infections in animals suggests that antibody or lymphocyte-mediated cytotoxicity directed against the HB Ag on the hepatic cell surface might be the damaging mechanism. Alternatively, a direct lytic action of the virus on liver cells is a possibility. Also by analogy with animal hepatitis, it is possible that Kupffer cells play a central role in regulating the replication of the virus, as mentioned above.

Non-specific Immunological Features in Viral Hepatitis

As with some other viral infections, non-specific depression of cell mediated immunity as shown by both skin-testing and *in vitro* tests of lymphocyte function occurs in acute viral hepatitis. As already mentioned, a defective cell mediated immune response to the HBs Ag could be responsible for the development of the carrier state, and it is known that the latter is more likely to be found in patients with impaired cell mediated immunity, e.g. lepromatous leprosy, Hodgkin's disease, Down's syndrome and uraemia. In addition, there are alterations in serum complement levels, immunoglobulin disturbances and elevated antibody titres to a variety of bacterial, viral and auto-antigens in viral hepatitis.

Interpretation of the low serum complement levels which may occur initially is complicated by the possibility of decreased synthesis by the damaged liver, and there may be subsequent over-production in response to low levels. IgM levels are frequently elevated in hepatitis A infections, but not in HBs Ag-positive infections, whereas IgG levels may be slightly elevated in both. There is also non-specific elevation of antibodies to gut-associated bacteria such as *E. coli* and to a variety of unidentified faecal antigens (Triger *et al.*, 1972; Almeida *et al.*, 1974). This probably results from the failure of Kupffer cells in the diseased liver to sequester antigens or from their abnormal release after liver damage. An antibody reacting with smooth muscle is present in the sera of a high proportion of patients with acute viral hepatitis, whether HBs antigen-positive or negative, and may indicate alteration of a component of liver cell membrane resembling smooth muscle actomyosin (Holborow, 1972).

Immunotherapy and Prophylaxis of Hepatitis B Infection

The possibility of using active and passive immunization to prevent hepatitis B infection is being intensively investigated. In one study, specific immune globulin to the HBs Ag and heat-inactivated HB Ag-positive serum has had a protective effect, inoculation preventing or attenuating subsequent infection and decreasing the carrier rate. Clinical trials are being undertaken, particularly in the newborn infants of mothers who are carriers of the HBs Ag, or who have had acute HB Ag-positive hepatitis during pregnancy. Specific immune globulin or transfer factor have been used to treat acute or chronic liver disease, but both are still to be evaluated.

Hepatitis A Infection

Viral particles 27 nm in diameter have been detected in the stools of acute phase HB Ag-negative hepatitis. These particles appear in the stools five days before elevation of the serum transaminase, and are probably identical with the particles detected in the livers of marmoset monkeys to which type A hepatitis has been transmitted (Lancet, 1975). The significance of these findings is still uncertain and caution is necessary in interpreting clumping of viral particles in stools by convalescent serum, since a variety of immune responses to non-pathogenic agents in stools has been reported following acute viral hepatitis.

CHRONIC PERSISTENT HEPATITIS

It is well known that a proportion of patients with viral hepatitis, including either virus A or virus B infections, continue to have symptoms and signs of liver disease for months or years after the onset. If liver biopsy shows only minor changes, such as cellular infiltration and expansion of the portal triads, the condition is known as chronic persistent hepatitis. Such cases do not show immunological abnormalities, smooth muscle antibodies being infrequent and immunoglobulins normal, or only marginally elevated. Although the hepatitis B antigen may persist in the serum, the prognosis is good. Cases showing bridging necrosis on biopsy or features of chronic aggressive hepatitis are indistinguishable from chronic active hepatitis, which is discussed below.

Since the discovery of the HB Ag, it has been recognized increasingly that some patients showing hepatomegaly or abnormality of liver function tests but without a history of acute viral hepatitis have had anicteric infections with hepatitis B. Subjects found on routine screening to have the hepatitis B antigen may or may not have evidence of hepatomegaly and liver dysfunction, and the liver biopsy shows changes which vary from normality or mild liver cell dysplasia to a frank chronic aggressive hepatitis with or without cirrhosis.

HB Ag-positive Chronic Active Hepatitis

It was realized before the discovery of the HB antigen that some cases of acute viral hepatitis progress to a chronic aggressive hepatitis or cirrhosis, and its use as a marker of hepatitis B infections has since shown that chronic active hepatitis or cirrhosis may also follow anicteric infection.

In cases which start with an acute disease resembling viral hepatitis, it has been possible to trace progression to an active cirrhosis with the HB antigen in the serum, and this implies persistence of the hepatitis B virus as the cause. The frequency with which the HB Ag is detected in the serum of patients with chronic active hepatitis or cirrhosis varies greatly in different parts of the world, and probably reflects geographical differences in the prevalence of the hepatitis B virus carrier state in the community. It is low in Great Britain and the United States, but high in central Europe, Africa and Asia (Wright, 1972).

There is as yet no direct evidence that hepatitis A can progress to chronic active hepatitis or cirrhosis.

Chronic Active Hepatitis of Unknown Aetiology

HB Ag-negative chronic active hepatitis is a form of progressive liver disease occurring predominantly in females and associated with a high frequency of multisystem involvement and immunological disturbances. About 15–20% of cases begin acutely and are indistinguishable from viral hepatitis, but in others the jaundice is mild though often persistent, with pronounced spider naevi and palmar erythema. It may be associated with other disorders which may have an immunological basis, such as ulcerative colitis, arthritis, arthralgia, fibrosing alveolitis, Sjögren's syndrome, glomerulonephritis, renal tubular acidosis and a variety of endocrine and haematological disorders. Liver function tests are usually grossly abnormal, but may fluctuate, their pattern being that of hepatocellular damage.

Established active cirrhosis may be seen on liver biopsy at the time of clinical presentation, but the characteristic lesion is a heavy infiltrate of plasma cells and lymphocytes, with liver cell destruction and loss of the limiting plate of hepatic lobules, which has given rise to the term "piecemeal necrosis". The response to corticosteroids may be initially good, but the prognosis is poor.

Immunological Abnormalities

Hyperglobulinaemia is a striking serological abnormality, and a proportion of patients give a positive LE cell test.

Circulating antibodies, notably anti-nuclear antibody (ANA) is present in the serum of over half the patients with chronic active hepatitis, and is often associated with high titre antibodies to smooth muscle. The smooth muscle antibodies sometimes show concomitant staining of renal glomeruli. Although often present at highest titres in chronic active hepatitis, smooth muscle antibody is not specific for this disorder, and is seen in other liver disease, acute viral infections such as infectious mononucleosis, and in some neoplastic disorders (Holborow, 1972).

DNA binding antibodies, originally thought to be specific for systemic lupus erythematosus, have recently also been reported in patients with chronic active hepatitis (Davis and Read, 1975). High-titre antibodies to a variety of antigens, including dietary and viral and bacterial antigens, have also been described. The significance of these is uncertain, the bacterial antibodies involved being against microorganisms which colonize the normal gut, but they may arise, as discussed above, following ineffective sequestration of gut-derived antigens by damaged Kupffer cells. The high-titre antibodies to measles, rubella and cytomegalovirus which are also found may represent release of antigen sequestered in Kupffer cells as a result of tissue damage, or persistent infection with these viruses.

Serum immunoglobulins, particularly IgG, are elevated in about 70% of patients with chronic active hepatitis, and to a lesser extent IgA and IgM levels. Low serum complement has also been reported but, as with acute viral hepatitis, it is not known whether this represents immune complex formation or impaired synthesis by the liver.

That genetic factors may be important is suggested by the high incidence of HLA-B1 and HLA-B8 antigens in HB antigen-negative chronic active hepatitis (MacKay and Morris, 1972).

Impairment of cell-mediated responses has been demonstrated in chronic active hepatitis by skin-testing with dinitrochlorobenzene and by lymphocyte stimulation with phytohaemagglutinin, and a decrease in the number of circulating T-lymphocytes has also been reported, but results are conflicting. Studies of cell-mediated immunity to autologous or heterologous liver tissue, using lymphocyte transformation, have also been inconclusive, but sensitization to human foetal and adult liver has been demonstrated by leucocyte migration inhibition. Two human liver-specific antigens active in the latter, one a lipoprotein which appears to be a normal constituent of the liver cell membrane and the other a soluble cytoplasmic antigen, have been identified by Meyer zum Büschenfelde and Miescher (1972). Repeated immunization of rabbits with a mixture of these antigens produces inflammatory lesions in the liver which closely resemble chronic active hepatitis.

Leucocyte migration inhibition by HBs antigen has been reported in patients with both antigen-negative and antigen-positive chronic active hepatitis, and on this basis the concept has been put forward that HB antigen-negative chronic active hepatitis represents an autoimmune response to hepatitis B virus infection (Eddleston and Williams, 1974). However, on clinical and epidemiological grounds this seems unlikely.

Recently, there have been reports of specific cytotoxicity of lymphocytes from patients with chronic active hepatitis against homologous or heterologous liver cells in tissue culture, or against rabbit hepatocytes. Factors in human serum which block this reaction have been described, and it has also been reported that rabbit liver-specific lipoprotein will block the reaction of patients' lymphocytes against rabbit hepatocytes. Blocking factors in the serum of patients with chronic active hepatitis or acute viral hepatitis, have also been described which inhibit stimulation by phytohaemagglutinin. The nature of these blocking factors and their significance have yet to be determined, but they may be immune complexes or lymphocytotoxins (Paronetto and Vernace, 1975).

PRIMARY BILIARY CIRRHOSIS

In its advanced form, primary biliary cirrhosis is associated with prolonged intrahepatic cholestasis, pruritis, jaundice, steatorrhoea, pigmentation of the skin, xanthomata, xanthelasma and hepatosplenomegaly. It occurs most commonly in middle-aged or elderly females. The onset is usually insidious, often with pruritis. Signs of hepatic decompensation or portal hypertension may not develop for years. Evidence of multisystem involvement is not as striking as with chronic active hepatitis, but it has been seen in association with scleroderma, the sicca syndrome and renal tubular acidosis.

The fibrosis in the liver is often patchy, the earliest and most striking lesions being in the portal triads, where there is an inflammatory infiltrate of lymphocytes, plasma cells and some eosinophils, causing destruction of septal and interlobular ducts. A granulomatous reaction may occur, both in the liver and in the draining lymph nodes, which may be enlarged.

There is often considerable overlap with features of chronic active hepatitis, particularly in the early stages, and Doniach and Walker (1969) have presented a unified concept of auto-immune hepatitis. The serum bilirubin and transaminase levels are usually only mildly elevated, and the most striking abnormality is in the alkaline phosphatase and cholesterol. Immunosuppressive drugs are ineffective.

Immunological Abnormalities

Circulating antibodies to smooth muscle and anti-nuclear factor are detected in a smaller proportion of patients with primary biliary cirrhosis than with chronic active hepatitis, and antibodies to bile ducts have been found, but are not specific for the disease. The immunoglobulin levels, predominantly IgM, are often raised, and IgM-containing cells have been demonstrated in the liver in relation to damaged bile ducts.

The most striking abnormality is an antibody reacting with mitochondria (AMA). This was described by Walker *et al.* (1965) and may be detected by complement fixation or by indirect immunofluorescence. With the latter technique, there is a granular pattern of staining, strongest with distal renal tubular cells, gastric parietal cells and thyroid acinar cells. The mitochondrial antibody is present in approximately 90% of patients with primary biliary cirrhosis (Walker *et al.*, 1965; Klatskin and Kantor, 1972), but is rare in extrahepatic obstruction, so that it has proved of value in the diagnosis of prolonged cholestatic jaundice. The frequency with which it occurs in chronic active hepatitis and cryptogenic cirrhosis varies from 12 to 25%, but the titres are usually lower, and it is rare in other forms of liver disease. The AMA cannot be related to clinical features or the stage of the primary biliary cirrhosis, is unaffected by immunosuppressive drugs, and falls only transiently after liver transplantation.

When liver biopsies have been performed on patients found to have a mitochondrial antibody on routine screening, evidence of early subclinical liver disease has been observed, but it is not known whether these lesions progress. There is an increased incidence of mitochondrial and other auto-antibodies in the relatives of patients with primary biliary cirrhosis (Feizi *et al.*, 1972). Berg *et al.*, (1969) have concluded that mitochondrial antibody reacts with a lipoprotein localized to inner mitochondrial membrane, particularly in the mitochondria of cells engaged in high energy activity. The AMA of primary biliary cirrhosis is distinguishable from other types of mitochondrial antibody, as well as from microsomal antibody (Rizzetto *et al.*, 1973) which occur in the sera of patients with syphilis or with a variety of auto-immune disorders with biologic false positive reactions for syphilis.

There is no evidence that the mitochondrial antibody plays a role in the pathogenesis of primary biliary cirrhosis, but the structure of mitochondrial inner membranes resembles that of the outer coats of some viruses and bacteria, raising the possibility that the antibody may be generated by cross-reacting unidentified microorganisms.

Patients with primary biliary cirrhosis show an even greater depression of delayed hypersensitivity reactions than patients with chronic active hepatitis. There is depression of skin sensitivity to both DNCB and tuberculin, and of lymphocyte transformation in response to phytohaemagglutinin and such patients show inhibition of leucocyte migration to liver-specific lipoprotein and biliary antigens, though to a lesser degree than patients with chronic active hepatitis (Miller *et al.*, 1972).

CRYPTOGENIC CIRRHOSIS

Cryptogenic cirrhosis is the commonest type of cirrhosis in Britain. It usually presents late with portal hypertension or hepatic decompensation. It is probably due to a variety of causes, including anicteric viral infection, but may also result from an auto-immune response, since anti-nuclear factor and smooth muscle antibody are present in 25 to 40% of cases.

ALCOHOLIC LIVER DISEASE

Alcohol-induced liver damage may be manifest as a fatty liver, as an alcoholic hepatitis with liver-cell necrosis and polymorpho-nuclear infiltration, or as an established cirrhosis. The development of cirrhosis depends on the average daily consumption of alcohol, and the duration of excessive intake. However, there is considerable individual variation in susceptibility to develop cirrhosis, which may in part be genetically determined.

There is no direct evidence that immunological mechanisms are concerned in the pathogenesis of the liver disease but there are some immunological features. Berenyi *et al.* (1974) showed depressed delayed hypersensitivity response to DNCB in 80% of patients with alcoholic liver disease. The PHA responsiveness of circulating lymphocytes does not differ from that in alcoholic patients without evidence of liver disease but a reduction in T-lymphocytes has been reported. Inhibition of leucocyte migration in response to antigens extracted from liver tissue of patients with alcoholic hepatitis is reported, and suggests that cell mediated immunity plays a part (Mihas *et al.*, 1975).

Immunoglobulins may be elevated in alcoholic cirrhosis as in other forms of chronic liver disease. In particular, there may be elevation of IgA (Feizi, 1968) but there is no significant increase in auto-antibodies.

HEPATIC DRUG SENSITIVITY

Many drugs may cause liver dysfunction, some by direct toxic effect, some indirectly due to metabolic idiosyncrasy, and some as a result of a hypersensitivity reaction. Evidence for the latter is generally circumstantial, and based largely on clinical observations. In hepatic drug hypersensitivity, the liver injury occurs in only a small proportion of patients taking the drug, is not dose-dependent and generally cannot be reproduced in experimental animals. There may be extra-hepatic manifestations of hypersensitivity, such as fever, skin rashes, arthritis and eosinophilia. Skin testing is usually negative and tests for antibody or for *in vitro* evidence of delayed hypersensitivity to the drug by the usual techniques are not helpful. Metabolic idiosyncrasies may predispose; for example Lal *et al.* (1972) have shown a predominance of slow acetylators among patients who developed liver damage on therapy with isoniazid and rifampicin.

TABLE 2

Classification of hepatic drug hypersensitivity reactions

Predominantly Hepatocellular	Predominantly cholestatic	"Mixed"
α-methyldopa	[a]Chlorpromazine (and other phenothiazines)	[a]PAS
Amitriptyline	[a]Chlorpropamide	Isoniazid
Phenytoin sodium	Tolbutamide	Sulphonamides
Tridione	Imipramine	[a]Sulphones
Propylthiouracil	Erythromycin estolate	Phenindione
Halothane	Thiouracil	Procainamide
methoxyflurane		
Oxyphenisatin	Chlordiazepoxide	Phenylbutazone

[a]Incidence 0·5–5%.

The types of liver injury are cholestatic, hepatocellular or mixed (Table 2). Apart from occasional eosinophilic infiltration of the liver, or granuloma formation, there are usually no histological indications of hypersensitivity.

Cholestatic Drug Hypersensitivity

Phenothiazines, in particular chlorpromazine, anti-thyroid drugs and oral hypoglycaemic agents, are the drugs most likely to cause this type of reaction. The jaundice due to chlorpromazine usually develops one to four weeks after administration of the drug, although it may occur after a single dose. Although re-administration of chlorpromazine results in a relapse in about half of the cases, the jaundice may fade despite continuance with the drug.

Hepatocellular Damage Due to Drug Sensitivity

A hepatitis-like reaction, indistinguishable clinically and histologically from viral hepatitis, may occur with a number of drugs, and is often severe and sometimes fatal. Such reactions have been reported with the monoamine oxidase inhibitors, other hydrazine derivatives such as phenelzine, and isoniazid, sulphonamides, phenindione and PAS. A bizarre picture called "pseudomononucleosis" has been seen with PAS therapy, in which the liver disease is accompanied by a glandular fever-like illness with lymphadenopathy and atypical lymphocytes in the blood.

Both alpha-methyldopa (Toghill *et al.*, 1974) and oxyphenisatin (Reynolds *et al.*, 1971) can cause chronic liver disease resembling chronic active hepatitis, with positive anti-nuclear antibody and LE cell formation. The activity of the liver disease regresses on withdrawing the drug. Alpha-methyldopa may also produce a Coombs positive haemolytic anaemia caused by an antibody with rhesus specificity. The drug itself does not appear to act as a hapten, and the precise mechanisms by which the anaemia and the auto-immune liver disease develop are unknown.

There has been much controvery over the reported association between post-operative hepatic necrosis and exposure to the anaesthetic agent halothane. That halothane may produce liver damage is well-documented in certain cases (Moult and Sherlock, 1975) and a recent study (Wright *et al.*, 1975) comparing the effects on liver function tests of halothane with a non-halothane anaesthetic suggests that a significant number of patients develop minor abnormalities after repeated exposures to the drug. Mortality due to halothane-induced liver injury appears to be extremely low.

It has been suggested that halothane-induced liver injury is based on a hypersensitivity reaction, since it may be associated with fever, rigors, eosinophilia and skin rashes. The liver histology shows features which are usually identical with those of viral hepatitis, although ultrastructural differences have been reported.

Paronetto and Popper (1970) reported increased lymphocyte transformation in response to halothane in 10 out of 15 patients, but other workers have failed to demonstrate any *in vitro* evidence of delayed hypersensitivity to halothane or its major metabolite trifluoracetate (Walton *et al.*, 1974).

Halothane metabolism in man leads to formation of higher molecular weight products which are more likely to act as haptens than halothane itself. Halothane or its metabolites may bind covalently to protein in the liver and Mathieu *et al.* (1974) recently induced delayed hypersensitivity in guinea-pigs given trifluoroacetate conjugated with guinea-pig albumin.

The finding of low-titre anti-mitochondrial antibodies by Rodriguez *et al.* (1969) in patients with halothane hepatitis supports an immunological basis for this condition, but others have obtained negative results. Anti-mitochondrial antibodies and liver damage have also been demonstrated experimentally in rats pre-treated with phenobarbitone following repeated exposure to halothane but it is doubtful whether this is an animal model of human halothane sensitivity.

IMMUNOLOGICAL FEATURES OF GASTROINTESTINAL AND LIVER TUMOURS

Skin tests show depressed cellular immunity to DNCB and a variety of other antigens in patients with gastrointestinal cancer. In addition, reduced PHA transformation of circulating lymphocytes and lymph-node lymphocytes from patients with gastrointestinal carcinomas supports the concept of impairment of cell mediated immunity in these conditions. Serum factors may be present in these patients that reduce lymphocyte transformation, and humoral antibody responses may be depressed.

Despite immunological suppression in gastrointestinal cancer it is possible to demonstrate tumour-specific immunity. Cellular immunity to tumour extracts has been shown by skin tests and by *in vitro* tests of leucocyte reactivity, and lymphocytes from patients with carcinoma of the colon may be cytotoxic to cultured autologous tumour cells. It is possible that serum factors (e.g. immune complexes) may block this immune response and thus enhance tumour growth and spread (see Chapter 28). A recent study has shown the presence of anti-IgG antibodies in patients with colonic carcinoma, and these may be capable of blocking the cytotoxic effect of anti-tumour antibody (Hartman and Lewis, 1974).

Immunotherapy

There have been attempts to enhance cellular immunity to gut neoplasms by means of immunotherapy. Cross-immunization with tumour cell extracts and transfusion of sensitized leucocytes thus obtained have produced some effects in patients with advanced colonic carcinoma. Alternatively, sensitized lymphocytes have been prepared by immunizing pigs with human tumour cells and removing the mesenteric lymph-nodes. Out of three patients with colonic carcinoma treated with suspensions of sensitized pig lymphocytes, two were reported to have made clinical responses.

Onco-foetal Antigens

Carcino-Embryonic Antigen

The discovery that carcino-embryonic antigen (CEA), a glyco-protein normally present in the digestive tract of the two to five month old foetus, re-appears in the blood of patients with carcinoma of the large bowel raised the possibility of a specific screening test for gastrointestinal cancer. The CEA is detected in the plasma by gel-diffusion or by radioimmunoassay. Although present in most cases of colono-rectal carcinomas, it also occurs in carcinoma of the pancreas and in a number of benign conditions including inflammatory bowel disease. The overlap of CEA levels in colonic carcinoma patients and in normal people is considerable, so that the usefulness of CEA measurement as a diagnostic test is limited. However, it may prove to be of value in follow-up of patients after colectomy for carcinoma of the colon if a rise in CEA level antedates clinical symptoms due to recurrence of the tumour.

Alpha-Foeto-Protein

The finding of alpha-foeto-protein in the serum of an adult is almost diagnostic of a hepatoma. This protein, an alpha-1-globulin, is present in foetal serum in high concentration but subsequently is detectable only in minute amounts. Following the discovery of elevated levels of alpha-foeto-protein in the serum of patients with primary hepato-cellular carcinomas, the value of this test in the diagnosis of hepatoma has become established. There is a marked geographical variation in positivity rates for alpha-foeto-protein in hepato-cellular cancer. Alpha-foeto-protein is detectable in the serum of approximately 30% of patients with hepatomas in the United Kingdom, compared with 87% in a series from Indonesia. Elevated levels are also reported in association with other tumours, in particular undifferentiated terato-carcinomas. By more sensitive techniques the antigen has been found in various other forms of liver disease including acute viral hepatitis. In the latter, the alpha-foeto-protein level generally parallels changes in transaminase levels, suggesting that it is in some way related to liver injury.

PANCREAS

Pancreatitis

Although a number of aetiological factors have been identified in both acute and chronic pancreatitis, the pathogenesis of these conditions remains obscure and it may be that immunological mechanisms are at least in part concerned. Many cases of pancreatitis are associated with alcoholism, biliary tract disease and malnutrition, but in some no such factors are evident.

Circulating antibodies to pancreatic tissue may appear in patients with pancreatitis but could well be secondary to pancreatic damage. Similarly, increased lymphocyte transformation in response to pancreatic tissue extracts in pancreatitis may be secondary. Raised immunoglobulin levels, in particular IgA, are found in a proportion of cases of calcific pancreatitis. A recent study demonstrating by immunofluorescence the presence of antibodies to pancreatic tissue in acute pancreatitis lends support to the view that auto-immune mechanisms may be involved (Lendrum and Walker, 1975).

Diabetes Mellitus and Auto-immunity

There is an increased incidence of auto-immune thyroid disease and pernicious anaemia amongst patients with diabetes mellitus and their first degree relatives. In addition, some 14% of patients with auto-immune adrenalitis are diabetic. As with thyrotoxicosis and idiopathic Addison's disease, the histocompatibility antigen HLA-B8 occurs more frequently amongst juvenile-onset insulin-dependent diabetics than in the normal population, raising the possibility that immune response (Ir) genes play a part.

Lymphocytic infiltration of the islets of Langerhans is present in some young diabetics though this appears to be transient. Nerup *et al.* (1971) demonstrated in diabetics T-cell sensitization to pancreatic antigen, using the leucocyte migration inhibition test. More recently, the presence of an islet-cell antibody detectable by immunofluorescence has been discovered in the sera of diabetic patients with other auto-immune disorders (Bottazzo *et al.*, 1974; MacCuish *et al.*, 1974) (see Chapter 12).

REFERENCES

Almeida, J., Gay, F. W. and Wreighitt, T. G. (1974). Pitfalls in the study of hepatitis A. *Lancet* **ii**, 748.

Bancroft, W. H., Mundon, F. K. and Russell, P. K. (1972). Detection of additional antigenic determinants of hepatitis B antigen. *J. Immunol.* **109**, 842.

Berenyi, M. R., Strauss, B. and Cruz, D. (1974). *In vitro* and *in vivo* studies of cellular immunity in alcoholic cirrhosis. *Am. J. Dig. Diseases* **19**, 199.

Berg, P. A., Roitt, I. M. Doniach, D. and Horner, W. (1969). Mitchondrial antibodies in primary biliary cirrhosis. III Characterisation of the inner membrane complement fixing antigen. *Clin. Exp. Immunol.* **4**, 511.

Bjørneboe, M., Prytz, H. and Ørskov, F. (1972). Antibodies to intestinal microbes in serum of patients with cirrhosis of the liver. *Lancet,* **i**, 58.

Blumberg, B. S. (1972). The nature of Australia antigen: Infections and genetic characteristics. *In* "Progress in Liver Disease" (eds. H. Popper and F. Schaffner), pp. 367–379, Grune and Stratton, New York.

Blumberg, B. S., Alter, H. J. and Visnich, S. (1965). A "new" antigen in leukaemia sera. *J. Am. Med. Assoc.* **191**, 541.

Bottazzo, G. F., Florin-Christensen, F. and Doniach, D. (1974). Islet-cell antibodies in diabetes mellitus with autoimmune polyendocrine deficiencies. *Lancet* **ii**, 1279.

Cantor, H. M. and Dumont, A. E. (1967). Hepatic suppression of sensitization to antigen absorbed into the portal system. *Nature (London)* **215**, 744.

Dane, D. S., Cameron, C. H. and Briggs, M. (1970). Virus-like particles in serum of patients with Australia-antigen associated hepatitis. *Lancet* **i**, 695.

Davis, P. and Read, A. E. (1975). Antibodies to double-stranded (native) DNA in active chronic hepatitis. *Gut* **16**, 413.

Doniach, D. and Walker, J. G. (1969). A unified concept of auto-immune hepatitis. *Lancet* **ii**, 813.

Eddleston, A. L. W. F. and Williams, R. (1974). Inadequate antibody response to HB Ag or suppressor T-cell defect in development of active chronic hepatitis. *Lancet* **ii**, 1543.

Feizi, T. (1968). Immunoglobulins in chronic liver disease. *Gut* **9**, 193.

Feizi, T., Naccarato, R., Sherlock, S. and Doniach, D. (1972). Mitochondrial and other tissue antibodies in relatives of patients with primary biliary cirrhosis. *Clin. Exp. Immunol.* **10**, 609.

Giles, J. P., McCollum, R. W., Bernston, L. W. and Krugman, S. (1969). Viral hepatitis—relationship of Australia/SH antigen to the Willowbrook MS-2 strain. *New Eng. J. Med.* **281**, 119.

Hartmann, D. and Lewis, M. G. (1974). Presence and possible role of anti-IgG antibodies in human malignancy. *Lancet* **i**, 1318.

Holborow, E. J. (1972). Immunological aspects of viral hepatitis. *Brit. Med. Bull.* **28**, 142.

Keraan, M., Meyers, O. L., Englbrecht, G. H., Hickman, R., Saunders, S. J. and Terblanche, J. (1974). Increased serum immunoglobulin levels following portacaval shunt in the normal rat. *Gut* **15**, 468.

Klatskin, G. and Kantor, F. S. (1972). Mitochondrial antibody in primary biliary cirrhosis and other diseases. *Ann. Intern. Med.* **77**, 533.

Krugman, S., Hoofnagle, J. H., Gerety, R. J., Kaplan, P. M. and Gerin, J. L. (1974). Viral hepatitis B, DNA polymerase and antibody to HB core antigen. *New Eng. J. Med.* **290**, 1331.

Lal, S., Singhal, S. N., Burley, D. M. and Crossley, G. (1972). The effect of rifampicin and isoniazid on liver function. *Brit. Med. J.* **i**, 148.

Lancet, Editorial (1975). Viral hepatitis updated. *Lancet* **i**, 1365.
Le Bouvier, G. L. (1971). The herogeneity of Australia antigen. *J. Infect. Dis.* **123**, 671.
Lendrum, R. and Walker, G. (1975). Serum antibodies in human pancreatic disease. *Gut* **16**, 365.
MacCuish, A. C., Barnes, E. W., Irvine, W. J. and Duncan, L. J. P. (1974). Antibodies to pancreatic islet cells in insulin dependent diabetics. *Lancet* **ii**, 1529.
Mackay, I. R. and Morris, P. J. (1972). Association of autoimmune active chronic hepatitis with HL-A1 and 8. *Lancet* **ii**, 793.
Magnius, L. O. and Espmark, J. A. (1972). New specificities in Australia antigen positive sera distinct from the Le Bouvier determinants. *J. Immunol.* **109**, 1017.
Mathieu, A., Di Padua, D., Mills, J. and Kahan, B. (1974). Experimental immunity to a metabolite of halothane and fluroxene: cutaneous delayed-type hypersensitivity. *Anaesthesiology* **40**, 385.
Mazzur, S., Falker, D. and Blumberg, B. S. (1973). Geographical variation of the "w" subtype of Australia antigen. *Nature New Biol.* **24**, 344.
Meyer zum Büschenfelde, K. H. and Miescher, P. A. (1972). Liver specific antigens: purification and characterisation. *Clin. Exp. Immunol.* **10**, 89.
Mihas, M. A., Bull, D. M. and Davidson, C. S. (1975). Cell-mediated immunity to liver in patients with alcoholic hepatitis. *Lancet* **i**, 951.
Miller, J., Smith, M. G. M., Mitchell, C. G., Reed, W. D., Eddleston, A. L. W. F. and Williams, R. (1972). Cell-mediated immunity to a human liver specific antigen in patients with active chronic hepatitis and primary biliary cirrhosis. *Lancet* **ii**, 296.
Moult, P. J. A. and Sherlock, S. (1975). Halothane-related hepatitis. *Quart. J. Med.* **173**, 99.
Nerup, J., Anderson, O. O., Bendixen, G., Egeberg, J. and Poulsen, J. E. (1971). Antipancreatic cellular hypersensitivity in diabetes mellitus. *Diabetes* **20**, 424.
Paronetto, F. and Popper, H. (1970). Lymphocyte stimulation induced by halothane in patients with hepatitis following exposure to halothane. *New Eng. J. Med.* **283**, 277.
Paronetto, F. and Vernace, S. J. (1975). Immunological studies in patients with chronic active hepatitis. Cytotoxic activity of lymphocytes to autochthonous liver cells grown in tissue culture. *Clin. Exp. Immunol.* **19**, 99.
Perrett, A. D., Higgins, G., Johnston, H. H., Massarella, G. R., Truelove, S. C. and Wright, R. (1971). The liver in Crohn's disease. *Quart. J. Med.* **40**, 187.
Rambaud, J. C., Boguel, C., Prost, A., Bernier, J. J., Le Quintrec, Y., Lambling, A., Nanon, F., Hurez, D. and Seligmann, M. (1968). Clinico-pathological study of a patient with Mediterranean type of abdominal lymphoma and a new type of IgA abnormality ("alpha chain disease"). *Digestion* **1**, 321.
Reynolds, T. B., Peters, R. L. and Yamada, S. (1971). Chronic active and lupoid hepatitis caused by the laxative oxyphenisatin. *New Eng. J. Med.* **285**, 813.
Rizzetto, M., Swana, G. and Doniach, D. (1973). Microsomal antibodies in active chronic hepatitis and other disorders. *Clin. Exp. Immunol.* **15**, 331.
Rodriguez, M., Paronetto, F., Schaffner, F. and Popper, H. (1969). Anti-mitochondrial antibodies in jaundice following drug administration. *J. Am. Med. Assoc.* **208**, 148.
Sabesin, S. M. and Koff, R. S. (1974a). Pathogenesis of experimental viral hepatitis (1). *New Eng. J. Med.* **290**, 944.
Sabesin, S. M. and Koff, R. S. (1974b). Pathogenesis of experimental viral hepatitis (2). *New Eng. J. Med.* **290**, 996.
Thomas, H. C., MacSween, R. N. M. and White, R. G. (1973). Role of the liver in controlling the immunogenicity of commensal bacteria in the gut. *Lancet* **i**, 1288.
Toghill, P. K., Smith, P. G., Benton, P., Brown, R. C. and Matthews, H. L. (1974). Methyldopa liver damage. *Brit. Med. J.* **iii**, 545.

Triger, D. R., Alp, M. H. and Wright, R. (1972). Bacterial and dietary antibodies in liver disease. *Lancet* **i**, 60.

Triger, D. R. and Wright, R. (1973a). Studies on hepatic uptake of antigen. 2. The effect of hepatotoxins on the immune response. *Immunology* **25**, 951.

Triger, D. R. and Wright, R. (1973b). Hyperglobulinaemia in liver disease. *Lancet* **i**, 1494.

Walker, J. G., Doniach, D., Roitt, I. M. and Sherlock, S. (1965). Serological tests in diagnosis of primary biliary cirrhosis. *Lancet* **i**, 827.

Walton, B., Simpson, B. R. and Strunin, L. (1974). Halothane hepatitis. *Anaesthesiology* **41**, 415.

Wright, R. (1972). Chronic hepatitis. *Brit. Med. Bull.* **28**, 120.

Wright, R., Eade, O. E., Chisholm, M., Hawksley, M., Lloyd, B., Moles, T. M., Edwards, J. C. and Gardner, M. J. (1975). Controlled prospective study of the effect on liver function of multiple exposures to halothane. *Lancet* **i**, 817.

20

Reproductive Medicine

KARL JOHANSEN

Advances in midwifery have allowed the weary obstetrician greater control over an intrinsically unpredictable speciality, giving him the opportunity to study its physiopathology in depth. At the same time it has become apparent that a study of immunological characteristics could open a new chapter in the fundamental science of reproductive physiology. The gulf between immunological theory and clinical practice remains wide, not because of any conflict but rather by virtue of the antithetical attitudes of the scientist and the obstetrician towards reproductive medicine.

This chapter attempts a rapprochement by crystallizing some of the theory in the clinical context. It is convenient to review briefly the physiological basis of human reproduction, before considering those obstetric disorders in which an immunological pathogenesis is known or believed to exist.

DEVELOPMENTAL PHYSIOLOGY

Spermatogenesis

The development of spermatozoa in the male testis begins after puberty under the influence of follicle stimulating hormone from the pituitary. There are three principal cell types in the testis. The spermatogonia, which line the seminiferous tubules, undergo division and differentiation into spermatozoa. Initially they pass through several stages becoming primary spermatocytes after about 32 days. These, which contain the normal diploid chromosome content, undergo reduction meiosis giving rise to secondary spermatocytes which are haploid, with either an X- or a Y-chromosome, and they in turn divide (equation meiosis) into spermatids which differentiate progressively into immature spermatozoa, the whole cycle taking some 64 days to complete. During differentiation spermatozoa are dependant for their nutrition upon the Sertoli cells of the seminiferous tubules. The third main testicular cell is the interstitial or Leydig cell, which secretes testosterone under the influence of pituitary luteinizing hormone (LH). Once fully developed the spermatozoa pass through the epididymis and vas deferens, and during this time mature further, developing the capacity for movement upon which their ultimate fertility depends (Israel, 1967).

Oogenesis

In the female the development of mature ova takes even longer, beginning during intra-uterine life at a time when the foetus is still under the influence of maternal hormones. In the embryo the ovary develops when the primordial germ cells migrate across the peritoneal cavity from the urogenital ridge, implanting themselves within the mesonephric mesenchyme which condenses in continuity with the ovarian ligament. These oogonia become enclosed by cells of the germinal epithelium forming follicles, whose number is greatest at the seventh month of intra-uterine life, diminishing thereafter. During the first few weeks of extra-uterine life the oogonia mature into primary oocytes, whose further development remains arrested at prophase until puberty. Subsequently a number of follicles are stimulated each month by pituitary follicle stimulating hormone (FSH). The growth of one of these accelerates, possibly as a result of its own intrinsic production of oestradiol, and this hormone, by positive feedback to the pituitary, causes the release of luteinizing hormone (LH), which apparently provokes rupture of the follicle and ovulation. It is at about this time that the first reduction meiosis takes place, giving rise to a secondary oocyte together with a polar body, which represents the residue of unused chromatin.

If the ovum is fertilized by a spermatozoon the secondary oocyte undergoes equation meiosis forming a second polar body and the ootid. The latter units with the sperm head forming the zygote which immediately undergoes its first cell division. This process normally takes place in the ampullary portion of the Fallopian tube, while further cell divisions take place during its transit to the uterine cavity. Pregnancy as a physiological state is generally assumed to begin only at the time of implantation of the blastocyst into the secretory endometrium, although there is evidence that in certain species the influence of the zygote on the maternal physiology may begin before implantation (Short, 1969).

Placentation

At the time of implantation the blastocyst consists of an inner cell mass destined to give rise to the embryo and an outer shell of cytotrophoblast from which the villi gradually develop, eroding the maternal venous sinuses of the decidua to create the chorio-decidual space. From the moment of implantation the cytotrophoblast secretes the hormone human chorionic gonadotrophin (HCG) in escalating quantities. The luteinizing action of HCG is apparently responsible for maintenance and enlargement of the corpus luteum of the maternal ovary, so that its secretion of oestrogen and progesterone also increases. As pregnancy progresses a cellular syncytium develops from the cytotrophoblast and becomes the predominant tissue in the placenta. Towards mid-pregnancy the cytotrophoblast becomes extremely attenuated and its production of HCG decreases. Consequently, the corpus luteum tends to regress and its hormone contribution decreases. By this time, however, the syncytio-trophoblast is capable of converting maternal steroid precursors to progesterone which is utilized by the foetal adrenal in the production of much greater amounts of oestrogens.

The syncytio-trophoblast also produces very large quantities of another important hormone, placental lactogen (HPL), also known as human chorionic somato-mammo trophic hormone (HCS). The functions of this hormone are uncertain but its close resemblance to the pituitary hormones, growth hormone (GH; syn. somatotrophin, STH) and prolactin (luteotrophic hormone, LTH), suggests that it may contribute to the rapid growth of the foetus *in utero*—which is achieved without acromegalic features developing in the mother—and to the development of the maternal breast. Many of these hormones influence various immunological processes of the pregnant woman.

Placentation occurs in virtually all mammals but there are wide histological variations between different species which are important when their immunological implications are considered. The mature human placenta as it appears following delivery is almost entirely composed of syncytio-trophoblast and supporting tissues which are of foetal origin. The maternal surface, however, is decidual in origin and is a thin layer enclosing the intervillous space hence its alternative name, the chorio-decidual space.

In man and, perhaps fortunately for those studying immunology, in rodents, placentation is of the haemochorial type with trophoblastic villi lying in the maternal blood which circulates through the chorio-decidual space. By contrast, in the pig, the foetal trophoblast fails to invade through the decidua so that the two lie in direct contact; the term "epithelio-chorial" is then applied. In carnivores the trophoblast invades further, touching the endothelium of the maternal capillaries (endothelio-chorial), while, in cattle it is separated by uterine connective tissue as well (syndesmo-chorial). One further variation is the haemo-endothelial placenta which is peculiar to certain species, including the rabbit, where the trophoblast, lying between the foetal vessels and maternal blood, is extremely attenuated or even absent (Boyd and Hamilton, 1970).

Transport of substances across the placenta between the maternal and foetal circulations depends on a variety of processes. Substances of low molecular weight, such as electrolytes, gases and water, cross rapidly by simple diffusion. The transfer of substances of higher molecular weight apparently depends on various active processes, which in the case of certain hormones involve intrinsic metabolic pathways through the cells of the trophoblast in the course of which conversion into different hormones takes place. Large molecules such as immunoglobulins cross by pinocytosis, and this will be considered in greater detail below.

Physiological Changes in Pregnancy

Pregnancy is accompanied by changes in physiological function in virtually every maternal system. Some are obvious, others more subtle, but all are governed by alterations in hormone and enzyme production in pregnancy. Of primary importance are the hormones produced by the foeto-placental unit, notably HCG and HCS, together with oestrogenic and progestational steroids and their metabolites.

The immunological characteristics of the mother are influenced by these changes. Alterations in the plasma proteins are among the more obvious of these. The fibrinogen titre rises to almost twice the non-pregnant level while the globulin fraction increases rather less. In compensation, *vis-á-vis* the plasma osmolality, the albumin level is reduced and the albumin/globulin ratio approaches unity. However, these serum levels are to some extent misleading because the total blood volume is about 25% greater. Thus the total plasma globulin rises by some 30–40% in pregnancy.

Within the globulin fraction the greatest increase is in the α and β proteins. Recent work has identified two components in both α_2 and β globulins which are apparently specific to pregnancy (Lin *et al.*, 1974). The precise identification of these pregnancy proteins is awaited with interest. By contrast, IgG, IgA and IgM show a slight decrease in concentration although the total amounts in the body increase considerably (Hytten and Leitch, 1971).

Transfer of Immunoglobulins

The extent to which these changes occur in the foetus depends upon placental transmission. It appears that, of all the plasma proteins, only the IgG fraction of the immunoglobulins is able to cross to any appreciable extent, a facility apparently conferred by the intrinsic structure of its Fc rather than its Fab portion (Ovary, 1974). The stage at which passage begins in normal pregnancy is uncertain but is at least as early as the 13th week, and the foetal immunoglobulin levels reach those of the maternal circulation after mid-pregnancy. The mechanism of transfer is by pinocytosis, the protein being first bound to appropriate receptors on the cell surface and then actively transported across the cytoplasm. By this means protection from intracellular enzymes is provided in transit and considerable selectivity achieved (see Fig. 1).

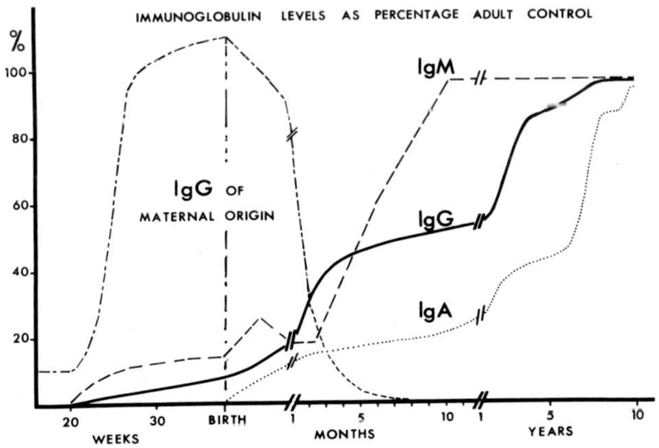

Fig. 1. A composite illustration of foetal, neonatal and infant serum immunoglobulin levels showing the maternal component of IgG. After Alford (1971).

The placental transfer of IgA and IgM is negligible, while foetal production is able to achieve blood levels about 10% of those in the maternal circulation. However, in response to intra-uterine infection, foetal production of IgM rises to unusually high levels. This offers an important diagnostic procedure to the clinician confronted by an inexplicably sick baby. The infections in which this effect is most conspicuous include cytomegalovirus, hepatitis, syphilis and rubella.

It has been inferred that the foetus produces minimal amounts of IgG before delivery, though this is difficult to assess because IgG is in dynamic equilibrium across the placenta, its distribution reflecting the homeostatic requirements and changing in response to the stresses of normal labour, when levels of both albumin and globulin in the umbilical cord blood are increased (Cochran and Good, 1974).

The transfer of maternal IgG to the foetus provides the newborn infant with passive immunity corresponding to that previously acquired by the mother. It may also be the source of pathogenic processes of which haemoytic disease of the newborn is the best known example. The concentration of maternal IgG in the neonate decreases rapidly in the first month, then more gradually, being scarcely detectable at the age of six months (Alford, 1971). By this time the baby's own immunological system has been exposed to external antigens and can manage without the maternal contribution.

In the newborn, additional protection may be afforded if maternal breast feeding is established, because immunoglobulins are actively secreted into both colostrum and milk. This is a particularly important source to the baby of IgA, though IgM and IgG are also secreted. The approximate amounts of these three proteins in colostrum the day after delivery are IgA:600 mg/dl, IgM:125 mg/dl, IgG:80 mg/dl, while the rate of transfer is roughly halved on successive days.

Changes in Other Immunological Factors in Pregnancy

The influence of pregnancy on factors which participate in immunological reactivity is poorly appreciated. On the one hand, alterations in the levels of hormones such as HCG and HPL are well recognized, but their immunological significance is not; on the other, the changes in factors which have an important immunological role, such as the complement system or lymphocyte behaviour, are not well documented.

The leucocyte count in peripheral blood increases during pregnancy by about 50%, but the rise is confined to polymorphs and lymphocyte levels scarcely alter. The increase in blood volume means that the populations of all types of white cells are much greater. Alterations in the morphology of the lymphocytes have been reported which are characterized by the appearance of cells with micronucleoli and a reduction in the proportion with ring-shaped nuclei. There is little change in the proportion of "activated" lymphocytes unless infection is also present (Knobloch *et al.*, 1975).

The effect of these changes on the response of the maternal system to infection seems to be relatively small. Pregnancy is a time when a woman is traditionally supposed to enjoy particularly good health but this may be an illusory effect of the cardiovascular changes and increased metabolic rate which endow her with a rosy complexion. In fact, the pregnant woman seems to be slightly more vulnerable to common infections. There is also a diminution in both the lymphocyte response and in the production of specific antibody in the face of both viral and bacterial infections.

Not all medical disorders are aggravated by pregnancy and some are renowned for the remissions which occur. These include certain conditions with auto-immune characteristics such as rheumatoid arthritis, but the pattern is variable, and some deteriorate or even begin in pregnancy. It is not known whether this reflects an inherent sensitivity to the higher circulating levels of corticosteroids or a change in the patient's immune responsiveness.

THE FOETUS AS AN ALLOGRAFT

The enigmatic success of the foeto-maternal allograft has intrigued biologists for many years although it has tended rather to be taken for granted by the clinician—at least until confronted by a woman with rhesus antibodies. It is important to draw a clear distinction between rhesus isoimmunization—which is mediated by immunoglobulins—and graft rejection which is accompanied by a local inflammatory reaction and is generally attributed to cell mediated immunity. Nevertheless, it is equally important to emphasize that, in purely practical terms, iso-immune disease is clearly rejection of an incompatible graft—albeit comparatively slowly. Moreover, our knowledge of what precisely is happening at the placental site in human pregnancy is extremely limited and, when the pregnancy graft fails, the macerated foetus or placenta provide poor material for study. Furthermore, it is possible that the presence of a pregnancy as a graft which is virtually inside the maternal vascular compartment may well influence the pattern of any rejection process.

Despite this, a variety of hypotheses have been proposed to explain the success which pregnancy normally enjoys (see Currie, 1969).

Foetal Antigenicity

The placenta forms a substantial, although selective, barrier between mother and foetus which is breached at some stage in most, if not all pregnancies allowing foetal cells to enter the maternal circulation. Foetal lymphocytes are a component of any vascular spillage and are known to be antigenically mature from early pregnancy. Perhaps of greater significance is the phenomenon of trophoblast deportation which was recognized in the last century. Its extent and potential importance have only recently been fully appreciated, for it is estimated that as many as 100,000 fragments of syncytium may be shed into the maternal circulation each day. The antigenicity of human trophoblast remains uncertain because it is difficult to obtain uncontamined cell samples, but it is likely that histocompatibility antigens of the HL-A system are present although they may be masked or deficiently expressed.

Irrespective of the source of antigenic stimulus it is known that histocompatibility antibodies may be formed by the mother from early pregnancy and that those which are IgG can cross the placenta and reach the foetal circulation. Recently, attention has focused on a number of possible ways whereby the potentially destructive maternal immune response is neutralized in a successful pregnancy.

Maternal Immunological Responsiveness

Studies of graft acceptance during pregnancy have been largely conducted in experimental animals where interpretation is simplified, and sometimes perhaps oversimplified, by the use of pure-bred strains. In general it has been found that paternal-to-maternal grafts are rejected more slowly during pregnancy. This unresponsiveness may persist after delivery and increase to the point of total graft acceptance after multiple pregnancies.

In seeking an explanation for this depression of maternal responsiveness a number of serum factors have been studied, although usually under *in vitro* conditions. The customary experimental model has involved the demonstration of interference with blast-transformation of human lymphocytes in mixed culture, induced by mitogens such as concanavalin A, phytohaemagglutinin or tuberculin.

By these techniques, immunological reactivity has been shown to be depressed by several hormones including human chorionic gonadotrophin (HCG) and somato-mammotrophin (HCS) which are specific to pregnancy. Similar properties have been attributed to oestrogens and progestogens, the output of which is greatly increased in pregnancy. However, these results must be interpreted cautiously because of the unphysiologically high hormone concentrations employed.

Suppression of lymphocyte transformation has been attributed also to a variety of serum proteins. These include α_2 macroglobulins and glycopeptides derived from these and other glycoproteins such as IgG and transferrin. The capability is apparently present in non-pregnant sera but is increased in pregnancy samples, in which raised levels of certain, possibly specific, α_2 macroglobulins are found. Whilst attempting to define more precisely the subfraction which is responsible, Jenkins (1974) reported a comparable effect in the sero-mucoid glycoprotein component.

It appears that serum from the baby may have similar properties and it has been suggested that the foetus itself may be the source of factors such as α-foetoprotein, which inhibit the maternal immune reaction. It is interesting, in this context, to recall that serum inhibitors of lymphocytic activity have been found also in a wide variety of diseases including carcinoma and tuberculosis. The implication of such immunological activity is therefore of great importance within the wider horizons of clinical medicine, so their further identification is awaited with keen interest.

Tolerance and Enhancement

Various hypotheses have been proposed, and their definitions periodically amended, to explain certain natural or experimental examples of altered immunological responsiveness. The concept of tolerance arose following the observation that binovular twin offspring of cattle, which share a common circulation, will subsequently tolerate indefinitely an interchange of grafts.

In this case the mutual tolerance was attributed to contact with the foreign antigen before the host's immune competence was fully developed. It is interesting that, although similar tolerance may be induced in adult experimental animals, it is perpetuated only if repeated exposure to small amounts of antigen is effected. The ease with which tolerance can be established varies considerably among different species, and is a facility which is usually lost completely by the end of pregnancy.

The continual bombardment of the mother with fragments of syncytiotrophoblast throughout pregnancy may achieve a form of induced tolerance, either by a "desensitizing" mechanism or by offering a buffer for the continual absorption of maternal antibody. Support for this concept is seen in the work of Ferrara *et al.* (1974), who showed that HLA unresponsiveness can be induced and maintained by weekly injections of whole blood.

The term "enhancement" has been evolved following observations that repeated heterospecific pregnancies in animals diminished the maternal reactivity to paternal skin allografts. It is defined as the delayed rejection of a graft resulting from the production by the host of antibodies specific to the transplanted tissue. The mechanism is that the antibody combines with antigen sites on the graft, impeding access by host lymphocytes (see Hellström *et al.*, 1969). This could account for some of the observations made in human pregnancy concerning the production of histocompatibility antibodies. Moreover, the variable deposition of antibody, or of an intermediate or alternative blocking factor, on the maternal placental surface would explain some of the conflicting histological interpretations that have been proposed. Alternatively, antibody might be preferentially absorbed by the syncytial fragments which are later shed into the maternal system.

One other aspect which deserves mention is the presence in amniotic fluid—and presumably in other foetal tissue fluids—of soluble HLA-like substances, quite distinct from those normally present in the maternal serum (Johnson, 1974). The significance of this finding is uncertain but if its antigenic nature were confirmed then it would seem likely that exposure of the mother to foetal antigens is a normal physiological event.

In summary, the human foetal allograft is apparently protected by several interdependent mechanisms. The placenta forms a mechanical barrier, the antigenicity of which is intrinsically low and may be modified further by adsorbed blocking substances. Maternal immunological responsiveness is depressed by circulating hormones and other factors, and is perhaps influenced by the establishment of a state of induced tolerance.

ISO-IMMUNE DISEASES IN PREGNANCY

Acknowledging that the foetus is an antigenically mature graft which has the capacity to initiate maternal rejection processes, it becomes easier to consider from a clinical standpoint a number of conditions where this might occur. Firstly it is convenient to review the known examples of histo-incompatibility such as ABO and rhesus iso-immunization.

Haemolytic disease of the newborn was long thought to reflect a maternal reaction against the baby, but early expectations that it resulted from ABO incompatibility were not fulfilled and it was not until the discovery of the rhesus factor that the true pathogenesis was appreciated. Now it is known that the ABO system may occasionally be implicated but there are still examples of neonatal haemolysis and, more particularly, of intra-uterine death from hydrops foetalis which cannot be attributed to either system and whose pathogenesis remains unexplained.

Erythrocyte antibodies

Rhesus (Rh) Iso-immunization

This condition results from leakage of erythrocytes from an Rh (D) positive baby into the circulation of an Rh (D) negative mother, usually at the time of delivery, though occasionally during pregnancy. Typically, the mother is sensitized at this stage, the production of antibody in significant amounts being provoked during the course of a subsequent incompatible pregnancy. The risk is almost eliminated if the foetus is ABO incompatible with the mother because any foetal cells are destroyed by maternal anti-A or B antibody; moreover 30% of susceptible women are apparently unresponsive. However 17% of Rh negative women have developed antibodies by the end of their second pregnancy (Worlledge, 1974). Passive administration of 100 mg anti-D IgG within 72 hours after any delivery will prevent the development of antibodies in 98% of Rh negative women. To eliminate failures, protection should also be offered to women following abortion, ectopic pregnancy or to those with a positive Kleihauer test after amniocentesis, or antenatal complications such as antepartum haemorrhage. A second dose of anti-D IgG is indicated if more than two foetal cells per low-power microscopy field remain in the maternal circulation following the first injection.

The mode of action is uncertain but protection is achieved by a dosage sufficient to neutralize a mere 5–10% of the D antigen sites present on the red cell surfaces.

Clinical Aspects of Rhesus Disease

The trend towards smaller families and the introduction of anti-D prophylaxis have largely eliminated rhesus iso-immunization as a major perinatal problem. The condition still appears sporadically in women sensitized before the introduction of protection or those for whom treatment with anti-D globulin has been overlooked. It is in these subjects that the more severe examples of iso-immunization occur so that the obstetrician and paediatrician, although becoming less familiar with its management, must remain alert to the problem.

All women should be screened for abnormal erythrocyte antibodies when they first attend hospital early in pregnancy, and again at 34–36 weeks gestation. Rhesus (D) negative women should also be checked at 26–28 weeks. These times are determined by the inevitable delay in receiving results and by the time required for antibodies to develop. At delivery umbilical cord blood must be taken, at least from the babies of Rh-negative women, and for this purpose a syringe should be used to avoid the contamination with Wharton's jelly which may occur if the cord is simply cut and drained. The sample should be sent for grouping and, in women with antibodies, for Coombs test, haemoglobin and bilirubin levels as well.

If a Kleihauer test is required the maternal sample should be taken within 12 hours of delivery and anti-D globulin given within 72 hours, after which a further Kleihauer test may be performed. Subsequent screening for antibodies is recommended about six months after delivery.

The management of women in whom antibodies have already developed calls for careful judgement and specialized facilities. A high (greater than 0·2 μg/ml) or rising antibody concentration is an indication for amniocentesis after ultrasonic placental localization. The severity of foetal involvement is reflected by the level of bile pigments in amniotic fluid measured by spectrophotometry, which is the most useful practical test. The interpretation of results requires considerable experience as does the decision whether to treat an affected foetus by intra-uterine transfusion or by termination of the pregnancy.

The clinical effects of iso-immunization range from nothing more than subclinical anaemia or jaundice in the newborn baby, through heart failure, oedema, and hepato-splenomegaly when haemolysis is severe, to intra-uterine death from hydrops foetalis, which in extreme cases may develop early in pregnancy. Severe rhesus iso-immunization may occasionally be a cause of recurrent intra-uterine death or habitual abortion. In such cases, plasmaphoresis has been used as an adjunct to other therapy (see Chapter 31).

Other Rhesus Antibodies

Haemolytic disease in the babies of Rh (D) positive women is uncommon but may result from the development of anti-c or anti-E antibodies. Although neither c nor E is as strongly antigenic as D, the development of antibodies against them is equally serious from a clinical standpoint. On rare occasions the presence of an anti-G antibody in an Rh negative woman may cause problems of interpretation but it is relatively insignificant from an obstetric standpoint.

ABO Haemolytic Disease

Naturally occurring anti-A and B iso-haemagglutinins are IgM immunoglobulins and so do not reach the foetus. The occasional development of IgG immune anti-A and anti-B haemolysins in women of blood group O may initiate foetal haemolysis and, although this only rarely necessitates emergency exchange transfusion of the neonate, the "topping-up" of babies with progressive anaemia is sometimes required. The mildness of this condition is attributed to the adsorption of maternal antibody by soluble and fixed blood group antigen in foetal tissues other than erythrocytes.

It is perhaps this effect which accounts for recurrent and otherwise unexplained first trimester abortions in a small proportion of patients who have anti-A haemolysins. This has not been reported with anti-B haemolysins perhaps because of their relative infrequency and the lesser immunogenicity of B antigen.

Other Antibodies

Anti-Kell immunization may cause foetal haemolysis but other unusual antibodies only rarely do so and virtually never pose a serious threat to the baby. However, their presence may influence the obstetric management of a patient and they should always be reported and their significance explained to the obstetrician so that precautions may be taken if and when the need for maternal blood transfusion arises.

Platelet antibodies

Iso-immune Thrombocytopenic Purpura

Approximately 20% of cases of neonatal thrombocytopenic purpura occur in the infants of haematologically normal mothers. A complement-fixing platelet iso-antibody is responsible, and this can be demonstrated in the maternal serum following delivery of an affected infant (Pearson *et al.*, 1964). The antibody, which cannot be detected by conventional platelet agglutination techniques, is active against not only the baby's but also the father's platelets, confirming its iso-antigenic nature. The antigen most commonly involved in the cases reported is Pl^{A1}, though antibodies to $PlGrLy^{B1}$ and $PlGrLy^{C1}$ are also recorded. There is no evidence of concurrent haemolysis or lymphopenia and no antibody activity demonstrable against erythrocytes. The HLA status of the families concerned was not explored.

The clinic outcome for the baby is as serious as that resulting from maternal auto-immunization (ITP). A generalized petechial rash develops within half an hour of delivery with ecchymoses over bony prominences. The jaundice which sometimes develops may reflect haemolysis in occult haematomas. The principal cause of death is from intracranial haemorrhage. The high perinatal mortality (10–20%) is a serious feature of both auto- and iso-immune conditions and early elective exchange transfusion is advisable in all affected infants.

Leucocyte Antibodies in Pregnancy

Leucocyte antibodies were demonstrated in animals by Metchnikoff and in humans were thought to be physiological. In the 1950s their relationship with blood transfusion and pregnancy was clearly established but there was little incentive to study these apparently non-pathogenic factors until the next decade, when impetus was given to research into histocompatibility by the development of organ transplantation.

The frequency with which antibodies may be found during or after pregnancy depends to a great extent on the techniques used. Leuco-agglutinins, for instance, are found in only 1% of women after their first pregnancy, their incidence rising sharply in the second and third but changing little thereafter. Variations between reported studies are attributable to sampling or to laboratory methods. By contrast, leucocytotoxins are more readily demonstrated in pregnancy and it is this group of antibodies, studied by methods based on that of Terasaki and McLelland (1964), which have permitted identification of the HLA system and are most widely studied in relation to pathological conditions in pregnancy. Other tests for cytotoxic antibodies, such as isotope release, are more sensitive and results lead one to suspect that, given the right test, antibodies of some sort may be found in virtually all incompatible pregnancies.

The HLA System

The degree of HLA compatibility between mother and foetus is variable although they are always isogeneic for two and sometimes for all four antigens. Nevertheless most foetuses are heterozygous for one and often both paternally derived antigens, the frequency depending to some extent on the incidence of particular antigens within the community, which itself reflects the prevalence of interrelated marriages.

A factor which compounds the intricate problems of the HLA system in pregnancy is that certain antigens are more effective than others in provoking production of cytotoxins. In an extensive survey, Tovey and Darke (1973) found that antibodies against HLA A28 B5, B27, Bw40 and Bw22 appear in pregnancy up to twenty times as often as expected. Conversely, anti-HLA A3 is present ten times less frequently than anticipated. This curious effect has not been explained, and contrasts sharply with the formation of HLA antibodies after tissue transplantation when those to first series antigens are generally stronger. It may imply that the sensitizing mechanism in pregnancy differs from that resulting from grafted maternal. For a fuller discussion of the HLA system see Chapter 29.

Lymphocytotoxins in Pregnancy

In contrast with Rhesus antibodies, lymphocytotoxins may be found as early as the tenth week, and even in the first pregnancy, increasingly towards term. Their incidence is variable but is about 10% in the first, 20% in the second and about 25% in subsequent pregnancies. Single or multiple HLA specificities may be established in about half of these sera, a further quarter being polyspecific and the remainder giving only a limited cytotoxic reaction. Occasionally antibody may disappear during pregnancy and recur afterwards, and *vice versa*. Inconsistencies may also be found if maternal sera are tested against both donor and paternal cells, but the greatest problem is that of cross-reactions within the system itself and it is clear that the test system remains far from ideal. However, it has permitted study of several aspects of pregnancy with reasonably consistent results.

It is clear that the ability to produce cytotoxins is present in all maternal age groups and that the antigenic stimulus offered by an early gestation which aborts is very weak by comparison with that of a term pregnancy. There do not appear to be correlations between the development of lymphocytotoxins and such unexplained obstetric complications as pre-eclampsia, abruptio placentae or intra-uterine death. Neither is there any clear association with foetal abnormalities or intra-uterine growth. Some of the earlier studies of these parameters took insufficient account of factors already known to be relevant to these conditions, such as maternal parity and foetal sex, but the suggestion that the male foetus might be more strongly antigenic than the female is unconfirmed. The significance of cytotoxins in patients with habitual abortion and in grand multipara and the coincidence, if any, between the formation of antibodies to particular HLA antigens and maternal ABO group remain obscure (Burke and Johansen, 1974).

By analogy with Rhesus disease or thrombocytopenia, depletion of lymphocytes in the neonate might be expected when the mother has circulating cytotoxins. That this does not seem to happen may be due to the rapid turnover of leucocytes or to the existence of a large pool of antigen in the tissues.

MATERNAL AUTO-IMMUNE DISEASES AFFECTING THE FOETUS

A number of pathological states are characterized by the presence of auto-antibodies in the circulation. When such a disease affects a woman in pregnancy and when the auto-antibody is an IgG immunoglobulin, its ability to cross the placenta may provoke clinical features in the baby, usually after delivery. The phenomenon was recognized in the babies of women with thyrotoxicosis long before its significance was appreciated. Latterly, a comparable effect has been noted in several other diseases, the clinic features being apparent only as long as the specific antibody remains in the baby's circulation (Scott, 1966).

Thyrotoxicosis

Long acting thyroid stimulator (LATS) is demonstrable in about one third of patients with thyrotoxicosis, notably those with exophthalmos. It is a feature of the more severe forms of hyperthyroidism and, since severely affected women tend not to ovulate, is uncommon in pregnancy. It is an IgG protein and as such may cross the placenta and cause signs of hyperthyroidism in the baby, which is affected in about 2% of pregnancies in thyrotoxic women.

Foetal involvement may be recognized *in utero* by the presence of tachycardia. Affected babies are of low birth weight and are often irritable following delivery. They tend to succumb to cardiac failure or from intractable diarrhoea and the perinatal mortality, if treatment is inadequate, is about 25%. The pattern of neonatal disease may be extremely variable because both LATS and antithyroid drugs cross the placenta. It is important to realize that if the maternal condition has been controlled by thyroid suppressant drugs the baby may appear unaffected at first, but develop symptoms several days later when the effect of medication has diminished. Another paradox is the appearance of toxicity in the baby of a woman who is euthyroid following thyroidectomy; this may be due to the persistence of LATS in her circulation.

Myasthenia Gravis

This uncommon disease was the first in which the mechanism of neonatal involvement was appreciated. Myasthenia gravis has little effect on pregnancy, except that the incidence of abortion may be increased. Similarly, the maternal symptoms are not aggravated by the pregnancy although their control may be more difficult. The baby is affected in up to 20% of cases and, as with thyrotoxicosis, the development of the full clinical picture may be delayed until the effect of maternal anticholinergic therapy wears off. The clinical features include apnoeic episodes in an inert, floppy baby which cries little and cannot suck. They may be reversed by use of drugs such as neostigmine. If a mildly affected baby is not treated there is a risk that it will develop an inhalational pneumonia because it cannot swallow properly and its respiration is depressed.

Idiopathic Thrombocytopenia Purpura (ITP)

The clinician's preoccupation with the maternal problems engendered by this disease may cause him to overlook the risks to the baby, which may be variably affected in up to 70% of cases with an overall perinatal mortality of 16%. The situation is influenced by the treatment the mother has received, such as splenectomy or cortico-steroids. Following splenectomy the mother may be free from purpura but may still have circulating platelet antibodies. Consequently, the baby may develop the typical purpuric rash after delivery, and is at risk from intracerebral haemorrhage.

Alternatively the mother may be receiving treatment with cortico-steroids, with variable efficacy. In pregnancy such medication should be started reluctantly, for it complicates the management of the mother in labour. The baby is shielded from the effects of maternal therapy by its ability to metabolize large amounts of steroids, and does not show systemic withdrawal effects after delivery although the risk of haemorrhage persists.

Auto-immune Haemolytic Anaemias

This heterogenous group of anaemias includes those mediated by "cold" and "warm" agglutinins (see Chapter 26). The former is usually an IgM antibody but the latter is often IgG and may cross the placenta. This possibility should be considered if the newborn of an affected mother develops unexplained haemolytic anaemia or jaundice. The condition is in any case uncommon in pregnancy partly owing to increasing reluctance to use drugs such as phenacetin or sulphonamides, often incriminated in its pathogenesis.

Systemic Lupus Erythematosus

The immunological effect on the baby of this serious illness in the mother is of little importance when contrasted with the risk of placental insufficiency and intrauterine death. In a small proportion of infants, a transient facial rash of the typical "butterfly" distribution may be seen.

Diabetes Mellitus

There have been occasional reports of temporary insulin-responsive diabetes in new born babies of non-diabetic mothers. It has been suggested that an immunoglobulin of maternal origin is responsible but there is as yet no clear explanation of this obscure disease.

Treatment of Auto-immune Neonatal Diseases

In many instances the condition is not harmful to the baby but, when an infant is seriously affected, as may be the case in thyrotoxicosis or myasthenia, a good response to drug therapy can be expected. Where this proves inadequate or is judged inappropriate, as for instance in ITP, the logical treatment is exchange transfusion. The distribution of IgG throughout the baby's tissue fluids may necessitate more than a single exchange although experience with rhesus disease suggests that more than two are rarely required.

REPRODUCTIVE DISORDERS WITH POSSIBLE IMMUNOLOGICAL FEATURES

Fertility and Infertility

The ability of erythrocyte antibodies to provoke abortion or intra-uterine death encourages the theory that they or other tissue antibodies could interfere with the earlier stages of pregnancy, fertilization or implantation. Were this so, then an unusual degree of paterno–maternal compatibility might be found among highly fertile couples. This possibility has been investigated extensively in respect of the ABO system and considerable supporting evidence produced.

The ABO System

It has been found that, in ABO incompatible matings, there is a deficiency in the numbers of group A and B babies born to group O women. Moreover, women of group AB appear to have slightly greater fertility (Behrman *et al.*, 1960). The mechanism by which this selection is achieved is debatable but studies in animals suggest that it operates before, rather than after implantation and that it may reflect the susceptibility of spermatozoa to cervical or uterine secretions.

In the case of the ABO system it is known that soluble A and B antigens are present in seminal fluid and may also be identified on spermatozoa although it is suggested that in the latter instance they are merely superficially adsorbed. IgM antibodies to both A and B antigens are naturally present in the blood but are not normally found in cervical mucus or uterine secretions, although IgA and IgG are. Consequently selection would not normally be expected to operate unless immune anti-A or B had arisen. Even so, spermatozoa are not always vulnerable to such antibodies and ABO incompatible pregnancies are frequently successful in their presence.

It is uncertain whether antigens such as the Rhesus factors are represented on spermatozoa, but even if they are, the existence of Rh antibodies in the female has no obvious effect on her ability to conceive.

The HLA System

There is some evidence that preferential selection of spermatozoa with particular characteristics may operate in other ways. A number of different antibodies have been demonstrated which are directed against sperm antigens. HLA antigens, for instance, are represented on the acrosomal cap of the sperm head, where they apparently express the haploid genome. On theoretical grounds they might well be susceptible to the anti-HLA activity of IgG lymphocytotoxins in the cervical mucus of parous women, when present. Were this so, then a proportion of women might be refractory to fertilization by spermatozoa bearing the paternal antigens to which they had been sensitized. The corollary is that an unusual degree of HLA compatibility should be present in couples of unusually high parity and *vice versa*. Evidence on this point, relating to the incidence of lymphocytotoxins in women of high and low parity has been conflicting and the results of more extensive family studies are awaited (Burke and Johansen, 1974).

Apart from the influence of these major histocompatibility factors, it is apparent that selective fertility may sometimes be achieved in other ways. Perhaps the most obvious is in respect of sex determination, which apparently operates in the case of occasional families in which the offspring through several generations are exclusively or predominantly of one sex. Sex-specific antibody systems have not as yet been identified in man, although they are present in animals (Ivanyi, 1970), and in mouse spermatozoa the H-Y antigen has been located on the acrosomal cap.

Studies of sex ratios in human pregnancy are difficult but many associations have been postulated (Stevenson and Bobrow, 1967), notably with the ABO system but also with the HLA system (Johansen *et al.*, 1974) though neither has been confirmed. Nevertheless a recent study of renal allograft survival showed better survival of male than female donor kidneys when the recipient was female—and especially if she was multiparous.

If a sex-specific histocompatibility system is confirmed in man it is likely that it would operate before implantation, probably as a result of the preferential union of particular sperms and ova according to immunological characteristics.

Other Sperm Antigen – Antibody Systems

Antibodies to spermatozoa were first found in the serum of some infertile men in 1954 and several types have since been distinguished depending on the method used for detection. With agglutination techniques separate reactive sites are found in the head, tail and tail extremity, whereas with fluorescent staining, distinct sites are seen in the acrosomal cap, equatorial segment, post-nuclear region, neck, mid-piece and main tail-piece. Other antibodies cause sperm immobilization, cytotoxicity or internal staining. Cross-reactivity between sperm antibodies and other tissues, such as brain or adrenal, has been demonstrated in a few instances but, in general, the specificity and nature of these sperm antigens remains undetermined (Hekman and Rumke, 1974).

Sperm antibodies formed against antigens of the head are mainly IgM whereas those against the tail tend to be IgG. The latter are sometimes present in the seminal fluid, usually in low concentration and only rarely in greater amounts than in the serum. Their clinical significance is uncertain, for agglutinins are present in many fertile men and often develop after vasectomy. However, their prevalence and titres among infertile men are greater, a factor which clinicians have attempted to rectify either by washing and re-suspending the husband's spermatozoa before artificial insemination or by occlusive techniques. It is difficult to assess the effectiveness of the latter but they have not been outstandingly successful.

The incidence of sperm antibodies in women shows a wide variation. Agglutinins have been reported in a high proportion of those with unexplained infertility. In general, there is a low incidence in unmarried women and in those who have had children. Paradoxically, agglutination has been demonstrated in up to 80% of pregnancy sera, leading to speculation about the possible role of sperm antibodies in providing natural or sometimes pathologically irreversible immunity to pregnancy.

A micro-agglutination technique has usually been employed in these tests, and the sera are not always diluted. Results have consequently been influenced by non-specific factors, such as β-macroglobulins and, possibly, leucocytotoxins, interference from which can be reduced by dilution. Until more precise techniques are available, uncertainty remains regarding the significance of results.

The potential importance of seminal antibody systems in the wider context of fertility control is not easy to predict but sperm antigens have an undoubted ability to induce a state of immune tolerance, as was demonstrated by Lengerová and Vojtíšková (1963) who found that rejection of syngeneic male to female skin grafts in mice could be delayed by repeated insemination of the recipient.

Whether spermatozoa are protected from the action of antibodies is not established but the admixture of seminal fluid and sperm is accompanied by changes in the immunological characteristics of the latter. The sperm acquire a coating of antigenic proteins of which lactoferrin from the seminal vesicles is the principal component; other antigens may also be contributed by prostate and epididymis.

Foetal Development

Abortion

Pregnancy becomes clinically recognizable by modern HCG antiglobulin tests about four weeks after implantation. Although a woman may be suspicious when she misses her first period, only those who are recording their basal temperature will have any confirmation at this stage. Thus the number of pregnancies which abort before six weeks of amenorrhoea is unknown—a problem clouding the validity of many studies of the subject. The incidence of clinically recognizable abortion is about 20–25% and probably over half of these result from developmental abnormalities—many with a chromosomal fault.

The blastocyst and embryo are remarkably resistant to all but the highest titres of rhesus antibodies in early pregnancy although ABO immunoglobulins may be a cause of abortion. There has been no extensive search for lymphocytotoxins in women with unexplained habitual abortion and contemporary studies are inconclusive. Little is known about the antigenicity of the human blastocyst under normal circumstances nor about possible mechanisms which may protect it against antibodies.

Foetal Abnormality

There is no evidence for a causal relationship between maternal ABO or Rh antibodies and foetal anomaly nor of any correlation with the presence of lymphocytotoxins, although insufficient notice may have been taken of other relevant factors such as maternal age, parity and foetal sex. It is unlikely that tissue antibodies would produce this type of damage, and probable that development would be retarded or prevented altogether.

Foetal Growth

Studies in laboratory mammals have produced results which are hard to interpret. Antigenically dissimilar matings in particular inbred strains apparently result in heavier placentae and bigger litters, despite the occurrence of smaller litters and lighter foetuses after maternal sensitization to paternal antigens.

In man it has been suggested that the drop in mean birth weight between first and subsequent pregnancies is compatible with an immunological cause. Early reports linking maternal lymphocytotoxins and low birth weight babies are unsatisfactory because they disregard foetal (gestational) age, sex and birth rank. However, in a recent study of over 1,000 births these factors were considered and no correlation found (Johansen, unpublished). In contrast, other authors have suggested that close HLA compatibility promotes higher foetal birth weights. More extensive study is required.

Intra-uterine Foetal Death: Runting

Runting, a graft-versus-host reaction arising when maternal lymphocytes cross the placenta to the newborn at delivery, is a feature of certain mammalian species but is not known in man. However, it has been reported on a few occasions following intra-uterine transfusion with allogeneic blood of a foetus with rhesus haemolytic disease (Lancet, 1974). The immunogenic potential of transfused lymphocytes may be destroyed by irradiation of the blood before infusion (3,000 rads), and this precaution has been recommended despite the rarity of the complication.

It is uncertain how runting is avoided in human pregnancy. Maternal lymphocytes are not generally demonstrated in the baby's circulation after delivery although foetal lymphocytes often reach the mother. It is likely that the foetus recognizes foreign cells and can mount an effective cytotoxic response from at least the 16th week, so in the normal course of events, such cells are eliminated. On the other hand this defence might be deficient and so lead to intra-uterine foetal death. Supporting evidence is sparse, for the macerated stillborn baby is not a fruitful source of information, but occasional reports of materno–foetal and foetal–foetal chimaerism (in twins) following abortion demonstrate the feasibility of such a mechanism.

Maternal Pathology

Pre-Eclampsia

The idea that this mysterious condition results from foeto–maternal incompatibility was first proposed by Dienst in 1905 following suggestions that foreign protein fragments such as syncytio-trophoblast in the maternal circulation might be responsible. The theory remains attractive because the histological changes in the spiral arteries of the placental bed resemble those in the vessels of rejected renal allografts. Moreover renal biopsies in women with pre-eclampsia reveal deposition of IgM, IgG and complement within the glomeruli and both afferent and efferent arterioles to an extent commensurate with the severity of the disease (Petrucco *et al.*, 1974). It seems likely that the lesion in the uterine spiral arteries (described as fibrinoid necrosis) is of a similar nature, but a detailed study is necessary. In this connection it is of interest to recall the observation that antibodies formed against placenta may also be active against human glomerular basement membrane.

Early reports of a correlation between pre-eclampsia and ABO blood group have been neither confirmed nor refuted. Recently, interest has revived in the observation that pre-eclampsia is more common in primigravidae—particularly if the foetus is male—leading to the suggestion that a Y-linked histocompatibility factor may be responsible.

The relationship between pre-eclampsia and iso-immunization is variable. Women with a rhesus-affected pregnancy are more prone to pre-eclampsia, but most studies of lymphocytotoxins have disregarded maternal age, parity and foetal sex when making comparisons. In their absence no correlation has yet been demonstrated (Johansen, unpublished). More pertinent, perhaps, will be the results of studies of materno–foetal HLA compatibility in pregnancies complicated by pre-eclampsia (Jenkins, 1974).

Abruptio Placentae

Although this obstetric catastrophe is thought to result from rupture of a spiral artery in the placental bed, its true aetiology is unknown. It has been widely, but incorrectly, supposed that there is a close association between placental abruption and hypertensive disease. There is no known relationship with any histocompatibility factor in man but there may be an oblique relationship between it and another immunological phenomenon, the Shwartzman reaction.

The Shwartzman Reaction

This is seen in rabbits receiving intravenous injections of gram-negative bacterial endotoxin. The normal animal survives the first such injection but dies if given a second dose after an appropriate interval. Pregnancy in some way sensitizes the animal, rendering it equally susceptible to the *first* injection (McKay, 1965). Post-mortem examination reveals a pattern of mixed renal tubular and cortical necrosis reminiscent of that found sometimes when human pregnancy is complicated by severe septic abortion or abruptio placentae. In the former there is an obvious source of endotoxin while in the latter it is possible that exsanguination leads to intestinal hypoperfusion, so that endotoxins from bacteria in the gut can enter the circulation. This hypothesis would explain the unusual vulnerability of pregnant women to these serious complications, but confirmation must await the development of a reliable laboratory test for the presence of endotoxin.

It is uncertain how endotoxin acts; the substance itself is a lipo-polysaccharide which is released from the cell wall on the death of a gram negative organism. It appears to interact with the C3 and C5 components of the complement system. Among other effects it increases capillary permeability and activates the clotting and fibrinolytic systems, producing disseminated intravascular coagulation. These features are not unique to endotoxin nor are they invariably present in women with septic abortion or abruptio. However, they occur sufficiently often to be classed among the most serious complications of those diseases, although frequently unrecognized by obstetricians.

The general Shwartzman reaction has been induced in experimental models not only by injection of endotoxin but also by feeding a diet with a high oxidized fat content. A similar effect has been demonstrated in rats given high doses of progesterone in late pregnancy. Death of the foetus and mother occurred in a high proportion, with signs of intravascular coagulation in kidneys, adrenals, liver and lungs. The similarities between this and the extreme eclamptic state in humans need no emphasis and lends force to arguments suggesting immunological factors in this disease. There is undoubtedly an urgent need for further research in this context, for the toxaemias of pregnancy are among the commonest and most intractable of problems in obstetrics today.

Hydatidiform Mole

Several features of trophoblastic diseases suggest that these conditions might have an immunological basis. Hydatidiform mole is thought to be more prevalent among closely related couples as shown by several studies of women having recurrent molar pregnancies and there is a report of a man whose two wives had trophoblastic diseases.

Approximately 80% of moles have a female karyotype (XX) and it has been observed that among women who develop chorionic carcinoma and who are of blood group A, the husband is ten times as likely to be of blood group O as A. This implies that trophoblastic proliferation is facilitated by an unusual degree of paterno–maternal compatibility. The HLA system has been investigated in this respect in patients with trophoblastic disease but no unusual compatibility or antigen combinations found (Bagshawe, 1974).

IMMUNOLOGICAL ASPECTS OF GYNAECOLOGICAL CANCER

It is widely thought that immunological factors are important in the development of, and resistance to a variety of neoplasms. Two tumours which have been extensively studied are chorion-epithelioma and breast carcinoma. In the case of the latter it has been suggested that the tumour is recognized as "non-self" by the host, even while still at the *in situ* stage. It is thought that the lympho–reticulo–endothelial (LRE) system may play a part in controlling tumour spread, and the degree of lymph node histiocytosis and of lymphoid infiltration of the tumour itself may reflect the ultimate prognosis (Black, 1974).

It was believed that a cellular response was absent in chorio-carcinoma but it is now apparent that a mononuclear cell reaction is present around both primary and secondary growths. More important, the response to chemotherapy is greater where the cellular reaction is more marked. *In vitro* studies have shown also that lymphocytes from the peripheral blood of patients with chorio-carcinoma may be cytotoxic towards cells from the tumour itself (Bagshawe, 1974).

The increase in lymphocytic activity in patients with other gynaecological carcinomas is reflected in the rise in IgA which occurs and by the cytotoxicity of the patient's serum and lymphocytes against tumour cells which is often demonstrable not only in breast tumours but also in cancer of the cervix, ovary and vulva (Onnis, 1974). The absence of similar patterns in advanced neoplasia may simply mean that tumour growth has been facilitated but it probably implies active interference with host defences by the production of specific factors by the tumour itself.

There have been three main trends in therapy in the light of these observations. The first is to question the wisdom of extensive resection of lymph nodes, many of which contain no metastases. In gynaecological practice the classical examples of radical surgery are Wertheim's hysterectomy for cervical carcinoma and radical vulvectomy. However it is interesting to recall that early descriptions of the former operation advised removal only of those lymph nodes which contain obvious tumour and this perhaps should still be the ultimate objective. However, the use of lymphangiography to discriminate between normal and affected nodes has proved disappointing.

The second trend has been to explore means of stimulating the host immune reaction with, amongst other things, tuberculin in the form of BCG immunization. Malignant melanoma is one tumour in which this largely experimental treatment has occasionally appeared to be effective, but overall results have been poor.

The third trend is to avoid, as far as possible, damage to the host's LRE system when treating a tumour with radiotherapy and chemotherapy. This is an automatic precaution in the case of the former but not of the latter, the dosage of antimitotic drugs tending to be controlled by observing the depression of leucocyte levels. Sufficient is now known of the differential effects of chemotherapeutic agents on lymphoid and tumour cell division cycles to enable a careful choice of regime to be made. In particular, continuous use of agents may be less beneficial than intermittent treatment (Goldie *et al.*, 1972).

The demonstration of tumour antibodies encourages hopes that serological tests may be developed which will permit the early detection of cancer, particularly of occult tumours such as those of the ovary which are often inoperable at the time of diagnosis. A number of serological specificities have now been identified as associated with tumours, including carcino-embryonic antigen (gut adenocarcinoma), α-foetoprotein (hepatoma), foetal sulphoglycoprotein (stomach), and tumour specific lipoprotein (Kitschke *et al.*, 1974), and further developments are awaited.

A totally opposite concept has been proposed to explain the invasive characteristics of tumour cells. Stafl and Mattingly (1972) have shown in cervical carcinoma that, whereas the erythrocyte antigens A and B are clearly present on cells from a benign or *in situ* lesion, they are absent once the tissue shows evidence of becoming invasive. The implication of this observation is that it is a loss of normal antigenicity rather than the development of new antigens that endows a tissue with malignant characteristics and enables invasion to occur.

OTHER IMMUNOLOGICAL ASPECTS OF REPRODUCTIVE MEDICINE

Pregnancy and Renal Transplantation

There have now been several reports of pregnancy in women who have received renal transplants, principally in North America but also in Europe. In general, women with anuria and uraemia who are entirely dependent on dialysis do not ovulate (there was an exceptional pregnancy in such a patient at the London Hospital in 1973). Those who have received renal transplants achieve normal blood urea levels and ovarian function is then likely to return. The ultimate prognosis must make pregnancy in these circumstances ill advised both because of the possible social problems and because of the risk of accelerating graft rejection, although this is probably less serious than might be expected (Golby, 1970). Transplant patients are often maintained on steroid drugs or azathioprine which makes the occurrence of pregnancy even more surprising. It has been suggested that azathioprine should be stopped during pregnancy because of the risk to foetal development, but this may increase the likelihood of renal graft rejection, and fears of danger to the foetus seem to be largely unfounded (Sciarra *et al.*, 1975).

Two particular factors are worth consideration. The first is that paternal antigens of the foetus may be incompatible with the graft; however, it is unlikely that tissue typing a woman's husband, as well as herself, before selecting a donor would ever be practicable. The second factor concerns blood transfusion. Transplant patients may be anaemic and the natural concern of the obstetrician is that transfusion may be required. However, it must be restricted to the absolute minimum and blood used which has been both grouped and tissue-typed against the graft, to avoid accelerating its rejection. For similar reasons transfusion of any woman receiving dialysis is generally discouraged.

Antibody Testing in Pregnancy

Syphilis

As well as routine blood grouping and antibody screening, it is customary to exclude maternal syphilis by a Wasserman reaction.

Unfortunately, false positive results are relatively common in pregnancy, so the interpretation of positive or dubious results sometimes requires clarification by other tests, such as the Reiter complement fixation or fluorescent treponemal antibody test. Nevertheless, these do not permit the distinction between syphilis and yaws or pinta to be made. Where there is still doubt about the result it is customary to treat the mother with a prophylactic course of penicillin. It is also necessary to screen the baby of any mother with a positive WR after birth, but this test must be delayed until six weeks after delivery to distinguish a true infection from the false positive resulting from residual maternal antibody.

Rubella

The advent of a reliable screening test for rubella enables the obstetrician to identify a recent infection when the mother books at hospital for her confinement. The presence of IgG antibody suggests previous exposure and implies resistance, whereas a high or rising titre of IgM indicates a recent infection, allowing the obstetrician the opportunity of advising the couple regarding termination of pregnancy to avoid the risk of foetal abnormality. A negative result means that the woman is susceptible to infection and should be offered active immunization after the pregnancy. Under no circumstances should rubella vaccine be administered during pregnancy or to any female who might be pregnant. The use of immune (anti-rubella) globulin in susceptible patients who have been exposed to infection is not to be recommended because it may fail to prevent a subclinical infection which could affect the baby (Macrae and Reid, 1968).

Hepatitis

Many blood transfusion centres routinely screen serum samples for hepatitis associated antigen. The management of pregnant women found positive presents certain problems, since current recommendations specify a degree of isolation or barrier nursing which is psychologically unsettling and may be unnecessary. The absence of any report of serum hepatitis in maternity staff despite their frequent exposure to large amounts of blood at the time of delivery implies that this may not be such a dangerous source of infection as has been suggested. Alternatively one might speculate that the virus is in some way modified during pregnancy.

Other Infections

Few other tests are employed routinely in obstetrical or gynaecological practice but antibody titres against *Brucella*, *Toxoplasma* and cyto-megaloviral antigens are required occasionally in women with habitual abortion.

Immunization Procedures in Pregnancy

Apart from rubella immunization, only smallpox vaccination is known to be dangerous to the foetus and it is positively contraindicated because of the risk of foetal vaccinia, which frequently causes intra-uterine death or abortion. Nevertheless foetal or neonatal infection with many other viruses has been reported, sometimes with results fatal or severely damaging to the foetus.

As a general rule immunization procedures which depend on the use of live or attenuated virus should be avoided during pregnancy unless the indications for its use are strong and have been carefully evaluated. Thus poliomyelitis and yellow fever immunization should be avoided whereas typhoid (TAB) and cholera are probably safe. In contrast, maternal immunization with tetanus toxoid should be recommended during pregnancy in parts of the world where neonatal tetanus infection is prevalent. The active immunization of the mother stimulates the production of IgG which is transferred to the foetus.

Hormone Assay in Reproductive Medicine

The advent of a dependable immunological pregnancy test has been a great asset to clinical practice, freeing countless small rodents and amphibians for better things. The test depends on the neutralization by maternal chorionic gonadotrophin (HCG) of an anti-HCG antibody raised in rabbits. In the absence of extraneous HCG, the antiserum agglutinates latex particles coated with HCG. If care is taken to follow the instructions implicitly the test is extremely reliable. False positives are rare and may relate to use by the patient of certain drugs, including those of the phenothiazine group. High levels of luteinizing hormone (LH), which cross-reacts with HCG, are occasionally found in post-menopausal women and may rarely give positive results.

In the last five years advances in radio-immunoassay have permitted a degree of sensitivity in the measurement of several hormones hitherto impossible. Among these are HCG—used in monitoring the treatment of patients with trophoblastic disease—and LH, the levels of which are much lower; antisera used in these assays often cross-react so the hormones are not always distinguishable. A similar problem has been encountered in discriminating HPL and prolactin although some departments now have specific antisera permitting the study of prolactin levels in pregnancy. Other tests for pituitary hormones such as FSH and thyroid hormones have simplified the investigations of amenorrhoea and of thyroid disorders in pregnancy.

Blood Transfusion

It is helpful to know a woman's blood group and complete antibody status from early pregnancy. This facilitates the management of patients for whom it might be difficult to obtain blood at short notice. Theoretically, group-compatible blood might then be given in an emergency with a greater sense of security. However, the risk that cross-matching might then be bypassed is too great for such a routine to be commended as standard practice.

The patient with persistent post-partum bleeding presents special problems. In most instances doubts arise regarding the patient's coagulation status and some continue to ooze despite assurances that this is normal. Obviously unresolved factors must be present in such cases which unfortunately are easily subjected to confused therapy, but problems in management can often be resolved by bedside consultation between the obstetrician and haematologist.

The role of unusual antibodies such as leucocytotoxins in patients with persistent haemorrhage is not known and few departments have the facilities to investigate this routinely. It is known however that they are present in the majority of patients, usually women, who have non-febrile, non-haemolytic transfusion reactions. Nevertheless, by their very nature, it is possible that these antibodies may interfere with platelet function. For example, a patient, who by chance was known to have an HLA B13 antibody, eventually required 30 units of blood because of persistent bleeding after hysterectomy for placenta percreta. She ultimately responded, but only after receiving platelet infusions from three non-HLA B13 donors. Obviously other explanations are possible, but this is simply one which deserves consideration in these worrying cases.

REFERENCES

Alford, C. A. (1971). Immunoglobulin determinations in the diagnosis of fetal infection. *Pediat. Clin. N. Amer.* **18**, 99–113.

Bagshawe, K. D. (1974). A review of some immunological relationships in trophoblastic neoplasia. "Immunology in Obstetrics and Gynaecology"*, pp. 287–291.

Behrman, S. J., Buettner-Janusch, J., Heglar, R. and Gershowitz, H. and Tew, W. L. (1960). ABO(H) blood incompatibility as a cause of infertility. *Am. J. Obstet. Gynaecol.* **79**, 847–855.

Billington, W. D., Elson, J., Jenkinson, E. J. and Searle, R. F. (1974). Antigenicity of the trophoblast. "Immunology in Obstetrics and Gynaecology"*, pp. 111–115.

Black, M. M. (1974). Immunology of breast cancer. "Immunology in Obstetrics and Gynaecology"*, pp. 292–296.

Boyd, J. D. and Hamilton, W. J. (1970). "The Human Placenta", Heffer, Cambridge.

Burke, J. and Johansen, K. (1974). The formation of HL-A antibodies in pregnancy. *J. Obstet. Gynaecol. Brit. Comm.* **81**, 222–228.

Cochran, T. E. and Good, W. (1974). The distribution of immunoglobulins and albumin between maternal and cord serum at delivery. *J. Obstet. Gynaecol. Brit. Comm.* **81**, 980–987.

Currie, G. A. (1969). "Foetal Autonomy:" A Ciba Foundation Symposium (Eds. G. E. W. Wolstenholme and Maeve O'Connor), pp. 32–58, J. and A. Churchill, London.

Ferrara, G. B., Tosi, R. M., Azzolina, G., Carminati, G. and Longo, A. (1974). HL-A unresponsiveness induced by weekly injections of small aliquots of whole blood. *Transplantation* **17**, 194.

Golby, M. (1970). Fertility after renal transplantation. *Transplantation* **10**, 201–205.

Goldie, J. H., Price, L. A. and Harrap, K. R. (1972). Methotrexate toxicity. *Eur. J. Cancer* **8**, 409–414.

Hekman, A. and Rümke, Ph. (1974). "Male Fertility and Sterility": Proceedings of the Serono Symposia, (eds. R. E. Mancini and L. Martini), Vol. 5, p. 249. Academic Press, London and New York.

Hellström, K. E., Hellström, I. and Brawn, J. (1969). Abrogation of cellular immunity to antigenically foreign mouse embryonic cells by a serum factor. *Nature* **224**, 914–915.

Hytten, F. E. and Leitch, I. (1971). "The Physiology of Human Pregnancy", p. 44. Blackwell Scientific Publications, Oxford.

Israel, S. L. (1967). "Diagnosis and Treatment of Menstrual Disorders and Sterility." 5th Edition, p. 500 *et seq.* New York. Hoeber Medical Division, Harper and Row.

Ivanyi, P. (1970). The major histocompatibility antigens in various species. *Curr. Top. Microbiol. Immunol.* **53**, 1–90.

Jenkins, D. M. (1974). Immunological aspects of pre-eclampsia/eclampsia. "Immunology in Obstetrics and Gynaecology"*, pp. 211–215.

Johansen, K., Festenstein, H. and Burke, J. (1974). Possible relationships between maternal HL-A antibody formation and fetal sex. *J. Obstet. Gynaecol. Brit. Comm.* **81**, 781–785.

Johnson, M. H. (1974). Foeto-maternal interactions. "Progress in Immunology". (Eds. L. Brent and E. J. Holborow), Vol. 2, pp. 400–403. North Holland Publishing Company.

Kitschke, H. J., Krebs, D. and Kleinhans, V. (1974). Purification of human tumour specific antigens from human ovarian cancers. "Immunology in Obstetrics and Gynaecology"*, pp. 301–304.

---

*"Immunology in Obstetrics and Gynaecology": Proceedings of the first international congress, Padua, (June, 1973) (Eds. A. Centaro and N. Narretti). Published by: Exerpta Medica, Amsterdam; American Elsevier Publishing Co. Inc., New York (1974).

Knobloch, V., Jouja, V. and Svobodova, M. (1975). Morphological changes in leucocytes in pregnancy. *Brit. J. Obstet. Gynaecol.* **82**, 146–150.

Lancet (1974). **1**, 718, Editorial.

Lengerová, A. and Vojtíšková, M. (1963). Prolonged survival of syngeneic male skin grafts in parous C57 Bl mice. *Folia Biol. (Praha)* **9**, 72–73.

Lin, T. M., Halbert, S. P., Keifer, D., Spellacy, W. N. and Gall, S. (1974). Characterisation of four human pregnancy associated plasma proteins. *Am. J. Obstet. Gynecol.* **118**, (2) 223–236.

Macrae, A. D. and Reid, D. (1968). Studies of rubella in pregnancy. Report of the public health laboratory service working party on rubella. *Brit. Med. J.* **3**, 203–206.

McKay, D. G. (1965). Disseminated intra-vascular coagulation, pp. 212–247, Hoeber Medical Division, Harper and Row, New York.

Onnis, A. (1974). Immunological implications of antimitotic chemotherapy. "Immunology in Obstetrics and Gynaecology"*, p. 297–300.

Ovary, Z. (1974). The structure of antibody molecules as related to transplacental passage. "Immunology in Obstetrics and Gynaecology"*, pp. 231–239.

Pearson, H. A., Shulman, N. R., Marder, V. J. and Cone, T. E. (1964). Iso-immune neonatal thrombocytopenic purpura. *Blood* **23**, 154–177.

Petrucco, O. M., Thompson, N. M., Lawrence, J. R. and Weldon, M. W. (1974). Immuno-fluorescent studies in renal biopsies in pre-eclampsia. *Brit. Med. J.* **1**, 473–476.

Sciarra, J. J., Toledo-Pereyra, L. H., Bendel, R. P. and Simmons, R. L. (1975). Pregnancy following renal transplantation. *Am. J. Obstet. Gynecol.* **123**, (4), 411–424.

Scott, J. S. (1966). Immunological diseases and pregnancy. *Brit. Med. J.* **1**, 1559–1567.

Short, R. V. (1969). Implantation and the maternal recognition of pregnancy. "Foetal Autonomy", a Ciba Foundation Symposium (eds. G. E. W. Wolstenholme and Maeve O'Connor), pp. 2–31. J. and A. Churchill, London.

Stafl, A. and Mattingly, R. F. (1972). Isoantigens ABO in cervical neoplasia. *Gynaecol. Oncol.* **1**, 26–35.

Stevenson, A. C. and Bobrow, M. (1967). Determinants of sex proportions in man. *J. Med. Gen.* **4**, 190–221.

Terasaki, P. I. and McClelland, J. D. (1964). Microdroplet assay of human serum cytotoxins. *Nature (London)* **204**, 998.

Tovey, G. H. and Darke, C. C. (1973). Some observations on the immune response to HL-A antigens in pregnancy. *Haematologia* **7**, 171–176.

Worrledge, S. M. (1974). "Blood and its Disorders". (Eds. R. M. Hardisty and D. J. Weatherall), pp. 714–762. Blackwell Scientific Publications, Oxford.

---

* "Immunology in Obstetrics and Gynaecology": Proceedings of the first international congress, Padua, (June, 1973) (Eds. A. Centaro and N. Narretti). Published by: Exerpta Medica, Amsterdam; American Elsevier Publishing Co. Inc., New York (1974).

21

Respiratory Disease

PETER COLE

The lung can be considered a gigantic filter handling approximately 10,000 litres of air and 7,000 litres of blood in each 24 hours. Within the airways the ciliary system, with its investing layer of mucus, traps and clears particles from the air which ventilates the lung, while distally, alveolar macrophages assist in such trapping.

In company with the skin and alimentary system, the lung is intimately related to the environment. It possesses a complex series of defence mechanisms against invasion and the sequelae of invasion by foreign antigens, whether living or inanimate, organic or inorganic. The outcome of such invasion depends upon the response of these mechanisms. Clearance of the antigen may in itself be defective or it may be accompanied by reactions which cause tissue damage.

IMMUNOLOGICAL REACTIONS IN THE LUNG

Immunological priming or sensitization through initial contact with antigen can set the scene for reactions which on subsequent exposure to that antigen may be protective or harmful to the host, or both. Those mediating protection are often termed immune, those causing host tissue damage are termed hypersensitivity reactions.

Protective Immunity

Although important non-immunological protection is mediated by mechanisms such as particle-trapping in the bronchial mucous secretions and their clearance by the ciliary "escalator", the cough reflex and non-specific scavenging of alveolar phagocytes, protective immunity is mediated by specific antibodies and cellular mechanisms. Specific immunity is concerned with protection against living material such as microorganisms, whereas inorganic material is cleared mainly by non-immunological mechanisms.

In the respiratory secretions immunoglobulin A (IgA) is the principal class of antibody. It is synthesized by the plasma cells surrounding the mucus glands and in the lamina propria of the respiratory tract and is secreted in dimer form with an additional peptide, the secretory piece. Evidence for the protective actions of secretory IgA is circumstantially strong (see Chapter 4) but there is still lack of direct evidence. The role of cell mediated immunity in respiratory disease is uncertain, but it probably plays a role in the host response to tuberculosis by lymphokine-mediated (Chapter 9) bactericidal activation of macrophages recruited to the site of infection. At the same time these reactions lead to tissue damage in the lung.

Hypersensitivity

In pulmonary medicine the commonest hypersensitivity states are those mediated by IgE (and occasionally by "short-term" IgG) antibodies acting in a cytophilic manner and causing release of mediators as part of a reaginic or anaphylactic response. In addition, damage may be caused by membrane-reactive, immune complex, T-cell and possibly other cellular mechanisms (see Chapters 1 and 10).

Although the word "hypersensitivity" conjures up the picture of an excessive reaction against antigen, it may take origin in a primary deficiency of specific protective immune mechanisms (e.g. secretory IgA). A possible example is the IgA deficiency which occurs in a significant proportion of patients who are prone to atopic disease (see Chapter 22).

In any disease of the lung in which immunological reactions may be occurring, it is important to examine the clinical and laboratory data, firstly for evidence whether the reaction is useful to the host and secondly for evidence of harm resulting.

MECHANISMS OF HYPERSENSITIVITY REACTIONS IN THE LUNG

The mechanisms of hypersensitivity reactions are dealt with fully in Chapter 10. Here their relationship to respiratory disease is considered.

Reaginic hypersensitivity is responsible in man for a complicated series of vascular, muscular and secretory responses when the antigen challenge is via the bronchial route, while the skin response to challenge (intradermal injection) is principally due to vascular changes.

Immune-complex mediated hypersensitivity is important since in a number of conditions (e.g. farmers' lung) it is a major pathogenetic factor. Because precipitation of complexes induced in antibody excess occurs very rapidly, the immune-complex reaction occurs at the entry site of the antigen and if the latter is inhaled the lung will be the organ involved. When soluble complexes form in antigen excess a systemic serum-sickness syndrome results with fever, rash, lymphadenopathy and arthropathy. Here also, the lung may be involved since the complexes may filter out in the pulmonary capillary bed. A role for immune complexes in the pathogenesis of lung disease is deduced principally from the following observations:

i. in farmers' lung, specific precipitating antibody can be demonstrated in over 80% of cases (Pepys and Jenkins, 1965);

ii. intradermal challenge of such patients with the suspected antigen provokes an immune complex (or Arthus) skin reaction at the site of the injection, consisting of erythema and brawny swelling about four to six hours after challenge. IgG antibody and complement have been demonstrated by immunofluorescence to be deposited around small blood vessels in the lesion, and the histology shows a polymorphonuclear leucocyte infiltration (Pepys *et al.*, 1968).

iii. Challenge by the endobronchial route in these patients causes a reaction at the challenge site, which is manifest clinically four to six hours after inhalation, sometimes as bronchoconstriction, but usually as a systemic response of fever, malaise, myalgia, neutrophil leucocytosis, dry cough, shortness of breath, widespread crepitations throughout the lungs, and a restrictive ventilatory defect, all characteristic of the disease itself.

The paradox that precipitating antibodies may be present in asymptomatic patients, e.g. farmers exposed to mouldy hay (Pepys and Jenkins, 1965) is explicable by the exposure being intermittent, albeit of high intensity. Few budgerigar fanciers are asymptomatic whilst possessing such antibodies, presumably because their exposure is continuous, although it may be of low intensity.

Delayed hypersensitivity to microbial products is an important clinical indication that contact with various infectious agents has occurred. This contact may have resulted in acquisition of immunity to the organism concerned, but it is not justifiable to equate delayed hypersensitivity to skin challenge with cell mediated immunity at the site of infection since the two may be separate entities. This aspect will be discussed more fully in the section on tuberculosis.

DISEASES CAUSED BY HOST RESPONSES TO ORGANIC DUSTS

There are three respiratory diseases whose pathogenesis is mainly hypersensitivity to organic matter entering the body, usually by inhalation. These are asthma, pulmonary eosinophilia and fibrosing alveolitis. Each individual's response to an antigen differs according to the balance struck between the properties of the particular antigen and the host's innate and acquired reactivity towards it. In all three diseases the host response depends upon the following properties of the antigen:

i. immunogenicity;
ii. particle size, determining where it is deposited (if less than 5μ diameter it will reach the alveoli);
iii. dose and intensity of exposure;
iv. duration; i.e. intermittent or continuous exposure.

The response also depends upon the reactivity of the host:

i. non-immunological, e.g. efficiency of clearance mechanisms;
ii. immunological; genetic (atopy, immune deficiency) and acquired (immuno-suppression by drugs etc.).

ASTHMA

Partial obstruction of the airways which is spontaneously or therapeutically reversible is termed asthma and may start at any age, may cause considerable socio-economic distress, and may be fatal. It is therefore important to diagnose and treat it effectively.

Asthma may be regarded as the abnormal response of a target organ (the bronchus) to one or more triggering factors. The division of asthma by Rackemann (1940) into extrinsic and intrinsic types still holds good (Turner-Warwick, 1974) as a useful clinical concept leading to a clearer understanding of pathogenesis and treatment. However, patients should not be forced into categories which they do not fit, and there are some whose pattern of asthma clinically and investigationally does not fall into either category. As with many other conditions there tends to be a spectrum between the two polar groups.

Extrinsic Asthma

This term implies bronchoconstriction due to an allergic reaction to antigens entering the respiratory tract from outside. Immunological support for such allergic mechanisms can usually be found, and understanding of the latter throws light on the pathogenesis and permits rational therapy. Intrinsic asthma implies bronchoconstriction due to a causal factor within the body, although it is also possible that this pattern of asthma may be a response to undetected external antigens. Information about the operation of allergic mechanisms in this group is scanty and indirect.

The pathogenesis of extrinsic asthma depends upon the prior sensitization of mast cells and basophils by heat-labile specific IgE antibody produced in response to specific antigen. On subsequent exposure this antibody combines with the antigen with resultant rapid release of mediator substances, histamine, slow reacting substance (SRS-A) and others, from the sensitized cells. Release of eosinophilic chemotactic factor (ECF-A) probably provokes the eosinophilia seen in the target tissues and their secretions.

Atopy

Some people suffer from extrinsic asthma because of an abnormal propensity to produce IgE antibodies which are normally stimulated only in small quantities by antigen exposure in every day life. This state of overreactivity to a wide range of antigens is termed "atopy" and clinically is manifest in the subject, and often in his first degree relatives, as a tendency to suffer from asthma, eczema, hay fever and rhinitis. The condition is important to identify because it has implications in treatment.

The pathogenesis of atopy is beginning to be understood with the realization that the portal of entry of antigens into the body is usually across natural barriers, such as the mucous membranes of the respiratory and gastro-intestinal tracts, and that secretory IgA antibody forms the principal specific defence mechanism of these barriers against invasion by antigens. Prospective studies of infants born into atopic families suggest that IgE production is greater, and development of eczema is more common, in those with temporary or persistent secretory IgA deficiency at a time when cow's milk is introduced into the diet. Evidence suggests that exclusion of this foreign protein by breast-feeding may reduce the incidence of the atopic state.

It is not understood why atopic persons may be totally unreactive with respect to one target organ e.g. nasal mucosa (rhinitis), yet perpetually suffering symptoms from another target organ e.g. bronchial smooth muscle (asthma). Exactly what determines the nature and site of response in atopic persons is unknown. Clinically it is important to bear this in mind because unless challenge tests to determine the antigens responsible for asthma are performed on the target organ involved in the disease, it is never absolutely certain which antigens are responsible, however strongly positive the skin prick test or nasal challenge test (useful as easy screening tests) may be.

It was recently recognized from results of passive transfer of human serum to monkey skin that IgE is not the only antibody capable of sensitizing mast cells and basophils; heat-stable IgG antibody is capable of performing this function in the short-term—and is therefore called short-term sensitizing IgG (STS-IgG) antibody. These antibodies have been found mainly in non-atopic subjects and seem to be of the IgG_4 subclass.

Intrinsic Asthma

This state of reversible airways obstruction (also termed cryptogenic asthma) in which there is neither clinical history nor skin prick test evidence of antigenic cause accounts for less than 10% of childhood asthmatics, but has a steadily increasing prevalence as age of onset of symptoms increases. About 80% of asthma beginning over the age of 60 is of the intrinsic type. Looked at another way, over 80% of cases of intrinsic asthma developed initial symptoms over the age of 30 years.

The pathology is identical to that seen in known allergic asthma—eosinophilic infiltration of the bronchial mucosa with thickened basement membrane and desquamation of the epithelium. The bronchial secretions contain eosinophils and in many cases a blood eosinophilia exists.

Immunology has little to offer in the investigation or treatment of these cases. Total immunoglobulin levels are within the normal range although increased amounts of IgE have been shown to be present on the surface of leucocytes by a technique measuring histamine release from the cells after challenge with anti-IgE. The specificity of this cytophilic IgE is unknown, but whether specific or non-specific, such cell sensitization could render mast cells and basophils more likely to discharge histamine when triggered by a range of non-allergic stimuli. The cytophilic IgE in these cases may also explain the efficacy of sodium cromoglycate (SCG) in this condition.

Occupational Asthma

Provocation tests simulating occupational exposure to chemical dusts, vapours and gases have indicated that asthma identical to that induced by common antigens may be triggered by these substances. There is little direct immunological evidence for an immunological pathogenesis of these reactions but the following observations make this likely:

i. only some exposed persons are affected;
ii. symptoms develop after a period of exposure and tend to worsen;
iii. symptoms are elicited by molecular amounts of substances (amounts causing no symptoms in unaffected persons, less than normally encountered at work, and less than effective as a non-specific irritant).

Examples of substances incriminated as causing reaginic and immune complex mediated asthmatic reactions are toluene di-isocyanates, used in manufacture of polyurethane products, and a variety of synthetic epoxy-resins. It is possible that some cases of asthma now thought to be intrinsic in type, may turn out to be immunological reactions to antigens not yet incriminated.

The main features of asthma are summarized in Table 1, the investigations relevant to every case of the disease are listed in Table 2, and a summary of therapy is given in Table 3.

Investigation of Asthma

A history of allergic provocation is a crucial piece of information and it is essential to take a very careful history of exposure to pollens, fungi, domestic pets, house dust, chemicals, drugs etc. and its relation to symptoms. A seasonal variation in symptoms is important as it may indicate allergy to pollens or moulds present in the air. A history of atopy suggests that further search for particular antigens as triggers of asthma will be unhelpful because of the high overall reactivity of the patient to a wide variety of antigens in small dose. A positive history is very often supported by the results of simple skin prick tests and provocation tests with relevant antigen(s).

TABLE 1

Summary of the clinical features of asthma

	Extrinsic		Intrinsic
	Non-atopic	Atopic	
CLINICAL SYMPTOMS	Dyspnoea with wheezing which may be associated with cough and sputum:		
	onset at any age; in response to one or two known antigens; often seasonal (depending on antigen)	onset often infancy/ childhood; in response to many antigens; part of atopic diathesis of eczema, rhinitis, asthma and food intolerance; often seasonal	onset usually after 20 years of age in non-atopic subject; no demonstrable antigens; perennial, may be associated with rhinitis; often worsened by aspirin
NATURAL HISTORY	May persist or lessen with age	Tend to "grow out of it"	Tends to worsen, requiring active measures
CLINICAL SIGNS	Normal between attacks, except for overinflated chest (A-P diameter increased) in chronic cases, but during episodes audible wheezes, rhonchi and prolonged expiratory phase present		
			may be nasal polyps very rarely may be a presentation of PAN
PATHOLOGY	Obstruction of airways by viscous mucus plugs, smooth muscle contraction and mucosal oedema. Hypertrophy of bronchial musculature and mucous glands with thickened basement membrane of the mucosa, and eosinophil infiltration		

PAN = Polyarteritis nodosa.

Skin Tests

Anaphylactic Reactions

The skin prick test with extracts containing common antigens provides useful corroborative evidence of allergy to antigens suggested by the clinical history. Positive reactions correlate well with history, results of provocation tests, and serological tests for specific IgE antibody.

The test consists of looking for a wheal and flare reaction in the skin ten minutes after gently but firmly pressing the skin of the forearm with a number 12 gauge hypodermic needle through a drop of the relevant antigen. The

TABLE 2
Summary of the investigation of asthma

	Extrinsic		Intrinsic
	Non-atopic	Atopic	
BLOOD eosinophils	Eosinophilia	Eosinophilia	Eosinophilia
ESR	Normal	Normal	Raised in PAN*
Total IgE	Raised	Raised	Normal
Precipitins to *Aspergillus*	Negative	Positive if broncho-pulmonary aspergillosis complicates	Negative
SPUTUM microscopy	Eosinophils in excess, Charcot-Leyden crystals (effete eosinophils), Creola bodies (columnar ciliated epithelial cell clumps from bronchial lining)		
Culture	Bacterial or viral infections are common causes of attacks of asthma		
CHEST X-RAY	Normal or transient bronchial thickening, with hyperinflation in chronic cases		
EXERCISE TEST	True "exercise-induced" asthma follows exercise; exercise usually exacerbates existing asthmatic attacks		
SKIN TESTS (PRICK)	Positive immediate and late responses: to one or two specific antigens provoking the asthma	to many antigens	Negative
LUNG FUNCTION TESTS	Airways obstruction reversible with bronchodilator therapy		
BRONCHIAL CHALLENGE	Positive immediate and late responses: to one or two specific antigens provoking the asthma	to many antigens	Negative

*PAN = Polyarteritis nodosa.

TABLE 3
Summary of treatment of asthma

	Extrinsic		Intrinsic
	Non-atopic	Atopic	
PROPHYLACTIC	Remove antigen(s) known to provoke asthma SCG	Reduce antigen "load" SCG	Prevent precipitating infections
SYMPTOMATIC	Bronchodilators as tablets, aerosols, suppositories, slow release tablets		
SPECIFIC HYPOSENSITIZATION	Often useful	Rarely useful	Inappropriate
SUPPRESSIVE	Corticosteroids as tablets or aerosols		

SCG = Sodium cromoglycate.

antigen is introduced into the superficial layers of the epidermis by a gentle lifting motion which should not puncture the skin, and which should be painless and readily accepted by children. A separate needle is used for each antigen and a control is included consisting of the vehicle in which the antigens are mounted. A positive result is a wheal and flare reaction to one or more antigen preparations, accompanied by a negative control test. The size of a reaction can be measured with a perspex "key" on which circles of known area are inscribed, but it should be remembered that the target organ being tested is skin, not bronchus, so that the size of a reaction may bear little relation to the actual severity of symptoms caused by the antigen elsewhere. The finding of a positive result is more important than the degree of positivity.

Before such tests are performed it is essential to ensure that the patient has taken no antihistamines for 24 to 48 hours. Corticosteroids do not affect results. It is unusual for skin tests to provoke any systemic effect except as described below under immune complex responses. Extracts of common antigens in use at present vary considerably in potency both between manufacturers and between different batches from the same manufacturer. There is an urgent requirement for standardization of such extracts.

What is true for skin holds good for nasal mucosa, another part of the body readily accessible for challenge tests, except that results are of much more significance for allergic rhinitis, since the organ tested is the target of the allergic response in life.

Immune Complex Reactions

It is well recognized that a sufficiently intense anaphylactic skin response may be followed by an immune complex reaction, with brawny swelling appearing around the test site after about four to six hours. This occasionally has a systemic counterpart of fever and malaise, which resolves spontaneously within 24 hours, or which can be blocked by corticosteroid if necessary. Immunofluorescent examination of such "non-immediate" skin test reactions has shown perivascular and vascular endothelial aggregates staining for IgG, IgM, IgA, and also complement, supportive evidence of their immune complex nature.

The significance of such late reactions is difficult to assess. Certainly, as will be seen later, in allergic bronchopulmonary aspergillosis complicating asthma this response is provoked by *Aspergillus* antigen, but in the context of uncomplicated asthma it is uncertain whether it is relevant to prolongation of the acute asthmatic attack into "status asthmaticus".

Bronchial Challenge Tests

The only proof that a particular antigen actually causes asthma is the reproduction of symptoms by inhalation. As such provocation tests may cause severe reactions they must be done only by experts, and respiratory function should be adequately monitored throughout. They should not be done as out-patient procedures.

Baseline documentation of physical signs, spirometry, temperature and differential blood count is initially obtained in response to inhalation of a buffered aerosol of the vehicle which will be used for the antigen challenge. The aerosol containing antigen is then administered for an initial period of one minute, at a dilution which produces no more than a 3 mm wheal on skin testing. If no response in the forced expiratory volume (FEV_1) occurs within 20 minutes a further two minute inhalation is allowed, followed by observation for ten minutes. If no reaction occurs after inhalation for a total of five minutes, ten-fold increasing dilutions are used. Symptoms, signs and spirometry are recorded at ten minute intervals for one hour, then at hourly intervals. Temperature is recorded hourly, and differential blood counts are taken at four, eight and twelve hours following challenge.

The results in a positive case will show an early (reaginic type) response (temporary fall in FEV_1 of $> 15\%$) and may additionally show a later reaction of immune complex type with a prolonged fall in FEV_1, and often fever and

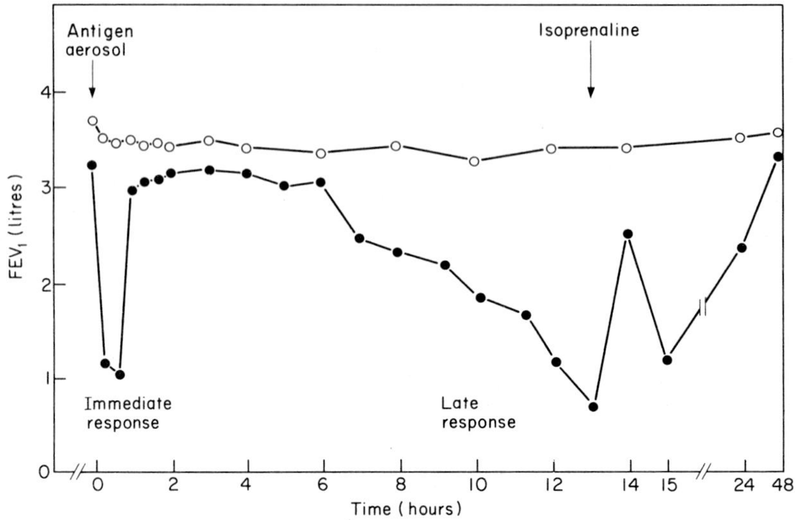

Fig. 1. A bronchial challenge test with dual asthmatic response.

leucocytosis (Fig. 1). The two responses seen in the same patient are termed a dual asthmatic response and occur in almost half the patients who give an anaphylactic response on bronchial provocation to extracts of the two house dust mites, *Dermatophagoides pteronyssinus* and *D. farinae*. Possible results of bronchial challenge tests are shown in Table 4.

The time course of the early reaction to provocation is closely related to that of the reaginic skin test reaction, suggesting that they have the same immunopathological mechanisms. Histamine, histamine-liberating agents, methacholine and a variety of non-specific stimuli elicit similar reactions when used experimentally, and it is known that such tissue mediators are released during the course of reaginic responses mediated by antibodies sensitizing mast cells and basophils. The inability of antihistamine drugs to block the reaginic type of asthma may be due to release of SRS-A as one of the tissue mediators, against which such drugs have no action. Antihistamines can block anaphylaxis in the guinea-pig however, because the bronchial smooth muscle in this species is insensitive to SRS-A, and the same drugs can block the reaginic skin test reaction in man presumably because skin is a different target organ to bronchial smooth muscle. Asthmatic attacks following the ingestion of aspirin, usually in asthmatics with an intrinsic pattern, may be explained by the observation that anti-inflammatory drugs (e.g. indomethacin) experimentally increase the release of SRS-A from sensitized human lung *in vitro*, despite blocking histamine and prostag-

TABLE 4
Significance of bronchial challenge tests

If history of response to antigen is	And skin test to that antigen is	Then bronchial challenge test will probably be	Clinical use
Positive	Positive	Positive	No advantage over skin test
Positive	Negative	Usually negative early response, but may be positive late response	May indicate immune complex basis for asthma
Negative	Negative	Usually negative early response, but may be positive late response	May indicate immune complex basis for asthma
Positive but *recent* initial exposure	Negative	Positive	Useful when initial exposure recent

landin release. The non-immediate asthmatic reaction to provocation is analogous in time course to the immune complex, complement-dependent skin test response to the relevant antigen. Likewise it may be accompanied by fever, malaise, myalgia and leucocytosis. This reaction is also blocked by corticosteroids.

Recently it has been recognized that there is a non-immediate response to antigen provocation which takes the form of a nocturnal fall in FEV_1 recurring for many nights after such a test. This cyclic phenomenon, which is unassociated with obvious asthmatic reaction during the day time, is obscure in its mechanism but is likely to be related to that responsible for the pronounced early morning "dip" seen in the FEV_1 of many asthmatics who experience more pronounced "tightness" in the early mornings.

Serology

Serum IgE measurements are generally unhelpful in that they add nothing (except a number) to the conclusion derived from skin tests, which is that there is a direct relationship between the number and intensity of immediate skin test responses and the serum level of IgE. It is to be expected that skin-test negative intrinsic asthmatics will have normal IgE levels, and that extrinsic asthmatics will have elevated levels. The finding of a very high total IgE in the serum may be useful in pointing to a common complication of asthma, allergic bronchopulmonary aspergillosis, but such levels are also common in parasitic diseases.

Specific IgE antibody measurements are potentially more useful but again merely put a value on the qualitative result of skin tests to specific antigens. One method of measurement, the immunochemical radio-allergosorbent test (RAST), is both sensitive and can deal with large numbers. It is expensive to run however, and has not replaced the simple, safe, and quick skin prick-test.

Management

This is summarized in Fig. 2. Although immunological manoeuvres are of help in extrinsic asthma, there is little of relevance to offer the intrinsic asthmatic apart from the administration of corticosteroids whose mechanism of action in this setting is far from clear.

Prevention of Exposure to Known Antigens

The perfect answer to allergic asthma would be to prevent the host coming into contact with the relevant antigen(s). This is extremely difficult to achieve in practice particularly in the case of antigens widely distributed in nature,

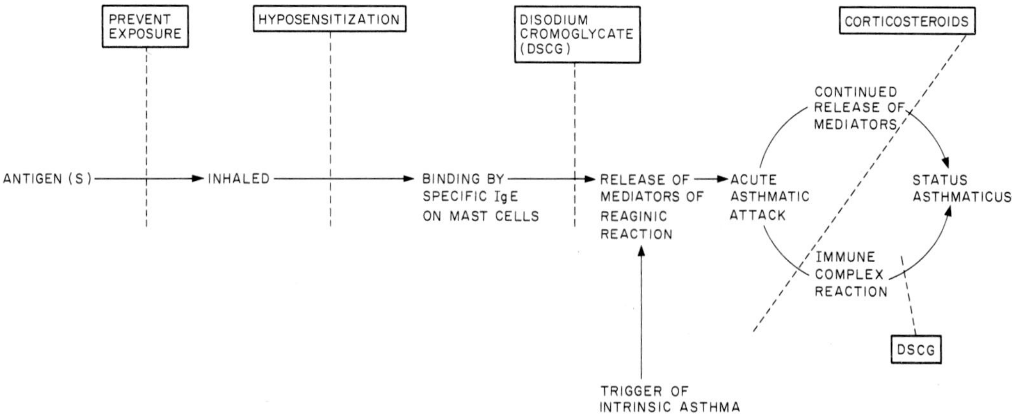

Fig. 2. Immunological relevance of treatment of asthma.

such as pollens. With seasonal antigens, patients will recognize from experience what they cannot do, where they cannot go, and at what times of year these prohibitions operate. The Asthma Research Council assists by publishing "pollen count" readings each day throughout the year—sometimes indicating a rise in count which gives warning of heavy exposure to come and allows the patient to make plans to avoid it by staying indoors, or to prevent its effects by the use of drugs.

With household antigens, the prevention of exposure is more practicable. House dust allergy, caused by the potent antigen, the housedust mite, can be reduced by careful domestic measures as detailed in Table 5.

TABLE 5

Environmental control in the management of asthma

1. Vacuum-clean house regularly
2. Dust with a damp cloth
3. Vacuum-clean mattress and pillows weekly
4. Wash blankets every two months
5. Enclose mattress in a large plastic bag and wipe weekly
6. Substitute foam pillows for feather ones
7. Do not keep domestic pets in the house

In atopic asthma, the antigens capable of inciting a reaction in the respiratory tract are so many and so varied that this form of prophylaxis is virtually useless.

Hyposensitization

When it is difficult to keep the patient apart from the relevant antigen, in that even molecular dosage is capable of eliciting reactions, it may still be possible to reduce the degree of reactivity of the host by a process of hyposensitization, thereby reducing the number and severity of attacks. The following criteria must be satisfied for the safe and effective use of this immunological technique:

i. frequent or severe asthma, resistant to other simple forms of therapy;
ii. asthma known to be due to one or, at most two, antigens. Hyposensitization to what amounts to a "soup" of antigens, as recommended by some advertising, is rarely if ever effective, and may be harmful;
iii. hyposensitization to seasonal antigens to be started before natural exposure begins;

iv. Adrenaline and antihistamines to be to hand in case of a reaginic reaction.

The practical procedure is to start by giving a parenteral injection of the antigen at extremely low concentration. If this causes no reaction then injections of gradually increasing concentrations of antigen are given at weekly intervals until the patient can tolerate the concentration that may be expected in normal life.

The mechanism accounting for successes by this procedure is thought to be the induction of "blocking" antibodies to the antigen of IgG class. The extremely low concentration of antigen employed initially is usually insufficient to cause a reaginic reaction, although there may be local side effects at the site of injection, but the gradually increasing concentration can induce sufficiently high affinity IgG antibodies to make it likely that subsequent exposure to antigen will result in the latter binding to these IgG antibodies which thereby block the IgE-mediated reaginic reactions. Because results are unpredictable it is possible that there are other mechanisms involved, such as decreased reactivity of basophil cells. The procedure can be effective as shown by definite improvement in symptoms in over 60% of grass pollen allergic subjects. There is less evidence for the effectiveness of hyposensitization to other antigens. In successful cases the effect appears to be related to total dosage. When specific IgE levels are measured they are found to rise at the beginning of treatment and then to fall as it progresses.

Sodium Cromoglycate (SCG)

This drug has revolutionized the treatment of extrinsic asthma particularly the atopic and exercise-induced varieties. It is strictly prophylactic and therefore must be taken regularly to obtain a satisfactory result. In the atopic patient with frequent attacks of asthma unresponsive to sympathomimetics this drug may allow return to a normal life. It is less useful in cases with few or intermittent attacks because it cannot be used as therapy for an existing attack and, unless such attacks are severe and unresponsive to other treatment, the continued use of the drug several times each day to prevent only rare attacks seems unjustifiable. Intrinsic asthmatics respond in similar numbers to the drug and therefore it is worth a trial in them since many will otherwise require corticosteroids. The socially crippling "exercise-induced" asthma, starting either towards the end of exercise or some minutes after it has terminated, is often blocked by SCG, so that a trial of the drug immediately before exercise is warranted.

SCG is marketed in two forms—plain capsules of the drug in a lactose base, and capsules compounded with isoprenaline. In most cases, but particularly in trials of therapy, it is preferable to use the plain variety because the isoprenaline in the compound may cause some relief from asthma which may be misinterpreted as a true response to SCG and lead to continuation of an expensive drug with little benefit. The compound capsule is used when attacks of coughing and wheezing follow SCG given alone due to the irritant effect of the powder. It is probably better in such cases to give plain SCG about ten minutes after an aerosolized bronchodilator has been administered. The drug is taken three or four times a day from a spinhaler and it is of paramount importance to ensure that the patient is actually *seen* to be taking it properly before assessing its affect. In the case of exercise-induced asthma the drug should obviously be taken prior to exercise.

The mechanism of action of SCG is unclear but it evidently intervenes after the reaction of antigen with cell-bound IgE, inhibiting the release of histamine and other mediators from sensitized mast cells, probably stabilizing the cell lysosomes via cyclic nucleotide control. Patients suffering asthmatic reactions apparently mediated by "short term" IgG antibody do not seem to benefit as much from SCG although it is too early to be sure of this. Non-immediate asthmatic reactions (immune complex reactions) can also be blocked by pre-treatment with SCG, as can be seen from provocation tests. The mechanism of action of the drug in this situation and also in prophylaxis of exercise-induced asthma is not clear.

Corticosteroids

These anti-inflammatory agents are ineffective in blocking reaginic type asthmatic reactions in the experimental situation, but can be shown to have a beneficial effect on naturally occurring asthma provided that one allows a time lapse of hours before judging the response. This probably reflects the fact that corticosteroids block immune complex mediated asthmatic reactions as seen in provocation tests.

Steroids used to be prescribed only when sympathomimetics, theophylline derivatives and SCG failed, because the side-effects from prolonged dosage outweigh the advantages of use until all other safer agents have been tried. Recently however, aerosolized corticosteroid has become available (beclomethasone dipropionate) which in normal dosage acts locally at the level of the bronchus without undergoing enough absorption to suppress the adrenal glands. Beclomethasone aerosol can thus be used in conjunction with other non-steroidal agents without dangerous side effects. Furthermore, the use of the aerosol in patients requiring systemic corticosteroids can reduce considerably the requirement for the latter, thereby lessening the risk of side effects. It appears that oro-pharyngeal candidiasis may occur unpredictably in the upper range of dosage, but the factors predisposing to this are undetermined.

Systemic corticosteroids are very often required to control intrinsic asthma. In these cases it may be possible to reduce dosage after starting the drug, but later the requirement for corticosteroids tends to increase. In extrinsic asthmatics whose disease is refractory to other agents, corticosteroids are indicated in sufficient dosage to control the wheezy breathlessness. The often quoted problem of whether to give a short course or continuous therapy ceases to exist if sufficient dosage is given to control these symptoms. It is always important, however, to try continually to reduce the dosage and not simply to accept that the patient "is on steroids" for good; the fluctuating course of the disease may allow complete weaning on occasions. During corticosteroid therapy of asthma it is important to continue supportive therapy with other agents. The regular and correct use of bronchodilators, SCG and aerosolized steroids may considerably reduce the oral corticosteroid requirement.

PULMONARY EOSINOPHILIA

This syndrome embraces all the causes of recurrent, transitory pulmonary radiographic shadows with concomitant blood eosinophilia, and usually excess eosinophils in the sputum. It may be classified into "extrinsic", in which an external cause is identifiable (fungi, drugs or parasites), and "cryptogenic" when none is found. The pulmonary shadowing is due to lung infiltration by cells, mainly eosinophils, and may be associated with asthma.

Drugs Causing Pulmonary Eosinophilia

Drugs known to cause pulmonary eosinophilia include nitrofurantoin, para-aminosalicylic acid (PAS), penicillin, sulphonamides, hydrallazine, aspirin, and hydrochlorothiazides as the most common. Wheezing is not a striking feature of this condition.

There is little known about the mechanisms operating to cause disease in these cases and it is rare (although described in the case of nitrofurantoin) for the disease to progress to fibrosis. Antibodies to the drugs can often be demonstrated in the serum of patients suffering from the disease, but as these can often be found in asymptomatic persons taking the drugs their significance is in doubt. Recently, T-lymphocyte sensitization to nitrofurantoin has been described in patients suffering from pulmonary eosinophilia due to this drug. Such cells have been shown to be cytotoxic for human lung fibroblasts in tissue culture; both these cellular reactions, and also exocytosis (active release) of lysosomal enzymes from normal alveolar macrophages, was potentiated by the presence of serum from patients suffering from the acute syndrome. This suggests a role for immune complexes formed between the drug and antibodies in such drug-induced syndromes.

Parasites Causing Pulmonary Eosinophilia

Pulmonary eosinophilia due to parasites has been termed "Loeffler's syndrome" and "tropical eosinophilia". Here again wheeze plays a small part in symptomatology which is usually self-limiting. Parasites causing this condition are many—in natives of the United Kingdom *Toxocara canis* and *T. catis* should be considered, although these parasites probably cause only a few cases. The diagnosis is established by a positive skin test to an extract of the parasite, and the presence of complement-fixing antibodies in the serum.

Allergic Bronchopulmonary Aspergillosis

The ubiquitous fungus *Aspergillus* is the cause of this form of pulmonary eosinophilia but *Candida*, *Phycomycetes*, *Blastomyces*, *Coccidioides*, and others may give rise to a similar condition especially outside the United Kingdom.

The host response to *Aspergillus* varies with the immunological reactivity of the patient, and the circumstances of exposure. The following responses may be seen:

i. extrinsic asthma due to a reaginic mechanism response in the atopic subject;

ii. pulmonary eosinophilia (allergic bronchopulmonary aspergillosis); intense antigenic stimulus in the atopic subject produced by saprophytic growth of the fungus in the bronchi;
iii. extrinsic allergic alveolitis; the response of the non-atopic subject to inhaled particles of organic dust;
iv. aspergilloma (a fungus "ball"); saprophytic growth of the fungus in a pre-existing cavity of the lung, usually in non-atopic persons;
v. invasive aspergillosis; progressive invasion of the lung by fungus seen in the immunosuppressed subject.

McCarthy and Pepys (1971a) showed that allergic bronchopulmonary aspergillosis occurs predominantly in atopic persons and is due to the growth of *Aspergillus fumigatus* within bronchi of medium size. They found it to be the commonest cause of pulmonary eosinophilia in the United Kingdom.

Clinical Features

The cardinal clinical features of the disease are given in Table 6. In the United Kingdom the diagnosis should be suspected strongly in any extrinsic asthmatic whose asthma worsens for no apparent cause and becomes refractory to treatment which was previously effective. Aspergillosis is the commonest complication of asthma in the United Kingdom excepting iatrogenic disease. Supportive evidence is a history of transient episodes of fever, pleurisy, sputum plugs, and bronchiectasis. The development of this condition often occurs in early winter when the *Aspergillus* spore count in the air rises. The natural history is of "flu-like" episodes lasting often for several weeks with worsening asthma which if untreated leads to clearly reversible airways obstruction.

Investigation

Skin Tests

Since this condition commonly complicates extrinsic asthma, immediate wheal and flare responses in the skin from prick test challenge with *A. fumigatus* antigen would be expected in virtually all patients, and this is the case. Furthermore, about one quarter of the patients show a later immune complex type of skin response to the antigen after the prick-test (Table 6) and virtually all patients show this if the challenge is more intense as with intra-

TABLE 6

Features of allergic bronchopulmonary aspergillosis during episodes

Clinical features	Autumn or winter exacerbation (spore count high) Asthma, often severe Fever Cough with purulent, often bloodstained, sputum containing firm plugs of fungus about 10 mm in size Pleurisy and pulmonary collapse/consolidation
Blood	Eosinophilia 500–2000/cm
Pathology	Sputum plugs contain eosinophils and fungal elements Eosinophils in alveolar spaces in areas of consolidation Bronchial wall changes as in asthma, but fungi may be seen with immunofluorescent evidence of immune complexes in proximal bronchial walls where there is bronchiectatic change No vasculitis
Skin tests to *A. fumigatus*	Early response in all cases Late response in 25% cases (prick method), or 100% cases (intra-cutaneous method)
Serology	Precipitating antibodies in most cases (concentrated serum)
Bronchial challenge	All show early asthmatic response Approximately 75% show a late asthmatic response } Dual response

cutaneous injection. Evidence that this skin response is mediated by immune complexes rests on its time relationship to the challenge, and the biopsy evidence showing oedema, polymorph infiltration, scanty eosinophils, and immunofluorescent staining of deposits (presumably immune complexes) of three immunoglobulin classes and complement in mononuclear cells, vascular endothelium and perivascular tissues (McCarthy and Pepys, 1971b).

There is a group of patients developing pulmonary eosinophilia due to *A. fumigatus* within a few years of (or occasionally preceding) the development of asthma at about the age of 30. About half of these patients show positive reactions to *A. fumigatus* antigen alone on the prick test (i.e. intrinsic type of asthma with supervening allergic bronchopulmonary aspergillosis).

Sputum

Culture of the sputum is unhelpful as the fungus is ubiquitous and may be cultured from many patients with chronic respiratory disease. In many cases of aspergillosis the fungus does not grow on routine culture media used to isolate fungi.

Microscopy of the cut sputum plugs show mycelia of *A. fumigatus* and eosinophils. At bronchoscopy, sputum plugs may be firmly adherent to the walls of proximal bronchi, owing to growth of the fungus into the latter, and dissection may precipitate bleeding.

Serology

The intensity of the antigenic stimulus generated by actual growth of fungus in the bronchial wall provokes the formation of precipitating antibodies in all cases. The concentration of precipitins is proportional to the intensity of exposure rather than to the severity of the clinical disease.

Precipitating antibodies can be demonstrated by the simple technique of double immunodiffusion in agar in which the patient's serum and *Aspergillus* extract are placed in adjoining wells in an agar plate and are allowed to diffuse towards each other, whereupon antibodies (precipitins) react with the antigens in the extract, forming lines of precipitation in the agar. It must be emphasized that demonstration of precipitins requires the use of a number of extracts which may contain antigens differing from those commonly used, and that about one third of cases will require three to four-fold concentration of serum. A quicker result can be obtained if counter-current immuno-electrophoresis is used.

Positive precipitin tests are seldom found in healthy persons and their incidence is less than 10% in patients with apparently uncomplicated asthma or other lung disease. With increasing intensity of stimulus by the fungus the host responds with production of a greater number of different precipitins against the various antigens of the fungus, and this is reflected in the test as a larger number of different precipitin lines. In allergic bronchopulmonary aspergillosis there are usually one to three lines in contrast to the extreme example of aspergilloma where the antigenic load of the fungus ball is so great that from 10 to 20 lines can often be seen. IgG, IgM and IgA classes are all represented in the precipitating antibodies.

Levels of specific IgE serum antibody to *A. fumigatus* rise, as shown by RAST tests, during episodes of allergic bronchopulmonary aspergillosis, as does the total serum IgE, and are higher in such patients than in prick test positive uncomplicated asthmatics.

Bronchial Provocation

This is usually unnecessary for the diagnosis of aspergillosis since the results of skin tests and serology give a definite answer in most cases, especially if the serum is concentrated before a negative result is accepted in the precipitin test. However, as in some patients with asthma, while the history of exposure and onset of symptoms may be strong, no supporting evidence is forthcoming from skin tests or serology and in such cases bronchial provocation may be helpful. If carried out with the precautions described above it does not cause radiological lung involvement.

Passive Cutaneous Anaphylaxis (PCA Reaction)

This research method has provided further evidence of the immune complex basis for development of the disease. Golbert and Patterson (1970) provoked early and late skin and bronchial responses (including pulmonary infiltration) in monkeys sensitized by passive transfer of serum from humans who had clinical evidence of aspergillosis with immediate hypersensitivity and precipitins to *Aspergillus*. Monkeys sensitized with serum from patients with only immediate hypersensitivity to the antigen, develop neither the dual reaction nor pulmonary infiltration.

Management

The same principles apply as in the treatment of asthma, for aspergillosis is invariably associated with asthma if it does not complicate pre-existing asthmatic disease. However, there are important differences.

Prevention of Exposure to Aspergillus

The patient should avoid barns, granaries and hay; but cannot avoid the ubiquitous distribution of this fungus in the air.

Hyposensitization is contraindicated because:

i. it is ineffective in practice
ii. local immune complex type reactions at the site of injection become unacceptably severe
iii. theoretically it could aggravate the disease by stimulating more antibodies contributing to immune-complex reactions.

Sodium Cromoglycate (SCG)

This drug inhibits the reaginic and immune complex components of the disease, as in asthma (Fig. 2), by blocking release of inflammatory mediators of anaphylaxis and tissue damage. However, it is usually ineffective in controlling symptoms completely.

Corticosteroids

These agents used systemically suppress the effects of the tissue-damaging mediators of the immune complex reaction and tend to prevent their release. They have little or no effect on the reaginic response (compare asthma, Fig. 2). The value of local aerosol corticosteroids in this condition is questionable. They are probably not as effective as by the systemic route because of the difficulty of achieving penetration to the site of immune complex deposition. Furthermore a high concentration of corticosteroid accumulating locally could theoretically lead to growth of other fungi (e.g. *Candida*).

Anti-fungal agents

These non-immunological weapons are ineffective largely because the fungus is ubiquitous and returns as soon as the drug (e.g. 5-fluorocytosine) is stopped. The drugs available cannot be used in the long-term and have undesirable side-effects in the short-term.

Bronchodilators

It may be inferred from the above that treatment of this condition is relatively simple, aiming to suppress symptoms with adequate dosage of specific or non-specific drugs. However, in practice there are many young patients in whom to suppress all symptoms and radiological signs large doses of corticosteroids would have to be used for long periods. As well as the side-effects of corticosteroids in the dosage necessary to suppress radiological evidence of the disease, one can never be sure that in the periods between X-rays there may not have been further fleeting shadows. The question is whether prolonged periods of fleeting shadows without symptoms produce irreversible damage to the lung, and in view of the role of immunopathology outlined above the likely answer is that they do. The physician is thus between the devil of corticosteroid toxicity and the deep blue sea of disease-mediated irreversible lung damage.

Cryptogenic Pulmonary Eosinophilia

This variety of pulmonary eosinophilia has been reviewed by McCarthy and Pepys (1973). It refers to the syndrome of fleeting radiographic lung shadows with blood eosinophilia when known causes have been excluded.

In childhood most cases occur in atopic subjects and are associated with pronounced asthma. It is likely that some unidentified antigen induces this syndrome but this has not been proven. In adults the situation is different because most cases occur in non-atopic subjects in whom an asthmatic component is present in only a proportion.

The following clinical features distinguish the syndrome from that of allergic bronchopulmonary aspergillosis:

i. it is more common in females;
ii. the patient is often very ill with high fever and marked dyspnoea;
iii. sputum plugs are rare;
iv. radiographic lung shadowing is more widespread and more peripheral;
v. lack of bronchial wall damage, therefore usually no bronchiectasis, lung shrinkage or fibrosis;
vi. raised ESR;
vii. hepatosplenomegaly and lymphadenopathy may be present.

The patients have normal, or only slightly raised, total IgE antibody levels in the serum. Rarely pulmonary vasculitis is seen, but it is uncommon for cryptogenic pulmonary eosinophilia to lead to polyarteritis nodosa.

The condition requires treatment with corticosteroids which, again in contrast with their effect in the pulmonary eosinophilia of aspergillosis (and in polyarteritis nodosa), dramatically improve the patient. It is often possible to wean such patients off corticosteroids without relapse.

FIBROSING ALVEOLITIS

This term embraces a group of conditions in which the alveolar walls become thickened and later fibrosed. They may be classified into two main groups.

Extrinsic Alveolitis. Hypersensitivity to known organic dusts whose size is usually less than 5μ, allowing penetration to the alveoli.

Cryptogenic Alveolitis. Of unknown cause and often associated with non-organ specific auto-antibodies.

Both conditions are uncommon, but they are of importance for two main reasons. First, many causal agents of extrinsic alveolitis are known and appropriate treatment can thus be given to patients with this type of disease to limit an otherwise potentially fatal condition. Second, the pathogenetic mechanisms of both types of disease are still undetermined, although more is known about the extrinsic variety, and their elucidation may increase understanding of the mechanisms provoking other granulomatous and fibrosing diseases.

The cardinal clinical features of the two conditions are summarized in Table 7, and the known causes of the extrinsic variety in Table 8. The extrinsic conditions are reviewed by Pepys (1969).

Investigation of Extrinsic Allergic Alveolitis

The diagnosis should be suspected in any person exposed to the antigens listed in Table 8 and suffering from respiratory symptoms. The presence of the other features of the condition (Table 7) will strongly support it. However, the circumstances of exposure of the host to antigens is an important factor in the mode of presentation of the disease. The more continuous and the lower the exposure dose (e.g. budgerigar fanciers lung), the more insidious the onset and progression of the disease, and therefore the more difficult it is to make the diagnosis if a good history of exposure at home or at work is not obtained. Intermittent exposure to large amounts of antigen (e.g. a pigeon-fancier cleaning his loft each week) results in the classical syndrome of acute symptoms appearing about four hours after exposure and resolving within 24 hours.

The absence of a history of exposure, especially associated with features shown in Table 7, supports a diagnosis of cryptogenic alveolitis as long as the main causes of widespread pulmonary fibrosis have been excluded.

Serology

The presence of precipitins to the suspected antigens strongly supports, but does not prove, the diagnosis of extrinsic alveolitis, since it is possible for an individual to produce precipitins without suffering disease. Almost all farmers suffering from exposure to mouldy hay have positive precipitin tests, but 20% of apparently normal farmers also produce precipitins to the antigen. Likewise a high percentage of asymptomatic poultry-breeders may have precipitins, yet most budgerigar fanciers with precipitins suffer from the disease.

TABLE 7
Clinical and laboratory features of fibrosing alveolitis

	Extrinsic	Cryptogenic
ONSET	Episodic following exposure to antigen, unless latter is continuous when onset will be insidious	Onset insidious
SYMPTOMS AND SIGNS	Dyspnoea without wheeze; cough with little sputum; fever, malaise, myalgia, anorexia; weight loss; fine rales throughout lung fields; later, tachypnoea, tracheal displacement and flattening of chest wall:	
	Finger clubbing unusual	Finger clubbing in $>60\%$
NATURAL HISTORY	Initial acute episodes following exposure merge into later insidious progression unless exposure to antigen terminated	Progression at varying rates
ASSOCIATED DISORDERS	Nil	May coexist with a "connective tissue" disorder
PATHOLOGY	Granulomata throughout alveolar and respiratory bronchiolar walls Multinuclear cells with inclusions Lymphocytes and plasma cells common Late progressive fibrosis of alveolar walls especially in upper lobes	Alveoli packed with mononuclear cells (desquamative pattern) Progressive fibrosis of alveolar walls (mural pattern) Both patterns may coexist
BLOOD	Initially WBC and ESR raised in acute episodes Precipitins to causal antigen	Initially γ-globulins and ESR raised Non organ specific auto-antibodies in about 60% of acute cases, less in chronic
TREATMENT	Prevent further exposure to antigen Corticosteroids if resolution incomplete Resolution poor once fibrosis occurs	Corticosteroids may improve a minority if given before established fibrosis Other immunosuppressants probably unhelpful
	Oxygen and the control of infection	

TABLE 8
Causes of extrinsic alveolitis

Source	Name of disease	Antigen
Mouldy hay	Farmer's lung	*Micropolyspora faeni* *Thermoactinomyces vulgaris*
Contaminated humidified air conditioning	—	*M. faeni* and *T. vulgaris*
Avian droppings	Bird fancier's lung	Avian serum protein
Mushroom compost	Mushroom worker's lung	Post-spawning compost
Mouldy cheese	Cheese worker's lung	*Penicillium casei*
Infected maple bark	Maple bark stripper's lung	*Cryptostroma corticale*
Mouldy bagasse	Bagassosis	*Thermoactinomyces sacchari*
Mouldy cork dust	Suberosis	*P. frequentans*
Infested wheat flour	Wheat weevil disease	*Sitophilus granarius*
Bovine and porcine pituitary snuff	Pituitary snuff-taker's lung	Heterologous serum protein
Animal food factory	Fishmeal worker's lung	Fish meal
Mouldy sawdust	Sequiosis	*Pullalaria pullulans*
Paper mill	Wood-pulp worker's lung	*Alternaria*
Mouldy malt and barley	Malt worker's lung	*Aspergillus fumigatus and A. clavatus*

The magnitude of the precipitin reaction is related to intensity of exposure, not to severity of clinical disease.

Skin Tests

The extrinsic variety usually occurs in non-atopic persons who may give reaginic or immune complex type skin test responses to the offending antigen, although extracts of the spores from mouldy hay often incite responses in unaffected persons. Intracutaneous tests may uncover positive immune complex type responses in cases where a prick test is negative.

Provocation Tests

When clinical features are inconclusive, or serology and skin tests unhelpful, provocation tests may confirm the diagnosis of extrinsic alveolitis. It is important to carry them out by simulating as exactly as possible the conditions encountered by the patient in daily life at his home or at work, using the actual substances he encounters and handling them in exactly the same way as they would be handled in normal life. In this way it is possible to discover causal antigens which might be missed by using standard extracts, or preparations thought wrongly to contain the antigen.

The usual result of such an inhalation test is an immune complex type of reaction which will reproduce symptoms of alveolitis—but in patients whose disease includes airways obstruction the asthma may be a part of the immune complex type of response.

Lung Biopsy

This should be done in all atypical cases who are in sufficiently good clinical condition to tolerate it safely, in order to determine whether the histological pattern is of the extrinsic type—because if it is, further search for an antigen must be made. The characteristic appearances are described in Table 7. In addition, immunofluorescent tests may show the presence of IgG and complement in the lesions.

Cryptogenic fibrosing alveolitis

This may be associated with the presence of rheumatoid arthritis, Sjogren's syndrome, systemic sclerosis, active chronic hepatitis, ulcerative colitis, polymyositis, renal tubular acidosis or Hashimoto's thyroiditis. As with intrinsic asthma, immunology has little to contribute to the diagnosis apart from the demonstration of certain autoantibodies.

IgM rheumatoid factor in low titre is found in about a quarter of cases, and about a half of these have clinical rheumatoid arthritis. Anti-nuclear antibody is found in a slightly higher percentage of cases and may be complement-fixing. Antibodies to single-stranded DNA can be demonstrated by precipitation using calf-thymus DNA preparations, but anti-lung antibodies demonstrated in complement-fixation or antiglobulin consumption tests are usually found to be non-organ specific.

Lymphocyte sensitization to DNA can occasionally be demonstrated using leucocyte migration inhibition tests, but the significance of this is unknown.

Immunofluorescent studies on lung biopsies have rarely shown immune complexes and the evidence for circulating immune complexes is inconclusive.

About one quarter of cases have circulating rheumatoid factors, sera may be anti-complementary and cryoblobulins are occasionally present.

Digital vasculitis occurs in association with complement-fixing antibodies in some patients, but no complement conversion or consumption has been demonstrated.

Management

Extrinsic alveolitis presents little problem in therapy if diagnosed early, because prevention of exposure to antigen, with or without temporary help from corticosteroids, results in cure. For the unfortunate sufferer from the cryptogenic variety, attempts to halt progress of the disease can be based only on the empirical use of corticosteroids or other immunosuppressive agents.

Immunopathogenesis of Fibrosing Alveolitis

Extrinsic

The evidence for immune complex reactions being implicated in the pathogenesis of this group of conditions is strong—the time course of the symptoms in relation to exposure, their sensitivity to corticosteroids, the presence of precipitating antibodies and positive immune complex type skin reactions. However, a characteristic feature of the histopathology of this condition is the presence of granulomas. These are commonly regarded as being part of a delayed hypersensitivity host reaction to antigen, but immune complexes may also stimulate granuloma production and could be responsible for the pathological features of the disease.

There are cases with an undoubted allergic basis where precipitins are not found. Delayed hypersensitivity reactions or the activation of complement by the alternative pathway (known to be produced by some antigens involved in this disease e.g. *Microsporum faeni*), or both, may be responsible for producing the disease in such cases. It is likely that fungal spores could produce granulomas by delayed hypersensitivity in a similar way to the granuloma-provoking action of *Schistosoma* antigen-coated particles when injected into animals sensitized to *Schistosoma*—a reaction which is passively transferable by lymphoid cells but not serum. The complex of antigens which composes a fungal spore may provoke several different host reactions according to whether they are particulate or diffusible.

A unifying concept proposed by Reed (1974) is that of "granulomatous hypersensitivity". Steps in the process may be:

i. ingestion of large amounts of organic dust by macrophages;
ii. granuloma formation due to the particulate state of the antigen, and depending on host reactivity;
iii. "adjuvant" effects on antibody production and delayed hypersensitivity to the antigens in the dust;
iv. re-exposure to the dust results in
   a. delayed hypersensitivity with lymphocyte infiltration and granuloma formation to particulate antigens, and/or
   b. formation of insoluble antigen–antibody complexes at equivalence or in antibody excess in the lung, where an unusually large amount of antibody has accumulated since it is the sole site of the reaction to inhaled dust. These complexes incite further granuloma formation by virtue of their persistence through insolubility and resistance to degradation by lysosomal enzymes in macrophages.

Cryptogenic

The pathogenesis of this, and other comparable states such as intrinsic asthma, is unknown. As evidence grows for viral triggering of other connective tissue diseases, e.g. systemic lupus erythematosus (Hughes, 1974), often on a genetic background, it is tempting to hypothesize that the respiratory conditions described above also have a viral basis.

DISEASES CAUSED BY HOST RESPONSES TO INORGANIC DUSTS

The mineral dust pneumoconioses have stimulated immunologists to determine what factors in the reactivity of the individual exposed to mineral dusts (such as asbestos, silica and beryllium) determine onset and progression of symptomatic lung disease (Turner-Warwick, 1973).

At the radiographic level, Caplan (1953) noted that coalminers with seropositive rheumatoid arthritis developed large lung nodules which often became confluent or cavitated. The histology of the nodules is identical with that of subcutaneous rheumatoid nodules, and, as in the latter, there are deposits of immunoglobulin, rheumatoid factor and complement present, as well as plasma cells in the neighbouring tissue (Pernis, 1968). Since then it has been shown that coalminers with progressive massive fibrosis, but without rheumatoid arthritis, often have rheumatoid factor in their serum and that this is more common in severely affected cases. Similar correlation with extent of disease has been found in studies of anti-nuclear antibodies in coalminers, but it appears that while either rheumatoid factor or anti-nuclear body may be present, both are rarely so.

Similarly, patients with asbestosis and silicosis (induced by exposure to relatively pure silica, e.g. sandblasters) have increased frequency of anti-nuclear antibodies. In asbestosis these are mainly IgM and in low titre, also showing a relation to age, whereas in silicosis higher titre, non-age dependent, IgG antibodies are found. The relationship of the host's immune responses to the predisposition to bronchial carcinoma and mesothelioma (in the case of asbestosis) and tuberculosis (in the case of silicosis) is undetermined.

DISEASES CAUSED BY HOST RESPONSES TO UNDETERMINED AGENTS

There is evidence, in some cases stronger than others, to suggest that in the following diseases a pathogenetic mechanism involves the triggering or suppression of immunological reactions by transmissible agents, usually on a stronger or weaker "background" of genetic predisposition. Depending on the latter, a given agent might be visualized as inciting a variety of host immunological responses, each or a combination of which might be responsible for the different conditions seen by the clinician. If this were the case it would be expected that many of these conditions would have some clinical and laboratory findings overlapping. One concept is that these conditions form a spectrum of disease.

Three important host responses to unknown agents—intrinsic asthma, cryptogenic pulmonary eosinophilia and cryptogenic fibrosing alveolitis—have for convenience already been described above under the heading "host responses to organic dusts" since each has a closely similar counterpart known to be incited in this way.

SARCOIDOSIS

This granulomatous disease is characterized pathologically by the presence of epithelioid cell granulomas without caseation in several organs.

Clinically, the commonest presentation is of bilateral hilar lymph node enlargement which resolves spontaneously within two years in about 90% of patients. Other clinical manifestations of the disease are erythema nodosum, febrile arthralgia and eye involvement. Pulmonary infiltration, which may be preceded or accompanied by bilateral hilar lymphadenopathy, is the most important of the common manifestations of the disease because the sequelae of pulmonary fibrosis may be disabling or fatal. Less commonly, the disease affects skin (lupus pernio, plaques and nodular infiltrations, subcutaneous nodules and erythema nodosum), bones, nervous system, heart, and kidneys (via defects in calcium metabolism).

Investigation

The above pattern of symptoms and signs, especially if occurring in a West Indian or an American Negro, make a diagnosis of sarcoidosis probable. Confirmation may be obtained by the following methods.

Tissue biopsy

Convenient sources are enlarged superficial lymph nodes, skin lesions and conjunctival follicles. Failing this, liver biopsy or lymph node biopsy obtained at mediastinoscopy may give positive findings.

Kveim Test

About 80% of active sarcoidosis cases respond with a granuloma at the site of intracutaneous injection of Kveim antigen (an extract of human sarcoid spleen). The skin site is biopsied after a 4–6 week period and any granulomas seen on microscopy are examined under polarized light to exclude induction by foreign bodies. Administration of corticosteroid agents during the period of the test, especially soon after injection, lessens the chance of a positive reaction in known sarcoid cases. The pitfalls of this test are the considerable variation in reaction seen with different lots of the same validated material and false positive reactions in individuals with diseases other than sarcoidosis (e.g. Crohn's disease and ulcerative colitis). Negative tests are common in long-standing disease.

Serology

There appears to be a general hyperreactivity of the antibody-producing system. Both IgM and IgA are raised in active disease, tending to diminish as remission occurs, but it should be remembered that there are racial differences in the level of serum gammaglobulin, the African Negro having especially high levels. Antibodies to specific antigens such as *Mycobacterium tuberculosis* and viruses are increased, as is also the specific antibody response to immunization (e.g. pertussis).

Cellular Immunology

Delayed hypersensitivity as manifest by skin reactions such as the Mantoux test, lymphocyte transformation to mitogen and specific antigen, and leucocyte migration inhibition by specific antigen, is depressed. This depression of delayed hypersensitivity apparently reflects an unusual type of T-cell depression, since reactivity may be restored by various manoeuvres *in vitro*. It is claimed that when Kveim reagent is used as antigen in *in vitro* tests, a positive response is obtained.

Pathogenesis

The defect in T-lymphocyte function in the peripheral blood may be due to one or more causes, amongst them blocking of the cells by a serum factor, trapping of immunocompetent lymphocytes in lymph nodes and other sites (thereby depriving the body of circulating component cells), and suppression of T-lymphocyte function by an infective agent. The hyperreactivity of the B-lymphocyte system implied by the presence of hypergammaglobulinaemia, could be due to the effects of an infective agent, or to the release of B-lymphocytes from suppressor T-lymphocyte control.

As these hypotheses are compatible with the presence of an infective agent it is interesting that evidence exists for a transmissible agent derived from Kveim material which can be passaged in mice (Mitchell and Rees, 1969). Persistence of such an agent might account for granuloma formation, T-lymphocyte suppression and hypergammaglobulinaemia.

PULMONARY VASCULITIS

In most diseases in which generalized vasculitis occurs (e.g. serum sickness, and systemic lupus erythematosus) it may involve the lung. However, it is interesting that in polyarteritis nodosa the widespread vasculitic lesions often spare the lung.

WEGENER'S GRANULOMATOSIS

This condition may be limited to the respiratory tract or may be widespread. It is characterized by necrotizing granulomas which commonly involve the lower respiratory tract but may affect any system of the body. Occasionally it is limited to the upper respiratory tract but usually there is associated glomerulonephritis and, uncommonly, widespread disseminated vasculitis.

The disease formerly carried a very bad prognosis but now, because of early diagnosis and treatment with corticosteroids and immunosuppressive agents, long remissions may be obtained and occasionally the disease may not recur.

The common glomerular lesion is one of focal glomerulonephritis, and coarse granular deposits of IgG and complement in the glomeruli may be demonstrated.

GOODPASTURE'S SYNDROME

This collection of symptoms and signs is characterized by glomerulonephritis and haemorrhagic pneumonia with recurrent haemoptysis, characteristically affecting young adult males. It is a rapidly progressive disease sometimes following an episode resembling a viral upper respiratory tract infection.

The condition carries a poor prognosis, but corticosteroids and immunosuppressive drugs may control the disease, and recently plasma exchange therapy has produced promising results.

The immunopathogenesis involves production and deposition of anti-basement membrane antibodies which can be seen as linear immunofluorescent staining for IgG and complement of the glomerular and alveolar basement membranes. Eluates from the glomeruli contain antibodies which bind to glomerular basement membrane and fix complement. Infused into monkeys, these antibodies produce severe glomerulonephritis.

SYSTEMIC LUPUS ERYTHEMATOSUS (SLE)

The pulmonary manifestations of this disease are recurrent pleurisy, pulmonary consolidation and atelectasis, diffuse and persistent micronodular infiltration of the lung fields on chest X-ray and "disappearing lungs". In the latter presentation the lung volumes on respiratory function testing and chest X-ray progressively diminish in volume. Renal involvement is uncommon with pleuropulmonary presentations of SLE, and the prognosis is relatively good.

In most presentations of SLE the Farr binding technique reveals double-stranded-DNA binding antibody, especially in active disease. In pleuropulmonary disease this is not the case, and, by contrast, precipitating antibody to single-stranded DNA is the common finding. It is important in such cases not to delay therapy on the basis of a low double-stranded DNA antibody binding result.

Lung biopsy shows evidence of IgG and complement in the alveolar walls on immunofluorescent staining, compatible with immune complex deposition in the lung. There is also evidence of delayed hypersensitivity as shown by lymphocyte sensitization to DNA, nucleo protein and whole nuclei, suggesting cell mediated mechanisms of tissue damage in addition to immune complex deposition.

RHEUMATOID LUNG

The lungs of patients with rheumatoid arthritis may be affected by pleurisy and pleural effusions, necrobiotic nodules, and fibrosing alveolitis. In coalminers with rheumatoid arthritis necrobiotic nodules may be extremely florid. These clinical patterns occur usually in persons with preexisting rheumatoid arthritis and rheumatoid factor, but rarely the nodules precede the arthritis, and in these cases rheumatoid factor appears concomitantly with the arthritis. There seems to be no relationship between the prevalence of fibrosing alveolitis complicating rheumatoid disease and the titre of rheumatoid factor.

Deposition of IgG and IgM has been seen, by immunofluorescence, in the alveolar walls. The absence of complement is puzzling but may be due to insensitivity of the technique used for its demonstration. It seems likely that in this condition, which resembles cryptogenic fibrosing alveolitis, immune complex deposition is a factor in pathogenesis.

DISEASES DUE TO DEFECTIVE HOST RESPONSE TO KNOWN INFECTIVE AGENTS

Respiratory infections are a common presentation of immune deficiency states in man. Where antibody production is defective, acute and chronic bacterial infections of the lungs, difficult to treat successfully with antibiotics, may be the first sign in childhood of a humoral immune deficiency (see Chapter 14). Cellular immune deficiencies may lead to respiratory infections with tuberculosis, viruses, fungi and *Pneumocystis carinii*. Defects in neutrophil killing (e.g. chronic granulomatous disease) predispose to chronic bacterial infections. Opsonin defects for specific organisms (e.g. staphylococci) may present with recurrent respiratory infections.

It is important for respiratory physicians to be aware that immune deficiencies may present within their practice. Recurrent infections, especially if slow to resolve when treated with antibiotics to which the organism is sensitive, may be the forerunner of a fatality; e.g. a child with recurrent respiratory infections, unrecognized as being due to immune deficiency, may subsequently die from a live virus vaccination.

CHRONIC RESPIRATORY INFECTIONS

Many patients with chronic expectoration of sputum, which may become infected at intervals, are suffering from chronic bronchitis due to smoking. There are however a few patients with this syndrome who have never smoked. Studies to determine the host defence defect leading to such recurrent infections, which often require continuous, or almost continuous, antibiotic therapy, reveal no obvious defect to account for the syndrome. Within this group are a few patients with selective IgA deficiency in serum and secretions, with lymphocytotoxins, or with serum blocking factor for lymphocyte responses. Except for fully developed hypogammaglobulinaemia, and possible IgA deficiency, it is doubtful whether these defects are responsible for the infections.

Until recently, the alveolar macrophage could not be studied in man because of its inaccessibility. The technique of fibre-optic bronchoscopy has allowed broncho-alveolar lavage to obtain these cells, and work is in progress to determine whether defective killing mechanisms in them may be responsible for some such infections.

TUBERCULOSIS

It is now clearly recognized that immunity to tuberculosis is separate from the possession of delayed hypersensitivity to the organisms responsible for the disease, although both may be the result of T-lymphocyte function. The evidence for this is as follows:

i. mice formerly infected but recovered from tuberculosis, when desensitized to the organism (i.e. with loss of delayed hypersensitivity skin reaction), still retain immunity to it.
ii. vaccination with mycobacterial RNA endows mice and guinea-pigs with immunity against the disease, but no delayed hypersensitivity develops, and no migration inhibition factor is demonstrable *in vitro*.
iii. rifampicin strongly suppresses the immune response of mice to live tubercle bacilli, but has no effect on the response to mycobacterial RNA vaccine.
iv. mice vary in response to vaccination with the tubercle bacillus according to strain; those exhibiting marked delayed hypersensitivity tend to be less resistant to infection with the organism.
v. likewise in man, there is an inverse relationship between delayed hypersensitivity and resistance to infection.

These observations suggest strongly that delayed hypersensitivity is dissociated from immunity to this organism. It seems that tuberculoprotein is instrumental in provoking delayed hypersensitivity, whereas mycobacterial RNA induces resistance.

It is hardly surprising that *Mycobacteria* can cause diseases of complexity since their cell wall components are potent adjuvants for the immune system. Relevant to host immunological responses in tuberculosis may be those in leprosy, where a spectrum of disease exists between two polar forms—a tuberculoid form, with a high degree of host resistance and delayed hypersensitivity, and a lepromatous form in which a mainly humoral response occurs. In man, a similar difference in responses to the tubercle bacillus may be seen. It is well known that some patients with severe disease of miliary type are anergic both in the Mantoux skin test and in ability to overcome the disease. *In vitro* studies show that anergy may be accounted for by two different mechanisms. The first is unavailability of sensitized lymphocytes in the peripheral blood (those which would traffic to the site of Mantoux test antigen in the skin) because of their trapping in lymph nodes or other sites. A second mechanism is the presence of serum factors blocking the ability of lymphocytes to respond to antigen.

Tubercle bacilli are finally disposed of by an intracellular killing mechanism in macrophages which have ingested them. Sensitized T-lymphocytes are required for the activation of macrophages to kill many intracellular organisms, possibly by release of lymphokines, and this is probably true also for *M. tuberculosis*.

REFERENCES

Caplan, A. (1953). Certain unusual radiological appearances in chest of coal-miners suffering from rheumatoid arthritis. *Thorax* **8**, 29.

Cochrane, C. G. (1971). Mechanisms involved in the deposition of immune complexes in tissues. *J. Exp. Med.* **134**, 75s.

Golbert, T. M. and Patterson, R. (1970). Pulmonary allergic aspergillosis. *Ann. Intern. Med.* **72**, 395.

Hughes, G. (1974). Systemic lupus erythematosus. *Brit. J. Hosp. Med.* **12**, 309.

McCarthy, D. S. and Pepys, J. (1971a). Allergic broncho-pulmonary aspergillosis. Clinical immunology. 1. Skin, nasal and bronchial tests. *Clin. All.* **1**, 261.

McCarthy, D. S. and Pepys, J. (1971b). Allergic broncho-pulmonary aspergillosis. Clinical immunology. 2. Skin, nasal and bronchial tests. *Clin. All.* **1**, 415.

McCarthy, D. S. and Pepys, J. (1973). Cryptogenic pulmonary eosinophilias. *Clin. All.* **3**, 339.

Mitchell, D. W. and Rees, R. J. W. (1969). A transmissible agent from sarcoid tissue. *Lancet* **2**, 81.

Pearson, R. S. (1973). Asthma in Barbados. *Clin. All.* **3**, 289.

Pepys, J. (1969). "Hypersensitivity Diseases in the Lungs due to Fungi and Organic Dusts." Karger, Basel.

Pepys, J. and Jenkins, P. A. (1965). Precipitin (F.L.H.) test in farmer's lung. *Thorax* **20**, 21.

Pepys, J., Turner-Warwick, M., Dawson, P. L. and Hinson, K. F. W. (1968). *In* "Proceedings of the Sixth International Congress of Allergology", p. 221. Montreal, ICS No. 162.

Pernis, B. (1968). *In* "silicosis". (Eds. Miescher, P. A. and Muller Eberhaid, H. J.), Vol. 1, p. 293, New York.

Rackemann, F. M. (1940). Intrinsic asthma. *J. Allergy* **11**, 147.

Reed, C. E. (1974). *In* "Progress in Immunology II", Vol. 4 (Clinical Aspects I), p. 271.

Turner-Warwick, M. (1973). Immunology of the respiratory tract. *Brit. J. Hosp. Med.* **9**, 19.

Turner-Warwick, M. (1974). Allergic disorders. *Medicine* **14**, 889.

22

Atopic Disorders

W. G. REEVES

The subject of atopy and the various disorders which different authors seek to include within it has for long been a contentious and confused area. Now that more is known about the pathological mechanisms involved and more accurate methods are available for clinical investigation it has become possible to look at each condition in turn to discover:

i. whether a reaginic mechanism of tissue damage (see Chapters 1 and 10) is responsible for the clinical findings.
ii. whether it occurs in response to a relatively normal level of exposure to the provoking antigen(s).
iii. whether it shows a significant association with other "atopic" disorders in affected individuals and their families, forming part of a constitutional "atopic trait".

It is the purpose of this chapter to show that the concept of atopy is still a useful one but that the term has to be used with great care—as defined below—and that some modification is necessary of certain traditional views which have often had only an empirical basis.

CONCEPT AND DEFINITION

The term atopy was first used by Coca and Cooke (1923) to describe those patients with a familial tendency to become sensitized to foreign materials and who demonstrated this in the form of hayfever and asthma. Their classification of hypersensitivity contrasted "normal" forms e.g. the dermatitis induced by contact with poison ivy, and serum sickness with "abnormal" forms which included atopic hypersensitivity. In 1925 Coca and Grove utilized the Prausnitz-Küstner test to show that this kind of response could be transferred by serum and gave the term "atopic reagins" to these factors. They were shown to be heat labile, non-precipitating, specific and long-lasting and were identified as a new class of immunoglobulin, IgE, in 1967 (Johansson and Berrich, 1967). Atopic disorders have always been considered in the framework of a reaginic mechanism (sometimes referred as to "anaphylactic" or "immediate" hypersensitivity). Although infantile eczema was not initially included, it has since become, in the minds of many allergists and immunologists, a typical atopic condition. Its only claim to such a categorization is that affected patients usually show elevated levels of serum IgE (mostly of undetermined specificity) and that they may also suffer from extrinsic asthma or hay fever. As discussed below, there is no direct evidence of a reaginic mechanism in so-called "atopic eczema". It is best therefore to refer to these associated disorders collectively as an "atopic syndrome" and reserve the term atopic disease or disorder for those in which the three criteria listed above can be fulfilled.

A familial tendency is often marked in atopic disease and the incidence of these disorders in Western society is of the order of 5 to 10% although this can reach a peak of 16% in children (Soothill, 1976). In view of the familial background and a reasonably clear understanding of the pathological mechanism involved it is, perhaps, surprising that we still lack a clear idea of its pathogenesis. Nevertheless there are several proposals for which evidence can be marshalled and these are discussed in a specific section below. Often it has been thought that atopic patients are distinguished from normals by a qualitative tendency to produce IgE antibody in response to antigen. Yet all normal individuals are capable of IgE production; the more so if antigen is given in a potent form and by a parenteral route (Greenert *et al.*, 1971). Despite such IgE production they may not, however, show any kind of atopic disorder. Much controversy has centred upon the difficulty of equating atopic status with reaginic hypersensitivity but it is more fruitful, at present, to consider the detectable differences as of a quantitative nature; bearing in mind that it is very likely that a qualitative abnormality is the underlying basis for this different order of reactivity. It has been well shown that certain conditions of environmental exposure have to be fulfilled before an underlying atopic trait becomes expressed in the form of symptoms and disease.

For these reasons it is best to define the atopic trait or tendency as follows:

The spontaneous tendency for an individual to produce high levels of IgE antibodies reacting with one or more common antigens in association with antigen-provoked disorders, in some or all of which a reaginic mechanism can be clearly identified.

Such a definition does not confuse atopic status with reaginic responsiveness and preserves the possibility that IgE and reaginic responses may have an important physiological counterpart (see below).

Clinical disorders which have an established reaginic basis and satisfy the criteria for atopy include: extrinsic allergic asthma, allergic rhinitis or hay fever, vernal kerato-conjunctivitis and some gastrointestinal reactions e.g. one form of milk allergy and the condition of allergic gastroenteropathy. Acute anaphylaxis and other manifestations such as urticaria and angioneurotic oedema, may occur in patients who do not have atopy although it is often alleged that acute anaphylactic reactions are more common in atopic patients. Infantile eczema is strongly associated with the above disorders and its occurrence is followed by a ten-fold increase in the subsequent incidence of asthma and hay fever (Stifler, 1965). The term "atopic eczema" is an unfortunate one but is probably best left undisturbed until a more satisfactory label (based on a clearer understanding of its pathological basis) can be put upon it. Several animal models of the atopic state have been described. Studies performed on a colony of beagles hypersensitive to ragweed have confirmed the similarity to human atopic disease (Schwartzman *et al.*, 1971).

A fact which has never been adequately explained is the remarkable individual variation with regard to the localization of atopic manifestations: some patients have only hay fever, some only asthma and some both. It is likely that the timing of the triggering antigenic experience is a particularly important variable in determining the nature of the subsequent atopic disturbance. This may take the form of undue exposure to antigen in the presence of a transient form of IgA deficiency or some kind of perturbation induced by infection e.g. with a respiratory tract virus (see below). Patients who are prone to both asthma and eczema may show a very interesting and thought-provoking relationship between exacerbations of these two conditions: as one gets worse the other often improves and vice versa. It has also been noted that the injection of histamine tends to induce wheezing without urticaria in asthmatic patients whereas it gives rise to urticaria without wheezing in patients prone to chronic urticaria (Szentivanyi, 1968). Now that reaginic processes can be specifically and effectively inhibited by sodium cromoglycate it is even more important to identify their existence in any clinical context and to distinguish them from other patterns of immunologically-determined tissue damage (see Chapters 1 and 10). The further study of reaginic hypersensitivity may also shed light on the possible physiological role for IgE and mediator cell degranulation in the normal operation of the immune response.

ATOPIC DISORDERS AND RELATED CONDITIONS

Hay fever

Charles Blackley first established the role of air-borne pollens in the production of seasonal "hay fever". The condition is characterized by nasal irritation with sneezing, nasal discharge and nasal obstruction although the relative contribution of these individual components may vary (Taylor, 1973). Some patients experience symptoms throughout the year—perennial rhinitis—and have been subdivided into allergic and vasomotor forms. There is little data to justify this distinction and a majority of these patients show raised IgE serum levels and positive cutaneous prick tests to relevant antigens and improve when treated with sodium cromoglycate. Skin tests can be unreliable and nasal provocation is the investigational method of choice where there is any doubt as to the nature or identity of the provoking antigen. A group of patients has been identified (Huggins and Brostoff, 1975) with allergic rhinitis and a clinical history suggestive of house-dust mite allergy but with negative skin tests and no detectable antigen-specific IgE in the serum. These patients do show positive nasal provocation tests and have specific IgE antibodies in their nasal secretions. Approximately one third of young adults suffering from grass pollen sensitivity also show a secondary or "late" form of nasal reactivity when studied by quantitative nasal provocation methods (Taylor, 1973). This suggests (as with some patients with extrinsic asthma) that other mechanisms may augment a purely reaginic picture in some patients. Cell mediated (delayed hypersensitivity) responses have also been identified in patients with summer hay fever (Brostoff and Roitt, 1969) although their presence is usually masked by the preceding reaginic hypersensitivity reaction.

Patients with allergic rhinitis may also show associated irritation of the eyes or "atopic conjunctivitis". This should be distinguished from vernal kerato-conjunctivitis (see below).

Extrinsic Asthma

Intermittent reversible airways obstruction, or asthma, can be brought about by a number of different processes. These are discussed in Chapter 21 and attention will only be directed here to that variety in which reaginic hypersensitivity plays a part. These patients tend to develop their asthma in relatively early life and often show an obvious seasonal pattern of exacerbation. The distinction from intrinsic asthma is on the basis of a higher serum IgE level, multiple positive cutaneous prick tests and positive bronchial provocation tests where applicable and relevant. These patients tend to have a peripheral blood eosinophilia although this is usually less marked than in intrinsic asthma. A significant proportion of such patients have a prior history of infantile eczema and many of them also suffer from allergic rhinitis. Provocation testing emphasizes the "immediate" or reaginic type of hypersensitivity and the response to sodium cromoglycate confirms the role of reaginic mediators in this condition. Children with "wheezy bronchitis" show an increased incidence of hay fever and positive cutaneous prick tests when compared to a control group and represent an important variant of classical extrinsic asthma (Williams and McNicol, 1969).

Although the very large majority of patients with extrinsic asthma can be considered to be "atopic" a small number may show a fairly specific form of extrinsic allergic asthma i.e. to a single kind of antigenic material without having any evidence to suggest an underlying atopic trait. An example of this is allergic bronchopulmonary aspergillosis which can occur in the absence of multiple positive prick tests and a history of other atopic disease (see page 727). It is difficult to categorize this last group as "atopic" which again emphasizes the quantitative rather than the qualitative difference between normal and atopic people although it is possible that antibodies of class other than IgE may be responsible for the asthmatic symptoms seen in these patients (Pepys and Hutchcroft, 1975).

There is evidence to suggest that reaginic antibodies can also be of class IgG (Parish, 1973). A heat-stable short-term sensitizing (STS) IgG antibody has been demonstrated in some patients with "immediate" extrinsic asthmatic reactions to the house-dust mite (Bryant *et al.*, 1973). These subjects are usually non-atopic and their reactions may not respond to sodium cromoglycate. Some asthmatic patients show a "late" pattern of reactivity in bronchial provocation tests in addition to an "early" component; may show a "late" skin reaction following prick testing and usually possess circulating precipitins. These late reactions are not necessarily associated with atopic status and the asthmatic attack which may not commence for some hours develops gradually and is only poorly responsive to inhaled bronchodilators although it is inhibited by corticosteroids. In some cases, sodium cromoglycate inhibits both the immediate and the late asthmatic reactions.

Although intrinsic asthma is not characterized by positive cutaneous prick tests or a history suggestive of provocation by external antigens, it is not uncommon for these patients to have nasal polyposis and when the polyp fluid is examined it is found to contain extremely high levels of IgE. No explanation for this finding has yet appeared.

"Atopic" Eczema

This is manifest either as infantile eczema or a generalized dermatitis in the adult. Infantile eczema usually begins by the sixth month of life and occurs predominantly in a flexural distribution. The serum level of IgE is raised, usually much higher than in extrinsic asthma or hay fever. The elevation of the IgE level tends to correlate with the extent of skin involvement. The serum IgG is also raised. Multiple positive cutaneous prick tests are the rule and dietary antigens are often represented.

Although this condition has often been called "atopic", histological examination gives little clue as to the existence of a reaginic mechanism underlying it. The characteristic changes are those of spongiosis with vascular dilatation and lymphocytic infiltration in the dermis, not unlike the changes seen in contact dermatitis—a condition due to cell mediated responses (see Chapter 23). Several workers have found evidence of a depression of cell mediated reactions in association with infantile eczema although this may well be a secondary effect of the inflammatory process rather than playing a pathogenetic role. Infantile eczema is more common in children who are not breast fed and this supports the notion that the failure to exclude orally ingested antigenic material at a key period of development may be important in the development of this condition. This is discussed further below.

Recent studies on the effect of orally administered sodium cromoglycate show considerable improvement in atopic eczema in which untoward responses to milk or eggs were frequently identified (Orr, 1976). It is likely, therefore, that a reaginic mechanism is involved in the pathogenesis of eczema although whether this event takes place in the gut or the skin is still not clear.

Urticaria is often thought of as an atopic condition but extensive studies have indicated that in only a very small minority can any allergic component be clearly identified (Champion *et al.*, 1969). Nevertheless, atopic patients do show an increased incidence of urticarial eruptions and mast cell degranulation in the skin can follow a variety of stimuli. Patients with intrinsic asthma as well as some with urticaria may show an exacerbation of their symptoms following the ingestion of aspirin and other analgesic substances. The chemical nature of the triggering substances varies widely and it is likely that these patients have an abnormality of prostaglandin metabolism rather than any kind of disturbed immunological response.

Vernal Kerato-conjunctivitis

This is a chronic inflammatory disorder of the conjunctiva which occurs predominantly in children and is often characterized by seasonal exacerbations; hence the synonym, spring catarrh. Symptoms include photophobia, irritability and itching of the eyes, thick mucoid discharge and reduction of visual acuity when keratitis is present (Rice and Jones, 1973). The large majority of these patients are atopic and show multiple positive skin tests to common antigens. The condition responds to corticosteroids as well as sodium cromoglycate (SCG). There is little other direct evidence for reaginic hypersensitivity although this seems very likely. The inflammatory infiltrate contains many eosinophils and IgE levels in tears are higher in patients with this condition.

Secretory Otitis Media

This, the commonest form of deafness in children, is characterized by a collection of fluid or mucus in the middle ear. It often develops after a "cold" or bouts of nasal congestion and the middle ear exudate contains very high levels of IgE when compared to the serum level in the same individuals (Phillips *et al.*, 1974). There is little other evidence, as yet, to suggest an underlying atopic abnormality.

Gastrointestinal Disturbances

Untoward responses to milk or milk components are the best documented form of gastrointestinal reaction in which a reaginic mechanism has been identified. The condition is usually seen in infancy on exposure to cows' milk products. Vomiting and/or diarrhoea occurs and eczema, urticaria and recurrent respiratory infections are often associated. There may be marked cutaneous hypersensitivity to contact with cows' milk. A family history of milk allergy is present in the majority. The commonest antigenic component of cows' milk to which reactivity can be demonstrated is β-lactoglobulin and 25% of infants with milk allergy have been shown to have IgE antibodies against it. These individuals show a favourable response to oral sodium cromoglycate (Freier, 1973). Other patients show complement activation after challenge feeding and an immune complex mechanism may play a part in these cases (Matthews and Soothill, 1970).

More than 50% of children with cows' milk induced diarrhoea have a flat jejunal mucosa and although symptoms have usually disappeared by the age of one year only 29% show a normal proximal jejunal mucosa at that time. There is also an increased likelihood of intolerance to other dietary antigens and about 10% subsequently develop coeliac disease (Kuitenen *et al.*, 1975). A syndrome characterized by oedema, growth retardation, extreme hypoalbuminaemia, hypogammaglobulinaemia, anaemia with eosinophilia and various atopic manifestations e.g. asthma, eczema and hay fever, has also been described (Waldmann *et al.*, 1967). Most of these patients gave a history of milk intolerance and responded to an elimination diet with or without corticosteroid therapy. Although fatal anaphylaxis has followed the administration of milk to allergic subjects the incrimination of untoward reactions to milk proteins in "cot death" is still uncertain.

Seasonal Nephrotic Syndrome

Although a tendency towards a seasonal incidence of the minimal change nephrotic syndrome has been known for some time, relatively few cases have been described in which there has been a clear-cut relationship between reaginic hypersensitivity and minimal change nephrosis (Reeves *et al.*, 1975). These patients usually have a strong personal and family history of atopic disorders related to grass pollen sensitivity. The seasonal relapse in their nephrotic syndrome coincides with the peak of the pollen season and with a rise in both total and pollen-specific serum IgE levels. IgE is not detectable in the glomeruli and it is possible that the proteinuria is a result of the direct action of mediators which increase vascular permeability in the glomerulus. It has also been shown that patients who are grass pollen sensitive and who possess the HLA-B12 histocompatibility antigen have a much greater risk of developing the steroid-sensitive nephrotic syndrome (Soothill, 1976).

OTHER DISORDERS ASSOCIATED WITH RAISED IgE LEVELS

Parasitic Infestation

Many kinds of parasitic infestation are associated with raised serum levels of IgE. Ascariasis, visceral larva migrans, intestinal capillariasis and filariasis are important examples and even higher levels occur in tropical pulmonary eosinophilia (Ezeoke *et al.*, 1973). This is not associated with any indication of reaginic tissue damage in man although the phenomenon of "self-cure" is well described in animals infected with *Nippostrongylus brasiliensis* (see page 761).

Skin Disease

Of the various bullous skin disorders, pemphigoid is particularly associated with a raised serum IgE level (Reeves *et al.*, 1977). One group has described the finding of linear deposition of IgE at the epidermal/dermal junction in pemphigoid but we have been unable to confirm this. Mycosis fungoides is also associated with raised levels although the mechanism is unknown.

Immunodeficiency Disorders

Raised levels have been demonstrated in Job's syndrome, a familial neutrophil chemotactic defect; hypogammaglobulinaemia associated with atopy; the Wiskott–Aldrich syndrome; the DiGeorge syndrome; various kinds of combined immunodeficiency and in Hodgkin's disease.

It is likely that further conditions will be incorporated under the "atopic" umbrella although this has been a fairly hazardous pursuit, to date. It is easy to confirm the atopic nature of a condition when the clinical history and provocation studies give a clear picture of immediate hypersensitivity and reaginic antibody can be demonstrated. In other, often more complex, disorders there may be no clinical evidence to support this. Attempts have been made to investigate such problems by immunofluorescent examination of biopsy material in order to see whether IgE is an important component of the diseased tissue. Eosinophils tend to stain non-specifically with fluorescein-conjugated proteins and this is probably the explanation for anomalous findings in studies in cows' milk allergy (Shiner *et al.*, 1975) and in proctitis (Heatley *et al.*, 1975). In any such study the quality and specificity of the reagents as well as the execution of the technique are of paramount importance and it is very easy to be misled due to methodological difficulties. The particular problems and their circumvention are well outlined in a recent publication (Brandtzaeg and Baklien, 1976).

INVESTIGATION OF ATOPIC DISORDERS

The taking of a relevant and detailed history is of especial value. Physiological studies are useful in determining a therapeutic baseline and eosinophil counts and immunoglobulin quantitation, including IgE, are often helpful. It is only relatively recently that the upper limit of the normal range for total IgE serum levels has been reduced to 200 units/ml following the analysis of a group of patients from which all individuals with possible quiescent atopic disease had been removed (Nye *et al.*, 1975). Appropriate target organ provocation tests, e.g. nasal and bronchial studies, may give a more specific diagnosis and cutaneous prick tests are often helpful in screening for the relevant antigen. Particular care should be taken to perform prick testing in a careful and reproducible fashion. The use of skin tests in diagnosis is reviewed by Pepys (1975b). Other specialized studies such as the measurement of antigen-specific IgE by the radio-allergosorbent test (RAST) or the red cell linked antigen antiglobulin reaction (RCLAAR) can be of value (Pepys, 1975a). Direct tissue studies for the detection of IgE are a demanding exercise and can give erroneous results as mentioned above.

THE PATHOLOGICAL MECHANISM

The process by which tissue damage is induced in the reaginic type of hypersensitivity has already been discussed in Chapter 10. In summary, the recognition part of the response consists of molecules of reaginic antibody (mostly of class IgE) which attach by their tail or Fc fragment to the surface of mediator cells. These are basophils in the peripheral blood and mast cells in extravascular tissues. The granules of these cells contain various mediators including histamine, slow-reacting substance of anaphylaxis (SRS-A), eosinophil chemotactic factor of anaphylaxis (ECF-A) and other substances which vary from species to species. When antigen combines specifically with reaginic antibody and crosslinks two adjacent molecules the surface membrane of the cell becomes triggered so that the cell degranulates and discharges the mediator contents into the surrounding tissue. The cell is not lysed and is able to regenerate its mediator potential. These mediators produce a local increase in capillary permeability and smooth muscle contraction. This is manifest in the skin as a weal and flare reaction, in the lungs as bronchospasm and in the nose as rhinorrhoea or obstruction. The biochemical sequence of events taking place between antigen combination with reaginic antibody and the extracellular release of mediators is now fairly well understood and involves an energy-requiring, calcium-dependent pathway modulated by cyclic nucleotide levels (Kaliner and Austen, 1975). Sodium cromoglycate does not prevent the combination of antigen but does block the release of mediators following that event. It seems to act directly on the metabolic processes involved in membrane transport (Orr, 1976) although an inhibitory effect on phosphodiesterase has also been postulated.

Although IgE is the predominant reaginic antibody there is evidence that a subclass of IgG, probably IgG4, is also able to sensitize mediator cells in a similar way (Parish, 1973). One of the unique characteristics of IgE molecules is that they are able to sensitize mediator cells for comparatively long periods, with a half-life of about 14 days. IgG reagins also attach via their Fc fragment and can trigger mediator release following contact with antigen although the sensitization effect is optimal at about 4 hours. Such antibodies are often found in sera containing precipitins but they do not mediate an immune complex type of injury, probably because of their inability to fix complement. Their importance has been confirmed in several clinical situations, e.g. milk allergy and extrinsic asthmatic reactions to the house dust mite.

Chapter 1 has discussed the reason for favouring the term "reaginic" over "anaphylactic" when describing this kind of immunopathological mechanism. The term anaphylaxis is often used loosely for a variety of acute immunological events, some of which can be caused by other mechanisms. Endotoxin shock, particularly in the dog, can give rise to a clinical picture not unlike acute anaphylaxis although this is known to act via a direct effect on complement. Mediator cell degranulation can occur as a consequence of complement activation via the effect of the "anaphylatoxins" C3a and C5a acting directly on basophils and mast cells (see Chapter 7). Although careful analysis has shown that the reaginic mechanism alone has considerable potential for host damage and demise there are augmenting factors derived from other mechanisms which may colour the final outcome, although the interrelationship between reaginic hypersensitivity and other mechanisms of tissue damage is still not entirely clear. "Late" forms of reactivity are sometimes seen in association with the reaginic or "early" forms in the skin, nose and bronchial tree, and in each case there is good evidence that these late reactions are due to an immune complex mechanism. It seems that a marked "late" reaction does not occur in the absence of an early response and it may be that a reaginic mechanism is a prerequisite for an immune complex type of response (Pepys, 1973).

Several lines of evidence suggest that the T-cell mechanism of tissue damage may be closely linked to reaginic hypersensitivity. The eosinophilia which develops in response to *Trichinella* infestation has a T-cell-dependent component (Walls *et al.*, 1971) and T-lymphocytes liberate chemotactic factors for both eosinophils and basophils when responding to antigenic stimulation. The possible role of T-cells and their factors in the regulatory control of IgE production is referred to in more detail on page 766. Basophils are present in the cellular infiltrate in contact dermatitis and to a lesser degree in the tuberculin response and during graft rejection, although their degranulation is much less marked in these situations than in reaginic responses (Richerson and Parker, 1974). Jones-Mote type "delayed" reactions may contain a large excess of basophils although there is evidence that much of the basophil accumulation may be antibody-mediated (Askenase *et al.*, 1976). Experimentally these different patterns of response can be induced by varying the mode and route of immunization.

The release of kallikrein from basophils after challenge with antigen or anti-IgE suggests a link with the plasma kinin generating system (Newball *et al.*, 1975). It has also been suggested that complement may be activated via the alternative pathway in IgE mediated reactions (Malley *et al.*, 1971) and other work indicates that various antigens commonly associated with the production of atopic disorders have a direct inactivating effect on complement (C3) independently of antibody (Berrens *et al.*, 1973).

PHYSIOLOGICAL SIGNIFICANCE OF THE REAGINIC MECHANISM

Most of the components of the immune system which bring about tissue damage have a clearly recognizable physiological role. This is not so for reaginic processes, although there are several possibilities.

Parasitic Infestation

Parasitic infestation is associated with some of the highest serum levels of IgE that have been detected. A role for IgE in the phenomenon of "self-cure" seen with *Nippostrongylus brasiliensis* infection in rats seems likely (Jarrett *et al*., 1968) although other work suggests that sensitized lymphocytes may also play a part (Dineen *et al*., 1973). IgE levels are generally higher in rural areas in countries where infestation is common (Johansson *et al*., 1968) and it is likely that such a reactive over-production of IgE is important in determining host immunity against parasitic infestation. Asthma and other atopic disorders are much less common in such communities (Godfrey, 1975) and *in vitro* evidence indicates that serum containing high levels of parasite-induced IgE is able to block mediator release by third-party specific antigen (Godfrey and Gradidge, 1976). It thus seems likely that atopic disease has only appeared as an important clinical problem following the reduction in man's parasite load. Helminth infection is able to potentiate the production of reaginic antibody non-specifically, although most experiments have involved the use of *B. pertussis* as an adjuvant and this may produce such effects of its own accord.

Extravascular Immunity

The concentration of each of the major immunoglobulin classes as well as that of the individual complement components is much lower in the extravascular compartment. The marked increase in capillary permeability which follows the release of IgE-triggered mediators and the almost invariable disposition of tissue mast cells along the adventitial surface of small blood vessels suggests that intermittent and local increases in capillary permeability may be of particular importance in compensating for these deficiencies. Foreign antigen which obtains entry into the extravascular tissues and which does not stimulate cell mediated immune responses may be only effectively dealt with by such a local boosting effect of intravascular components.

Interrelationship with Immune Complex Reactions

The importance of vaso-active amines in determining the localization of circulating immune complexes has been known for some years and, in the rabbit at least, this effect has been shown to be mediated by a factor released from sensitized basophils which then gives rise to amine release from platelets (Cochrane, 1971). The frequent co-existence of "early" and "late" reactions in the skin, nose and bronchial tree further suggests an interrelationship between reaginic and immune complex mechanisms. This may be a further reflection of the mechanism proposed above i.e. that reaginic processes produce a local boosting effect of extravascular immunity and that this dual effect is most evident in extravascular sites such as the interstitial areas of the dermis and the nasal and bronchial mucosae.

The clinical features of partial forms of hypogammaglobulinaemia also help to reinforce this view. Lone IgA or IgE deficiency is not necessarily associated with recurrent respiratory tract infection whereas this is very common in patients who have a deficiency of both IgA and IgE (Polmar *et al.*, 1972). This might be explained if IgG is unable to function optimally in this site when there is a deficiency of the interrelating mechanism.

Induction of Immunity

IgE-forming plasma cells predominantly occur in the regional lymph nodes as well as the respiratory and gastrointestinal mucosa (Tada and Ishizaka, 1970). Mast cells are also well represented in lymphoid tissue (Selye, 1965). The production of small amounts of IgE during the early phase of normal immune responses suggests that IgE may have a physiological role associated with the inductive phase of the immune response. The nature of any such involvement is, as yet, a complete mystery, for relatively trivial responses have tended to be overshadowed by the more gross reactions seen in atopic disease and parasitic infestation. It may be that the marked changes in permeability (to cells as well as colloid) displayed by the post-capillary venules surrounding the lymphoid follicles may be determined by alterations in local mast cell function triggered by surface IgE.

Atopy and Cancer

Several authors have suggested that there is an inverse relationship between the incidence of atopic disease and cancer in individual patients. This has been looked at in some detail more recently and has not been substantiated. The role of IgE in immune surveillance against neoplastic transformation is thus entirely hypothetical at the present time.

THE PATHOGENESIS OF THE ATOPIC TRAIT (Fig. 1)

The identification of reaginic antibody as IgE in 1967 (Johansson and Bennich, 1967) as well as the acquisition of detailed knowledge of the metabolic processes by which the mediator cell degranulates (Kaliner and Austen, 1975) have greatly enhanced our understanding of this mechanism of tissue damage. It is therefore possible to postulate what the constitutional defect might be in subjects who exhibit an atopic trait. Several proposals have been made and these will be reviewed in turn. It is worth emphasizing that an atopic trait or overt atopic disorder is not synonymous with the presence of an elevated

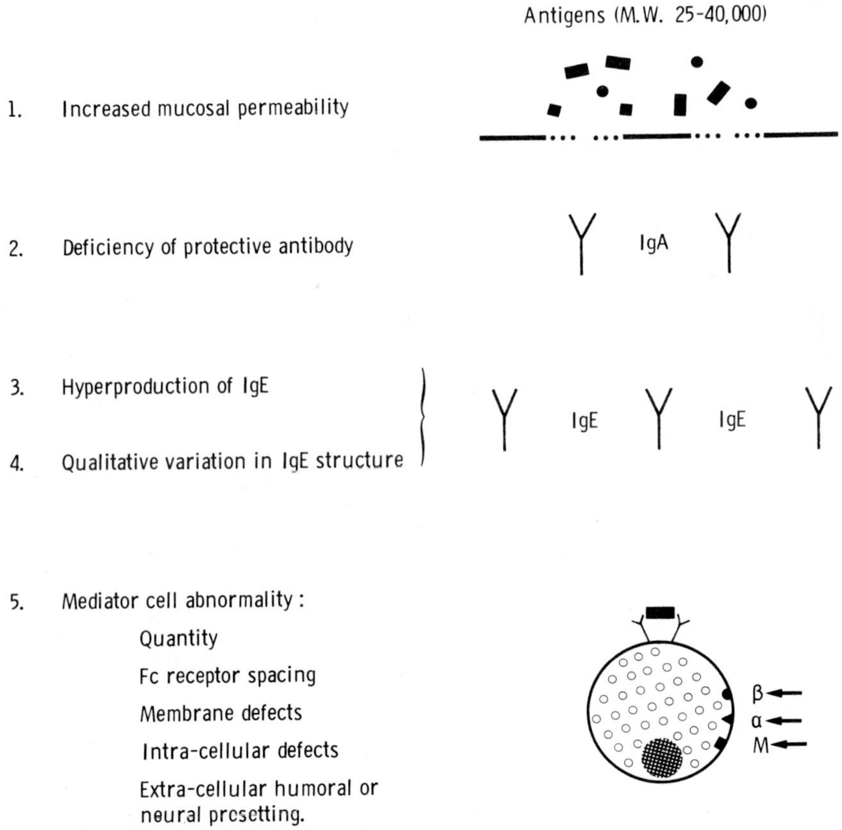

Fig. 1. Possible sites for the atopic lesion (β, α and M, refer to β and α adrenergic and muscarinic receptors respectively).

level of reaginic antibody. Greenert *et al.* (1971) immunized 42 non-atopic volunteers with multiple doses of ragweed extract for periods of six months to two years. They were able to detect specific reaginic reactivity to ragweed antigen in these patients although none developed symptoms during the succeeding ragweed pollen season.

Mucosal Permeability

Various workers have suggested that the propensity which atopic patients show for developing untoward responses to airborne and ingested antigens may result from the presence of abnormal mucosal permeability to these materials. The antigens that are commonly incriminated in atopic disorders show a fairly restricted molecular weight range of 25–40,000 daltons. This is an unusually narrow range of molecular size for antigens in general and may be relevant to the nature of the underlying defect. It may, however, merely indicate the size of particle which can cross normal mucous membranes irrespective of the end-result. Atopic patients respond similarly to normal individuals when antigens are administered parenterally although differences can be detected when immunization is performed intranasally even when a high molecular weight material such as keyhole limpet haemocyanin is used (Salvaggio *et al.*, 1969). Measurement of the transfer of radio-iodinated albumen across the nasal mucosa into the blood has shown a marked difference in the degree of uptake between patients with "quiescent" atopic rhinitis and normals (Buckle and Cohen, 1975) although no increase in nasal transport was seen in patients with extrinsic asthma. It has also been shown that non-atopic patients with rhinitis do not become sensitized after intranasal administration of antigen.

It is obviously difficult to be certain that any abnormality present in the atopic patients is not a secondary rather than a primary feature of the disease. In another study the production of an indirect form of Prausnitz-Kustner test, in which a reaginic serum was injected into the skin followed by intranasal challenge with antigen, failed to show a difference in nasal absorption between atopic and normal individuals (Kontou-Karakitsos *et al.*, 1975).

Deficiency of Protective Antibody

Several reports have indicated an increased frequency of IgA deficiency in atopic patients (Kaufman and Hobbs, 1970; Soothill, 1976). Such deficiency may only be present in early life and in one series IgA deficiency at three months was strongly associated with the development of atopic symptoms within the first year, although the IgA levels had become higher than those of a normal population by twelve months of age (Taylor *et al.*, 1973). A prophylactic regime of breast feeding combined with the reduction of contact with potent sources of environmental antigens seems to have prevented the development of eczema in the offspring of allergic parents (Soothill, 1976).

Intranasal immunization with tetanus toxoid is followed by lower antigen-specific IgA and higher antigen-specific IgE levels in the nasal secretions of atopic versus normal subjects (Butcher *et al.*, 1975). That antigen-specific IgA prevents the absorption of antigen across the mucosal surface in the respiratory tract has been definitively shown by injecting a fortuitously antigen-specific mouse IgA myeloma protein into the rat respiratory tract prior to intratracheal injection of radio-iodinated antigen (Stokes *et al.*, 1975) and a similar effect can be demonstrated in the gastrointestinal tract.

It appears, therefore, that atopic patients often show a relative deficiency in IgA production in mucosal surfaces and that this is often associated with a relative over-production of IgE antibody. If prolonged periods of immunization e.g. during successive pollen seasons, occur then intermittent and often high levels of IgE may be detected in the serum. Atopic patients have also been shown to have higher levels of circulating antibodies following the ingestion of bovine serum albumin (Barrick and Farr, 1965) and patients with IgA deficiency also show an increased spontaneous incidence of precipitins to bovine serum and milk proteins (Tomasi and Katz, 1971).

Primary Hyperproduction of Reaginic Antibody (IgE)

The concept of "hypersensitivity" has always implied an inherent over-production of immunological factors. A body of evidence now exists to support a genetic basis for atopic reactivity and the production of high levels of IgE antibodies (Levine, 1973). More specifically, a close correlation has been found between IgE antibody production to a specific antigen associated with ragweed and the histocompatibility type HLA-B7 (Goodfriend *et al.*, 1973). Such a link may be obscured with more complex antigens and other work has demonstrated that the distribution of total serum IgE levels in atopic and non-atopic populations is governed by autosomal recessive genes (Marsh *et al.*, 1974). Heterozygotes for the autosomal recessive gene which determines cystic fibrosis also show an increased incidence of atopic disorders and positive cutaneous prick tests (Warner *et al.*, 1976). The markedly raised levels of IgG4 antibody seen in some patients with cystic fibrosis suggests that this may be an IgG rather than an IgE-mediated effect (Shakib *et al.*, 1976).

Quite apart from any primary genetic control of IgE production there is also impressive evidence of controlling influences mediated by specific populations of lymphoid cells and possibly by other classes of antibody e.g. IgG. Tada *et al.* (1975) have performed an elegant series of experiments in the rat on IgE production to a chemical derivative of an extract of *Ascaris*. They have found that the IgE response is considerably enhanced by various methods which deplete the number of T-cells (e.g. X-irradiation, thymectomy and splenectomy, and treatment with anti-thymocyte serum). They have also been able to study the nature of this regulation (i.e. suppression) of IgE production and have identified a soluble factor produced by T-lymphocytes, which is not immunoglobulin in nature, has a molecular weight of between 35–60,000 and shows a marked "carrier" specificity (q.v.). They also identify a helper factor which is immunoglobulin like, having a molecular weight of 100–200,000 and which likewise shows carrier specificity. Although their system involves the use of two components which may themselves potentiate IgE responses non-specifically i.e. *Ascaris* antigen and *B. pertussis* as adjuvant, it is possible that a similar state of affairs operates in man. Several clinical studies have attempted to demonstrate the existence of T-cell deficiency in patients with atopic disease but where this has been suggested by impaired delayed hypersensitivity responses in the skin, reduced T-cell numbers or impaired responses to phytohaemagglutinin it is still possible that these may be secondary manifestations of the atopic disorder. It is nevertheless possible that the underlying genetic factor in atopic disease operates via T-cell control of IgE responses.

Qualitative Differences in IgE

In a study involving the measurement of total serum IgE levels with a radial immunodiffusion technique, Houri *et al.* (1972) noticed that the sera from some patients with atopic disease showed double rings of precipitation. They postulated that these two rings represent different forms of IgE and found that if a serum which initially produced only one ring was incubated with nasal secretion derived from the same patient after a specific positive provocation test, then two rings of precipitation were seen. They suggest that one form of IgE is of local origin and the other is a different form present in the circulation. It is also possible that one form represents IgE complexed with a specific anti-globulin (see below) or that the IgE has undergone some kind of aggregation or denaturation.

It has also been suggested that the strength of binding, or avidity, of the IgE molecule for the mediator cell might be abnormally high in patients with atopic disorders. There is no direct evidence for this but a qualitative difference in the behaviour of peripheral blood basophils from extrinsic and intrinsic asthmatics when subjected to anti-IgE has been observed (Assem *et al.*, 1971). It was found that despite the lower serum IgE levels in intrinsic asthma, the cells taken from these patients discharged increased amounts of histamine on challenge with anti-IgE. If this indicates an increased amount of IgE coating the basophils in intrinsic asthma in the presence of a much lower serum level it also implies an increased avidity of binding. These workers also showed, however, increased histamine release in intrinsic asthmatics with anti-IgG and it is possible to explain their results on the basis of a cellular abnormality which determines a lower threshold for mediator release via either kind of antibody.

Anti-globulins

The presence of anti-IgE activity has been demonstrated in the sera of patients with atopic disorders (Williams *et al.*, 1972). An increased incidence has been found in atopic patients although this could well be a secondary effect following the frequent and persistent aggregation of IgE molecules, similar to the anti-globulin formation which occurs in rheumatoid arthritis and chronic infection.

Mediator Cell Abnormalities

Local variation in the numbers of mast cells between different tissues and between individuals has been suggested as an explanation for the atopic diathesis as well as the variation in the location of the target organ but there are no histometric findings to support this. The restricted molecular weight range for "atopic" antigens could be explained on the basis of the spacing of the Fc receptors on the surface of mediator cells. Mediator cell degranulation occurs when two adjacent IgE molecules are bridged by antigen (or anti-IgE). However, the fact that IgE on the surface of mediator cells can be shown to patch and cap in a similar manner to the surface immunoglobulin on lymphocytes is against fixed spacing between Fc receptors, although there may be a standard arrangement of IgE molecules in the resting state.

More attention has been directed to possible abnormalities which may lie between triggering of the mediator cell and its degranulation. β-Adrenergic substances, e.g. isoprenaline, act via a receptor enzyme, adenyl cyclase, to increase the intracellular concentration of cyclic adenosine monophosphate (cyclic AMP). This effect is associated with the inhibition of many aspects of cell function including mast cell degranulation (Kaliner and Austen, 1975). On the other hand (as discussed below) stimulation with either α-adrenergic or cholinergic agents is associated with enhanced mediator release (Fig. 2). Similar modulating influences also apply to the bronchial smooth muscle cell (Schultze *et al.*, 1973).

The annual dinner of the Rocky Mountain Allergy Society in 1962 was marked by Szentivanyi's exposition of the "β-adrenergic theory" of the atopic abnormality (Szentivanyi, 1968). This proposal attempted to explain collectively the abnormalities in both extrinsic and intrinsic asthma and was based on evidence derived from animal models such as the "hypothalamically-imbalanced" anaphylactic guinea-pig and *B. pertussis*-induced hypersensitive states in mice and rats. In support of this view was the fact that blockade of adrenergic β-receptors gives rise to increased reactivity to various mediator substances such as histamine and also increased bronchial reactivity to methacholine and relevant antigens in patients with seasonal rhinitis who have no previous history of asthma. Although an increase was not detected in normal patients using conventional methods a change is seen when normal individuals are studied in the whole body plethysmograph.

Others have suggested that α-adrenergic receptors are of especial importance in atopic disease and that their over-stimulation may give rise to an identical pattern to β-blockade (Palmer *et al.*, 1974). α-Receptor stimulation has been associated with a fall in cyclic AMP levels (Kaliner and Austen, 1975) as well as an elevation in the level of cyclic guanosine monophosphate (cyclic GMP) (Haddock *et al.*, 1975). This effect is not blocked by atropine and thus is not mediated directly via cholinergic receptors. The exact nature of the alpha adrenergic receptor and its interaction with the cyclic AMP and GMP pathways is unclear (Fig. 2).

Irritant receptors in the smaller airways react to a wide variety of stimuli to produce vagally-mediated bronchoconstriction (Empey *et al.*, 1976). Evidence in dogs suggests that much of the bronchoconstrictor response to antigen is mediated via the parasympathetic nervous system and can be blocked by atopine or by cooling the vagus. Histamine can stimulate the irritant receptors directly and may provide the link between mast cell degranulation

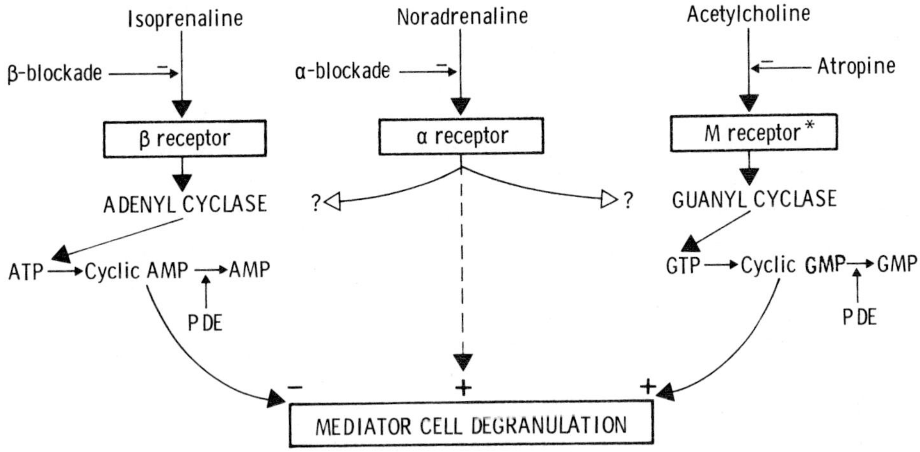

Fig. 2. Modulating pathways for effector cell function e.g. mediator cell degranulation (*M = muscarinic).

and the involvement of cholinergic pathways (Gold, 1973). These receptors show a lower threshold and a greater severity of response in asthmatic patients and it has been suggested that such receptors become "sensitized" during infections of the respiratory tract. Increased bronchial reactivity to aerosols of histamine and citric acid has been demonstrated in normal subjects during the course of viral infection (Empey *et al.*, 1976) and some viruses, e.g. rhinoviruses, influenza and respiratory syncytial viruses are more prone to cause asthmatic episodes (Minor *et al.*, 1976).

Figure 2 shows some of the known interrelationships between α- and β-adrenergic and cholinergic pathways which modulate cell function. Although such an analysis helps to explain the mode of action of many of the currently available therapeutic agents, e.g. isoprenaline, salbutamol, indoramine, atropine and theophylline derivatives, it is impossible to tell whether any of the observed alterations in these pathway components are the cause or effect of atopic disorders. No doubt a further selection of postulated defects will appear as other cyclic nucleotides (e.g. CMP and IMP) are found to be of importance in the control of cell function.

In so far as a number of different abnormalities can be detected simultaneously in atopic patients even when in a quiescent phase it is likely that one is looking at several aspects of a highly perturbed system. It seems unlikely that a defect in this area is going to explain the genetic basis for the atopic trait. Discordant identical twins for asthma have been studied (Falliers *et al.*, 1971): the asthmatic twins showed various abnormalities e.g. reduced lymphocyte adenyl cyclase activity and increase membrane APT-ase whereas the normal twins did not. A further complication is the demonstration that antigen can induce bronchoconstriction in a sensitized animal when it has only obtained access to the most superficial parts of the bronchial epithelium (Richardson *et al.*, 1973). With peroxidase as antigen in sensitized guinea-pigs, electron microscopy did not show any penetration of the antigen into epithelial or endothelial layers. As mast cells are situated beneath the basement membrane of the epithelium it is unlikely that their degranulation is a primary phenomenon. Nerve endings are located between the bronchial epithelial cells and it is possible that antigen induced bronchoconstriction follows antigen–antibody combination in the superficial part of the bronchial epithelium with irritant receptor stimulation giving rise to bronchoconstriction with secondary mast cell degranulation. The bronchial lymphoid tissue may also have a role in these rapid and relatively superficial events (Bienenstock *et al.*, 1973).

Prostaglandins have been shown to have potent effects on bronchial tone: the E-series relax and $F_{2\alpha}$-constricts. These effects may also operate via adenyl and guanyl cyclase receptor enzymes (Patel, 1975). The constrictor effect of $PGF_{2\alpha}$ is increased 8,000-fold in asthmatic versus normal patients and the serum levels of both E and F prostaglandins have been shown to be higher in asthmatics in addition to a higher F/E ratio (Nemoto *et al.*, 1976). This has suggested that there may be an underlying abnormality of prostaglandin metabolism in asthma such as a reduction in prostaglandin dehydrogenase activity or an abnormality of prostaglandin synthetase. However, prostaglandin levels are influenced by various non-specific factors such as stretching of the lung and there is no definitive evidence to favour a primary abnormality as yet.

Various proposals for the abnormality in atopy have thus been proposed but in many of them there is no clear evidence that the observed abnormalities are primary rather than secondary to the atopic disorder. Of them all, the well established deficiency in secretory antibody is most likely to have a definitive role in determining atopic responses in conjunction with genetically determined variations in IgE production (Fig. 3). Such a view has to be seen in the evolutionary context of man's development for, in more primitive surroundings, he shows considerably elevated levels of IgE production in response to parasitic infestation. It is possible that the reduction in this source of IgE stimulation has led to inappropriate production of IgE to other environmental antigens. Whatever the primary cause the importance of adrenergic and cholinergic pathways in modulating the response should not be underestimated. It is still possible that the not infrequent development of bronchial and nasal atopic reactivity following virus or other infection may be due to an underlying trait becoming manifest after cholinergic or other receptors have become preset or "sensitized" to discharge at a lower threshold.

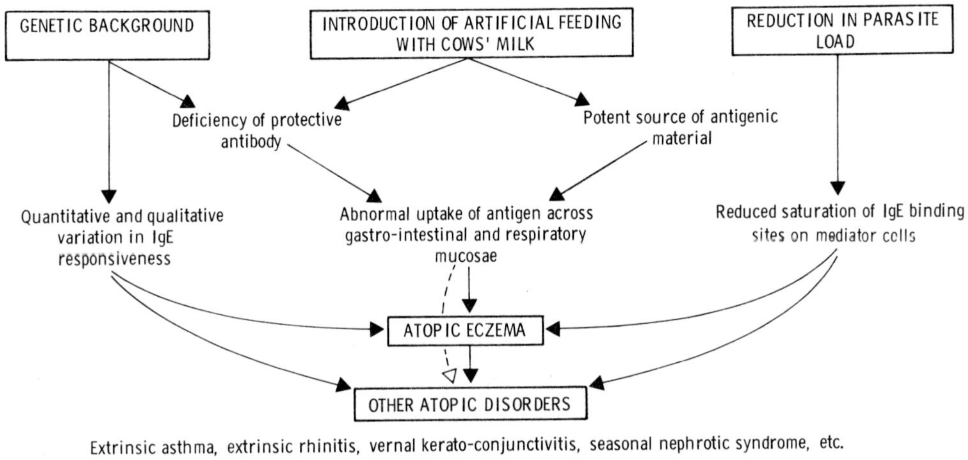

Fig. 3. A sequence for the pathogenesis of the atopic trait.

In view of the evidence in twins (cited above) it should be possible to determine the relative contribution of these various factors in a prospective study of the offspring of atopic parents. This is already being studied from an immunological point of view (Soothill, 1976) and the longer term results are awaited with interest.

MANAGEMENT OF ATOPIC DISORDERS

Great strides have been made in recent years concerning the therapeutic manoeuvres available for the control of atopic disorders. The advent of safe and sophisticated β-adrenergic stimulators as well as the discovery of sodium cromoglycate have had an impressive impact on the morbidity of extrinsic asthma. Although systemic corticosteroids are usually kept in reserve for the treatment of extrinsic asthma and are of doubtful value in hay fever, the use of steroid aerosols in the management of both these conditions has given rise to significant improvement in the absence of adrenal suppression.

Antigen Avoidance

Environmental elimination of the offending antigen should be achieved wherever possible e.g. animal danders and dietary antigens. However, for the large majority of sufferers there is no relief from the ill-effects of the pollen season short of a major sea voyage. The control of contact with provoking antigens may be of more value in early life where it seems to reduce the development of eczema in atopic offspring (Soothill, 1976).

Hyposensitization

Although hyposensitization was introduced in the early part of this century (Noon, 1911) little advance has been made in understanding the underlying mechanism or in determining the most relevant clinical indications for its use. It has been most successful in the treatment of asthma and hay fever associated with hypersensitivity to pollens and has had some success in the control of house dust mite reactions. It is very unlikely to be effective in the presence of multiple positive challenge tests to different antigens and even with "monovalent" reactivity a course of hyposensitization injections may have to be abandoned because of the appearance of increasingly severe symptoms. Hyposensitization is much less in demand for the management of extrinsic asthma now that sodium cromoglycate, selective β_2 agonists and corticosteroid aerosols are available. It is still used in the management of allergic hay fever and has been effectively administered via the nasal route (Mehta and Smith, 1975) although intranasal corticosteroid aerosols and/or sodium cromoglycate are likely to reduce the necessity for its use.

Success in systemic hyposensitization is usually attributed to the development of "blocking" antibody of IgG class. Although antigen-specific IgG and IgE levels show parallelism in seasonal hay fever, treated patients show a rise in IgG and a more marked fall in IgE levels during hyposensitization (Ishizaka and Ishizaka, 1973). The fall in IgE occurs after a delay of up to six months and may be preceded by an initial rise. Most of the increase in antigen specific IgG is located in the subclass IgG4 (Devey *et al.*, 1976) although the level of increase does not seem to correlate with the degree of clinical improvement.

"Blocking" activity has been assessed by passive transfer tests performed in the patient's own skin as well as by *in vitro* methods involving the measurement of histamine release from leucocyte preparations. In both situations little correlation has been found between the levels of blocking activity and the degree of symptomatic improvement (Lichtenstein *et al.*, 1971). It is feasible that negative modulation of the specific IgE response takes place via a central mechanism involving the development of suppressor T-cells and their factors as described in the studies performed in the rat (Tada *et al.*, 1975).

Adrenergic Agents

Adrenergic agents have been the mainstay of the management of acute asthma since the administration of subcutaneous adrenaline was introduced in 1910. The development of isoprenaline aerosols provided a more suitable day-to-day means of controlling intermittent bronchospasm but a marked increase in the mortality of asthmatic patients experienced during the 1960s (Speizer *et al.*, 1968) was attributed to isoprenaline aerosol abuse, particularly in patients who had developed status asthmaticus. The development of more specific β_2 adrenergic stimulators e.g. salbutamol and terbutaline, which lack any β_1 stimulatory effect on the heart, has largely removed this problem. The use of α blockers has not met with the same degree of success although their administration has been shown to inhibit antigen-provoked bronchospasm (Patel and Kerr, 1975).

Anti-cholinergic Agents

Increased interest in the importance of vagal pathways in the production of antigen-induced bronchospasm has resurrected the occasional use of atropine, usually in conjunction with β_2 stimulators, in the management of asthma. Potential disadvantages are the tendency to suppress bronchial secretion and other unpleasant side-effects. More promising anti-cholinergic analogues are under active study (Hoffbrand, 1975). Surgical denervation of the lungs has also been tried in severe cases of asthma with mixed results. Regeneration of both afferent as well as efferent pathways can occur within a few months of operation (Edmonds *et al.*, 1971) and thus its application is extremely limited.

Theophylline Derivatives

Aminophylline and its derivatives are effective in the control of antigen-induced bronchoconstriction although they do not act via adrenergic or cholinergic receptors. Instead, their site of action is inhibition of the phosphodiesterase which metabolizes cyclic nucleotides such as cyclic AMP. Theophylline derivatives show synergism with β-stimulators in the control of bronchial tone. Theophylline does not seem to act on the phosphodiesterase which breaks down cyclic GMP to the same degree (Shephard, 1973).

Sodium Cromoglycate (Intal)

The discovery that sodium cromoglycate was an effective agent in the control of antigen-induced reaginic hypersensitivity has transformed the management of extrinsic asthma (Pepys, 1973). It is not steroid-like and acts independently of adrenergic or cholinergic pathways, yet it prevents mediator cell degranulation despite combination of antigen with surface IgE. Although it has a potent effect on mast cells it does not act similarly on circulating basophils. Its predominant mode of action is thought to be via an effect on cell membrane transport mechanisms and ionic processes (Orr, 1976) although inhibition of phospholipase A and an inhibitory effect on phosphodiesterase have also been postulated (Taylor *et al.*, 1974).

Although it does not seem to be as effective in intrinsic asthma it has been shown to inhibit the bronchoconstriction following aspirin challenge in aspirin sensitive subjects (Basomba *et al.*, 1976). Intal has also been used for the control of allergic rhinitis and as eye-drops has been shown to be of value in the management of vernal kerato-conjunctivitis (Rice and Jones, 1973).

Antihistamines

Despite the fact that histamine is the major inflammatory mediator liberated during mast cell degranulation, the use of antihistamines has not been successful in the control of atopic disease. They are of no value in extrinsic asthma and although they may help to control symptoms in allergic hay fever the drowsiness which they induce is often an unacceptable side-effect. Their anti-pruritic effect is of value in eczema. Their lack of efficacy has been explained on the basis of failure to achieve a sufficient concentration of the drug at the extravascular site at which histamine acts when this is so closely approximated to the site of its release from the mast cell. Most antihistamines used thus far antagonize H_1 receptors such as those in bronchial smooth muscle and it is possible that H_2 antagonists e.g. burimamide, may produce different effects in the lung e.g. on the cholinergic receptors which histamine is known to stimulate.

Corticosteroids

The administration of systemic corticosteroids is often life-saving in the management of intrinsic asthma and may be required on a less permanent basis during periods of exacerbation in extrinsic asthma. Nevertheless, it does produce untoward side-effects and strenuous efforts are made to keep the dose and the consequent adrenal suppression down to an absolute minimum. The use of ACTH and its synthetic analogues can help to alleviate this problem and intermittent dosage e.g. on alternate days is a further useful manipulation. The introduction of potent steroid aerosols e.g. betamethasone, has almost removed the problem of adrenal suppression and these are now in general use in the management of hay fever and extrinsic asthma (Hiller and Milner, 1975). Their use in the lung has been complicated by *Candida* infection of the upper respiratory tract although this is an infrequent problem.

Much of what has been said thus far does not apply to the management of "atopic" dermatitis. Here adrenergic and cholinergic blocking agents are not applicable and preparations of Intal analogues are only just beginning to be tried. Antigen avoidance may help e.g. if dietary factors are identified, but apart from attempts to maintain a cool and moist skin there is little else to offer apart from the administration of topical corticosteroids. This is given initially as a 1% hydrocortisone cream, or alternatively, a more potent fluorinated preparation e.g. beclomethasone. Systemic steroids are not used. It is important to avoid smallpox vaccination in patients with eczema as this may be followed by the potentially fatal complication—Kaposi's varicelliform eruption.

Considerable advances have been made in the management of hay fever and extrinsic asthma in the last few years and it is likely that similar agents will become available for the control of non-respiratory atopic disorders in the near future. Prophylactic measures are already being tried in patients who may be supposed to have an atopic trait and the identification of the exact site of the biochemical lesion in atopy is the next goal in the analysis of this complex group of disorders. If, as seems likely, this turns out to be an immunological rather than a pharmacological defect (Fig. 3), and one of relative impairment of immune function or control, then it is possible that specific measures to potentiate the regulatory aspects of the immune response will be able to correct the underlying abnormality.

REFERENCES

Askenase, P. W., Haynes, J. D. and Hayden, B. J. (1976). Antibody-mediated basophil accumulations in cutaneous hypersensitivity reactions of guinea-pigs. *J. Immunol.* **117**, 216.

Assem, E. S. K., Turner-Warwick, M., Cole, P. and Shaw, K. M. (1971). Reversed anaphylactic reaction of leucocytes in intrinsic asthma. *Clin. All.* **1**, 353.

Barrick, R. H. and Farr, R. S. (1965). The increased incidence of circulating anti-beef albumin in the sera of allergic persons and some comments regarding the possible significance of this occurrence. *J. All.* **36**, 374.

Bascomba, A., Romar, A., Peláez, A., Villalmanzo, I. G. and Campos, A. (1976). The effect of sodium cromoglycate in preventing the aspirin-induced bronchospasm. *Clin. All.* **6**, 269.

Berrens, L. and Van Rijsvijk-Verbeek, J. (1973). Inactivation of complement (C3) in human sera by atopic allergens. *Int. Arch. All. App. Immunol.* **45**, 30.

Bienenstock, J., Johnston, N. and Perey, D. Y. E. (1973). Bronchial lymphoid tissue. *Lab. Invest.* **28**, 686.

Buckle, F. G. and Cohen, A. B. (1975). Nasal mucosal hyperpermeability to macromolecules in atopic rhinitis and extrinsic asthma. *J. All. Clin. Immunol.* **55**, 213.

Brandtzaeg, P. and Baklein, K. (1976). Inconclusive immunohistochemistry of human IgE in mucosal pathology. *Lancet* **1**, 1297.

Brostoff, J. and Roitt, I. M. (1969). Cell-mediated (delayed) hypersensitivity in patients with summer hayfever. *Lancet* **II**, 1269.

Bryant, D. H., Burns, M. W. and Lazarus, L. (1973). New type of allergic asthma due to IgG "reaginic" antibody. *Brit. Med. J.* **4**, 589.

Butcher, B. T., Salvaggio, J. E. and Leslie, G. A. (1975). Secretory and humoral immunologic response of atopic and non-atopic individuals to intra-nasally administered antigen. *Clin. All.* **1**, 33.

Champion, R. H., Roberts, S. O. B., Carpenter, R. G. and Roger, J. H. (1969). Urticaria and angio-oedema—a review of 554 patients. *Brit. J. Derm.* **81**, 588.

Coca, A. F. and Cooke, R. A. (1923). On the classification of the phenomena of hypersensitiveness. *J. Immunol.* **8**, 763.

Coca, A. F. and Grove, E. (1925). Studies in hypersensitiveness XIII. A study of the atopic reagins. *J. Immunol.* **10**, 445.

Cochrane, C. G. (1971). Mechanisms involved in the deposition of immune complexes in tissues. *J. Exp. Med.* **134**, 75s.

Devey, M. E., Wilson, D. V. and Wheeler, A. W. (1976). The IgG subclasses of antibodies to grass pollen allergens produced in hay fever patients during hyposensitisation. *Clin. All.* **6**, 227.

Dineen, J. K., Ogilvie, B. M. and Kelly, J. D. (1973). Expulsion of Nippostrongylus brasiliensis from the intestine of rats. *Immunology* **24**, 467.

Edmunds, L. H., Graf, P. D. and Nadel, J. A. (1971). Reinnervation of the reimplanted canine lung. *J. Appl. Physiol.* **31**, 722.

Empey, D. W., Laitinen, L. A., Jacobs, L., Gold, W. M. and Nadel, J. A. (1976). Mechanisms of bronchial hyper-reactivity in normal subjects after upper respiratory tract infection. *Am. Rev. Resp. Dis.* **113**, 131.

Ezeoke, A., Pereira, A. B. V. and Hobbs, J. R. (1973). Serum IgE elevation with tropical eosinophilia. *Clin. All.* **3**, 33.

Falliers, C. J., de Cardoso, A., Bane, H. N., Coffey, R. and Middleton, E. (1971). Discordant allergic manifestations in monozygotic twins: genetic identity versus clinical, physiologic, and biochemical differences. *J. All.* **47**, 207.

Freier, S. (1973). Paediatric gastro-intestinal allergy. *Clin. All.* **3** (Suppl.), 597.

Godfrey, R. C. (1975). Asthma and IgE levels in rural and urban communities of the Gambia. *Clin. All.* **5**, 201.

Godfrey, R. C. and Gradidge, C. F. (1976). Allergic sensitisation of human lung fragments prevented by saturation of IgE binding sites. *Nature* **259**, 484.

Gold, W. M. (1973). Cholinergic pharmacology in asthma. *In* "Asthma". (Ed. K. F. Austen and L. M. Lichtenstein), Academic Press, New York and London.

Goodfriend, L., Lapkoff, C. B. and Marsh, D. G. (1973). Ragweed pollen antigen Ra5: Isolation, chemical properties and genetic basis for its cutaneous activity in man. *J. All. Clin. Immunol.* **51**, 81.

Greenert, S., Bernstein, I. L. and Michael, J. G. (1971). Immune responses of non-atopic individuals to prolonged immunisation with ragweed extract. *Lancet* **II**, 1121.

Haddock, A. M., Patel, K. R., Alston, W. C. and Kerr, J. W. (1975). Response of lymphocyte guanyl cyclase to propranolol, noradrenaline, thymoxamine and acetylcholine in extrinsic bronchial asthma. *Brit. Med. J.* **2**, 357.

Heatley, R. V., Rhodes, J., Calcraft, B. J., Whitehead, R. H., Fifield, R. and Newcombe, R. G. (1975). Immunoglobulin E in rectal mucosa of patients with proctitis. *Lancet* **II**, 1010.

Hiller, E. J. and Milner, A. D. (1975). Betamethasone 17 valerate aerosol and disodium cromoglycate in severe childhood asthma. *Brit. J. Dis. Chest* **69**, 103.

Hoffbrand, B. I. (Ed.) 1975). The place of parasympatholytic drugs in the management of chronic obstructive airways disease. *Postgrad. Med. J.* **51**, Supp. 7.

Houri, M., Mayer, A. L. R., Houghton, L. E. and Jacobs, D. (1972). Correlation of skin, nasal and inhalation tests with the IgE in the serum, nasal fluid and sputum. *Clin. All.* **2**.

Huggins, K. G. and Brostoff, J. (1975). Local production of specific IgE antibodies in allergic-rhinitis patients with negative skin tests. *Lancet* **II**, 148.

Ishizaka, K. and Ishizaka, T. (1973). Role of IgE and IgG antibodies in reaginic hypersensitivity in the respiratory tract. *In* "Asthma". (Ed. K. F. Austen and L. M. Lichtenstein), Academic Press, New York and London.

Jarrett, E. E. E., Jarrett, W. F. H. and Urquhart, G. M. (1968). Quantitative studies on the kinetics of establishment and expulsion of intestinal nematode population in susceptible and immune hosts. *Parasitol.* **59**, 625.

Johansson, S. G. O. and Bennich, H. (1967). Immunological studies of an atypical (myeloma) immunoglobulin. *Immunology* **13**, 381.

Johansson, S. G. O., Mellbin, T. and Vahlquist, B. (1968). Immunoglobulin levels in Ethiopian pre-school children with special reference to high concentrations of immunoglobulin E (IgND). *Lancet* **I**, 1118.

Kaliner, M. and Austen, K. F. (1975). Immunologic release of chemical mediators from human tissues. *Ann. Rev. Pharmacol.* **15**, 177.

Kaufman, H. S. and Hobbs, J. R. (1970). Immunoglobulin deficiencies in an atopic population. *Lancet* **II**, 1061.

Kontou-Karakitsos, K., Salvaggio, J. E. and Mathews, K. P. (1975). Comparative nasal absorption of allergens in atopic and non-atopic subjects. *J. All. Clin. Immunol.* **55**, 241.

Kuitunen, P., Visakorpi, J. K., Savilahti, E. and Pelkonen, P. (1975). Malabsorption syndrome with cow's milk intolerance. *Arch. Dis. Child.* **50**, 351.

Levine, B. B. (1973). Genetics of atopic allergy and reagin production. *Clin. All.* **3** (Suppl.), 539.

Lichtenstein, L. M., Norman, P. S. and Winkenwerder, W. L. (1971). A single year of immunotherapy for ragweed hay fever. *Ann. Int. Med.* **75**, 663.

Malley, A., Baecker, K. and Birger, D. (1971). The role of complement in allergen-reagin mediated histamine release from monkey lung tissue. *Proc. Soc. Exp. Biol. Med.* **136**, 341.

Marsh, D. G., Bias, W. B. and Ishizaka, K. (1974). Genetic control of basal serum immunoglobulin E level and its effect on specific reaginic sensitivity. *Proc. Nat. Acad. Sci.* **71**, 3588.

Matthews, T. S. and Soothill, J. F. (1970). Complement activation after milk feeding in children with cow's milk allergy. *Lancet* **II**, 893.

Mehta, S. B. and Smith, J. M. (1975). Nasal hyposensitisation and hay fever. *Clin. All.* **5**, 279.

Minor, T. E., Dick, E. C., Baker, J. W., Ouellette, J. J., Cohen, M. and Reed, C. E. (1976). Rhinovirus and influenza type A infections as precipitants of asthma. *Am. Rev. Resp. Med.* **113**, 149.

Nemoto, T., Aoki, H., Ike, A., Yamada, K., Kondo, T., Kobayashi, S. and Inagawa, T. (1976). Serum prostaglandin levels in asthmatic patients. *J. All. Clin. Immunol.* **57**, 89.

Newball, H. H., Talamo, R. C. and Lichtenstein, L. M. (1975). Release of leukocyte kallikrein mediated by IgE. *Nature* **254**, 635.

Noon, L. (1911). Prophylactic inoculation for hay fever. *Lancet* **I**, 1572.

Nye, L., Merrett, T. G., Landon, J. and White, R. J. (1975). A detailed investigation of circulating IgE levels in a normal population. *Clin. All.* **5**, 13.

Palmer, K. N. V., Gaddie, J. and Skinner, C. (1974). Alpha-adrenoceptor-blocking drugs in asthma. *Brit. Med. J.* **4**, 409.

Parish, W. E. (1973). A human heat-stable anaphylactic or anaphylactoid antibody which may participate in pulmonary disorders. *In* "Asthma". (Ed. K. F. Austen and L. M. Lichtenstein), Academic Press, New York and London.

Patel, K. R. (1975). Atropine, sodium cromoglycate and thymoxamine in $PGF_{2\alpha}$-induced bronchoconstriction in extrinsic asthma. *Brit. Med. J.* **2**, 360.

Patel, K. R. and Kerr, J. W. (1975). Effect of alpha receptor blocking drug, thymoxamine, on allergen induced bronchoconstriction in extrinsic asthma. *Clin. All.* **5**, 311.

Pepys, J. (1973a). Disodium cromoglycate in clinical and experimental asthma. *In* "Asthma". (Ed. K. F. Austen and L. M. Lichtenstein), Academic Press, New York and London.

Pepys, J. (1973b). Immunopathology of allergic lung disease. *Clin. All.* **3**, 1.

Pepys, J. (1975a). Atopy. *In* "Clinical aspects of Immunology". Third Edition. (Ed. P. G. H. Gell, R. R. A. Coombs and P. J. Lachmann), Blackwell, Oxford.

Pepys, J. (1975b). Skin tests in diagnosis. *In* "Clinical Aspects of Immunology". Third Edition. (Ed. P. G. H. Gell, R. R. A. Coombs and P. J. Lachmann), Blackwell, Oxford.

Pepys, J. and Hutchcroft, B. J. (1975). Bronchial provocation tests in etiologic diagnosis and analysis of asthma. *Am. Rev. Resp. Dis.* **112**, 829.

Phillips, M. J., Knight, N. J., Manning, H., Abbott, A. L. and Tripp, W. G. (1974). IgE and secretory otitis media. *Lancet* **II**, 1176.

Polmar, S. H., Waldmann, T. A., Balestra, S. T., Jost, M. C. and Terry, M. D. (1972). IgE in immunologic deficiency diseases. *J. Clin. Invest.* **51**, 326.

Reeves, W. G., Camerson, J. S., Johansson, S. G. O., Ogg, C. S., Peters, D. K. and Weller, R. O. (1975). Seasonal nephrotic syndrome. *Clin. All.* **5**, 121.

Reeves, W. G., Allen, B. R. and Marriott, D. W. (1977). (In press.)

Rice, N. S. C. and Jones, B. R. (1973). Vernal kerato-conjunctivitis: an allergic disease of the eyes of children. *Clin. All.* **3** (Suppl.), 629.

Richardson, J. B., Hogg, J. C., Bouchard, T. and Hall, D. L. (1973). Localisation of antigen in experimental bronchoconstriction in guinea pigs. *J. All. Clin. Immunol.* **52**, 172.

Richerson, H. B. and Parker, D. (1974). Jones-Mote reactions. *Prog. Immunol.* **II**, 3, 373.

Salvaggio, J. E., Castro-Murillo, E. and Kundur, V. (1969). Immunologic response of atopic and normal individuals to keyhole limpet hemocyanin. *J. All.* **44**, 344.

Schultz, G., Hardman, J. G. and Sutherland, E. W. (1973). Cyclic nucleotides and smooth muscle function. *In* "Asthma". (Ed. K. F. Austen and L. M. Lichtenstein), Academic Press, New York and London.

Schwartzman, R. M., Rockey, J. H. and Halliwell (1971). Canine reaginic antibody. *Clin. Exp. Immunol.* **9**, 549.

Selye, H. (1965). "The Mast Cells". Butterworth, London.

Shakib, F., Stanworth, D. R., Smalley, C. A. and Brown, G. A. (1976). Elevated serum IgG_4 levels in cystic fibrosis patients. *Clin. All.* **6**, 237.

Sheppard, H. (1973). Phosphodiesterase inhibitors and analogs of cyclic AMP as potential agents for the treatment of asthma. *In* "Asthma". (Ed. K. F. Austen and L. M. Lichtenstein), Academic Press, New York and London.

Shiner, M., Ballard, J. and Smith, M. E. (1975). The small-intestinal mucosa in cow's milk allergy. *Lancet* **I**, 136.

Soothill, J. F. (1976). Some intrinsic and extrinsic factors predisposing to allergy. *Proc. Roy. Soc. Med.* **69**, 439.

Speizer, F. E., Doll, R. and Heaf, P. (1968). Observations on recent increase in mortality from asthma. *Brit. Med. J.* **1**, 335.

Stifler, W. C. (1965). A 21-year follow-up of infantile eczema. *J. Paediat.* **66**, Supp. 166.

Stokes, C. R., Soothill, J. F. and Turner, M. W. (1975). Immune exclusion is a function of IgA. *Nature* **255**, 745.

Szentivanyi, A. (1968). The beta adrenergic theory of the atopic abnormality in bronchial asthma. *J. All.* **42**, 203.

Tada, T. and Ishizaka, K. (1970). Distribution of γE-forming cells in lymphoid tissues of the human and monkey. *J. Immunol.* **104**, 377.

Tada, T., Taniguchi, M. and Takemori, T. (1975). Properties of primed suppressor T-cells and their products. *Transp. Rev.* **26**, 106.

Taylor, B., Norman, A. P., Orgel, H. A., Stokes, C. R., Turner, M. W. and Soothill, J. F. (1973). Transient IgA deficiency and pathogenesis of infantile atopy. *Lancet* **II**, 111.

Taylor, G. (1973). Allergic diseases of the upper respiratory tract. *Clin. All.* **3** (Suppl.), 639.

Taylor, W. A., Francis, D. H., Sheldon, D. and Roitt, I. M. (1974). The anti-anaphylactic actions of disodium cromoglycate, theophylline, isoprenaline and prostaglandins. *Int. Arch. All. App. Immunol.* **46**, 104.

Tomasi, T. B. and Katz, L. (1971). Human antibodies against bovine immunoglobulin M in IgA deficient sera. *Clin. Exp. Immunol.* **9**, 3.

Waldmann, T. A., Wochner, R. D., Laster, L. and Gordon, R. S. (1967). Allergic gastro-enteropathy—a cause of excessive gastro-intestinal protein loss. *New Eng. J. Med.* **276**, 761.

Walls, R. S., Basten, A., Leuchars, E. and Davies, A. J. S. (1971). Mechanisms for eosinophilic and neutrophilic leucocytoses. *Brit. Med. J.* **3**, 157.

Warner, J. O., Norman, A. P. and Soothill, J. F. (1976). Cystic fibrosis heterozygosity in the pathogenesis of allergy. *Lancet* **I**, 990.

Williams, H. and McNicol, K. N. (1969). Prevalence, natural history, and relationship of wheezy bronchitis and asthma in children. An epidemiological study. *Brit. Med. J.* **4**, 321.

Williams, R. C., Griffiths, R. W., Emmons, J. D. and Field, R. C. (1972). Naturally occurring human antiglobulins with specificity for E. *J. Clin. Invest.* **51**, 955.

23

Skin Disease

B. R. ALLEN and W. G. REEVES

Studies on the biology of skin have yielded important immunological advances. For example, the work which Medawar's group began in the 1940s on the phenomenon of pigment spread led to a fundamental understanding of transplantation immunity and the confirmation of Burnet's prediction of neonatally-induced tolerance (Billingham, 1974). Similarly, the use of grafts of hamster cheek pouch "skin" has defined the role of lymphatic drainage in the process of sensitization and the importance of "privileged sites" in unresponsive states.

The skin has also featured as a testing ground for many diverse immunological hypotheses: from Edward Jenner's bold inoculation of James Phipps with small-pox virus to Carl Prausnitz' demonstration of reaginic antibody in the serum of Kustner; from studies of the effects of hypnosis on delayed hypersensitivity to the demonstration that bridging of two adjacent IgE molecules is required for mast cell degranulation. The involvement of the skin in systemic immunological reactions was described in 1905 by Von Pirquet and Schick in their treatise on "serum sickness" and more recently a characteristic rash has been recognized as an important feature of graft-versus-host disease.

Dermatological nomenclature is complex and often confusing. A clearer understanding of the underlying mechanisms is gradually producing a rationalization of what has often been a "Linnaean" approach. And, as such knowledge accumulates, it is obvious that immunological processes are frequently involved in dermatological disease. In this chapter we discuss those areas of dermatology where immunology has something relevant to say.

Normal Structure and Function

Although there are local variations the division of the epidermis into basal, prickle, granular and horny layers is universal. The cells proliferate from the basal layer which sits on the basement membrane at the epidermal/dermal junction. The desmosomes between the cells are linked to cytoplasmic tonofibrils and hold the epidermal cells together. They may also function in transporting nutrients between the cells, for the epidermis is an avascular tissue.

The basement membrane has two components:

i. A superficial basal lamina between 500 and 1,000 nm in width. It can only be seen in the electron microscope and is attached to the basal epidermal layer by hemidesmosomes.
ii. A deeper reticular lamina which contains reticulin fibres (unit fibrils of collagen) surrounded by an amorphous mucopolysaccharide ground substance. This layer can be seen in the light microscope when special stains are used, either for reticulin (e.g. silver impregnation methods) or for the mucopolysaccharide matrix (e.g. PAS techniques).

Under normal conditions the basal lamina probably acts as a semi-permeable membrane allowing the transport of nutrient materials from the capillary loops in the dermal papillae across into the epidermis. The situation in the skin is comparable to that in the renal glomerulus where endothelial and epithelial basal laminae become opposed back-to-back for transport purposes. This greatly facilitates the transport and deposition of immunological material, a fact which is already well recognized in glomerulonephritis.

The dermis is much less well defined and regular. Its outer part containing the capillary loops and loose connective tissue is often referred to as the papillary layer; the deeper reticular layer showing more dense connective tissue with some muscle, appendages and larger vessels. Mast cells occur in the dermis in a perivascular distribution.

The vascular supply to the dermis is complex. The reticular layer contains an irregular deep plexus with arteries of 50–100 μ in diameter. These subdivide to give a subpapillary plexus from which the capillary loops (about 15 μ in diameter) arise. These loops arcade into the dome of the dermal papillae approximating to the basement membrane of the epidermis. There is usually one capillary loop per papilla. The capillaries drain into two anastomosing venous plexuses in the superficial and deep dermis. Arteriovenous anastomoses, as well as other factors, can produce marked changes in differential flow through the superficial and deep vessels. Superficial and deep lymphatic collection systems exist in the dermis but their functional significance is poorly understood.

Antibody Transport

Little is known about the quantitative aspects of transport across the epidermal/dermal interface or the factors which affect it. Although the deposition of immunological material in the region of the basement membrane may show patterns of diagnostic value in various skin diseases it may occur non-specifically where there is telangiectasia of the cutaneous vessels as in rosacea. The amount of immunoglobulin (particularly IgG) present in the dermis is considerably increased in almost any inflammatory disease of the skin. There may be special factors controlling the access of circulating antibody to the basement membrane and the epidermis. Ultraviolet irradiation abolishes the normal resistance to immunoglobulin transfer into the epidermis and this effect is largely due to the response of the papillary microcirculation. It is likely that a small amount of antibody gets across normally but unless it has a specificity for material within the basement membrane or the epidermis, it passes through into the outer layers and is shed along with the outer part of the horny layer.

Methods of Investigation

Skin Testing

Cutaneous challenge with antigen and other *in vivo* cutaneous studies are discussed in Chapter 21.

Biopsy Examination

Conventional histological examination is often helpful but advances in knowledge of immunologically determined disorders have been made by using specific immunohistochemical techniques to localize abnormal deposits within biopsy material. Most of this work has been done using fluorescein-conjugated antisera although peroxidase-labelling is also used and is of especial value in the electron microscope.

Direct Immunofluorescence

The *direct* immunofluorescent (IF) technique involves the examination of biopsy material using directly conjugated antisera. The tissue for examination must not be placed in formalin but should be snap frozen immediately in liquid nitrogen after suitable orientation on metal foil. Cryostat sections are then treated with specific conjugated reagents for each kind of material sought e.g. IgG, IgA, IgM, C3, Clq, fibrinogen, etc. Antisera for IgD, IgE and other complement components are also used although, as with all such reagents, valid results depend on the exact specificity of the antiserum. If there is any doubt, it should be checked by careful testing, using an immunofluorescence or passive haemagglutination system. Immunodiffusion is not sufficiently sensitive to exclude non-specificity in a reagent used in an immunofluorescent system.

Indirect Immunofluorescence

Certain tissues, e.g. guinea-pig lip or rat oesophagus, can be used as a convenient skin substrate for the detection of skin-reactive antibodies in the sera of patients by the indirect IF technique. This involves incubating cryostat sections of the frozen tissue with the test serum and, after washing, reacting the product with fluorescein-conjugated antisera against the various kinds of human antibody that may have become bound to antigens present in the normal tissue.

Other Serum Studies

The detection of other auto-reactive antibodies is of value in several disorders which involve the skin e.g. lupus erythematosus and rheumatoid arthritis, and these conditions are discussed in detail elsewhere.

Estimation of serum immunoglobulins (IgG, IgA, IgM) and complement (e.g. C3 and C4) levels is often helpful. IgE levels are particularly high in atopic eczema and they are often raised in pemphigoid and possibly other bullous disorders. Estimation of the Cl esterase inhibitor is important in the diagnosis of hereditary angioneurotic oedema.

A full screen of immunoglobulin, complement, lymphocyte and neutrophil function is only necessary when an immunodeficiency disorder is suspected.

Specific Cell Mediated Responses

Little *in vitro* work has been done on cellular responses in skin diseases because of the great difficulties involved in defining and preparing the antigens relevant *in vivo*. Intracutaneous or patch tests are still the most useful although they must be used with caution in the investigation of drug hypersensitivity (see below). One system in which *in vitro* methods mirror *in vivo* testing is with sensitization to dinitrochlorobenzene (DNCB). The haptenic nature (see Chapter 5) of the pure chemical may be overcome by linking it to lymphocyte membranes and then using a lyophilized product as the antigenic stimulus in a lymphocyte culture system.

BULLOUS DISORDERS

The primary blistering disorders, in which vesicles or bullae occur as an essential part of the disease process, are few in number but immunological studies have made a significant contribution to our knowledge of them. Some of the immunological findings are summarized in Table 2 (page 789).

Pemphigus

All disorders which correctly include the word pemphigus in their title have in common clinical and histological disintegration of the epidermis. In benign familial pemphigus (Hailey-Hailey disease) this results from a congenital epidermal defect. In other forms (pemphigus vulgaris, pemphigus vegetans, pemphigus foliaceus or erythematosus and Brazilian pemphigus) immunological abnormalities are found.

Direct Immunofluorescence

Biopsies should be taken from an area adjacent to a fresh blister or a fresh erosion if mucous membrane is examined. Direct immunofluorescence shows a pattern of IgG and complement deposition in the intercellular region of the epidermis giving rise to a "chicken-wire" appearance (Fig. 1). The precise antigen is unknown. No distinction has yet been made in the pattern of deposition between one kind of pemphigus and another.

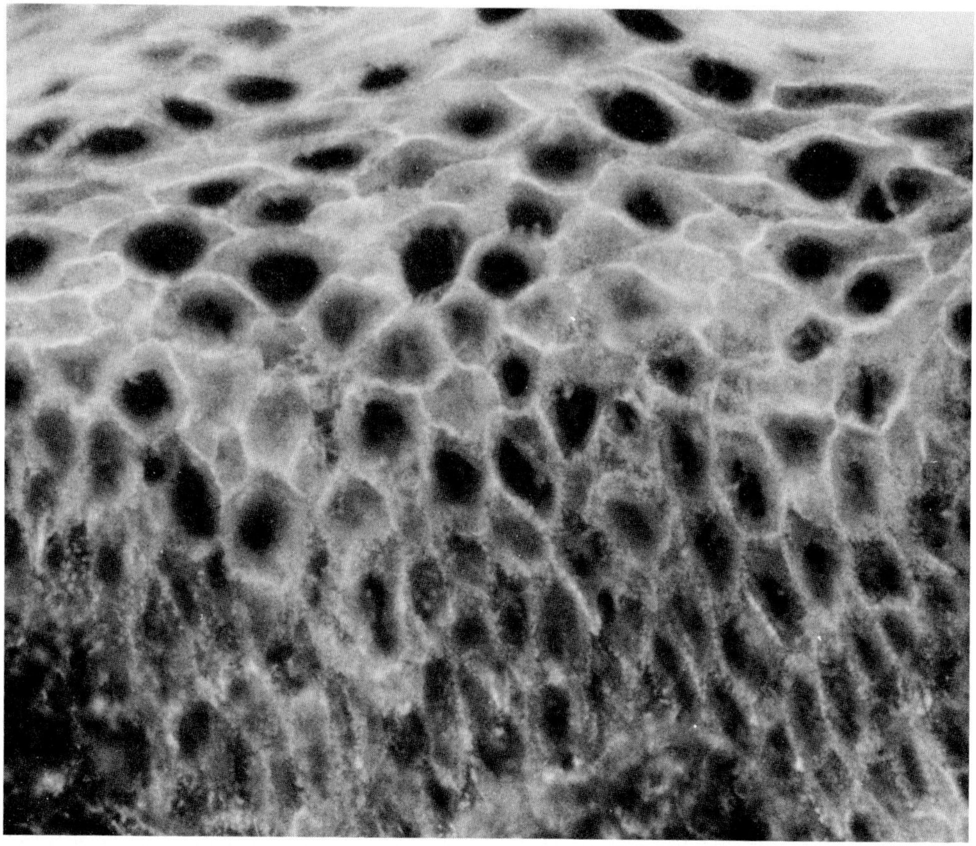

Fig. 1 (a). Direct and indirect immunofluorescence in pemphigus: intercellular "chicken-wire" pattern of deposition of IgG detected by direct examination of biopsy of pemphigus skin.

Serum Findings

In nearly all active cases, indirect immunofluorescence shows the presence of an antibody which combines with the intercellular region of stratified squamous epithelia producing a pattern virtually identical to that seen on direct immunofluorescence. In mild cases, the titre may be low and it is advisable, for diagnostic purposes, to take a skin biopsy for direct immunofluorescence as well. The amount of antibody fluctuates with disease intensity and may drop to undetectable levels during treatment. The experimental induction of

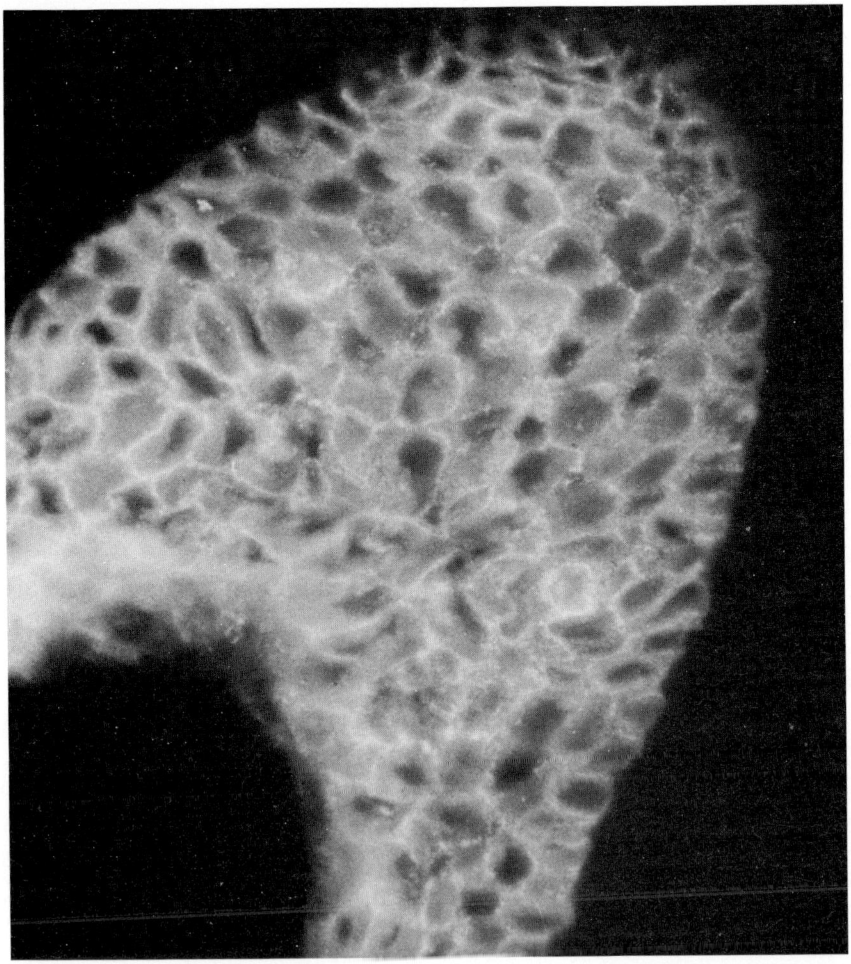

Fig. 1 (b). Indirect examination for the detection of circulating IgG reactive with the intercellular material of guinea-pig lip epidermis.

lesions in apparently normal skin following UV irradiation is probably due to the increased leakage of antibody from the papillary circulation.

It is probable that a rise in titre precedes an exacerbation. Patients in whom the antibody level remains high during treatment may be expected to relapse when it is withdrawn. The highest levels are found in patients with Brazilian pemphigus. The antibody usually reacts with stratified squamous epithelium derived from various species but the degree of species and tissue specificity does vary and human, monkey or rat oesophagus will demonstrate a minority of antibodies which are negative with guinea-pig lip.

Differential Diagnosis

Intercellular immunofluorescent staining is confined to pemphigus and other conditions in which pemphigus-like antibodies (PLA) are found are listed in Table 1. Characteristically, these antibodies are present in low titre and direct immunofluorescence is negative.

Significance of Intercellular Antibodies

The localization of the antibody between the epidermal cells—which under light microscopy are acantholytic—and the direct relationship with disease activity are strongly in favour of a causal relationship. It is likely that the weaker reactions of pemphigus-like antibodies arise as secondary phenomena. In burns, for example, PLA are not detectable until two weeks after the initial episode and gradually disappear over the succeeding few weeks. They are detected in a minority (15–50%) of patients.

It is not clear why some pemphigus antibodies fail to react with skin sections from various sources (including man) in the indirect test although readily detectable using the stratified squamous epithelium of primate or rat oesophagus. The most likely explanation is that antigen density varies between these tissues and that on direct examination skin fixation is seen only after

TABLE 1
Conditions associated with pemphigus-like antibodies (PLA)

Burns
Myasthenia gravis[a]
Thymoma[a]
Lepromatous leprosy
Drug eruptions:
Penicillin
Phenylbutazone
Penicillamine[a]
Phenophthalein
Practolol

[a] A pemphigus-like disorder has occasionally been reported in association with these conditions.

TABLE 2

Patterns of antibody deposition or reactivity in skin diseases

	Direct immunofluorescence		Serum antibodies	
	Lesional skin	Non-lesional skin	Skin reactive	Other specificities
Pemphigus	I-C	I-C	I-C	—
Pemphigoid	BM	BM	BM	—
Cicatricial pemphigoid	BM	—	—	—
Juvenile pemphigoid	—	—	—	—
Dermatitis herpetiformis	—	papillae/BM	—	reticulin
Herpes gestationis	BM	—	±	—
Erythema multiforme	—	—	—	—
Lichen planus	BM	—	—	—
Porphyria	BM	BM[a]	—	—
Discoid lupus	BM	—	—	nuclei
Systemic lupus	BM	BM[a]	—	nuclei and DNA
Systemic sclerosis	—	—	—	nuclei and RNA
Cutaneous vasculitis	In and around blood vessels		—	—

I-C, intercellular zone of epidermis; BM, basement membrane zone.
[a] Indicates when this may only be positive in light-exposed skin.
The individual types of antibody, complement and fibrin that may be present and their patterns of deposition are of particular value in distinguishing between these various disorders. Each pattern is discussed more fully in the text.

considerable local concentration of the antibody. It is also possible that, *in vivo*, free antigen is present in the intercellular space.

Pemphigoid

Pemphigoid was distinguished from pemphigus in 1953 when Lever recognized that the blister was occurring beneath, and not in, the epidermis. Its demarcation from dermatitis herpetiformis, which often shows a similar histological change has become possible using immunological techniques (Fig. 2).

Direct Immunofluorescence

Direct immunofluorescence shows deposition of IgG and complement in the basement membrane zone of the epidermal/dermal junction (Fig. 2). It is usual to take the biopsy from the area adjacent to an intact fresh blister. If the blister itself is examined, complement deposition is usually seen on both the base and roof of the blister cavity.

Uninvolved skin, as well as skin from eczematous areas which frequently precede the blisters, often shows immunoglobulin deposition, but its reliability for diagnostic purposes has not yet been fully assessed.

Serum Findings

In over 80% of active cases of pemphigoid, circulating antibody to the basement membrane zone of stratified epithelium can be detected. This antibody, which is usually IgG, but occasionally IgM or IgA as well, appears to be almost specific for this disease. For diagnostic purposes, if the antibody is detected by indirect immunofluorescence, further investigation is unnecessary but, as 20% of patients have no detectable circulating antibody, it is better to carry out a skin biopsy for direct immunofluorescence as well.

Blister Fluid

In comparison with other serum proteins, complement levels are reduced in blister fluid. This implies utilization within the blister space (Jordan *et al.*, 1973).

Differential Diagnosis

Cicatricial pemphigoid, lupus erythematosus and herpes gestationis also give rise to IgG or complement deposition in the basement membrane zone (Table 2). In lupus erythematosus the deposits tend to be coarse and irregular

(Fig. 3), in contrast to the thin, linear staining seen in pemphigoid. Ultrastructural studies with immunoperoxidase techniques show that in pemphigoid the antibody deposit is between the basal cells and the basal lamina of the basement membrane, whereas in lupus the deposits occur on the dermal side of the basal lamina (Schaumburg-Lever *et al.*, 1975). Patients with cicatricial pemphigoid may have similar direct IF findings to those with pemphigoid, but do not appear to have circulating antibody.

Significance of Immunoglobulin Deposition

The relationship of immunoglobulin deposition to the site of the blister and the consumption of complement within the blister are in favour of the antibody being of significance in the process of blister formation. Against this must be weighed the fact that patients in remission may have circulating antibody levels as high as those found when their disease was active.

There are no clues at present as to why these patients develop antibodies against of their cutaneous basement membrane although in another basement membrane antibody disease (Goodpasture's syndrome—see Chapter 17) there are circumstantial links with influenza virus and exposure to petrochemicals. The eczematous reaction which may precede the development of blistering in pemphigoid might conceivably be triggered by an environmental agent which provokes what appears to be an auto-immune response.

Patients with bullous pemphigoid often have a particularly high serum IgE level. It does not seem to be due to associated atopic disease and the mechanism is unclear (Reeves *et al.*, 1977). IgE deposition has been reported to occur in the basement membrane zone of skin biopsies from a minority of patients with pemphigoid (Provost and Tomasi, 1974) although we have not been able to confirm this finding

Cicatricial Pemphigoid (Benign mucous membrane pemphigoid)

This is a condition of the skin and some mucosal membranes in which subepidermal blisters are followed by chronic erosions and scars. The eyes are nearly always involved. It is a rare disease and a clear pattern of immunological findings has not yet emerged. Most reports indicate that involved skin and mucous membrane show IgG and complement deposits but uninvolved skin and mucous membrane are normal. Circulating antibody has rarely

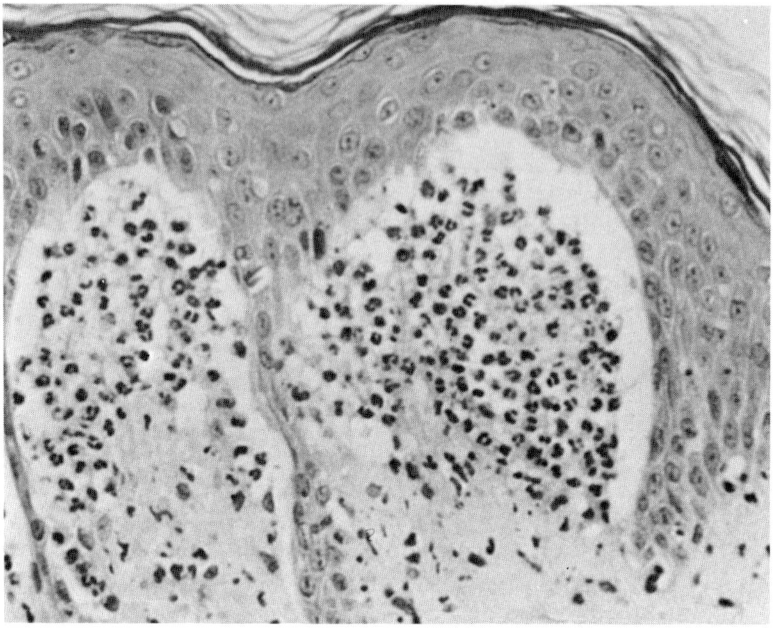

(a)

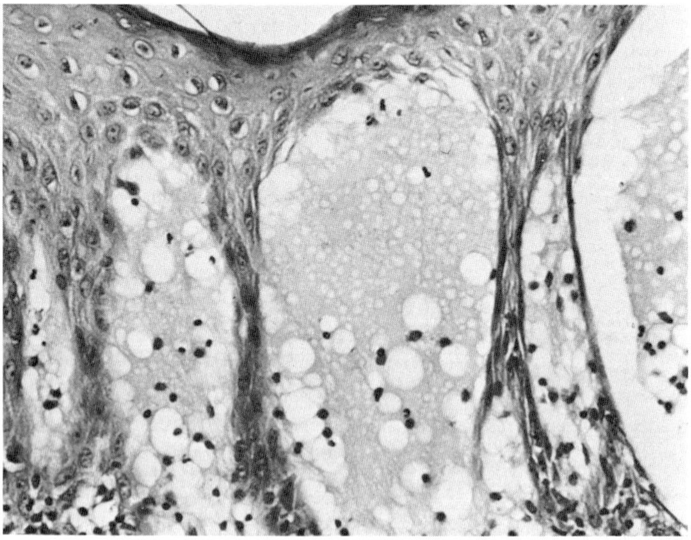

(b)

Fig. 2. Histological and immunofluorescent findings in dermatitis herpetiformis and pemphigoid: (a) H and E of dermatitis herpetiformis skin, (b) H and E pemphigoid skin.

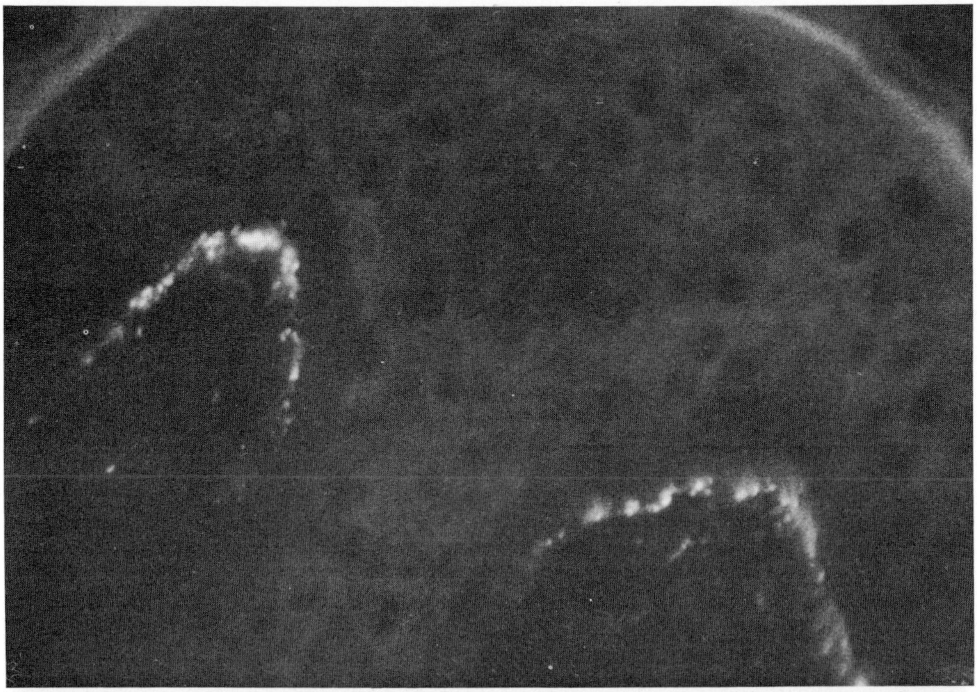

(c)

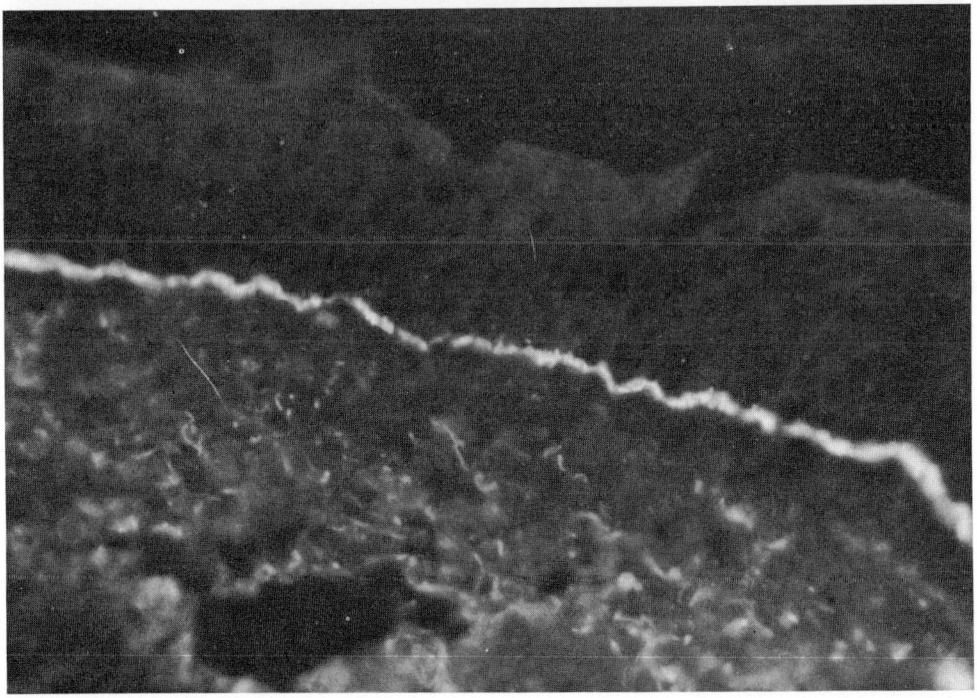

(d)

Fig. 2. (c) granular deposition of IgA in the apices of dermal papillae of DH skin (direct immunofluorescence), (d) linear deposition of C3 along the epidermal/dermal junction in pemphigoid skin (direct immunofluorescence).

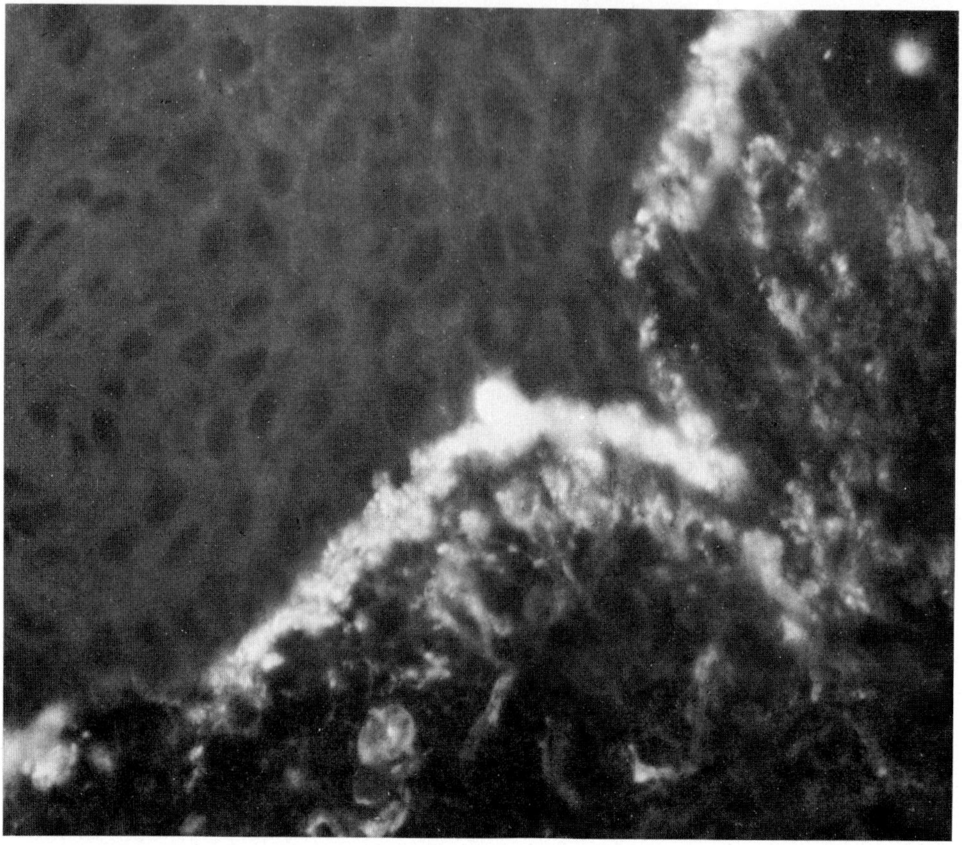

Fig. 3. Coarsely granular deposition of immunoglobulin (IgM) at the epidermal/dermal junction of clinically normal skin in systemic lupus.

been found, and the presence of a highly species or organ specific antibody cannot be excluded.

Juvenile Pemphigoid

This is a self-limiting disorder of childhood in which subepidermal blisters appear, especially on the genitalia and face. It has been variously classified as a form of pemphigoid or dermatitis herpetiformis. Immunological studies show it to be neither. No circulating antibodies have been found and there is no basement membrane zone staining. Dermatitis herpetiformis does occur in children, however, and detection of IgA in the dermal papillae can be used to differentiate it from juvenile pemphigoid.

Dermatitis Herpetiformis (DH)

The lack of distinctive differences between the histological changes in DH and pemphigoid led some authorities to regard them as variants of the same disease. However, the immunological findings indicate that this is not the case. Dermatitis herpetiformis also has a strong association with subtotal villous atrophy of the small intestine although clinical malabsorption is unusual. Fry *et al.* (1973) have shown that clinical remission and ultrastructural improvement of the skin lesions can follow a prolonged gluten-free diet.

Direct Immunofluorescence

Granular or fibrillar deposits of IgA are found in the dermal papillae of clinically uninvolved skin. C3 can also be detected at the same site and usually in the absence of earlier complement components suggesting fixation of complement by the alternative pathway (see Chapter 7). Less commonly IgA is deposited in a linear fashion along the line of the epidermal/dermal junction and this may be confined to the papillae or may be continuous. These two patterns of deposition may occur alone or in combination. Sometimes other classes of antibody e.g. IgM and IgG, are also found. Ultrastructural studies have shown that the antibody is localized to the dermal side of the basal lamina and is often mostly within the dermis itself. Treatment with dapsone does not appear to influence the presence of IgA in the skin although C3 may disappear. Rather surprisingly, active lesions do not show the deposits. Biopsies should, therefore, always be taken from uninvolved skin.

Serum Findings

There are no consistent abnormalities in the sera of patients with DH and attempts to demonstrate a circulating antibody against the basement membrane zone have failed. A minority, however, have other circulating antibodies.

Anti-reticulin antibodies were described by Seah *et al.* (1971) in 17% of 29 patients with DH. They are of class IgG and IgA and show a specificity for collagenase-resistant fibres of connective tissue. The same antibody was detected in 36% of 31 patients with adult coeliac disease and has been found in Crohn's disease. The titre is lower in patients on a gluten-free diet. This antibody has been shown to cross-react with gluten although the degree of chemical similarity between gluten and reticulin has yet to be determined.

Seah *et al.* also reported finding anti-nuclear antibodies in one third of their patients with DH and an increased incidence of anti-thyroid antibodies has been described.

Diagnosis

In the past, DH has been diagnosed in many patients with troublesome pruritic eruptions which were not sufficiently distinctive to allow another credible label to be attached. The discovery of the various immunological abnormalities has allowed the application of more precise diagnostic criteria even in the absence of typical blisters. Seah and Fry (1975) found IgA in the normal skin of all patients with DH and conclude that the diagnosis should not be made in its absence.

Significance of the Immunological Findings

The most striking difference between pemphigus, pemphigoid and DH is that in the first two the pattern of antibody fixation seen in a biopsy can be reproduced by incubating the patient's serum with a normal skin section, but not in dermatitis herpetiformis in which, despite the consistent finding on direct IF, nothing comparable is seen in the indirect test. The usual restriction of the deposited immunoglobulin to class IgA is also a specific feature and suggests that it originates from the gut. The relationship of DH to gluten ingestion and subtotal villous atrophy points to the involvement of an extrinsic antigen. The frequent localization of the skin antibody to the papillary regions and the lack of skin-reactive material in the indirect test suggest that circulating antigen–antibody complexes are involved.

Evidence for circulating complexes has been obtained by Mowbray *et al.*, 1973. Dapsone—the drug of choice in DH—blocks the effect of experimentally-induced immune complex disease without affecting antibody production. This fits with the fact that in treated patients with DH the skin lesions clear but the IgA remains. The low incidence of anti-reticulin antibodies in DH suggests either that this antibody does not belong to the primary antigen–antibody system involved or that in a majority of patients most of the antibody is present in the form of complexes so that free antibody is not detectable. The fact that anti-reticulin antibody has been completely removed by absorption with gluten extracts suggests more than a peripheral involvement. Although the reticulin antibody always includes IgG, IgA is also present in 64% of cases. It is conceivable that dimeric secretory IgA of molecular weight 380,000 forms complexes with reticulin antigen of a size which preferentially deposit in the papillary vessels of the skin.

The definitive experiment of eluting the deposited IgA from the skin, and testing it for anti-reticulin activity has not yet been done. It is puzzling why some people with gluten-sensitive enteropathy develop coeliac disease and others dermatitis herpetiformis.

Epidermolysis Bullosa Acquisita

This is an exceedingly rare disorder in which excessive skin fragility develops during adult life and results in subepidermal blisters of similar appearance and distribution to those seen in the autosomal dominant dystrophic form of epidermolysis bullosa. In a recent case we have demonstrated a broad linear band of IgM in the basement membrane zone together with large clumps in the upper dermis and lower epidermis reminiscent of the findings in bullous lichen planus. Gibbs and Minus (1975) describe a case with direct immunofluorescence findings similar to those found in pemphigoid.

Herpes Gestationis

This uncommon bullous disorder occurs during pregnancy and usually clears rapidly in the puerperium. It is highly likely to recur during subsequent pregnancies and has been observed pre-menstrually and as a result of progestogen administration.

Carruthers and Black (1975) described three cases in which C3 was detected as a linear band in the basement membrane zone on direct immunofluorescence. In two of the cases IgG was demonstrated. No circulating antibody against the basement membrane zone was detected but the sera of two of the patients contained a circulating factor capable of depositing complement on the basement membrane zone of normal skin.

Toxic Epidermal Necrolysis (TEN, Lyell's Disease)

Occasionally a child infected with a phage type 71 staphylococcus develops generalized erythema, tenderness of the skin and a loss of cohesion between the epidermis and the underlying dermis. Certain drugs, especially butazones, sulphonamides and barbiturates may produce a similar reaction in adults. The split is in the lower epidermis in staphylococcal TEN and is subepidermal in drug-induced cases. A comparison has been made between this condition and experimentally induced graft-versus-host reactions in mice but an immunological basis for TEN in humans has not been convincingly demonstrated.

Erythema Multiforme and Stevens-Johnson Syndrome

Erythema multiforme may follow a number of different stimuli e.g. drugs and infections. There is usually a delay of 10–20 days although in the recurrent form this may be shortened to a few days or even hours. Herpes simplex, mycoplasma, psittacosis and orf are some of the more common triggering infections and herpes simplex lesions are often associated with the recurrent form of erythema multiforme. The cellular infiltrate in the skin is mostly lymphocytic and the appearances often resemble vasculitis. The skin lesions may be papular, giving the "iris" or target lesions or may be bullous in type. The latter form may be associated with oral and genital ulceration as part of the Stevens-Johnson syndrome, which can also include bronchitis or pneumonitis, diarrhoea and fever. Uveal and corneal involvement as well as renal, neurological and myocardial problems have been described and there is often transient polyarthritis.

Various microbial antibodies may rise in titre in different patients during attacks e.g. those against herpes simplex virus (HSV), influenza A, psittacosis virus, *Mycoplasma* and *Histoplasma*, and simplex virus or *Mycoplasma pneumoniae* have been cultured from the blister fluid. Injection of HSV intradermally into a patient who had recurrent Stevens-Johnson syndrome following simplex lesions was followed 48 hours later by the appearance of bullous lesions at the site of the injection and also elsewhere on the skin. Serum immunoglobulin levels do not seem to be raised although complement levels may fall during attacks. Skin-reactive antibody has not been detected by either direct or indirect immunofluorescent techniques (Table 2).

Corticosteroids are of value in controlling attacks. When recurrent episodes are a problem, the prompt application of idoxuridine to preceding herpetic lesions may reduce their severity or incidence.

Aphthous Ulceration and Behcet's Syndrome

Aphthous ulcers affect more than 10% of the population at some time whereas the symptom-complex of Behcet's syndrome is fairly uncommon. In addition to oral and genital ulceration this may include iridocyclitis, neurological disturbances, cutaneous involvement e.g. erythema nodosum, erythema multiforme and pustular lesions, arthropathy usually confined to the larger joints, intestinal involvement and thrombophlebitis.

Various infective factors have been implicated but no convincing proof has yet appeared. A recent study established the high incidence of villous atrophy of the jejunal mucosa in recurrent aphthous ulceration and demonstrated a beneficial effect from treatment with a gluten-free diet (Ferguson *et al.*, 1976). The lesions show intense perivascular infiltration with lymphocytes and monocytes initially, followed by a polymorphonuclear reaction. Occasionally fibrinoid necrosis is seen and vascular lesions, more often in Behcet's syndrome. Serum and salivary IgA levels are often raised and antibodies to saline homogenates of oral mucosa have been detected in patients with recurrent aphthous ulceration as well as in Behcet's syndrome. The same antigenic preparation will also stimulate blood lymphocytes from both groups of patients (Lehner, 1975). Lehner has also shown that the degree of lymphocyte reactivity, unlike the antibody levels, correlates with the clinical activity of the disease and this and other evidence suggests that cell mediated responses are of particular importance. Many patients have a family history of aphthous ulceration but there are no clues, as yet, to indicate why a minority develops the more widespread form of this disease.

ECZEMATOUS DISORDERS

Unless otherwise qualified the terms eczema and dermatitis are synonymous. They are used to describe a pruritic, erythematous, scaling eruption characterized histologically by an inflammatory reaction and intra-epidermal oedema (spongiosis).

Contact Eczema / Contact Dermatitis

The work of Frey and co-workers (Frey, 1974) showed that eczema could be produced by a cellular hypersensitivity reaction to a topically applied antigen. By implication it was also shown that, however good the epidermal barrier, many substances can be absorbed and act as haptens.

Clinical Aspects

The prevalence of contact dermatitis is difficult to assess since its occurrence is influenced by geographical and industrial factors as well as by prescribing habits. Some antigens e.g. mercury and sulphonamides have become less of a problem because of decreasing use. Others have been recognized as potent sensitizers and, like the hair dye paraphenylamine diamine, have been replaced by less harmful alternatives.

Geographical factors are important. In the United States allergy to *Rhus* (poison ivy and poison oak) is common but is a rarity in Europe where *Primula obonica* replaces it as the commonest plant antigen.

Chrome dermatitis is common amongst building workers but its frequency varies with the quantity of chrome in the local cement and, to a certain extent, the temperature and humidity of the environment. Nickel dermatitis is commoner in women than men. Sensitization is usually caused by direct contact of the metal against the skin but secondary patches of eczema are frequently found distant from the site of contact. Cobalt is an almost universal contaminant of nickel and this can explain the occasionally negative patch tests in an apparently nickel sensitive patient.

Rubber dermatitis is also common. The trouble lies not with the latex itself but the many stabilizers which are used in the vulcanization process and the relevant antigen varies from one kind of rubber to another.

Topical medicaments, such as neomycin, antihistamines and local anaesthetics are a major cause of contact eczema. The effect is enhanced when the skin on which they are applied is damaged. Manufacturers have recognized the problem of possible sensitivity to the components of otherwise harmless ointments e.g. lanolin base and the preservative parabens, and attempts have been made to restrict their use.

Removal of the antigen is the first step in management. When patch tests are indicated they must be applied when the dermatitis is quiescent. During the active phase, false positive reactions are frequent and true positives may cause a recrudescence. Avoidance of nickel objects by a patient with nickel dermatitis usually results in the rapid resolution of both primary and secondary lesions. At the industrial level the concept of "antigen replacement" has now become accepted. Continuous surveillance is necessary as the frequent introduction of new chemicals presents fresh hazards.

Factors Influencing the Production of Contact Eczema

Chemicals vary in their ability to produce sensitivity. Some, such as dinitrochlorobenzene (DNCB) produce sensitivity in all normal people. Others are so weak that there are only a handful of authenticated reports of sensitivity. Clinical experience has identified most of the potent sensitizers in our environment but the "maximization test" devised by Kligman and Wooding (1967) has proved useful in identifying potential antigens.

To be fully effective the antigen must be applied to the epidermal surface. Slightly damaging the epidermis by abrasion or freezing may enhance the effect but sensitization is much less likely to occur following intradermal or subcutaneous injection. Ingestion of the antigen may produce a flare-up in cutaneous sites already sensitized but rarely causes eczema in previously unexposed subjects. In experimental animals prefeeding has been used as a method of preventing topical sensitization.

The ability to mount a T-cell response decreases with age and is depressed in debilitated patients. In normal people individual variation in reactivity is greatest with the less potent antigens. Genetic factors are almost certainly important and family studies have shown an increase in the incidence of sensitivity in the close relatives of allergic patients. Experimental animals can be bred to produce either sensitivity or resistance to antigens. Metal sensitivity in guinea-pigs can be inherited as a simple Mendelian dominant.

The problems of contact eczema in atopic subjects is discussed below.

Methods of Investigation

Patch testing is the only method currently available for routine assessment of patients suspected of having contact eczema. Despite being subjective in interpretation patch tests can give reliable results. Some skill is required in assessing them and careful attention must be given to the concentration and vehicle for each test substance used since irritant reactions and sensitization by the patch test itself must be avoided. Cross-sensitivity between antigens is common and false conclusions may be drawn if this is not borne in mind.

The techniques and problems involved in patch testing are discussed by Cronin and Wilkinson (1973).

Medenica and Rostenberg (1971) distinguish histological differences between the reactions caused by DNCB as an irritant and as a sensitizer. The irritant reaction causes a cleft at the epidermal/dermal junction and cell necrosis with a dermal infiltrate of polymorphonuclear leucocytes. Spongiosis and secondary lysosomes appear only during regeneration. However, in the allergic reaction they are seen as the first change; without clefting or cell death and the dermal infiltrate consists mainly of lymphocytes and monocytes. The histological changes in established contact eczema often show a mixed and more chronic picture than is seen experimentally. Dvorak and Mihm (1972) have shown that when special fixation and staining methods are used, a substantial infiltrate of basophil leucocytes can be seen, following the initial perivascular accumulation of lymphocytes. Later, eosinophils also appear. These findings parallel the Jones-Mote reaction (cutaneous basophil hypersensitivity) in animals.

Although a number of methods exist for studying cell mediated responses *in vitro*, none has proved generally applicable to the analysis of contact dermatitis or drug hypersensitivity (Reeves and Trounce, 1971). The main difficulty relates to lack of information regarding the identity of the antigenic material formed *in vivo* after combination of the sensitizing chemical or hapten with host material. In such "hapten-carrier" systems (see Chapter 4) there is a strict requirement for the conjugated carrier material in the assay system.

Levis *et al.* (1975) have surmounted this problem in DNCB sensitivity by coupling the hapten to red cells or leucocytes to form a particulate complex. Their studies in man show a convincing correlation between cutaneous reactivity and the response of leucocytes in culture to the conjugated antigen. They also find that although lymphokine production is not detectable during a primary response to DNCB it is observed after rechallenge. Earlier, Delescluse and Turk (1970) showed that *in vitro* cytotoxicity could be generated by lymphocytes from DNFB-sensitized guinea-pigs in the presence of DNFB-conjugated red cells. There is no reason why a similar approach should not be used for many other sensitizing agents once a conveniently conjugated form of the hapten can be found.

Photoallergic Contact Eczema

Sometimes the action of light is necessary before contact eczema is produced. Light causes chemical change in certain compounds leading to formation of antigens which then cause contact eczema in the usual way. The chemical change can be induced *in vitro*, so it is more accurate to describe this condition as contact eczema to phototransformation products.

A decade ago a world wide epidemic was caused by the addition of salicylamide derivatives as antiseptics to toilet soaps. This example is now only of historical interest but similar photosensitivity has been noted to several currently-used antiseptic and antifungal agents such as fentichlor and buclosamide.

To detect photosensitivity and determine the activating wavelength of light the technique of photopatch testing has been developed (Osmundson, 1969). After application of a patch test for 48 hours in the usual way the area is irradiated with light of known wavelength and intensity. The reaction is compared with control areas which have been either patch tested but not irradiated or irradiated but not pretreated with a patch test.

Autosensitization

When severe eczema affects one area it is common for a diffuse but milder eczematous eruption to appear on other parts of the body. This may occur irrespective of the cause of the original eczema and has been called an absorption or autosensitization eruption. In some cases, the eruption may be due to absorption of a substance applied topically to which the patient has become sensitized but in most cases no external factor is evident.

Parish *et al.* (1965) detected antibodies capable of agglutinating particles coated with skin extracts in four out of eighty-one patients with eczema. The antibodies were detectable only when the disease was active and disappeared during remission. The serum from three of the patients also showed a cytotoxic effect when incubated with fresh skin. Thus, antibodies may have a role in "autosensitization" eczema.

Atopic Eczema / Atopic Dermatitis

Atopic disease is discussed more generally in Chapter 22. Although atopic eczema occurs much more commonly in patients who have a personal or family history of other "atopic" disorders there is very little evidence to suggest that an anaphylactic, IgE-mediated mechanism is responsible for its production.

It is a symmetrical eczematous disorder which most often presents before the age of twelve months. A frequent observation is that when a child has both atopic eczema and extrinsic asthma, the severity of the two conditions often shows an inverse relationship. The eczema can clear completely during a bad attack of asthma.

Ichthyosis vulgaris and keratosis pilaris (follicular keratosis) are common associations of atopic eczema and these patients may develop a specific kind of cataract. In atopic eczema, the existence of paradoxical vascular responses have been demonstrated by a number of different techniques. Their persistence in the microscopically normal skin of atopic eczema patients makes it possible that they have a primary role in this disease.

The histological changes are by no means suggestive of a reaginic mechanism and often it is difficult to distinguish them from those of contact eczema. The dermal blood vessels are dilated and there is oedema and a perivascular infiltrate which consists mostly of lymphocytes although mast cells and eosinophils may be numerous.

Various workers have found that delayed hypersensitivity responses to a number of antigens (e.g. PPD, mumps, trichophyton and candida) are depressed when compared with those of suitable control subjects, and an inability to become sensitized to DNCB has also been described. Some have found an impaired *in vitro* response to non-specific mitogens, such as phytohaemagglutinin (PHA), and decreased T-cell numbers. In the absence of a prospective study of "pre-atopic" patients it is difficult to know whether these changes are primary or secondary. It is possible that this apparent "anergy" or T-cell impairment might be a sequel to persistent antigenic stimulation within the skin although an atopic type of eczema is associated with several immunodeficiency disorders, e.g. the Wiskott-Aldrich syndrome and ataxia-telangiectasia, in which there is primary T-cell deficiency. There is also an increased incidence of other partial forms of immunodeficiency in "atopic" patients, notably indifferent IgA and IgG production and this too may have a role, related or unrelated to a T-cell defect, in the pathogenesis of atopic eczema.

The most striking immunological finding is the marked increase in serum and sweat IgE levels seen in this condition. The degree of elevation mirrors activity of the disease and the serum levels are usually much higher than those seen in extrinsic allergic asthma or allergic rhinitis. This may be a secondary phenomenon resulting from an inordinate antigen challenge via the skin. If so, it would help to explain the high IgE levels seen in bullous pemphigoid.

There is also a possible link between reaginic T-cell mechanisms, as suggested by the descriptions of the Jones-Mote reaction or cutaneous basophil hypersensitivity (Dvorak and Mihm, 1972).

DRUG ERUPTIONS

Adverse drug reactions are of several types. Toxic and side-effects are the commonest and are usually well-recognized for a particular drug. Idiosyncratic or hypersensitivity responses are more difficult to diagnose and to distinguish from each other. The former relate to individual variations in biochemical constitution; the latter are, by definition, those reactions where immunological mechanisms are responsible although proof of that fact may be difficult to obtain (Reeves and Trounce, 1971).

Reactions to aspirin, in the form of asthma or urticaria, are difficult to characterize. Some have proposed an immunological basis but the evidence is now overwhelmingly in favour of a biochemical idiosyncrasy. There is a striking lack of chemical specificity among the various substances, including aspirin, which may trigger an attack in an individual patient.

Lupus-like rashes and anti-nuclear antibodies (ANA's) may follow administration of a number of drugs, including hydrallazine, procaine amide and practolol. With hydrallazine there is evidence that patients who acetylate the drug at a slower rate are more prone to develop a lupus syndrome. Thus, although the end result may have an immunological basis the primary reason for this kind of drug reaction is probably biochemical.

As with contact eczema many of the causative drugs may function as haptens. They or their metabolites conjugate *in vivo* with host proteins to form a complete antigen which it may be impossible to characterize. Although any drug may cause a skin eruption some do this more often than others. Table 3 lists some of the more frequent culprits and the kinds of eruption seen. Usually only a small percentage of patients show hypersensitivity to a particular drug. An exception is patients with infectious mononucleosis who have been treated with ampicillin virtually 100% of whom develop a morbilliform rash. It is not clear whether this is immunologically determined, but rechallenge after recovery usually gives negative results.

The Investigation of Drug Hypersensitivity

This is still a most unrewarding exercise in most patients and clinical suspicion is, all too often, the safest and most accurate basis for diagnosis. Skin testing is

TABLE 3

Drug eruptions: clinical types and commoner causes

Eruption	Causes
Maculo-papular	Many drugs especially antibiotics Para-aminosalicyclic acid Gold Allopurinol
Urticarial	Antibiotics, especially penicillins Foreign sera Toxoids
Lichenoid	Gold Antimalarials Thiazide diuretics
Purpuric	
(a) non-thrombocytopenic	Carbromal
(b) thrombocytopenic	Sedormid[a] Novobiocin
Fixed drug eruption	Phenolphthalein Tetracycline
Exfoliative dermatitis	Gold and other heavy metals Barbiturates Sulphonamides
Toxic epidermal necrolysis	Sulphonamides Butazones Barbiturates

[a] No longer available as a therapeutic agent.

unwise as negative results may occur in the presence of systemic hypersensitivity and positive results can have serious consequences.

Many people have endeavoured to find an *in vitro* test suitable for general application to the diagnosis of drug hypersensitivity (Reeves and Trounce, 1971) but there is no clear answer to this problem as yet. A solution is unlikely to appear until more is known about the chemistry of hapten conjugation *in vivo* and the process of sensitization. Nevertheless, some laboratory methods have a limited application. Where a drug can be linked to red cells, passive haemagglutination can be used to detect specific antibody. A more sophisticated version of this, the red cell linked antigen antiglobulin reaction (RCLAAR) has been used to detect antibodies of different immunoglobulin classes, against penicillin, penicillamine and some other agents. Where a reaginic mechanism is thought to be responsible as in urticaria or anaphylaxis, the detection of drug specific IgE antibody alone can be of value. If the relevant drug can be linked to suitable inert particles then this antibody can be measured by the radioallergosorbent test (RAST).

The problem is far more difficult when T-cell responses are involved. The requirement for carrier as well as hapten specificity, already referred to on page 802, militates against attempts to create *in vitro* parallels. It is possible that the approach used by Levis *et al.* (1975), will be more generally applicable. The spontaneous conjugation of hapten to the surface proteins of lymphocytes may explain the surprisingly specific results obtained with *in vitro* lymphocyte stimulation in gold and nickel hypersensitivity.

In some drug eruptions it is possible that at least part of the pathology may be related to formation of skin-reactive antibodies. Van Joost (1974) has demonstrated the presence of circulating antibodies reactive with basal cells of the epidermis in seven out of 42 patients with drug eruptions. He postulates that some drugs may complex with epidermal cells to form potent antigens. If this is so it gives a further clue to the location of important carrier molecules *in vivo*.

URTICARIA AND ANGIO-OEDEMA

The formation of urticarial weals is due to localized vasodilatation, increased capillary permeability and perivascular oedema. This may be brought about by irritant or pharmacological factors acting directly on blood vessels or via the release of mediators from cutaneous mast cells. In other instances the release of inflammatory mediators from mast cells is determined by immunological means. This may occur either as part of a reaginic response when antigen combines with specific IgE antibody on the mediator cell surface, or following the activation of complement with the production of active fragments i.e. C3a, C5a and C567 (see Chapter 7) which cause mast cell mediator release independently of IgE. Complement activation is triggered in both membrane-reactive and immune complex mechanisms (see Chapters 1 and 10) although urticaria is most often associated with the latter mechanism and has long been recognized as a feature of serum sickness. Angio-oedema occurs where there is subcutaneous extension of the same process and this is usually confined to the eyelids, lips and tongue.

A large number of different clinical types of urticaria have been described by dermatologists and allergists, often based on dubious distinguishing criteria. Nevertheless, there are differences, and the relatively simple classification used here is based on the extensive work of Champion and his colleagues (Table 4). The most striking feature is the large majority of patients (79%) in whom no aetiological factor could be identified.

TABLE 4
Clinical types of urticaria and angio-oedema

Clinical types	Percentages of cases seen
Allergic urticaria	3·1
Physical urticaria	17·0
Pregnancy urticaria	0·5
Hereditary angio-oedema	0·4
Urticaria and/or angio-oedema of unknown aetiology	79·1

Adapted from Champion *et al.*, 1969.

Allergic Causes

These include inhaled antigens e.g. pollens, foods and drugs. Asprin, which may produce its effect by pharmacological means, has been found to exacerbate 21% of cases of urticaria and it is unlikely that it is functioning as an antigen in this context.

Insect bites often cause urticaria and two separate mechanisms are often involved. The injected material may contain vasoactive substances, and a subsequent allergic response may considerably prolong the reaction giving the typical picture of "papular urticaria".

Physical Urticaria

This includes: (i) "cholinergic" urticaria, where exertion and heat provoke attacks, (ii) dermographic and pressure urticaria, (iii) solar urticaria and (iv) cold urticaria. The last of these may occur in association with immunological disturbances such as cryoglobulinaemia, systemic lupus, paroxysmal cold haemoglobulinaemia and the presence of cold agglutinins.

Urticaria which recurs in pregnancy is rare and little is known about the underlying mechanisms. In some forms of urticaria, especially the physical varieties, the lesions clear within minutes. In others—often those associated with deeper weals, individual lesions may last for days. In most cases the histological changes are simply those of oedema although accumulations of eosinophils are commonly seen some hours after the onset of a lesion. Older lesions may stain and become purpuric and the histological picture may then show striking cellular infiltration as well as other changes of leucocytoclastic vasculitis. In such cases direct immunofluorescence usually shows the presence of complement, and often antibody, in the walls of the dermal blood vessels.

Hereditary Angio-oedema

Sir William Osler established the hereditary form of angio-oedema as a distinct entity in 1888. It is transmitted as an autosomal dominant and is associated with a deficiency in the C1 esterase inhibitor (see Chapter 7). Attacks usually start in childhood and subsequently occur at irregular intervals. The tissue swellings may be large and firm and are not usually associated with urticaria. They do not itch but may be painful. The gut or respiratory tract may be involved in an attack and this can occur in the absence of cutaneous involvement. Abdominal pain or intestinal obstruction may suggest a surgical emergency although the radiological changes are typical of localized oedema. When oedema occurs in the larynx or pharynx there is a grave risk of respiratory obstruction.

Attacks can be controlled by the prompt administration of fresh plasma, and prophylaxis with ε-aminocaproic acid or its analogue, tranexamic acid, significantly reduce their incidence. These agents are plasmin inhibitors and may also have effects on other enzyme systems which trigger activation of C1.

Other Associations of Urticaria

Patients with atopic disease are particularly prone to develop urticarias, usually of an allergic nature. Other diseases which are less commonly associated include systemic lupus, juvenile rheumatoid arthritis, inherited amyloidosis, myelo-proliferative and lympho-proliferative disorders and other kinds of neoplasia (Warin and Champion, 1974). In several of these conditions there is good evidence of the presence of circulating antigen–antibody complexes and these may well be responsible for the production of intermittent urticarial lesions.

Investigation

Specific tests can be used to identify physical urticaria and assay of the C1 esterase inhibitor, particularly if there is associated angio-oedema, is extremely important in diagnosis of the hereditary form. Routine skin testing for allergy is of little help although an unexpected cause may be uncovered in an occasional case. Where the lesions are more chronic, biopsy and immunofluorescent examination will detect the small minority of cases that have an underlying vasculitis.

The chief enigma is the 79% or so of cases in which no definitive cause can be identified. Urticaria and angio-oedema will continue to be clinical prolems until more light is shed on this silent majority.

CUTANEOUS VASCULITIS

Inflammation developing in or around cutaneous vessels occurs in a wide variety of conditions. Classification is almost impossible at the clinical level but attempts have been made on the basis of the size of vessel involved and the nature of the cellular infiltrate (Ryan and Wilkinson, 1972). Table 5 includes some of the more important types listed according to infiltrate alone.

In the first group an intense infiltrate is seen and nuclear debris or "dust" is evident in the acute stages. This has given rise to the term *leucocytoclastic vasculitis* which is often used as a synonym for "allergic" or necrotizing vasculitis when the disease is confined to the skin. An unusual variant is *erythema elevatum diutinum* in which the disease is remarkably localized and persistent, and histologically there is marked capillary proliferation in addition to a leucocytoclastic picture. An association with polyarthritis has been described.

The Arthus Phenomenon and Serum Sickness

The Arthus phenomenon provides a striking experimental parallel to many clinical forms of vasculitis. After the local injection of soluble antigen (e.g.

TABLE 5

Types of cutaneous vasculitis

POLYMORPHONUCLEAR INFILTRATE	
	"Allergic vasculitis"
	Erythema elevatum diutinum
	Henoch-Schonlein purpura (anaphylactoid purpura)
	Rheumatoid vasculitis
	Polyarteritis nodosa and variants e.g. hypersensitivity angiitis
	Superficial migratory thrombophlebitis (Behcet's syndrome)
LYMPHOCYTIC INFILTRATE	
	Erythema nodosum
	Paraproteinaemias
	Some drug eruptions
	Lupus erythematosus
	Perniosis (chilblains)
GRANULOMATOUS INFILTRATE	
	Wegener's granulomatosis
	Giant cell arteritis
	Erythema induratum (Bazin's disease)

horse serum) into an animal that has been previously immunized a reaction develops which usually culminates in extensive emigration of neutrophils from vessels, gross oedema and segmental necrosis of venules and arterioles. Later lymphocytes, macrophages and eosinophils may predominate. Immunofluorescent techniques demonstrate the formation of antigen–antibody complexes within the walls of the blood vessels, resulting in complement fixation and the generation of chemotactic factors for the various kinds of infiltrating cell. A necrotizing arteritis also develops in experimental serum sickness coincident with the formation of antigen–antibody complexes within the circulation.

Immunological Findings

Clinical studies have demonstrated the presence of immunoglobulin, complement and various kinds of antigenic material within and around the walls of blood vessels of patients with cutaneous vasculitis (Fig. 4). Immunoglobulin deposition is more commonly found in lesions containing a mononuclear

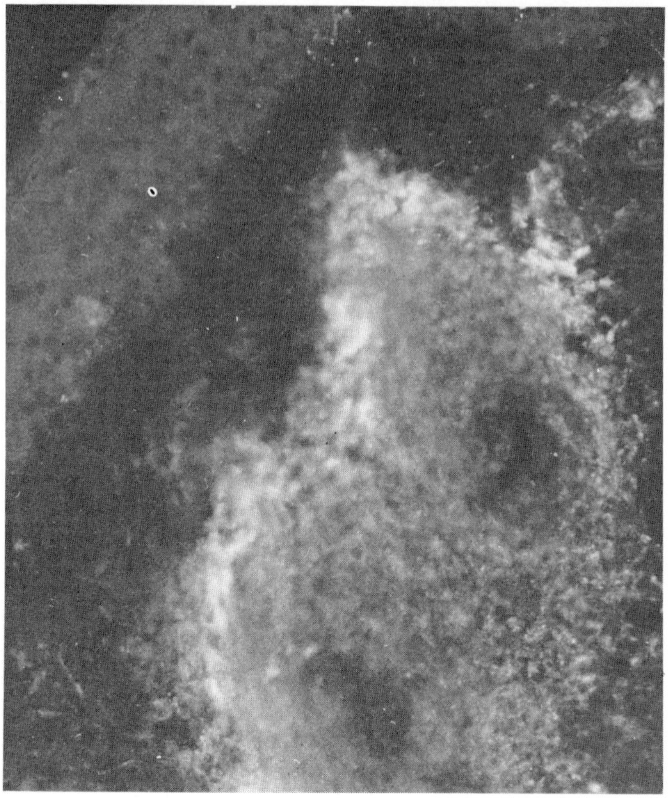

Fig. 4. Perivascular deposition of complement (Clq) in the dermis of a patient with cutaneous vasculitis (direct immunofluorescence).

cell infiltrate although C3 occurs more frequently in the neutrophil vasculitis group (Parish, 1971). This discrepancy may reflect different stages in the natural history of a very closely related group of disorders. More recently it has become clear that antibody and complement are often present in the walls of blood vessels contained within the areas of clinically normal skin of patients with leucocytoclastic vasculitis. Although these blood vessels do not show cellular infiltrate, this can be readily precipitated by the intradermal injection of histamine (Braverman and Yen, 1975). Several workers have stressed that once a lesion has developed both antibody and complement many disappear within 24–48 hours. This disappearance is almost certainly due to the ingestion and digestion of complexed material by the infiltrating cells. Thus a biopsy for immunofluorescent examination should always be taken from clinically normal skin or from a recently developed lesion. A number of factors affect the deposition and biological behaviour of antigen–antibody complexes *in vivo* (Cochrane, 1971) and it is not yet clear what the important variables are in patients with cutaneous vasculitis.

So far, antigenic material derived from streptococci, staphylococci, *M. tuberculosis* and *Candida* has been demonstrated in vasculitis lesions. Hepatitis-associated antigen has been detected in polyarteritis nodosa, and this and a number of other antigens have been detected together with antibody and complement in some forms of glomerulonephritis (Chapter 17).

Cryoglobulins of the mixed variety are often detectable when there are plentiful circulating complexes. In addition there are now several more sensitive techniques for the detection of soluble circulating complexes e.g. anti-complementary activity and assays involving C1q binding, macrophage uptake and the inhibition of K-cell killing. None of these is entirely specific but they usually give positive results in cutaneous vasculitis. In a recent study Andrews *et al.* (1975) detected circulating complexes in both neutrophilic and lymphocytic forms of cutaneous vasculitis. There was poor correlation between the degree of skin deposition and the positivity of a battery of tests for circulating complexes. Hypocomplementaemia is unusual unless the vasculitis is associated with systemic lupus or with severe forms of rheumatoid arthritis.

Henoch-Schonlein Purpura (Anaphylactoid Purpura)

The presence of a rash which may contain erythematous, urticarial and purpuric elements in association with joint, gut and sometimes renal involvement merits separate consideration. It predominantly affects children but can occur at any age and the histological changes in the skin are those of a leucocytoclastic vasculitis. Antibody and complement have been detected in the lesions in some cases and in one patient, who also had a deficiency of the second component of complement, *Mycoplasma* was detected in the serum (Sussman *et al.*, 1973).

Polyarteritis Nodosa

This is discussed in detail in Chapter 11.

Erythema Nodosum

The development of painful erythematous nodules on the legs which fade to leave a flat bruise-like lesion is a well-recognized complication of a number of disorders, many of them infective in origin. Often this picture develops 7–14 days after an upper respiratory tract infection. Arthralgia occurs in more than 50% of cases.

The infiltrate is predominantly lymphocytic and the degree of vascular damage is much less. If examined initially, neutrophils predominate and antibody has been detected in the lesions. *Erythema nodosum leprosum* is a more severe variety seen in lepromatous leprosy in which the lesions may ulcerate and there are other manifestations of a serum sickness-like disorder. This condition has every appearance of a pure immune complex reaction. The predominant cell is polymorphonuclear and antibody and complement can be readily demonstrated in the lesions. This is in keeping with the fact that lepromatous (in contrast to tuberculoid) leprosy is characterized by considerable depression of cell mediated immunological responses.

Erythema Induratum

This is another nodular form of vasculitis predominantly affecting the lower legs, but which runs a more chronic course and may ulcerate. Histologically there is intense vascular inflammation with frequent granulomata. The variant described by Bazin responds well to anti-tuberculous therapy whereas in the milder Whitfield variety, which is associated with venous stasis, there are few clues regarding the presence or role of an antigenic stimulus.

Pyoderma Gangrenosum

This condition is not usually classified as a form of vasculitis but circumstantial evidence suggests that it is. The lesions may complicate active ulcerative colitis or rheumatoid arthritis and tend to mirror the activity of the primary disease. In the former they may follow on the erythema nodosum-like lesions and are dramatically improved by colectomy. Although there have been few immunological studies so far, the clinical and histological features suggest that local involvement of immune complexes or of bacterial endotoxin may be the trigger for production of these lesions. The pathological process closely resembles the Schwartzman reaction, where it is known that endotoxin has a direct effect on complement, platelets and neutrophils without necessarily involving antibody in the process.

SYSTEMIC IMMUNOLOGICAL DISEASE AND THE SKIN

Lupus Erythematosus

Although about 80% of cases of systemic lupus (SLE) have a rash at some stage, cutaneous involvement is often clinically undetectable and when it is apparent it tends to show a more varied pattern than that seen in the discoid form (DLE). There is still some dispute regarding the exact relationship between these two conditions. It looks as if only 5% or less of patients with DLE eventually develop the systemic form despite the fact that they often have serological abnormalities (Rowell, 1972).

Immunofluorescent examination of the skin has proved useful in distinguishing the two conditions and also in establishing a diagnosis of DLE when other causes of lymphocyte infiltration of the skin have to be considered e.g. Jessner's lymphocytic infiltration and polymorphic light eruption.

Direct Immunofluorescence

Coarse granular deposits of immunoglobulin (IgG, and often IgA and IgM in addition) as well as complement are present along the epidermal/dermal junction in the lesions of both DLE and SLE and in the clinically uninvolved but light exposed skin of patients with SLE (Fig. 3). The deposits are on the dermal side of the basal lamina (Wolff-Schreiner and Wolff, 1974) in contrast with the linear staining seen at and immediately above the basal lamina in bullous pemphigoid. Again in contrast to pemphigoid, indirect immunofluorescence is negative apart from the frequent presence of anti-nuclear antibody. Occasionally, a less coarse and more continuous "stippled" pattern is seen, and this is more common in patients who have been treated with corticosteroids although such treatment can cause the pattern to regress completely. Conditions in which basement membrane zone staining is seen on direct immunofluorescence are listed in Table 2. Of these, only pemphigoid gives a positive result in the indirect test. Jessner's lymphocytic infiltration and polymorphic light eruption both give negative results on direct immunofluorescence.

The almost invariable presence of anti-nuclear antibody (ANA) in the serum of untreated patients with SLE and the existence of abnormal levels of DNA binding by SLE sera, as well as the presence of circulating complexes, suggest that the coarse granular material deposited at the epidermal/dermal junction should contain DNA/anti-DNA complexes. However, elution studies in both discoid and systemic LE have not always confirmed this (Van Joost, 1973) and the fact that a considerable amount of virus material has been eluted from the glomeruli of NZB/W mice with an advanced disease which resembles SLE suggests that other antigen–antibody systems may be important. Certainly patients with SLE have elevated levels of antibody against a wide variety of microorganisms, including many viruses, and it is possible that any complexed antibody in the circulation may non-specifically deposit in the skin particularly in areas that are light exposed. SLE, its animal model, and their likely pathogenesis are discussed more fully in Chapter 11.

Serum Findings

The LE cell test has now outlived its usefulness in favour of detection of anti-nuclear antibody (ANA) by indirect immunofluorescence and the measurement of DNA binding by modifications of the Farr technique. Fluctuations in the level of DNA binding and of serum complement give some indication of changes in activity of the condition in individual patients.

Systemic Sclerosis

In systemic sclerosis (systemic scleroderma) the skin histology is identical with that found in morphoea (localized scleroderma) although the two conditions are clinically distinct. Immunological abnormalities have only rarely been reported in adult morphoea, although in the childhood linear form, ANA is present in about 20% of cases and antibody to native DNA also. In systemic sclerosis ANA is present in 60–80% of cases and the pattern of staining is usually speckled or nucleolar, unlike the diffuse homogeneous or peripheral ring patterns characteristic of systemic lupus. DNA-binding levels are normal but it is of particular interest that Alarcon-Segovia *et al.* (1975) have shown that these patients have high titre anti-RNA antibodies.

Deposits of immunoglobulin and complement are not detectable in the skin unless a telangiectatic area is studied when a "false positive" but mild degree of staining may be seen.

Several variants of systemic sclerosis have been described and two will be mentioned here.

Thibierge-Wissenbach (CRST) Syndrome

Calcinosis, Raynaud's phenomenon, Sclerodactyly and Telangiectasia are all manifestations of systemic sclerosis but it has been suggested that patients with this particular combination of features show a more benign course. Be that as it may, it is unlikely that this group is immunologically distinct.

Mixed Connective Tissue Disease

Under this heading, Sharp *et al.* (1972) described a group of patients whose predominant features were: arthralgia, swelling of the hands, Raynaud's phenomenon, lymphadenopathy, myositis and abnormal oesophageal motility. All the patients had high titre speckled ANA reacting with an extractable nuclear antigen (ENA) of RNA type. In contrast to most cases of systemic sclerosis they show a good response to corticosteroids.

While the nature of the primary disorder remains obscure there is little profit in detailed clinical subdivision. The finding of virus particles on electron microscopy (EM) and evidence that some form of RNA may function as an antigen suggests that systemic sclerosis and its variants may turn out to have as rich an immunopathology as systemic lupus.

Dermatomyositis

Although both polymyositis and dermatomyositis have a positive association with neoplastic disease, not all cases develop overt malignancy. Some studies have demonstrated immunological responses against striated muscle and others against tumour extracts. Several studies have found virus-like particles on EM of affected tissues. It remains to be seen whether these represent the cause or an effect of the disease and what their exact identity may be.

Immunoglobulin is not detected in the skin lesions unless an area of telangiectasia is biopsied. Serological findings are usually non-specific.

Rheumatoid Arthritis

Patients with rheumatoid bands and nodules are usually positive for rheumatoid factors and ANA. Their presence may precede the development of arthritis by several years. Likewise, digital necrosis—as evidenced by pin-point infarcts in the finger tips and around the nails—is also associated with more active disease. Table 6 lists the various cutaneous manifestations. Direct immunofluorescence does not reveal immunoglobulin or complement at the epidermal/dermal junction and this finding can be of help in distinguishing this condition from systemic lupus. Arteritic lesions may appear as purpuric or necrotic areas which may break down and ulcerate. Leg ulcers are usually gravitational or arteritic and are more commonly found in Felty's syndrome of arthritis, splenomegaly, lymphadenopathy and leucopenia.

TABLE 6
Cutaneous manifestations of rheumatoid arthritis

Subcutaneous nodules
Subcutaneous linear bands
Vasculitic changes:
digital necrosis
arteritic lesions
leg ulcers
Livedo reticularis
Maculo-papular eruption
Pyoderma gangrenosum

A characteristic maculo-papular eruption is seen in 25% of children with Still's disease but only rarely in adult rheumatoid. Pyoderma gangrenosum (page 814) occurs less commonly than in ulcerative colitis.

Hypocomplementaemia is a rare finding in rheumatoid arthritis but low complement levels are commonly found in the synovial fluid of involved joints together with immune complexes and large numbers of polymorphonuclear leucocytes. Although not all the skin changes may be explained on the basis of immune complex damage it is very likely that this is the cause when vasculitic features or pyoderma gangrenosum supervene.

CUTANEOUS INFECTION

The intact skin presents an efficient barrier to pathogenic organisms but once a breach in the surface has occurred the mechanisms of defence are chiefly those of the immunological system. Usually a percutaneous infection remains localized and is short-lived unless (i) a particularly virulent organism is involved e.g. *Streptococcus pyogenes* or *Clostridium tetani*, (ii) a large area of skin is affected e.g. patients with burns or various dermatoses e.g. extensive atopic eczema or (iii) there is an immunological or nutritional defect e.g. chronic mucocutaneous candidiasis or Norwegian scabies. Much of our present knowledge regarding the delicate balance between cutaneous defence on the one hand, and microorganisms present in or on the skin on the other, is based on studies of bacterial and fungal infection. Viruses may be much more successful in surviving inoculation through the skin and hepatitis B (especially via tattooing), herpes simplex, smallpox and rabies are well-defined examples. The cutaneous manifestations of immunodeficiency states, especially those involving defects of cell mediated immunity, may not always have the overt appearance of clinical infection. Various examples have been described where cutaneous ulceration or hypertrophic lesions, often virus-induced, are prominent. Such a possibility should be considered in the presence of atypical persistent or recurrent skin lesions. Infectious and parasitic diseases are covered in Chapter 13 but a few selected infections of the skin are discussed here.

Leprosy

Lepromatous and tuberculoid leprosy represent the two extremes of immunological response to the lepra bacillus (Turk and Bryceson, 1971).

The lesions of lepromatous leprosy contain innumerable bacilli, most of them surviving within histiocytes. Lymphocytes are virtually absent and the lepromin test is negative. In tuberculoid leprosy bacilli are scanty and cell mediated immunity is intact, with an intense lymphocytic reaction and a positive lepromin test. Between these two extremes lie a large number of patients with borderline and indeterminate leprosy in whom cell mediated immunity is present but not as strongly as in tuberculoid leprosy. In most of these patients the lepromin test is positive but it is not a diagnostic test, for 90% of normal Mantoux positive people also show a positive reaction to lepromin.

Many patients with lepromatous leprosy have a positive Mantoux and thus the impaired cell mediated response appears to be specific for the lepra bacillus. Humoral antibody production in these patients is high despite the lack of a T-cell response, whereas in tuberculoid leprosy it is low. Treatment may cause a patient with lepromatous leprosy to move towards the tuberculoid end of the spectrum and produce a "reversal reaction" with infiltration of the lesions by lymphocytes. Clinically, the patient may develop a severe peripheral neuritis and erythema nodosum leprosum.

Tuberculosis

In someone without acquired immunity to tuberculosis the inoculation of bacilli into the skin produces a shallow ulcer known as a tuberculous chancre. As immunity develops the ulcer heals but may be followed by an area of lupus vulgaris. This chronic scaling lesion is characteristic of secondary spread in a person with high immunity and is often ignored for many years. If tubercle bacilli are inoculated directly into the skin of a person who already has a high level of immunity, a slowly-growing verrucous lesion known as "warty tuberculosis" occurs.

Syphilis

Although the primary lesion has few immunological connotations it does not develop again upon reinfection unless adequate treatment has been given at the earliest stage of the initial attack.

The clinical features of secondary syphilis are very suggestive of a systemic immunological disturbance e.g. rash, fever, arthralgia, lymphadenopathy, splenomegaly and proteinuria. Histologically the skin may show intense perivascular infiltration with lymphocytes and plasma cells, and immunoglobulins and complement have been detected in the kidneys.

Tertiary syphilis has an abundance of immunological features—not least the various auto-antibodies which may co-exist (e.g. rheumatoid factor) with the specific response to *Treponema pallidum*. The granulomatous involvement of the skin may resemble tuberculosis quite closely although the degree of vascular involvement is usually much greater in syphilis. It is difficult to demonstrate the presence of the treponeme in the tertiary lesions and the auto-immune response may have a role in determining their chronicity.

Fungal Infections

Dermatophytes

Little is known about the factors which limit the spread of superficial fungal infections. There is strong circumstantial evidence that resistance occurs for it is rare to find second infections with *T. verrucosum* (cattle ringworm) or in children with tinea capitis. No naturally-occurring antibody directed solely against dermatophytes has been detected but serum is fungistatic as are certain fatty acids derived from sebum. Anthropophilic fungi excite very little reaction in the skin and it is probable that no form of lasting resistance develops against them.

The trichophyton skin test is not useful diagnostically although claims have been made that the severity and frequency of positive reactions is higher in infected patients.

Chronic Mucocutaneous Candidiasis

Candida albicans is not pathogenic under normal circumstances and is present in the gut of 75% of normal adults. Chronic candida infection occurs in various kinds of immunodeficiency disorder—notably those associated with abnormalities of cellular immunity. In some instances the defect may be a partial one. The different patterns of immunological reactivity have been classified by Valdimarsson *et al.* (1973). Some cases may respond well to the administration of iron.

Pityriasis Versicolor

This condition is caused by a yeast-like organism and is more common in hot climates and in patients on corticosteroids.

Virus Infections

Some viruses (e.g. those of the herpes group) persist indefinitely within the body after a primary infection and may give rise to subsequent lesions when certain factors encourage their reappearance.

Herpes Simplex

Most people experience mild or subclinical infection in early life but a minority continue to get recurrent local lesions which usually occur on the lips and face. Attacks may be triggered by sunlight, menstruation, minor respiratory tract infections, pneumococcal pneumonia, meningococcal infection and malaria. Partial defects in cell mediated responses have been described in a minority of such patients. Patients with atopic dermatitis, pemphigus and some other skin disorders may show a particularly severe reaction to a primary infection with herpes simplex in the form of Kaposi's varicelliform eruption. Widespread vesicles occur and the condition can be fatal. A similar situation may follow smallpox vaccination in such patients.

Herpes Zoster

Shingles almost always occurs in patients who have had chicken-pox in the past. The virus persists in the posterior root ganglia and it is probably only when the circulating antibody level has fallen with time that the virus lesions reappear in a segmental distribution. There is also a high incidence of clinical zoster infections in association with various kinds of lymphoma and leukaemia, and both simplex and zoster infections are a hazard for patients on immuno-suppressive regimes.

Molluscum Contagiosum

This is caused by a pox virus and is probably more common in atopic subjects. It is more severe in patients on immunosuppressive drugs.

Pityriasis Rosea

The sequence of a "herald patch" followed by a widespread secondary eruption and the rarity of further attacks suggest an infective origin with an immunological response. A viral aetiology has yet to be proved.

Skin Disease due to Arthropods

Stings

The immediate pain of a bee or wasp sting is due to the release of histamine, kinins and other pharmacologically active substances. A few people, probably less than one per cent, react to antigens in the venom and produce a more severe immediate IgE-mediated reaction which in rare circumstances may result in anaphylactic shock. There is usually, but not always, adequate warning of impending trouble in the form of increasingly severe local reactions.

Bites

Bites from insects give rise to the eruption known as papular urticaria. The bite itself is often painless but irritation followed by a weal occurs within a few minutes. A delayed hypersensitivity reaction produces a more chronic irritating papule two days later.

It has been shown experimentally that although a reaction does not follow the first bite by a particular insect, the host becomes sensitized to antigens in the saliva. The degree of sensitivity shows considerable variation between individuals. After very frequent exposure tolerance may develop with the loss of both types of reaction.

Scabies

During the first month of infestation the mite, which burrows at the base of the horny layer, does not produce a clinical or histological reaction. Thereafter pruritus develops with increasing severity and a careful examination of the burrow shows an inflammatory papule at the point where the mite was twenty-four hours previously. Histologically there is a polymorphonuclear response in the early stages but later the infiltrate is more lymphocytic. Second infestations are rarely seen because itching is almost immediate and the parasite is quickly removed. Patients who have had scabies in the past demonstrate an immediate weal and flare reaction to injections of mite extracts and their serum gives a positive Prausnitz-Kustner reaction. This immunological response and the itching which results from it are crucial factors in limiting spread of the mite. Where either is absent an overwhelming infestation, known as Norwegian scabies, may occur.

NEOPLASIA AND THE SKIN

Warts

These common and benign epidermal tumours have several features which suggest that immunological responses play a part in their restriction and eventual elimination. They are caused by infection with a virus of the papova group which gets into the nuclei of the epidermal cells following inoculation into the skin. Hyperplasia of all the epidermal layers is seen in addition to marked hyperkeratosis. Genital (or accuminate) warts show different histological features from common or plantar warts and may be associated with infection with an antigenically distinct strain of virus which is thought to be transmitted by sexual contact.

Circulating antibodies (IgG and IgM) are detectable against wart virus in most cases and are most readily detectable when the warts are disappearing. In an animal model Allison (1966) showed that circulating antibody prevented the formation of new tumours but did not cause established tumours to regress. Warts often undergo spontaneous remission and cell mediated responses seem to be more effective in eliminating them. Greenberg *et al.* (1973) were able to clear warts by painting them with dinitrochlorobenzene when the patients had previously been systemically sensitized to this substance.

Immunological defects can be associated with generalized and resistant warts and this is most often seen in patients who are on immunosuppressive regimes or in patients with chronic leukaemia or lymphoma.

Pre-malignant Conditions

Mycosis Fungoides

In its earliest stage this may appear as a patchy eczema or one of the more specific pre-mycotic lesions e.g. parapsoriasis or poikiloderma. The eczematous patches are often quite dark in colour, may itch intensely and tend to enlarge gradually over a period of years. Histologically the skin is infiltrated with a mixed population of cells, lymphocytes, histiocytes and reticulum cells predominating. Immature large "mycosis cells" containing indented nuclei are often seen. These show some similarities with the Sézary cell (see below) and like them, probably belong to the T-cell population.

Later on tumours develop in previously infiltrated areas. Although a few patients eventually develop leukaemia or a lymphoma, other organs are usually not involved. Many patients die of causes other than their skin disease.

No striking immunological abnormalities have been detected thus far. Immunoglobulin levels and antibody formation are grossly normal although high IgE levels have been recorded. DNCB reactivity has been shown to be intact.

Local Malignancy

Squamous Cell Carcinoma

Some tumours have been described at the site of previous herpes simplex infections and there is evidence that ultraviolet light can transform the infectious form of the herpes simplex virus—HSV type I—into the oncogenic HSV type II. The latter type has also been linked to cervical carcinoma.

Carcinoma of the skin is one of the commonest tumours seen in immunosuppressed transplant recipients and 90% of affected patients develop clinical or serological evidence of herpes virus infection. Squamous-cell carcinoma is also an occasional complication of chronic granulomas, such as syphilis, lupus vulgaris and leprosy and can also be a sequel to various forms of chronic ulceration, infection and scarring.

Basal-cell Carcinoma

Although this tumour ulcerates early, it only very rarely metastasizes—unlike the squamous lesion. Both tumours show an inflammatory reaction which is often lymphocytic in type.

Malignant Melanoma

This tumour may develop *de novo* in normal skin, from a pigmented naevus or mole, or from either of two pre-malignant pigmented lesions, the melanotic (or Hutchinson's) freckle or pre-cancerous melanosis.

A degree of lymphocytic reaction is seen in both pre-malignant forms and is also evident in established malignant melanoma. Specific immunological reactivity can be demonstrated in most cases, either as antibody or sensitized lymphocytes or both, although the exact significance of these responses in terms of the natural history of the tumour is still unclear.

Occasionally a pigmented naevus develops a halo of depigmentation and undergoes spontaneous resolution. Antibody directed against the cytoplasm of malignant melanoma cells has been demonstrated in the sera of such cases. It is not found in the sera of patients with other pigmentary disturbances, apart from malignant melanoma itself. Thus, a "halo naevus" may represent the acute rejection of a naevus which has just undergone malignant change.

Malignant melanoma is a very unpredictable tumour and spontaneous regression occurs in a small minority of cases. In many instances the tumour activity fluctuates without any very obvious clinical reason and in view of this it is of paramount importance that any attempts at therapeutic modification of the disease be conducted in a controlled manner with randomized allocation of patients to control and test groups. There are now many reports of the effects of immunotherapeutic regimes on the course of this disease and although individual or uncontrolled reports may suggest that considerable benefit can be achieved there is still a shortage of valuable information on this point.

By analogy with immunotherapy in other conditions (see Chapters 28 and 31) and from some evidence based on treating malignant melanoma itself, it looks as if contact immunotherapy (in which irradiated tumour cells are mixed with BCG) may give the best results. This can produce untoward effects and more information is needed before the optimum dose and form of administration can be determined. Several trials in progress may help in answering these questions.

Immunotherapy is only likely to be of value once the primary tumour has been removed and the patient made putatively "tumour-free". In cases with recurrent or widespread tumour the chemotherapeutic agent dacarbazine (DTIC) may help to control the disease when further surgical intervention is inappropriate.

Systemic Malignancy

Acanthosis Nigricans

There is almost always an underlying adenocarcinoma or lymphoma although the skin changes can be present for as long as five years before the internal tumour is diagnosed. The histology does not suggest an immunological process but little has been done to investigate this possibility.

Sézary Syndrome

This condition is characterized by the development of a pruritic erythoderma in association with infiltration of the dermis by atypical mononuclear cells. Lymphadenopathy is often present and the patients usually develop leukaemia, lymphoma or other malignancy within a short period of time.

The infiltrating cells are large and have PAS positive vacuoles within their cytoplasm. Similar cells are also found in blood and lymphoid tissue. These cells have been shown to form rosettes with sheep red blood cells and to lack surface immunoglobulin, and are thus thought to belong to the T-cell lineage. Although it is not clear why these cells should preferentially localise in the dermis it has been shown that intensive leucaphoresis can produce a dramatic reduction in the degree of infiltration (Edelson *et al.*, 1974).

MISCELLANEOUS DISORDERS

Lichen Planus

The characteristic papules develop insidiously in middle life and clear spontaneously within a few months. Itching is a common feature and lesions may develop following skin trauma (Koebner phenomenon). Histologically there is intense infiltration of the dermis with lymphocytes and a few histiocytes, which form in a narrow band beneath the epidermis. The basal layer shows necrotic change and the degenerating epidermal cells give rise to the characteristic hyaline or colloid bodies which tend to lie in clusters just beneath the epidermis together with pigment-containing macrophages. Occasionally bullous lesions develop in which the infiltrate has become separated from the epidermis.

No definitive cause has been established although there is evidence to incriminate viruses and drugs in the pathogenetic process. There is now an impressive list of drugs which can produce a lichen planus-like eruption, including gold, anti-malarials and thiazide diuretics, and some cases have developed after exposure to colour developer containing substituted para-phenylene diamines. Patch tests are usually positive in these latter cases and although the initial reaction is usually eczematous, it can progress to a lichenoid pattern. Although Van Joost (1974) has detected antibodies reacting with the basal cells in various forms of drug reaction he did not find this in the three cases of lichenoid eruptions included in his series. Thus, circumstantially, the available evidence is in favour of a cell mediated mechanism of basal cell damage. Direct contact between the infiltrating cells and the damaged basal cells is not necessary in view of the variety of inflammatory and cytotoxic mediators that T-lymphocytes release when they become activated.

Direct immunofluorescent examination of lichen planus lesions usually gives positive results for IgM and fibrinogen, in, or adjacent to, the colloid bodies. Occasionally there are patches of linear deposition of these components at the basement membrane close to the lesions. The deposition of IgG, IgA, C3 and C4 has also been observed and although these components are less commonly found they are also mostly localized to the sub-epidermal bodies (Fig. 5). Uninvolved skin is usually negative (see Table 2). Neither the presence of colloid bodies nor their staining with reagents for immunoglobulin and fibrinogen is specific for lichen planus (Abell *et al.*, 1975) and similar findings can be seen in discoid lupus, eczema and various other dermatoses. Nevertheless the immunofluorescent findings in conjunction with conventional histology are usually sufficient for diagnostic purposes. Several workers have been impressed by the lack of correlation between the numbers of colloid bodies detected on light microscopy and the much greater numbers of fluorescent sub-epidermal bodies seen when the tissue is examined by specific immunofluorescence. It may be that the eosin and PAS negative bodies represent a less mature stage in the development of classical colloid bodies but that these are still able to bind and localize antibody and fibrinogen.

Although immunological factors undoubtedly have a role in the natural history of lichen planus it is unlikely that we shall appreciate their exact significance until the relevant antigens are identified. This in turn will allow analysis of the cell mediated immunological response by *in vitro* methods.

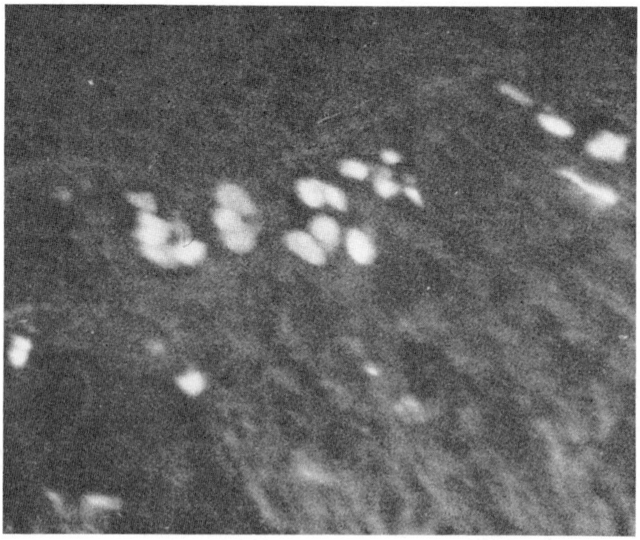

Fig. 5. Fluorescing sub-epidermal "colloid" bodies in lichen planus (direct immunofluorescence for IgA).

Further study of the antigen-specificity of the bound antibody by elution and subsequent testing in an indirect system will decide whether the antibody becomes localized for entirely non-specific reasons or whether it is primarily involved in the disease process. On present evidence the latter seems unlikely.

Psoriasis

Antibody and complement can be detected in psoriatic scales but as antibodies reacting with the stratum corneum have been found in all normal sera by a variety of techniques (Krogh, 1973) it is unlikely that antibody formation is related to the primary cause of the condition. The serum level of these antibodies falls during exacerbations of various skin diseases including psoriasis and pemphigus and is not clear whether they are irrelevant cross-reacting hetero-antibodies or whether they have a physiological role in relation to skin shedding. It is likely that the migration of neutrophil polymorphs is mediated via complement-derived chemotactic factors produced during antibody fixation in the stratum corneum. Abnormality of the papillary circulation may be the primary event, giving rise to very greatly enhanced permeability across into the epidermis.

Porphyria

Disorders of porphyrin metabolism which result in an excess of circulating porphyrinogens or porphyrins produce photosensitivity. Cutaneous hepatic porphyria (CHP, porphyria cutanea tarda) and erythropoietic protophyria (EPP) are the two most frequently seen in Great Britain.

Tuffanelli *et al.* (1973) studied forty-one patients with various forms of porphyria including thirty-two with CHP and five with EPP. Ten of the patients with CHP were in remission. In almost every case IgG deposits were found in, and adjacent to, blood vessels and at the epidermal/dermal junction in light exposed skin and less frequently in unexposed skin as well. The differences between the various types of porphyria were quantitative rather than qualitative.

The significance of these findings is mainly in pointing to the site at which the porphyrins, in combination with sunlight, produce the maximum damage. Any localization of antibody is probably a non-specific event.

Alopecia Areata

There are several reasons to suspect that alopecia areata has an immunological basis. The infiltrate around the hair follicles is mainly lymphocytic; steroids produce a remission and there is an increased incidence of vitiligo and other diseases in which auto-antibodies are present. Smooth muscle, thyroid, adrenal and parietal cell antibodies all show increased incidence and it has been suggested that alopecia areata itself results from the formation of an antibody to matrix cells (Thies, 1966).

Vitiligo

In the depigmented patches of vitiligo melanocytes are absent, or reduced in number, and an auto-immune cause for their destruction has been suggested. In support of this is an association between vitiligo and thyroid disease, pernicious anaemia and Addison's disease, but so far immunofluorescence studies of affected skin have been negative. In the early stages of the disorder some of the lesions may have a red elevated margin which histologically shows infiltration with lymphocytes, further supporting the idea of a destructive immunological process.

In the Vogt-Kayanagi syndrome extensive vitiligo and poliosis (patchy loss of hair pigmentation) of rapid onset are associated with uveitis, meningitic symptoms, deafness and alopecia areata. This may represent an abnormal response to a viral infection.

Partial Lipodystrophy

Rarely, a progressive loss of subcutaneous fatty tissue may occur. This often develops in childhood and may follow a measles infection. In its partial form it has a characteristic distribution which usually mirrors the distribution of the measles rash. Several patients with this condition have also been found to have mesangiocapillary glomerulonephritis, hypocomplementaemia and the presence of a circulating C3 activator (Peters *et al.*, 1973). The partial lipodystrophy, and probably the hypocomplementaemia, can antedate the renal disease by many years. Thus the development of this disorder seems to be yet another example of an immunodeficient response to infection.

REFERENCES

Abell, E., Presbury, D. G. C., Marks, R. and Ramnarain, D. (1975). The diagnostic significance of immunoglobulin and fibrin deposition in lichen planus. *Brit. J. Derm.* **93**, 17.

Alarcon-Segovia, D., Fishbein, E., Garcia-Ortigoza, E. and Estrada-Parra, S. (1975). Uracil specific anti-RNA antibodies in scleroderma. *Lancet* **i**, 363.

Allison, A. C. (1966). Immune responses to shope fibroma virus in adult and new-born rabbits. *J. Nat. Cancer Inst.* **36**, 869.

Andrews, B. S., Cains, G., McIntosh, J., Petts, V. and Penny, R. (1975). Circulating complexes in human cutaneous vasculitis. Work presented at the European Immunology Meeting, Amsterdam, September 1975.

Arbesman, C. E., Wypych, J. I., Reisman, R. E. and Beutner, E. H. (1974). IgE levels in sera of patients with pemphigus or bullous pemphigoid. *Arch. Derm.* **110**, 378.

Billingham, R. E. (1974). Reminiscences of a "transplanter". *Transplant. Proc.* Suppl. 1, **6**, 5.

Braverman, I. M. and Yen, A. (1975). Demonstration of immune complexes in spontaneous and histamine-induced lesions and in normal skin of patients with leucocytoclastic angiitis. *J. Invest. Derm.* **64**, 105.

Carruthers, J. A. and Black, M. M. (1975). Immunological findings in herpes gestationis. *Brit. J. Derm.* **93**, Suppl. 11, 17.

Champion, R. H., Roberts, S. O. B., Carpenter, R. G. and Roger, J. H. (1969). Urticaria and angio-oedema—a review of 554 patients. *Brit. J. Derm.* **81**, 588.

Cochrane, C. G. (1971). Mechanisms involved in the deposition of immune complexes in tissues. *J. Exp. Med.* **134**, 755.

Cronin, E. and Wilkinson, D. S. (1973). Contact dermatitis. *In* "Recent Advances in Dermatology". (Ed. A. Rook), Churchill-Livingstone, London.

Delescluse, J. and Turk, J. L. (1970). Lymphocyte cytotoxicity: a possible *in vitro* test for contact dermatitis. *Lancet* **ii**, 75.

Dvorak, H. F. and Mihm, M. C. (1972). Basophilic leucocytes in allergic contact dermatitis *J. Exp. Med.* **135**, 235.

Edelson, R., Facktor, M., Andrews, A., Lutzner, M. and Schein, P. (1974). Successful management of the Sézary syndrome. *New Eng. J. Med.* **291**, 293.

Ferguson, R., Basu, M. K., Asquith, P. and Cooke, W. T. (1976). Jejunal mucosal abnormalities in patients with recurrent aphthous ulceration. *Brit. Med. J.* **1**, 11.

Frey, J. R. (1974). Contact sensitivity: induction, tolerance, desensitization. *Int. Arch. All. App. Immunol.* **46**, 806.

Fry, L., Seah, P. P., Riches, D. J. and Hoffbrand, A. V. (1973). Clearance of skin lesions in dermatitis herpetiformis after gluten withdrawal. *Lancet* **i**, 288.

Gibbs, R. B. and Minus, H. R. (1975). Epidermolysis bullosa acquisita with electron microscopical studies. *Arch. Derm.* **111**, 215.

Greenberg, J. H., Smith, L. and Katz, R. M. (1973). Verrucae vulgaris rejection: a primary study of contact dermatitis and cellular immunity response. *Arch. Derm.* **107**, 508.

Van Joost, Th. (1973). An attempt to identify the nature of immunoglobulin-complement deposits in the skin in lupus erythematosus. *Brit. J. Derm.* **89**, 15.

Van Joost, Th. (1974). Incidence of circulating antibodies reactive with basal cells of skin in drug reactions. *Acta Dermatovener, Stockholm* **54**, 183.

Jordon, R. E., Day, N. K., Sams, W. M. and Good, R. A. (1973). The complement system in bullous pemphigoid. I. Complement and component levels in sera and blister fluids. *J. Clin. Invest.* **52**, 1207.

Kligman, A. M. and Wooding, W. M. (1967). A method for the evaluation of irritants on human skin. *J. Invest. Derm.* **49**, 78.

Krogh, H. K. (1973). Antibodies to stratum corneum in man. *In* "Immunopathology of the skin: Labelled antibody studies". (Ed. E. H. Beutner, T. P. Chorzelski, S. F. Bean and R. E. Jordon), Dowden, Hutchinson and Ross Inc., Stroudsberg, Pennsylvania.

Lehner, T. (1975). Immunological aspects of oral disease. *In* "Clinical Aspects of Immunology". Third Edition. (Ed. P. G. H. Gell, R. R. A. Coombs and P. J. Lachmann), Blackwell, Oxford.

Levis, W. R., Whalen, J. J. and Powell, J. A. (1975). Studies on the contact sensitization of man with simple chemicals. III. Quantitative relationships between specific lymphocyte transformation, skin sensitivity and lymphokine activity in response to dinitrochlorobenzene. *J. Invest. Derm.* **64**, 100.

Medenica, M. and Rosenberg, A. (1971). A comparative light and electron microscope study of primary irritant contact dermatitis and allergic contact dermatitis. *J. Invest. Derm.* **56**, 259.

Mowbray, J. F., Hoffbrand, A. V., Holborow, E. J., Seah, P. P. and Fry, L. (1973). Circulating immune complexes in dermatitis herpetiformis. *Lancet* **i**, 400.

Osmundsen, P. E. (1969). Photopatch testing. *Trans. St John's Hosp. Derm. Soc.* **55**, 160.

Parish, W. E. (1971). Studies on vasculitis. I. Immunoglobulins, β_1C, C-reactive protein and bacterial antigens in cutaneous vasculitis lesions. *Clin. All.* **1**, 97.

Parish, W. E., Rook, A. and Champion, R. H. (1965). A study of auto-allergy in generalised eczema. *Brit. J. Derm.* **77**, 479.

Peters, D. K., Williams, D. G., Charlesworth, J. A., Boulton-Jones, J. M., Sissons, J. G. P., Evans, D. J., Kourilsky, O. and Morel-Maroger, L. (1973). Mesangio-capillary nephritis, partial lipodystrophy and hypocomplementaemia. *Lancet* **ii**, 535.

Provost, T. T. and Tomasi, T. B. (1974). Immunopathology of bullous pemphigoid. Basement membrane deposition of IgE, alternate pathway components and fibrin. *Clin. Exp. Immunol.* **18**, 193.

Reeves, W. G., Allen, B. R. and Marriott, D. W. (1977). (In press).

Reeves, W. G. and Trounce, J. R. (1971). The problem of drug hypersensitivity. *Guy's Hosp. Rep.* **120**, 245.

Rowell, N. R. (1972). Lupus erythematosus, scleroderma and dermatomyositis. *In* "Textbook of Dermatology". Second Edition. (Ed. A. Rook, D. S. Wilkinson and F. J. G. Ebling), Blackwell, Oxford.

Ryan, T. J. and Wilkinson, D. S. (1972). Cutaneous vasculitis (angiitis). *In* "Textbook of Dermatology". Second Edition. (Ed. A. Rook, D. S. Wilkinson and F. J. G. Ebling), Blackwell, Oxford.

Schaumburg-Lever, G., Rule, A., Schmidt-Ullrich, B. and Lever, W. F. (1975). Ultrastructural localisation of *in vivo* bound immunoglobulins in bullous pemphigoid. *J. Invest. Derm.* **64**, 47.

Seah, P. P. and Fry, L. (1975). Immunoglobulins in the skin in dermatitis herpetiformis and their relevance in diagnosis. *Brit. J. Derm.* **92**, 157.

Seah, P. P., Fry, L., Hoffbrand, A. V. and Holborow, E. J. (1971). Tissue antibodies in dermatitis herpetiformis and adult coeliac disease. *Lancet* **i**, 834.

Sharp, G. C., Irwin, W. S., Tam, E. M., Gould, R. H. and Holman, H. R. (1972). Mixed connective tissue disease—an apparently distinct rheumatic disease associated with a specific antibody to an extractable nuclear antigen (ENA). *Am. J. Med.* **52**, 148.

Sussman, M., Jones, J. H., Almeida, J. D. and Lachmann, P. J. (1973). Deficiency of the second component of complement associated with anaphylactoid purpura and presence of mycoplasma in the serum. *Clin. Exp. Immunol.* **14**, 531.

Thies, W. (1966). Vergleichende histologishe Untersuchungen bei Alopecia areata und narbig-atrophisierenden Alopecian. *Arch. Klin. Exp. Derm.* **227**, 541.

Tuffanelli, D. L., Epstein, J. H. and Epstein, W. L. (1973). Cutaneous porphria. *In* "Immunopathology of the Skin". (Ed. E. H. Beutner, T. P. Chorezelski, S. F. Bean and R. E. Jordon), Dowden, Hutchinson and Ross, Inc. Pennsylvania.

Turk, J. L. and Bryceson, A. D. M. (1971). Immunological phenomena in leprosy and related diseases. *Adv. Immunol.* **13**, 209.

Valdimarsson, H., Higgs, J. M., Wells, R. S., Yamamura, M., Hobbs, J. R. and Holt, P. J. L. (1973). Immune abnormalities associated with chronic muco-cutaneous candidiasis. *Cellular Immunol.* **6**, 348.

Warin, R. P. and Champion, R. H. (1974). Urticaria. Saunders, Philadelphia.

Wolff-Schreiner, E. and Wolff, K. (1973). Immunoglobulins at the dermal/epidermal junction in lupus erythematosus: ultrastructural investigations. *Arch. Derm. Res. Forsch.* **246**, 193.

24

Muscle Disease

ROGER DAWKINS

From an immunological point of view skeletal and cardiac muscle possess many features in common. They share a number of tissue-specific antigens and immunization with either type may lead to both myositis and myocarditis. In polymyositis and myasthenia gravis there may be cardiac as well as skeletal muscle involvement. Smooth muscle, on the other hand, appears to be less closely related in terms of immunological cross-reactivity and involvement in experimentally induced and human diseases.

This chapter will be concerned with diseases which predominantly affect skeletal muscle. Diseases affecting cardiac muscle are dealt with in Chapter 16.

STRUCTURE AND FUNCTION OF MUSCLE

The basic unit of skeletal muscle is the myofibril as shown in Fig. 1. Each myofibril contains alternating bands best seen with polarization or phase contrast microscopy. The segments between successive Z lines are referred to as sarcomeres. Each sarcomere contains an A or anisotropic band consisting of thick filaments and bisected by the H zone within which there is a fine M line. The I band consists of the non-overlapped thin filament and is bisected by the Z line. Thick filaments consist of myosin and a relatively small amount of C protein. The M protein may be important in maintaining the orientation of thick filaments. Myosin has a molecular weight of approximately 500,000 daltons and is 1,200 Å in length. The structure is reminiscent of IgG in that there are two heavy and two light chains. These light chains, of about 22,000 daltons, occur in the heavy meromyosin fragment obtained by proteolytic digestion and are closely associated with the portion of the molecule responsible for binding to actin. In addition, the heavy meromyosin fragment

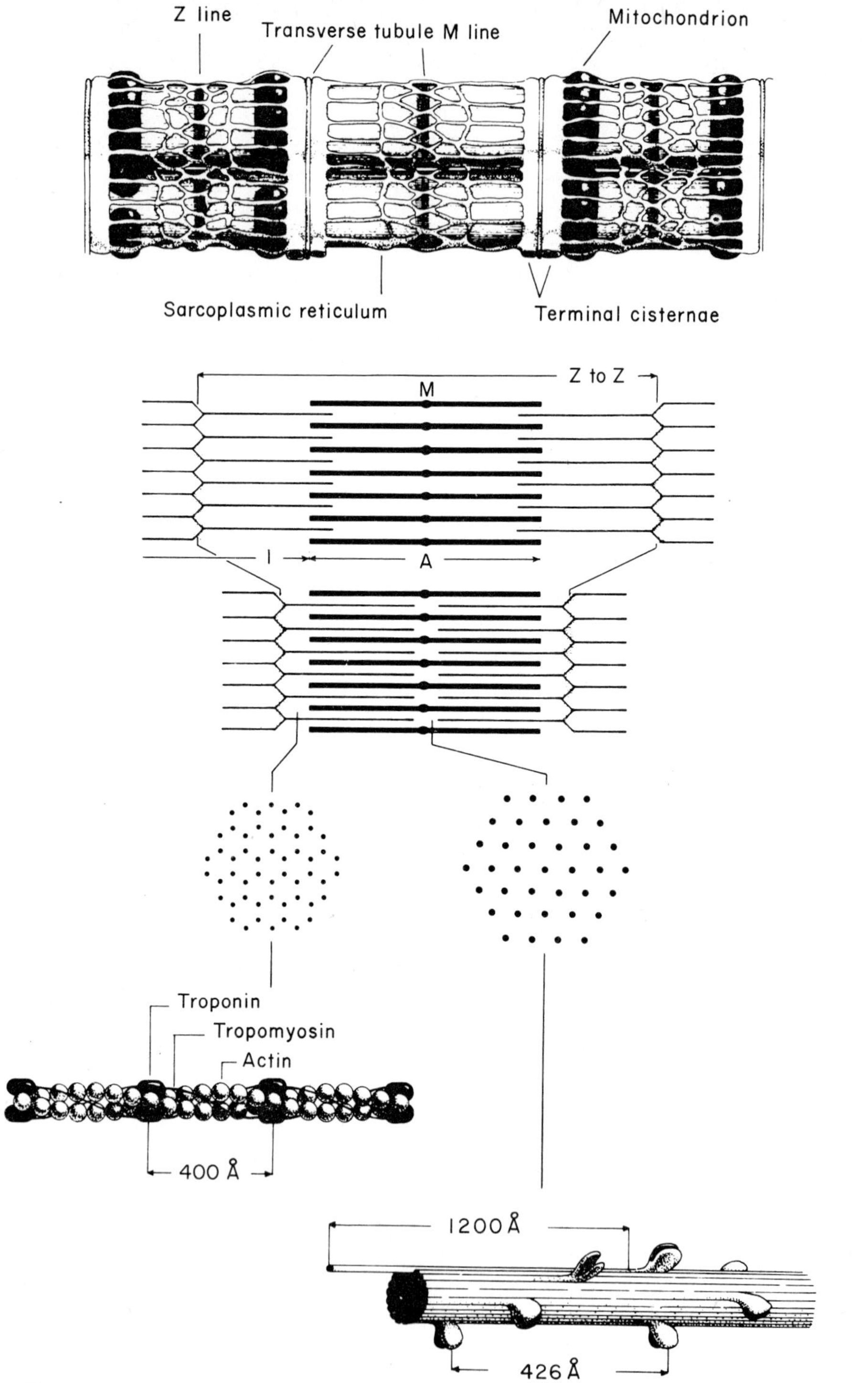

Fig. 1. The myofibril of skeletal muscle together with diagrams of relaxed and contracted sarcomeres. Cross-sections through the I band and the H zone indicate the arrangement of the thick and thin filaments. The postulated molecular structure of these filaments is also shown.

possesses ATPase activity. The thin filament consists of actin, tropomyosin and troponin as illustrated in Fig. 1. Further data on the proportion and situation of these proteins are given in Table 1.

TABLE 1
Composition of myofibrils

Protein	Approximate proportion	Site
Myosin	60	A
Actin	20	I
Tropomyosin	4	I
Troponin	3	I
α-actinin	2	Z
C protein		A
M protein		M

After Ebashi in Bourne (1973) and Gergely in Walton (1974).

Myofibres are made up of myofibrils lying side by side with sarcomeres in register. Mitochondria and sarcoplasmic reticulum are found between myofibrils with sarcolemma encircling the entire myofibre. The transverse tubular system traverses the surface of the myofibril at the A-I junction (in man but not all species) and appears to provide continuity between the sarcolemma and the sarcoplasmic reticulum. Outside the carcolemma there is loose connective tissue containing capillaries and known as endomysium. Denser connective tissue or perimysium separates bundles of myofibres and thick fascia or epimysium surrounds these bundles to complete the whole muscle.

Myofibres are innervated by motor nerves which terminate at neuromuscular junctions. On stimulation of the nerve there is release of acetyl choline which then reacts with a specific receptor to produce a depolarization wave which passes along the fibre. Individual sarcomeres are thought to be activated via the transverse tubular system and the sarcoplasmic reticulum which in turn releases calcium. In this way the rapid spread of excitation from neuromuscular junction to sarcomere and the coordination of contraction of multiple sarcomeres is explained. The mechanism of coupling between the depolarization wave and the release of calcium ions from the sarcoplasmic reticulum is not understood. However the calcium released is thought to interact with the calcium binding component of troponin. In this way the resting inhibition of troponin over actomyosin ATPase may be overcome so that actin–myosin cross-bridges form and the thin filaments move into the A band according to the sliding filament model. Relaxation occurs when calcium is pumped back into the sarcoplasmic reticulum with resultant inhibition of actomyosin ATPase.

Until recently muscle was considered to be a relatively stable tissue but it is now known that there is a rapid turnover of its components and a very substantial capacity for regeneration. *In vitro* studies have shown that the progenitor cell of muscle, the mononucleated myoblast, proliferates rapidly until a certain cell concentration is achieved. Thereafter there is a dramatic and almost synchronous fusion of myoblast with myoblast to form multinucleated myotubes. Further myoblasts may fuse with myotubes but nuclear division does not occur within the latter. Contractile proteins may be seen within myoblasts by immunological and ultrastructural methods but organized sarcomeres are not normally seen until after the formation of myotubes. Once such sarcomeres are present myotubes grown *in vitro* may contract but orderly contraction appears to be a consequence of later innervation. Regeneration of mature muscle is thought to be a consequence of the break-down of myofibres with the formation of nucleated fragments which can then divide. Alternatively injury may lead to stimulation of resting subsarcolemmal mononucleated satellite cells which may then fuse to form myotubes and ultimately myofibres. By these mechanisms mature muscle may be replaced within a matter of weeks of injury.

The immunology of skeletal muscle has been studied largely as a consequence of attempts to understand the structure and function of sarcomeres although, more recently, the lessons learnt have been fruitfully applied to the study of human disease. By immunofluorescence with antisera raised against partially purified contractile proteins, much of the localization referred to in Table 1 has been demonstrated or confirmed. The antibodies used have shown considerable cross-reactivity with cardiac muscle but the antigens concerned appear to be tissue-specific. The antimuscle antibodies found in patients with myasthenia gravis produce similar staining patterns to those found with experimental antisera and also show tissue specificity for skeletal muscle, heart and thymic myoid cells.

Antibody has also been produced against the acetyl choline receptor and as discussed below a syndrome simulating myasthenia may be produced experimentally. Unfortunately there is very little information concerning the antigenic nature of the conducting system including the transverse tubules.

From the point of view of immunologically-mediated human disease, muscle may be considered as a functional unit composed of antigenically distinct components namely, the neuromuscular junction, the conducting tubular system and the contractile proteins. The immunology of nerve is considered elsewhere but it is clear that a variety of processes may lead to malfunction of muscle due to seemingly selective involvement of nerves. Similarly in immunologically-mediated vasculopathies there may be symptomatic muscle disease as a consequence of the vasculitis. In the present chapter only processes which involve muscle itself will be considered in detail.

The structure and function of cardiac muscle is less relevant to the present purpose but it is noteworthy that it shows a number of differences which may be of practical importance in clinical immunology. Mitochondria are more numerous and this probably explains the intense and distinct pattern found when anti-mitochondrial antibody is applied to cardiac muscle. A number of biochemical differences have been demonstrated which might explain the more subtle antigenic differences between skeletal and cardiac muscle but it should be emphasized that there is considerable cross-reactivity of serology in diseases apparently mediated by immunological mechanisms.

In smooth muscle the contractile proteins resemble those of skeletal and cardiac muscle in some respects but their spatial organization and antigenicity appear to be different. Serologically, a degree of cross-reactivity can be demonstrated but this aspect has been poorly investigated and immunologically-mediated diseases which involve skeletal muscle do not appear to be associated with affection of smooth muscle.

EXPERIMENTAL AUTO-ALLERGIC DISEASE OF MUSCLE

Immunization of experimental animals with skeletal muscle in Freund's adjuvant leads to production of generalized myositis characterized by segmental necrosis and evidence of humoral and cell mediated immunity against various components of muscle (Dawkins, 1975). Not surprisingly, various antibodies are produced by immunization with crude muscle but a major pattern demonstrated by immunofluorescence is I band staining. With respect to cell mediated immunity, hypersensitivity to tropomyosin, and perhaps myosin, has been demonstrated by a migration inhibition method in guinea-pigs. If both humoral and cell mediated reactions are to be explained in terms of one particularly immunogenic antigen it would be tempting to implicate tropomyosin. Other antigens are clearly immunogenic also, since the sera of animals with experimental autoallergic myositis stain the M line and parts of the A band as well as the I band. One complication in the interpretation of these additional patterns is the fact that thick and thin filaments may not be stained where they have interacted. Competition between antimyosin and actin for myosin-binding sites is suggested by the demonstration that antibody may prevent contraction of glycerinated fibres.

Important features of experimental myositis in relation to human disease are the self-limited nature of the myositis, perhaps reflecting non-repeating sensitization, and intense regenerative activity. Most evidence suggests that T-cell mechanisms are predominant in the pathogenesis of the myositis but more work is required to determine the significance of the antibodies which have been demonstrated. Serum creatine kinase can be used as an index of disease activity and presumably reflects necrosis of fibres and release of cytoplasmic enzymes.

Immunization with skeletal muscle may lead to myocarditis as well as myositis, but there is no evidence of involvement of smooth muscle. Immunization with cardiac muscle leads to myocarditis and may be associated with involvement of skeletal muscle.

Immunization with thymus has been reported to induce an inflammatory lesion of the thymus associated with electromyographic changes suggestive of myasthenia gravis. It has been suggested that the thymus may release an inhibitor of neuromuscular transmission variously known as thymin or thymopoietin (Goldstein and Schlesinger, 1975).

This work has achieved considerable prominence but its relevance to human disease is far from clear. Apparently more significant is the work initiated by Patrick and Lindstrom (1973) which shows that immunization of rabbits with acetyl choline receptor leads to a clinical picture resembling myasthenia gravis. This has been reproduced by others in a variety of species and appears to hold great promise as a model. However the immunological features of the disease have yet to be defined.

Muscle may be involved in immunological processes not directed at muscle components themselves. Thus forty years ago it was shown that an intense myositis could be produced by immune complexes presumably as a consequence of their non-specific phlogistic effect.

POLYMYOSITIS

Polymyositis is generally considered to encompass a rather heterogeneous group of conditions characterized by the presence of weakness due to inflammatory myopathy. In the presence of skin lesions the designation dermatomyositis is used. Some patients have a coexistent neoplasm, and there may be associated features which are characteristic of connective tissue disorders such as systemic lupus erythematosus and systemic sclerosis.

Definition

No completely satisfactory definition exists in spite of many attempts to provide one. A major difficulty is the lack of precise correlation between clinical and histological features. Inflammatory changes occur in the muscle of patients with diseases such as rheumatoid arthritis and myasthenia gravis and there appears to be no qualitative difference between these lesions and those seen in the presence of the clinical features of polymyositis. Given these circumstances there seems little prospect of a rigorous definition or classification until the spectrum of polymyositis can be classified on an aetiological basis. In the meanwhile the following criteria are the most satisfactory.

Criteria

i. Objective evidence of symmetrical weakness of proximal muscle groups developing over weeks to months with an excess of weakness over wasting. The weakness must be relatively "fixed" in that only minor variations occur by the hour or the day.
ii. Systemic and/or local evidence of necrosis of skeletal muscle where systemic evidence includes elevated serum creatine kinase, aldolase and/or other muscle enzymes and local evidence consists of myofibre necrosis or regeneration implying previous necrosis.
iii. Systemic and/or local evidence of inflammatory disease where local evidence consists of interstitial and/or perivascular mononuclear infiltration.

These three criteria must show a temporal relationship. If they do, they can be used to indicate the presence of a chronic inflammatory condition leading to muscle necrosis and weakness without paying excessive attention to variable histological and clinical features. However, it is important to consider the possibility of infectious, neurogenic, genetic, metabolic, endocrine, toxic and physical disorders which may produce some of the features referred to above.

Incidence

The overall incidence (including subtypes) appears to be approximately five per million per year and most cases occur in the fifth and sixth decade. The male/female ratio is approximately 1:2. Familial occurrence is rare.

Clinical Features

As indicated above the term "polymyositis" as currently employed includes a heterogeneous group of conditions. The following description refers to "pure" polymyositis as it occurs in the adult. Reference to subtypes and associated features will be deferred until later sections.

The predominant clinical feature is symmetrical sustained weakness of proximal muscle groups. Characteristically there is relative sparing of distal groups and complete sparing of facial and extra-ocular musculature. Although symptomatic involvement is generally maximal in the shoulder and pelvic girdles, there may also be severe weakness of spinal, cervical and respiratory muscles. Dysphagia is also common. The weakness is generally progressive but some fluctuation may occur. There may be sufficient fatiguability to suggest a myasthenic component but this is superimposed upon relatively sustained weakness which shows minimal diurnal variation.

In the absence of associated synovitis, pain and tenderness are not prominent features. In the more acute cases muscle aching may be a relatively major symptom but even in these cases weakness tends to predominate. Wasting may be seen in some patients and especially those with slowly progressive disease but one feature of polymyositis is the relative excess of weakness over wasting. Muscle swelling may be seen in the fulminant case but this is relatively unusual.

Associated Phenomena

Dermatomyositis

About one-third of patients with the syndrome described above have distinctive skin lesions. Elements which justify the designation dermatomyositis are: (i) heliotrope rash with a lilac discoloration of the upper eyelids and dusky erythema of the face; (ii) skin oedema and erythema which can be bright red or purplish involving the face, neck, shoulders, arms and upper chest; (iii) periungual erythema and even haemorrhage associated with red, shiny, peeling skin of the fingers; and (iv) erythema, with or without scaling, over extensor surfaces such as the posterior neck, elbows, knuckles, knees and ankles. Other patterns of skin involvement may be seen but these appear to be less characteristic and it is doubtful whether they should be considered sufficient for a diagnosis of dermatomyositis. In general, the features described coexist with the "pure" polymyositis syndrome at one time or another but they may precede clinical evidence of muscle involvement and may disappear although muscle involvement remains. In some instances the scaly erythema is replaced by atrophic and telangiectatic lesions in the same distribution.

The pathological and prognostic implications of the typical skin involvement are not entirely clear although they are a particular feature of juvenile dermatomyositis in which systemic angiopathy is generally found. It is possible that they also reflect some form of vasculopathy in adult patients but this has never been demonstrated clearly. In adults the typical dermal features may be associated with a more rapid course and with the frequent coexistence of neoplasia.

The term "sclerodermatomyositis" has been used to refer to those patients with polymyositis and sclerodermatous changes. The problem of overlap with systemic sclerosis will be considered further below but the use of this term is unnecessarily confusing.

Associated Neoplasia

Some patients with polymyositis have an associated neoplasm which may become clinically apparent before or after the diagnosis of polymyositis. The frequency of this association remains uncertain (Bohan and Peter, 1975). It is generally said that approximately one-fifth of adults will be found to have a tumour at some time but the proportion is substantially higher in older age groups and especially males. The type of tumour varies considerably and larger studies suggest that different types of neoplasm are distributed approximately in accordance with their distribution in the population as a whole. An exception to this rule might be the more frequent occurrence of lymphoid tumours, especially thymoma.

Unfortunately there are no clearly established criteria which allow the physician to decide whether a full tumour work up is indicated in a patient presenting with uncomplicated polymyositis. Advanced years, male sex, the presence of dermatomyositis and dysphagia and a relatively rapid course with a poor response to prednisone have been taken as indications of increased risk of underlying neoplasia.

Features of the Connective Tissue Diseases

The pure syndrome of polymyositis described above bears little resemblance to the connective tissue disorders, but superadded features such as sclerodactyly, Raynaud's phenomenon and synovitis are sufficiently common to suggest there may be some overlap. It is clear that polymyositis as defined above may occur in patients with obvious additional evidence of systemic lupus erythematosus, systemic sclerosis, rheumatoid arthritis, fibrosing alveolitis and Sjögren's syndrome. It is also clear, however, that these disorders may be associated with inflammatory changes in muscle which do not justify the designation polymyositis. Similarly, features such as dermatitis, scleroderma and synovitis may be associated with polymyositis without sufficiently justifying a diagnosis of systemic lupus erythematosus, systemic sclerosis or rheumatoid arthritis.

A concept of distinct overlap syndromes is of little value until it has been demonstrated that there are significant implications in terms of natural history and response to therapy. Meanwhile, it is preferable to diagnose and treat one or more of these diseases as distinct entities and to use qualifications such as "polymyositis together with synovitis" if there is insufficient evidence to establish two firm diagnoses. It has been suggested that the chance of an underlying neoplasm may be less in patients with an associated connective tissue disease or even isolated features such as Raynaud's phenomenon, sclerodactyly and synovitis but this important difference requires confirmation.

Visceral Involvement

As indicated above various viscera may be involved in patients with polymyositis. Thus there may be myocarditis, serositis, pneumonitis and perhaps gastrointestinal involvement but features such as hepatitis or nephritis do not occur. The myocarditis could represent cross reactivity between skeletal and cardiac muscle but some of the visceral involvement may be due to a systemic angiopathy of the type which occurs in children.

Pathology

In most cases histopathology reveals the presence of necrotizing myositis. Typically, there is myofibre necrosis with phagocytosis of necrotic debris by macrophages, and interstitial inflammatory changes. Mononuclear cells predominate but the infiltrate is often sparse with some concentration around vessels. A predominance of neutrophils or eosinophils and the presence of granulomas or epithelioid cells should lead to consideration of other inflammatory myopathies. On occasion, extensive necrosis may be seen with minimal inflammatory infiltrate but more commonly there are discrete foci of necrosis with adjacent mononuclear infiltration. At times these foci are particularly concentrated at the periphery of muscle fascicles. Perifascicular atrophy in the absence of adjacent necrosis of inflammation is a common subsidiary finding. Regeneration is suggested by cytoplasmic basophilia and the presence of central vesicular nuclei with prominent nucleoli in otherwise intact fibres.

In addition to these changes there may be evidence of vasculitis or ischaemia but these changes are common only in juvenile dermatomyositis (see below) and in adults should lead to suspicion of polyarteritis and related disorders. Other less specific features such as fibrosis, fatty replacement and extensive variation in fibre size may be seen in the more chronic cases.

In a few cases biopsy reveals no abnormality even when there is good other evidence of an inflammatory necrotizing myositis e.g. elevated serum enzymes and systemic evidence of inflammation. Although this may be due to inadequate sampling and although careful selection of the biopsy site based on clinical and electrographic data may reduce the proportion of negative biopsies, positive histopathology cannot be considered a *sine qua non* for the diagnosis.

The histopathology of the skin involvement in dermatomyositis is generally held to be variable and of little diagnostic value. Direct immunofluorescence is generally negative but we have seen junctional deposition of IgG in the involved skin of a patient with the typical finger lesions of dermatomyositis, no other features to suggest systemic lupus erythematosus, but accompanying Sjögren's syndrome and fibrosing alveolitis. Myocarditis may also occur.

Electron microscopy of skeletal muscle has not revealed diagnostic changes, only those predictable from light microscopy. Vascular changes such as capillary necrosis and basement membrane reduplication have been reported but the significance is uncertain. Similarly, particles resembling viruses have been demonstrated in some cases and recently Coxsackie virus has been isolated in some. It is not clear whether viruses are relevant to the pathogenesis of polymyositis as a whole or whether they are found only in virally-induced myositis mimicking polymyositis.

The most useful biochemical estimations in polymyositis are serum creatine kinase, transaminases and aldolase. There is no direct relationship between the levels of these enzymes, and occasionally they may all be normal even in cases with proven necrotizing myositis. Some workers suggest that urinary creatine may be a more sensitive index of necrosis of muscle. In cases with extensive myolysis there may be myoglobinuria. The erythrocyte sedimentation rate is moderately elevated in perhaps half the cases but elevations of more than 40–50 mm (Westergren) per hour suggest the possibility of an associated neoplasm or connective tissue disease.

Electromyography

Electromyography may reveal patchy non-specific changes suggesting a myopathy. These comprise small amplitude, short duration and at times polyphasic motor unit potentials. When these changes are associated with spontaneous fibrillation potentials, positive sharp-waves and pseudomyotonic discharges the electromyographic findings are more specific. These latter features are attributed to involvement of the terminal innervation of muscle fibres but conventional nerve conduction studies are usually normal.

Immunology

For more than a decade polymyositis has been considered to be an autoimmune disease although until recently there has been little substantial evidence in support of this concept. Early claims that anti-nuclear factor, rheumatoid factor and hypergammaglobulinaemia were common, probably reflect the association with diseases such as systemic lupus erythematosus and rheumatoid arthritis. Patients with pure polymyositis without associated connective tissue disease do not have an increased prevalence of auto-antibodies. Furthermore, hypo- or eu-gammaglobulinaemia is usual and hypergammaglobulinaemia should lead to consideration of other diagnoses. In a study of twenty patients with pure polymyositis or dermatomyositis 50% were found to have borderline low or distinctly low serum IgG and/or IgM concentrations (Dawkins, 1975). It is noteworthy that polymyositis has been reported in association with gross hypogammaglobulinaemia including genetically determined varieties.

Autoantibodies against muscle have never been demonstrated convincingly in polymyositis. There was some confusion in the past due to the ability of normal serum to bind to muscle by non-immunological mechanisms, and the fact that some normal and other individuals possess heterophile antibodies which react with the interstitium of skeletal muscle of some species. This appearance on immunofluorescence may be produced by treating human muscle with serum containing high titre isohaemagglutinins.

Anti-myoglobulin antibodies have been described but have yet to be confirmed. Skin testing and immunofluorescence studies have been interpreted as indicating the presence of antibody to associated tumours but no convincing data are forthcoming.

Complement levels are generally said to be normal in polymyositis. With respect to CH_{50} this appears to be true irrespective of dermal or vascular involvement (as for example in juvenile dermatomyositis) although, not surprisingly, we have seen depressions in patients with associated systemic lupus erythematosus. It has been claimed that C3 may be depressed in 10–20% of patients with pure polymyositis or dermatomyositis but there was no relationship to CH_{50}. A patient with an apparently genetically-determined deficiency of C2 has been reported (Leddy *et al.*, 1975). One group has reported finding immunoglobulin and complement in vessel walls in polymyositis and various other myopathies but there was no histological evidence of associated inflammatory or necrotizing lesions (Whitaker and Engel, 1972).

It may be concluded that at present there are no serological abnormalities which characterize polymyositis and no convincing evidence that serological mechanisms lead to necrotizing myositis. This does not exclude the possibility that humoral immunodeficiency may be a factor in its pathogenesis.

Studies of the cell mediated immune status of patients with polymyositis have failed to reveal evidence of deficiency. Deficiency can occur after immunosuppressive therapy, anti-tumour therapy and conceivably in the presence of associated diseases but so far there is nothing to indicate that cell mediated defects precede the development of polymyositis. One case with low T- and B-cell numbers has been reported but the patient had an undifferentiated adenocarcinoma and died within three weeks. In our series T-cell deficiency has not been apparent.

Evidence of a cell mediated reaction directed against muscle has been reported by numerous groups using a variety of different assays which allow the detection of cell mediated cytotoxicity to muscle grown *in vitro* (Dawkins, 1975). The precise nature of this reaction is unclear but it is presumed to reflect direct T-cell cytotoxicity. Further work is required to exclude the possibility of antibody dependent cytotoxicity and to show unequivocally that the reaction is directed against a muscle-specific antigen. In the meanwhile it is of interest that lymphocyte mediated myotoxicity falls to normal with immunosuppressive therapy.

Classification

In spite of many attempts at classification of polymyositis there is no simple scheme of value in practice. Until more is known about the significance of the skin lesions and until there is unanimity about the specificity of the different forms of skin involvement, there seems no real value in separating polymyositis into cases with dermatomyositis and cases without dermal lesions. More important would appear to be a category of patients with typical dermal lesions who have yet to develop myositis i.e. dermatomyositis *sine* myositis, since there is no evidence that their disease has the same natural history as polymyositis (including true dermatomyositis). Nor is there evidence that these cases require therapy. Juvenile dermatomyositis, however, appears to be an important subclass of polymyositis and its distinctive features justify a separate designation. In children polymyositis is almost always associated with the typical dermal features, and solid tumours, if not all tumours, do not occur with increased prevalence. Calcinosis and contractures are common complications as are features reflecting the systemic angiopathy.

At present there is little merit in subgrouping patients with an associated neoplasm since the neoplasm may appear some years after presentation with polymyositis and there is no satisfactory method of predicting which patients belong to this group prior to the appearance of the neoplasm. Furthermore the natural history and therapy of these patients is substantially affected by the type and extent of the associated tumour.

Some workers have attempted to define a group which includes patients with a second diagnosis of connective tissue disease. Since the type of disease may vary and, since it remains to be shown that this group is in any way homogeneous, such subgrouping appears premature. Furthermore it has not been demonstrated that these patients require different therapy from those without a second diagnosis. At this stage it appears more appropriate to consider polymyositis as an essentially muscle-specific process and to treat other associated features independently as required.

Differential Diagnosis

As indicated above, the diagnosis of polymyositis rests upon satisfying the criteria given and to this end every patient in whom polymyositis is suspected requires careful clinical examination of muscle power, determination of serum creatine kinase, aldolase and transaminase and tests, such as erythrocyte sedimentation rate, which might reflect systemic evidence of inflammatory disease. In patients with weakness of the deltoid or quadriceps groups muscle biopsy should be taken from one of these sites. In cases with clinical involvement of relatively inaccessible muscle, the deltoid and quadriceps may be biopsied together, but in some instances it is helpful to perform electromyography beforehand and to biopsy the site contralateral to the area of greatest electromyographic involvement. The actual site of needle insertion should not be biopsied because focal necrosis may be induced by this means. Determination of serum immunoglobulins, complement and auto-antibodies assist in detecting associated conditions. Other investigations may be helpful in certain circumstances. A barium swallow may reveal changes compatible with involvement of the striated muscle of the upper third of the oesophagus and electrocardiography may show ST-T wave changes compatible with the presence of myocarditis.

With this approach it should be possible to determine whether or not a patient has polymyositis but it is always important to consider the following differential diagnosis.

i. Muscular dystrophy. The presence of a family history, the distribution of wasting and weakness and the slowly progressive course generally allow ready distinction between dystrophy and polymyositis. However, these conditions may be histologically similar in some cases and there may be some response to prednisone in dystrophy.
ii. Endocrine myopathy, especially thyroid and steroid myopathies. These can sometimes create confusion so that thyroid function tests and thyroid auto-antibodies should be determined. Steroid myopathy is a particular problem in patients who have received corticosteroid therapy since steroids may suppress the inflammatory components of polymyositis whilst inducing weakness particularly of the quadriceps group. In hypothyroidism substantial elevations of creatine kinase may be seen.
iii. Metabolic myopathy, especially those associated with changes in serum potassium or calcium levels. Lipid storage diseases should also be considered.
iv. Toxic myopathy, including alcohol and drugs.
v. Infective myositis, including viral e.g. post-influenza and parasitic e.g. toxoplasmosis.
vi. Neurogenic atrophy. This can be difficult to exclude because of the relative non-specificity of electromyographic changes and because serum creatine kinase concentrations may be increased in long-standing cases.

vii. Polymyalgia rheumatica and giant-cell arteritis. These will be considered further below.

viii. Granulomatous myopathy, see below.

ix. Other myopathies associated with connective tissue disorders. Inflammatory changes including focal nodular myositis may be found in association with rheumatoid arthritis and other connective tissue disorders but in most cases these changes are not associated with necrosis and weakness. In such cases, confusion arises if disproportionate attention is paid to the muscle biopsy. Real difficulty may be encountered when the patient is found to have a compatible lesion in muscle together with proximal muscle weakness due to associated joint involvement, neurogenic lesions or steroid therapy. A particular vacuolar form of myopathy has been described in systemic lupus erythematosus but the significance and specificity of the observed changes is uncertain (Pearson and Currie, 1974).

x. Myasthenic myopathy. This will be discussed further below. Polymyositis can complicate thymoma with and without myasthenia gravis.

xi. Carcinomatous myopathy and cachexia. Considerable confusion has been created by the use of these terms. They are probably appropriate in cases where there is muscle wasting and weakness without inflammatory changes. Although such features may sometimes be due to a neuropathy, the pathogenesis of any primary involvement of muscle is completely uncertain.

Treatment

In the presence of the syndrome described, conventional therapy consists of relatively high dose prednisone in the first instance. Histological evidence of myositis in the absence of clinical weakness is not an accepted indication for such therapy. Similarly, even in the presence of typical dermal lesions, dermatomyositis is not considered to be an indication for high dose (if any) corticosteroid therapy if evidence of polymyositis *per se* is lacking.

Before commencing steroid therapy it is important to consider the possible effects on associated disease e.g. systemic sclerosis, myasthenia gravis. In the presence of a treatable tumour it may be desirable to treat the tumour first since occasionally some improvement may be seen after surgical excision. Furthermore, there may be situations where prednisone might have a particularly detrimental effect on the tumour itself.

Once the decision to use high dose prednisone has been taken the patient should be started on at least 40–80 mg prednisone daily. This dosage should be maintained for at least two months or until there is objective evidence of response. The dose can then be reduced but it is important to avoid rapid decrements because exacerbations may result. Muscle enzyme activities in serum may be of some value in monitoring dosage but these can be affected by other factors such as exercise and intramuscular injection. After gradual reduction many patients can be maintained at near physiological levels of corticosteroids but rarely is it possible to withdraw treatment altogether. Alternative dosage regimens of prednisone therapy are recommended by some workers but adequate controlled studies have not been performed. The relatively recent use of alternate day therapy remains to be evaluated. Fluorinated corticosteroids should be avoided because of their reported propensity to induce steroid myopathy.

In the event of steroid resistance, azathioprine, cyclophosphamide or methotrexate have been used. Again, as with steroids, proper controlled studies have not been performed. One group with considerable experience has recommended the use of intravenous methotrexate (Metzger *et al.*, 1974). In view of the serious side-effects of this treatment in psoriasis, and because it is unknown whether it can be tapered off, methotrexate should probably be reserved for steroid–refractory polymyositis.

In addition to the above mentioned therapy, designed principally to treat necrotizing myositis, there may be a role for other treatment of associated features. Topical steroids may be of value in treatment of the skin lesions of dermatomyositis. Physiotherapy can help in cases with contractures but is generally not prescribed during the more acute stages of the disease.

SARCOIDOSIS (GRANULOMATOUS MYOPATHY)

Pathologically, muscle is involved in approximately half of all patients with sarcoidosis. Clinically, the proportion is very much less. Three patterns of symptomatic involvement are recognized (Douglas *et al.*, 1973; Gardner-Thorpe, 1972): (i) acute myositis with pain and tenderness; (ii) palpable nodules in muscle; and (iii) chronic myopathy with a clinical picture resembling muscular dystrophy. Neuropathies may be associated and can lead to difficulties in diagnosis. In almost all cases organs other than muscle will be found to be involved. The more acute cases respond to prednisone therapy.

MYASTHENIA GRAVIS

Myasthenia gravis is fundamentally different from polymyositis and the other conditions referred to above in that the pathogenesis involves a defect of neuromuscular transmission leading to excessive fatiguability. Since specific pathological characteristics have never been demonstrated, the disease must be defined in clinical, electrophysical and pharmacological terms.

Definition

There is excessive fatiguability whereby exercise or sustained muscle tension leads to rapidly increasing weakness with substantial recovery after rest. Electrophysiologically a decrement in action potential can be demonstrated after repetitive stimulation. The clinical and electromyographic features are reversed by administration of anticholinesterase therapy. Thus, the defect appears to involve a failure of neuromuscular transmission due to a functional deficiency of acetylcholine. The precise nature of this deficiency remains uncertain but most evidence is consistent with a post-synaptic lesion due to inhibition of binding between acetylcholine and the acetyl choline receptor.

Incidence

The incidence of myasthenia gravis is approximately 2–3 per million per year although higher estimates have been made. A prevalence figure of 1 per 50,000 is widely accepted. As in the case of polymyositis there is evidence of genetic factors in pathogenesis and there are epidemiological grounds for separating juvenile and adult myasthenia gravis.

Females are affected more commonly than males (approximately 3:1) with a peak age incidence in early adulthood. In patients over 50 years males predominate. In some respects the epidemiological data are reminiscent of systemic lupus erythematosus.

Clinical Features

Onset may be insidious but is often sudden after an infection or emotional disturbance. Characteristically excessive fatiguability affects predominantly ocular and bulbar musculature, and ptosis, diplopia and dysphagia are common symptoms. More generalized involvement of muscle is not uncommon but there is usually more involvement of proximal than distal groups. Respiratory involvement is an important feature of more severe cases.

Symptoms are generally worse as the day progresses and fluctuate considerably from day to day. Intercurrent infections and emotional stress may lead to striking deterioration. Other frequent symptoms in myasthenia gravis can be largely explained on the basis of associated diseases as discussed below.

Mention should be made of neonatal myasthenia which occurs in the babies of mothers with myasthenia gravis. Myasthenia persists for a period of days or weeks and is followed by complete recovery.

Pathology

For many decades it has been appreciated that inflammatory lesions may be found in skeletal muscle. The best known form of these consists of "lymphorrhages" or interstitial clusters of lymphocytes but similar clusters may occur in connective tissue diseases and apparently other conditions. Serial sectioning has demonstrated that "lymphorrhages" probably represent focal myofibre necrosis; in some instances, the myositis may be pronounced and may mimic exactly the changes of florid polymyositis. This is especially so in patients with an associated thymoma. In other patients only atrophic changes, especially of Type II muscle fibres, suggest neurogenic atrophy. Such changes may reflect chronic functional denervation but other factors could be involved in their pathogenesis.

Perhaps the most outstanding pathological feature of myasthenia gravis is the finding of abnormalities within the thymus in approximately 80% of all patients. These range from so-called thymic hyperplasia in which there is hypercellularity of the medulla to frank germinal centre formation. The gland may be grossly enlarged as compared with the size expected at the relevant age. These changes, however, are by no means specific for myasthenia gravis and may be seen in auto-immune thyroiditis, systemic lupus erythematosus and other disorders thought to reflect auto-immunization.

The second most common thymic abnormality in patients with myasthenia gravis is thymoma, seen in up to 30% and particularly common in elderly males. The histological features of the thymoma are rather variable as is the biological behaviour of the tumour. Distant metastases are distinctly uncommon but local invasion is a relatively frequent occurrence. Most commonly, however, the tumour remains encapsulated and is readily removed without apparent recurrence. It has been reported that there may be hyperplastic changes in the adjacent non-neoplastic thymus.

Other pathological features of myasthenia can be largely accounted for in terms of the associated diseases which occur.

Electrodiagnosis

Electromyography is of some value in characterizing the disorder of neuromuscular transmission in myasthenia gravis and in making the distinction between this condition and the myasthenic syndrome of Eaton and Lambert (see Adams, 1975; Walton, 1974). However with routine methods, negative results may be obtained in as many as 20–50% of patients with myasthenia gravis depending on the mucles tested. Unfortunately the most accessible muscles for studying neuromuscular transmission are rarely involved in early or mild cases. A number of methods have been used in attempts to increase diagnostic sensitivity, including raising the temperature of the limb, inducing a period of temporary ischaemia in the limb, and attempting to demonstrate post-tetanic facilitation, but the greatest promise appears to lie in single fibre electromyography.

Immunology

In 1960 Simpson suggested that myasthenia gravis may be an auto-immune disease involving the neuromuscular junction and possibly other tissues (Simpson, 1974). Evidence in support of this hypothesis included the frequent association between myasthenia gravis and features or diseases thought to reflect auto-immunity. The occurrence of neonatal myasthenia made it appear likely that there is an antibody which in some way interferes with the action of acetylcholine at the neuromuscular junction. Also in 1960, Strauss and Nastuk demonstrated that a proportion of patients with myasthenia gravis possess an anti-muscle antibody (Strauss *et al.*, 1960) and that some patients may have hypocomplementaemia (Nastuk *et al.*, 1960). The anti-muscle antibody was shown by immunofluorescence to bind to muscle itself rather than to the neuromuscular junction.

Initially it was thought that anti-muscle antibody reacts with the A band of the sarcomere. Later, however, it was shown that I rather than A bands are stained and further work by Strauss revealed that most, if not all, sera actually bind to the I band. Our own studies have highlighted the effects of sarcomere length on the overall staining pattern and show that staining of the A-I junction is often associated with I band staining (Fig. 2). On the basis of these findings it appears that there are at least two antibodies: one reacting with actin, tropomyosin, troponin or some other component of the thin filament and the other reacting with some as yet unidentified antigen in the A-I junction. Further work is required to determine whether or not the latter is related to the transverse tubular system or whether it is the same thin filament component responsible for I band staining. Immunoperoxidase methods have been applied with only limited success but have shown predominant staining of the I rather than the A band. They also suggest that there is binding to the sarcoplasmic reticulum. Until the antigenic specificity of the antibody(s) has been defined, the designation anti-striational appears preferable to anti-myosin, anti-A or anti-I as used in the past.

Other features which have been shown by immunofluorescence include cross-reactivity with cardiac muscle and thymic myoid cells. In the heart there is striational staining very similar to that seen in skeletal muscle, but in addition there tends to be peripheral accentuation in staining which can closely mimic the subsarcolemmal staining seen with the post-cardiotomy syndrome and rheumatic fever, especially if fixation is poor and striational staining is overlooked. The myoid cell staining may also be striational especially if the substrate is thymus of lower vertebrates. Homogeneous staining of the heads or bodies of the myoid cell accords with the distribution of contractile protein as shown ultrastructually. Some have interpreted cardiac and myoid cell cross-reactivity as evidence for variety of antibodies in myasthenia gravis but the data are consistent with the view that these tissues share a contractile protein antigen with skeletal muscle. Immunofluorescence has shown that the antibody is IgG in class and can fix complement *in vitro*. For routine screening purposes, rat heart can be included in a composite block used to detect anti-nuclear factor, anti-parietal cell, anti-smooth muscle and other antibodies. If heart staining is seen, the serum can be tested on human heart for detection and classification of the antibodies found in the post-cardiotomy syndrome and in rheumatic fever, and the serum can also be titrated on glycerinated skeletal muscle fibres. If sections of snap frozen tissue only are used problems can arise due to artefactual disruption of striations, and to non-specific staining by heterophile and other antibodies (Figs. 3, 4, 5 and 6).

It has been said that serum must be tested at high dilution (such as 1/64) because normal serum can stain at lower titres. Clearly the screening level is

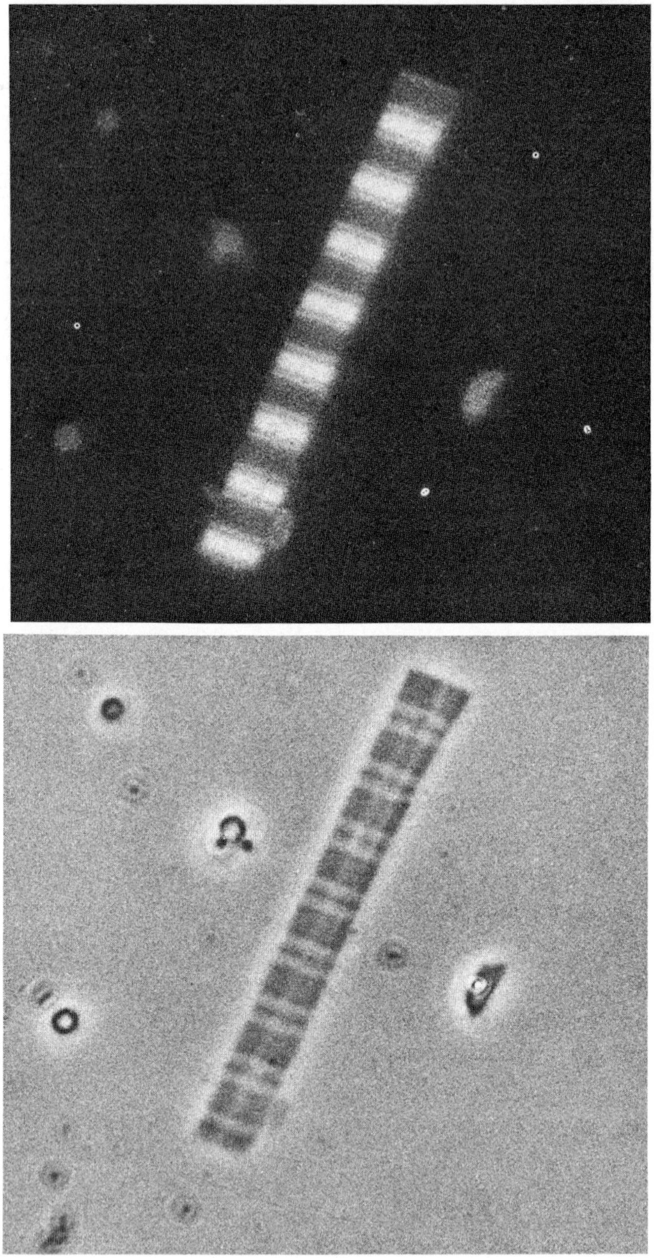

Fig. 2. Glycerinated guinea-pig muscle fibres (a) stained with serum from a patient with myasthenia gravis by indirect immunofluorescence (b) same fibre under phase contrast. The wide fluorescent band is the I band, with a narrow fluorescent band at the AI junctions on either side. The A band is not fluorescent.

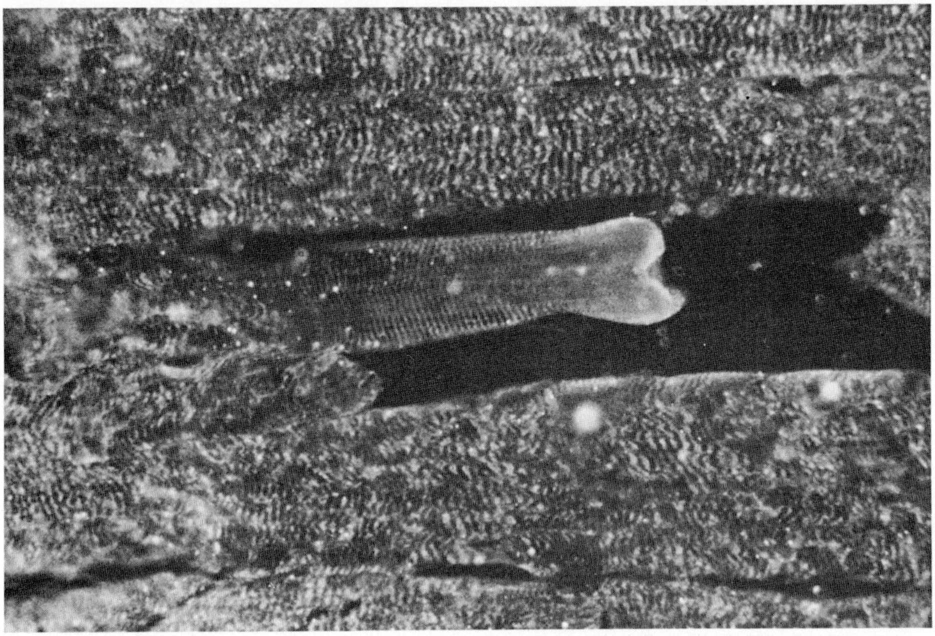

Fig. 3. Guinea-pig skeletal muscle in frozen section. Pattern is that seen with the anti-striational (anti-muscle) antibody found in association with thymoma and/ or myasthenia gravis. Note the effect of sarcomere shortening as seen in an area of artefactual super-contraction.

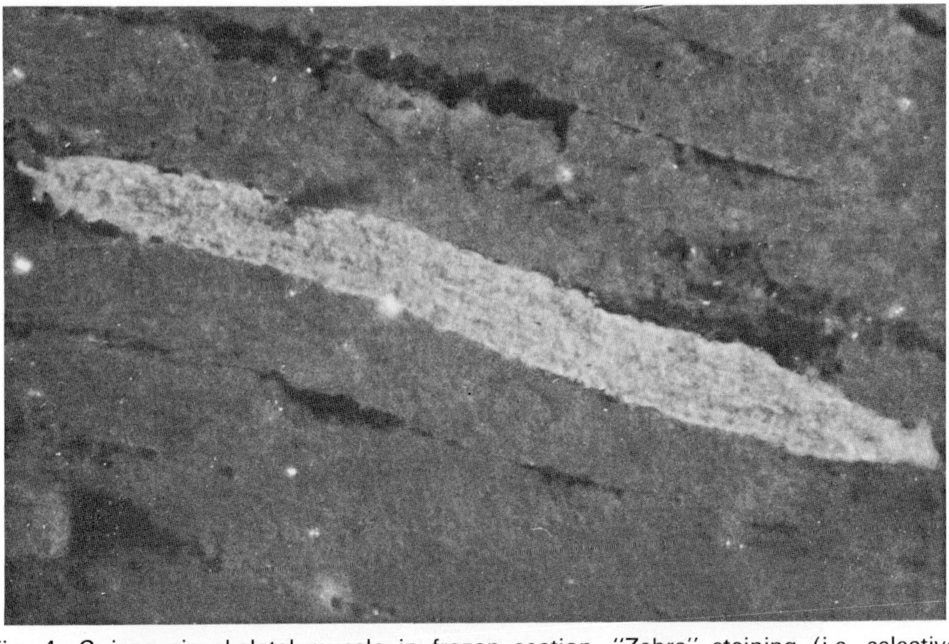

Fig. 4. Guinea-pig skeletal muscle in frozen section. "Zebra" staining (i.e. selective staining of certain muscle fibre types) is present. This pattern has no known diagnostic significance. Contrast with striational pattern (Fig. 3).

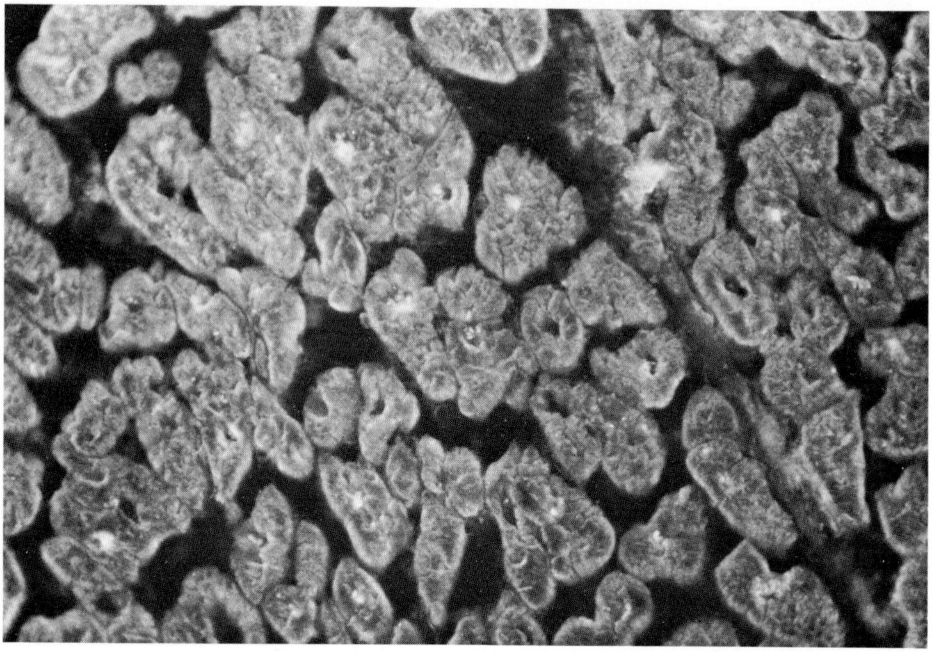

Fig. 5. Human heart. Sarcoplasmic staining with peripheral accentuation i.e. subsarcolemmal–subsarcoplasmic pattern as seen in rheumatic fever and the post-cardiotomy syndrome. Myasthenic sera can produce a similar appearance but striational staining is readily seen in longitudinal sections or when skeletal muscle fibres are used.

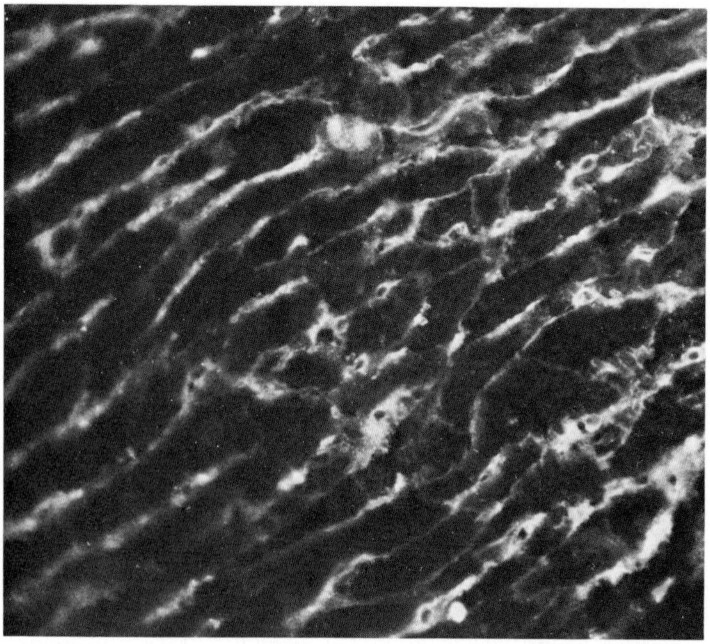

Fig. 6. Rat heart. Heterophile pattern to contrast with peripheral sarcoplasmic staining (Fig. 5). A similar pattern may be seen on skeletal muscle substrates. Although the heterophile antibody may occur after transfusion it is of no known diagnostic significance.

affected by a multitude of variables including substrate, optics and conjugate dilution, and these factors can be adjusted to allow screening at the dilution used for antinuclear factor and other antibodies (e.g. 1/5 or 1/10). We have not found undue staining with normal serum although some non-specific binding occurs partly because of reactivity between the Fc fragment and the I band.

By immunofluorescence, approximately 30% of all patients with myasthenia gravis have striational antibody. This rises to 90% (in our experience, virtually 100%) in patients with associated thymoma and approximately 25% of patients with a thymoma without obvious myasthenia gravis also have the antibody. Thus the antibody appears to be associated with the thymoma rather than with neuromuscular block *per se*. Its greatest usefulness is in indicating which patients need a thorough search for a thymoma as opposed to thymic hyperplasia. Patients with thymoma may have some form of auto-immune muscle disease unrelated to the presence of myasthenia or thymic hyperplasia.

Other methods have been used to detect anti-muscle antibodies. By haemagglutination using crude actomyosin (undoubtedly contaminated with other contractile proteins), antibody may be demonstrated in patients positive by immunofluorescence but also in a small proportion with either borderline or negative immunofluorescence. Immunodiffusion has also been used but may detect different antibodies e.g. "antimyosin".

Thus although anti-muscle antibody(s) demonstrated by immunofluorescence or haemagglutination may be useful for detection of patients with a thymoma, there is no evidence to suggest that the antibody is involved in the pathogenesis of neuromuscular block. Further evidence that these anti-muscle antibodies are unrelated to the presence of myasthenia *per se* comes from the work of Oosterhuis *et al.* (1966) which shows that there is no relationship between development of neonatal myasthenia and placental transfer of anti-muscle antibody. Accordingly the search for other auto-antibodies has continued. It has been claimed that patients with myasthenia gravis possess an anti-neuronal antibody but this has been refuted. More recently Almon *et al.* (1974) have reported that myasthenics may possess a serum factor (apparently IgG) which binds to the acetyl choline receptor. Further work on this is urgently required since it appears to be the most promising lead with regard to myasthenia itself.

Auto-antibodies other than anti-muscle antibody are common irrespective of whether there is a thymoma. Anti-nuclear factor, anti-thyroid (microsomal) and anti-parotid duct antibodies occur in approximately 30% of all patients. Anti-smooth muscle, anti-parietal cell, anti-mitochondrial and anti-reticulin may also occur with increased frequency but it has yet to be shown that such increases are statistically significant. The anti-nuclear factor is generally homogeneous or peripheral in type and occasionally double-stranded DNA binding may be found to be increased by the Farr assay. Speckled or nucleolar anti-nuclear antibody occurs in approximately 6% of all patients.

Hypocomplementaemia in myasthenia gravis may be related to activity but substantial fluctuations appear to be more characteristic than consistently low levels. Its nature has not been elucidated; C3, C4 and CH_{50} may be depressed but no clear pattern has emerged. The clinical significance of these findings is also unknown but they may relate in some way to the anti-acetyl choline receptor antibody. Hypocomplementaemia does not correlate with the presence of anti-muscle antibody.

Cell mediated immune competence appears to be normal in myasthenia gravis. Even after thymectomy many years previously we have been unable to demonstrate a defect in terms of response to ubiquitous antigens, PHA transformation or T-cell numbers. Evidence for specific cell mediated immunity directed against muscle has been reported (Dawkins, 1975). There may be inhibition of leucocyte migration by crude muscle antigens and it is claimed this is especially so in patients with anti-muscle antibody. The lymphocytes of some of the latter are cytotoxic to muscle, but the majority of patients with myasthenia gravis appear quite normal in this respect. Thus there may be both humoral and cell mediated auto-immunization against muscle in patients with thymoma but such hypersensitivity is unrelated to the presence of neuromuscular block. Studies with the acetyl choline receptor suggest that there may be cell mediated immunity parallel to the putative anti-receptor antibody (Abramsky *et al.*, 1975).

In contrast with evidence indicating that cell mediated competence is normal there are a number of reports of humoral immune deficiency associated with myasthenia gravis. Thus there may be mild to moderate hypogammaglobulinaemia together with reduced titres of isohaemagglutinins and antibodies against common organisms. In addition there is some evidence of poor responses to antigenic challenge with *S. typhi* and tetanus toxoid. It is relevant that humoral immune deficiency is a well known association of thymomata.

Recent work has demonstrated an association between myasthenia gravis and HLA antigens (Feltkamp *et al.*, 1974). Considering all patients there is an association with HLA-B8 but this is especially so in the younger females with thymic hyperplasia. In the older males with associated thymoma there may be an increase in the incidence of HLA-A2 but this remains controversial.

Associated Phenomena

Auto-immune Disease

As suggested by the high prevalence of anti-nuclear factor and other auto-antibodies some auto-immune disorders are associated with myasthenia gravis. Autoimmune thyroid disease, including Hashimoto's and Graves' disease occurs in as high as 20%. These associations are clinically important because of the influence that thyroid dysfunction has on the management of myasthenia gravis. Since deviation from the euthyroid state makes control of myasthenia particularly difficult, it is important to screen for thyroid auto-antibodies and to evaluate thyroid function. Systemic lupus erythematosus may also be associated with myasthenia gravis and/or thymoma. In the presence of antinuclear factor and hypocomplementaemia, SLE must be considered even if characteristic clinical features are lacking. Anti-DNA binding may be elevated in the absence of clinically obvious renal lupus. For these reasons it can be difficult to exclude a diagnosis of SLE, but every attempt should be made to do so before introducing prednisone therapy (see below). Other auto-immune diseases have also been found in association with myasthenia gravis but do not appear to be as important in statistical or therapeutic terms.

Thymic Hyperplasia

Although this is the most common feature associated with myasthenia gravis it is noteworthy that it may also occur with other auto-immune diseases in the absence of neuromuscular block. Its pathogenesis and significance remains uncertain. It has been suggested that excision or irradiation of a hyperplastic thymus may lead to beneficial effect in systemic lupus erythematosus but the data are meagre and provide no real support for the possibility that thymic hyperplasia in some way leads to these auto-immune processes. It appears equally likely that thymic hyperplasia is the consequence of some unidentified process which leads to auto-immune disease. It may be relevant that the hyperplastic thymus is reported to contain B-cells as well as T-cells and that mixed lymphocyte reactivity can be demonstrated between thymic and peripheral blood lymphocytes.

Thymoma

Myasthenia gravis is only one of an impressive list of disorders which may be found together with thymoma (Souadjian *et al.*, 1974). Cytopenias (including red cell agenesis and pancytopenia), hypogammaglobulinaemia and polymyositis are probably the best known but pemphigus, systemic lupus erythematosus, autoimmune thyroid disease and coeliac disease may also be associated. In addition patients with thymomata appear to have an increased frequency of carcinomas arising in other tissues.

Red cell agenesis has been attributed to the presence of an auto-antibody which reacts with red cell precursors. Improvement may be seen after removal of the thymoma.

Hypogammaglobulinaemia has been reported in association with thymoma in at least 25 cases. The histopathology of the thymoma varies, and immunological function also appears to vary, some patients having features suggesting impairment of cell mediated as well as of humoral immunity. The pathogenesis of the lesion is unknown. There has been no adequate study of immunological function in patients presenting with a thymoma and features other than overt clinical immunodeficiency.

Differential Diagnosis

Because of the rather distinctive clinical picture with predominant involvement of certain muscle groups, there is generally little difficulty in establishing a definite diagnosis of myasthenia gravis. Pharmacological confirmation is helpful although it should be emphasized that false positive responses can be obtained with anti-cholinesterase and it is necessary to include a placebo control. One approach to the standard edrophonium (tensilon) test is to quantify some form of weakness in terms of the number of repetitive movements or of ventilatory function and after an interval to allow recovery, to administer intravenous saline. Tests are then repeated and, after the same interval for recovery, 10 mg of edrophonium chloride is administered intravenously over 30 seconds. The tests are then repeated and any additional symptoms recorded. In myasthenia gravis there should be improvement between 1 and 5 minutes after the injection unless the patient has been overtreated with cholinergic therapy. Significant responses are sometimes found in disorders with fixed weakness e.g. polymyositis, so that the test is of real value only in confirming a clinical diagnosis and in determining whether or not anticholinesterase therapy is likely to be beneficial.

The major specific syndrome to be distinguished from myasthenia gravis is the Eaton-Lambert syndrome. This occurs in patients with oat cell carcinoma of the lung and very rarely other conditions. It is characterized by maximal involvement of proximal limb musculature and sparing of extra ocular muscles. There is usually no significance response to tensilon and electromyography reveals a marked incremental response on repetitive nerve stimulation rather than the typical decremental response of myasthenia gravis.

Treatment

Before commencing drug therapy it is important to consider the possibility of associated disease, discussed above. It may be possible to distinguish the neuromuscular block as separate from associated features such as thyrotoxic myopathy, polymyositis or the direct effects of an invasive thymoma, and to treat each condition separately.

For the neuromuscular block, initial therapy should be with anti-cholinesterases. Different workers vary in preference but one established regime is to use pyridostigmine, starting with 30–60 mg at 4–8 hourly intervals. Depending on response at different times of day, the dosage and frequency can be varied and it may be possible to use sustained release 180 mg capsules alone or in combination. It is important to appreciate that neuromuscular junctions at different sites vary in sensitivity so that some muscle groups may be adequately treated whilst others are over-treated. Since a cholinergic crisis may lead to weakness it is imperative to evaluate deterioration in muscle power carefully before increasing the dosage of anti-cholinesterase therapy. Atropine can be of value in treating cholinergic effects such as abdominal cramps.

Other forms of drug treatment therapy include spironolactone and potassium supplements, but the most important appears to be corticosteroid therapy. Initial usage of adrenocorticotrophic hormone suggested that, although some benefit could be seen, there was often a phase of deterioration. Corticosteroid therapy appeared to have little advantage but it has recently been reported that alternate-day prednisone may be given with relative impunity and frequently with substantial benefit. Low-dose prednisone with gradual increments has also been recommended.

A major consideration in therapy relates to the role of thymectomy. There is no universal agreement as to the precise indications and even to effectiveness but most agree that thymectomy should be considered at some stage in essentially all cases. It has been said that the best response is seen in young females with thymic hyperplasia but existing data are difficult to interpret and there is evidence that the greatest benefit is seen after excision during "early" disease. There is little doubt that thymectomy should be advised if the disease is generalized and severe and not readily controlled with anti-cholinesterases. Because myasthenia gravis may remit completely, and because some patients do very well after an initial period of anti-cholinesterase therapy, some believe it unwise to perform thymectomy in patients without a thymoma unless a trial of medical management has failed. Others argue for earlier thymectomy by a transcervical approach which avoids many of the hazards of thoracotomy. In patients with a thymoma most agree that excision should be undertaken. Since the behaviour of the tumour is unpredictable and since it can be locally invasive, if not metastasizing, thymectomy should be performed even if the myasthenia gravis is minimal. One of the major difficulties in evaluating the results of thymectomy is that apparent response may be delayed for weeks, months or even years. In these circumstances it is possible that the myasthenia has remitted for incidental reasons. Another difficulty is the problem of removing all of the thymus and it is often said that a poor response may reflect the persistence of aberrant gland. Further work is clearly required to resolve these issues.

If control has not been achieved with anti-cholinsterase therapy and thymectomy, prednisone appears to be the drug of choice.

Pathogenesis

There is little doubt that the neuromuscular block of myasthenia gravis is due to some humoral agent which interferes with neuromuscular transmission, presumably by inhibiting the reaction between acetyl choline and the acetyl choline receptor. In view of the epidemiology, the frequency of multiple auto-antibodies and the association with HLA-B8, Simpson's auto-immune hypothesis has gained increasing favour and it is generally accepted that an auto-antibody to the acetyl choline receptor would explain many of the observed features of the disease. The demonstration that myasthenia may be induced experimentally by immunizing with purified receptor (Patrick and Lindstrom, 1973) provides strong additional support. Furthermore there is now good evidence that patients with myasthenia gravis are hypersensitive to a receptor antigen. Preliminary reports of identification of an IgG antibody which reacts with the receptor are encouraging but there is no convincing evidence yet that this antibody is actually responsible for the neuromuscular block.

Many issues remain to be clarified. These include the relationship to thymic hyperplasia, the possible benefit of thymectomy and the significance of hypocomplementaemia and immune deficiency. It is of interest that myasthenia gravis can develop during penicillamine therapy given for rheumatoid arthritis (Bucknall *et al.*, 1975). We have also seen one patient who developed myasthenia gravis and thymic hyperplasia and anti-acetylcholine receptor antibody whilst receiving penicillamine for Wilson's disease. Furthermore, we have seen anti-striational antibody develop in 6 of 34 patients treated with penicillamine for rheumatoid arthritis. Penicillamine is known to lead to a reduction in serum immunoglobulin levels so that it is possible that it induces some subtle form of humoral immunodeficiency which allows the development of myasthenia gravis.

It remains to consider the significance of the anti-muscle antibody. As pointed out above, this antibody provides a useful means of screening for the presence of a thymoma associated with myasthenia gravis but it has never been shown to play a role in pathogenesis. Existing evidence suggests that it reflects auto-immunization against components of the sarcomere rather than the neuromuscular junction. It therefore appears more relevant to the myositis which is associated with thymoma and myasthenia.

POLYMYALGIA RHEUMATICA—TEMPORAL ARTERITIS

Polymyalgia rheumatica is a poorly defined entity which affects the middle-aged and elderly. Clinically it is characterized by the presence of diffuse and generally symmetrical muscle pain and stiffness in the absence of weakness and wasting. The erythrocyte sedimentation rate is elevated but other tests such as serum creatine kinase and muscle biopsy are normal. This combination suggests that the disease is due to inflammatory changes involving the interstitium or the attachment of muscle without any direct involvement of muscle parenchyma. The pathogenesis is unknown but it has been suggested that vascular antigens may be involved since lymphocyte transformation studies have shown evidence of hypersensitivity to crude homogenates of blood vessels (Hazelman *et al.*, 1975).

The differential diagnosis includes polymyositis but the distinction is generally straightforward. More difficulty is experienced in patients with early rheumatoid arthritis or its variants since there may be considerable pain and tenderness at a time when there is little evidence of true synovitis. Other causes of myalgia which should be considered include neuropathies, McArdle's syndrome and various forms of vasculitis. Endocrine conditions including hypercalcaemia, Addison's disease and hypothyroidism can also lead to poorly localized myalgia but again the distinction is generally straightforward if these conditions are carefully considered.

The major importance of polymyalgia rheumatica is probably that it is one form of presentation of giant cell arteritis and this condition can be extremely difficult to exclude with any confidence. In the absence of giant cell arteritis it is usual to treat polymyalgia with anti-inflammatory therapy or low dose corticosteroids and the response is often dramatic. If giant cell arteritis is suspected, however, high dose corticosteroid therapy is advisable although the precise indications remain somewhat controversial. Giant cell arteritis is discussed in Chapter 11.

RHEUMATIC FEVER

The immunology of cardiac diseases is discussed in Chapter 16.

Although histological evidence of skeletal muscle involvement is recognized in rheumatic fever this is of minimal significance clinically. The heart reactive antibody found in rheumatic fever cross-reacts with skeletal muscle and could lead to confusion in the laboratory (Nicholson *et al.*, 1975). Although the pattern of staining is subsarcolemmal or diffuse in skeletal as well as cardiac muscle and although there is no true striational staining, the superimposition of fluorescence and I band refractility can produce a superficial resemblance to the anti-striational antibody found in myasthenia gravis. Similarly the heterophile antibody which stains the interstitium of cardiac and skeletal muscle has sometimes been misinterpreted as indicating sarcolemmal staining and therefore rheumatic fever or the post-cardiac injury syndromes. Illustrations of these staining patterns are given in Figs 5 and 6.

ACKNOWLEDGEMENTS

I am grateful to Drs J. B. Peter and F. L. Mastaglia for valuable material and Miss J. Peers and Mr H. Upenieks for Fig. 1.

REFERENCES

Abramsky, O., Aharonov, A., Webb, C. and Fuchs, S. (1975). Cellular immune response to acetylcholine receptor-rich fraction in patients with myasthenia gravis. *Clin. Exp. Immunol.* **19**, 11–16.

Adams, R. D. (1975). "Diseases of Muscle", 3rd Ed., Harper Row, New York and London.
Almon, R. R., Andrew, C. G. and Appel, S. H. (1974). Serum globulin in myasthenia gravis: inhibition of α-bungarotoxin binding to acetylcholine receptors. *Science* **186**, 55–57.
Bohan, A. and Peter, J. B. (1975). Polymyositis and dermatomyositis: a critical review. *New Engl. J. Med.* **292**, 344–403.
Bourne, G. H. (1973). "The Structure and Function of Muscle. Volume III Physiology and Biochemistry". Academic Press, New York and London.
Bucknall, R. C., Dixon, A. St. J., Glick, E. N., Woodland, J. and Zutshi, D. W. (1975). Myasthenia gravis associated with penicillamine treatment for rheumatoid arthritis. *Brit. Med. J.* **i**, 600–2.
Dawkins, R. L. (1975). Experimental autoallergic myositis, polymyositis and myasthenia gravis: autoimmune muscle disease associated with immunodeficiency and neoplasia. *Clin. Exp. Immunol.* **21**, 185–201.
Douglas, A. C., Macleod, J. G. and Matthews, J. D. (1973). Symptomatic sarcoidosis of skeletal muscle. *J. Neurol. Neurosurg. Psychiat.* **36**, 1034–1040.
Feltkamp, T. E. W., Van den Berg-Loonen, P. M., Nijenhuis, L. E., Engelfriet, C. P., Van Rossum, A. L., Van Loghem, J. J. and Oosterhuis, H. J. G. H. (1974). Myasthenia gravis, autoantibodies and HL-A antigens. *Brit. Med. J.* **i**, 131–133.
Gardner-Thorpe, C. (1972). Muscle weakness due to sarcoid myopathy. *Neurology* **22**, 917–928.
Goldstein, G. and Schlesinger, D. H. (1975). Thymopoietin and myasthenia gravis: neostigmine-responsive neuromuscular block produced in mice by a synthetic peptide fragment of thymopoietin. *Lancet* **ii**, 256–259.
Hazelman, B. L., MacLennan, I. C. M. and Esiri, M. M. (1975). Lymphocyte proliferation to artery antigen as a positive diagnostic test in polymyalgia rheumatica. *Ann. Rheum. Dis.* **34**, 122–7.
Leddy, J. P., Griggs, R. C., Klemperer, M. R. and Frank, M. M. (1975). Hereditary complement (C2) deficiency with dermatomyositis. *Am. J. Med.* **58**, 83–90.
Metzger, A. L., Bohan, A., Goldberg, L. S., Bluestone, R. and Pearson, C. M. (1974). Polymyositis and dermatomyositis: combined methotrexate and corticosteroid therapy. *Ann. Intern. Med.* **81**, 182–189.
Nastuk, W. L., Plescia, O. J. and Osserman, K. E. (1960). Changes in complement activity in patients with myasthenia gravis. *Proc. Soc. Exp. Biol. Med.* **105**, 177–184.
Nicholson, C. G., Dawkins, R. L., Macdonald, B. L. and Wetherall, J. D. (1975). A classification of anti-heart antibodies: differentiation from a heterophile antibody. *Clin. Immunol. Immunopath.* (in press).
Osterhuis, H. J. G. H., Feltkamp, T. E. W. and Van der Geld, H. R. W. (1966). Muscle antibodies in myasthenic mothers and their babies. *Lancet* **ii**, 1226–7.
Patrick, J. and Lindstrom, J. (1973). Autoimmune response to acetylcholine receptor. *Science* **180**, 871–872.
Pearson, C. M. and Currie, S. M. (1974). *In* Walton, J. N. (1974).
Simpson, J. A. (1974). *In* Walton, J. N. (1974).
Souadjian, J. V., Enriquez, P., Silverstein, M. N. and Pépin, J-M. (1974). The spectrum of diseases associated with thymoma. *Arch. Intern. Med.* **134**, 374–379.
Strauss, A. J. L., Seegal, B. C., Hsu, K. C., Burkholder, P. M., Nastuk, W. L. and Osserman, K. E. (1960). Immunofluorescence demonstration of a muscle binding complement fixing system. *Proc. Soc. Exp. Biol. Med.* **105**, 184–191.
Walton, J. N. (1974). "Disorders of Voluntary Muscle", 3rd Edition, Churchill, Livingstone.
Whitaker, J. N. and Engel, W. K. (1972). Vascular deposits of immunoglobulins and complement in idiopathic inflammatory myopathy. *New Engl. J. Med.* **286**, 333–338.

ADDITIONAL READING

Aharonov, A., Abramsky, O., Tarrab-Hazdai, R. and Fuchs, S. (1975). Humoral antibodies to acetylcholine receptor in patients with myasthenia gravis. *Lancet* **ii**, 340–2.

Eisenberger, B. R., Kuda, A. M. and Peter, J. B. (1974). Stereological analysis of mammalian skeletal muscle: I. soleus muscle of the adult guinea-pig. *J. Cell Biol.* **60**, 732–754.

Lennon, V. A., Lindstrom, J. M. and Seybold, M. E. (1976). Experimental autoimmune myasthenia gravis: cellular and humoral immune responses. *Ann. N.Y. Acad. Sci.* **274**, 283.

Lindstrom, J., Lennon, V., Seybold, M. and Whittingham, S. (1976). Experimental autoimmune myasthenia gravis and myasthenia gravis: biochemical and immunochemical aspects. *Ann. N.Y. Acad. Sci.* **274**, 254.

25

Neurological Disease

R. A. C. HUGHES and S. LEIBOWITZ

Various factors modify the way in which immunological processes can affect nervous tissue. In the central nervous system (CNS) the most important of these is the blood–brain barrier which restricts the entry of both antibody and antigen and limits their diffusion into the intercellular space. This is exemplified by the low immunoglobulin levels in the cerebrospinal fluid (CSF) compared with interstitial fluid elsewhere. The nervous system also lacks organized lymphoid structures and contains few lymphocytes. To mount an immune reaction antibody and/or sensitized cells must enter the CNS from the blood stream. These limitations are more apparent than real since they only apply to the brain under normal conditions. Once an inflammatory lesion is established, whether due to infection or hypersensitivity, these barriers become modified. Antibody, complement, lymphocytes and macrophages enter the central nervous system and immunological reactions can then proceed much as in any other tissue. Increased vascular permeability also permits antigens to reach the lymphoreticular organs via the blood stream. The absence of conventional lymphatic channels probably delays rather than prevents an immune response. The brain has been considered to be an immunologically privileged site but this is a relative rather than an absolute state. Reactions to tumours, grafts, viruses and other antigens do occur, although they are often muted and frequently delayed.

In one respect the CNS is more, rather than less, vulnerable to immunological tissue damage. This is in its exquisite sensitivity to anoxia and the consequences of oedema. All immunological reactions involve some degree of vascular damage and in the brain the effects of severe inflammatory oedema are frequently more serious than in other tissues and often irreversible.

IMMUNOGLOBULINS IN THE CENTRAL NERVOUS SYSTEM

The intercellular fluid of the central nervous system contains extremely low levels of plasma proteins, including the immunoglobulins. It forms the internal environment of the closely packed cells of the brain and is contained in minute channels which communicate with the CSF. Electron microscopic studies have shown that the fluid in the ventricles and the subarachnoid and intercellular space constitutes a single compartment. The composition of the CSF thus reflects that of the fluid in direct contact with neural cells and their processes.

The bulk of the cerebrospinal fluid is formed from the plasma by the choroid plexus. Water, electrolytes and protein diffuse from the choroid vessels into the interstitial tissue of the plexus. An ultrafiltrate of this interstitial fluid then passes across the choroidal basement membrane and epithelium into the ventricles. The meningeal vessels also make a significant contribution and a similar filtrate enters the intercellular space via the cerebral capillaries. In this way a protein concentration of 7500 mg/100 ml in the plasma is reduced to 20–40 mg/100 ml in the CSF, a reduction of about 250:1. Smaller molecules such as albumin cross the barrier with greater facility and the immunoglobulin albumin ratio of the serum is much higher than that of the CSF.

Estimates of the CSF IgG level vary slightly with the method used but the range is generally given as 1–4 mg/100 ml. This represents about 4–11% of the total protein. The IgA concentration is 0·0–0·4 mg/100 ml. IgD, IgE and IgM are undetectable in normal cerebrospinal fluid.

CSF Immunoglobulins in Disease

Raised immunoglobulin levels in the CSF may be due to 1) increased levels in the serum, 2) increased permeability of the blood–brain barrier, or 3) local synthesis of antibody within the nervous system (Heremans, 1966; Laterre, 1973; Lumsden, 1972).

Raised levels secondary to an increase in serum antibody are seen in the paraproteinaemias where the occurrence of paraprotein bands identical to those in the serum is a common finding. The majority are IgG or IgA myelomas. In macroglobulinaemia the abnormal band probably consists of light chains or a monomeric 7S variety of IgM as neither the larger 19S IgM nor the higher polymers of IgA can pass the intact blood/CSF barrier. It is possible that some increase in CSF immunoglobin levels also occurs in association with polyclonal increases in circulating antibody in conditions such as chronic infections, some auto-allergic disorders and some forms of liver disease, but little information is available on this point.

In conditions associated with enhanced permeability of the blood–brain barrier CSF antibody levels are elevated in proportion to the increase in total protein and there may be little or no percentage increase. Thus the IgG level may rise well above the normal upper limit of 5 mg/100 ml without constituting more than 11% of the total protein concentration. IgA may also increase and IgM may appear in the CSF. These changes may be found in many infections such as acute bacterial meningitis, viral meningitis and encephalitis, and acute poliomyelitis (Table 1). A similar pattern can also be seen in chronic inflammatory conditions, including tuberculous meningitis as well as in primary or secondary intracranial malignancies. An increase in total protein and immunoglobulin levels also occurs in cerebrovascular disease, even in the absence of frank haemorrhage; in diabetes with or without overt neurological complications; and in a variety of non-infective inflammatory conditions such as systemic lupus erythematosus (Table 2). An increase in vascular permeability is usually inferred by noting the fairly normal Ig/total protein ratio although in some cases it has been possible to obtain direct evidence by measuring the rate at which radiolabelled protein injected intravenously enters the cerebrospinal fluid.

A CSF protein pattern very similar to that due to increased permeability may be found in the fluid below a lesion obstructing the subarachnoid space. This occurs in obstructive hydrocephalus or below a spinal block due to any cause. The fluid below the obstruction contains an increase in immunoglobulin as well as total protein. The meningeal vessels normally contribute to the formation of the CSF and the composition of this transudate approximates more closely to that of the serum than does the choroid plexus ultrafiltrate. When the flow of CSF is obstructed the fluid below the site of obstruction is entirely meningeal in origin and therefore contains higher levels of serum protein including immunoglobulin.

Antibody Synthesis in the CNS

Under pathological conditions antibody may be synthesized locally within the CNS and an isolated or disproportionate increase in CSF immunoglobulin levels is seen in several disorders. Multiple sclerosis and subacute sclerosing panencephalitis (SSPE) provide two of the most striking examples but many chronic and subacute inflammatory diseases of the nervous system

TABLE 1

Typical CSF changes in meningitis

	Appearance	Cells per µl	Protein g/l	IgG g/l	Glucose mmol/l	Comment
Normal	clear colourless	0–5	<0·4	0·01–0·04	2·8–4·6	
Bacterial	usually cloudy	polymorph pleocytosis	increased	increased	decreased	
Tuberculosis	clear or cloudy	mixed pleocytosis	increased	increased	decreased	may be normal in earliest stages
Viral	clear or opalescent	lymphocyte pleocytosis	mildly increased	normal or increased	usually normal	
Cerebral abscess	clear	mixed	normal or increased	normal or increased	normal	LP dangerous
Carcinomatous	clear	often normal	increased	normal or increased	decreased	neoplastic cells identifiable

TABLE 2

Typical CSF changes in other neurological disorders

	Cells per µl	Protein g/l	IgG		Comment
			g/l	% Total protein	
Spinal block	usually normal	> 1·0	increased	normal	
Multiple sclerosis	lymphocyte pleocytosis (25%)[a]	slightly increased	increased (67%)[a]	increased (67%)[a]	oligoclonal increase in γ-globulin (95%)[a] raised CSF/serum measles antibody ratio
Guillain–Barré syndrome	normal	usually increased	increased	increased	
SLE	increased (30%)[a]	slightly increased (50%)	increased	increased	low C4 levels
Spongiform encephalopathies (e.g. Jakob–Kreutzfeldt disease)	normal	normal	normal	normal	

[a] Percentage of patients showing this change.

show a similar pattern. These include neurosyphilis, chronic lymphocytic choriomeningitis, trypanosomiasis, tuberculous meningitis and brain abscess. Even in acute bacterial meningitis local antibody production may be superimposed on an increase in vascular permeability. This increase in the proportion of immunoglobulin to total protein in the CSF may occur in patients with normal or near normal levels of total protein, as in multiple sclerosis, or associated with a markedly raised protein level as in many cases of neurosyphilis. Radiolabelled IgG has been injected into patients with multiple sclerosis and subacute sclerosing panencephalitis and the rate of its accumulation in the CSF measured. In both cases the CSF immunoglobulin level in these patients could not possibly be explained by transfer across the blood–brain barrier. Further confirmation was provided by the observation that the antibody in the CSF of these patients is not only increased but also of relatively restricted heterogeneity. When the CSF proteins of patients with multiple sclerosis are separated by agar or starch gel electrophoresis, discrete bands may be identified in the globulin region. The pattern differs markedly from that in the serum. Similar oligoclonal restriction has been observed in SSPE, the Guillain–Barré syndrome and neurosyphilis. In SSPE and multiple sclerosis it has also been observed that the ratio of κ to λ light chains in the CSF may differ from that in the serum. The implication of these findings is that antibody may be produced locally in neurological disease and is frequently derived from a limited number of plasma cell clones.

IgA and IgM may also be formed in the nervous system. A striking instance of the latter is that of a seventeen-year-old boy with combined immunodeficiency and a chronic progressive encephalopathy. He had IgM in the CSF although it was undetectable in the serum. When detectable, the appearance of IgM in the CSF usually precedes that of both IgG and IgA. In some diseases e.g. syphilis and trypanosomiasis, IgM levels remain high in the chronic phase. In both diseases there is evidence to suggest that some of this antibody is produced within the nervous system.

In most of the diseases mentioned above lymphoid cells in varying degrees of differentiation are found within the CNS. Lymphocytes and plasma cells may be found in the meninges, CSF or in perivascular accumulations of inflammatory cells. In cerebral trypanosomiasis, a special type of vacuolated plasma cell, the "morular cell" of Mott is present in the CSF. Direct evidence that lymphoid cells from the CNS are able to form antibody is that lymphocytes from the CSF of patients with multiple sclerosis are capable of synthesizing immunoglobulin in tissue culture (Cohen and Bannister, 1967).

HYPERSENSITIVITY IN THE NERVOUS SYSTEM

Reaginic Type Reactions

We know very little about immediate-type hypersensitivity in the nervous system. The cerebral vessels respond to histamine and it must be assumed that they are involved to some degree in systemic anaphylactic shock, although the effect is imperceptible against the general background of respiratory and circulatory failure. Local cerebral anaphylaxis has never been convincingly demonstrated in experimental animals or in man.

Mast cells are found in the meningeal connective tissue, the choroid plexus and the walls of the large cerebral blood vessels. They are also present in the epineurium and perineurium of the peripheral nerves.

Although reaginic reactions probably do occur in the meninges they are unlikely to take place in the brain parenchyma itself.

There have been reports of transient encephalopathies accompanied by urticaria and other manifestations of anaphylaxis. There have also been cases of encephalopathy following vaccination (against influenza and poliomyelitis) in which cerebral manifestations appeared so rapidly as to suggest an immediate-type reaction. In all these formal proof of reaginic hypersensitivity is lacking.

Direct Effects of Antibody

The low levels of antibody which are present in the extravascular space make it unlikely that circulating antibody to neural antigens is capable of initiating immunological damage within the CNS. High titres of circulating antibody to myelin components, such as the encephalitogenic basic protein or galactocerebroside, may be present in the serum of experimental animals without evidence of neurological disease. The one exception is antibody to antigens present in the vascular endothelium. Massive cerebral damage can be produced in guinea-pig brains by the intra-arterial injection of antisera to the Forssman hapten, which is an endothelial component. This does not mean that antibody to neural elements cannot play a role in established disease. In experimental allergic encephalomyelitis, it is conceivable that once the vascular barrier has been breached by the cell mediated auto-immune reaction to myelin, the presence of circulating antibody may have an important role in the pathology. This might take the form of a damaging cytotoxic effect, a protective blockade of cell mediated damage i.e. "enhancement" or an effect on the phagocytosis of myelin debris.

Similar considerations apply in the case of auto-antibody to neural components in man. So far only one has been investigated in any detail. This is the complement-dependent demyelinating factor described by Bornstein (1969). It has been found in the serum of patients with multiple sclerosis as well as some other neurological diseases but its role in pathogenesis is uncertain.

Immune Complex Lesions

The therapeutic administration of foreign serum may give rise to neurological as well as systemic disease. Rarely the former may predominate or even be the sole manifestation.

In the early days of serum therapy intrathecal injections were occasionally given, sometimes resulting in massive necrosis of the brain and spinal cord. Thus both serum sickness and the Arthus reaction may cause lesions in the nervous system. The basic pathology in both forms of immune complex disease is a fibrinoid necrosis of the small vessels. Similar lesions are present in acute haemorrhagic leucoencephalitis although there are no other positive pointers towards an immune complex pathogenesis. Some of the neurological manifestations of connective tissue disorders may be due to damage via immune complexes. Polyarteritis nodosa may affect the central as well as the peripheral nervous system and a rather different kind of vascular damage in the basal ganglia may be responsible for the choreic complications of rheumatic fever.

In experimental animals with serum sickness it has been shown that immune complexes and complement may be deposited in the choroid plexus as well as the renal glomerulus. Similar deposits have been detected in patients with systemic lupus erythematosus. It is possible that the neurological manifestations in this disease might be explained in this way and may cause subtle changes in the CSF. This does not explain the alterations in cerebral function.

As yet there are few neurological diseases which can be attributed to immune complex deposition with any degree of certainty. Nevertheless, further investigation may prove this to be an important aspect of immunopathology in the nervous system.

Cell Mediated Immunity

The most clearly understood hypersensitivity reactions in the nervous system are those due to cell mediated immunity. Since antigens cannot be injected into the brain without injuring tissue and disrupting the blood–brain barrier, direct experimentation is difficult to interpret. Two alternative experimental models—both involving cell mediated immunity indirectly—have been skilfully exploited and analysed. The first of these is experimental allergic encephalomyelitis (EAE), an auto-immune reaction to myelin. The second comprises a group of acute viral diseases of which acute lymphocytic chorio-meningitis in mice has proved the most instructive. EAE provides a model for a cell mediated reaction to a normal brain component. Hypersensitivity in viral disease illustrates the nature of the response to extrinsic antigens. The most significant finding to emerge from these investigations is that the basic pattern of the reaction is much the same in both.

Delayed hypersensitivity reactions in the nervous system produce an acute disseminated meningo-encephalomyelitis. The main histological feature is the accumulation of mononuclear cells, lymphocytes, macrophages and occasional plasma cells. There is also an increase in vascular permeability with protein extravasation and oedema. In the closely packed brain parenchyma this takes the form of perivascular cuffing and cerebral oedema. In the meninges the cellular accumulations are more diffuse and mononuclear cells enter the subarachnoid space. In hyperacute disease polymorphonuclear cells may also be present and there may be vascular necrosis.

It is often assumed that the immunological reaction to myelin can easily be distinguished from that to an extrinsic antigen by the occurrence of demyelination, but the degree of demyelination in EAE may be minimal and demyelination may occur in association with viral disease, as can be seen in the lesions of canine distemper. Whether the myelin destruction in the latter is due to the direct action of the virus, to delayed hypersensitivity to viral antigens or to the triggering of an auto-immune reaction against the myelin sheath is uncertain. The fact remains that it is not possible at present to distinguish cell mediated reactions to extrinsic antigens from those to myelin components by the presence or absence of demyelination. This is an important and unsolved problem in such human demyelinating diseases as post-vaccinial encephalomyelitis.

Increased vascular permeability is an important element in all delayed hypersensitivity reactions. In the CNS the vascular changes are of major importance in the development of the neurological signs. In both experimental allergic encephalomyelitis and hypersensitivity to viruses it is probably the cerebral oedema rather than cytotoxicity, inflammatory cell accumulation or demyelination which determines the symptomatology and the clinical course of the disease.

EXPERIMENTAL ALLERGIC ENCEPHALOMYELITIS

Experimental allergic encephalomyelitis (EAE) demonstrates clearly the effects of an auto-immune reaction against CNS antigens. It is produced by injecting animals with CNS tissue with adjuvant. The severity of the illness depends on the species used and the nature of the encephalitogenic emulsion. Animals may have histological lesions with no overt disease, transient illness after a latent period of 10 to 14 days or a rapidly fatal severe disease. The course is always acute and monophasic, unlike the chronic relapsing course of multiple sclerosis with which it is so often compared. Even before the appearance of neurological signs infiltration of lymphocytes and macrophages and leakage of immunoglobulin into the CNS parenchyma can be detected. Substantial perivascular collections of inflammatory cells form round the vessels of the brain and spinal cord and there is some loss of myelin immediately outside these cuffs (Figs. 1 and 2). The transient nature of the illness in some animals, in spite of persistent severe perivascular infiltration, suggests that the amount and rate of accumulation of oedema are important factors in producing the neurological deficit.

Encephalitogenic Antigens

The encephalitogenic component of central nervous tissue has been localized to the acid-extractable cationic basic protein of myelin (Dunkley and Carnegie, 1974). It is difficult to obtain a truly homogeneous preparation of basic protein, which may represent a family of closely related proteins. Nevertheless, the fragment of human and bovine basic protein responsible for producing EAE in the guinea-pig has been identified by enzyme digestion of the whole protein as:

(Ser—Arg-) Phe—Ser—Trp—Gly—Ala—Glu—Gly—Gln—Arg or Lys

This has been confirmed by showing that the identical synthetic peptide is also encephalitogenic. Investigation of analogues of this peptide showed that the N-terminal serine and arginine residues were not necessary, and that the essential components are tryptophan and glutamine and arginine or lysine separated by any four amino acid residues i.e.:

– – Trp – – – – Gln, Arg or Lys

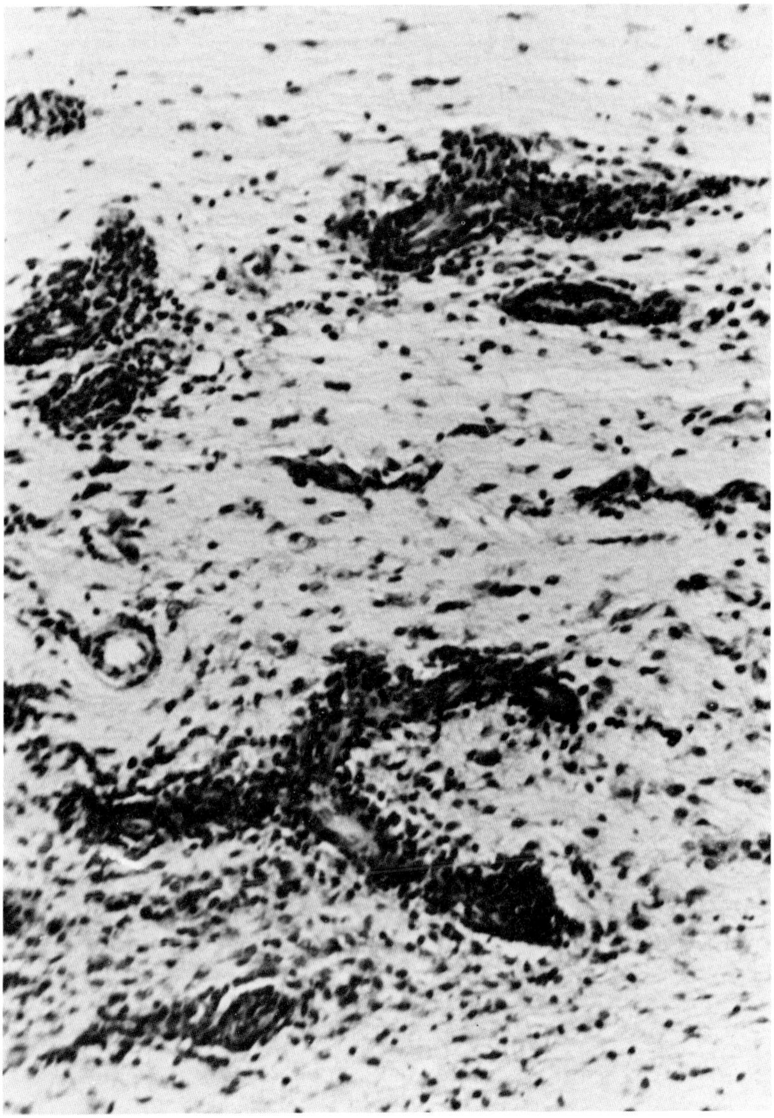

Fig. 1. Experimental allergic encephalomyelitis in the rabbit. Vessels surrounded by inflammatory cells forming a cuff and infiltrating the parenchyma. Cresyl violet. ×130.

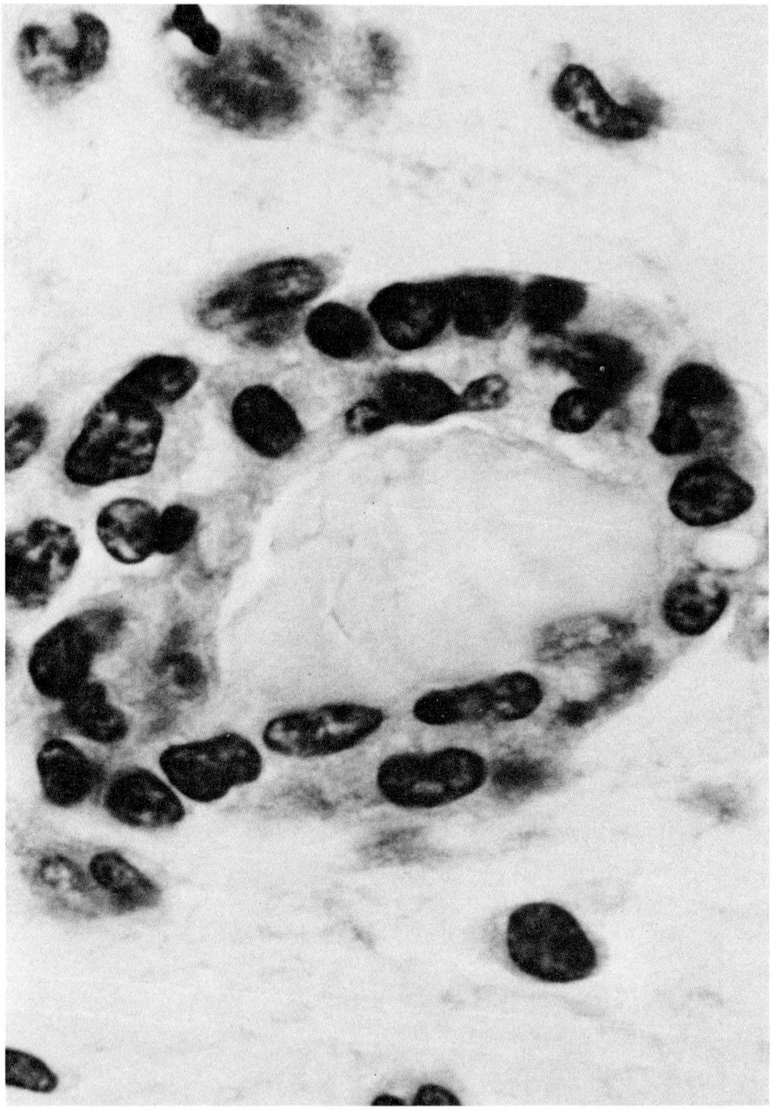

Fig. 2. Experimental allergic encephalomyelitis. High power view of perivascular cuff of inflammatory cells. H and E. ×1280.

While this part of human and bovine basic protein is the most encephalitogenic in guinea-pigs, the encephalitogenic fragment is not constant from species to species. For instance, the C-terminal region of the whole molecule is encephalitogenic in monkeys and yet another fragment has such an activity in the rat. We have no information as to which component is encephalitogenic in man.

Detailed knowledge about the chemical specificity of EAE is now accumulating rapidly and has given rise to some intriguing attempts to protect animals from EAE by immunization with chemically modified basic proteins. Chemical modification of the vital tryptophan residue with 2-hydroxy-5-nitrobenzyl bromide produces a compound which is not encephalitogenic but protects guinea-pigs from developing EAE in response to a subsequent challenge with unmodified basic protein.

Cellular Responses

A cell mediated immune reaction of the delayed hypersensitivity type is regarded as the major factor in the production of EAE because it can be transferred from animal to animal with lymphocytes but not with serum. The importance of T-cell rather than B-cell responses is suggested by the development of EAE in bursectomized agammaglobulinaemic chickens but not in thymectomized birds with depressed cell mediated immunity. This conclusion is supported by the occurrence of delayed hypersensitivity skin reactions to homologous basic protein in guinea-pigs shortly before the appearance of the disease. Under ordinary conditions there is a reasonable correlation between positive *in vitro* tests associated with cellular immunity, lymphocyte transformation and macrophage migration inhibition, and the occurrence of EAE.

A complicating feature is that the encephalitogenic properties of basic proteins can be dissociated from the responses they elicit in conventional tests of cellular immunity. Guinea-pigs immunized with synthetic encephalitogenic peptides develop EAE but do not show cellular immunity to whole basic protein by skin testing, lymphocyte transformation or macrophage migration inhibition. Conversely guinea-pigs immunized with the non-encephalitogenic 2-hydroxy-5-nitrobenzy bromide treated basic protein show cellular immunity to untreated basic protein by all these criteria and yet do not develop EAE (Spitler *et al.*, 1972). These experiments suggest that the encephalitogenic determinant is a different part of the basic protein molecule from that producing these other manifestations of cell mediated immunity.

The Role of Antibody

Antibodies to myelin, basic protein and galactocerebroside have been demonstrated by many techniques during the course of the disease. In rats antibody against basic protein produced in the course of EAE is directed largely against parts of the molecule other than the main encephalitogenic determinant (McFarlin *et al.*, 1975). EAE serum also contains complement dependent 7S antibody which demyelinates cultures *in vitro* (Bornstein, 1969). The antigen responsible is not basic protein but may be galactocerebroside (Fry *et al.*, 1974). EAE serum has been shown to block polysynaptic conduction in CNS tissue cultures (Bornstein, 1969). A major role for antibody in the production of disease is unlikely because EAE can be induced with minute doses of basic protein which produce no detectable antibody, cannot be transferred with serum, and can be produced in agammaglobulinaemic chickens. Nevertheless demonstration that EAE is a function of T-cells by transfer of purified sensitized T-cells has not yet been attempted.

Host Susceptibility

There is great variation in susceptibility to EAE between species and between strains within species. Guinea-pigs develop florid EAE with small doses of encephalitogen whereas rats and mice are relatively resistant. Genetic studies of EAE in different rat strains have shown that susceptibility is inherited as a Mendelian dominant character closely linked but not identical with the major histocompatibility locus. More recently it has been shown that the susceptible Lewis strain gives positive skin tests and lymphocyte transformation and MIF production tests for cell mediated immunity, and also produces antibody to the fragment of basic protein which is encephalitogenic in rats, while the resistant Brown Norway strain does not react in any of these ways (McFarlin *et al.*, 1975). These results suggest that susceptibility to EAE is dependent on a gene which controls all types of immune response to myelin basic protein.

Prevention of the Disease

Antiserum to whole CNS inhibits the disease in rats if given during the latent period after injection of the encephalitogenic emulsion and before the development of the disease. This is not a very powerful effect and cannot be demonstrated after neurological signs have appeared. Attempts to protect guinea-pigs from EAE with lymphocytes from resistant donors have been unsuccessful, but it is interesting that in rats repeated transfers of sensitized lymphocytes produce successively less severe disease. This might be interpreted as due to protective cells preventing the encephalitogenic effect of the subsequent transfers. The development of EAE in monkeys and guinea-pigs has been prevented by the intravenous injection of basic protein. It is possible that basic protein is released during the induction of EAE and eventually reaches a level at which the immune response is suppressed.

Whether the termination of EAE is due to an active inhibitory immune response or exhaustion of a supply of sensitized cells is an unsolved problem. When ways of treating comparable human disease are being considered, it may be of more practical value to know that EAE can be treated effectively with steroids, immunosuppressive drugs like cyclophosphamide and with anti-lymphocyte serum.

EXPERIMENTAL ALLERGIC NEURITIS

Experimental allergic neuritis (EAN) is the peripheral nervous system counterpart of EAE. In 1955 Waksman and Adams injected rabbits with an emulsion of peripheral nerve and adjuvant and produced an illness consisting of weakness and ataxia with subsequent recovery, with the histological appearance of an extensive polyneuritis. This experimental model closely resembles the Guillain–Barré syndrome (Arnason, 1971).

Relevant Antigens

The neuritogenic determinant resides in the myelin fraction and by analogy with EAE might be expected to be a basic protein. Bovine peripheral nerve myelin contains two basic proteins. One of these is similar to the CNS myelin basic protein A1 and is both neuritogenic and encephalitogenic.

Another basic protein P11 with a different amino-acid sequence and a molecular weight of 14,200 daltons is absent from CNS myelin and is purely neuritogenic (Abramsky *et al*., 1975a).

The earliest pathological events in EAN are passage of lymphocytes and mononuclear cells through the walls of the vasa nervorum, aggregation of these cells around the vessels and demyelination of the surrounding nerve fibres. At the ultrastructural level there is retraction of myelin from the nodes and penetration of macrophage processes through the Schwann cell basement membrane, and into the myelin sheath. At sites in close relation to macrophages and lymphocytes, the myelin disintegrates and forms bubbles. Electron microscopic studies suggest that cells, and particularly macrophages, are important in the breakdown of myelin.

Mechanisms of Damage

Cell mediated immunity is more important than humoral antibody in EAN as in EAE. EAN is transferable by intravenous injection of sensitized lymphocytes into irradiated rabbits and by intraneural injection of lymphocytes in rats. During the course of the disease lymphocyte transformation in response to whole peripheral nerve or isolated basic protein and MIF production with basic protein is demonstrable. Antibodies to peripheral nerve basic protein, which cross-react with CNS basic protein, are also detected. Complement-dependent antibodies which demyelinate cultures of peripheral nerve ganglia are demonstrable but the myelinotoxic effect of lymphocytes is more impressive than that of serum. It is doubtful whether any of the demonstrated antibodies have much pathogenetic significance because anti-peripheral nerve serum does not appear harmful *in vivo* even when injected directly into the nerve.

Course of the Disease

The disease is monophasic and relatively mild compared with EAE. Animals usually recover completely. The pathological appearances suggest a more chronic process with concurrent evidence of remyelination and persistent inflammatory cell infiltration. As in EAE, there must be an effective mechanism capable of inhibiting the auto-immune response and preventing progressive neuritis and death. Previous injections of nerve in saline before injection of the neuritogenic emulsion protect animals from developing EAN in response to subsequent immunization with nerve in adjuvant. The fact that antiserum to nerve prevents the myelinotoxic action of sensitized lymphocytes *in vitro* suggests that antibody may inhibit the production of EAN, as has been suggested in EAE (Arnason, 1971). Steroids and immunosuppressive drugs have not been tried in EAN, but by analogy with EAE they might be expected to prevent it or reduce its severity.

Two naturally occurring forms of peripheral neuropathy deserve consideration in relation to EAN and as possible models of the Guillain–Barré syndrome. Dogs may develop coon-hound paralysis, an acute polyneuritis with inflammatory lesions and segmental demyelination resembling EAN, about 14 days after being bitten by a raccoon. No virus has yet been isolated and immunological studies have not been done. Chickens with fowl paralysis (Marek's disease) develop a generalized lymphoma with infiltration and demyelination of peripheral nerves. The disease is due to a herpes virus which can be found in the Schwann cells. Most of the lymphocytes in the nerve are T-cells and the disease is made worse by bursectomy. The cause of Marek's disease is clearly the herpes virus, but the cause of coon-hound paralysis is unknown. The peripheral neuritis in both is so similar that an EAN-like mechanism seems likely.

IMMUNITY TO VIRUSES IN THE CENTRAL NERVOUS SYSTEM

The nervous system is unique in presenting a barrier to the entry of viruses as well as the agents of immunity, such as antibody, lymphocytes and inflammatory cells. Within the brain virus diseases show a wide variation in pattern, reflecting both the nature of the organism and the character of the immune response. The spectrum extends from acute meningoencephalitis at one end to persistent, "slow" and latent infection at the other.

Routes of Entry of Viruses

The majority of viral infections in the CNS enter the brain via the blood stream. Apart from a few special cases such as rabies, the modern view is to regard them as complications of systemic infection rather than as neurotropic in the classical sense (Johnson and Mims, 1968a, b). The main defences therefore lie outside the nervous system. Many of the common viruses including mumps, chicken pox, measles and herpes simplex are spread by the respiratory route. Others such as the enteroviruses, which include poliomyelitis, are primarily infections of the gastrointestinal tract. The arborviruses on the other hand are directly injected into the blood stream by insect bites. All these must run the gauntlet of the general body defences before reaching the brain.

The poliovirus, for example, has to survive humoral and cellular immunity in the gut, lymphoid tissue and blood stream. It must then proliferate (at primary and secondary sites) and maintain a degree of viraemia sufficient to breach the CNS barrier.

Viruses in general may enter the brain across the cerebral capillaries, infecting adjacent glia or neurones, or involve the choroid plexus and enter the CSF. This formidable array of defences explains why infection of the brain is a rare event despite the large number of potential pathogens.

Subsequent Events

Once inside the nervous system the reaction it evokes depends upon the behaviour of the virus. If it enters a susceptible cell and persists without replicating or producing cytopathic effects an inflammatory response does not follow. In the closely packed brain parenchyma it may even spread from cell to cell without perceptible reaction. On the other hand proliferation of virus and destruction of the infected cell results in an acute inflammatory reaction to the breakdown products, and may also give rise to cell mediated immunity which releases virus. In either case there is a complete breakdown of the barrier which normally excludes the effectors of the immune response from the CNS. The virus is then exposed to the action of antibody, complement components, macrophages and lymphocytes. Similar consequences may follow expression of viral coded antigen on the host cell surface.

The Immunological Response

The protective effect of inflammation due to specific sensitization has been demonstrated in several animal models. One of the most convincing is Sindbis virus infection in mice. Intracerebral inoculation of the virus is followed by an inflammatory reaction which correlates with a decline in the viral content of the brain. Cyclophosphamide inhibits inflammation and allows the virus to flourish. Both the inflammatory reaction and the ability to inhibit viral replication can be restored by the transfer of lymph node cells from immunized animals. Serum antibody is ineffective and so is transfer of cells from normal animals. These experiments indicate that cell mediated reactions play an important role in viral immunity in the brain. Their effect is to release the virus from its protected environment in the interior of the cell and to generate an inflammatory reaction which brings the full weight of cellular and humoral immunity to bear across the CNS barrier.

With certain viruses delayed hypersensitivity may prove harmful, converting a relatively innocuous infection into a potentially lethal disease. The most striking instance is that of lymphocytic choriomeningitis infection in the mouse (Cole and Nathanson, 1974). In nature, mice may harbour the virus for life and mothers transmit it across the placenta to their offspring, which become carriers harbouring the virus in the cells of the brain, spleen and other tissues. Viral antigen can be demonstrated by immunofluorescent staining in the neurones and the glia. Despite this the animals have no neurological disease. They remain perfectly healthy, although a proportion may develop glomerular disease in later life due to the accumulation of antigen, antibody complexes in the renal glomerulus. The virus itself is harmless and the immune response minimal. The viral antigens appear to induce a state of partial or low grade tolerance.

In the adult, intracerebral inoculation of the virus does not lead to tolerance or a carrier state, but to an acute meningo-encephalitis. This is not due to the virus itself, but to a cell mediated immune reaction to viral antigens. The disease can be prevented or inhibited by immunosuppressive drugs, neonatal thymectomy and anti-lymphocyte serum. These animal models demonstrate very clearly that immunological reactions, and cell mediated responses in particular, may damage as well as protect. In some cases they provide immunity, in others they merely compound the injury and hypersensitivity may itself constitute a major part of the disease.

Examples in Man

Hypersensitivity is thought to play a role in a number of important viral diseases in man. Foremost among these are the acute disseminated encephalomyelitides which may follow some common viral infections or vaccination (Weiner *et al.*, 1973). They occur with acute exanthematous diseases such as measles, varicella or rubella, and after influenza. Typically the disease follows 4–11 days after the appearance of the rash and is characterized by an acute encephalomyelitis with perivenular accumulations of inflammatory cells and demyelination. A similar condition may occur as a rare complication of vaccination against smallpox. A number of features suggest that the lesion may be due to hypersensitivity. The first is the time interval between the acute exanthem and the onset of neurological disease. The second is the histological similarity of lesions due to quite different viruses and the fact that inclusion bodies or other morphological indications of viral infection are lacking (Fig. 3). It has also proved difficult to recover virus from affected brain.

Despite these indications there is no direct evidence of hypersensitivity and it is still uncertain whether this acute demyelinating lesion is due to sensitivity to viral antigens, to auto-immunity to components of the myelin sheath or to the direct action of the virus itself.

The Role of Immunodeficiency

Defects of cell mediated immunity predispose to viral infections, including those affecting the nervous system (Allison, 1972). Such defects are found in the Swiss-type combined immunodeficiency, ataxia telangectasia and in the Wiskott–Aldrich and Di George syndromes. They also occur secondarily in Hodgkin's disease, and following cancer chemotherapy or immunosuppressive treatment for transplantation. In all these conditions recurrent virus infections may occur. Measles, cytomegalovirus, vaccinia, herpes simplex (HSV) and herpes zoster (HZV) are among those which may involve the nervous system.

Herpes Viruses

The most interesting of these infections are those, such as HSV and HZV, which are due to the reactivation of a latent virus. In both diseases there is evidence that the virus remains latent in the ganglia of the peripheral and cranial nerves. Reactivation results in the passage of the virus down the sensory axon with the development of an associated skin eruption. The mechanism of reactivation is unknown. However, its occurrence in immunodeficiency states suggests that imperfect responses play a part in the breakdown of equilibrium between virus and host.

Evidence on the role of antibody is contradictory. In man there is little correlation between the serum level of neutralizing antibody to HSV and recurrence of the disease. In experimental lesions in mice, on the other hand, IgG antibody inhibits the reappearance of infectious virus.

Multi-focal Leucoencephalopathy

An extremely rare disease of the brain which has also been attributed to immune depression is progressive multi-focal leucoencephalopathy. This is a

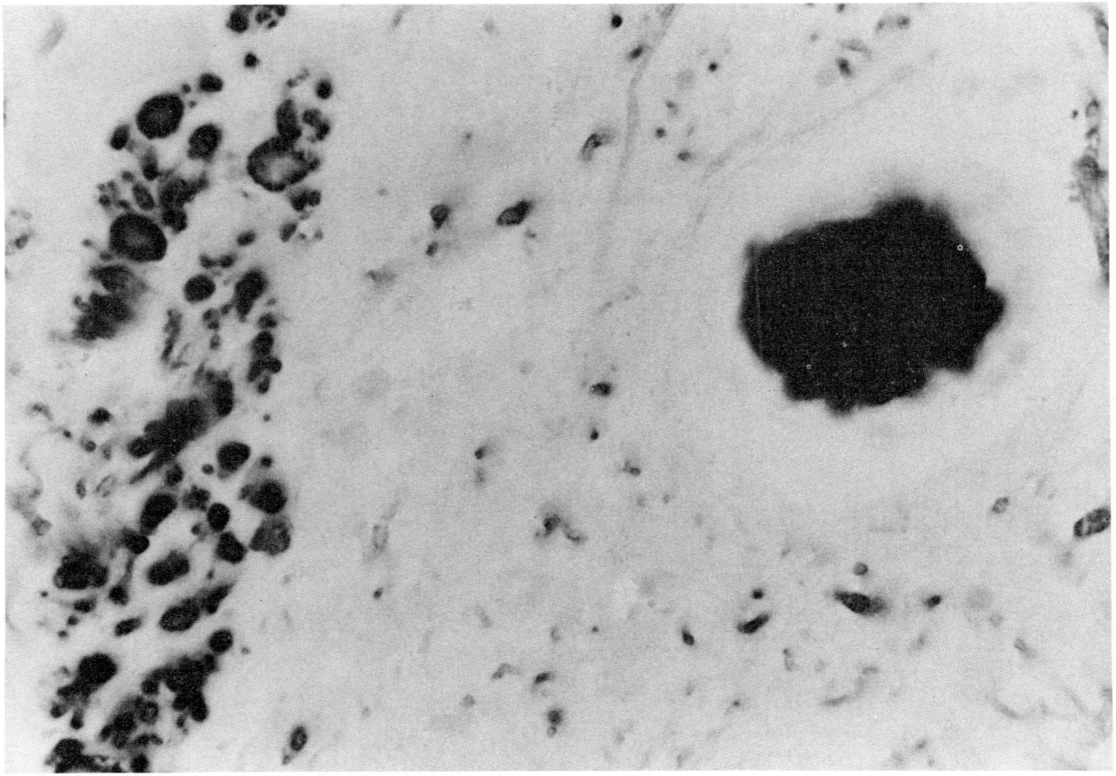

Fig. 3. Post-infectious demyelination in man. Acute disseminated encephalomyelitis. Normal myelin (left). Vessels (dark lumen, right) surrounded by area of demyelination. Loyez. ×320.

fatal demyelinating disease occasionally seen complicating lymphoreticular disorders such as Hodgkin's disease, lymphosarcoma or leukaemia, or following immunosuppressive therapy. It is characterized by a progressive course and a multi-focal neurological deficit. Areas of demyelination are found associated with intranuclear inclusion bodies in the oligodendrocytes. Two types of papovavirus, JC and SV40, have been isolated from the lesions and papovavirus has been identified in the inclusions on electron microscopy. Cytosine arabinoside has recently been reported to be a helpful therapeutic agent.

Measles Virus

The common measles virus provides the most striking example of the way the pattern of disease may be affected by the nature of the immune response. The EEG findings in the acute disease of childhood show that a mild cerebral disturbance frequently occurs and it is likely that the virus commonly enters the brain. Occasionally this may cause an acute disseminated encephalomyelitis. Very rarely, the virus appears to survive in some form and subsequently gives rise to a progressive fatal disease in childhood or late adolescence. This condition, subacute sclerosing panencephalitis (SSPE) is associated with an inflammatory cell infiltration, loss of neurones, gliosis and demyelination. Inclusion bodies may be present in both neurones and glia, and measles virus has been identified on electron microscopy and isolated from the brain. Important diagnostic features are the high titres of anti-measles antibody present in the serum and the CSF. The colloidal gold curve is paretic. Immunoglobulin levels in the CSF are raised and on electrophoresis discrete bands may be detected. It has been shown that this represents oligoclonal synthesis of anti-measles antibody in the CNS.

Despite high levels of serum antibody cell mediated responses to measles antigen are reduced in this disease (Valdimarsson *et al.*, 1974). This deficiency is accompanied by a varying degree of anergy to other common antigens. It has therefore been suggested that the persistence of the virus in SSPE is due to a defect in the capacity of the patient to generate cell mediated reactions to the measles virus. However, there is as yet no general agreement on the status of cell mediated immunity in this disease and it may well be that the disease is due to an incomplete or abnormal form of the measles virus. If this is the case the general state of anergy found in this disease may be a secondary phenomenon. A transient depression of cell mediated immunity is known to accompany many viral infections, including measles.

Slow Viruses

The most extreme form of indolence of viral behaviour in the CNS is represented by the "slow viruses". The term was coined by Sigurdsson in his studies on visna infection in sheep in order to distinguish them from the more familiar chronic and latent agents. They are characterized by a long asymptomatic incubation period, followed by a protracted slowly progressive clinical phase, often terminating in death. They include the scrapie agent and visna virus in sheep and Kuru and Jakob–Kreutzfeldt disease in man. The identification and isolation of the virus under these conditions presents considerable technical difficulties and it is probable that the list of human diseases due to viruses of this type will be extended, possibly to include multiple sclerosis.

Kuru and Jakob–Kreutzfeldt disease are spongiform encephalopathies. The pathological lesions are restricted to the nervous system, primarily to the grey matter of the brain. They consist of neuronal vacuolation, astrocytic hypertrophy and proliferation and intracellular status spongiosus. There is little or no inflammatory reaction and no immune response to either of the two viruses has yet been detected. It seems that immune reactivity is completely lacking or minimal and that it plays little or no part in the causation of or protection against diseases due to slow virus infection.

MULTIPLE SCLEROSIS

Immunological, virological, biochemical and other hypotheses about the aetiology of multiple sclerosis (MS) have all had and still have their proponents. The appearance of lymphocytes in the early plaque, the manufacture of IgG within the CNS, and the recent discovery of an association with histocompatibility antigens, possibly linked to immune response genes, support an immunological hypothesis.

The chronic, inert plaque with massive gliosis, loss of myelin and no inflammatory cells gives no hint of a past immunological reaction (Fig. 4). The earliest lesions of MS are rarely available for study, but show scanty cuffs of lymphocytic and macrophage infiltration round veins. Such an inflammatory response is by no means specific, since similar appearances are seen in EAE, in viral encephalitis and in areas adjacent to gliomas. The leading edge of the established, but still active, lesion is characterized by lipid-laden phagocytic cells, loss of myelin basic protein and increased concentrations of proteolytic enzymes; lymphocytes are still present, but few. IgG and to a

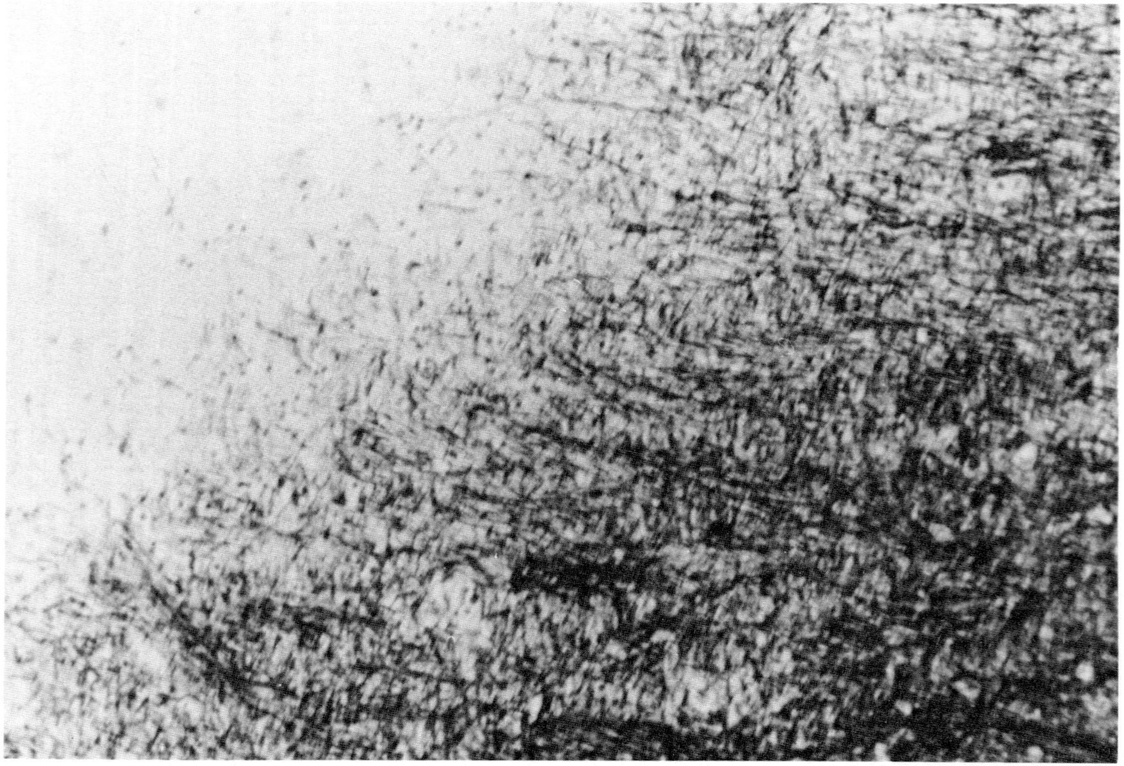

Fig. 4. Multiple sclerosis. Margin of plaque showing normal myelin (right) and area of demyelination (left). Luxol-blue. ×130.

lesser extent IgM and complement can be detected in the peripheral rim of such plaques by staining fresh unfixed post-mortem tissue with fluorescein-labelled antisera.

CSF Changes

The impossibility of obtaining biopsy material during the course of MS has focussed attention on the CSF and some interesting observations have emerged. In about 25% of patients the CSF cell count is greater than 5 per μl, the upper limit of the normal range, and increased counts are more common in relapse than remission. The cells are mostly lymphocytes but lipid-laden macrophages, plasma cells and neutrophils have also been detected in the centrifuged CSF deposit (Lumsden, 1972). There is a very approximate correlation between increased cell count and raised CSF protein and IgG.

The total CSF protein is raised in 25–50% of all patients, irrespective of the stage of the disease. Levels are usually less than 60 mg/100 ml and if greater than 100 mg/100 ml cast doubt on the diagnosis. The IgG level is usually raised out of proportion to the rise in total protein level, suggesting that it is locally produced within the CNS (Lumsden, 1972). The identification of a paretic Lange colloidal gold curve is merely a less sophisticated and less sensitive way of identifying the elevated IgG level.

The characteristic immunological profile of the CSF is a normal or slightly elevated cell count, a normal or slightly elevated total protein, a raised IgG level and a negative test for syphilis. Of 145 patients with such findings, 74% had clinically established MS at the time of puncture. Of the remainder, one-third proved on follow-up to have developed MS, nearly two-thirds remained undiagnosed but with MS still a possible diagnosis, and less than 4% had other neurological diseases (Bergman and Gilland, 1968). A similar profile is seen in SSPE, but this does not enter the clinical differential diagnosis.

Comparisons between the CSF IgG level and stage or activity of the disease show that the IgG is elevated from the first clinical manifestations and this persists as a plateau throughout the disease even during prolonged remissions. Patients with multiple attacks or lesions at multiple sites tend to have higher IgG levels (Lumsden, 1972).

Genetic Background

An increased proportion of patients with MS bear the serologically defined histocompatibility antigens HLA-A3 and HLA-B7 and the lymphocyte-defined antigen HLA-DW2. In a study of 1,000 patients and a similar number of controls, 35·8% carried HLA-A3 compared with 28·8% controls: HLA-B7 was carried by 35·3% compared with 26·0% controls, and HLA-A3 and B7 by 9·21% compared with 6·34% controls (Bertrams and Kuwert, 1974). These differences though small are significant. The differences in prevalence of the HLA-DW2 antigen are much more impressive: 70% of 28 unrelated patients carried this antigen compared with 16% of the normal population. Furthermore a crude retrospective clinical analysis suggested that the patients with the HLA-DW2 determinant had more rapidly progressive disease than those without (Jersild *et al.*, 1973a). By contrast with the now discredited association between blood group O and MS, the association between the disease and these histocompatibility antigens is of considerable theoretical interest because of the probability that genes controlling immune responses are closely related to the loci coding for the histocompatibility antigens. In animals, immune response genes controlling susceptibility to various autoimmune diseases, including EAE in rats, have been mapped into the region of the major histocompatibility locus. The association with HLA-DW2 is so strong that its determination might sometimes be of diagnostic value. The association with this and other antigens may go some of the way towards explaining the peculiar racial and geographical distribution of MS because HLA-A3 and HLA-B7 antigens are rare in populations where MS is rare. It also supports the conclusion of a genetic susceptibility to the disease which is one interpretation of the documented and not uncommon occurrence of familial cases of MS. The risk of developing MS is 20 times greater in the sibs and 12 times greater in the parents of an affected patient than the risk in the general population.

Immunological Mechanisms

A spectrum of histological appearances exists from animal EAE, through post-rabies vaccine encephalomyelitis to acute multiple sclerosis (Adams and Leibowitz, 1969). This has provided the basis for an autoimmune theory of MS and has stimulated a large body of research, but direct evidence of autoimmunity to components of CNS tissue is still fragmentary. Antibodies to crude brain extracts and a variety of lipid and protein antigens have been looked for but not found (Lumsden, 1972). Antibodies to the encephalitogenic basic protein have not been convincingly demonstrated by a haemagglutination technique or radioimmunoassay. The few reports of conventional skin testing with basic protein have been negative. Even in EAE, skin tests with homologous basic protein give only weakly positive results, which are maximal soon after immunization and decrease sharply after the onset of clinical signs. *In vitro* tests of lymphocyte sensitization by various modifications of the lymphocyte transformation technique have given conflicting results but the balance of this evidence suggests that there is a mild degree of sensitization to basic protein which may or may not be specific for MS. A suggestion that CSF contains an antigen to which the lymphocytes of patients with MS respond in a transformation test has been refuted. Most recently Sheremata and colleagues (1974) have claimed that migration inhibition factor (MIF) (see Chapter 9) is produced by patient's lymphocytes in response to a purified basic protein preparation and that MIF production is greater just before or after an acute relapse than during remission. Although the analogy with EAE has laid the emphasis of research on cell mediated responses to basic protein, it is not certain that this is the most important or only antigen involved.

The leukocyte migration inhibition test has been used to show that MS and other patients are sensitized to a synaptosome preparation of brain lacking any basic protein (Alvord *et al.*, 1974). These difficult tests and the complex antigens involved require further definition before the implications become clear and are a long way from providing a diagnostic tool.

An even more complex *in vitro* test of immunity has been much discussed in relation to MS. Caspary and Field claim that in the presence of myelin basic protein lymphocytes, from certain patients, produce a factor slowing migration of guinea-pig macrophages in an electrophoretic field. This index of "sensitization" gave positive results not only in MS but in a wide range of neurological cases and also in patients with cancer (Field and Caspary, 1972). The diagnostic interpretation and theoretical significance are therefore uncertain.

Myelinotoxic antibodies like those detectable in EAE which demyelinate rodent myelinated CNS cultures *in vitro* are also found in MS. These antibodies have aroused considerable interest because of the prominence of primary demyelination in MS. They have been detected in "active" but not "inactive" MS, but are not specific for demyelinating disease, being found in non-demyelinating conditions such as motor neurone disease at least as frequently. MS serum is reported, like EAE serum, to contain complement-dependent factors which reversibly block polysynaptic conduction in CNS tissue cultures but this effect is not specific to MS (Bornstein, 1969).

The Viral Hypothesis

One working hypothesis is that MS is due to a virus infection. A childhood infection with a prolonged latent period before the development of disease manifestations would fit many of the epidemiological data and some of the properties of the known "slow viruses". The histological appearances of MS are however quite unlike those of any of the recognized CNS slow virus infections such as SSPE or kuru. Filamentous intranuclear inclusions in brain cells of patients with MS resemble the nucleocapsids of a paramyxovirus, but are probably merely altered chromatin strands. There are reports of the passage of a virus resembling either parainfluenza or measles to monkey cells in tissue culture, but others have obtained negative results (Barbosa and Hamilton, 1973) so that further information is required before this issue can be properly judged.

One well documented fact relevant to the viral hypothesis is that MS patients have higher titres of antibody to measles in their serum than properly matched controls. Their siblings have titres intermediate between the MS patients and their controls. The antibodies in the serum are partly IgM, and IgG antibodies are found in the CSF significantly more often than in other neurological conditions. In some patients the serum/CSF antibody ratio was low, suggesting that antibody to measles is being synthesized in the CNS, rather than diffusing passively from the blood (Norrby *et al.*, 1974). Although interest has focussed on measles, antibody titres to herpes simplex, herpes zoster, rubella and mumps have also been found to be raised in MS compared with controls. Titres to EB virus and parainfluenza are normal. Patients with MS appear to lack normal cell mediated immunity to measles as shown by the inability of their lymphocytes to produce MIF in the presence of measles antigen. According to Utermohlen and Zabriskie (1973) this decreased cell mediated immunity is confined to measles, but Ciongoli (1973) finds a similar reduction in reactivity to parainfluenza, mumps and rubella as well as measles although the response to tuberculin was not different from that of controls. The significance of increased humoral and decreased cellular immunity to measles virus is still a matter for speculation.

The relevance of much previous work on measles and other viruses is called in question by the recent identification of a replicating agent in the brain, spleen and serum of patients with MS which will cause depression of the polymorphonuclear leukocyte count in mice. It also inhibits growth of a mouse fibroblast cell line in tissue culture. It seems to be a previously unidentified particle of viral type between 25 and 50 nm in size, i.e. smaller than measles or influenza but bigger than polio virus. It is not present in the CNS or serum of patients with other neurological diseases. Neutralizing antibodies to this "multiple sclerosis-associated agent" have been demonstrated in MS patients and their relatives but not in encephalitis patients nor generally in controls with no contact with MS. Interestingly these antibodies are found in the blood of East Africans in whom MS is rare. One interpretation of these data would be that early childhood infection with this agent is asymptomatic but later infection leads to persistence of the agent and development of MS in susceptible people (Henle *et al.*, 1975). Intensive research is in progress to confirm and extend the data on which these conclusions are based.

Therapeutic Manoeuvres

The simultaneous development of the auto-immune and viral hypotheses has led to the extraordinary situation where some clinicians are currently trying the effect of massive immunosuppression while others are trying to stimulate immunity with transfer factor. It is to some extent accepted that short courses of ACTH are helpful in speeding recovery from attacks of retrobulbar neuritis and MS, although they do not affect the long-term sequelae. Short courses of prednisone have been thought helpful on the basis of clinical impression but have not been proven under controlled conditions or by comparison with ACTH. It is debatable whether any improvement has its explanation in terms of immunosuppression or of a non-specific effect on conduction in demyelinated nerve.

Long-term prednisone and ACTH treatment are not superior to placebo. Azathioprine and 6-mercaptopurine have been tried for acute relapses and also as maintenance treatment but without obvious benefit. In one controlled study anti-lymphocyte globulin (ALG) with ACTH was found to prolong the duration of remission compared with ACTH alone (Seland *et al.*, 1974). An uncontrolled trial of massive immunosuppression with cortisone, azathioprine, ALG and thoracic duct drainage has been reported to have a favourable effect on the course of the disease (Ring *et al.*, 1974); the results of a controlled trial are awaited with interest and also with some apprehension because of the possible formidable side-effects.

Arguing from analogy with the suppression of neurological signs by intravenous injections of basic protein in EAE, Campbell and colleagues (1973) treated 64 MS patients with weekly intramuscular injections of 5 mg crude human basic protein. The most striking fact to emerge was that 21 patients did not complete the trial: there was no convincing difference between the treated and the untreated groups during the period of double-blind observation. At the other end of the scale, trials of treatment with transfer factor have been initiated on the basis of the apparent cellular unresponsiveness to some paramyxoviruses in MS (Jersild *et al.*, 1973b), but the results are not yet available.

GUILLAIN–BARRÉ SYNDROME

Immunological studies have been more rewarding in the Guillain–Barré syndrome (GBS) than in any other disease of the nervous system. The eponymous title is preferred because it is widely used and is always applicable whereas "acute post-infective polyneuritis" is not appropriate if there has been no preceding infection. Furthermore it does not prejudge aetiological problems as would the designation "acute auto-immune polyneuritis" or even "acute idiopathic polyneuritis". It consists clinically of an acute monophasic neuropathy affecting motor, sensory and autonomic nerves for which no known cause can be found; it varies in intensity from mild paresis of limb muscles to tetraplegia with cranial nerve involvement and respiratory failure. The disease usually evolves to its maximum intensity in less than three weeks and most patients recover completely in about 6 months although some are left with a persistent neurological deficit and about 10% die (Marshall, 1963; Prineas, 1970).

Infective Agents

About half the patients have a history of illness, often a respiratory tract infection, about 10 days before the onset of neuropathic symptoms but no infective agent has been consistently cultured from the nerves or CSF or implicated by a rise in antibody titre. In a few patients with a similar clinical picture a definite history or serological evidence of a recent identified virus infection such as measles, rubella, chicken pox, herpes zoster, mumps, influenza and herpes simplex may be obtained. These all share in common the possession of an envelope containing host antigens. These viruses are well equipped to stimulate an auto-immune reaction but other viruses, not coated with host antigen, such as ECHO-9, Coxsackie B5 and infectious hepatitis are also reported to be associated with the GBS (Arnason, 1971). A similar peripheral neuropathy, often accompanied by clinical and EEG evidence of encephalopathy (which is not usual in GBS) may occur in infectious mononucleosis with a positive Paul–Bunnell test and serological evidence of EB virus infection or cytomegalovirus infection. Reports have also appeared of the association of GBS with mycoplasmal infection.

The GBS may sometimes follow surgery or hyperthermic treatment and a similar condition is occasionally seen in association with carcinoma and lymphoma (Arnason, 1971).

Comparison with Experimental Allergic Neuritis (EAN)

The strongest evidence linking GBS and EAN is that rabies vaccination with desiccated rabbit nervous tissue infected with rabies virus was sometimes followed by a neurological disorder characterized not by the better known encephalomyelitis but by a polyneuropathy. The inoculum used for the vaccination contained rabbit spinal roots as well as cord and the acute neuropathy which followed closely resembled GBS both clinically and pathologically. This vaccination unwittingly provided an example of human EAN. The antigen responsible for the post-rabies vaccine neuritis is not known. It has even occurred after vaccination with suckling mouse brain harvested nine days after birth and thus expected to contain no myelin and therefore to lack encephalitogenic or neuritogenic potential.

Immunological Features

Post-mortem studies show diffuse perivascular infiltration throughout the peripheral nerves from the spinal roots to the most peripheral nerve twiglets. The infiltration is associated with segmental demyelination with relative preservation of axons. The sympathetic nerves are also involved. There are no changes in the CNS beyond those secondary to peripheral nerve damage. The pathological changes indicate a process directed against myelin in preference to axons, a specificity which could readily be explained by an immunological mechanism. Ultrastructural studies have shown the same process of myelin breakdown as in EAN–myelin invasion and ingestion by macrophage processes and vesicular breakdown of myelin. An important feature is that myelin breakdown is not observed in the absence of cellular infiltration, which favours involvement of cell mediated rather than humoral mechanisms.

Associated immunological disease is not usually recognized in GBS but careful study may reveal evidence of a mild glomerulonephritis. In all of eight renal biopsies from patients with GBS a mixture of proliferative and membranous changes were found (Rodriguez-Iturbe *et al.*, 1973). Nephrotic syndrome due to deposition of immunoglobulin and C3 on the glomerular basement membrane has been described in association with chronic or recurrent forms of neuropathy but not with typical acute GBS. A normal cell count and a raised CSF total protein concentration are characteristic but not invariable features of GBS. The CSF protein often does not rise until one or two weeks after the onset of symptoms of neuropathy and in some otherwise typical cases raised values are never obtained. Elevation of the protein is said to depend on whether the spinal roots are involved. Most series have a few cases with slightly increased numbers of lymphocytes in the CSF. The protein in the CSF consists largely of albumin, but with a modest rise in the proportion of IgA, IgG and perhaps IgM. As in MS the rise in the proportion of immunoglobulin is thought to be due to local production in the nervous system, not diffusion from the blood.

During the acute phase of GBS increased numbers of large mononuclear cells resembling spontaneously transformed lymphocytes are present in the circulating blood. During the acute stage lymphocyte transformation has been demonstrated *in vitro* in the presence of crude peripheral nerve extract, peripheral nerve basic protein and probably brain basic protein. There is disagreement about the duration for which this test remains positive. Knowles *et al.* (1969) found that transformation still occurred months or years after the onset but Behan and colleagues (1970) found that transformation did not occur in the later stages.

Tests of leukocyte migration inhibition and MIF production by lymphocytes also indicate sensitization to human peripheral nerve. According to Sheremata and colleagues (1974) the MIF production test with a peripheral nerve extract is positive in the early but not the late stage and negative in other neuropathies. A few positives are found in MS and stroke cases. According to Paty and colleagues (1974) the MIF production test is also positive in many patients with carcinoma and in patients with chronic idiopathic neuropathy. A few patients have persistently positive tests for months or years after the acute episode, particularly if there is persistent disease. Abramsky *et al.* (1975b) reported three cases of GBS in which they found evidence of sensitization to the neuritogenic peripheral nerve basic protein PIL, but not to the other peripheral nerve basic protein P2 or to the CNS basic protein.

Lymphocytes from patients with GBS in the presence of either human sciatic nerve or human brain basic protein inhibit the migration of guinea-pig macrophages in an electrophoretic field (Caspary *et al.*, 1971). This complex test gives results which often conflict with those of other tests of immunity, possibly because of its extreme sensitivity, and these findings await confirmation.

The role of serum factors has been explored surprisingly little. Serum IgG and IgM and occasionally IgA are raised in some but not all series. Melnick (1963) found low titres of complement-fixing antibody to crude saline extracts of human peripheral nerve in 50% of 38 cases of GBS during the acute stage, but in none of eight cases following recovery. Tse and colleagues (1971) demonstrated antibody attaching to nerve fibres by the indirect immunofluorescent technique during the acute stage in four of six cases of GBS.

It was mostly IgG, but sometimes IgM and occasionally IgA. The fluorescence outlined the axon in a ring and was interpreted as due to staining of myelin. Attempts to demonstrate antibodies to myelin in the GBS have been bedevilled by the fact that normal serum produces similar staining and the possibility that the membrane stained may be axonal and not myelin. It is surprising that conventional antibodies to peripheral nerve are not more readily demonstrated in the GBS in view of the positive *in vitro* tests of lymphocyte sensitization to peripheral nerve and its basic protein.

Sera from many patients with GBS are toxic to the myelin of dorsal root ganglion cultures. These sera produce reversible, complement-dependent destruction of myelin with sparing of axons. On EM the disintegrating myelin shows separation of its lamellae and eventual disruption into vesicles in the absence of macrophages, rather different from the ultrastructural appearances of demyelination in the GBS. This myelinotoxic serum factor is also not specific because it is found less often in other forms of neuropathy, with CNS disease and occasionally in normal individuals (Cook *et al.*, 1971). Lymphocytes from GBS patients also have myelinotoxic properties (Arnason *et al.*, 1969).

Direct immunofluorescent staining has been used to show IgM and complement lying along the myelin sheaths of patients with GBS, but whether this represents non-specific leakage due to local vasculitis or indicates a pathological role for IgM in the production of the disease is not known.

Therapeutic Aspects

If immunological mechanisms are as important in GBS as the similarities between EAN and the human disease suggest, immunosuppression might be expected to be a valuable form of treatment. Steroid therapy however is of doubtful benefit: some authors claim that steroids produce more rapid recovery, or at least speed the onset of improvement, without affecting the total disease duration (Prineas, 1970). Others have found no difference between steroid-treated and untreated patients. In a recent series the disease lasted longer in the steroid-treated than the untreated patients (Goodall *et al.*, 1974). These observations were made retrospectively over long periods of time so that the answer to the question whether steroids are helpful in GBS still awaits a prospective controlled trial. Cytotoxic immunosuppressive drugs have been used in occasional cases of GBS with apparent benefit but no controlled data are available. On the other hand GBS sometimes occurs in transplant patients fully immunosuppressed with prednisone and azathioprine.

Some patients with chronic neuropathy have clinical, physiological and histological resemblances to acute GBS. There are two poorly differentiated subgroups. In one there are recurrent attacks of neuropathy, each of which behaves like the acute attack of GBS. These cases are rare and relapse after GBS proper occurs in less than 5% of patients. Patients with a relapsing course are often particularly responsive to steroids. In the second group the neuropathy is slowly progressive over weeks or months without relapses or remissions, although these too may sometimes be steroid-responsive. In both chronic and relapsing neuropathy, lymphocytic infiltration may be found in nerve biopsies, with evidence of remyelination including Schwann cell proliferation causing "onion-bulb" formation and palpable hypertrophy of nerves. Detailed immunological assessment might allow a more rational classification of these interesting disorders.

NEUROLOGICAL COMPLICATIONS OF SYSTEMIC DISEASE

Many systemic disorders with an immunological basis have an important neurological component, often presenting with and sometimes remaining confined to the nervous system. Polyarteritis nodosa (PAN) may affect the CNS causing cerebral infarction or myelopathy. A peripheral neuropathy, usually a mononeuritis multiplex may develop and focal infarction of the muscles can occur. Detailed post-mortem study of one patient with a neuropathy showed degeneration of nerve fascicles increasingly severe in the distal parts of the nerve and corresponding to the distribution of a necrotizing vasculitis of the epineurial vessels (Dyck *et al.*, 1972).

In immune complex cryoglobulinaemia a symmetrical mixed motor and sensory neuropathy is not uncommon and is due to a small vessel vasculitis.

Giant cell, temporal or cranial arteritis is a characteristic form of vasculitis, differing from PAN in histological detail, and occurring exclusively over the age of 55. It causes inflammation of branches of the external carotid, that portion of the internal carotid which traverses the skull, and the ophthalmic and vertebral arteries. The sedimentation rate (ESR) is almost invariably elevated and the diagnosis can usually be confirmed by examination of a superficial temporal artery biopsy. Because of the high risk of blindness due to involvement of ophthalmic artery branches, treatment with steroids should be started immediately the clinical diagnosis is made. The prominent symptoms and signs are headache and visual loss but general malaise, weight loss, joint pains and sometimes peripheral neuropathy indicate a systemic illness. The histology, elevation of the ESR, steroid responsiveness, and association with polymyalgia rheumatica are pointers to an immunological process which may be directed against a component of elastic tissue in the arterial wall (Wilkinson, 1976).

Some rare neurological conditions resemble the Wegener's granulomatosis end of the PAN spectrum. Pseudotumour of the orbit, an inflammatory granuloma causing proptosis, ophthalmoplegia and optic nerve affection, usually occurs in isolation but may be associated with systemic disease typical of PAN and is usually associated with an elevated ESR (Jellinek, 1969). In the superior orbital fissure syndrome described by Tolosa (1954) and Hunt and colleagues (1961) transient painful ophthalmoplegia with sensory loss in the first trigeminal division was shown in the single post-mortem examination to be due to granulomatous infiltration of the cavernous segment of the internal carotid artery and the surrounding nerves (Tolosa, 1954). An elevated ESR and positive LE cell tests were found in about half of one series of similar cases of painful ophthalmoplegia (Mathew and Chandy, 1972) although it seems likely that more than one pathological entity is included within the "superior orbital fissure syndrome". Cases with features of both this syndrome and orbital pseudotumour are described. Both conditions respond dramatically to steroids and, by analogy with Wegener's granulomatosis, azathioprine is also used.

The immune complex vasculitis associated with serum sickness may be complicated by a peripheral neuropathy with particularly painful lesions involving branches of the brachial plexus. Serum sickness is now rare but similar brachial plexus neuropathy is still observed and often called "neuralgic amyotrophy". About one-third of cases follow a non-specific upper respiratory tract infection, infectious mononucleosis, surgery or immunization and the remainder have no recognized precipitant. The neurological signs usually indicate patchy involvement of the brachial plexus affecting more than one nerve, the suprascapular and circumflex nerves and nerve to serratus anterior being sites of predilection (Tsairis and Dyck, 1972). Recovery eventually occurs in 80% of cases. There is no definitive proof of the involvement of immune complexes in the development of this condition.

Neurological manifestations are common in systemic lupus erythematosus (SLE), occurring in 59% of 150 patients and being responsible for death in 20% of 53 cases (see Table 3). The pathological basis of the mental disorders and cerebral syndromes which are the commonest neurological manifestations appears to be multiple infarction and haemorrhage round small capillaries and arterioles, with swollen endothelial cells and only occasional sparse lymphocytic infiltration. Large vessel vasculitis and fibrinoid necrosis, typical of polyarteritis, are infrequent (John and Richardson, 1968). It is probable that the cerebral syndromes are the result of small vessel vasculitis which has partly resolved by the time of post-mortem examination. The CSF shows a raised protein in about 50% of cases and less often a pleocytosis, a paretic Lange curve and a proportionately raised IgG (Johnson and Richardson, 1968). Immunoglobulin deposits have been demonstrated between the

TABLE 3
Neurological manifestations of SLE

Mental disorders—depression, psychosis, confusional state
Epilepsy
Hemiplegia
Movement disorders—especially chorea
Intracranial hypertension
Optic nerve lesions
Cranial nerve palsies
Myelopathy
Peripheral neuropathy
Myasthenia gravis
Polymyositis

choroid plexus cells and the capillary basement membrane by post-mortem immunofluorescent staining. A low CSF C level assayed by a haemolytic technique was detected in all of 11 cases of SLE with neuropsychiatric involvement, while the C level was normal in patients with SLE without CNS manifestations, as well as in normal subjects and in all but five of 55 patients with other neurological disease (Petz *et al.*, 1971).

A condition described as "lupoid sclerosis" has been defined in which there are some clinical features resembling multiple sclerosis and some serological features resembling an SLE-like disorder. The abnormal immunological tests in the group of six cases on which this "syndrome" is based consisted of a positive anti-nuclear antibody, positive LE cell tests, a raised serum IgM, a false serological reaction for syphilis and positive mitochondrial antibody (Fulford *et al.*, 1972). Further clinico-pathological data to confirm this as a separate entity have not yet appeared.

NEUROLOGICAL DISORDERS ASSOCIATED WITH MALIGNANT DISEASE

Non-metastatic neurological disorders are relatively common in association with carcinoma, occurring in 7% of one large unselected series and in 16% of men with carcinoma of the lung. These disorders include cerebellar, spinal cord, peripheral nerve and muscle syndromes and neuromuscular conduction disorders or combinations of these. Pathological studies in some cases of pure sensory or mixed sensory and motor neuropathy have shown perivascular lymphocytic infiltration in peripheral nerves and dorsal roots. In some cases of sensory neuropathy with carcinoma of the bronchus, antibodies to brain (but not peripheral nerve) antigens were detected by complement-fixation and indirect immunofluorescent techniques (Alvord, 1965). A study with the MIF production test showed sensitization to peripheral nerve in patients with neuromuscular syndromes due to carcinoma, and also in those with carcinoma and no clinical or electrophysiological evidence of such disorder, and with "idiopathic polyneuritis" but not with other neurological disease (Paty *et al.*, 1974). These studies of small numbers of patients provide evidence of an immunological response to nervous tissue antigens in some, but leave unanswered the main question whether the response is merely a secondary effect or an important causative mechanism.

Similar neurological disorders occur in only 2% of cases of reticulosis, where opportunistic infections and pressure effects from tumour growth are the common causes of cerebral, spinal and root syndromes.

The immunological disorders associated with plasma cell dyscrasias cause several neurological syndromes. The presence of plasma cells and paraprotein in the CSF may help in the diagnosis of compression or infiltration of the spinal cord or roots by myeloma deposits. Peripheral neuropathy occurs in about 5% of cases of myeloma and may respond to irradiation of a solitary primary tumour. The neuropathy may be due to infiltration with tumour, degeneration without evident infiltration or diffuse amyloid deposition in the peripheral nerves although the latter is rare. Carpal tunnel syndrome due to deposition of amyloid in the flexor retinaculum is more common and is relieved by surgical decompression.

Diffuse neuropathy and the carpal tunnel syndrome occur only in those forms of primary sporadic amyloidosis associated with paraproteins in the serum or Bence–Jones protein in the urine. In these cases the amyloid material contains deposits of abnormal light chain protein. Neuropathy does not occur with primary sporadic amyloidosis in the absence of paraproteins or in secondary amyloidosis. Paraproteins are also not a feature of hereditary amyloid neuropathies (Benson *et al.*, 1975).

Waldenström's macroglobulinaemia may also be accompanied by a neuropathy, in some cases due to amyloid deposition, in others to infiltration by tumour cells, and in others to degeneration without evident infiltration. IgM has been identified along the myelin sheaths in nerve biopsies from some such patients. Many of the earlier cases categorized under this heading may in reality have been due to a mixed cryoglobulinaemia (see Chapter 26).

The most striking neurological complications of Waldenström's macroglobulinaemia are directly due to the increased viscosity of the blood which retards the retinal and cerebral circulation leading to retinal exudates and haemorrhages, cerebral and brainstem ischaemic episodes, postural hypotension and coma which can be corrected or prevented by plasmapheresis. Symptoms appear when the viscosity reaches about 4 to 7 times that of water (normal blood viscosity is 1·4 to 1·7 times). IgM complexes with clotting factors predispose to cerebral haemorrhage. The peripheral neuropathy and deafness which also occurs in this condition are not clearly related to the increased plasma viscosity (Solomon, 1965). IgG myelomas, particularly IgG_3, occasionally cause hyperviscosity syndromes.

CEREBRAL TUMOURS

About one-third of gliomas are found at post-mortem to be surrounded by a rim of brain parenchyma containing perivascular lymphocytic infiltration which may be quite prominent. Although this suggests the occurrence of an immunological reaction against the tumour, little useful clinical immunological information has yet emerged. It has been theorized that the development of a glioma is due to the failure of an immunological surveillance mechanism, and the brain as an immunologically privileged site might be expected to be a site of predilection for neoplasia. It was mentioned at the beginning of this chapter that the brain is only relatively privileged in this respect. Experimental solid tissue grafts are rejected, albeit more slowly than grafts at other sites (Ridley, 1971). Human astrocytomas possess surface antigens which are unique to astrocytomas and gliomas and not shared by normal brain (Coakham, 1974) and which might be expected to be immunogenic. Attempts to stimulate immunity by inoculation with autologous tumour tissue produce precipitating antibodies reacting with antigens specific to glioma or astrocytoma but have not produced tumour regression (Ridley, 1971).

A disproportionately large number of neoplasms occurring in immunosuppressed transplant recipients affect the brain. Of 24 mesenchymal tumours reported from over 5,000 transplant recipients, 11 were in the brain, 8 being confined to it. They occurred between 5 months and 4 years after transplantation: lack of fever helped to differentiate them clinically from abscess and meningitis which might be a difficult diagnosis in a transplant recipient. All the brain tumours found were primitive reticulum cell tumours (reticulum cell sarcomas or microgliomas). This is an extraordinarily high incidence of this type of tumour which constitutes only 1% or less of all cerebral tumours in most reported series (Schneck and Penn, 1971). It is not known whether the neoplasia arises *in situ* in the brain or reaches the brain by blood-borne spread. It may be that the combination of systemic immunosuppression and the relatively immunologically privileged site combine to permit the development of these tumours.

REFERENCES

Abramsky, O., Teitelbaum, D., Webb, C., and Arnon, R. (1975a). Neuritogenic and encephalitogenic properties of the peripheral nerve basic proteins. *J. Neuropath. Exp. Neurol.*, **34**, 36–46.

Abramsky, O., Webb, C., Teitelbaum, D. and Arnon, R. (1975b). Cell-mediated immunity to neural antigens in idiopathic polyneuritis and myeloradiculitis: clinical-immunologic classification of several autoimmune demyelinating disorders. *Neurology*, **25**, 1154–1159.

Adams, C. W. M. and Leibowitz, S. (1969). The general pathology of demyelinating diseases. *In* "The Structure and Function of Nervous Tissue", (ed. G. H. Bourne), pp. 309–382. Academic Press, New York and London.

Allison, A. C. (1972). Immune responses in persistent virus infections. *J. Clin. Path.* **25**, Suppl. 6, 1–7.

Alvord, E. C. (1965). Brain antigens and antibodies. The possible relationship between carcinomatous and experimental allergic neuro-encephalomyelitides. *In* "Remote Effects of Cancer on the Nervous System", (eds R. L. Brain and F. H. Norris), pp. 188–203. Grune and Stratton, New York.

Alvord, E. C., Hsu, P. C. and Thron, R. (1974). Leukocyte sensitivity to brain fractions in neurological diseases. *Arch. Neurol.* **30**, 296–299.

Arnason, B. G. W. (1971). Idiopathic polyneuritis and experimental allergic neuritis. *In* "Immunological Disorders of the Nervous System", (ed. L. P. Rowland), pp. 156–177. Williams and Wilkins, Baltimore.

Arnason, B. G. W., Winkler, G. F. and Hadler, N. M. (1969). Cell-mediated demyelination of peripheral nerve in tissue culture. *Lab. Invest.* **21**, 1–10.

Barbosa, L. H. and Hamilton, R. (1973). Virological studies with multiple sclerosis brain tissues. *Lancet* **1**, 1415–1417.

Behan, P. O., Lamarche, J. B., Feldman, R. G. and Sheremata, W. A. (1970). Lymphocyte transformation in the Guillain–Barré syndrome. *Lancet* **1**, 421.

Benson, M. D., Cohen, A. S., Brandt, K. D. and Cathcart, E. S. (1975). Neuropathy, M components and amyloid. *Lancet* **1**, 10–12.

Bergmann, L. and Gilland, O. (1968). Monosymptomatic gamma globulin elevation in CSF as an indicator of multiple sclerosis. *Acta Neurol. Scand.* **44**, 228.

Bertrams, J. and Kuwert, E. (1974). HL-A segregation analysis in multiple sclerosis. *Lancet* **2**, 43–44.

Bornstein, M. B. (1969). Anti-neuroglial and anti-neuronal cell factors in experimental allergic encephalomyelitis and multiple sclerosis. *Int. Arch. Allergy Appl. Immun.* **36**, Suppl. 574–586.

Campbell, B., Vogel, P. J., Fisher, E. and Lorenz, R. (1973). Myelin basic protein administration in multiple sclerosis. *Arch. Neurol.* **29**, 10–15.

Caspary, E. A., Currie, S., Walton, J. N. and Field, E. J. (1971). Lymphocyte sensitization to nervous tissues and muscle in patients with Guillain–Barré syndrome. *J. Neurol. Neurosurg.* **4**, 179–181.

Ciongoli, A. K., Platz, B., Dupon, B., Svejgaard, A., Fog, T. and Jersild, C. (1973). Lack of antigen response to myxoviruses in multiple sclerosis. *Lancet* **2**, 1147.

Coakham, H. (1974). Surface antigen(s) common to human astrocytoma cells. *Nature* **250**, 328–330.

Cohen, S. and Bannister, R. (1967). Immunological synthesis within the central nervous system in disseminated sclerosis. *Lancet* **1**, 366.

Cole, G. A. and Nathanson, N. (1974). Lymphocytic choriomeningitis. *Prog. Med. Virol.* (Slow Virus Diseases), **18**, 94–108.

Cook, S. D., Dowling, P. C., Murray, M. R. and Whitaker, J. N. (1971). Circulating demyelinating factors in acute idiopathic polyneuropathy. *Arch. Neurol.* **24**, 136–144.

Dunkley, P. R. and Carnegie, P. R. (1974). Isolation of myelin basic proteins. *In* "Research Methods in Neurochemistry" (eds N. Marks and R. Rodnight), Vol. 2, pp. 219–245. Plenum Press, New York.

Dyck, P. J., Conn, D. L. and Okazaki, H. (1972). Necrotizing angiopathic neuropathy. Three dimensional morphology of fiber degeneration related to sites of occluded vessels. *Mayo Clin. Proc.* **47**, 461–475.

Field, E. J. and Caspary, E. A. (1972). Cellular sensitization studies in multiple sclerosis: application of macrophage electrophoresis method. *In* "Multiple Sclerosis", (eds E. J. Field, T. M. Bell and P. R. Carnegie), pp. 50–61. North Holland Publishing Co., Amsterdam and London.

Fry, J. M., Weissbarth, S., Lehrer, G. M. and Bornstein, M. B. (1974). Cerebroside antibody inhibits sulfatide synthesis and myelination and demyelinates in cord tissue cultures. *Science* **183**, 540–542.

Fulford, K. W. M., Caterall, R. D., Delhanty, J. J., Doniach, D. and Kremer, M. (1972). A collagen disorder of the nervous system presenting as multiple sclerosis. *Brain* **95**, 373–386.

Goodall, J. A. D., Kosmidis, J. C. and Geddes, A. M. (1974). Effect of corticosteroids on course of Guillain–Barré syndrome. *Lancet* **1**, 524–526.

Henle, G., Koldovsky, U., Koldovsky, P., Henle, W., Ackermann, R. and Haase, G. (1975). Multiple sclerosis-associated agent: neutralization of the agent by human sera. *Infect. Immun.* **12**, 1367–1374.

Heremans, J. F. (1966). The proteins of cerebrospinal fluid. *In* "Molecular Biology of Human Proteins" (eds. H. E. Schultze and J. F. Heremans), pp. 732–761. Vol. 1, Elsevier, Amsterdam.

Hunt, W. F., Meagher, J. M. Lefever, H. E. and Zeman, W. (1961). Painful ophthalmoplegia. Its relation to indolent inflammation of the cavernous sinus. *Neurology* **11**, 56–62.

Jellinek, E. H. (1969). The orbital pseudotumour syndrome and its differentiation from endocrine exophthalmos. *Brain* **92**, 35–58.

Jersild, C., Fog, T., Hansen, G. S., Thomsen, M., Svejgaard, A. and Dupont, B. (1973a). Histocompatibility determinants in multiple sclerosis with special reference to clinical course. *Lancet* **2**, 1221–1225.

Jersild, C., Platz, P., Thomsen, M., Hansen, G. S., Svejgaard, A., Fog, T., Ciongoli, A. K. and Grob, P. (1973b). Transfer factor therapy in multiple sclerosis. *Lancet* **2**, 1381–1382.

Johnson, R. T. and Mims, C. A. (1968a). Pathogenesis of viral infections of the nervous system. I. *New England J. Med.* **278**, 23–30.

Johnson, R. T. and Mims, C. A. (1968b). Pathogenesis of viral infections of the nervous system. II. *New England J. Med.* **278**, 84–92.

Johnson, R. T. and Richardson, E. P. (1968). The neurological manifestations of systemic lupus erythematosis. A clinico-pathological study of 24 cases and review of the literature. *Medicine* **47**, 337–369.

Knowles, M., Saunders, M., Currie, S., Walton, J. N. and Field, E. J. (1969). Lymphocyte transformation in the Guillain–Barré syndrome. *Lancet* **2**, 1168–1170.

Laterre, E. C. (1973). The normal protein in cerebrospinal fluid. I. *Clin. Lab.* **3**, 736–763.

Laterre, E. C. (1974). The normal protein in cerebrospinal fluid. II. *Clin. Lab.* **4**, 540–566.

Lumsden, C. E. (1972). The proteins of cerebrospinal fluid. *In* "Multiple Sclerosis", 2nd ed. (eds Douglas McAlpine, Charles E. Lumsden and E. M. Acheson), pp. 333–432. Churchill Livingston, Edinburgh and London.

McFarlin, D. E., Hsu, S. C-L., Slemenda, S. B., Chou, F. C-H. and Kibler, R. F. (1975). The immune response against myelin basic protein in two strains of rat with different genetic capacity to develop experimental allergic encephalomyelitis. *J. Exp. Med.* **141**, 72–81.

Marshall, J. (1963). The Landry–Guillain–Barré syndrome. *Brain* **86**, 55–66.

Mathew, N. T. and Chandy, J. (1972). Painful ophthalmoplegia. *J. Neurol. Sci.* **11**, 243–256.

Melnick, S. C. (1963). 38 cases of the Guillain–Barré syndrome: an immunological study. *Brit. Med. J.* **1**, 368–373.

Norrby, E., Link, H. and Olsson, J-E. (1974). Measles virus antibodies in multiple sclerosis. *Arch. Neurol.* **30**, 285–292.

Paty, D. W., Campbell, M. J. and Hughes, D. (1974). Carcinomatous neuropathy: 2. Immunological studies. *J. Neurol. Neurosurg. Psychiat.* **37**, 142–151.

Petz, L. D., Charp, G. C., Cooper, N. R. and Irvin, W. S. (1971). Serum and CSF complement and serum antibodies in systemic lupus erythematosus. *Medicine* **50**, 259–275.

Prineas, J. (1970). 1. Polyneuropathies of undetermined cause. *Acta. Neurol. Scand.* **46**, Suppl. 44.

Ridley, A. (1971). Clinical significance of immunopathological mechanisms in diseases of the nervous system. *Clin. All.* **1**, 311–342.

Ring, J., Seifer, T., Lob, G., Coulin, K., Angstwurm, H., Frick, E., Brass, B., Mertin, J., Backmund, H. and Brendel, W. (1974). Intensive immunosuppression treatment of multiple sclerosis. *Lancet* **2**, 1093–1096.

Rodriguez-Iturbe, B., Garcia, R., Rubio, L., Zabala, J., Maros, G. and Torres, R. (1973). Acute glomerulonephritis in the Guillain–Barré syndrome. Report of 9 cases. *Ann. Intern. Med.* **78**, 391–395.

Schneck, S. A. and Penn, I. (1971). De novo brain tumours in renal-transplant recipients. *Lancet* **1**, 983–986.

Seland, T. P., McPherson, T. A., Grace, M., Lamoureux, G. and Blain, J. G. (1974). Evaluation of antithymocyte globulin in acute relapses of multiple sclerosis. *Neurology* **24**, 34–40.

Sheremata, W., Cosgrove, J. B. R. and Eylar, E. H. (1974). Hypersensitivity to basic myelin protein and multiple sclerosis. *New Engl. J. Med.* **291**, 14–17.

Sheremata, W. A., Rocklin, R. E. and David, J. R. (1974). Cellular hypersensitivity in Guillain–Barré syndrome. *Can. Med. Ass. J.* **110**, 1245–1247.

Solomon, A. (1965). Neurological manifestations of macroglobulinaemia. *In* "The Remote Effects of Cancer on the Nervous System", (eds W. R. Brain and F. Norris), pp. 112–124. New York.

Spitler, L. E., von Muller, C. M., Fundenberg, H. H. and Eylar, E. H. (1972). Experimental allergic encephalomyelitis: dissociation of cellular immunity to basic protein and disease production. *J. Exp. Med.* **136**, 156–174.

Tolosa, E. (1974). Periarteritic lesions of the carotid siphon with the clinical features of a carotid infraclinoidal aneurysm. *J. Neurol. Neurosurg. Psychiat.* **17**, 300–302.

Tsairis, P. and Dyck, P. J. (1972). Natural history of brachial plexus neuropathy. *Arch. Neurol. Chicago* **27**, 109–117.

Tse, K. S., Arbesman, C. E., Tomasi, T. B. and Tourville, D. (1971). Demonstration of anti-myelin antibodies by immunofluorescence in Guillain–Barré syndrome. *Clin. Exp. Immunol.* **8**, 881–887.

Utermohlen, V. and Zabriskie, J. B. (1973). A suppression of cellular immunity in patients with multiple sclerosis. *J. Exp. Med.* **138**, 1591–1596.

Valdimarsson, H., Agnarsdottir, G. and Lachmann, P. J. (1974). Cellular immunity in sub-acute sclerosing panencephalitis. *Proc. Roy. Soc. Med.* **67**, 1125–1129.

Weiner, L. P., Johnson, R. T. and Herndon, R. M. (1973). Viral infections and demyelinating diseases. *New Engl. J. Med.* **24**, 1103–1110.

Wilkinson, I. M. S. (1976). Giant cell arteritis. *Brit. J. Hosp. Med.* **15**, 154–161.

Wisniewski, H. M., Brostoff, S. W., Carter, H. and Eylar, E. H. (1974). Recurrent experimental allergic polyganglioradiculoneuritis. *Arch. Neurol.* **30**, 347–358.

26

Haematological Disorders

D. L. BROWN

It would be impossible to give a totally comprehensive account of the immunology of diseases of the blood since virtually all the lymphoid, polymorphonuclear and mononuclear phagocytic systems have at least one blood-borne phase. Instead certain specific topics have been chosen for this chapter, particularly those in which the principal immunopathology can be recognized from examination of the blood.

The first and major section deals with auto-immune and drug-induced damage to red cells, platelets and neutrophils. The second section deals with rather selected topics in which the immunological recognition of the disease rests primarily on examination of circulating cells or serum; these topics are cryoglobulinaemia, infectious mononucleosis, the leukaemias and lymphomas and finally, a "near immunological" aberration of red cells involving the complement system, paroxysmal nocturnal haemoglobinuria.

AUTO-IMMUNE HAEMOLYTIC ANAEMIA

The auto-immune haemolytic anaemias (AIHA) present many of the diagnostic problems of other auto-immune diseases, though in many respects they are the most accessible of this group of disorders to investigation and demonstrate most clearly that the auto-antibody is the agent responsible for the immunological damage; in this case the accelerated destruction of circulating red cells.

Essential for the diagnosis is the demonstration of:

1. a shortened autologous red cell survival and,
2. the presence of an auto-stimulated antibody with or without complement on the red cells detected by the direct antiglobulin test (DAT).

These minimal criteria can in most circumstances be expanded by supporting evidence as follows:

i. the eluted auto-antibody possesses specificities directed at antigens intrinsic to the mature red cells;
ii. an antibody of similar specificity can be demonstrated in the serum;
iii. the auto-antibody eluted from the red cells or present in the serum will sensitize phenotypically identical allogeneic red cells (i.e. derived from another donor) and shorten their survival *in vivo*;
iv. the patient's sensitized red cells are destroyed *in vitro* either by complement mediated lysis or through erythrophagocytosis by neutrophils and cells of the mononuclear phagocytic series, monocytes and macrophages. In the case of cold auto-antibodies, autologous rosettes may form between washed red cells and peripheral blood lymphocytes at 37°C;
v. the destruction of the sensitized red cells can be localized *in vivo* to a particular site in the reticulo-endothelial system i.e. the liver or spleen.

In a proportion of cases the diagnosis cannot be established by any of the criteria listed above. In extreme cases neither antibody nor complement can be demonstrated on the red cells and the only evidence of an auto-immune pathogenesis for the haemolysis are the presence of acquired red cell spherocytosis and rapid splenic sequestration of red cells.

It is possible that in some of these cases the red cells are destroyed in the spleen in a lymphocyte mediated cytotoxicity reaction, but there is little or no evidence for this at present and a more plausible explanation is that the amount of sensitizing antibody is below the limits of detection (see below). In other instances the red cells can be shown to be complement-coated in the absence of antibody. However, the presence of complement alone does not in itself constitute evidence for AIHA, since the red cells of primates, including man, exhibit immune adherence. This means they adhere to particles or immune complexes which have fixed C3, the third component of complement. Red cells which have reacted with complexes in this manner acquire a "spurious" complement coating which does not necessarily shorten survival of these cells *in vivo*. This may account for the observation that approximately 8% of patients admitted to hospital show a weakly positive DAT of the complement-only type. Another often-quoted reason for a positive DAT is that some antisera are not monospecific and contain contaminating antibodies such as anti-transferrin which agglutinates reticulocytes.

Treatment with the anti-hypertensive agent α-methyldopa may produce a haemolytic anaemia which mimics AIHA in every respect. The drug apparently elicits a true auto-antibody, though how it does this is still unexplained. The majority of drug-induced immune haemolytic anaemias arise either from drugs adsorbed on the red cell membrane and behaving as extrinsic antigens or from adsorbed immune complexes. Dacie (1951) showed that the auto-immune haemolytic anaemias, on the basis of the clinical presentation and the thermal characteristics of the antibody, fall into two groups. These are the warm antibody type, in which the auto-antibody is optimally bound at 37°C, and the cold antibody type in which the antibody is optimally bound at 4°C and has a characteristic maximum thermal amplitude usually well below 37°C. 70% of cases of AIHA are of the warm type and 30% of the cold type.

There is some dispute about what proportion of cases of AIHA are symptomatic or secondary and what proportion truly idiopathic or primary. In several large European series 45–70% of cases are idiopathic at presentation and the majority remain so even after several years observation. The American experience is different in that less than 20% are idiopathic. In both, however, the common associations of secondary AIHA are lymphoma, Hodgkin's disease, chronic lymphocytic leukaemia, auto-immune disease such as SLE and a variety of infections.

Warm AIHA

Clinical Findings

The mode of presentation in secondary cases is influenced by the primary disorder. Idiopathic cases often present with flu-like prodromal illnesses and fever, or more insidiously with the symptoms of anaemia such as weakness, lassitude, dizziness, dyspnoea, cardiac failure or oedema. The commonest presenting signs are splenomegaly, jaundice and hepatomegaly. Lymphadenopathy is less commonly found. Purpura may occur in the 20% of cases of AIHA associated with thrombocytopenia (Evan's syndrome). When haemolysis is very intense there are certain characteristic appearances in the peripheral blood morphology. Marked anisocytosis arises from the presence of large numbers of reticulocytes derived from macronormoblastic erythrocyte precursors in the bone marrow and the presence of large numbers of spherocytes among the mature red cell population. The neutrophil count may be high, often exceeding 20,000/μl and the platelet count may also be elevated.

The idiopathic disease had a very high mortality (40%) before the advent of steroid therapy. At the present time the appropriate use of prednisolone, splenectomy and azathioprine has reduced the mortality to 10–20%. Deaths rarely occur from the direct effects of haemolysis but rather from complications such as thrombosis or infection. The prognosis in secondary cases reflects the underlying primary disease. Relapse followed by remissions may occur at intervals of months or years. Some patients go on to an apparent "cure" with permanent disappearance of the auto-antibody from the red cells and the serum.

Antibodies on the Red Cells in Warm-type AIHA

The antibody on the red cell membrane is most simply detected by the direct antiglobulin test using class specific anti-Ig antisera. IgG is present in about 85% of cases (Table 1), often in the presence of complement; IgA is uncommonly present with or without IgG, while IgM is rarely if ever detected.

TABLE 1

Warm-type AIHA; incidence of immunoglobulin class on the red cells

	%
IgG only	36
IgG + complement	44
IgA only	3
IgA + IgG	3
Complement only	9
Negative	6

After Dacie and Worlledge (1975).

The IgG antibody is not monoclonal, though tests for kappa and lambda light chain frequency show wide deviations from the normal serum κ/λ ratio of 2/1, indicating that the warm antibodies are not fully polyclonal but partially restricted. The IgG subclass incidence is shown in Table 2.

Only IgG and IgA of the immunoglobulin classes can be eluted from the red cell membrane for further characterization. IgM and complement (C3 or C4) are not elutable.

In a small proportion of cases immunoglobulin cannot be detected on the red cells by the DAT. The limits of sensitivity of this test under optimal conditions are 250–500 molecules of IgG/red cell. One great disadvantage of the test is the requirement for repeatedly washed red cells. Bound antibody tends to elute during washing and the loss is high if the avidity of the bound antibody is low. The loss is exaggerated if the washing fluid is not buffered to pH 7·2–7·4. These factors may account for the virtual failure to detect warm-type IgM antibodies and for the many apparently negative results where IgG antibodies are suspected.

TABLE 2

IgG subclass in warm-type AIHA

%	1	2	3	4
50–70	+	–	–	–
8–14	+	–	+	–
10–14	+	+	–	–
10–20	–	–	–	–

After Engelfriet *et al.* (1974) and Dacie and Worlledge (1975).

Two similar techniques have recently been introduced in an attempt to increase the sensitivity of the antiglobulin test.

i. An antiglobulin consumption test in which residual antiglobulin was measured by its ability to bind to IgG and fix complement after partial absorption by the washed test red cells (Gilliland, 1971).
ii. An antiglobulin consumption test in which the residual antiglobulin lyses IgG-coated sheep red cells after partial absorption by the washed test red cells (Rosse *et al.*, 1974).

It appears that the useful detection range for both tests is from 50–500 molecules/red cell. Unsensitized washed red cells have less than 50 IgG molecules. (Above 500 molecules/red cell the simple DAT should be positive.)

Correlations between rate of haemolysis and amount of bound IgG are disappointingly poor when comparisons are made between different patients. Nevertheless for a given patient, treatment with steroids results in a reduction in the average number of bound IgG molecules and a fall in the haemolytic rate. No satisfactory explanation can be given for the poor correlation between patients though a number of factors influence haemolysis which cannot easily be assessed, such as reticulo-endothelial function or the relative proportion of opsonic (i.e. phagocytosis-promoting) IgG subclasses in the auto-antibody. On the latter point there is firm evidence that only subclasses IgG_1 and IgG_3 show appreciable opsonizing activity.

Specificity of Eluted Warm Auto-antibodies

Eluted antibodies suitable for characterization are IgG or IgA, and the majority of these are of anti-Rhesus specificity. In a third of cases the specificity can be well defined by agglutination patterns against panels of red cells of known Rh phenotype. The commonest specificities determined by this method are anti-e and anti-Ce. If Rh_{null} cells, i.e. cells lacking all CDE antigens and the LW antigen, are included in the panel, some apparent anti-Rh specificity is found in 40–80% of cases, although these include auto-antibodies reacting outside the Rh-system. Some eluates which fail to react with Rh_{null} cells may have more subtle specificities than is at first apparent. It is now recognized that Rh_{null} cells have an aberrant U antigen and abnormalities of the Ss system. In the light of this it is clear that some warm auto-antibodies have anti-U or anti-LW specificities. Warm auto-antibodies of other specificities such as anti-Kell, anti-Jk^a and anti-Fy^a have also been described on rare occasions. Non-specific eluates may also be tested with En^{a-} cells. These very rare red cells have a greatly reduced sialic acid content and diminished electrophoretic mobility. They behave serologically rather like enzyme treated red cells. If non-specific eluates are tested with En^{a-} cells 80% show some anti-En^{a-} specificity.

Antibodies in the Serum in AIHA

Auto-antibody is usually detected in the serum, though its avidity may be markedly lower than the auto-antibody bound to the red cells. For this reason an attempt is made to increase its uptake in the indirect antiglobulin test (IAT) by using enzyme-treated (papainized) red cells. The use of papainized red cells may also reveal the presence of warm haemolysins i.e. auto-antibodies causing complement mediated lysis at 37°C. These haemolysins, which are usually present with warm IgG auto-antibodies, are invariably IgM and without recognizable blood group specificity. The patient's red cells are found to be coated with IgG and complement *in vivo*, but it is not certain that the complement is fixed by the warm haemolysins nor what role the haemolysins play in red cell destruction. Very rarely, haemolysins are present which agglutinate and lyse normal red cells at 37°C. These, in contrast with haemolysins reacting with papainized red cells, may cause intense intravascular red cell destruction with severe anaemia, haemoglobinaemia, haemoglobinuria and jaundice.

Symptomatic Variants of Warm Type AIHA

AIHA is a frequent complication of systemic lupus erythematosus (SLE). The incidence of a positive DAT without haemolysis is high (20–40%) and with overt haemolysis is 5–10% in most series. The auto-antibody may show some anti-Rh specificity in that it is unreactive with Rh_{null} cells, but the presence of complement, C3 and C4, on the red cells suggests that a complement-fixing antibody of a non-specific type is also present. Rarer associations of warm-type AIHA are with ulcerative colitis, rheumatoid arthritis and chronic active hepatitis. Evan's syndrome is the appearance of ITP (idiopathic thrombocytopenic purpura) and AIHA in the same individual. Either condition may precede the other by months or years and regress at a different rate. It is, therefore, uncertain whether the auto-antibody sensitizing the platelets is of the same specificity as that sensitizing the red cells. ITP in its unassociated forms is further discussed below.

Warm type AIHA may occur in children at any age from the early neonatal period. At least five cases occurring within the first years of life have been treated by thymectomy in attempts to control the haemolysis after unsuccessful steroid therapy and splenectomy. Four of these infants rapidly recovered and have not relapsed, though it is not clear how thymectomy helped to bring about a remission. It will be of major interest to follow up these early thymectomy patients to see whether thymus-dependent lymphocyte functions can be maintained throughout adult life. A number of cases of childhood AIHA have been associated with immunity deficiency, particularly X-linked hypogammaglobulinaemia. There is an association between cytomegalovirus infection and AIHA in young children aged 2–12 years. The series reported comprised a clinically heterogeneous group, though half the cases had evidence of hypogammaglobulinaemia, particularly IgA deficiency. The most severe cases had, in addition, complications such as neutropenia and lymphadenopathy.

The common findings were some degree of immunity deficiency and lymphoid tissue abnormalities associated with a progressive virus infection. IgA deficiency is the only common immunoglobulin abnormality found in adult patients with idiopathic AIHA. Since it is the commonest isolated immunoglobulin deficiency in the adult population its significance in AIHA is uncertain. The association of AIHA with malignancy of the lymphoreticular system is well recognized. Warm-type AIHA complicates chronic lymphocytic leukaemia in 10–15% of cases and Hodgkin's disease in 2–5% of cases.

Associations with tumours are rather less common. Thymoma with or without myasthenia gravis has been described with AIHA. An unusual but well-established association of warm-type AIHA is with ovarian tumours or dermoid cysts. The antibodies are usually IgG and of recognizable anti-Rh specificity. In at least two cases the antibody has been present at higher concentrations in the tumour tissue or cyst fluid than in the plasma, suggesting that this is the active site of synthesis. Removal of the tumour, often combined with splenectomy, has in all cases been curative.

Cold Type AIHA

The two types of cold auto-antibody give rise to two different clinical syndromes. These are cold haemagglutinin disease (CHAD) and paroxysmal cold haemoglobinuria (PCH) respectively.

Cold haemagglutinin Disease

Clinical Features

The chronic idiopathic form of the disease commonly first presents between 40–70 years in males and females. It may have an insidious onset with anaemia weakness and lassitude or may present acutely with haemoglobinaemia, haemoglobinuria and jaundice. Raynaud's phenomenon may be a prominent feature and is caused by agglutination of red cells with stasis of blood in capillary beds at exposed skin sites such as the ears, nose and fingers. The cold agglutinating antibody usually has a maximum thermal range of 28–32°C, consequently there is seasonal variation in the severity of the disease with exacerbations in winter and amelioration during the summer. Prolonged exposure to moderate cold reduces skin temperatures to 20–25°C. Raynaud's phenomenon usually develops at this point, whereas systemic reactions appear only after the patient has returned to a warm environment. Rigors, fever, haemoglobinaemia or jaundice may occur.

Some cases show little seasonal variation in the incidence of haemolytic attacks while others have a chronic persistent haemolytic anaemia with few acute exacerbations on exposure to cold. The latter category includes rare individuals with high thermal range cold antibodies agglutinating at temperatures as high as 37°C. These patients, paradoxically, often have only moderate haemolysis. Several factors seem to account for this apparent paradox. Complement levels (CH_{50}) are often very low and it seems that a major degree of hypocomplementaemia protects against acute haemolytic episodes. In addition, complement activation frequently fails to progress to lysis for reasons poorly understood. Sub-lytic complement fixation *in vivo* leads to the coating of red cells with early complement components, especially C4 and C3. If the red cells escape destruction by C3 mediated opsonic adherence and phagocytosis, then both C4 and C3 decay *in vivo* to inactive forms, which interfere with the further uptake of antibody and complement. Most of the circulating red cells in patients with high thermal range cold antibodies acquire resistance to haemolysis by this mechanism.

Many chronic cases of CHAD survive for many years. However, if left untreated their haemagglutinating antibody titres progressively rise and the clinical features become more pronounced and troublesome. A small proportion develop lymphoma after several years of "benign" CHAD and become indistinguishable from the secondary cases, except that the malignancy may progress much more rapidly. Secondary cases of CHAD are associated with neoplasia of the lymphoid tissue, particularly lymphoma and reticulum cell sarcoma and the clinical presentation reflects the primary disorder.

Other secondary forms of CHAD occur as an acute benign complication of certain infections. The best documented is that following atypical pneumonia caused by *Mycoplasma pneumoniae*. A high thermal range cold agglutinin develops 2–3 weeks after the onset of illness in many cases. Haemolysis is rare and when present occurs only at the peak of the antibody response, which lasts a few days. Haemoglobinaemia and haemoglobinuria are less common in the acute form than in the chronic form and the only signs of haemolysis may be anaemia and jaundice. Rarely, however, the haemolysis is severe enough to be associated with renal failure. Raynaud's phenomenon does not seem to be a feature of acute CHAD.

High thermal range cold agglutinins of anti-i specificity also occur in infectious mononucleosis, although the incidence varies widely in different outbreaks. Overt haemolysis is very uncommon, perhaps because of the relative insusceptibility of adult I red cells to the anti-i cold antibody. When haemolysis does occur, however, it clinically resembles that seen in *Mycoplasma pneumoniae* infections. Other infectious agents e.g. adenoviruses, have also been associated with acute forms of cold haemagglutinin disease.

Antibodies in CHAD

Chronic CHAD is caused by the monoclonal proliferation of an abnormal B-cell line. Most of the abnormal lymphocytes are in the bone marrow or the peripheral lymphoid tissues and the cells secrete large amounts of highly homogeneous cold antibody. The cold antibodies are usually IgM antibodies of anti-I specificity, though occasional examples are of anti-i specificity. Some examples of IgA or IgM cold antibodies agglutinate all human red cells and are known as either anti-Sp or anti-Pr. When the haemolytic symptoms first develop the anti-I IgM is usually present in sufficient quantities to be detectable as a compact band on electrophoresis migrating in the slow β-position. Amounts of monoclonal protein present range from 70–2,000 mg/100 ml. Almost all the IgM in the patient's plasma is cold agglutinin and the concentration rises progressively over a period of several years if the patient is not treated. Evidence for homogeneity of the proteins is supported by extensive physico-chemical data. The light chains are commonly kappa only and rarely lambda only. If kappa they tend to belong to a kappa subgroup $V_{\kappa}III$. Antisera prepared against the cold agglutinins will, after appropriate absorption, recognize μ-chain subgroup specificities or even individual or idiotypic specificities. For example one common anti-idiotypic serum recognizes 73% of cold agglutinins of anti-I specificity. The antibodies have the typical thermal characteristics of cold agglutinins with agglutination titres at 4°C of 8,000–128,000 against group O adult red cells. Titres fall progressively as avidity falls at higher temperatures and each cold agglutinin has a characteristic maximum thermal amplitude, usually 28–32°C but sometimes extending to 37°C. Cord blood red cells carrying the i-antigen are only weakly agglutinated by the antibody.

The antibody is weakly lytic. Lysis can be demonstrated monophasically at 20–23°C or biphasically by alternately cooling to 4°C and then rewarming to 37°C. Lysis is enhanced with enzyme treated cells, but in all cases agglutination titres are higher than lytic titres. Abnormal lymphocytes may be present in the peripheral blood. Although the presence of these cells may suggest the development of a lymphoma, in some cases the lymphocytes may be actively sensitized, since a proportion of peripheral blood lymphocytes rosette with adult red cells at 4°C in a reaction which can be inhibited by soluble I-antigen.

The cold agglutinins in the acute secondary cases are usually of anti-I specificity in *Mycoplasma pneumoniae* infections and anti-i in infectious mononucleosis, though rarer specificities are sometimes reported, for example anti-N, anti-M and anti-IT. The antibodies are polyclonal, distinguishing them from the idiopathic variety, though the κ/λ ratio is abnormal, suggesting some restriction of heterogeneity. Some cold antibodies in infectious mononucleosis appear to be of a more complex composition. A cold-reacting IgG antibody of anti-i specificity binds to red cells; an agglutinating IgM anti-IgG then reacts with the bound IgG, in the manner of rheumatoid factor.

The Red Cell in CHAD

In chronic CHAD the DAT is always positive and in acute CHAD is positive at the peak of haemolysis. The red cells only react with anti-complement sera and detailed analysis of these reactions shows that C4 and C3 are present. The C3-coating on the circulating cells is the haemolytically and opsonically inactive form known as C3d. The significance of this observation appears to be that the red cells acquire a complement coating through the continuous weak interaction of the cold agglutinin with red cells at temperatures around 20–30°C. For reasons not fully understood complement fixation is arrested at the C3-step and the active form of bound C3 known as C3b decays to C3d through the action of the plasma inactivator of C3b (see Chapter 7). The major antigenic fragment (A) of C3b is lost, leaving a weaker antigenic determinant (D) on the C3d part of the molecule. It is this D-determinant of C3d that is detected by agglutination with anti-C3 sera when the DAT is carried out with the red cells of patients with CHAD. Most anti-C3 sera can be used since they react with both A and D determinants.

Paroxysmal Cold Haemoglobinuria (PCH)

The clinical features of PCH have been recognized for many years as a result of its dramatic and highly characteristic presentation. The chronic form of PCH was a classical complication of congenital syphilis and in some individuals episodes of haemolysis were observed and recorded for several years. Few cases of PCH are seen now, and appear as a rare complication of measles, mumps, chickenpox, infectious mononucleosis or other undiagnosed "flu-like" illnesses. Unlike the chronic syphilitic form, the virus-associated illness is transient, appearing after 2–3 weeks of illness and rapidly disappearing as the titre of the Donath–Landsteiner antibody of PCH falls. The haemolytic attacks are usually more severe than those associated with CHAD and a single paroxysmal episode may destroy up to 40% of the circulating red cells. There appear to be several reasons for this. The antibody is highly lytic but has a low thermal range usually not exceeding 10–17°C. Complement levels are consequently normal until extreme skin cooling occurs.

Complement fixation is then initiated in the cold peripheral capillaries and completed as the cells return to the central circulation. Since the antibody is not a powerful agglutinin, peripheral stasis is not marked. The result is that relatively large numbers of red cells pass through the cold areas and become sensitized. These same cells rapidly return to the warm central circulation where lysis occurs throughout the period of cold exposure. Rigors, fever, haemoglobinaemia, and neutropenia occur at this stage. Later during re-warming, jaundice, haemoglobinuria and neutrophilia develop. At this stage spherocytes appear for the first time in the peripheral blood.

The Antibody in PCH

The cold antibody of PCH is the classical biphasic haemolysin first described by Donath and Landsteiner in 1904. This D–L antibody is an IgG antibody of anti-P specificity, i.e. it will lyse all except the rare pp and pk red cells. The biphasic characteristics of the lytic reaction are a consequence of the antibody's very low maximum thermal amplitude of 10–17°C. Fixation of C1 and C4 occurs at 4°C and so initiates complement fixation. When the incubation temperature is raised to 25–37°C complement fixation progresses through to lysis. It is usually possible to produce slow monophasic lysis of red cells by the D–L antibody at 15–25°C. The antibody is so weakly agglutinating in saline, even at 4°C, that its detection on red cells is best carried out by washing the red cells in the cold and carrying out the DAT at 4°C. For a few hours after a paroxysmal attack the patient's red cells are agglutinable by an anti-C3 serum.

Aetiology and Pathogenesis of AIHA

Auto-antibody is clearly implicated in the pathogenesis of the majority of cases of AIHA and the pattern of haemolysis *in vivo* depends on the type of coating the red cells acquire.

IgG-only Coatings (Warm-type AIHA)

If complement is not fixed by the IgG auto-antibody, red cell destruction occurs without lysis at restricted sites in the reticulo-endothelial system, particularly in the spleen. Inability to fix complement is a characteristic of auto-antibodies of anti-Rh specificity including the auto-antibodies associated with methyl-dopa therapy. At present the most plausible explanation for the inability to fix complement is that the Rh antigenic sites are too far apart to allow a pair of IgG molecules to bind within a critical minimum distance of one another on the red cell membrane. Pairing or doublet formation of IgG antibodies is required for fixation of C1.

In the absence of complement fixation, red cells which have been lightly coated with IgG are removed from the circulation by interaction between the Fc ends of the red cell bound IgG and Fc-receptors on cells of the mononuclear phagocytic series (Fig. 1). These interactions take place most readily in the red pulp of the spleen where the red cells come into close proximity with fixed and free macrophages in the Bilroth cords. Within this specialized sequestration tissue red cells are either phagocytosed whole or partially fragmented. It is believed that surface fragmentation by removing proportionately more red cell membrane than red cell volume progressively converts

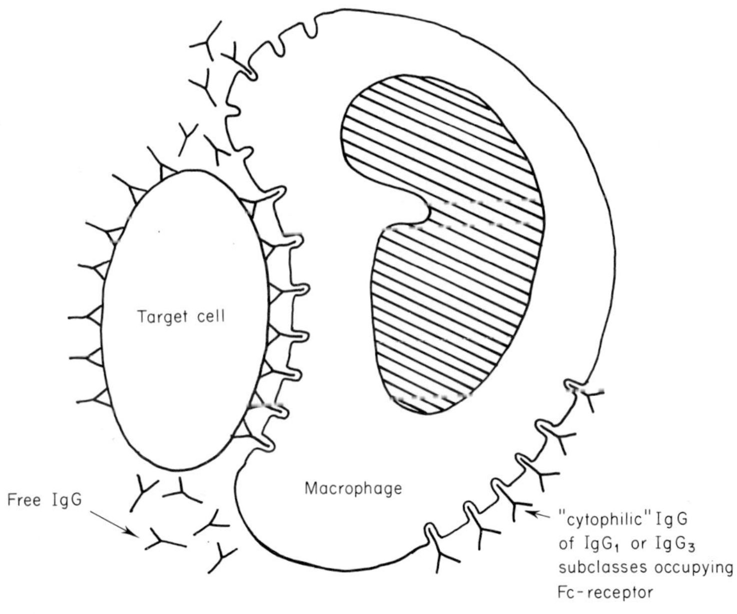

Fig. 1. Interaction between a target red cell coated with IgG and a cell of the mononuclear phagocytic series. The phagocytic cell possesses Fc-receptors which can be occupied by free immunoglobulin of the IgG_1 or IgG_3 subclasses. This cytophilic IgG may be displaced from the Fc receptors by the array of IgG molecules coating the target cell. Immune (opsonic) adherence follows and may finally result in erythrophagocytosis. IgM (19S macroglobulin form) is not cytophilic or opsonizing and takes no part in this reaction.

the biconcave red cell into a spherocytic shape. Increasing spherocytosis decreases red cell deformability and successive passages through the red pulp may eventually sphere the cell sufficiently to prevent it crossing the venous sinus walls to return to the general circulation, since the effective gap between endothelial cells in the sinus walls is only 2–3 μm. Outside the environment of the spleen, the binding of the Fc-piece of IgG with Fc receptors on monocytes or hepatic macrophages (Kupffer cells) is less easily achieved, since the sites are competed for and occupied by free-circulating IgG (Fig. 1). The result is that hepatic sequestration of IgG-coated red cells or phagocytosis by peripheral blood monocytes occurs only if the IgG-coating is high, perhaps 5,000–15,000 molecules/red cell. Of the four IgG subclasses, only two, IgG_1 and IgG_3, are significantly sensitizing or opsonic and take part in the Fc–Fc receptor interactions discussed above.

Complement Coatings

Fixation of complement increases the haemolytic rate by antibody in most circumstances. This is particularly so for IgM antibodies which have no capacity to react via Fc–Fc receptor interactions with cells of the mononuclear phagocytic system. IgM antibodies, therefore, have no inherent opsonizing potential unless they fix complement. Nevertheless, there are rare examples of non-complement fixing agglutinating antibodies which bring about non-lytic red cell destruction, perhaps by the trapping effect of intravascular agglutination.

There are two types of complement mediated red cell destruction. The first is complement lysis. Intravascular haemolysis liberates red cell membrane ghosts and haemoglobin into the plasma and the ghosts are cleared from the circulation by Kupffer cells in the liver. This type is seen following chilling in CHAD and PCH when complement levels are high and not limiting for lysis. A more subtle form of complement mediated red cell destruction occurs when the complement cascade fails to complete to lysis but is arrested at an intermediate stage after C3-fixation. There is no entirely satisfactory explanation at present why this happens, though it may be related to (i) the lability of some active complement component, (ii) imbalanced consumption of C5–7 or (iii) to over-action of the C3b-inactivator which destroys the "haemolytic" activity of bound C3.

Red cells which have acquired a coating of opsonically-active C3(C3b) are removed at sites throughout the RES by adherence to C3b-receptors on monocytes, macrophages and neutrophils (Fig. 2). Erythrophagocytosis may follow, or surface adherence to the cytoplasmic membrane of the phagocytic cell may result in red cell fragmentation. The C3b-receptor sites of phagocytic cells "recognize" C3b but not native C3 in the plasma or the breakdown products C3c and C3d. The most important implication of this for receptor function is that unlike the Fc-receptor, which is readily blocked by IgG immunoglobulin, the C3b receptor is uninhibited by native C3. C3b-coated red cells freely interact with C3b-receptor sites throughout the circulation and are predominantly sequestered in the liver, the reticulo–endothelial organ with the highest blood flow and largest number of macrophages. The selective environment of the spleen is therefore not a special requirement for C3b-coated red cells. However, the presence of a powerful C3b-inactivator introduces a slight complication to the system. Red cells which escape phagocytosis in the reticulo–endothelial system eventually return to the circulation, as the

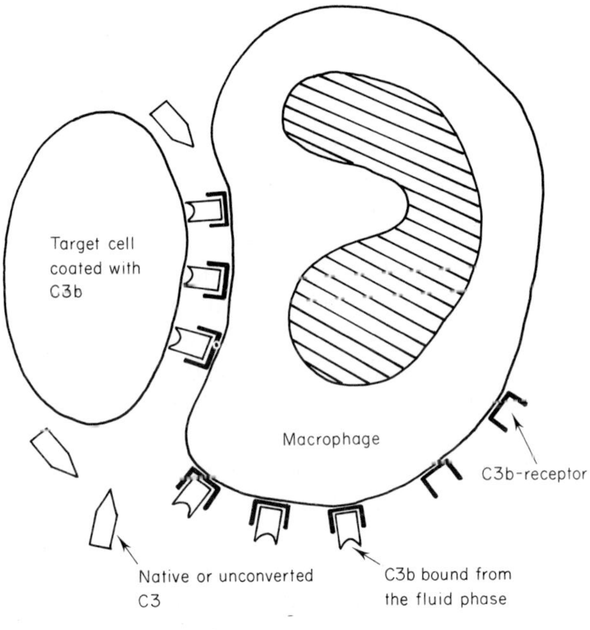

Fig. 2. Interaction between a target red cell coated with C3b and either a cell of the mononuclear phagocytic series or a neutrophil. The C3b coating has been fixed by either an IgG or an IgM antibody. C3b receptors cover the phagocytic cell. These receptors cannot be occupied or blocked by native unconverted C3, though they may be occupied by C3b activated in the fluid phase. Immune (opsonic) adherence follows interaction between the C3b-coated red cell and the phagocytic cell. Whether or not phagocytosis follows may depend on (i) maturity or degree of activation of the macrophage (ii) the surface density of receptors or (iii) the amount of C3b on the target cell.

C3b is inactivated. The inactivator destroys C3b–C3b receptor interaction by cleaving the molecule into a C3d fragment which remains attached to the red cell and a C3c fragment which is lost into the plasma. The opsonic activity of C3b is therefore of limited half-life *in vivo* and red cells which escape phagocytosis may return to the circulation coated with C3d. It is likely that complement-fixation in CHAD at 25–37°C often occurs at such a low intensity that any C3b formed is inactivated to C3d before the red cells are sequestered at all. Red cells may gradually accumulate a coating of C3d by such a mechanism. It is this C3d coating which reacts relatively weakly with most anti-C3 sera in the DAT in complement-fixing AIHA.

The concept of failure of self-tolerance is central to any discussion of the aetiology of AIHA. However, since no direct studies have been attempted in man to determine whether tolerance to red cell auto-antigens really exists, or, even assuming its existence, whether it is selectively abrogated in AIHA, any views on the subject tend to be highly speculative and are usually based on an understanding of tolerance mechanisms obtained from experimental systems.

Three main groups of auto-antibodies need to be accounted for:

i. IgG antibodies of anti-Rh specificity.
ii. Acute cold antibodies of anti-I, anti-i or anti-P specificity.
iii. Chronic "monoclonal" antibodies of anti-I specificity.

There are several forms of tolerance or hyporeactive states (see Chapter 2), and it would be inappropriate to discuss all of them here. Tolerance may result from destruction of antigen reactive cells, a phenomenon known as clonal elimination. Since potentially reactive cells are thought to be permanently removed by clonal elimination, it might be expected to be a highly stable form of tolerance. However, there is increasing evidence that some forms of tolerance are active processes in which potentially reactive cells must be kept in a continually suppressed state.

Optimum doses of soluble antigen are required to trigger T- or B-cells. Any wide deviation from the optimum range may result in failure to react or tolerance. An excess of soluble antigen can result in "high zone" tolerance affecting both B- and T-cell populations. B-cells with their high antigen–receptor density can normally be made tolerant only under high zone conditions and they may quickly recover if the antigen is eliminated. Tolerance is induced in T-cells, on the other hand, not only under high zone conditions, but also by subimmunogenic amounts of antigen (low zone tolerance).

There is evidence in man that tolerance to certain self-antigens is maintained only at the T-cell level and that the B-cells are not in a tolerant state but are potentially capable of responding to thymus-dependent antigens with the appropriate T-cell help if T-cell tolerance can be broken. It is possible that tolerance to self Rh-antigens is of this type since some characteristics of the antigen would not make it a good B-cell tolerogen; (i) the "dose" of antigen is small (ii) it is only present on red cells and the total number of antigenic sites probably does not exceed 50,000–60,000 per cell (iii) it is not present in a soluble form in the plasma or secretions and does not have a repeating polysaccharide structure which would favour induction of B-cell tolerance. In this respect the Rh system can be contrasted with the ABO, Ii and Lewis blood group systems. Repeating carbohydrate determinants are present on the red cell membrane, in a soluble form in the plasma and in some individuals in saliva, gastric juice and milk. A major weakness of any hypothesis that tolerance to Rh-antigens is maintained at the T-cell level is that it could equally well be applied to many other blood group antigens to which auto-antibodies are rarely if ever elicited. The Rh auto-antibodies commonly show partial specificity for the weaker Rh-antigens such as C, c or e and rarely for the immunogenic antigen D. This apparent anomaly is consistent with the observation that powerful immunogens under one set of conditions can behave as tolerogens under different conditions, and raises the possibility that firm tolerance to the weaker Rh-antigens is never properly established in early life in some individuals.

In model carrier-hapten systems, escape from established T-cell tolerance towards a carrier can be achieved by immunizing with a cross-reacting carrier molecule. It is believed that this recruits T-cell help and circumvents the primary T-cell tolerance so allowing B-cells to produce antihapten antibody. Mechanisms of this type may be relevant to the appearance of auto-antibodies following infections by microorganisms. In particular, it may account for the rise in titre and thermal range of anti-I in acute CHAD and the appearance of anti-i in infectious mononucleosis. The presence of I-like antigen in *Mycoplasma pneumoniae* is disputed, though the intact organism has a high affinity for the red cell membrane and appears to be capable of "fusion" to the red cell in the manner of Sendai virus.

An even less well understood function of T-cells or a T-cell subpopulation is the capacity to exert suppressor function either on helper T-cells or on B-cells. There is some uncertainty about the target for the suppressor effect. In experimental animals, tolerance to xenogeneic red cells can only be established if T-cells are present. The tolerant state is an active one in that it is maintained despite the inherent capacity of the B-cells to respond by antibody formation and, moreover, the tolerance can be transferred to other animals by antibody free T-cells. One essential requirement therefore seems to be a competent T-cell subpopulation able to suppress other lymphocyte functions. The development of anti-red cell auto-antibodies in NZB mice occurs at a time when thymus-dependent lymphocyte functions are prematurely waning. Studies in the NZB mouse indicate that loss of T-cell suppressor activity is a critical factor in escape from tolerance. The relevance of this model system to man is far from clear, though the development of auto-antibodies in children with virus diseases such as cytomegalic inclusion disease, mumps, measles, or chickenpox is an interesting association, since there is often evidence of T-cell anergy or more complex immunodeficiency in these infections.

Hypotheses about T-cell helper or T-cell suppressor function in relation to auto-allergy may not be entirely incompatible with one another, and it is conceivable that the homeostasis of self-tolerance is an active process controlled by the balance between these two functions. However, until more information is available about tolerance in man, it would be inappropriate to speculate more about the aetiology of AIHA.

Treatment of Warm-type AIHA

The presence of markedly spherocytic red cells and a positive DAT with clinical evidence of haemolysis is sufficient to initiate treatment. It is important to attempt to establish whether the AIHA is idiopathic or secondary at an early stage, and in particular to exclude diseases such as SLE or lymphoma. Secondary cases should be suspected if the red cell coating is IgG + complement rather than IgG only.

Steroids

Steroid therapy is the standard treatment for warm-type AIHA and should not be delayed. Prednisone or prednisolone are commenced at 60–80 mg/day in divided doses. There seems to be no advantage in giving very much higher doses as has been recommended from time to time, and even the dose of 60–80 mg should be administered only for 5–6 days.

The dose is reduced step-wise to 20 mg/day within 6–8 days. The rate of reduction from this level should then be much slower, reducing to 2·5–10 mg/day over a period of several weeks. Of patients with idiopathic warm-type AIHA, 80–90% go into remission on this regime, the majority within 8–12 days. Remission is heralded by stabilization of haemoglobin concentration and haematocrit. The elevated bilirubin level falls and as the haemoglobin concentration reaches near-normal levels the reticulocyte count falls. Serum auto-antibody titres measured by the IAT fall progressively over several weeks and quantitative tests show that the mean number of red cell bound antibody molecules falls. However, this reduction of bound antibody is not readily detected by the DAT, which may remain positive for months or years, often without detectably weakening. The reason for this is not entirely clear, though it is possible that antibody of rather high avidity can be continuously transferred to younger red cells.

The persistence of splenomegaly or of lymphadenopathy after complete haematological remission are indications for a careful search to exclude Hodgkin's disease or lymphoma.

Ten to twenty per cent of patients either fail to go into remission or can be maintained in remission only on an unacceptably high dose of steroids. For these patients either splenectomy or immunosuppressive drugs should be considered. Either of these courses of action may be necessary if one of the complications of steroid therapy develops, such as osteoporosis, myopathy, psychosis, gastrointestinal bleeding or perforation.

Blood Transfusion

Packed red cells or whole blood should be given to maintain the patient in a clinically stable state. The necessity for transfusion needs to be stressed, especially where the antibody has no demonstrable specificity and all donor red cells are incompatible. Although it might seem doubtful here whether blood should be given, blood should be screened for compatibility and the least incompatible blood given, since if the donor red cells react more weakly than the patient's red cells with the serum antibody some benefit may be expected. If the antibody has definable anti-Rh specificity for example anti-e, then compatible blood, in this case R_2R_2 (cDE/cDE) is given.

Immunosuppressive Therapy

Azathioprine is, hitherto, the most widely used immunosuppressant in warm-type AIHA. It is given at a dose of 1·5–2·5 mg/kg/day, usually with little evidence of bone marrow depression though neutropenia is a risk. It can be usefully combined with steroid therapy to reduce the maintenance dose of the latter when unacceptably high. The steroids should not be reduced too soon, since the onset of effect of azathioprine is slow and usually takes 2–3 weeks.

Immunoglobulin levels should be regularly measured in patients receiving long-term azathioprine as they tend to fall.

Antilymphocyte globulin (ALG) may have a role as an immunosuppressive agent in AIHA, though there is little experience with it so far. This is true of auto-immune disease in general. One reason for the cautious use of the ALG preparations available has been the potential risk of inducing or promoting tumours, particularly those of the reticulo-endothelial system although statistical analysis of the limited data available suggests that this risk is no greater with ALG than for other immunosuppressive agents. Isolated reports of its successful use in secondary AIHA suggest that it can have a therapeutic effect. Practical drawbacks to ALG are its high cost and the development of allergic reactions through sensitization to horse globulins. Attempts have been made to overcome the problem of sensitization in patients who have never previously received horse proteins by making them tolerant by giving large doses of deaggregated horse globulin before attempting ALG therapy.

Splenectomy

Patients with warm-type AIHA who have failed to respond to or have only partially responded to steroids may be considered for splenectomy. The most favourable indications that splenectomy will be of value are as follows:

i. an IgG-only DAT;
ii. a spherocytic peripheral blood red cell morphology;
iii. evidence from radioactive studies with labelled red cells of selective splenic uptake estimated by surface counting or scanning of the liver and spleen;
iv. steroid-resistant splenomegaly.

The spleen is often removed in secondary cases either for biopsy material to aid the diagnosis or to "stage" Hodgkin's disease. When the red cell DAT is of the IgG + complement type, splenectomy is likely to be less beneficial and after splenectomy there may be as rapid, though now hepatic, destruction of red cells as before. The overall correctness of the preoperative prediction of benefit is 40–60%. Splenectomy is contra-indicated in children with warm-type AIHA less than 6–8 years old. Splenectomy in children for reasons other than uncomplicated trauma results in a substantial risk of major bacterial infection, particularly with encapsulated organisms such as the pneumococcus and *Haemophilus influenzae*. The risk is also present in adults if anaemia persists after splenectomy. Children should receive penicillin V as long-term prophylaxis against gram positive organisms if splenectomy has been performed. Patients in whom splenectomy has failed to ameliorate the haemolysis are at risk from further complications. Severe anaemia seems to "drive" the precursor cells of the bone marrow unselectively, so that the patient often has a neutrophilia and a mild thrombocytosis. Splenectomy without remission of the haemolytic rate may exaggerate such thrombocytosis, raising the platelet count to 600–1,000 × 10^3/μl. This group of patients are at considerable risk from thromboembolism.

Treatment During Pregnancy

There have been a number of reports of the successful treatment of pregnant patients with AIHA. High dose steroids and azathioprine have been given without harming the foetus. If remission of the AIHA occurs on steroids alone the dose of steroids should probably not be reduced below 20 mg/day until after delivery, when it can be slowly brought down over several weeks to 2·5–10 mg/day.

Treatment of Cold-type AIHA

Patients with acute infection-associated CHAD or PCH require no treatment except warmth and bed rest unless anaemia is severe enough to merit blood transfusion. Blood is best given as packed cells, or red cells suspended in saline to avoid transfusing complement and the cells should be pre-warmed in a coil passed through a 37°C water bath before they enter the patient.

The long-term management of idiopathic CHAD is less satisfactory. Steroid therapy and splenectomy are of little or no value, since most of the red cell destruction occurs either by intravascular lysis or by hepatic sequestration. The most widely used immunosuppressive agent is chlorambucil given at a dosage of 2–4 mg/kg daily. The aim is to depress the serum IgM level, which is a direct reflection of the amount of circulating cold agglutinin and by this manoeuvre to raise the haemoglobin concentration and reduce the amount of C3 on the circulating red cells as measured by the DAT. Agglutinin and lysin titres should also fall, though the clinical and haematological improvement may take many weeks. The risks of long and continued chlorambucil therapy are as for other alkylating agents and include neutropenia, depression of IgA and IgG levels, infection and the possible induction of lymphomas.

A technique which has not so far been completely evaluated may prove to be particularly useful in chronic CHAD. Of the cold agglutinin IgM, 70–90% is in the intravascular space, and therefore accessible to removal by plasmaphoresis using a continuous-flow blood cell separator (see Chapter 31). In a single session it is possible to exchange 5,000 ml of plasma and remove 75–85% of the intravascular IgM. Since the IgM synthesis rate by the abnormal lymphoid cells is independent of the serum IgM level, removing the intravascular IgM pool does not increase the synthesis rate by positive feedback. Initial studies of this plasmaphoresis technique indicate that the IgM level can be kept at an acceptable level by treatment every 5–6 weeks. The technique is less applicable to the removal of IgG antibodies because (a) 30–50% of the IgG is in the extravascular space, and (b) high affinity antibody will be firmly bound to red cells at 37°C.

Drug-induced IHA

Overt immune haemolytic anaemia (IHA) can arise from the administration of drugs and present with a clinical and serological picture virtually indistinguishable from AIHA. The distinction can usually, but not always, be made by showing that the drug is able to damage both autologous and allogeneic red cells in appropriate combination with an antibody of anti-drug specificity. Withdrawal of the drug usually results in rapid remission of IHA. Rechallenge of the patient with the drug after full haematological remission results in relapse within a few days. This step is generally unethical and is inadvisable unless there is genuine confusion as to the drug involved and it is therapeutically desirable to continue it. Alpha-methyl dopa is the prototype of several drugs which cause IHA by a mechanism which does not involve the interaction of the drugs with red cells in the circulation and the normal rules for demonstrating the involvement of the drug in IHA do not apply here.

Three main types of drug-induced IHA can be defined on the basis of the mechanism of sensitization of the red cells:

i. adsorption of drug-antibody complexes from the plasma to circulating red cells;
ii. stable haptenic-binding of the drug to circulating red cells;
iii. drug-induced auto-antibody formation to "normal" red cell antigens.

Adsorption of Drug-antibody Complexes

The largest group of drugs causing IHA are found under this heading (Table 3) and the list continues to grow as new drugs are added to it from time to time.

TABLE 3
Drugs causing IHA by immune complex formation

Stibophen
Para-aminosalicylic acid
Isoniazid
Quinine
Quinidine
Melphalan
Phenacetin
Pyramidon
Sulphonamides
Chlorpromazine
Tolbutamide
Dipyrone
Rifampicin
Tetracycline
Insulin

The requirements for the reaction *in vitro* are (i) the presence of the drug; (ii) a source of fresh human complement; and (iii) ABO compatible human red cells. The most widely accepted explanation for the reaction which follows are that (i) antibody to the drug is present in the plasma; (ii) this is usually IgM and complement fixing; (iii) a drug-antibody complex forms which "loosely" adsorbs onto the red cell membrane where complement activation occurs; (iv) activation of complement in close proximity to the red cell membrane results in the deposition of C4 and C3. If enzyme-treated or PNH red cells are used complement-dependent haemolysis may occur. *In vivo*, the effects of complement fixation by the complexes may be more severe. In 60–70% of cases administration of the drug is promptly followed by intravascular haemolysis, haemoglobinaemia and haemoglobinuria. Acute renal failure is a well documented complication. The DAT usually does not reveal either IgM or IgG on the red cells, though there are strong reactions with anti-complement sera.

It is not clear why certain drug–antibody complexes have a predilection to bind to red cells. The avidity is rather low, since washing the red cells usually removes the complex. In some cases where the IgM antibody is powerfully complement fixing, it is conceivable that the complex binds to red cells via the interaction of complex fixed C3b and the immune adherence (C3) receptor present on most primate red cells including man. However, a more likely explanation is that complex absorption precedes the fixation of complement. The red cells are thought to lyse *in vivo* by a "bystander" reaction. Complement is activated in close proximity to the red cell membrane and the "lytic phase" complement component complexes $C\overline{567}$ or $C\overline{567, 8, 9}$ are generated in the fluid phase. From here, by their contagious behaviour, they diffuse to the red cell membrane and cause lysis.

Stable Haptenic Binding of the Drug to Circulating Red Cells

Only penicillin and cephalosporin act in this manner and most of the information about the reactions leading to drug-induced IHA have come from extensive studies with penicillin. Penicillin is a chemically active molecule capable of stable covalent binding to plasma proteins and membrane-associated proteins. Once bound, it cannot be washed off, unlike the drug-antibody complexes described above. Serological reactions with anti-penicillin antibodies can only be performed against penicillin-coated red cells either obtained from patients or artificially coated *in vitro*. A great deal of interest has centred on the chemical alteration of penicillin required to enable it to bind in a haptenic form. The major haptenic determinant is the benzyl-penicilloyl group (BPO), though several minor haptenic forms have been described among which the benzyl-penaldic acid group is commonly quoted.

IHA due to penicillin only develops if patients receive very large doses (8–20 mega-units/day) for several weeks. High penicillin blood levels are achieved and the red cells become coated in the circulation. Antibodies to BPO are common and by sensitive tests can be shown to be present in more than 90% of normal individuals. The high incidence probably reflects the ubiquitous distribution of the drug. Most of the antibody in the normal population is IgM, but IgG antibodies may also be present. There appears to be no correlation between either of these two antibodies and the level of IgE anti-penicillin antibody which is responsible for the reaginic type of reaction to penicillin. Patients receiving large doses of penicillin develop high titres of IgG antibodies in addition to haemagglutinating IgM, but even in this group only about 3% develop IHA.

Red cell destruction by the IgG antibody is usually non-lytic and is effected by splenic sequestration, though patients have been reported with IgM antibodies who have developed severe haemoglobinaemia and haematuria. Continued administration of penicillin irrespective of the main antibody class can lead to severe anaemia requiring blood transfusion.

Cephalothin is the only other antibiotic to cause haemolytic anaemia by a mechanism similar to that of penicillin, and cephalothin is of further immunological interest in that it is sufficiently closely related to penicillin for anti-penicillin antibodies to cross-react with cephalothin-coated red cells. In addition, cephalothin apparently has the curious property of combining with red cell membranes and altering them in such a way that many plasma proteins such as albumin, IgA, α_1-antitrypsin, α_2-macroglobulin and fibrinogen as well as IgG and IgM immunoglobulins and complement are adsorbed non-immunologically. This phenomenon can result in false positive DATs and these will be particularly confusing if the anti-Ig sera are not strictly monospecific.

Drug-induced Auto-antibody Formation to Normal Red Cell Antigens

Alpha-methyldopa induced IHA is the commonest form of drug-related IHA described, and the commonest cause of a positive DAT without haemolysis due to drugs. L-dopa, structurally related and mefenamic acid, structurally unrelated, also cause positive DATs and very occasional haemolytic anaemia in the same manner as α-methyldopa.

Of patients receiving methyldopa therapy for more than three months 10–36% eventually develop a positive DAT, and the highest incidence occurs with the highest dosages (more than two g/day). A latent period of 3–6 months always seems to be required even when the drug is given a second time. The incidence of overt IHA is much lower than the incidence of a positive DAT and in most series is only 0·5–1·0%. The DAT progressively weakens after drug withdrawal, but may not completely disappear for many months. Recovery from IHA is usually more rapid, though some patients require blood transfusion and steroids.

The serology of the auto-antibodies which appear in methyldopa-induced IHA is virtually identical with that seen in warm-type AIHA where the antibody is IgG-only and of anti-Rh specificity. Eluates from patients' red cells react with all Rh-antigen bearing cells, sometimes with sufficient variation in the strength of the reaction with known Rh-phenotypes to allow a partial definition of anti-Rh specificity, e.g. anti-e, to be made. In many instances, however, it is only possible to prove a relationship to the Rh-system by failure of the antibodies to react with Rh_{null} and Lw-negative red cells. This lack of specificity seems to apply particularly to the serum auto-antibody.

No satisfactory explanation has yet been given for the development of what appear to be typical warm-type IgG auto-antibodies during methyldopa therapy. It seems unlikely that the drug behaves as a hapten since experiments have failed to show convincingly that it binds to red cells either by itself or in combination with antibody. The suggestion has been made that it combines with the red cell membrane during maturation in the bone marrow in such a way that it subtly alters the Rh-antigenic determinants and renders them antigenic, but again, evidence for such a concept is weak. Yet another possibility is that the drug acts centrally on the immune system in such a way that it removes restraints which hold potentially auto-reactive cells in a tolerant state. This hypothesis is untested.

Paroxysmal Nocturnal Haemoglobinuria (PNH)

The justification for including PNH in a group of immunological blood disorders rests on the evidence that PNH red cells show a greatly enhanced susceptibility to complement mediated lysis due to a still largely unexplained intrinsic abnormality of the red cell membrane. A detailed account of the haematological associations of PNH is outside the scope of the chapter and so will not be given.

Clinical Features

Only a minority of patients who develop PNH present with classical repeated episodes of nocturnal or post-nocturnal haemoglobinuria. In many cases the onset of haemolysis is insidious and overt attacks of haemoglobinaemia, haemoglobinuria and jaundice may only be precipitated from time to time by episodes of stress such as infections, immunizations, surgery or exercise. Abdominal pain is common and seems to be due to multiple venous thromboses in the intestinal and mesenteric circulation. Venous thrombosis is a common complication at other sites particularly in the liver, spleen and lungs, possibly because these are the sites of clearance of lysed red cells from the circulation. Although many ingenious clinical studies have been performed to determine the cause of PNH, at present there is no entirely plausible explanation for the cyclical nocturnal haemolysis and most of the evidence about the nature of the red cell abnormality has come from *in vitro* studies.

Defect in vitro

Several tests have been devised to detect the PNH abnormality with greater or lesser precision. All are based on the generation of the lytic (C5–9) phase of the complement activation cascade by either the classical or alternative (properdin) pathways (see Chapter 7) and then observing the excessive lytic effect of C5–9 on PNH red cells as compared with normal red cells.

In the *acid lysis test* complement is activated in the "fluid-phase" of virtually neat serum by lowering the pH of the final reaction mixture to 6·5–6·8. If the Mg^{++} ion concentration is sufficient the alternative pathway fires spontaneously and the PNH red cells lyse. The classical pathway is not required since the reaction takes place in Ca^{++} free medium and in serum devoid of C2 and C4. In contrast the reaction does require the components of the alternative pathway, which are properdin, Factor D and Factor B. At physiological pH, activators of the alternative complement pathway such as CVF (cobra venom factor) and particulate inulin lyse PNH red cells at low serum dilutions, i.e. 50–90% serum. Two other tests, the *cold lysis test* and the *sucrose lysis test*, depend on the generation of complement activation via the classical pathway through C142. In the cold lysis test PNH red cells are directly damaged by a lytic IgM cold antibody of anti-I specificity and enhanced lysis can be demonstrated compared with normal cells. In the sucrose lysis test the ionic strength of the serum is reduced to half normal by addition of 6% sucrose in water. Under these conditions it is believed that some IgG immunoglobulin aggregates and binds to red cells where it fixes complement via the classical pathway.

The common factor in the *in vitro* tests is the generation of the terminal lytic phase of the complement cascade, C5–9, in close proximity to red cell membranes, C$\overline{567}$, the activated form of C5, C6 and C7 and possibly C$\overline{567,89}$ (the complete terminal sequence) are activated in the ambient serum or "fluid phase" around the complement fixation site. In the fluid phase the terminal complement sequences are contagious and can attach to any lipid bilayer within a critical diffusion distance, effectively only a few microns, before they become inactive. C$\overline{567}$ can attach to PNH red cells by this contagious effect whether or not the cells were the original site of complement activation, whereas normal human red cells are relatively insensitive to this effect of C$\overline{567}$. PNH red cells also take up more purified C5 and lyse more efficiently when C6–9 are added. The underlying red cell membrane abnormality responsible for the greater sensitivity to complement lysis is unknown.

Varying proportions of patients' red cells (0–60%) show the PNH abnormality. This proportion may vary with the state of the disease and usually declines to zero as the patient recovers. In some cases the red cell populations are more complex and a third group of red cells may be present with characteristics intermediate between normal and PNH red cells. PNH-like red cells can be prepared from normal human red cells *in vitro* by treating them with reduced glutathione (GSH). It has also been found that normal guinea-pig red cells resemble PNH red cells *in vitro* in their high degree of sensitivity to C5–9, though the red cells do not haemolyse *in vivo*. At least a proportion of the platelets and neutrophils of patients with PNH show the same complement sensitivity indicating that the abnormality arises at the haemopoietic stem cell level.

THROMBOCYTOPENIC PURPURA

Clinical Features

A number of clinical syndromes are associated with severe thrombocytopenia due to the immunological destruction of circulating platelets. *Chronic* ITP (idiopathic thrombocytopenic purpura) is considered to be a true auto-immune disease in that the onset is insidious without prodromal signs. *Acute* ITP may not be an auto-immune disease since more than 80% of cases are associated with or follow infections, particularly rubella, pertussis, measles, mumps and chickenpox. Acute ITP also occurs predominantly in young children aged 2–12 years. When ITP is associated with AIHA in Evan's syndrome it seems to be a true auto-immune disease as it may also be in association with SLE, lymphoma and rheumatoid arthritis. The allergic drug-induced thrombocytopenias arise as a result of platelet damage by drug-antibody complexes.

Few physical signs are present in chronic ITP apart from those directly associated with a low platelet count such as petechiae, ecchymoses, bleeding from gums and mucous membranes, menorrhagia and hypochromic anaemia. Spontaneous bleeding is not usually a problem until the platelet count falls below $40–60 \times 10^3/\mu l$. In acute ITP there is rapid onset of haemorrhagic signs often associated with rash, fever, lymphadenopathy or mild splenomegaly. A small percentage (1·0%) of patients with acute or chronic ITP develop intracranial bleeding, usually a subarachnoid haemorrhage. The commonest drugs which cause allergic thrombocytopenia are listed in Table 4.

The bone marrow appearances are variable in ITP, though a characteristic finding in the chronic disease is the presence of large numbers of immature megakaryocytes and very few free platelets in a hypercellular marrow. Infants born of mothers with ITP commonly have thrombocytopenia at birth since the IgG auto-antibody crosses the placenta. The antibody seems to be species specific rather than allospecific since it readily sensitizes the platelets of all infants. Spontaneous recovery from the thrombocytopenia occurs as the maternal IgG is catabolized. There is usually improvement within 3–4 days, though platelet transfusions may be required. A rare form of acute ITP occasionally follows large blood transfusions and is associated with the platelet

TABLE 4
Drugs causing ITP

Quinine
Quinidine
Chlorothiazides
Sulphonamides
Rifampicin
Digitoxin
Diphenylhydantoin
Methyldopa
Acetazolamide
Chlorpropamide

antigen Zw^{a}. In four out of five cases the patients were reported to be Zw^{a-b+}. Within 4–5 days of transfusion the patients made the iso-antibody anti-Zw^{a} which destroyed the donor platelets. But within a further 3–4 days the recipients' platelets were also destroyed by anti-Zw^{a} or antibody very close in specificity to it. The mechanism is obscure though it appears that exposure to antigen Zw^{a} elicits a crossreacting antibody which temporarily breaks tolerance and destroys Zw^{a-b+} platelets.

Disorders which should be considered in the differential diagnosis of ITP and drug-induced thrombocytopenia are;

i. DIC (disseminated intravascular coagulation) distinguished by the presence of clotting factor abnormalities and increased fibrin degradation products;
ii. TTP (thrombotic thrombocytopenic purpura) distinguished by renal and neurological involvement, by the presence of fragmented red cells in the peripheral blood and by biopsy evidence of a disseminated vasculitis;
iii. Haemangioma, distinguished by the evident vascular abnormality and by the presence of fragmented red cells in the peripheral blood.

Serology of ITP

ITP is caused by an IgG auto-antibody which sensitizes autologous platelets and accelerates their destruction *in vivo*. The platelets are removed without lysis by sequestration in the mononuclear phagocytic system. Estimates of the number of platelet-bound IgG molecules indicate that sensitization is light, about 500–1,000 molecules/platelet. Sequestration is predominantly in the spleen and *in vitro* studies support this observation, viz.,

i. production of anti-platelet antibodies by splenic explants and
ii. phagocytosis of platelets by splenic leucocytes.

There are several problems associated with the serological identification of auto-antibodies to autologous platelets. Many patients, particularly those with chronic ITP, may have received multiple platelet transfusions and as a result developed allo-antibodies, some of anti-HLA specificity. The presence of allo-antibodies makes interpretation of reactions difficult since test platelets from an unrelated donor, which may be reactive with the allo-antibodies, are often required as indicator cells in the search for serum auto-antibodies. Attempts to wash patient or donor platelets present another problem. It may be difficult to obtain sufficient platelets in a thrombocytopenic individual. It is difficult to wash platelets free of all plasma since the platelet resembles a sponge and plasma may be trapped in the platelet open canalicular system. Platelets also tend to aggregate spontaneously if they are centrifuged. This can only be prevented by washing at pH 6·5–6·7 in ACD or calcium-free Tyrode's buffer or by washing on a Sepharose-4B column. Aggregation inhibitors such as AMP are also sometimes employed to reduce spontaneous aggregation. If aggregation does occur it is virtually indistinguishable from agglutination. The result is that detection systems based on agglutination are rarely successful in ITP.

Tests on the Patient's Platelets

A two-stage antiglobulin consumption test has been used to detect platelet bound IgG. Although this test has been partly successful it cannot distinguish allo- from auto-sensitization and may fail because the number of bound IgG molecules may be very low. Attempts to demonstrate membrane bound IgG by fluorescent-labelled antiglobulin are difficult to interpret because of the low level of sensitization.

Tests on the Patient's Serum

These seem more successful provided sensitization of the indicator platelets by allo-antibodies can be excluded. Two tests in particular seem promising:

i. measurement of PF3 (platelet factor 3) release from donor platelets damaged by sensitization with the patient's plasma. In one series significant shortening of the PF3 dependent clotting time was found in 65% of cases of ITP and in 78% of cases of SLE, though many of the latter patients were not thrombocytopenic at the time they were tested;

ii. release of ^{3}H-serotonin or ^{3}H-adenine from donor platelets which have been labelled by prior incubation with the radioactive markers. Significant release above control values occurred in 60% cases of ITP.

Serology of Drug-induced Thrombocytopenia

In drug-induced thrombocytopenia an "anti-platelet" antibody is frequently demonstrable in the plasma. Platelet aggregation by the antibody occurs only in the presence of the drug and platelet lysis may occur if complement is present. The alternative mechanisms proposed for platelet damage are similar to those used to account for red cell damage in drug-induced IHA. The drug or a metabolite may have a high natural affinity for platelet membranes and act as a hapten against which the antibody is directed. The main objection to this is that high concentrations of drug should be able to inhibit the reaction by "hapten inhibition", but in cases where it has been tested, inhibition is not usually observed. The other proposed mechanism is that the drug, possibly linked to a serum protein, combines with antibody in the plasma to form immune complexes which are bound to the platelet. This mechanism may be the most usual one since it has been established that human platelets carry an Fc-receptor and are aggregated by IgG containing immune complexes. Whether or not lysis takes place may depend on the efficiency with which the later complement components (C5–9) are activated to cause the "bystander" lysis phenomenon. Rifampicin induced thrombocytopenia is representative of this type of allergic thrombocytopenia. The antibody may be IgM or IgG and in some instances fixes complement.

Antibody detected in the patient's plasma disappears during challenge with the drug and this may be accompanied by profound though temporary thrombocytopenia. This procedure should not be deliberately carried out as an aid to diagnosis.

Treatment of ITP

Of patients with acute ITP, 80%, usually children, recover spontaneously without therapy. If steroids are given they should be used to treat presenting haemorrhagic symptoms rather than the low platelet count which reflects the balance between platelet production and peripheral consumption. Platelet consumption in ITP occurs not only by immune destruction but also as in normal individuals by physiological utilization of platelets in maintaining the endothelial lining of vessels. 40–80 mg prednisolone are given in divided daily doses. Haemostatic improvement may be apparent within 24–48 hours and the platelet count usually rises after 5–8 days in patients who are going to respond. The dose of prednisolone is lowered to 20 mg/day as soon as possible then slowly tailed off to 5–10 mg/day over 8–12 weeks. Seventy per cent of cases of acute ITP and 30% of chronic cases, improve on this regime, though the platelet count does not return to normal in all patients showing clinical improvement.

Splenectomy should be considered where steroid therapy is ineffective or where symptoms return as soon as attempts are made to lower the dose. The overall response to splenectomy in patients who have failed to respond to steroids is 40–60%. In some cases where there is symptomatic improvement following splenectomy, the platelet count may rise within 24–72 hours to levels as high as $10^6/\mu l$, in others the platelet count responds temporarily only to fall again within a few weeks. From 30 to 50% of patients fail to benefit at all from splenectomy in which case the introduction of an immunosuppressive drug such as azathioprine or possibly cyclophosphamide may make it possible to reduce the steroid dose to an acceptable level. The only treatment normally required in drug-induced allergic thrombocytopenia is to stop the offending drug as soon as it has been identified.

NEUTROPENIAS AND AGRANULOCYTOSIS

A large number of drugs, of which the major groups only are listed in Table 5, cause neutropenia or agranulocytosis though it has not always been demonstrated that immune mechanisms are the cause. The auto-immune nature of idiopathic forms of neutropenia may be even more difficult to establish. This is because most serological tests have to be carried out on the patient's serum against donor leucocytes and as in the case of platelet auto-immunity there is always a possibility that allo-antibodies are present following repeated whole blood transfusions, leucocyte transfusions or pregnancy. There have been a number of reports of IgM or IgG leucoagglutinins or leucocytoxins in patients'

TABLE 5
Drugs associated with neutropenia and agranulocytosis

Amidopyrine
Phenacetin
Phenylbutazone
Phenothiazines
Sulphonamides
Anti-thyroid drugs
Anti-histamines
Gold salts
Chloramphenicol

sera but their identification as true auto-antibodies as distinct from allo-antibodies by tissue-typing techniques has not usually been performed. Sensitive serological methods such as the antiglobulin consumption test have not contributed a great deal to understanding the condition; though in SLE, up to 70% of patients in some series have shown a positive test. A major drawback of the antiglobulin consumption test is that it may be positive with cells carrying surface adherent IgG-containing immune complexes.

In the drug-associated neutropenias there is sometimes more direct evidence that immune mechanisms are operating. The onset of neutropenia may be of acute onset, usually after the drug has been taken for 2–3 weeks and there is a pattern of remission and relapse as the drug is correspondingly withdrawn and reintroduced. Leucoagglutinins may be demonstrable only in the presence of the drug and it appears, by analogy with drug-induced thrombocytopenia, that the neutrophils are reacting with drug-containing immune complexes. Polymorphs may react nonspecifically with circulating complexes during acute drug challenge. This is manifest as a profound neutropenia due to the margination and trapping of neutrophils at certain sites such as the pulmonary capillaries. Neutropenias of this type are usually transient if the immune complexes are eliminated and are promptly followed by a reactive neutrophilia. However, if the drug is continuously absorbed into the circulation in the presence of excess antibody, exhaustion of the circulating and bone marrow neutrophil pools may eventually occur. Such a loss of mature neutrophils may account for the bone marrow appearance often seen in acquired neutropenias and called "maturation arrest". Granulocyte precursors, the myeloblasts and the promyelocytes are present in normal numbers but the myelocytes, metamyelocytes, and mature neutrophils are absent. This selective loss of the mature bone marrow granulocyte pool due to excessive peripheral consumption is in contrast with the effects of direct toxic damage to intracellular metabolism which damages all cells including precursor cells and result in complete agranulocytosis.

IMMUNOLOGICAL ASPECTS OF THE LEUKAEMIAS AND LYMPHOMAS

Two aspects of the leukaemias and lymphomas are of particular immunological interest now and will be considered in this section. These are: (a) the use of immunologically determined membrane markers to characterize the cell type; and (b) the immunological competence and reactivity of patients with leukaemia or lymphoma.

Membrane Markers

Chronic Lymphocytic Leukaemia (CLL)

CLL is the best characterized malignant leukocyte proliferation because of its homogeneity and accessibility. Abnormal B cells derived from a single clone accumulate in the blood and encroach upon the peripheral lymphoid tissue and bone marrow. The cells rosette with EAC (C3b) and EA (IgG), bind IgG-containing complexes or aggregated IgG, and carry membrane immunoglobulin (mIg). So, like normal B-cells, they possess Fc and C3 receptors and have endogenously derived mIg. Studies with fluorescein labelled anti-heavy chain and anti-light chain sera show that the mIg is usually IgM alone or IgM and IgD. The light chain type is $>90\%$ kappa-only or $>90\%$ lambda-only and not of mixed type. CLL cells have been observed with surface IgG or IgA carrying both kappa and lambda light chains. At least some of these anomalous examples can be accounted for by surface absorbed polyclonal antibody resulting either from host recognition of leukaemia-associated antigens or from the absorption of immune complexes by the lymphocyte Fc receptors.

Further evidence of the true clonal restriction of the CLL cell comes from the demonstration of allelic exclusion for Gm markers on the mIg and from their ability to give rise to anti-idiotype antibodies to determinants exposed on the mIg.

The cells do not transform with PHA (phytohaemagglutinin) or with PWM (poke-weed mitogen) though it has been reported that they transform and take up tritiated thymidine in the presence of LPS (lipopolysaccharide), a powerful B-cell mitogen. In some cases the mIg has antibody-like activity, e.g. anti-Forssman, anti-I or rheumatoid factor activity.

CLL cells show some unusual characteristics compared with normal B-cells. Capping of membrane markers with fluorescein-labelled divalent antibody is incomplete at 37°C and seems to result in coarse aggregates of surface fluorescence. This apparent failure to cap may be related to the observation that CLL cells have only 10% of the normal B-cell light chain sites (9,000 v. 90,000 in one study). There also seems to be defective uropod formation suggesting that CLL cell mobility is abnormal. A further abnormality is the marked discrepancy found in individual CLL patients between the numbers of Fc and C3 rosettes, with one marker often greatly outnumbering the other. On the rather rare occasions when lymphoblastic transformation takes place *in vivo*, it is reported that the lymphoblasts faithfully retain the markers of the original CLL cells. There have been isolated reports of CLL in which the abnormal lymphocytes typed as T-cells. However, it is clear that most examples of CLL are neoplastic proliferations of B-cells of a fixed degree of maturation in a lineage which extends to the Ig-secreting plasma cells of myeloma.

Other B-cell Line Proliferations

The cells of *Waldenström's macroglobulinaemia* are a pleomorphic lymphoid proliferation of greater maturation than the lymphocytes of CLL. The cells carry both IgM and IgG as mIg and secrete monoclonal 19S IgM. The abnormal lymphocytes of chronic cold haemagglutinin disease (see p. 918), though not in the strict sense malignant, are probably closely related to these cells. *Burkitt's lymphoblastic leukaemia* is a very rare clinical variant of acute lymphoblastic leukaemia (ALL) though the cells type as B-cells with mIg (IgM and IgD) and carry a single light chain type. *Hairy cell leukaemia* is another rare B-cell variant with surface IgM and/or IgD and variable proportions of Fc and C3 receptors. The cells transform with LPS but not with

PHA and like other malignant human B-cell lines they have been grown successfully in culture. They show no K cell-like activity. Lymphocyte markers in *lymphoma* have been less extensively studied than in CLL. Well-differentiated lymphocytic lymphoma and nodular lymphoma appear to be monoclones of B-cells and carry B-cell markers. However, a few examples type as T-cells or "null" cells. Typing of *reticulum cell sarcoma* reveals an even more heterogenous group in which no one cell is dominant and at present there is a poor correlation between histological and immunological classification.

Acute Lymphoblastic Leukaemia (ALL)

ALL cells from about half the cases studied form E-rosettes. They also sometimes react with anti-T cell sera of heterologous origin. Clinical impressions indicate that ALL with this T-cell like lymphoblast is a distinct entity since it occurs in older children, mainly boys and is often associated with a thymic mass. It appears to be a more aggressive form of the disease with higher leucocyte counts and shorter remissions than the ALL of early childhood. This form of the disease is more frequently associated with a "null" cell. Other examples of ALL are less easily typed and have features of both T- and B-cells.

At least one example of ALL has been established in culture as a lymphoblastoid line and has been shown to maintain T-cell markers in culture. This is an unusual example in that most lymphoblastoid lines are of B-cell origin. ALL cells do not normally respond to PHA or other mitogens.

Sézary Syndrome

This is an unusual condition showing an association of erythroderma, skin infiltration by lymphocytes and pruritus. The circulating lymphocytes rosette with sheep E, transform with PHA and have no EA or EAC receptors neither do they possess mIg. It therefore types as a T-cell leukaemia and usually runs a chronic course over several years. The EM morphology of the Sézary cells with their deeply indented nuclei is also highly characteristic.

Immunological Reactivity in Leukaemias and Lymphomas

The role of host immune responses in limiting the proliferation of leukaemic cells is still uncertain, particularly concerning the relative significance of cell mediated cytotoxic reactions versus humoral immunity. Many experimental situations have been recorded in which the optimum reactivity of one system may interfere with or "block" the activity of the other. The possibility that this occurs in patients has added to the uncertainty of the relevance of host immunity to the limitation of leukaemic spread. It is also far from clear to what extent leukaemia-associated antigens can be expressed on the surface of cells of different leukaemic types and to what degree the host can recognize them to mount an effective immunological attack. In the "natural" untreated state most of these neoplasms are rapidly lethal and no effective host-induced limitation occurs. It therefore seems that one of the main aims should be to encourage immunological reactivity by the host after the bulk of the tumour has been removed by chemotherapy or irradiation in the hope that the few remaining leukaemic cells will be removed by specific mechanisms.

The following evidence suggests that some immunological recognition of the leukaemic cell surface can take place and points to areas where further immunological investigations should be concentrated.

i. Delayed hypersensitivity skin reactions can be elicited in patients to autologous blast cell membranes.
ii. An MLR (mixed lymphocyte reaction) can be elicited with patients' lymphocytes against leukaemic cells. In some studies this MLR attenuates or disappears during remission. This has been interpreted as correlating with elimination of tumour tissue since persistence of the MLR occurs in patients who are soon to relapse.
iii. Lymphocytes which are cytotoxic to leukaemic cells in the cell mediated non-antibody dependent reaction have been found in patients with ALL.
iv. Eluates from leukaemic cell membranes can sensitize leukaemic cells of the same type from another individual and kill these cells *in vitro* in a cytotoxic reaction with anti-heavy chain sera and rabbit complement. The eluates will not sensitize other leukaemic cell types for this reaction.
v. Rabbits immunized against Raji cells, a human lymphoblastoid line, make antibodies which lyse other human lymphoblastoid lines and some leukaemic blast cells, suggesting immunological recognition of a common antigen.
vi. Certain acute leukaemias in animals and man may be related to infection with C-type RNA viruses. An antigen formed on human leukaemic cells (mainly myeloid or myelomonocytic) cross-reacts with a major structural protein of a C-type virus isolated from woolly monkeys and with the C-type virus associated with gibbon-ape leukaemia. Reverse

transcriptase activity, cellular evidence of the presence of endogenous RNA viruses, has been isolated from the leukaemic cells of AML (acute myeloid leukaemia), AMML (acute myelomonocytic leukaemia), CML (chronic myeloid leukaemia) and possibly CLL but not from normal or PHA-stimulated lymphocytes. This observation supports the view that some leukaemia-associated antigens may be virally determined.

Nonspecific Reactivity and Immunocompetence

Late in the clinical progression of the lymphoproliferative and myeloproliferative disorders a common pattern of infection tends to appear due predominantly to marrow damage and neutropenia. In contrast immunological reactivity as measured by antibody formation and delayed hypersensitivity may be well preserved and it seems that the neutropenia alone accounts for the severe systemic infections. These infections are mainly septicaemias caused by common pathogens such as *Pseudomonas aeruginosa*, *Klebsiella*, *Proteus*, *E. coli*, staphylococci and streptococci. Patients particularly at risk are those with long periods of neutropenia, and many infections arise from organisms normally present on the skin or in the gut.

Antibiotic sterilization of the gut may help to reduce the incidence of bacterial infection, but this in turn predisposes to fungal infection. The commonest infections in ALL and AML after antibiotic therapy are disseminated candidiasis and pulmonary aspergillosis with pneumonia and abscess formation.

Early in the course of the disease specific types of infection may be due to selective impairment of T or B cell function. In *Hodgkin's disease* virus infections occur with abnormally severe cytopathic effect. Particularly common are herpes zoster, disseminated herpes simplex, varicella and cytomegalovirus infection. Patients with Hodgkin's disease also seem particularly susceptible to fungal disease of which histoplasmosis, candidiasis, and cryptococcal infections are good examples. Infections by mycobacteria are also frequent. Several factors may account for this particular susceptibility, though it is only in stage III and stage IV Hodgkin's disease that a significant degree of immunological hyporeactivity is observed and then only in about 25% of patients. Lymphopenia may be present in the peripheral blood and thoracic duct lymph and there may be selective T cell depletion in peripheral lymphoid tissue. One result of loss of T cell function is loss of delayed-type skin responses to common antigens. These include SK-SD, candida, mumps, dermatophytin and tuberculin. PHA transformation and ^{14}C-leucine uptake by peripheral blood lymphocytes are also depressed. In addition there is recent evidence of suppression of the MLR of normal allogeneic cells by irradiated lymphocytes taken from patients in relapse. The suppression is reversible and disappears during remission. One interpretation of these results is that the effects are due to the accumulation of large numbers of suppressor T-cells during relapse. Macrophage function both as reticulo–endothelial cells and in thymus dependent antibody responses seems to be normal in Hodgkin's disease. In contrast to the apparent reduction in T-cell function in some cases of stage III and stage IV Hodgkin's disease, specific antibody formation, immunoglobulin levels, and B-cell marker levels in the peripheral blood seem well preserved even late in the disease.

T-cell "suppression" or "anergy" to delayed type responses is not typically seen in CLL or lymphoma. Here hypogammaglobulinaemia is the most troublesome early complication and affects about 30% at presentation. It is reflected in an increased susceptibility to upper respiratory tract infections, pneumonia and pulmonary aspergillosis.

In the acute leukaemias, ALL, AML and AMML the main problem is bone marrow replacement and defective neutrophil function. Markers for B-cells are low in the peripheral blood in ALL at the onset of disease but rise during remission.

INFECTIOUS MONONUCLEOSIS

Clinical and Pathological Features

Infectious mononucleosis (IM) is an almost invariably benign acute viral illness associated with infection by the Epstein–Barr virus (EBV). This is considered to be a virus of the herpes group with an icosahedral capsid and a DNA core. IM presents clinically as malaise, headache, sore throat and fever and the commonest physical findings are a localized or generalized lymphadenopathy and an exudative tonsillitis or pharyngitis. The pathology arises from the replication of the virus in B-lymphocytes without any overt cytopathic effect. All the peripheral lymphoid tissue is involved to some extent particularly the tonsils, lymph nodes, spleen and liver, which become infiltrated by pleomorphic lymphocytes. Occasional large reticulum cells are present in the infiltrates and some of these may be identical with the Reed–Sternberg cell of Hodgkin's disease. Lymphoproliferation is particularly striking in the lymph nodes and the greater part of this seems to be accounted for by the increased cellularity of the paracortical zones which fill with T-cells. In contrast, follicle enlargement and increased activity of germinal centres are not as marked. During the acute phase of the disease atypical and highly pleomorphic lymphocytes appear in the blood often in sufficient numbers to produce an absolute lymphocytosis of 4–10,000/μl. The bone marrow appearances, rather surprisingly, remain normal throughout the course of the disease. Only in rare instances has IM been shown to be other than a benign self-limiting disease. For example there has been one description of a family in which some members had an unusual T-cell defect, where infection with EBV resulted in a malignant lymphoma-like B-cell proliferation.

Relationship to EBV Infection

Only individuals seronegative for EBV can develop infectious mononucleosis. One complication in the diagnosis is the very large number of subclinical infections. Seroconversion occurs in childhood in poor unhygienic environments, in a manner similar to that observed with poliomyelitis, but is delayed in advanced clean environments until late adolescence. Prior to infection no antibody to EBV capsid antigen can be demonstrated but this appears after 5–10 days and the IgG antibody persists long after the peak titre and may still be detectable after several years. Its presence does not suggest recent infection unless the titre is rapidly rising or falling.

Direct person to person transmission of EBV has not been observed or performed experimentally in volunteers since the disease is unpleasant and potentially dangerous. However, seroconversion has occurred in patients receiving blood containing the viral capsid antigen which was presumably infective.

EBV is present in lymphoblastoid cell lines grown from donors who have had IM but the virus cannot usually be isolated directly from throat washings in the acute phase, though it has been reported that immunosuppression of patients for renal transplantation leads to renewed oropharyngeal excretion of EBV.

The Lymphocytes in IM

The majority of atypical lymphocytes in the peripheral blood type as T-cells, but both T- and B-cells increase in absolute number up to 5–10 times normal.

There is also a striking increase in the spontaneous uptake of tritiated thymidine by peripheral blood lymphocytes and as measured by autoradiography the normal background level of less than 0·2% rises to 5–9% in IM.

Recent work has shown that B-cells carry a receptor for EBV and that the virus replicates in B-cells which transform into cells capable of sustained growth as lymphoblastoid lines in culture. This transforming activity can be recovered from patients during the acute phase of the illness and will "infect" normal lymphocytes from seronegative individuals and allows these lymphocytes to grow as a lymphoblastoid line. It would appear that the B-cells in all individuals who are sero-positive contain EBV in the persistent carrier state. An *in vivo* corollary of the tissue culture experiments is the growth of lymphocytes from patients with IM in immunosuppressed animals as heterotransplants. In neonatal hamsters receiving ALG these heterotransplants proliferate into lethal lymphoma-like or leukaemia-like states. The abnormal cells carry a stable human karyotype and express human and EBV determinants on their surface.

Evidence that IM lymphocytes carry unique determinants on their surface comes from the observation that convalescent lymphocytes taken 3–9 months after the acute illness will react in the MLR with mitomycin-treated or irradiated lymphocytes taken during the acute illness. Although this reaction as originally described was most marked using allogeneically different combinations, it also works with autologous combinations and the reaction does not depend on the EBV antigens or on HLA differences. It seems clear that EBV replicates in B-cells, causes proliferation of these cells, and results in the expression of membrane neoantigens. It has been suggested that this stimulates an allogeneic-like reaction in the T-cell population which in turn reacts with the B-cell population and eventually terminates the abnormal proliferation perhaps by a direct T-cell dependent cytotoxic reaction.

Antibody Stimulation in IM

The classical Paul–Bunnell reaction as modified by Davidsohn detects the non-Forssman IgM heterophil agglutinin. The antibody appears during the acute phase of the disease and disappears within a few weeks without switching to a sustained IgG response. The heterophil agglutinin remains the most useful antibody for the diagnosis of the acute illness and has not been superseded by the more complex serological tests for the EBV specific antibodies some of which appear only transiently during the acute phase and some of which are sustained. The nature of the membrane antigen against which the heterophil agglutinin is directed is still unknown, though the antibody can be elicited in another primate species, the squirrel monkey, by inoculation with EBV transformed lymphoblasts. Paradoxically, it does not appear in Burkitt's lymphoma, which is the other EBV-containing B-cell lymphoproliferative disease of man.

Lymphocytotoxins are present in about half the cases of IM early in the disease. They are IgM cold antibodies. The majority seem to be of uncomplicated anti-I or anti-i specificities and are cytolytic in the presence of rabbit complement. There seems to be little support now for the view that some lymphocytotoxins in IM are specific for T- or B-cell subpopulations, though they may cause confusion in the typing of lymphocytes by providing a spurious membrane-bound μ-chain coat.

Smooth muscle auto-antibodies are common in IM. Other auto-antibodies such as rheumatoid factor and the Donath–Landsteiner antibody have been described. Antinuclear antibodies may appear transiently, but the incidence of other common auto-antibodies such as mitochondrial, microsomal and reticulin antibodies is not increased.

CRYOGLOBULINAEMIA

Clinical Features

The signs and symptoms of cryoglobulinaemia arise from the circulatory disturbances caused by the intravascular precipitation or gelation of immunoglobulins in the cold. Three types of cryoglobulins have been described (Table 6) on the basis of the characteristics of the primary abnormal globulin. These are, (a) *type I* monoclonal cryoglobulins with no recognizable antibody specificity and an inherent tendency to cryoprecipitate if the plasma concentration is high; (b) *type II* monoclonal anti-IgG antibodies, which only cryoprecipitate after forming immune complexes and; (c) *type III* polyclonal anti-IgG antibodies, rather like rheumatoid factors which only cryoprecipitate after formation of immune complexes. These are principally found in auto-immune states.

Type I Cryoglobulins

These may, in order of frequency, be IgM, IgG, IgA or rarely Bence Jones proteins. Only occasional examples of monoclonal cryoglobulinaemia appear

TABLE 6
Cryoglobulinaemia

	Type I	Type II	Type III
Incidence (%)	25	25	50
Specificity	Monoclonal no specificity	Monoclonal anti-IgG	Polyclonal anti-IgG
Class	IgM IgG IgA Bence Jones	IgM IgG IgA	IgM
Symptoms and presentation	Raynaud's phenomenon Vascular sludging and occlusion	Vascular purpura Vasculitis	Vascular purpura Vasculitis
Associated diseases	Myeloma macro-globulinaemia	Macroglobulinaemia Lymphoproliferative disorders Sjögren's syndrome	Auto-immune[a] e.g. SLE, PAN Sjögren's syndrome Lymphoproliferative disorders

[a] Approximately 30% of type III cryoglobulinaemias are idiopathic. After Brouet *et al.* (1974).

to be idiopathic or "essential", the majority are produced by abnormal plasma cells or B-cells in macroglobulinaemia or myeloma. Symptoms tend to occur late in the course of the disease at a time when the level of cryoglobulin is already high in the plasma, usually in the range 5–30 mg/ml.

Perhaps because of this, the dominant symptoms in type I cryoglobulinaemia are due to hyperviscosity and sludging of the cryoprecipitates in vessels rather than the more marked inflammatory effects caused by immune complexes in type II and III cryoglobulinaemia. Vascular purpura, Raynauds' phenomenon, thrombosis, haemorrhage, ulceration and gangrene are the most frequent clinical abnormalities.

Type II Cryoglobulins

These are of the mixed type, where monoclonal proteins of anti-IgG specificity combine at comparatively low avidity with IgG at 37°C and secondarily acquire cryoprecipitating characteristics (see below). As in Type I, IgM is the commonest monoclonal protein followed by IgG and IgA. The antibody reacts with determinants on the Fc-piece of IgG and specificity may be restricted to single IgG subclasses e.g. IgM anti-IgG_1 or anti-IgG_2. In this respect they differ from rheumatoid factors which react with both homologous and heterologous IgG. When IgG is the antibody it is frequently IgG_3 anti-IgG_1 or anti-IgG_2. Kappa greatly predominates over lambda as the monoclonal light chain type. The main reported clinical associations of type II cryoglobulinaemia are with chronic lymphocytic leukaemia, lymphoma, Sjögren's syndrome and rheumatoid arthritis, though some, like type I, are associated with myeloma and macroglobulinaemia. There appears to be a greater tendency to develop inflammatory disease such as diffuse vasculitis or glomerulonephritis in patients with mixed cryoglobulins, though most of the evidence is anecdotal.

Hypogammaglobulinaemia has been described in Sjögren's syndrome arising from the interaction of a monoclonal IgM anti-IgG with the patient's immunoglobulin. Cryoglobulins were formed only with subclasses IgG_1, IgG_2, and IgG_4 and the reduction in the plasma levels of these IgG subclasses to about 10% of normal was mainly accounted for by increased catabolism. IgG_3 was uninvolved and so spared.

Type III Cryoglobulins

These are usually polyclonal IgM "rheumatoid-like" factors which react with polyclonal IgG or IgA molecules of undetermined specificity. However, in some instances, the IgG or IgA "antigens" in the cryoprecipitating complexes carry recognizable specificities of their own such as anti-I cold agglutinins, anti-nuclear factors, heterophile antibodies or lymphocytotoxins. In some cases it is possible to show that the cryoprecipitate is enriched relative to the plasma with antibody of defined specificity. This has been shown for anti-nuclear factors and for lymphocytotoxins. A large proportion of cases (30%) are idiopathic while the remainder are associated with auto-immune disease such as SLE, PAN, Sjögren's syndrome, rheumatoid arthritis, lymphoma or haemolytic anaemia. In addition, low levels of mixed polyclonal cryoglobulins occur usually without symptoms in many infections, of which examples are syphilis, leprosy, trypanosomiasis, SBE, post-streptococcal nephritis, infectious mononucleosis, cytomegalic inclusion disease and tropical "big spleen" disease.

It is not entirely clear what part complement activation plays in the development of lesions in the associated vasculitis or renal damage, though low levels of C1, C4, and C2 have been reported in all three types of cryoglobulinaemia at the time of exacerbation of attacks. Cold urticaria which is an occasional manifestation of cryoglobulinaemia may be a complement-dependent phenomenon. It has also been reported that some cryoglobulins particularly in SLE may require Clq for cryoprecipitation.

Test for Cryoglobulins

Blood is collected and clotted in glass at 37°C. The serum is separated from the clot by spinning at 4,000 g and the clear serum left at 4°C overnight in a calibrated tube. The volume of cryoprecipitate can be measured the following morning, though completion of cryoprecipitation may take 72–96 hours. Cryoprecipitates are washed at 4°C. The cryoprecipitate can be analysed for immunoglobulin content by immunoelectrophoresis and quantitated by standard techniques. The individual components of the cryoglobulin are separated by G-200 gel-filtration, at pH 4·5 in 0·2M acetate buffer. Rheumatoid factor activity can be assayed by the FII latex test.

Mechanism of Cryoprecipitation

Cryoprecipitation is apparent as a flocculate or crystal precipitate or as gelation of the serum. Monoclonal type I cryoglobulins precipitate as a result of direct interaction between whole immunoglobulin molecules. Molecular fragments of immunoglobulins such as $F(ab')_2$, Fab and $(\mu Fc)_5$ lose the cryoprecipitating characteristics of the intact molecule. More is known about the cryoprecipitation of type II cryoglobulins. Cold precipitation depends on the formation of small complexes of rather critical size, in which the IgM molecule is pentavalent or more, while the IgG molecule, the antigen, is univalent. Complexes of the type $IgM(IgG)_{5-10}$ form at 37°C and the AgAb binding constant is virtually unaffected by temperature change. Three dimensional lattice formation is not possible with complexes of this type, in contrast to conventional AgAb complexes where the antigen possesses two or more determinants. It appears that cryoprecipitation is an intrinsic property of these small complexes once they have formed. On cooling the viscosity of the serum increases quite abruptly at a critical temperature which for many cryoglobulins falls within the range 32–28°C. In this respect cryoprecipitation is reminiscent of anti-I cold haemagglutination. The amount of precipitate can often be increased by lowering the ionic strength or increasing the purity of the cryoprotein by isolating it from whole serum.

REFERENCES

Atkinson, J. P. and Frank, M. M. (1974). Studies on the *in vivo* effects of antibody. Interaction of IgM antibody and complement in the immune clearance and destruction of erythrocytes in man. *J. Clin. Invest.* **54**, 339.

Brouet, J.-C., Clauvel, J.-P., Dannon, F., Klein, M. and Seligman, M. (1974). Biologic and clinical significance of cryoglobulins. *Am. J. Med.* **57**, 775.

Brown, D. L. (1974). The behaviour of phagocytic cell receptors in relation to allergic red cell destruction. *Series Haemat.* **7**, 348.

Dacie, J. V. (1951). Differences in the behaviour of sensitized red cells to agglutination by anti-globulin sera. *Lancet* **ii**/954.

Dacie, J. V. and Worlledge, S. M. (1975). Autoallergic blood diseases. In "Clinical Aspects of Immunology". 3rd ed. (eds P. G. H. Gell, R. R. A. Coombs, and P. J. Lachmann), p. 1149. Blackwell Scientific Publications, Oxford.

Engelfriet, C. P., Borne, A. E. G. Kr. V. D., Beckers, D. and van Loghem, J. J. (1974). Auto-immune haemolytic anaemia: Serological and immunochemical characteristics of the auto-antibodies: Mechanisms of cell destruction. *Series Haemat.* **7**, 328.

Garratty, G. and Petz, L. D. (1975). Drug-induced immune haemolytic anaemia. *Am. J. Med.* **58**, 398.

Gilliland, B. C., Leddy, J. P. and Vaughan, J. H. (1970). The detection of cell-bound antibody on complement-coated human red cells. *J. Clin. Invest.* **40**, 898.

Grey, H. M. and Kohler, P. F. (1973). Cryoimmunoglobulins. *Sem. Haemat.* **10**, 87.

Jensen, K. G. and Killman, S. A. (eds). Paroxysmal nocturnal haemoglobinuria. *Series Haemat.* **5**, 3–145.

Miescher, P. A. (1973). Drug-induced thrombocytopenia. *Sem. Haemat.* **10**, 311.

Pirofsky, B. (1969). "Autoimmunization and the Autoimmune Haemolytic Anaemias", p. 313. Williams and Wilkins, Baltimore.

Rosse, W. F. (1974). The detection of small amounts of antibody on the red cell in autoimmune haemolytic anaemia. *Series Haemat.* **7**, 358.

Rosse, W. F., Adams, J. P. and Thorpe, A. M. (1974). The population of cells in paroxysmal nocturnal haemoglobinuria of intermediate sensitivity to complement lysis: Significance and mechanism of increased immune lysis. *Brit. J. Haemat.* **28**, 181.

Salmon, S. E. and Seligman, M. (1974). B-cell neoplasia in man. *Lancet* **ii**, 1230.

Seligman, M. (1975). Membrane cell markers in human leukaemias and lymphomas. *Brit. J. Haemat.* **31**, 1.

Worlledge, S. M. (1973). Immune drug-induced haemolytic anaemias. *Sem. Haemat.* **10**, 327.

Weens, J. H. and Schwartz, R. S. (1974). Etiologic factors in autoimmune haemolytic anaemia. *Series Haemat.* **7**, 303.

Worlledge, S. M. (1974). Immune haemolytic anaemias. *In* "Blood and Its Disorders", eds R. M. Hardisty and D. J. Weatherall), p. 714. Blackwell Scientific Publications, Oxford.

27

Monoclonal Proteins

PAUL CARTER

The first well documented record of a case of multiple myeloma was made in 1850 by MacIntyre, who described a "case of mollities and fragilitas ossium accompanied with urine strongly charged with animal matter". Earlier, Dalrymple had described the microscopic features of the osseous lesions in a patient in whose urine Bence Jones discovered a "hydrated deutoxide of albumin".

Since then tumours of immunoglobulin producing cells (immunocytomas) have become widely recognized as entities, and their association with abnormal serum and urinary globulins well known. Laboratory studies of the abnormal proteins can be of help to clinicians in the diagnosis, prognosis and management of patients with these disorders. Such studies are the subject of this chapter.

THE SYNTHESIS OF NORMAL IMMUNOGLOBULINS

A detailed account of the synthesis and structure of normal immunoglobulins is given in Chapter 4, but a brief recapitulation will be useful here. Normal plasma cells in marrow and lymphoid tissue synthesize complete immunoglobulins. Large polyribosomes produce large (heavy) polypeptide chains, and shorter (light) polypeptide chains are synthesized on smaller polyribosomes. Four polypeptide chains, two heavy and two light, are then assembled and carbohydrate is incorporated by the Golgi apparatus before the intact immunoglobulin molecule is released from the cell. The synthesis of heavy and light chains is well balanced. Under normal conditions a very small excess of light chains is synthesized, and about 2–3 mg of polyclonal free light chain is filtered into the urine per day.

Heavy chains differ in physical and chemical properties, and immunoglobulins are classified as IgG, IgA, IgD, IgE and IgM on the basis of these differences. Normal serum immunoglobulins of classes IgG, IgA, IgD and IgE are monomers of the basic four chain unit (Fig. 1), while those of class IgM are pentamers. Light chains are of two types, kappa and lambda, which are common to all classes of immunoglobulins, although each immunoglobulin molecule contains light chains of a single type only. In normal human serum 70% of the immunoglobulin molecules are type κ and 30% type λ.

CELL CLONES AND PARAPROTEINS

Normal immunoglobulins of all classes are heterogeneous, migrating with widely differing mobilities on electrophoresis. Since immunocytomas are probably tumours derived from single cells (Waldenström, 1962), it follows that the immunoglobulin products of all the cells in a given tumour, whether intact molecules or only parts of them, have a common and unique protein structure. These homogeneous tumour products from a given patient all migrate with the same mobility on electrophoresis, appear as discrete bands when stained, and are termed "paraproteins".

Some immunocytomas synthesize only complete immunoglobulin molecules while others produce immunoglobulin fragments, either alone or in addition to the complete molecules; the significance of this is discussed later. By far the commonest fragments synthesized are free, complete light chains, of molecular weight about 22,000. Being of low molecular weight, they are filtered into the urine, where they are commonly found as dimers. Such free light chains are termed Bence Jones proteins. It is very much rarer to find tumours which synthesize free heavy chains and, when present, they usually synthesize incomplete ones. These heavy chain products, unlike other monoclonal proteins, may not appear as discrete bands on electrophoresis. This may be due to the formation of a series of polymers or to post-synthetic alterations in the molecules.

The finding of paraproteins in patients with malignant immunocytomas is, however, not invariable; although only 1% of patients with myelomatosis do not synthesize detectable paraproteins (Hobbs, 1975), many extra-medullary plasmacytomas are not associated with the presence of paraproteins, and most patients with malignant lymphomas have no detectable monoclonal protein.

DETECTION AND CHARACTERIZATION OF PARAPROTEINS

The association of paraproteins with immunocytomas may be used as the basis of investigations which can help in the diagnosis and monitoring of the underlying lesions. Serum, ascitic and cerebrospinal fluid may all be analysed for the presence of complete immunoglobulin paraproteins, and urine may be tested for the presence of low molecular weight fragments, such as Bence Jones proteins. Where body fluid paraprotein studies are inconclusive, marrow tumour cells may be investigated for immunoglobulin surface markers (Hobbs, 1967), although this is rarely necessary.

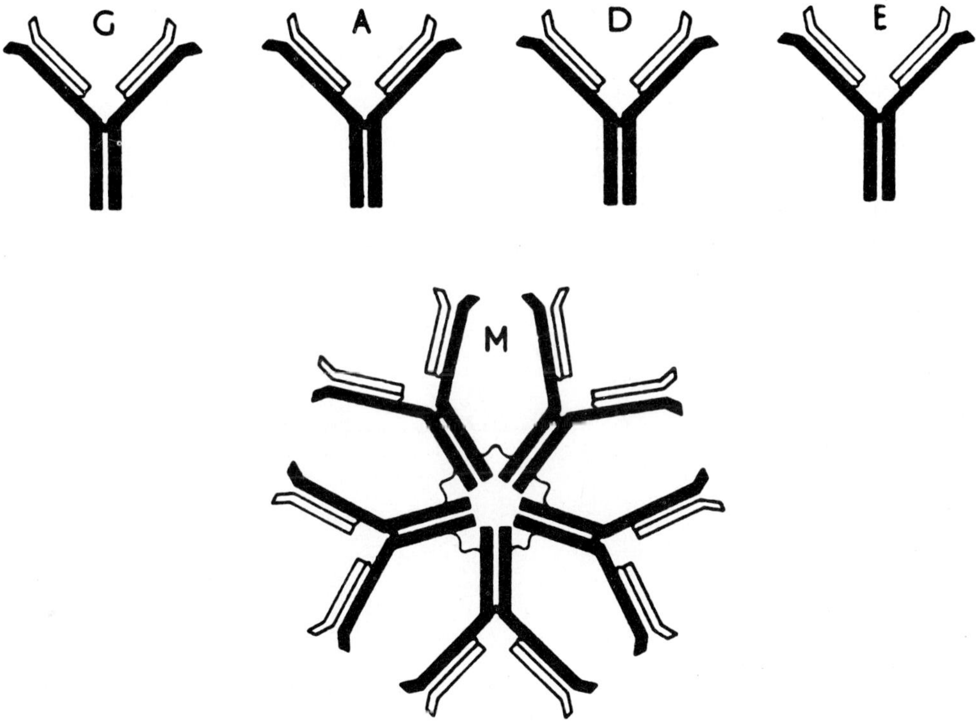

Fig. 1. Basic structure of the main immunoglobulin classes, showing light chains (unshaded) and heavy chains (shaded).

Zone Electrophoresis

Paraproteins are usually detected either by agar or cellulose acetate electrophoresis (Fig. 2), and characterized by immunoelectrophoresis of serum and urine (Fig. 3). Electrophoresis may be used to quantitate the amount of paraprotein present if the proportion of dye bound to the paraprotein on the stained strip is compared with the total amount of dye bound to all fractions, and with the total protein concentration of the sample. Urine must be concentrated up to 300-fold before electrophoresis, and this is conveniently performed by vacuum extraction through a collodion membrane. With this technique, Bence Jones protein can be detected in amounts above about

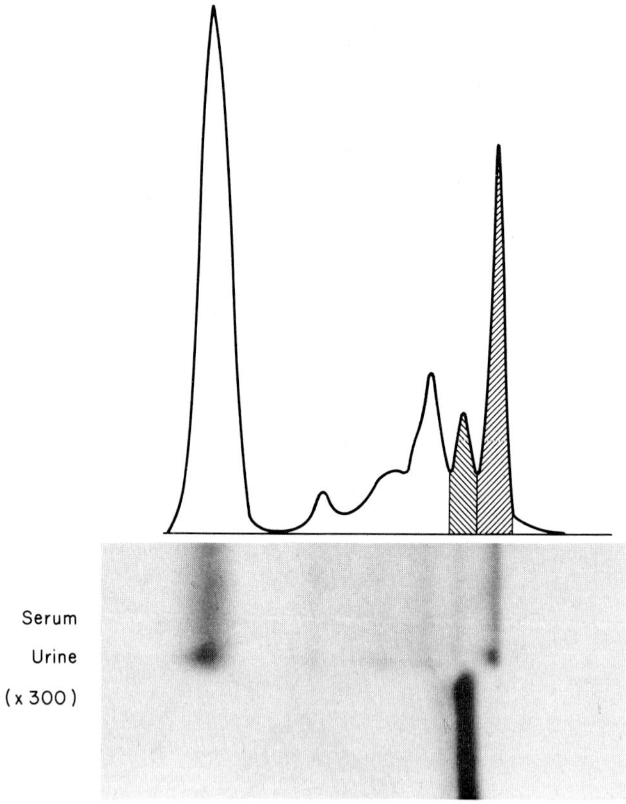

Fig. 2. Cellulose acetate electrophoresis of serum and of urine, concentrated 300 times, from a patient with a serum paraprotein and Bence Jones proteinuria. There is some retention of Bence Jones protein in the serum.

6 mg/litre. By contrast, serum paraproteins can only be detected by electrophoresis above a level of about 2 g/litre in unconcentrated samples. The techniques available have recently been reviewed by Kohn (1973).

Immunoelectrophoresis

The suspected presence of a paraprotein may be confirmed by demonstrating abnormal reactions between specimen and antisera on immunoelectrophoresis. Precipitin arcs may be bowed or split in the presence of a paraprotein (Fig. 3), and Bence Jones proteins, because of their low molecular weight, diffuse rapidly through agar and usually form precipitin arcs within two hours of adding antisera to the plate at room temperature. Antisera against free light chains, now commercially available, may be used to confirm the presence of Bence Jones proteins.

Immunoelectrophoresis also allows identification of the class and type of the abnormal immunoglobulin. In the presence of monoclonal rheumatoid

Anode

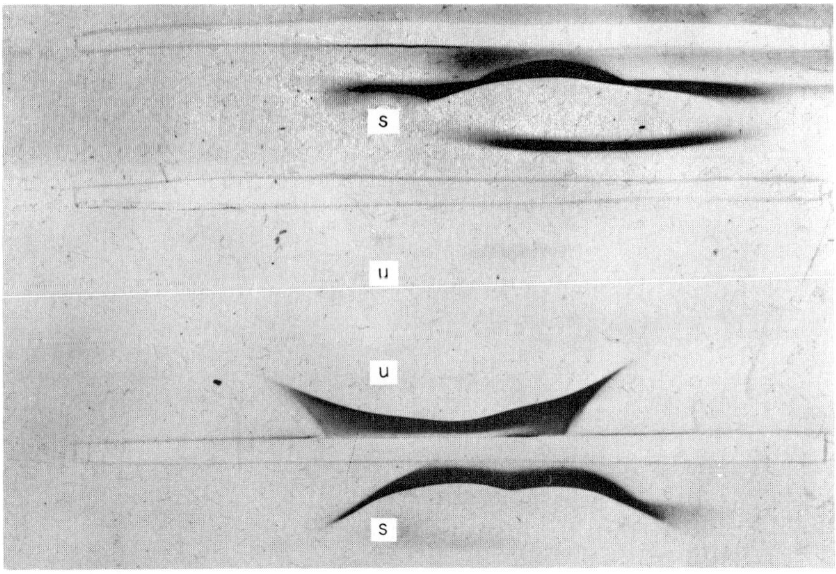

Anti - γ

Anti - k

Anti - λ

Fig. 3. Immunoelectrophoresis of serum (s) and concentrated urine (u) from the same patient as in Fig. 2, against anti-γ, anti-κ and anti-λ antisera. There is an IgGλ paraprotein in the serum; type λ Bence Jones proteinuria and retention of some Bence Jones protein in the serum.

factors, however, typing of the paraprotein may be difficult owing to the presence of IgG bound to the monoclonal protein. In the Medical Research Council's first myeloma trial 55% of the patients had an IgG paraprotein, 26% had an IgA paraprotein, 19% had Bence Jones proteins only, about 1% had two paraproteins and less than 1% had an IgD paraprotein (MRC, 1973).

It must be stressed that performing immunoelectrophoresis and interpreting the results requires experience. It is very easy for inexperienced workers to produce artefacts by poor technique and to misinterpret the findings.

The detection of Bence Jones proteins by chemical methods is not reliable. Even though the Bradshaw ring test for urinary globulins is the best of these,

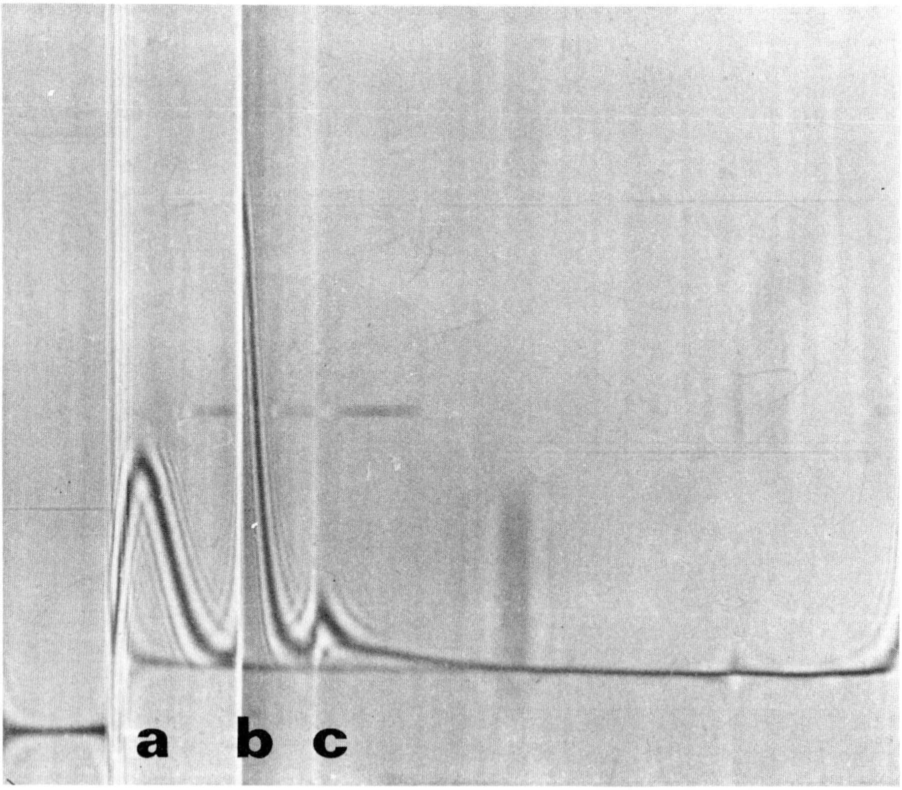

Fig. 4. The ultracentrifugal pattern obtained at 60,000 revs for 300 sec with the serum of a patient with an IgM paraproteinaemia. There is a 27S component (c) and a large 19S peak (b) in addition to the normal 4·5 and 7S peak (a). By courtesy of K. B. Cooke.

it fails to detect about 1 in 20 demonstrable by concentration and electrophoresis.

Detection of IgM Monomers and Complexes

An IgM paraprotein, detected by immunoelectrophoresis, may be further investigated to determine the molecular size of the abnormal protein. Monomeric (7S) IgM and complexes larger than the normal pentameric (19S) molecule, may be demonstrated by passing the samples through a thin layer of G-200 Sephadex (Carter and Hobbs, 1971) or by ultracentrifugation. The ultracentrifugal behaviour of human macroglobulins is characteristic and Fig. 4 shows the pattern obtained with a serum containing both a 19S IgM paraprotein and a larger 27S complex. The significance of the presence of 7S IgM and large IgM complexes is discussed below.

Immunoselection Techniques

Free heavy chains, unlike other monoclonal proteins, may either form a broad band on electrophoresis, or more rarely no band may be visible. The detection of these proteins relies on immunoelectrophoretic patterns showing a component reacting with antisera to the IgG, IgA or IgM heavy chains, designated γ, α and μ respectively, but reacting with antisera to neither κ nor λ-type light chains.

The sample is electrophoresed through a zone of agarose containing antisera to both κ and λ-type light chains which precipitate all the intact immunoglobulins (Gale *et al.*, 1974). Free heavy chains, however, continue to migrate anodally towards another zone of agarose containing antisera to the appropriate heavy chains, and precipitin peaks are formed. Figure 5 shows the reactions produced by normal controls and samples containing free α-chains.

A similar technique may be used to detect free light chains in unconcentrated urine samples above a level of about 3 to 5 mg/l. Although positive results must be shown to be Bence Jones protein by electrophoresis of a concentrated sample, negative results are conclusive.

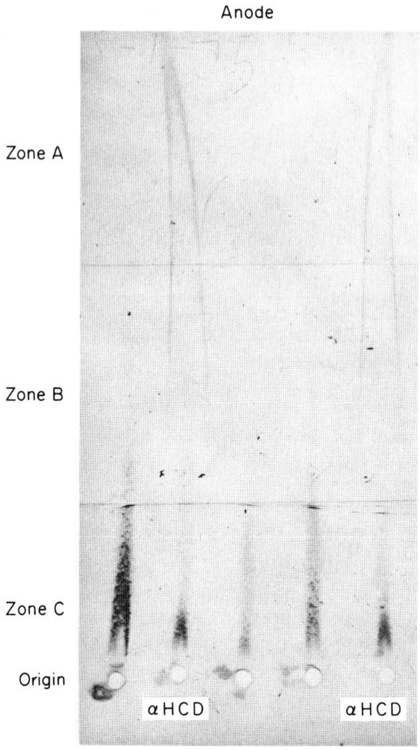

Fig. 5. Immunoselection plate showing preciptin arc formation between anti-α chain antiserum (present in zone A), and sera from both normals and two patients with αHCD (heavy chain disease). The specimen origin wells are in zone C (nearest the cathode) which contains antisera against both κ- and λ-chains. Zone B is plain agarose.

CLINICAL SIGNIFICANCE OF PARAPROTEINAEMIA

Population Studies

Although the incidence of paraproteinaemia in a normal population has been reported as high as 1% over the age of 50 and 3% over the age of 70 (Hällén, 1966), a recent survey of nearly 10,000 blood donors by Kohn and Srivastava (1973), found a much lower overall incidence of 0·2%. This incidence rose with age to a peak of 0·6% in subjects aged 61–62 (the oldest group in the series). The different incidences of paraproteinaemia in these two series illustrates the difficulties of comparing different populations, even when both are "normal".

Most paraproteins in "normal" populations seem to be associated with benign conditions but this is not so for paraproteins found in hospital patients. The final diagnoses in 691 hospital patients with serum paraproteins of any immunoglobulin class are shown in Table 1. 74% of the patients

TABLE 1

The final diagnoses in 691 hospital patients in whom serum paraproteins of any immunoglobulin class were detected

Diagnosis	No. of patients	Incidence (%)
Malignant	515	74
myelomatosis	422	
malignant lymphoma	33	
Waldenström's macroglobulinaemia	32	
extramedullary plasmacytoma	20	
chronic lymphocytic leukaemia	5	
α-chain disease	3	
Benign	158	23
no associated pathology	112	
pathology but no malignancy	46	
Uncertain	18	3

After Hobbs (1969a).

had malignant immunocytomas, myeloma being the commonest, and 23% had benign conditions. The incidence of underlying diseases varied between different groups of patients, and in another series, benign conditions were found in 30% of the patients (Cooke, 1969). For comparison, the final diagnoses of 204 patients in whom only IgM class paraproteins were found are shown in Table 2.

The reported incidence of paraproteinaemia with malignancies other than immunocytomas varies between 7 out of 2,000 patients (Osserman, 1958) and 63 out of 1,108 patients (Martin, 1970). The former is no more than the incidence for an age matched population without paraproteinaemia.

Benign Conditions

Essential paraproteinaemia was the term used by Waldenström (1952) to describe paraproteinaemia in patients without overt malignancy. This group

TABLE 2

The final diagnoses in 204 patients in whom IgM serum paraproteins were detected

Diagnosis	No. of patients	Incidence (%)
Malignant	163	80
malignant lymphoma	76	
Waldenström's macroglobulinaemia	58	
myeloma	10	
plasmacytoma	6	
chronic lymphocytic leukaemia	7	
carcinoma (only)	6	
Benign	21	10
no associated pathology	9	
pathology but no malignancy	12	
Uncertain	20	10

includes patients without detectable pathology and also those with pathology other than malignancy. In a survey of 69 cases of essential paraproteinaemia (Cooke, 1969), gastrointestinal tract and liver diseases accounted for nearly half the patients. Rheumatoid arthritis, systemic lupus erythematosus, ankylosing spondylitis, sarcoid, tuberculosis and Henoch Schönlein purpura were other diagnoses in this series.

Although paraproteins associated with these groups of patients are usually persistent, they may occasionally appear only as a transient finding.

Malignant Conditions

Paraproteins are also associated with a wide range of malignant immunocytomas of which myeloma is the commonest.

Multiple Myeloma

Multiple myeloma (Fig. 6) is commonly associated with paraproteinaemia, usually of class IgG, IgA or IgD. Rarely, it may be associated with IgM paraproteins, and only six cases of IgE myeloma have been reported so far in the world literature.

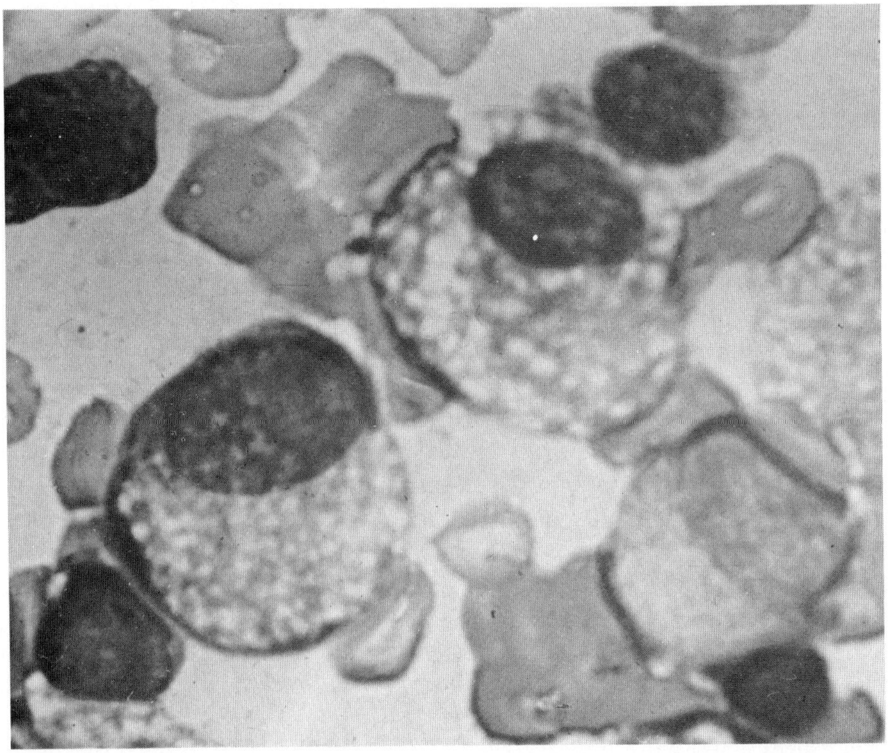

Fig. 6. Abnormal plasma cells, showing very vacuolated cytoplasm, in a marrow smear from a patient with myelomatosis (By courtesy of Professor J. Humble).

The skeletal lesions vary between diffuse plasma cell infiltration, in which all marrow is replaced by confluent small tumour nodules, and, less commonly, multiple plasmacytomas of the skeleton with apparently normal intervening bone marrow. There is considerable bone destruction giving rise to the lytic lesions seen on X-ray, and discrete plasma cell tumours may be accompanied by the local deposition of amyloid. The skeleton is usually extensively involved in the disease and even areas free of osteolytic lesions on X-ray may show sheets of myeloma cells on microscopy. Extraskeletal spread of the tumour occurs in about 65–70% of cases (Pasmantier and Azar, 1969).

Less common forms of this disease are (i) osteosclerotic myeloma, which may be localized to only one region of the skeleton, whilst the rest shows the more typical appearance, (ii) disseminated non-osteolytic myeloma, in which immature and frequently bizarre myeloma cells infiltrate both peripheral tissues and skeleton but without causing masses or osteolysis, and (iii) solitary myeloma. These are most probably unusual forms of presentation of myelomatosis rather than separate entities, unlike extramedullary plasmacytoma (Wiltshaw, 1969). They have unpredictable natural histories, and may remain localized for several years. Most solitary lesions do eventually disseminate, however, and spread has been reported as long as seventeen years after the initial diagnosis (Wiltshaw, 1969).

Rarely myeloma may be associated with plasma cell leukaemia.

Extramedullary Plasmacytoma

These tumours may be associated with paraproteins of any class. The majority of tumours diagnosed as such probably represent either extraskeletal spread from undetected myelomas or inflammatory non-malignant plasma cell granulomas. True extramedullary plasmacytomas are rare and arise particularly in the upper respiratory and gastrointestinal tracts. They often spread to local lymph nodes and frequently produce bony lesions.

Waldenström's Macroglobulinaemia

This is a slowly growing generalized malignancy associated with the presence of an IgM paraprotein. It invades lymph nodes, which become enlarged but retain their basic architecture, the spleen, which may also become enlarged, and the bone marrow. The infiltrate comprises lymphoid cells, often indistinguishable from mature lymphocytes, and cells which are intermediate in appearance between lymphocytes and plasma cells. In lymph nodes there is often a lymphocytic infiltration of the capsule and pericapsular adipose tissue.

Malignant Lymphoma

These rapidly growing tumours (Fig. 7) may cause massive enlargement and architectural destruction of both lymph nodes and spleen due to infiltration with lymphoid cells. Occasionally they are associated with paraproteinaemia, usually of class IgM. Histological appearances of these tumours are very variable and have recently been discussed by Bennett (1974), who stresses that the plasmacytoid differentiation found in Waldenström's macroglobulinaemia may also be seen in many diffuse malignant lymphomas.

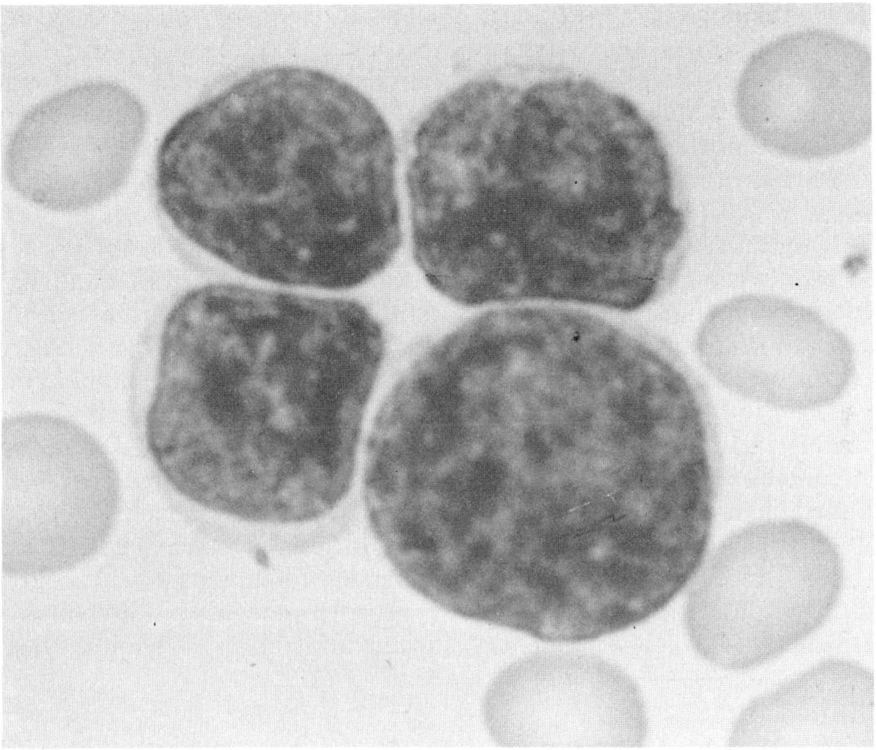

Fig. 7. Lymphocytes in a marrow smear from a patient with a malignant lymphoma.

Chronic Lymphatic Leukaemia

Occasionally paraproteins, usually of class IgM, are found in patients with chronic lymphocytic leukaemia; they may be a terminal feature in long-standing disease. In addition, a condition analogous to plasma cell leukaemia may be associated with an IgM paraprotein in which up to 10% of the circulating lymphocytes are precursors of IgM producing cells.

Heavy Chain Diseases

Heavy chain disease (HCD) was first described by Franklin *et al.* (1964) in a patient with a disorder characterized by the production of γ-heavy chains only. Most cases of γ-HCD have lymph node involvement, although of variable histological appearance. The most frequent finding is a diffuse pleomorphic infiltration by lymphocytes, plasma cells and eosinophilic and reticulum cells. The appearance of bone marrow smears is often similar to that found in Waldenström's macroglobulinaemia. Osteolytic lesions have never been reported. The natural history of the disease varies between that of a malignant tumour and that of a long-lasting, possibly benign, condition.

Alpha-chain disease (α-HCD), associated with the synthesis of α-chains only, is more common and was first recognized in 1968 (Rambaud *et al.*). There is diffuse mesenteric lymph node enlargement, with diffuse and massive proliferation of mature plasma cells, lymphocytes and reticulum cells in the lamina propria. In most cases this is invasive with secondary villous atrophy and crypt sparsity. There is a minimal involvement of other lymphoid organs and there are no osteolytic lesions visible on X-ray. The disease probably represents a condition primarily affecting the secretory IgA system, occurs mainly in young adults and children, and is usually seen in patients from the Mediterranean area, South America and the Far East.

Mu-chain disease, associated with the synthesis of μ-heavy chains only, is very rare. Three μ-HCD patients have been described with slowly progressive chronic lymphocytic leukaemia and hepatosplenomegaly but no lymph node enlargement. The marrow smears showed infiltration of lymphocytes and plasma cells.

ASSESSMENT OF THE UNDERLYING DIAGNOSIS

Laboratory results help to assess whether the underlying lesion is benign or malignant. The incidence of some laboratory findings in 112 patients with benign immunocytomas, who had been followed for at least 5 years, and 517 patients with malignant immunocytomas, diagnosed by biopsy, is shown in Table 3.

If the paraprotein is class IgM the presence of 7S monomeric units is of diagnostic importance (Carter and Hobbs, 1971). The incidence of 7S IgM and Bence Jones proteinuria in 117 patients with a variety of diseases associated with IgM paraproteins is shown in Table 4. It can be seen that 7S IgM occurs more frequently in the more malignant conditions but in benign conditions was found in only 4 out of 45 patients with primary cold haemagglutinin disease.

In patients with paraproteinaemias low levels of other immunoglobulin classes are suggestive of an underlying malignant lymphoma whilst a high

TABLE 3

The incidence of some laboratory findings in 112 patients with benign immunocytomas, followed for at least 5 years, and 517 patients with malignant immunocytomas, diagnosed by biopsy

Biochemical findings	No. of patients (incidence, %) Benign disorders	Malignant diseases
Immunoglobulin fragments	0	434 (84)
Reduction in normal immunoglobulins	11 (10)	506 (98)
Serum paraprotein concentration greater than 10 g/litre	17 (15)	475 (92)
Increase in paraprotein concentration with time	1 (1)	96 out of 97 untreated patients (99)

After Hobbs (1971).

TABLE 4

The incidence of monomeric (7S) IgM and Bence Jones proteinuria in 117 patients with a variety of diseases associated with IgM paraproteins

Diagnosis	No. of patients Total	7S IgM present	Bence Jones proteinuria
Myeloma	3	2	3
Malignant lymphoma	33	15	33
Waldenström's macroglobulinaemia	25	5	24
Chronic lymphocytic leukaemia	1	0	0
Primary cold haemagglutinin disease	45	4	4
Rheumatoid arthritis	1	0	0
Benign	9	0	0

serum IgG concentration is often associated with Waldenström's macroglobulinaemia. In the latter it is thought that the IgM paraprotein may interfere with the function of phagocytic cells, allowing a greater incidence of intercurrent infection, and a consequent immunoglobulin response.

Other useful investigations include examination of bone marrow smears and peripheral blood films, X-rays, especially of the axial skeleton, and, if possible, tissue biopsies. A low haemoglobin and high serum calcium suggest the presence of a malignant condition.

MODES OF PRESENTATION OF PATIENTS WITH PARAPROTEINAEMIAS

Patients with paraproteinaemia present in two main ways. Symptoms may be due to the presence of the tumour itself or be related to the presence of the paraprotein. A third group of patients are detected by chance before presenting clinically, either because a paraprotein has been found by electrophoresis, or because of a high ESR, lymph node enlargement or splenomegaly.

The proportion of cases in each of these categories varies with the underlying lesion. Patients with myeloma or malignant lymphoma usually present

TABLE 5

The modes of presentation and final diagnoses in 204 patients in whom IgM serum paraproteins were detected

		Final diagnosis			
Mode of presentation	No. of patients	Waldenström's macroglobulinaemia	Malignant lymphoma	Other malignant disease	Benign diseases or unknown
1. Symptoms due to the tumour:					
non-specific symptoms	46	3	35	8	—
frank presentation of tumour	17	4	9	4	—
symptoms due to its anatomical position	5	—	1	4	—
haemorrhage from tumour	1	—	—	1	—
TOTAL	(69)				
2. Symptoms due to the paraprotein:					
(a) Physical properties					
hyperviscosity syndrome	36	27	6	3	—
epistaxis only	6	2	2	1	1
due to cryoglobulinaemia	4	1	2	—	1
due to amyloid deposits	2	1	1	—	—

TABLE 5—contd.

Mode of presentation	No. of patients	Final diagnosis: Waldenström's macroglobulinaemia	Malignant lymphoma	Other malignant disease	Benign diseases or unknown
(b) Activity or affinity of paraprotein:					
cold haemagglutinin disease	13	—	3	1	9
neurological syndromes	10	1	4	—	5
rheumatoid arthritis	5	1	1	—	3
hyperlipidaemia	1	—	1	—	—
TOTAL	(77)				
3. Accidental discovery:					
paraprotein found by electrophoresis	41	11	9	6	15
a high ESR	14	6	—	1	7
lymphodenopathy or splenomegaly	3	1	2	—	—
TOTAL	(58)				
OVERALL TOTAL	204	58	76	29	41

with symptoms due to the tumour, whereas in patients with Waldenström's macroglobulinaemia, symptoms are usually due to the paraprotein. To illustrate these various groups, the modes of presentation and final diagnoses of 204 patients in whom IgM serum paraproteins were detected are shown in Table 5.

Symptoms Due to the Tumour

The common non-specific symptoms of malignant disease such as weight loss and malaise may occur in patients with any malignant disorder associated with paraproteinaemia. A malignant lymphoma may first become clinically obvious either as lymph node enlargement (Fig. 8) or as deposits in the skin.

Symptoms may be due to the anatomical position of the tumour. Such symptoms include bone pains, due to either tumour deposits or crush fractures

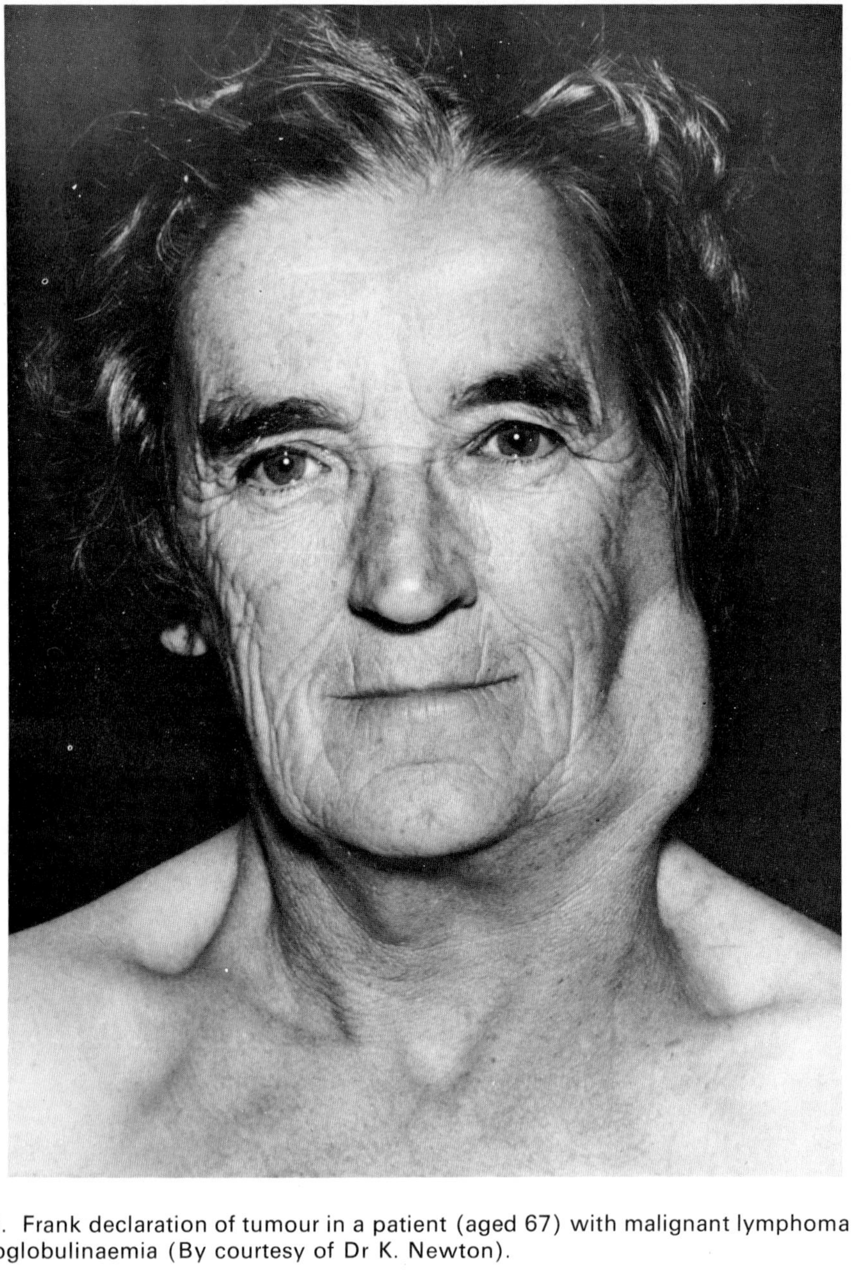

Fig. 8. Frank declaration of tumour in a patient (aged 67) with malignant lymphoma and macroglobulinaemia (By courtesy of Dr K. Newton).

of vertebrae. These commonly occur in patients with myelomatosis (Fig. 9). Non-bony deposits may also cause symptoms. Patients with α-HCD often present with intestinal obstruction due to intestinal lymphadenopathy, and we have seen a case presenting with weakness in the legs due to an intrathecal plasmacytoma.

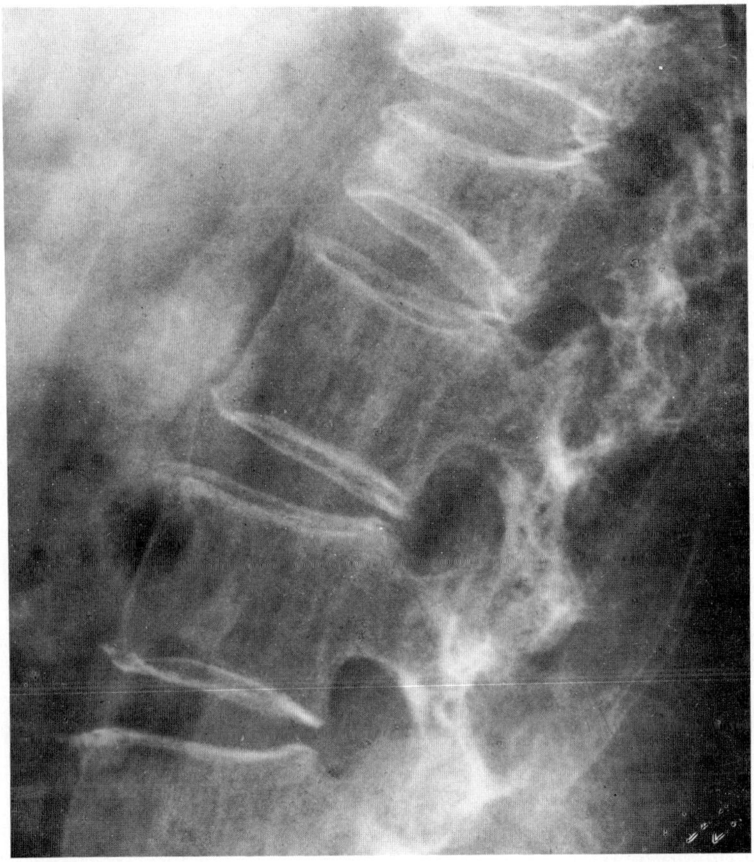

Fig. 9. Compression fractures of vertebrae in a patient with myelomatosis and spinal deposits of tumour.

Less commonly, the presenting symptom may be haemorrhage from a tumour, especially from a soft tissue plasmacytoma. This may occur in the upper respiratory or, less commonly, gastrointestinal tract as in one of our cases with a pelvic plasmacytoma who presented with rectal haemorrhage.

Symptoms Due to the Paraprotein

Symptoms caused by the paraprotein may be due simply to its presence, as in the "hyperviscosity syndrome", or to some specific activity or affinity which it possesses, as in patients with cold haemagglutinin disease; the range of symptoms is indicated in Table 5.

Symptoms Due to the Presence of Paraprotein

Hyperviscosity Syndrome

High serum concentrations of paraprotein, by increasing blood viscosity, may cause heart failure and breathlessness. Other symptoms which may be associated with hyperviscosity and can occur either together with heart failure or alone, include severe flushing and lethargy, reduction of vision due to retinal haemorrhages (Fig. 10), and epistaxis and other bleeding manifestations. Symptoms due to hyperviscosity are seen in many patients with IgM paraproteinaemias but only very occasionally in patients with myeloma. IgM paraproteins produce hyperviscosity because of their high molecular weight (about 1,000,000), their spatial configuration and their virtual confinement to the intravascular pool. IgG paraproteins, particularly of subclass 3, sometimes cause similar signs and symptoms (Capra and Kunkel, 1970); IgA paraproteins are a much rarer cause.

Large (27S) IgM complexes may be detected by ultracentrifugal analysis in the serum of patients with IgM paraproteinaemias. There is, however, no simple relationship between this finding and the occurrence of hyperviscosity symptoms. It may be that these large complexes are either acid-dissociable or covalently bound aggregates.

Cryoglobulinaemia

Paraproteins of any class may precipitate in the cold. If this occurs above about 21°C, it may cause Raynaud's phenomenon or even peripheral gangrene. If the cryoglobulin is an IgG paraprotein it is usually of subclass 2 or 3 (Virella and Hobbs, 1971). These monoclonal cryoproteins are often associated with skin eruptions which are characteristically flat and sometimes show central necrosis.

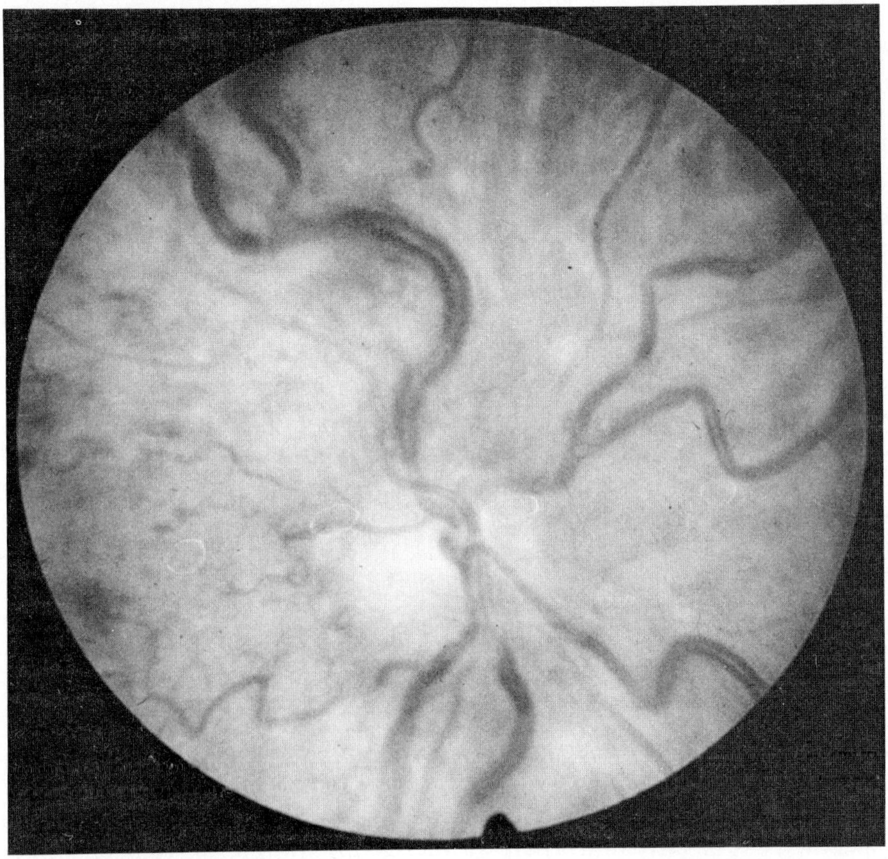

Fig. 10. Engorged veins and haemorrhages in the retina of a patient with macroglobulinaemia who presented with the symptoms of hyperviscosity.

Protein Deposition

Although most malignant immunocytomas associated with paraproteinaemia synthesize complete immunoglobulin molecules, many synthesize free light chains either as well as the complete molecules or alone, and these are excreted by the kidney as Bence Jones proteins. In addition, a small number of clones secrete light chain fragments or even half molecules (Hobbs, 1971). These incomplete products may cause clinical symptoms either by their deposition in the tissues or by the blockage of renal tubules due to the filtration of large amounts of free light chain through the kidney.

Another associated type of protein deposition is amyloidosis which may show itself as renal disease, bilateral carpal tunnel syndrome, heart failure, thrombosis, malabsorption or macroglossia. In a series of 115 patients with all types of amyloidosis (Hobbs, 1973), paraproteins were detected in 42% and 37% had Bence Jones proteinuria. The incidence of amyloid in all patients with paraproteinaemia is, however, lower and has been noted in 33 out of a series of 1,300 patients (Hobbs, 1973). Although the ratio of κ to λ-type light chains in normal immunoglobulin is 2:1, amongst the paraproteins associated with amyloid in this series the ratio was 1·25:1. Patients producing only Bence Jones proteins account for 45% of cases where amyloid is associated with immunocytomas, and in these cases the amyloid contains a component, B-protein, which is identical with the variable portion of the light chain of the coincident paraprotein (Glenner *et al.*, 1971).

Whether the symptoms associated with amyloid can be considered as simply due to the presence of paraproteins, however, is debatable since Bence Jones proteins show affinity for the very tissues in which amyloid is deposited (Osserman *et al.*, 1964a). In other words, it is possible that the deposition of amyloid represents a specific reaction of the paraprotein.

Symptoms Due to Paraprotein Activity or Affinity

Serum paraproteins appear to be structurally normal antibodies and although the specificity is usually unknown, an increasing number have been shown to have specific activity against one of a wide range of antigens. Examples are two cases described by Seligmann; one a patient with a history of rheumatic fever who developed myeloma with a paraprotein with antistreptolysin activity (Seligmann *et al.*, 1968), and the other a patient who, 30 years after two injections of unpurified horse serum, developed myelomatosis with an IgG paraprotein with activity against horse α_2-macroglobulin (Seligmann *et al.*, 1973).

Since Kritzmann and co-workers (1961) described an IgM paraprotein with rheumatoid factor activity, there has been an increased detection of paraproteins associated with myelomas as well as Waldenström's macroglobulinaemia which exhibit auto-antibody activity. The reasons for this are not clear, although there are several possibilities. It may be that in patients who develop these proteins there are areas of inflammatory reaction with tissue damage leading to exposure of previously concealed auto-antigens against which antibody synthesis becomes directed. The monoclonal proliferation of such an antibody-producing cell would result in the presence of a paraprotein with auto-antibody activity. In many cases, however, it remains in doubt whether such activities represent primary specific properties of the paraproteins or simply cross-reactions from other, unknown antigens. The more common paraprotein auto-antibody activities are discussed below.

Cold Haemagglutinins

Some of the commonest of such auto-antibodies are those which cause cold haemagglutinin disease (CHAD). Patients with CHAD may present either with severe acrocyanosis on exposure to the cold, or with the symptoms of chronic anaemia. The paraprotein is usually IgM type κ, and the underlying lesion may be either benign or malignant, such as a malignant lymphoma. The paraprotein reacts with components of erythrocyte membranes, usually the I antigen, and less commonly the i antigen. Table 6 shows our findings in a series of 19 patients with CHAD in whom IgM serum paraproteins were detected.

TABLE 6

The modes of presentation, serum antibody activities and final diagnoses in 19 patients with cold haemagglutinin disease (CHAD) in whom IgM serum paraproteins were detected

Mode of presentation	Serum antibody activity	Final diagnosis	No. of patients
CHAD an incidental finding	anti-i	malignant lymphoma	4
	anti-I	malignant lymphoma	2
CHAD the presenting feature	anti-I	primary CHAD	8
	anti-I	malignant lymphoma	3
	unidentified	primary CHAD	1
	unidentified	carcinoma (only)	1

Rheumatoid Factor Activity

There is a high reported incidence of paraproteins with rheumatoid factor activity (Meltzer *et al.*, 1966). These paraproteins with activity against IgG immunoglobulins, are usually of IgM class, although occasionally they are IgG or IgA, and are often detected by their ability to form cryoprecipitates.

In about 10% of patients with IgM monoclonal rheumatoid factors (Cooke, personal communication), IgM–IgG complexes in the serum are identifiable as acid-dissociable 22S complexes detected by ultracentrifugal analysis (Cooke and Apsey, 1971).

Anti-lipoprotein Activity

A number of cases of multiple myeloma have been described with hyperlipidaemia and xanthomata (Potter, 1971), and we have seen these features in one patient with a diagnosis of malignant lymphoma. Such findings may be due to activity by the paraproteins against lipoproteins. It is also interesting that four out of 16 patients with Gaucher's disease had IgG paraproteins (Pratt *et al.*, 1968).

Anti-factor VIII Activity

Antibody activity against antihaemophiliac globulin (factor VIII) has occasionally been found in serum from patients with either myelomatosis or a macroglobulinaemia (Perkins *et al.*, 1970).

Anti-nervous Tissue Activity

Lastly, in our recent series of patients with IgM paraproteins, 15 out of 204 had neurological symptoms in the absence of hyperviscosity or evidence of amyloid, usually peripheral neuropathies, and this was the cause of presentation in 12 of the patients. Fluorescent antibody studies have shown marked paraprotein activity against a wide range of nervous tissue antigens, especially those in axonal and glial tissues, in sera from 39 of the 63 patients with IgM paraproteinaemia studied in this series and in all but one of the patients with neurological symptoms (Fig. 11). No similar findings have been observed in over 150 patients with IgG or IgA paraproteins or in patients with polyclonal rises in IgM level (Carter *et al.*, in press). Whether these patients have presented because of a primary specific activity of paraprotein against nervous tissue—the paraproteins reflecting monoclonal responses to nervous tissue antigens exposed by some other process as discussed earlier—or whether the findings are simply due to a cross-reaction from some other, unidentified antigens is still not clear. Paraprotein activity against other tissues, such as smooth muscle, has also been observed.

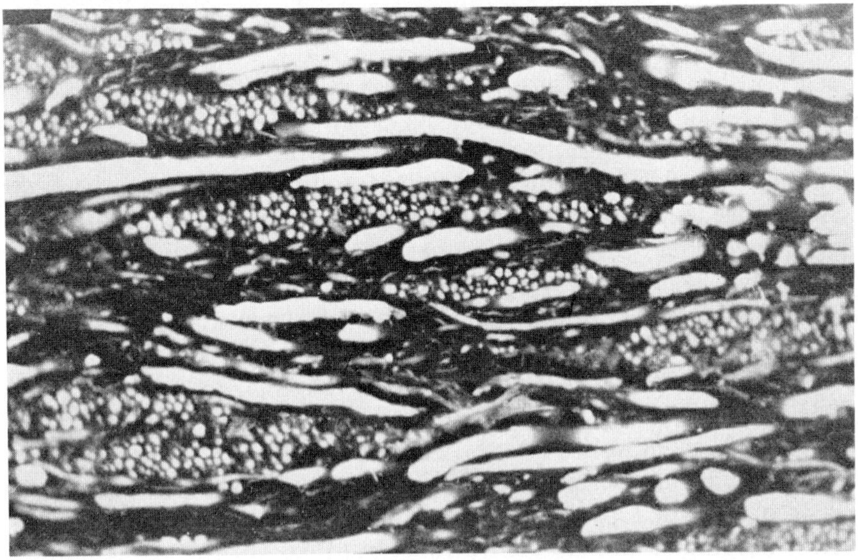

Fig. 11. Anti-axonal activity found in the serum of a patient with macroglobulinaemia who presented with a peripheral neuropathy, and detected by a fluorescent antibody "sandwich" technique. Reactions between serum and axons, cut both longitudinally and transversely, are seen as white areas. (By courtesy of Professor B. W. Lacey.)

Patients may also present in other ways. Symptoms may be due to renal failure associated with hypercalcaemia, particularly in the presence of myelomatosis, or to an increase in intercurrent infections in patients with low serum immunoglobulins especially if the diagnosis is myelomatosis or malignant lymphoma.

RELATIONSHIP BETWEEN SERUM PARAPROTEIN CONCENTRATION AND TUMOUR MASS

Paraprotein studies are of value in assessing the size of the underlying immunocytoma. Although the size of the immunocytoma at the time of clinical presentation is of no prognostic value, in patients receiving chemotherapy assessment of tumour size by serum paraprotein studies, as discussed below, allows monitoring during therapy.

Studies on experimental plasmacytomas in mice show that tumour weight is proportional to the turnover rate of the associated paraprotein (Nathans *et al.*, 1958). Tumour weight and serum paraprotein concentrations are also related (Osserman *et al.*, 1964b), and Fakhri and Hobbs (1970) showed a direct relationship between serum paraprotein concentrations and the number of ascitic plasmacytoma cells in mice. In addition to this, *in vitro* studies on marrow have shown that the amount of paraprotein synthesized by human myeloma cells is relatively constant both for different cultures and for the same culture over a period of time, at about $0{\cdot}5$ to $3{\cdot}4 \times 10^{-11}$ grams of paraprotein per myeloma cell per day (Salmon and Smith, 1970). The quantity of paraprotein synthesized in a given patient, and consequently the serum concentration, is therefore a function of the mass of tumour present (Salmon and Smith, 1970; Salmon *et al.*, 1971).

The relationship between serum paraprotein concentration and tumour mass is, however, not a simple one irrespective of immunoglobulin class, since the half lives of some classes of immunoglobulins *in vivo* vary with serum concentration (Schultze and Heremans, 1966). The daily rates of catabolism of the intravascular mass of IgG_3, IgA and IgM probably do not vary with changing serum concentrations, but those of IgG_1, IgG_2 and IgG_4 increase as the serum concentration rises (Salmon, 1973). Despite this difficulty, estimations of serum paraprotein concentration in patients with myelomatosis help to assess tumour size, except in the 1% of cases where paraprotein synthesis cannot be detected by serum electrophoresis.

Very little information is available on the relationship between serum paraproteins from other immunocytomas and tumour mass, but experience with patients with Waldenström's macroglobulinaemia suggests that it is similar to that in myelomatosis.

The average serum paraprotein concentrations in cases with myelomatosis, at the time of clinical presentation due to the tumour, are shown in Table 7. Such a wide range of serum IgM paraprotein levels are found at the time of presentation in patients with monoclonal IgM diseases that figures for this are more difficult to assess. They vary from below 10 g/litre in patients presenting either because of the tumour or because the paraprotein exhibits a specific activity, such as cold haemagglutination, to over 50 g/litre in patients presenting with symptoms of hyperviscosity. Nevertheless, some patients in the latter group may have serum paraprotein levels considerably lower than 50 g/litre, and some in the former group may have levels higher than 10 g/litre.

Allowing for *in vivo* turnover, a serum concentration of IgA paraprotein of 28 g/litre indicates a tumour mass of about $4{\cdot}6 \times 10^{11}$ cells, or about a kilogram of tumour. Calculations for IgG and IgD paraproteins, allowing for different turnover rates at different serum concentrations agree well with this figure. Similar estimates of tumour mass at the time of clinical presentation are quoted both for patients with myelomas with paraproteins of classes IgG, IgA and IgD and for a case of IgE paraprotein (Salmon *et al.*, 1971).

TABLE 7

Average serum paraprotein concentration found in patients with myelomatosis at the time of clinical presentation

Paraprotein class	Average serum concentration (g/litre)
IgG_1, IgG_2, and IgG_4	43
IgG_3	35
IgA	28
IgD	14
	Average urinary excretion (g/24 hr)
Bence Jones proteinuria only	5·4

Examination of 230 bone marrow smears taken from patients with myelomatosis at the time of clinical presentation showed that on average, 33% of marrow was replaced by tumour cells (Hobbs, 1971). Since it has been estimated that the average weight of bone marrow in a 70 kg patient is 3·2 kg (Mechanik, 1926), this also suggests the presence of about a kilogram of tumour at the time of presentation.

THE KINETICS OF TUMOUR GROWTH

Although there is agreement on the validity of calculations of the average amount of immunocytoma present at the time of clinical presentation, the mode of growth of immunocytomas to this size is the subject of debate.

Gompertzian Kinetics

Using a "sandwich" radioimmunoassay technique to investigate paraproteins secreted by fresh myeloma cells *in vitro* Salmon *et al.* (1969), studied 70 myeloma patients over a period of 2–4 years. Their findings suggest that while, initially, tumour growth occurs very rapidly, the rate slows as the tumour enlarges. Thus although the doubling time of the tumour at the time of clinical presentation may be 4–6 months, initially it might be as short as 1–3 days (Sullivan and Salmon, 1972). It has been argued that the growth of all animal tumours may better fit a Gompertzian growth curve (Laird, 1964) such as that described by Sullivan and Salmon than a first order kinetic model where growth is continuously exponential; this would imply that myelomata take only 1–2 years to develop from a single cell to a tumour which may cause symptoms. Support for this concept is given by the appearance of paraproteins within weeks of antigenic challenge in patients developing monoclonal responses to such severe infections as hepatitis, or to bone marrow transplantation (Salmon, 1973).

First Order Kinetics

By contrast, the growth of ascitic plasmacytomas in mice is continuously exponential up to a tumour size of 10^8 cells (Fakhri and Hobbs, 1970). Observations made on 94 untreated patients with progressing myelomatosis out of nearly 1,000 in MRC myeloma trials, also support the idea of a constant rate of growth over a wide range of tumour mass (Hobbs, 1967).

The median doubling time for IgA myelomas at presentation is 6·3 months (Hobbs, 1969b), and for IgG myelomas about 6 months (Salmon and Smith, 1970). Assuming a constant rate of growth, 21 years would be required for an IgA myeloma to develop from one cell to a kilogram of tumour (Hobbs, 1971), and about 33 years for an IgG myeloma (Hobbs, 1969c). The validity of such extrapolation is supported by the findings in some patients in the MRC trial who have become refractory to treatment. Their serum paraprotein levels, and therefore tumour sizes, have been observed to increase at a rate identical to that prior to therapy, even though the serum levels and tumour masses were then much higher.

There is much other evidence in favour of very long preclinical periods in these diseases, although some of it is circumstantial:

i. clinical recurrence of disease has been reported as long as 17 years after the removal of a solitary plasmacytoma (Wiltshaw, 1969);
ii. accidental detection of paraproteins has been reported in patients 15 to 24 years before the clinical emergence of myelomas associated with the same paraproteins (Nørgaard, 1971);
iii. six patients in the MRC myeloma trial were detected by accidental

discovery of a paraprotein as much as 8 years before the clinical declaration of tumours associated with these same proteins;

iv. one patient, already mentioned, developed an IgG myeloma with paraprotein antibody activity against horse α_2-macroglobulin over 30 years after an injection of unpurified horse serum (Seligmann *et al.*, 1973). It is, however, possible that growth of this malignant immunocytoma started considerably after the date of the antigenic challenge.

In most of the above patients a tumour could not have evolved in the time suggested by Gompertzian growth kinetics.

It is most likely that either type of kinetics applies in individual cases. In some patients the tumour growth rate will almost certainly slow as the mass enlarges, because of reduction of blood supply at the centre, but it may be that, because of their diffuse nature, many myelomas are not subject to the same limitations of growth as more discrete tumours.

MONITORING TUMOUR MASS DURING THERAPY

Responses to Therapy

The average survival of one series of patients with myelomatosis, before the introduction of alkylating agents such as melphalan and cyclophosphamide, was 17 months from the onset of symptoms (Farhangi and Osserman, 1973). In other series less than 50% of untreated patients with myelomatosis have survived a year from clinical presentation (Feinleib and MacMahon, 1960; Innes and Newall, 1961). In 6–12 months after clinical presentation there would be a further one to two doublings in tumour mass from $4{\cdot}6 \times 10^{11}$ to about $1\text{–}2 \times 10^{12}$ cells, or about 3 kilograms of tumour. This would cause bone marrow failure, although if areas other than those usually occupied by red marrow are invaded, larger masses of tumour may be tolerated.

Other types of malignant immunocytoma may run a less malignant course, and untreated cases of Waldenström's macroglobulinaemia may survive many years after presenting clinically. The natural history of these tumours, is, however, very variable.

The introduction of chemotherapy has, by reducing the size of tumour masses, markedly increased the survival of patients with myelomatosis after clinical presentation. This longer survival may also be due in part, however, to earlier diagnosis, to better general management, and to improved techniques in biochemical monitoring of the effects of chemotherapy. In the first

MRC myeloma trial 45% of the patients were alive after two years and 11% after five. Much longer average survival has been claimed for other series (Farhangi and Osserman, 1973), although it is difficult to compare results when different populations are involved.

Monitoring Reductions in Tumour Mass

Observations on MRC myeloma trial patients over 9 years indicate that, if both serum and urine are investigated, paraprotein concentrations may be used as a monitor of the response of tumour size to treatment in 98% of patients (Hobbs, 1975). In 2% of patients, however, tumours apparently continue to enlarge without a corresponding rise in serum paraprotein concentrations. Experience with patients with macroglobulinaemia suggests a similar correlation.

Many criteria have been used to define the responses of tumours to chemotherapy. We use those propounded by the Chronic Leukaemia Taskforce of the National Cancer Institute (cited in Snapper and Kahn, 1971) which include the observation of at least 50% reduction in both serum paraprotein concentration and Bence Jones proteinuria compared to the levels found at the time of clinical presentation. By these criteria 82% of patients in the first MRC myeloma trial responded to chemotherapy.

Allowing for the differing *in vivo* turnover of the various immunoglobulin classes and subclasses, the rate of fall of serum paraprotein concentration varies among patients with myelomatosis who respond to chemotherapy (Fig. 12). In a study on 167 patients, 107 patients (64%) showed a slow reduction (a fall of the original serum paraprotein level by at least 50%, but only after three months from the start of chemotherapy), 30 patients (18%) showed a rapid reduction (a fall of the original paraprotein level by at least 50% within three months), 25 patients (15%) showed little change, and 5 patients (3%) showed a continually increasing paraprotein level (Hobbs, 1969c). These responses to therapy of patients with myelomas producing detectable Bence Jones proteins only show a similar pattern.

Kinetics of Tumour Reduction

Whatever the speed of response to chemotherapy as estimated by serum paraprotein concentrations, reduction in *size* of immunocytomas has been shown to fit Gompertzian kinetics (Sullivan and Salmon, 1972). The rate of

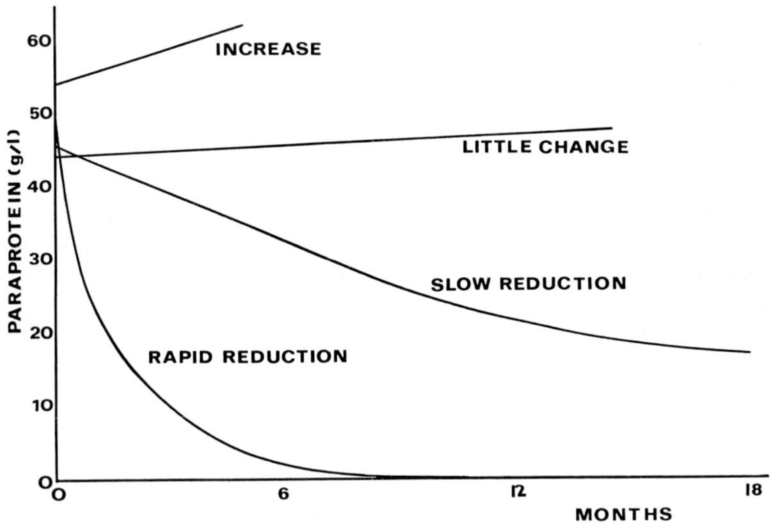

Fig. 12. Changes in serum IgG_1 paraprotein concentrations in four representative patients with myelomatosis and with similar initial serum levels of paraprotein, during chemotherapy. "Slow reduction" indicates a paraprotein level falling below 50% of the initial level after three months from the start of chemotherapy, and "rapid reduction" indicates a paraprotein level falling below 50% of the initial level within three months. (Reproduced by courtesy of *J. Clin. Path.*)

tumour regression falls as the mass decreases. Eventually a "plateau" tumour mass is reached which may be stable for months or even years.

There are a number of possible explanations for this phenomenon. Sullivan and Salmon (1972) suggest that as the tumour size reduces, so the proportion of dividing cells in the tumour increases, and that the "plateau" tumour size reflects a balance between an increased tumour cell death due to chemo therapy and an increased tumour cell birth due to an expanded proliferating compartment. They suggest that this pattern of tumour regression would be expected with drugs such as the currently used cytotoxic agents, which kill a constant fraction of tumour cells. Other possible explanations of the kinetics of tumour reduction are that these cytotoxic drugs may select subclasses of the tumour which are more resistant to their action, or that, since these agents are only active against dividing cells, the "plateau" phase represents a proportional expansion of the non-proliferating compartment.

If the amount of tumour present during the "plateau" phase is such that the amount of paraprotein synthesized is too low to be detected by electrophoresis, monitoring this phase of the disease is not possible by usual methods, and an increase in tumour size can be detected only when paraprotein concentrations again reach those visible by electrophoresis.

Serum paraproteins became undetectable during treatment in 21 of 258 patients in the first MRC myeloma trial. 9 of these are alive and well at the time of writing and form more than half of the 17 currently surviving patients from this trial. Admission to the trial ended in 1968.

Unfortunately there is not such detailed information about the response to therapy of paraproteinaemias other than myelomas. Few patients have yet been entered into the MRC macroglobulinaemia trial, but this should give similar detailed information on patients with monoclonal IgM diseases.

CAUSES OF THERAPEUTIC FAILURE

Although a high proportion of patients with myelomatosis initially respond to chemotherapy, about half the patients die within two years of clinical presentation.

There are many causes of death. These were not related to the myeloma in 7 out of a series of 145 patients and only indirectly related to it in another 11 patients (Hobbs, 1971). Of the remaining 127 cases, 40 died because of failure to respond to chemotherapy, and 87 relapsed and died despite an initial response.

This last group of patients accounted for 60% of the deaths in this series, and we should consider the behaviour of the tumours which became refractory to therapy after an initial response. This is summarized in Table 8.

In "simple" escape, the serum paraprotein level, and therefore tumour growth, increases at a rate identical to that before the onset of therapy, and in "growth rate" escape the rate of rise of both is greater than that before therapy.

There are a number of manifestations of increased tumour growth:

i. most commonly there may be an increased rate of synthesis by the tumour of Bence Jones protein only;
ii. there may be an increased rate of rise in serum concentration of the same serum paraprotein initially present;
iii. the paraprotein which increases during treatment may be different from that present before chemotherapy was started.

Each type of growth rate escape has only been observed in patients in the MRC studies six months or more after the start of cytotoxic therapy. It may be

TABLE 8

The modes of escape from treatment in 87 patients with myelomatosis in whom the tumours became refractory to therapy despite an initial response. "Simple" escape is when the serum paraprotein concentration, and therefore tumour growth, increases at a rate identical to that before the onset of therapy and "growth rate" escape is when the rate of rise of these is greater than before therapy

Modes of escape	No. of patients		Incidence (%)	
Simple	47		55	
Growth rate	37		42	
with Bence Jones protein only		30		35
with the same paraprotein		2		2
with a different paraprotein		5		5
Development of a further malignancy	3		3	
malignant lymphoma		2		2
monocytic leukaemia		1		1

that the treatment either selects or perhaps even generates faster growing elements from the original clone. Hobbs (1971) suggests that since current cytotoxic agents act on DNA they may actually cause mutations, and therefore favours the second theory. Moreover, "fingerprint" studies on both the original and on the paraproteins appearing during treatment may show changes in only one peptide due, perhaps, to single amino acid substitutions (Hobbs, 1975). Such changes could be explained by one point alteration of single DNA codons.

Alternatively, escape from therapy may be due to the development of another type of malignancy, such as malignant lymphoma or monocytic leukaemia. The risk of this during treatment with cytotoxic agents has been shown to increase after 5 years of chemotherapy (Osserman, 1969). When a diagnosis of malignant immunocytoma has been clearly established, the risks associated with long term chemotherapy are acceptable. However, when the underlying lesion may be a benign immunocytoma, it is probably best not to start cytotoxic therapy before the diagnosis is more certain.

LABORATORY ASSESSMENT OF PROGNOSIS

By investigating patients at the time of clinical presentation and during the course of treatment the value of many parameters and investigations in helping to form a prognosis has been assessed. Some findings, although of diagnostic value, are of no prognostic significance in patients with myelomatosis, as shown in Table 9 (Peto, 1971). It is interesting that the concentration of serum paraprotein, and therefore the tumour mass, at the time of presentation was found to be of *no* prognostic value in patients who subsequently received chemotherapy.

TABLE 9

Findings at the time of clinical presentation of patients with myelomatosis, later treated with chemotherapy, which have no prognostic significance

Investigation performed	Features of no prognostic significance
Radiology	Lytic lesions wedging or collapse of vertebrae osteoporosis
Serum or plasma analysis	calcium concentration alkaline phosphatase concentration uric acid concentration paraprotein concentration
Blood analysis	total leucocyte count platelet count

Findings at Presentation

Parameters, measured at the time of clinical presentation, which are of prognostic value are shown in Table 10. Why they help prognosis is not fully explained although there are several possibilities.

Both a high plasma urea concentration and heavy non-Bence Jones proteinuria indicates renal damage, and a low haemoglobin concentration may indicate pre-existing bone marrow suppression which will limit the effectiveness of cytotoxic chemotherapy.

It has been argued that Bence Jones proteinuria indicates the presence of a more dedifferentiated and faster growing tumour than in cases without it, (Hobbs, 1969c). Biochemical dedifferentiation of the tumour product may parallel the dedifferentiation of the tumour itself and experience with the detection of any immunoglobulin fragment in patients with myeloma (Hobbs, (1971) or with monoclonal IgM diseases (Carter and Hobbs, 1971) supports this view. Indeed, those immunocytomas which synthesize Bence Jones proteins only are associated with very poor prognoses (MRC, 1973). The type of Bence Jones protein is also of prognostic importance. The median length of survival from the time of clinical presentation of 22 patients in the first MRC myeloma trial with tumours which produced λ-type Bence Jones proteins only was 5 months, whereas that of 31 patients with tumours which produced κ-type Bence Jones proteins only was 2 months.

TABLE 10

Findings at the time of clinical presentation of patients with myelomatosis, later treated with chemotherapy, which are independently of prognostic significance

Findings	Percentage length of survival, relative to the average for all patients
Serum albumin (g/litre)	
above 30	140
20–29	90
below 19	60
Serum urea (mmol/litre)	
below 6·7	170
6·7–13·0	90
above 13·0	30
Non Bence Jones proteinuria (g/litre)	
below 0·4	130
above 0·4	60
Bence Jones proteinuria (g/litre)	
below 0·1	140
above 2·0	30
Haemoglobin (g/100 ml)	
above 10·0	200
7·5–9·9	90
below 7·5	50

If nephrotic syndrome is excluded, there is a striking correlation between serum albumin concentrations found at the time of clinical presentation and the subsequent length of survival of patients with myelomatosis (Fig. 13). The reasons for this correlation, which occurs independently of other factors, are not fully understood, for low serum albumin concentrations are found in a wide range of both benign and malignant diseases (cited in Zilva and Pannall, 1975). It has been shown that in tissue culture, normal cells pinocytose albumin in small regular droplets, and that malignant cells engulf albumin in larger, less regular droplets (Cohen *et al.*, 1961). A low serum albumin found at the time of presentation, and due to neither protein loss nor hepatic disease, might therefore indicate consumption of albumin by the tumour, though why this correlates with prognosis is not clear.

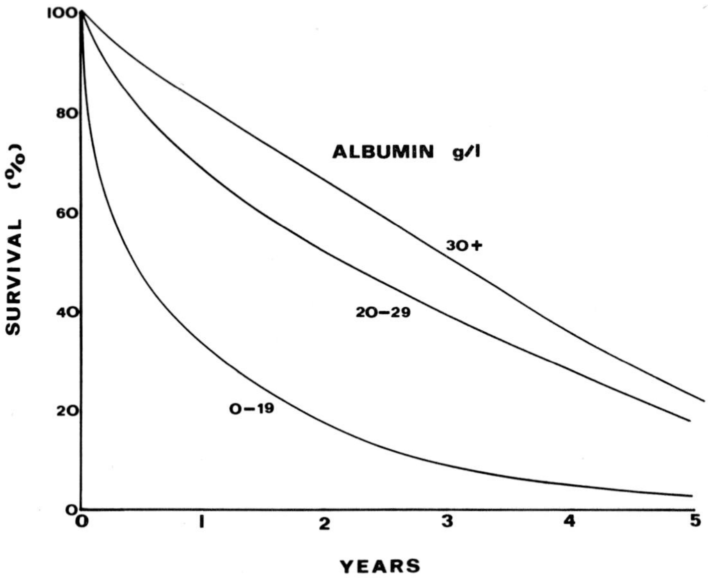

Fig. 13. Surivival rate of patients in the first MRC myeloma trial related to whether the serum albumin concentration found at the time of admission to the trial was below 19 g/litre, between 20 and 29 g/litre, or over 30 g/litre. (Reproduced by courtesy of *J. Clin. Path.*)

Nature of Response to Therapy

Apart from the findings at the time of clinical presentation, the rate of response of the paraprotein concentration and tumour mass to chemotherapy, as previously defined, also correlates with subsequent survival (Hobbs, 1969c). Figure 14 shows this correlation for 167 patients in the first MRC myeloma trial. It can be seen that the longest survivals were in patients whose initial response to therapy was slow, whereas that of patients who responded rapidly was little better than those who failed to respond at all. It may be that tumours which respond slowly to chemotherapy have a low proportion of dividing cells while those responding rapidly have a higher proportion.

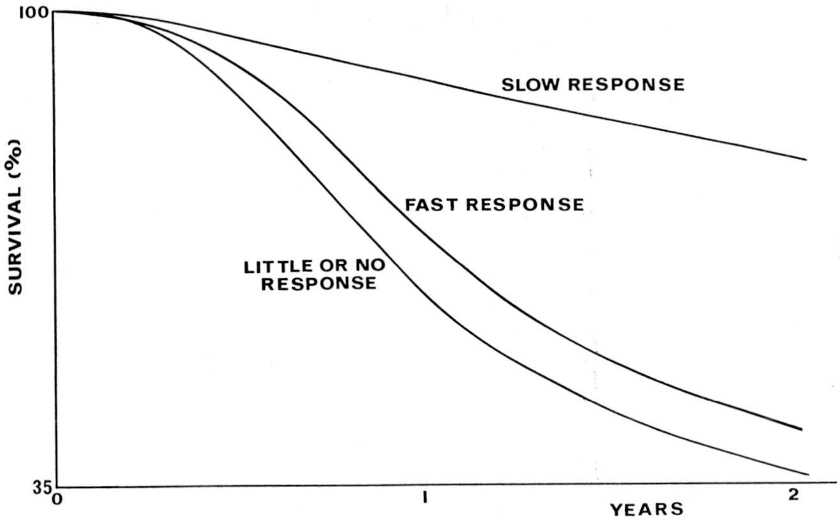

Fig. 14. Survival rate of 167 patients in the first MRC myeloma trial related to whether their response to chemotherapy was fast (paraprotein concentration falling to half initial level within three months, 30 patients), slow (paraprotein concentration falling to half initial level but not within three months, 107 patients), or whether they showed little or no response to therapy (30 patients). (Reproduced by courtesy of *J. Clin. Path.*)

The Histological Diagnosis

Histological examination of tissue biopsies can also be of diagnostic, and therefore of prognostic help. Patients with Waldenström's macroglobulinaemia may survive for many years, whilst the expected survival of those with malignant lymphoma or myeloma is much shorter.

The prognosis in patients with either solitary plasmacytoma or HCD is difficult to assess because of the variable nature and histories of these disorders.

CONCLUSIONS

To summarize the current views on paraproteins (Hobbs, 1971):

i. they are the products of single clones of cells which may follow benign or malignant courses;

ii. serum concentrations reflect the mass of the underlying immunocytoma both during the natural history of the disorder and, within the limitations already discussed, during tumour reduction by chemotherapy;
iii. incomplete immunoglobulins, such as Bence Jones proteins or monomeric (7S) IgM are produced by tumours more malignant than those producing only complete immunoglobulins.

Patients with disorders associated with paraproteinaemia may present with a wide range of symptoms, referable to either the tumour, especially in cases with myeloma and malignant lymphoma, or to the presence of the protein, particularly in patients with diseases associated with macroglobulinaemia.

Laboratory findings may help in both diagnosis and prognosis. Findings either at the time of clinical presentation, such as serum albumin and urea levels, haemoglobin level and the presence of Bence Jones or other proteins in the urine, or during treatment, such as the rate of response of serum paraproteins to chemotherapy may be of prognostic value.

The value of monitoring immunocytomas by investigations of serum and urine paraproteins has been clearly established. However, more sensitive techniques are required to monitor tumours if paraprotein is undetected by current techniques. The use of polyclonal antisera in immunochemical techniques, such as radial immunodiffusion (Fahey and McKelvey, 1965), to detect very low levels of paraproteins, is unsatisfactory owing to the differing reactivities of monoclonal proteins from different patients. It may be possible, however, to produce idiotypic anti-paraprotein antisera and to monitor each patient's paraprotein with antiserum specifically reactive against it.

Because immunoglobulins have relatively long half-lives patients with malignant immunocytomas need only be investigated at three-monthly intervals. Increase in Bence Jones proteinuria and rises in serum paraprotein levels during treatment should be carefully investigated. The possible development of malignant diseases, such as malignant lymphoma, must be borne in mind, especially after five years of chemotherapy. In patients without apparent malignant disease follow up studies should be performed every 6–12 months.

Only by the use of sensitive biochemical monitoring of the response to therapy will the best survival rates be achieved.

ACKNOWLEDGEMENTS

I would particularly like to thank Dr J. F. Zilva, Mr K. B. Cooke and Professor J. R. Hobbs for their considerable advice and helpful criticism during the preparation of this chapter, and the staff of the Westminster Hospital Protein Laboratories for their scientific contributions to the contents.

I would also like to thank Mr K. B. Cooke, Professor B. W. Lacey, Professor J. Humble and Dr K. Newton who contributed illustrations.

REFERENCES

Bennett, M. H., Farrer-Brown, G., Henry, K. and Jelliffe, A. M. (1974). Classification of the non-Hodgkin's lymphomas. *Lancet* **2**, 405–406.

Capra, J. D. and Kunkel, H. G. (1970). Aggregation of γG_3 proteins: Relevance to the hyperviscosity syndrome. *J. Clin. Invest.* **49**, 610–621.

Carter, P. M. and Hobbs, J. R. (1971). Clinical significance of 7S IgM in monoclonal IgM diseases. *Brit. Med. J.* **2**, 260–261.

Carter, P. M., Lacey, B. W. and Hobbs, J. R. (in press). Macroglobulinaemia associated with neurological symptoms. *Proc. Roy. Soc. Med.*

Cohen, S., Beiser, S. M. and Hsu, K. C. (1961). Immunohistochemical study of the uptake of serum proteins by neoplastic liver cells. *Cancer Res.* **21**, 1510–1512.

Cooke, K. B. (1969). Essential paraproteinaemia. *Proc. Roy. Soc. Med.* **64**, 777–778.

Cooke, K. B. and Apsey, M. E. (1971). Dissociation studies on a naturally occurring 22S Rheumatoid Factor. *In* "Protides of the Biological Fluids", Proceedings of the 18th Colloquium, Bruges, 1970 (ed. H. Peeters), pp. 351–354. Pergamon Press, Oxford.

Fahey, J. L. and McKelvey, E. M. (1965). Quantitative determination of serum immunoglobulins in antibody-agar plates. *J. Immunol.* **94**, 84–90.

Fakhri, O. and Hobbs, J. R. (1970). The serum paraprotein level related to the number of plasmacytoma-5563 cells in C3H mice. *Brit. J. Cancer* **24**, 395–397.

Farhangi, M. and Osserman, E. F. (1973). The treatment of multiple myeloma. *Sem. Haem.* **10**, 149–161.

Feinleib, M. and MacMahon, B. (1960). Duration of survival in multiple myeloma. *J. Nat. Cancer Inst.* **24**, 1259–1269.

Franklin, E. C., Löwenstein, J., Bigelow, B. and Meltzer, M. (1964). Heavy chain disease. A new disorder of serum γ-globulins. *Am. J. Med.* **37**, 332–350.

Gale, D. S. J., Versey, J. M. B. and Hobbs, J. R. (1974). Rocket immunoselection for detection of heavy chain diseases. *Clin. Chem.* **20**, 1292–1294.

Glenner, G. G., Terry, W., Havada, M., Isersky, C. and Page, D. (1971). Amyloid fibril proteins: proof of homology with immunoglobulin light chains by sequence analyses. *Science* **172**, 1150–1151.

Hällén, J. (1966). Discrete gammaglobulin (M-) components in serum. Clinical study of 150 subjects without myelomatosis. *Acta Med. Scand.* Suppl. 462, 127 pp.

Hobbs, J. R. (1967). Paraproteins, benign or malignant? *Brit. Med. J.* **3**, 699–704.

Hobbs, J. R. (1969a). Paraproteins. *Proc. Roy. Soc. Med.* **62**, 773–776.

Hobbs, J. R. (1969b). Immunochemical classes of myelomatosis. *Brit. J. Haematol.* **16**, 599–606.

Hobbs, J. R. (1969c). Growth rates and responses to treatment in human myelomatosis. *Brit. J. Haematol.* **16**, 607–617.

Hobbs, J. R. (1971). Immunocytoma of Mice and Men. *Brit. Med. J.* **2**, 67–72.

Hobbs, J. R. (1973). An ABC of amyloid. *Proc. Roy. Soc. Med.* **66**, 705–710.

Hobbs, J. R. (1975). Monitoring myelomatosis. *Archs Int. Med.* **135**, 125–130.

Innes, J. and Newall, J. (1961). Myelomatosis. *Lancet* **1**, 239–245.

Kohn, J. (1973). The laboratory investigation of paraproteinaemia. *In* "Recent Advances in Clinical Pathology", Series VI, Ch. 20, pp. 363–401.

Kohn, J. and Srivastava, P. C. (1973). Paraproteinaemia in blood donors and the aged: Benign and Malignant. *In* "Protides of the Biological Fluids", 20th Colloquium (ed. H. Peeters), pp. 257–261. Pergamon Press, Oxford.

Kritzman, J., Kunkel, H. G., McCarthy, J. and Mellors, R. C. (1961). Studies of a Waldenström type macroglobulin with rheumatoid factor properties. *J. Lab. Clin. Med.* **57**, 905–917.

Laird, A. K. (1964). Dynamics of tumour growth. *Brit. J. Cancer* **18**, 490–502.

MacIntyre, W. (1850). Case of mollities and fragilitas ossium accompanied with urine strongly charged with animal matter. *Med. Chir. Soc. Trans.* **33**, 211–232.

Martin, N. H. (1970). The paraproteinaemias. *Brit. J. Hosp. Med.* **3**, 662–666.

Mechanik, N. (1926). Untersuchungen uber das Gewicht des Knockermarkes des Menschen. *Z. Gesamte Anat.* Abt. 1. **79**, 58–99.

Medical Research Council (1973). Part 1. Analysis of presenting features of prognostic importance. *Brit. J. Haematol.* **24**, 123–139.

Meltzer, M., Franklin, E. C., Elias, K., McCluskey, R. T. and Cooper, N. (1966). Cryoglobulinaemia—a clinical and laboratory study II. Cryoglobulins and rheumatoid factor activity. *Am. J. Med.* **40**, 837–856.

Nathans, D., Fahey, J. L. and Potter, M. (1958). The formation of a myeloma protein by a mouse plasma cell tumour. *J. Exp. Med.* **108**, 121–130.

Nørgaard, O. (1971). Three cases of multiple myeloma in which the preclinical asymptomatic phases persisted throughout 15–24 years. *Brit. J. Cancer* **25**, 417–422.

Osserman, E. F. (1958). Natural history of multiple myeloma before radiological evidence of disease. *Radiology* **71**, 157–174.

Osserman, E. F., Takatsuki, K. and Talal, N. (1964a). Multiple myeloma I. The pathogenesis of "amyloidosis", *Sem. Haemat.* **1**, 3–85.

Osserman, E. F., Rifkind, R. A., Takatsuki, K. and Lawlord, P. (1964b). Studies of morphogenesis and protein synthesis in three mouse plasma cell tumours (X 5563, ADJ.PC-6C, ADJ.PC-20). *Ann. N. Y. Acad. Sci.* **113**, 627–641.

Pasmantier, M. W. and Azar, H. A. (1969). Extraskeletal spread in multiple plasma cell myeloma. A review of 57 autopsied cases. *Cancer* **23**, 167–174.

Perkins, H. A., MacKenzie, M. R. and Fudenberg, H. H. (1970). Haemostatic defects in dysproteinaemias. *Blood* **35**, 695–707.

Peto, R. (1971). Urea, albumin and response rates. *Brit. Med. J.* **2**, 324.

Potter, M. (1971). Myeloma proteins (M-components) with antibody-like activity. *New Engl. J. Med.* **284**, 831–838.

Pratt, P. V., Estren, S. and Kochwa, S. (1968). Immunoglobulin abnormalities in Gaucher's disease; report of 16 cases. *Blood* **31**, 633–640.

Radl, J. (1970). Light chain typing of immunoglobulins in small samples of biological material. *Immunology* **19**, 137–149.

Rambaud, J. C., Bognel, C., Prost, A., Bernier, J. J., Le Quintrec, Y., Lambling, A., Danon, F., Hurez, D. and Seligmann, M. (1968). Clinico-pathological study of a patient with "Mediterranean" type of abdominal lymphoma and a new type of IgA abnormality ("Alpha chain disease"). *Digestion* **1**, 321–336.

Salmon, S. E. (1973). Immunoglobulin synthesis and tumour kinetics of multiple myeloma. *Sem. Haemat.* **10**, 135–147.

Salmon, S. E. (1974). "Paraneoplastic" syndromes associated with monoclonal lymphocyte and plasma cell proliferation. *Ann. N. Y. Acad. Sci.* **230**, 228–239.

Salmon, S. E. and Smith, B. A. (1970). Immunoglobulin synthesis and total body tumour cell number in IgG multiple myeloma. *J. Clin. Invest.* **49**, 1114–1121.

Salmon, S. E., Mackey, G. and Fudenberg, H. H. (1969). "Sandwich" solid phase radioimmunoassay for the quantitative determination of human immunoglobulins. *J. Immunol.* **103**, 129–137.

Salmon, S. E., McIntyre, O. R. and Ogawa, M. (1971). IgE myeloma. Total body tumour cell number and synthesis of IgE and DNA. *Blood* **37**, 696–705.

Schultze, H. E. and Heremans, J. F. (1966). "Molecular Biology of Human Proteins", Ch. 2, pp. 63–170. Elsevier Publishing Co., Amsterdam.

Seligmann, M., Danon, F., Basch, J. and Bernard, J. (1968). IgG myeloma-cryoglobulin with anti-streptolysin activity. *Nature, Lond.* **220**, 711–712.

Seligmann, M., Sassy, C. and Chevalier, A. (1973). A human IgG myeloma protein with anti α_2 macroglobulin antibody activity. *J. Immunol.* **110**, 85–90.

Snapper, I. and Kahn, A. (1971). "Myelomatosis. Fundamentals and Clinical Features". Ch. 28, pp. 293–319. S. Karger, Basel.

Sullivan, P. W. and Salmon, S. E. (1972). Kinetics of tumour growth and regression in IgG multiple myeloma. *J. Clin. Invest.* **51**, 1697–1708.

Virella, G. and Hobbs, J. R. (1971). Heavy chain typing in IgG monoclonal gammopathies with special reference to cases of serum hyperviscosity and cryoglobulinaemia. *Clin. Exp. Immunol.* **9**, 973–980.

Waldenström, J. (1952). Abnormal proteins in myeloma. *In* "Advances in Internal Medicine". Vol. V (eds. W. Dock and I. Snapper), p. 398. The year book Publ. Inc., Chicago.

Waldenström, J. (1962). Monoclonal and polyclonal gammopathies and the biological system of gammaglobulins. *Prog. Allergy* **6**, 320–348.

Wiltshaw, E. (1969). The natural history of extramedullary plasmacytoma. M.D. Thesis University of London, 118 pp.

Zilva, J. F. and Pannall, P. R. (1975). "Clinical Chemistry in Diagnosis and Treatment". 2nd ed. Lloyd-Luke, London.

VI

Malignancy and Transplantation

28

Malignant Disease

GRAHAM CURRIE

Cancer has long been regarded as an autonomous process, the inexorable and unrestricted progression of a delinquent tissue mass flourishing in a wholly favourable host milieu. There are, however, several features of human tumours which suggest that this concept of tumour autonomy is defective. For example, the demonstration of hormone-dependence of tumours of the breast and prostate implies that important host-tumour interactions may play a role in moderating the biological behaviour of at least some tumours. Furthermore, many tumours are not biochemically autonomous. It is known, for instance, that some leukaemia cells require exogenous asparagine and will die in an asparagine-free environment whereas, under similar conditions, the normal cells are unaffected. This has led to the introduction of L asparaginase as a therapeutic agent in leukaemia. Indeed the use of enzymes for the selective depletion of essential nutrients, currently under intense scrutiny, may well provide substantial advances in tumour chemotherapy in the near future.

In 1906 Paul Ehrlich had introduced the concept of "athrepsis" to explain experimentally induced resistance to tumour growth. The immunity which developed was, he alleged, due to the depletion of nutrients essential for tumour growth. This view was subsequently and rightly discarded in favour of more conventional immunological explanations. Since these early days the possible role of immunological responses in resistance to the development, growth and dissemination of malignant tumours has received much attention with the emphasis laid, not unnaturally, on the potential value of immunological manipulations in therapy.

ANTIGENICITY OF TUMOURS

The presence of specific antigens on tumours had been hinted at by much of the early work. Clowes and Baeslack (1905) had encountered animals in which spontaneous regression of transplanted tumours was a common event. When rechallenged with cells from the same tumour line such animals showed heightened resistance and this sort of experimentation led to a boom in tumour immunology. Indeed, the first ten years of this century were probably the heyday of human cancer immunotherapy. However, despite an enormous literature recounting exhaustive and detailed experimentation there is little or no evidence for any beneficial effects produced by such manipulations. Subsequently (1929) Woglom in a splendidly critical survey pointed out the defects in the experimental work and the lack of success of the clinical escapades and effectively brought this subject to a standstill. His major point concerning the animal experimentation was the absence of genetic homogeneity in the experimental animals. In other words, tumour transplantation from one individual animal to another was merely an exercise in graft rejection and could not hope to detect tumour specific antigens or reactions to them.

In 1943, Gross, recognising the deficiencies of earlier experiments by workers such as Clowes and Baeslack (1905), carried out a similar experimental protocol, but in the then newly developed C3H strain of inbred mice. He induced sarcomas with methylcholanthrene and these were subsequently transplanted by intradermal inoculation. About 20% of the intradermal tumours grew for a while and then regressed. Gross was then able to show that these "regressor" mice were resistant to challenge with the same tumour line. C3H mice develop spontaneous mammary tumours and in the mice resistant to the sarcoma, spontaneous mammary tumours developed at the expected rate. He concluded that the resistance to tumour growth was immunologically specific and by inference provided evidence for the existence of specific tumour antigens. Foley (1953) drew similar conclusions after challenging inbred mice whose tumours had been surgically excised. Prehn and Main (1957) were able to confirm these results and at last the existence of tumour-specific antigens was proven beyond dispute.

Tumour-specific resistance to challenge can be evoked by amputation of a tumour-bearing limb, excision of the tumour, by ligation of the tumour or by pretreatment of the animals with irradiated tumour cells. Antigens detected by such methods are known as tumour-specific transplantation antigens (TSTA). Such TSTAs can be detected on most experimental tumours so far examined. Indeed development of these neo-antigens may be an essential feature of the malignant cell.

In man, however, evidence for the existence of similar antigens is less direct and is in many ways less convincing. *In vitro* techniques can allow the detection of specific antigens on human tumour cells and of specific reactions to them in tumour-bearing patients. While there is as yet little evidence that antigens detected by such assays are acting as the targets for immunologically-mediated rejection processes there is considerable optimism about the possible manipulation of such host immune responses for therapeutic purposes.

ROLE OF IMMUNITY IN HOST RESISTANCE

Before the immunological treatment of cancer can become a rational activity we will need to know a great deal more about the role of immunological mechanisms in tumour biology. Is there a role for immunological responses to such TSTA in host resistance to tumour growth? There is undoubtedly some form of host resistance to tumour growth but the precise contribution of immunological mechanisms to this resistance is at present unclear. This question can be approached by examining the effects of immunosuppression. In man the inadvertent transplantation of malignant cells with renal allografts into immunosuppressed recipients has occasionally led to rapid growth and dissemination of the donor's malignant cells. Cessation of immunosuppressive treatment in such patients has in some cases led to the rejection of the engrafted tumour. This unfortunate situation has little direct relevance to tumour immunity but it does illustrate that malignant cells, albeit allogeneic, are capable of unrestricted growth in the absence of normal immunological responses and are susceptible to rejection by the processes responsible for transplantation immunity.

In experimental animals the effects of immunosuppression on the growth of syngeneic tumours are variable. There is a remarkable lack of consistent evidence concerning the effects of immunosuppression on the growth of primary tumours and what evidence there is lacks conviction. Increased growth of primary tumours has occasionally been described but the overall effects are in no way striking. However, there is abundant and convincing evidence that immunosuppression can accelerate or even evoke the appearance of metastatic disease. Indeed a tumour, curable by surgical means, may, when inoculated into an immunosuppressed host, become incurable. Although the primary tumour may be successfully excised the host will die with metastatic disease. In a hamster lymphoma Gershon and Carter (1970) have shown that anti-lymphocyte serum treatment can promote the appearance of metastases. Similar treatment of mice bearing spontaneous mammary carcinomas leads to extensive metastases. Whole body irradiation will also promote the development of metastatic disease in a variety of animal model systems (Carnaud *et al.*, 1974; Vaage, 1973; Globerson and Feldman, 1964) and chronic drainage of the thoracic duct in tumour-bearing rats will provoke the development of extensive metastases. In their studies of this model system, Proctor *et al.* (1973) have shown that the metastasis-inhibiting properties of the lymph were associated with humoral rather than cellular factors.

Regression of Human Tumours

These observations suggest that specific immunological responses to tumour cells may have considerable significance for the clinical management of human cancer. Primary tumours constitute a mechanical problem and can, by and large, be dealt with by mechanical methods. It is in the development of metastatic disease that tumour immunity may have its greatest impact on clinical cancer medicine.

There is now every reason to believe that in animals at least specific immunological reactions may contribute to the resistance of the host to tumour growth and dissemination. Can such a conclusion be drawn for human cancer? An experimental approach to human tumours requires novel assay methods as transplantation techniques are both technically difficult and ethically dubious.

Anecdotal observations of the natural history of cancer patients have frequently implied the presence of host resistance but none of these allows conclusions to be drawn about the mechanisms of such resistance. For example, there are many reports of the spontaneous regression of human tumours (Everson and Cole, 1966). The highest incidence of such regressions is seen in neuroblastoma, hypernephroma, choriocarcinoma and in malignant melanoma, but there is no evidence from this sort of study that such regressions are immunologically determined. Other phenomena such as spontaneous differentiation are commonly seen in tumours such as neuroblastoma and may have little or no immunological foundation. In some diseases, notably breast carcinoma, patients may survive for up to 20 years or more following diagnosis and treatment of a primary carcinoma and then develop metastases with no evidence of further intervening primary lesions. If a tumour can remain dormant for such long periods it is tempting to invoke an immunological explanation.

The prevalence of some cancers, found at post-mortem is much higher than their overall clinical incidence. In neuroblastoma, for example, the ratio of post-mortem prevalence to clinical incidence is about 40:1. Similar observations have been made in prostatic and thyroid carcinomas. This implies that in otherwise normal healthy people, tumours are developing and regressing all the time. Occasionally complete disappearance of metastatic tumour has been reported following surgery, most frequently in cases of hypernephroma with lung metastases. Again, there is no direct evidence to incriminate immune reactions in these regressions but in the current climate of opinion the temptation to do so is almost overwhelming. In cases of malignant melanoma with multiple cutaneous deposits the extremely variable behaviour of each individual deposit would argue in favour of some form of host defence mechanism. Often such deposits regress completely while others are developing. In this type of extensive disease, usually confined to a single limb, the lesions can often remain apparently static for long periods of time (Bodenham, 1968).

Dramatic regressions of Burkitt's lymphoma have been seen after a single dose of a cytotoxic agent and this is not what one might have anticipated from the known effects of chemotherapy. A similar dramatic phenomenon occurs more consistently in gestational choriocarcinoma. It is of interest that both Burkitt's lymphoma and choriocarcinoma are tumours in which there is every reason to assume that immune reactions to tumour cells are important factors in their natural history.

During spontaneous regression of cutaneous deposits of malignant melanoma, Handley (1907) reported abundant infiltration by round cells. Indeed, many types of primary malignant tumour are known to be infiltrated by lymphocytes, macrophages and plasma cells, Furthermore, sinus histiocytosis of the draining lymph nodes has been described by Black *et al.* (1954). All the cell types found in such reactions are known to participate in the rejection of allogeneic tissues. There is also some evidence that these reactions may show a positive correlation with prognosis, i.e. a tumour showing regional node histiocytosis or round cell infiltration may well have a better prognosis than one without. However, in patients with advanced disease such reactions tend to disappear suggesting that if immunological reactions are involved then advanced tumour growth must be a manifestation of their failure. Elston (1969) has shown that in gestational choriocarcinoma there is a correlation between round cell infiltration of the tumour and prognosis. Thompson (1972) has reported similar findings in primary cutaneous malignant melanoma in Europeans, whereas Little (1972) was unable to detect such a correlation in Australia. In breast carcinoma Hamlin has described (1968) an extensive study which reveals a positive correlation between prognosis and a histological grading method which incorporates intensity of reactions around a tumour and in the regional nodes. Round cell infiltration of tumours has also been described in cases of neuroblastoma (Lauder and Aherne, 1972).

SPECIFIC IMMUNOLOGICAL RESPONSES TO TUMOUR CELLS

What evidence can be provided to support the contention that immunological mechanisms play a significant role in host resistance? In experimental animals the presence of TSTA on the surface of tumour cells is beyond dispute and the tumour-bearing host responds to these antigens by the production of circulating antibodies and cytotoxic mononuclear cells. Using a variety of immunological manoeuvres animals can be rendered resistant to challenge with tumour cells and in some instances the growth of established tumours can be slowed at least by such manoeuvres. Furthermore in such experimental animal systems there are some correlations between the immunological responses of the host and the natural history of the tumour, correlations which suggest that specific immunity may be a significant feature of host resistance, although it must be borne in mind that these correlations are of a somewhat tenuous nature.

In man the situation is less clear cut. In the animal models resistance to syngeneic tumours closely resembles allograft immunity and appears to be a predominantly cell-associated reaction which can be adoptively transferred with sensitized lymphoid cells but not with serum.

A variety of methods has been employed in cancer patients to detect tumour-specific cell-mediated immune responses. It must be emphasized that all these methods are technically complex and the results from most of them are at present of dubious significance, especially in view of their poor reproducibility in different centres. Many methods have been employed and will not be examined in any detail. However, there is an overall pattern of results emerging from the currently chaotic literature. Most of the assays provide data which suggest that cancer patients show specific immunological reactions to their own tumour cells. The pattern of specificity detected by these assays is, however, different from that found in animal model systems. The tumour antigens detectable by such methods on human tumour cells show a histogenic pattern of cross-reactivity, i.e. tumours derived from a given tissue seem to have similar antigenic configuration. Such antigens have been called "neo-histotypic" antigens. Chemically-induced tumours in experimental animals, on the other hand, have on their surfaces "private" or "idiotypic" individually specific antigens and so far no counterpart to these antigens has been reported with any degree of confidence in human cancer. This discrepancy between animal and human tumours is significant, for the individually specific TSTA are known to function as the targets for immunological rejection processes.

The cross-reacting antigens detectable on human tumours may not function in this way and in consequence may represent an irrelevant epiphenomenon which is neither associated with host resistance nor a suitable target for immunotherapy.

CONCOMITANT IMMUNITY AND ESCAPE

In experimental animals the injection of tumour cells into sites distant from an established primary tumour can reveal immunologically specific resistance to challenge. This form of resistance was termed concomitant immunity by Bashford (1908). The detection of specific resistance in a tumour-bearing animal is arguably the most vivid demonstration of specific immunologically mediated host resistance. In general, concomitant immunity shows two very important features. Firstly, it is readily detected early in the natural history of a primary tumour and tends to fade with progressive tumour growth. Secondly, there are dramatic variations in resistance to challenge in different sites in the body, e.g. it is well expressed when the tumour challenge inoculum is given intradermally or intravenously but is much weaker when the host is challenged by a subcutaneous dose of tumour cells. From the large number of animal models which have been studied there is a body of evidence which suggests that the disappearance of concomitant immunity is associated with dissemination of tumour. In other words, the development of metastatic disease occurs at the same time as the failure of detectable concomitant immunity. It is still not totally clear whether this association represents a causal connection.

Tumours are antigenic and the host can respond to them. This situation represents a paradox which implies the existence of what Woodruff (1964) has called "immunological escape", i.e. there must be routes by which a tumour evades destruction by host responses. The failure of concomitant immunity with progression of a tumour would seem to represent the most significant experimental manifestation of escape. Considerations of the potential value of immunotherapy in the treatment of tumours must by definition focus on those mechanisms responsible for escape, for if the tumour can escape the attentions of the host then it may similarly evade damage by whatever form of therapeutic attack is employed. Escape would seem to operate in two biologically distinct phases. The development of a malignant cell clone present initially as a microscopic nidus, and its subsequent development into a clinical detectable mass, implies the existence of "local escape".

The subsequent development of distant metastases with the failure of concomitant immunity can be regarded as a manifestation of "systemic escape". While the mechanisms responsible for the escape of tumours remain obscure it is apparent that it is a complex event and there may be many contributory factors. The possible routes of escape have been reviewed in detail elsewhere (Currie, 1974).

Specific Humoral Factors and Escape

Specific antibodies reacting with TSTA on the surface of tumour cells are exceptionally difficult to detect and consequently are often thought to contribute little to host resistance. Indeed at one stage it was believed in some quarters that humoral immunity was harmful and that antibodies block cell mediated immunity. Kaliss (1958) showed that the injection of antibody could facilitate the growth of allografted tumours which would otherwise have been rejected. He called this phenomenon "immunological enhancement" and showed that it could be exploited to prevent the rejection of normal tissue and organ allografts. It is important to remember, however, that there is no unequivocal evidence to show that specific anti-TSTA antibodies can enhance the growth of experimental syngeneic tumours. Nevertheless, the demonstration of allograft enhancement helped to propagate the idea that humoral responses to a tumour are in some way protective, capable of blocking cell-associated cytotoxic reactions and that B-cell responses to a tumour should be regarded as a bad thing. Despite a remarkable lack of evidence it became established dogma that T-cell responses to a tumour were beneficial and that B-cell responses were harmful. This notion gained most of its support from the studies described by Hellström and Hellström (1969).

Blocking Antibody

These authors demonstrated that the serum of tumour-bearing animals could block in an immunologically specific manner the anti-tumour cytotoxic activity of specifically sensitized lymphoid cells. Despite a singular lack of evidence, this serum activity became widely known as blocking antibody and the "protective" role of humoral responses in tumour immunology was generally regarded as a major mechanism in the immunological escape of tumours and a suitable target for immunotherapeutic attack.

However, closer scrutiny suggests that this blocking antibody concept is defective. Histological examination of the lymph nodes draining a tumour indicate that plasma cell reactions are seen only early in the growth of a tumour and that with escape of the tumour they disappear from the nodes (Black *et al.*, 1954). If the production of blocking antibody was associated with tumour progression then the opposite result would have been anticipated. Patients with severe defects in antibody synthesis such as Bruton hypogammaglobulinaemia show an increased incidence of malignant disease, hardly the result to be anticipated from the blocking hypothesis. Furthermore, Lewis and his colleagues (1969) detected specific antibodies to malignant melanoma in patients with early or localized disease and showed that these antibodies disappeared when dissemination occurred. But perhaps the most significant refutation of blocking antibody comes from the studies of Thompson and Linna (1973). They employed avian reticulo-endotheliosis virus in chickens. This virus induces tumours in both liver and spleen which are rapidly fatal. Following surgical thymectomy of the chickens they observed, as expected, accelerated tumour growth. However when they removed the bursa of Fabricius (abolishing antibody responses) they similarly found rapid growth and a higher incidence of tumours. This observation indicates that humoral responses are important in resisting tumour growth and that they cannot readily be incriminated in a blocking role as being responsible for protection of the tumour. Proctor, Rudenstam and Alexander (1973) had earlier suggested that humoral responses can play a major role in the prevention of metastatic disease. They demonstrated that prolonged drainage of thoracic duct lymph would promote the development of disseminated disease in rats bearing fibrosarcomata. This development of metastases could be prevented by returning the lymph plasma but not the lymphocytes, indicating that a humoral factor in the lymph plasma was responsible for preventing metastases. This factor, thought but not proven to be antibody, was immunologically specific in its effects.

Hellström and her colleagues (1971) introduced more complications into this field by their detection of a de-blocking factor, also thought to be antibody. This material antagonized the blocking factor found in patients' sera and was characteristically found in the sera of disease-free treated patients. At about the same time the blocking antibody concept was modified by the studies of Sjögren *et al.* (1971) who suggested that immune complexes were responsible for blocking effects.

In experimental animals immunized against a tumour, specific anti-TSTA antibodies can be detected in their sera. In animals bearing progressive tumours these antibodies are absent. Furthermore, as Baldwin and his co-workers (1973) have shown, "blocking" activity is present in the tumour-bearing sera but absent from post-amputation "immune" sera. In this system then there is a clear negative correlation between the presence of antibodies and "blocking" activity.

Further evidence for the bankruptcy of the blocking antibody concept was provided by the demonstration of co-operation between antibodies and unsensitized lymphoid cells. Möller (1965) had earlier shown that such normal lymphoid cells lyse target cells in the presence of specific antibody. This antibody-dependent cellular cytotoxic (ADCC) effect, also known as K cell damage can be detected in xenogeneic, allogeneic and even syngeneic combinations and seems to represent an exquisitely sensitive assay system for the detection of antibody and for the quantitative analysis of the effector cells, known as K (or killer) cells. Specific anti-tumour antibodies can be detected at high titres in the sera of rats during the early phases of tumour growth. With progressive tumour growth the disappearance of this tumour specific antibody coincides with the failure of concomitant immunity and the development of metastases (Basham and Currie, 1974).

Although the role of antibody in humorally mediated specific suppression of immunological effector mechanisms during tumour growth has been effectively disproven by all the above evidence there is clearly a need for an alternative hypothesis to explain the various forms of specific abrogation of cell mediated reactions which have been encountered in studies of tumour immunity.

Blocking Antigen

When the peripheral blood lymphocytes of cancer patients are added to cultured tumour cells of the specific histological type, damage to the target cells will occur over a period of 48 hours. The serum of patients with active disease will inhibit this cytotoxic activity in a specific manner. Currie and Basham (1972) have studied this serum-inhibitory activity and have shown that the site of inhibitory activity is the lymphocyte and not the target cell. Subsequent studies went on to show that the responsible material in the serum of patients with active disease is probably soluble tumour-specific antigen. In those patients with disseminated disease this antigen appears to be free in the serum whereas in patients with localized disease it is probably complexed with specific antibody.

Antigen Shedding

When maintained in tissue culture, tumour cells will spontaneously shed TSTA into the culture medium and there is evidence to suggest that there is a relationship between shedding and malignancy in that tumours which spontaneously metastasize appear to shed more TSTA than those that do not (Currie and Alexander, 1974). The release of TSTA in a soluble form into the extracellular fluid could provide a means of escape for the tumour, allowing it to evade cytotoxic host responses. Such a smokescreen of soluble antigenic determinants may have an important biological role in "local escape" allowing minute foci of primary or secondary tumours to develop without attracting the hostile attentions of host effector mechanisms. There are several ways in which TSTA could be released from a tumour into the extracellular fluid. By (a) spontaneous shedding, perhaps a consequence of the rapid turnover of glycocalyceal components, by (b) the local release of hydrolytic enzymes, (c) as a consequence of tumour cell necrosis or even (d) as a response to an immunological reaction to the tumour. It is not clear at the moment how such TSTA determinants are liberated from cells.

Although undoubtedly an over-simplification, the immunological escape of tumours could be explained by the shedding of antigens. In the development of a primary tumour the local tissue fluid could become flooded by soluble TSTA where it could combine with and possibly neutralize both specific effector cells and humoral antibody. This local escape would be associated with detectable concomitant immunity in other sites. Systemic escape could then occur when soluble TSTAs, shed by the growing primary tumour, overwhelm (and paralyse) the regional draining lymph nodes and emerge via the lymph into the systemic circulation. Presumably at this stage the TSTA will be present in the form of immune complexes but eventually the humoral antibody response would become overwhelmed until the TSTA are present in a free form in the circulation. This phase would obviously be associated with systemic escape, manifest as the failure of concominant immunity and the development of metastases.

MACROPHAGES AND HOST RESPONSE

In recent years so much attention has been focused on specific immunological reactions to TSTA as a major mechanism involved in host resistance that alternative explanations have been neglected. In experimental animals the evidence supporting the involvement of such specific reactions depends upon the demonstration of tumour-specificity in immunization and rechallenge experiments. In animals bearing tumours, procedures designed to abrogate such specific reactions can show effects on tumour growth, especially on the development of metastases. However none of these procedures (irradiation, thymectomy, anti-lymphocyte serum) restrict their effects to specific immunological responses; they could well have other effects. Specific cell-associated reactions have not unnaturally occupied the limelight and many workers have documented the existence of such reactions in tumour-bearing animals and patients. There is, however, no unequivocal evidence that such cell mediated responses to TSTA are a significant limiting factor in host resistance. Indeed there is an appreciable body of evidence which singularly fails to show correlations between, say, specifically cytotoxic lymphocytes and disease status.

Examinations of the cellular content of tumours so far suggest that lymphocytes are not a major host-cell component. Evans (1972) in examining the cellular content of animal tumours has shown that macrophages are the predominant host cell resident in a growing tumour mass. Furthermore quantitative estimations of the macrophage content of such tumours have revealed significant correlations with the *in vivo* biological behaviour of the tumours. Large numbers of macrophages are characteristic of highly immunogenic tumours and only low numbers present in tumours of low immunogenicity. Furthermore low numbers of macrophages are found in tumours which spontaneously metastasize and the presence of large numbers of macrophages is a favourably prognostic feature in all the animal tumours so far examined. A single cell suspension obtained from a highly immunogenic tumour by enzymatic dissociation can contain up to 60% macrophages, recognisable by both morphological and functional criteria.

The correlation between macrophage content and biological behaviour is retained when the host is "immunosuppressed", i.e. a reduction in macrophage content is associated with an increased metastatic capacity. The presence of large numbers of macrophages in a tumour is also associated with the failure of macrophage responses in other sites. Delayed hypersensitivity reactions and the inflammatory response following intraperitoneal injection of oyster glycogen are both suppressed in rats bearing highly immunogenic macrophage-rich tumours. The defective delayed hypersensitivity reactions can be corrected by the inoculation of normal macrophages. Although the reasons for the macrophage defect have not yet been elucidated its existence represents yet another correlation between macrophage infiltration of the tumour and *in vivo* behaviour. This macrophage response to tumours appears to be the only measurable and biologically relevant correlate of host response yet described and obviously implies that macrophages may be a significant if not the most significant cell type involved in the restraints imposed by the host on the growth of a tumour. Eccles and Alexander (1974) have indicated that the accumulation of macrophages in a tumour is part of a response to tumour antigens and that it is probably, in contemporary jargon, T-cell dependent. Although their accumulation may be in response to specific immunological reactions the tumour macrophages themselves may not show immunologically specific effects. The generation of the macrophage response to a tumour is immunologically specific but its functional expression may not be. Such observations suggest that we need to understand the functional capacity of macrophages in the host response to malignant cells. *In vitro* studies have indicated that macrophages may play several distinct roles in the efferent limb of an anti-tumour response and these will be mentioned briefly.

Functional Cooperation with Lymphocytes

Macrophages play a major, if passive, role in a variety of immunological reactions. Lymphocyte blastogenesis following exposure to specific antigen, the mixed lymphocyte reaction and primary *in vitro* antibody responses all depend upon the presence of macrophages. The macrophages play a role which has no immunological specificity, but seems to have a regulatory function. Their presence in low numbers is necessary for these responses to occur but in high numbers has a suppressor function. Indeed they may play a significant part in controlling the immune response. They seem to carry out both their facilitating and inhibiting roles by releasing supernatant factors.

In studies of immunity to syngeneic tumours the conversion of sensitized T-lymphocytes to "activated" killer T-cells requires the presence of macrophages. The macrophages themselves are not the effector cells yet their presence is necessary for the *in vitro* generation of effector cells. This phenomenon has been detected in rats bearing a syngeneic sarcoma, in which thoracic duct lymphocytes although sensitized are not cytotoxic unless normal macrophages are added (S. Denham, to be published). Similar observations have been made in patients with a variety of solid tumours (Currie, to be published). In view of the relative absence of lymphocytes from the tumour mass in most rat sarcomata studied it seems improbable that the massive macrophage infiltration of highly antigenic tumours is related to this co-operative activity.

It seems likely that they are playing a more direct role in inhibiting tumour cell growth and survival.

Specifically Armed Macrophages

Evans and Alexander have shown (1970) that under appropriate conditions macrophages can acquire the capacity to damage tumour cells in an immunologically specific manner. In the model system studied such macrophages, known as "armed" macrophages, could be detected in specifically sensitized animals in the absence of detectable lymphocyte or serum-mediated effects. Furthermore, such "armed" macrophages could be produced *in vitro* by the addition of specifically sensitized lymphocytes to cultures of normal macrophages and the "arming" of the macrophages was subsequently shown to be dependent upon the production of a cell-free factor by the lymphocytes. This substance was called specific macrophage arming factor (SMAF). Specifically armed macrophages were detectable in both allograft rejection and in response to a syngeneic tumour. Such armed macrophages were subsequently employed with some limited success as immunotherapy in an experimental animal model. However, as Evans and Alexander (1970) demonstrated, once an armed macrophage contacts the appropriate specific antigen a dramatic change occurs. The macrophages lose their immunological specificity and acquire the ability to damage a wide variety of target cells. The armed macrophage is unlikely to be a commonly encountered cell in a tumour-bearing individual since the presence of persistent antigen would ensure their prompt and continuous "activation" to the non-specifically cytotoxic state. If tumour macrophages are contributing to host responses by damaging malignant cells then it is probable that they are in this "activated" state and that their effects are not restricted by immunological specificity.

Activated Macrophages

When peritoneal exudate macrophages obtained from rodents are activated by a variety of stimuli they acquire the capacity to inhibit the growth of tumour cells in tissue culture. Such activated macrophages can be obtained from animals bearing chronic infections (Hibbs *et al.*, 1971), by the addition of specific antigen to "armed" macrophages, by exposure to T-cell products (lymphokines) or by the addition of agents such as endotoxin or double-stranded RNA to normal macrophages *in vitro*. In the latter experiments, described by Alexander and Evans (1971), minute doses of bacterial endotoxin added to cultured mouse macrophages bestowed upon them powerful growth inhibitory properties when they were subsequently tested against a range of mouse tumour cells. This growth inhibitory effect shows no evidence of specificity, and in all probability does not involve any form of specific immunological event. Furthermore Hibbs (1973) went on to show that the toxic effects of activated macrophages were only manifested on transformed cells. Normal cells were unaffected. He indicated that the anti-tumour activity of activated macrophages necessitated close cellular apposition and that the damaging interaction occurred at the meeting of cell surfaces between macrophages and the tumour cells. This tumour-selective action of activated macrophages has also been examined in the author's laboratory (Currie and Basham, to be published) and the following points can be made. Firstly the effect of activated macrophages on the tumour cells is a lethal event; the tumour cells are lysed over a period of 48 hours. These experiments also confirmed the apparent tumour-selectivity of the toxic action of the macrophages. In the presence of a high concentration of serum in the test system the lytic effect requires close cell contact between effector and target but in low serum concentrations is mediated by a macrophage product released into the medium. This material, not yet identified, named or even given a spurious acronym, is labile and is inhibited by serum. The biological basis for a tumour discriminating factor released by activated macrophages is obscure at present but such an observation could have considerable significance giving the macrophage the necessary equipment for it to play a role in a non-immunological form of surveillance against neoplastic cells. Furthermore the possible implications of such tumour selectivity and its mediation by a cell-free material for therapy are obvious.

The activated macrophage would seem to represent an elegant mechanism for the host to resist the growth of tumours and perhaps may be a suitable pathway for the development of therapeutic techniques aimed at inducing *in vivo* activation. This could be accomplished in two distinct ways.

Immunological Activation

The repeated administration of a potent antigen could be expected to result in the development of large numbers of activated macrophages. The use of agents such as BCG or *Corynebacterium parvum* may well operate in this way. Although initially employed as non-specific boosters of specific anti-tumour immunity their value in inducing macrophage activation *in vivo* may represent the major prospect for the use of such agents.

Direct Biochemical Activation

Agents such as bacterial endotoxins, lipid A, double stranded RNA (either synthetic or naturally occurring) or pyran copolymer will activate macrophages *in vitro*. Whether this is a direct biochemical effect on the cell or merely represents another form of immunological activation against a background of pre-existing immunity is unclear. Most evidence currently favours the direct biochemical effect. In experimental animals such macrophages can be shown to have anti-tumour activity but unfortunately they are all extremely toxic agents having effects on small blood vessels (Parr *et al.*, 1973) via which most of their anti-tumour activity is exerted. However, their activity on macrophages does make a contribution to their anti-tumour effects. Once the biochemical pathways underlying macrophage activation have been determined, it may become possible to devise less toxic pharmacological agents with macrophage-activating properties for use in therapy.

CLINICAL IMMUNOTHERAPY

The promise of immunotherapy remains unfulfilled after over 80 years of effort. It is easy to discount the early failures by stating that the pioneers did not have our sophisticated understanding of immunological processes. But that is too easy. Despite the complexity and sophistication of modern immunology none of the practical procedures being advocated and tested represents a significant advance over the work of, say, Hericourt and Richet (1895) or Coca *et al.* (1912).

A detailed historical review of clinical immunotherapy is both beyond the scope of this chapter and would represent a depressing series of failures. It has in any case been reviewed at length elsewhere (Southam, 1961; Currie, 1972).

Animal models of immunotherapy are also few and far between and indicate the relative ineffectiveness of such procedures when compared to, say, chemotherapy. Indeed most models in which experimental immunotherapy yields positive results are so artificial as to be irrelevant to clinical practice. Many different forms of immunotherapy are possible but few are practicable.

The potential methods are shown in Table 1, and it is of interest to note that most have been tested at one time or another and have been found to be of little or no clinical value.

TABLE 1
Potential methods of immunotherapy

	Specific	Non-specific
ACTIVE	Tumour cell vaccines or antigen preparations ± helper determinants	BCG, Corynebacteria. Reticulo-endothelial antisera. Levamisole
PASSIVE	Specific antisera alone or as a carrier for isotopes and cytotoxic drugs	Normal serum components, e.g. complement
ADOPTIVE	Sensitized lymphocytes or products from them. Armed macrophages	Normal lymphoid cells. GVH disease
	Other methods	
	Intralesional BCG—Topical DNCB. Coley's toxins—Endotoxin, double stranded RNA. Viral oncolysis—Lytic viruses with specificity for tumour cells.	

From a brief glance at the current oncology literature it is obvious that immunotherapy has become *de rigueur*. Several modes of immunotherapy currently occupy the limelight and these will be briefly described.

Intralesional Immunotherapy

In his now classic review Woglom (1929) concluded that injecting agents directly into a tumour was

> ". . . too much like shooting a rabbit in his hutch. For reasons which should be obvious, the rules of the game require that a cure exert its action without having been introduced into the growth itself."

The inoculation of a variety of agents into a cutaneous tumour can undoubtedly lead to its destruction. The injection of, say, living BCG (Bacillus Calmette-Guerin) into a tumour nodule can result in a catastrophic inflammatory reaction which frequently (but not always) leads to regression of that nodule or its replacement by an ulcerated granuloma. There are even occasional reports of the regression of some uninjected deposits especially in malignant melanoma. However, this effect is uncommon and can hardly be used as a justification for the use of intralesional BCG as a form of systemic treatment. Regression of local nodules can also be induced by the inoculation or application of other agents such as vaccinia virus or dinitrochlorobenzene. Similar results can be obtained by the use of diathermy or the application of corrosive chemicals. The regression of inoculated lesions or the application of corrosive chemicals. The regression of inoculated lesions following intralesional BCG is currently being held up as a success for immunotherapy. While it can on occasion be effective in a cosmetic sense, in that it can sometimes ablate cutaneous metastases it is difficult to see any great clinical value in the procedure unless it can be shown to prolong the survival of the patients. So far, there is no controlled evidence that intralesional immunotherapy can do this. Indeed when compared to the best form of therapy in current use its effect are less than exciting. In malignant melanoma, a favourite stamping ground for intralesional treatment, chemotherapy, although enjoying very limited success, seems to do much better than any form of local manipulation of skin lesions.

Non-specific "Immunostimulation"

There are many agents, derived mainly from microorganisms, which when inoculated into animals, can induce a variety of immunologically non-specific effects. Most of these agents, such as BCG, *Corynebacterium parvum*, zymosan, etc., are stimulants of the reticulo-endothelial system, having their most pronounced *in vivo* effects on macrophages. Macrophage function *in vivo* is heightened by these agents and is manifested by both qualitative and quantitative changes. Increased clearance of injected colloids, enhanced proliferation and activation of macrophages and splenomegaly can be readily detected in rodents. However, such treated animals also show increased resistance to heterologous infections, transplantable tumours and skin allografts. These effects can be accounted for by macrophage-mediated phenomena but closer examination shows that specific immunological reactions are also accentuated. In experimental models agents such as *Corynebacterium parvum* have been shown to "sensitize" tumours to the effects of irradiation and chemotherapy. Such observations have led to the enthusiastic deployment of these agents as "immunotherapy" for the treatment of cancer patients although their postulated mode of action remains unclear. BCG is the most commonly used. The main reasons for its popularity would seem to be its ready availability, its relative lack of toxicity and ease of administration rather than any considerations of effectiveness. Literally hundreds of clinical trials of BCG have been performed and so far there is a paucity of incontrovertible controlled data to suggest any significant anti-tumour activity. All of the properly controlled trials so far reported show clear-cut negative results. Suggestions for clinical benefit are almost inevitably obtained from uncontrolled studies. Furthermore, few trials have attempted to compare BCG with the current best form of therapy. Of the published controlled studies of BCG in the treatment of cancer the following are representative and have all failed to detect any evidence of clinical benefit. In childhood acute lymphoblastic leukaemia two separate trials of BCG for the maintenance of remission have given unequivocally negative results (Medical Research Council, 1971; Heyn *et al.*, 1973). In Burkitt's lymphoma the use of BCG had no detectable therapeutic effect (Ziegler and Magrath, 1973) and in patients with disseminated breast cancer being treated with cytotoxic chemotherapy the addition of BCG treatment was without beneficial effect (Nemato *et al.*, 1975). The appearance of each negative controlled trial is usually greeted (by the proponents of BCG) by criticisms of the strain of BCG employed, its dosage and its mode of administration and that new trials of different strains, dosage, etc. are needed. To conduct innumerable clinical trials of BCG to cope with all such possible criticisms is unlikely to be a fruitful exercise. A more logical step would seem to be the examination of the grounds for establishing such trials in the first place, to find out what it is we expect BCG to do to the patients and then to develop methods for detecting such effects. Often the reasons for performing such trials are less than scientific. "It is worth trying, just in case" or "It is simple, is unlikely to do any harm and just conceivably might do some good" are phrases commonly heard in an oncology clinic. Such motives are inadequate and are unlikely to lead to success without a modicum of divine intervention.

There has in recent years been an intensive search for chemically defined compounds with immunostimulatory properties; for the introduction of such agents could allow the elegant manipulation of immunological responses to become a practical reality. One compound which has been receiving much attention of late is levamisole (2,3,5,6-tetrahydro-6-phenyl imidazo (2, 1-b) thiazole. This agent, used originally for the treatment of parasitic worm infestations, has been shown to have some limited effects on the immunological reactivity of experimental animals. In tumour models it is alleged to act rather like an adjuvant by increasing the effectiveness of specific active immunotherapy (Spreafico *et al.*, 1975). A recent clinical trial of levamisole in the treatment of lung cancer claims significant beneficial effects (Study Group for Bronchogenic Carcinoma, 1975). Close scrutiny of this study shows that if these effects are real they are very slight, there being no effect on death rate in the treated patients. However, the attention being given to this drug is a significant advance in the field since it has helped to focus our attention on a search for chemically-defined agents capable of influencing immunological reactivity.

Specific Active Immunotherapy

The use of tumour cells as an immunogenic stimulus for immunotherapy was first attempted in 1902 (Von Leyden and Blumenthal) and has been a mainstay ever since. In experimental systems the administration of X-irradiated cells can have therapeutic effects, i.e. if given within one day of a minute tumour inoculum. Given at later times, to animals with established tumours, it is almost invariably ineffective and can be positively detrimental, presumably by producing a situation of "antigen overload". In recent years this approach has been employed in man, especially in view of the important observations of Haddow and Alexander (1964). These authors demonstrated that immunization with tumour cells could cause an increase in the radiosensitivity of primary chemically-induced rat sarcomata. This study led to a controlled trial of specific active immunization of patients with glioblastoma multiforme as an adjunct to radiotherapy. Autologous tumour material was used as the vaccine (Bloom *et al.*, 1973). This was a well controlled study with a long follow-up period and it unequivocally demonstrated a lack of therapeutic effect. However, the possible value of this form of immunization as an adjunct to other forms of cytoreduction is still being evaluated. In disseminated malignant melanoma an active immunization protocol, designed by reference to *in vitro* assays of tumour-specific immunological responses, has been combined with cytotoxic chemotherapy (Currie and McElwain, 1975). Although an as yet uncontrolled trial, the results of this pilot study indicate a marked increase in the incidence of objective tumour regression, although significant prolongation of life has probably not yet been achieved.

Other Forms of "Immunotherapy" Currently in Vogue

In designing an immunotherapy protocol innumerable assumptions have to be made. One such assumption, unsupported by any clear cut evidence, is that the growth of a tumour and its escape from host restraint is associated with (or even due to) a defect in cell mediated immune responses although the nature of any such defect (qualitative or quantitative) is unclear. It is also assumed that this undefined defect can be restored by the administration of sensitized lymphoid cells and that this hoped-for restoration will be therapeutic. The administration of large numbers of sensitized lymphoid cells (e.g. from "cured" patients) can, however, be hazardous. If given in small numbers they will be promptly rejected and if given in large numbers they will attack the host and this sorry state of affairs is recognizable as graft-versus-host (GVH) disease. While there is a little evidence that GVH disease can itself inhibit the growth of tumours its development can be lethal and may not permit the desired adoptive transfer of specific immunity. To overcome this problem, considerable effort is being expended to examine lymphocyte products or extracts as possible replacements for the intact living cell.

Transfer Factor

Lawrence and Landy (1969) have described a substance of low molecular weight which is readily obtained from peripheral blood leucocytes and which is alleged to transfer specific immunological information. It is in many ways a remarkable molecule if all that is said about it is true. It is supposed to transfer cell mediated responses only and is reputed to be quite specific in its effects. It operates, functionally at any rate, like antigen but is reputed to be antigen-free. That a molecule as small as 2,000 daltons can encode and transfer detailed and complex immunological information is surprising. Indeed this material is surprising in more ways. It is reputed to be undetectable in experimental animals, man being the only species in which it is readily found. However, it must be borne in mind that there are alternative explanations for the effects of transfer factor. It could conceivably be a hormone-like material whose function is to permit or stimulate T-cell function and that its immunological specificity is illusory and can be explained by quantitative effects, i.e. by heightening cell mediated responses in a totally non-specific manner it may allow the detection of a response formerly too weak to be detected by the tests employed. Such an effect could appear to be immunologically specific. No completed controlled trials of transfer factor have yet been described although the anecdotal reports of its beneficial effects in chronic mucocutaneous conditions are very impressive. Currently it is being tested as immunotherapy in a variety of human tumours including osteogenic sarcoma.

Immune RNA

In studies of adoptive cellular immunotherapy of rats bearing chemically induced tumours, Alexander and his colleagues (1967) demonstrated immunologically specific therapeutic effects using nucleic acid extracts of sensitized lymphoid cells. Most of this extract consisted of RNA and the assumption was made that specific informational RNA from lymphocytes can transfer immunity. These early observations have since been confirmed by other groups and lymphocyte RNA extracts are at present being tested for immunotherapeutic effects.

CONCLUSIONS

A brief and somewhat sceptical examination of the achievements of immunotherapy to date reveals a startling lack of success. However it is such a potent idea, such an exciting concept, that it cannot be simply set aside. We require a firmer scientific basis for what is happening in the clinic, to transform an unrewarding series of random escapades into a rational form of clinical science.

The explosive growth of tumour immunology, apart from holding out the carrot of immunotherapy has even more significant implications. The detection of specific immunological reactions to TSTA indicates the existence of biochemically distinct structures on the surface of tumour cells. The major scientific promise of tumour immunology would seem to be as a probe to examine the surface of tumour cells and seek out the Achilles' heel of the malignant process as a possible target for chemotherapeutic attack. In addition, the manipulation of immunologically-mediated host resistance could well play a significant role in combination with other forms of cytoreductive treatment in the overall management of cancer patients.

REFERENCES

Alexander, P. and Evans, R. (1971). Endotoxin and double stranded RNA render macrophages cytotoxic. *Nature, New Biol.* **232**, 76.

Alexander, P., Delorme, E. J., Hamilton, L. D. G. and Hall, J. G. (1967). Effect of nucleic acids from immune lymphocytes on rat sarcomata. *Nature* **213**, 569.

Baldwin, R. W., Price, M. R. and Robins, R. A. (1973). Inhibition of hepatoma-immune lymph-node cell cytotoxicity by tumour-bearer serum and solubilized hepatoma antigen. *Int. J. Cancer* **11**, 527.

Basham, C. and Currie, G. A. (1974). Development of specific cell-dependent antibody during growth of a syngeneic rat sarcoma. *Brit. J. Cancer* **29**, 189.

Bashford, E. F. (1908). "Third Scientific Report Imperial Cancer Research Fund." Taylor and Francis, London.

Black, M. M., Opler, S. R. and Speer, F. D. (1954). Microscopic structure of gastric carcinomas and their regional lymph nodes in relation to survival. *Surg. Gynec. Obstet.* **98**, 725.

Bloom, H. J. G., Peckham, M. J., Richardson, A. E., Alexander, P. and Payne, P. M. (1973). Glioblastoma multiforme: a controlled trial to assess the value of specific active immunotherapy in patients treated by radical surgery and radiotherapy. *Brit. J. Cancer* **27**, 253.

Bodenham, D. C. (1968). A study of 650 observed malignant melanomas in the South-West region. *Ann. Roy. Coll. Surg. Eng.* **43**, 218.

Carnaud, C., Hoch, B. and Trainin, N. (1974). Influence of immunologic competence of the host on metastases induced by the 3LL Lewis tumor in mice. *J. Nat. Cancer Inst.* **52**, 395.

Clowes, G. H. A. and Baeslack, F. W. (1905). Further evidence of immunity against cancer in mice after spontaneous recovery. *Med. News* **87**, 968.

Coca, A. F., Dorrance, G. M. and Lebredo, M. G. (1912). Vaccination in cancer. A report of the result of the vaccination therapy as applied in 79 cases of human cancer. *Z. Immun. Exp. Ther.* **13**, 546.

Currie, G. A. (1972). Eighty years of immunotherapy: a review of immunological methods used for the treatment of human cancer. *Brit. J. Cancer* **26**, 141.

Currie, G. A. (1974). *In* "Cancer and the Immune Response." E. Arnold, London.

Currie, G. A. and Alexander, P. (1974). Spontaneous shedding of TSTA by viable sarcoma cells: its possible role in facilitating metastatic spread. *Brit. J. Cancer* **29**, 72.

Currie, G. A. and Basham, C. (1972). Serum mediated inhibition of the immunological reaction of the patient to his own tumour: a possible role for circulating antigen. *Brit. J. Cancer* **26**, 427.

Currie, G. A. and McElwain, T. J. (1975). Active immunotherapy as an adjunct to chemotherapy in the treatment of disseminated malignant melanoma; a pilot study. *Brit. J. Cancer* **31**, 143.

Eccles, S. A. and Alexander, P. (1974). Macrophage content of tumours in relation to metastatic spread and host immune reaction. *Nature* **250**, 667.

Ehrlich, P. (1906). Experimentalle carcinomstudier an maüsen. *Arb. Inst. Exp. Ther. Frankfurt* **1**, 77.

Elston, C. W. (1969). Cellular reaction to choriocarcinoma. *J. Path.* **97**, 261.

Evans, R. (1972). Macrophages in syngeneic animal tumours. *Transplantation* **14**, 468.

Evans, R. and Alexander, P. (1970). Co-operation of immune lymphoid cells with macrophages in tumour immunity. *Nature* **228**, 620.

Everson, T. C. and Cole, W. N. (1966). "Spontaneous Regression of Cancer." W. B. Saunders, Philadelphia.

Foley, E. J. (1953). Attempts to induce immunity against mammary adenocarcinoma in inbred mice. *Cancer Res.* **13**, 578.

Gershon, R. and Carter, R. L. (1970). Facilitation of metastatic growth by antilymphocyte serum. *Nature* **226**, 368.

Globerson, A. and Feldman, M. (1964). Antigenic specificity of benzo (a) pyrene-induced sarcomas. *J. Nat. Cancer Inst.* **32**, 1229.

Gross, L. (1943). Intradermal immunization of C3H mice against sarcoma that originated in animal of same line. *Cancer Res.* **3**, 326.

Haddow, A. and Alexander, P. (1964). An immunological method of increasing the sensitivity of primary sarcomas to local irradiation with X-rays. *Lancet* **1**, 452.

Hamlin, I. M. E. (1968). Possible host resistance in carcinoma of the breast: a histological study. *Brit. J. Cancer* **22**, 383.

Handley, W. S. (1907). The pathology of melanotic growths in relation to their operative treatment. *Lancet* **1**, 927.

Hellström, I. and Hellström, K. E. (1969). Studies on cellular immunity and its serum mediated inhibition in Moloney-virus-induced mouse sarcomas. *Int. J. Cancer* **4**, 587.

Hellström, I., Hellström, K. E., Sjögren, H. O. and Warner, G. A. (1971). Demonstration of cell-mediated immunity to human neoplasms of various histological types. *Int. J. Cancer* **7**, 1.
Hericourt, J. and Richet, C. (1895). De la serotherapie dans le traitment du cancer. *C.r. Hebd. Seances Acad. Sci.* **121**, 567.
Heyn, R., Borges, W. and Joo, P. (1972). BCG in treatment of acute lymphocytic leukaemia. *Proc. Am. Ass. Cancer Res.* **14**, 45.
Hibbs, J. B. (1973). Macrophage nonimmunologic recognition: target cell factors related to contact inhibition. *Science* **180**, 868.
Hibbs, J. B., Lambert, L. H. and Remington, J. S. (1971). Tumor resistance conferred by intracellular protozoa. *J. Clin. Invest.* **50**, 45a (Abstr.).
Kaliss, N. (1958). Immunological enhancement of tumor homografts in mice: a review. *Cancer Res.* **18**, 992.
Lauder, I. and Aherne, W. (1972). The significance of lymphocytic infiltration in neuroblastoma. *Brit. J. Cancer* **26**, 321.
Lawrence, E. S. and Landy, M. (1969). "Mediators of Cellular Immunity." Academic Press, New York and London.
Lewis, M. G., Ikonopisov, R. L., Nairn, R. C., Phillips, T. M., Hamilton Fairley, G., Bodenham, D. C. and Alexander, P. (1969). Tumour-specific antibodies in human malignant melanoma and their relationship to the extent of the disease. *Brit. Med. J.* **3**, 547.
Little, J. H. (1972). *In* "UICC Proceedings of the International Cancer Conference." P. 107. Government Printers, Sydney.
Möller, E. (1965). Contact-induced cytotoxicity by lymphoid cells containing foreign isoantigens. *Science* **147**, 873.
Medical Research Council (1971). Treatment of acute lymphoblastic leukaemia. *Brit. Med. J.* **4**, 189.
Nemato, T., Rosner, D. and Dao, T. (1975). Proceedings of the XIth International Cancer Conference. (In press.)
Parr, I., Wheeler, E. and Alexander, P. (1973). Similarities of the anti-tumour actions of endotoxin lipid A and double-stranded RNA. *Brit. J. Cancer* **27**, 370.
Prehn, R. T. and Main, J. M. (1957). Immunity to methylcholanthrene-induced sarcomas. *J. Nat. Cancer Inst.* **18**, 769.
Proctor, J. W., Rudenstam, C. M. and Alexander, P. (1973). A factor preventing the development of lung metastases in rats with sarcomas. *Nature* **242**, 29.
Sjögren, H. O., Hellström, I., Bansal, S. C. and Hellström, K. E. (1971). Suggestive evidence that the "blocking antibodies" of tumor-bearing individuals may be antigen-antibody complexes. *Proc. Nat. Acad. Sci. USA* **68**, 1372.
Southam, C. M. (1961). Applications of immunology to clinical cancer. Past attempts and future possibilities. *Cancer Res.* **21**, 1302.
Spreafico, F., Lecchi, A., Mantovani, A., Poggi, A., Franchi, G., Anaclerio, A. and Garattini, F. (1975). Characterization of the immunostimulants levamisole and tetramisole. *Eur. J. Cancer* **11**, 555.
Study Group for Bronchogenic Carcinoma (1975). Immunopotentiation with levamisole in resectable bronchogenic carcinoma: a double-blind controlled trial. *Brit. Med. J.* **3**, 461.
Thompson, P. G. (1972). VIII International Pigment Cell Conference. Proc. Abst. IUAC, Sydney.
Thompson, K. D. and Linna, T. J. (1973). Bursa-dependent and thymus-dependent "surveillance" of a virus-induced tumour in the chicken. *Nature, New Biol.* **245**, 10.
Vaage, J. (1973). Influence of tumor antigen on maintenance versus depression of tumor-specific immunity. *Cancer Res.* **33**, 493.

Von Leyden, V. E. and Blumenthal, F. (1902). Vorlautige mittheilungen uber einige ergebnisse der krebsforschung auf der 1. medizinischen klinik. *Dt. med. Wschr.* **28**, 637.
Woglom, W. H. (1929). Immunity to transplantable tumors. *Cancer Rev.* **4**, 129.
Woodruff, M. F. A. (1964). Immunological aspects of cancer. *Lancet* **2**, 265.
Ziegler, J. L. and Magrath, I. T. (1973). BCG immunotherapy in Burkitt's lymphoma: preliminary results of a randomized clinical trial. *Nat. Cancer Inst. Monogr.* **39**, 199.

29

Transplantation

J. BRADLEY

The first real understanding of the immunology of transplantation developed during the Second World War when attempts were made to skin-graft victims of extensive burns. In 1943 Medawar, in order to elucidate the problems of skin grafts, examined the survival of skin-grafts in the rabbit and established that the rejection of allografts had an immunological basis (Medawar, 1958). It was observed that if the rabbit had been pre-sensitized to the donor tissue a skin transplant was subjected to an accelerated rejection process, the time of rejection being about six days instead of the usual time for a first graft of approximately ten days.

The same manifestations of rejection and accelerated rejection were found to occur in organ transplants and although the techniques of vascular surgery had been available since the 1950s, it soon became apparent that more than this was needed to ensure success. The work of Gorer and Snell (Snell, 1953) elucidating the histocompatibility system (H2) in the mouse and its relationship to tissue transplantation, together with the observations by Amos that serum obtained after allogeneic skin-graft rejection would agglutinate donor lymphocytes, were significant advances in the development of transplantation immunology.

Hume performed nine cadaveric kidney transplants between 1951 and 1953 but renal function was adequate only for a limited time although one recipient survived for six months. Soon afterwards, Merrill *et al.* (1956) demonstrated the technical feasibility of routine renal transplantation by transplanting kidneys between identical twins. The next major development was the discovery of potent forms of immunosuppression. Schwartz and Damashek showed that 6-mercaptopurine was a good immunosuppressive agent in rabbits and Calne observed that azathioprine would prolong the life of renal allografts in dogs.

HISTOCOMPATIBILITY ANTIGENS

The ABO antigens are important in transplantation but none of the other red cell groups appear to influence acceptance of tissue grafts, with the possible exception of the P-system.

ABO-System

The ABO blood group system is important in transplantation since incompatibility may produce hyperacute rejection of kidney and skin grafts, although not of liver grafts. Ceppellini *et al.* (1969) found that immunization of recipients with blood group substances A and B was highly effective in producing a white graft type of rejection of skin. Pre-immunization of an O-recipient with blood group substance A induces rejection of skin not only

TABLE 1
Acceptability of mismatch for tissue transplant in ABO and rhesus system

O to non O	acceptable
A to non A	dangerous
B to non B	dangerous
AB to non AB	dangerous
Rh^- to Rh^+	acceptable
Rh^+ to Rh	relatively acceptable

from Group A but also from Group B individuals. This suggests that the O-recipient does not distinguish between the galactosamine and galactose terminal sugars which respectively characterize the side-chains of Group A and Group B substances. Blood group P antigens are expressed on some tissues apart from blood and may also exert an effect on graft survival (Ceppellini, 1971).

The Histocompatibility Region in Man

The antigens on nucleated cells are called tissue or histocompatibility antigens and are present also on platelets but rarely on mature human red blood cells.

Early work on transplantation demonstrated the inheritance of these antigens but the histocompatibility gene loci are much more complex than appeared a few years ago. The major histocompatibility region contains distinct SD (serologically defined) loci, and LD (lymphocyte defined) loci (Fig. 1). They are situated on the sixth chromosome in man and between the first and second human leucocyte antigen (HLA) (SD) loci a third HLA locus has recently been recognized.

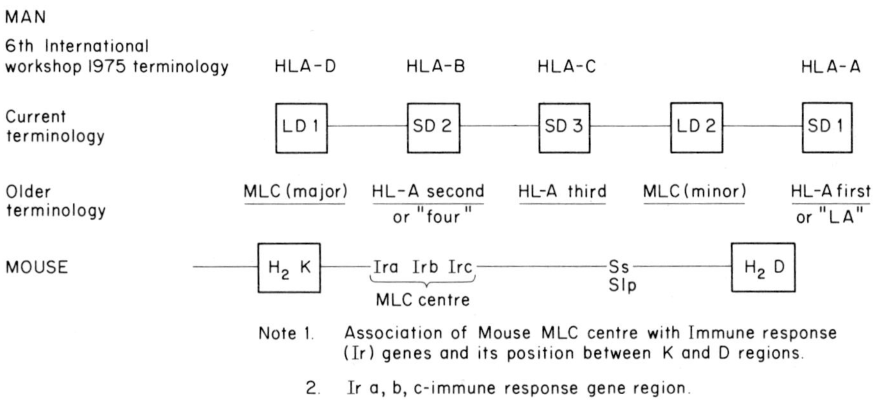

Fig. 1. Histocompatibility regions for man and mouse.

The HLA-System

Determination of HLA-type depends upon the detection of the antigens by serological means, hence the term "serologically defined" (SD) sites. These antigens are determined by two segregant series of alleles belonging to two closely-linked genetic loci. For each locus there are multiple co-dominant alleles. The HLA-genes are inherited on a pair of autosomal chromosomes, half being paternal and half maternal. Typing an individual defines only the phenotype but family studies define the genotype (Fig. 2). Antigens determined by SD loci are described by various terms:

i. the HLA (human leucocyte antigens) are antigens which are well defined and internationally recognized.
ii. other less well defined antigens at each locus are commonly given numbers preceded by W, indicating they have been provisionally established at histocompatibility workshops.

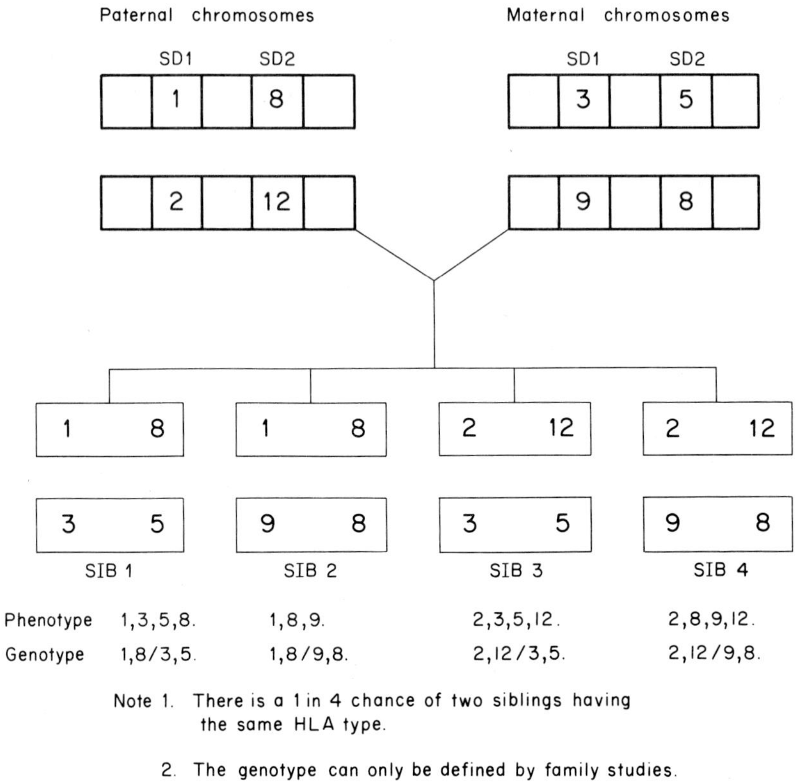

Fig. 2. Histocompatibility typing: Family distribution of HLA-antigens.

HLA-antigens are present on most human nucleated tissue cells, but the amount probably varies as much as it does in the comparable H2 system in the mouse (Table 2). HLA antigens are detected with specific antisera obtained from the following sources: (1) parous women who have become immunized by foetal leucocytes and have developed antibodies to paternal histocompatibility antigens, (2) by planned immunization of volunteers with skin-grafts or with leucocyte injections from unrelated donors, (3) from transplanted patients who have rejected their grafts and have developed anti-donor antibodies, (4) from patients who have received blood transfusions. The most useful sera are monospecific and the first two sources are more likely to produce these.

The first (SD 1 or "LA") and the second (SD 2 or "4") loci are well characterized. The gene frequencies for known antigens total 0·98 for SD 1

TABLE 2

Histocompatibility antigens on tissues: H2 antigens in the mouse

Spleen	Greatest amount (100%)	+ + + +
—		
Liver		+ + +
Lymph node		
—		+ +
Thymus		
Lung		
Adrenal		
Kidney		
Red cells		
Brain		
—		
Testis	↓	+
Skeletal muscle	Least amount (2–0·2%)	

and 0·97 for SD 2 but individual frequencies vary in different races (Table 3). The cross-over frequency (i.e. the frequency of exchange of genes between homologous chromosomes taking place at meiosis between the two loci) is 0·5–1%. Pronounced linkage disequilibrium has been found between some antigens of SD 1 and SD 2 which means that particular combinations of genes at the different loci occur together more often than might be expected on the basis of gene frequencies alone. Examples are the association of 1 and 8 and 3 and 7. The third locus (SD 3) has so far been shown to have four antigens whose gene frequencies total 0·5.

In general, typing the lymphocyte is the most convenient method of determining HLA-type. The method of choice uses cytotoxicity as a marker and a micro-method has been developed to conserve monospecific antisera. Agglutination and complement fixation tests are now rarely used for typing lymphocytes, but for typing platelets complement fixation is the method of choice.

Techniques for lymphocyte microcytotoxicity vary but the basic method is the same (Table 4). Lymphocytes are obtained from either fresh heparinized of defibrinated blood or from spleens or lymph nodes. They are separated from peripheral blood by centrifugation on a Ficoll–Hypaque density gradient or sometimes by sedimentation with dextran and filtration through nylon wool. Spleen or lymph nodes are gently teased to produce a suspension of cells and if necessary Ficoll–Hypaque gradient centrifugation is used to obtain a lymphocyte suspension. Lymphocytes prepared in one of these ways are mixed with antiserum and complement and incubated at 37° or

TABLE 3
Distribution of HLA-antigens in different races

HLA	Caucasians (%)	Arabs (%)	Japanese (%)	Eskimos (%)	Africans (%)
A1	30	28	0	2	12
A2	50	40	48	29	26
A3	25	22	3	3	12
A9	15	22	60	90	25
AW23	2	3	0	1	13
A10	6	9	26	1	45
AW25	3	0	4	1	2
AW26	2	0	26	1	42
A11	11	13	10	3	1
AW33	22	30	42	4	69
A29	10	7	1	1	39
AW30	3	15	0	0	13
AW31	6	0·6	14	14	0
AW32	5	4	0	0	9
A28	8	16	4	25	22
B5	9	36	42	30	14
B7	25	4	10	3	24
B8	25	13	0	3	6
B12	35	12	13	3	26
B13	5	3	1	0	3
BW35	12	8	27	14	15
BW40	15	9	36	36	12
B14	8	8	0	1	14
BW15	10	2	14	40	10
BW16	7	14	12	1	3
BW17	7	9	2	1	27
B18	7	10	1	0	24
BW21	5	15	2	1	6
BW22	7	8	18	1	5
B27	6	5	1	21	1
W4	60	65	66	67	65
W6	70	81	91	95	81

After joint report of fifth international histocompatibility testing workshop in histocompatibility testing (1972). Munskgaard, Copenhagen.

room temperature. The cytotoxic effect of antibodies is detected by cell death as estimated by cell swelling and staining with trypan blue or eosin, by phase contrast microscopy, or by release of a fluorescent label. Rabbit complement is sometimes used with the addition of fresh human serum. Such tests take two or three hours to perform. In order that reference may be made

TABLE 4
HLA-typing—lymphocytotoxicity test (micro-method)

HLA antisera	Obtained from multiparous women and immunized volunteers (usually immunized by skin grafts).
Antigen	Viable lymphocytes from peripheral blood spleen or lymph node.
Method	1–2 μl antiserum 1–2 μl lymphocytes (containing 2,000–4,000 cells) and complement (usually two-thirds rabbit and one-third human serum mixed) 0·5 μl 1% trypan blue

1 μl $2\frac{1}{2}$% gluteraldehyde in saline added after 15 min allows results to be read and checked after several days.

to lymphocytes from the recipient, from the donor or from typed individuals in the future, cells may be stored frozen in liquid nitrogen or its vapour. For this dimethylsulphoxide is used as a cryoprotective agent and a controlled rate of cell freezing is necessary to retain high viability (over 90%) for weeks or months.

The LD System

The LD or lymphocyte determinant loci code for determinants which clicit a proliferative response in mixed lymphocyte culture (MLC). In 1961 Schrek and Donnelly noticed a number of large cells with prominent nuclei and nucleoli in a culture consisting of a mixture of blood taken from two patients. Subsequently Bain *et al.* (1964) observed lymphocyte proliferation when blood leucocytes from immunogenetically different normal donors were mixed in culture, whereas mixed cultures of cells from identical twins showed no proliferation and from closely related individuals only slight proliferation. It was possible by microscopical examination to count the number of cells proliferating or transforming, but greater speed and reliability was achieved by measuring incorporation of radioactive metabolic precursors into newly formed nucleic acids. The observation that 28% of sibling mixtures failed to stimulate DNA synthesis suggested that this response is genetically determined and an expression of antigenic similarity or dissimilarity. Some MLC tests between HLA-identical siblings show evidence of stimulation, i.e. the combinations are HLA-identical but MLC non-identical. The percentage has been reported to be as little as 2% or as much as 33%.

It is known that pronounced lymphocyte proliferative activity is induced by the major MLC locus LD 1. This is located outside the region of the three SD loci but close to the second SD locus. LD 2, which elicits a weaker proliferative response, may be sited between SD 1 and SD 3 (Eijsvoogel, 1974). There is polymorphism at the major MLC locus (LD 1) but about 10% of SD identical unrelated individuals also are LD identical, since their lymphocytes do not stimulate each other when incubated together in mixed lymphocyte culture. This indicates linkage disequilibrium between SD 2 and LD 1. Typing for LD determinants is at present much less advanced than for SD determinants. It is performed by using lymphocytes from individuals of known LD constitution as the stimulator cells in unilateral mixed lymphocyte cultures. For lymphocytes to act merely as stimulator cells they have to be X-irradiated or inactivated by mitomycin. If the cells being typed (the responder cells) fail to proliferate, then the LD determinants of the stimulator cell are present in the responder cell (Table 5). This form of typing suffers from the disadvantage that several days are needed for lymphocyte culture.

There may also be other membrane antigens by which cells are destroyed in cell mediated lysis (CML). Although family and population studies suggest that in cell mediated lysis the specificities are those of the serologically determined antigens predominantly of the second locus, there is other evidence both in mice and men, of separate CML specificity.

Histocompatibility-linked specific immune response (Ir) genes

The capacity to form specific immune responses reflects an ability to recognize individual specific antigens as immunogens and is governed by genes

TABLE 5
Lymphocyte determinant (LD) typing

Typing cell (Homozygous)	Unknown cell	Increase in DNA synthesis	MLC type of unknown cell
H/H_{mit}	X	0	H/H or H/A
H/H	X_{mit}	0	H/H
H/H_{mit}	X	+	H not present
H/H	X_{mit}	+	H/H or H not present

H. Lymphocyte determinant H expressed on one chromosome.
A. Lymphocyte determinant A expressed on one chromosome.
mit. Cell inactivated either by mitomycin or X-irradiation.
\+ Lymphocytes proliferation increased, i.e. stimulated.
0 Lymphocyte not stimulated.

located in the genome in close relationship to genes which code for histocompatibility specificities. This has now been demonstrated in mice, rats, guinea-pigs, and rhesus monkeys. These genes are known as the histocompatibility linked immune response or Ir genes (Fig. 1).

TABLE 6
Examples of clinical associations of disease and HLA

	HLA type	Frequency (%)	Controls[a] (%)
Allergy to ragweed	B7	50	20
Ankylosing spondylitis	B27	96	4
Hodgkin's disease	Bw35	28–33	9–18
Gluten enteropathy	B8	88	22
Multiple sclerosis	B7	35	25
Reiter's disease	B27	88	8
Systemic lupus erythematosus	Bw15	46	8
	B8	33	16

[a] Selected normal population for investigation.

ALLOGRAFT REJECTION

Role of Lymphocytes

A role for lymphocytes in primary (first set) allograft rejection was inferred when Billingham, Brent and Medawar (1954) observed that after first set skin allografts proliferative responses were present in the regional lymph nodes, and at a later stage in the spleen. They found that accelerated (secondary or second set) rejection of skin grafts was obtained by injecting lymph node cells from a mouse which had received a graft of the same tissue. At the same time Mitchison (1954), studying in mice the rejection of allogeneic sarcoma grafts found that rejection of the tumour was accelerated by active immunization, and that accelerated tumour rejection was induced in a normal mouse which had received lymph node fragments from an animal inoculated with the tumour. These experiments demonstrated association of the rejection process, immunological memory and lymphocytes.

Examination of the lymph node draining a skin graft reveals that two to five days after grafting, large pyroninophilic cells are present in the lymph node cortex; similar changes are seen after allografts. These cells lack endoplastic reticulum and contain an abundance of polyribosomes. Similar changes have been observed in small lymphocytes during graft versus host reactions. In the medulla of the lymph node there is also an increase in the number of plasma cells and at a later stage an increase in the number of germinal centres can be observed. Injection of tritiated thymidine into the base of rabbit skin allografts daily from the second to seventh day after transplantation demonstrates the presence of large lymphoid cells which have incorporated the label and are therefore undergoing DNA synthesis. Examination of the efferent lymph from the draining lymph nodes shows that the number of lymphocytes is substantially increased and that the usual 5–10% of large basophilic cells present in the lymph from a resting node has increased up to 40%. Two-thirds of these large cells in the efferent lymph also show evidence of active DNA synthesis.

These changes point to involvement of lymphocytes in the rejection of allogeneic tissue and further evidence confirms that allograft rejection is initiated by lymphocytes. If an almost lethal dose of whole body irradiation is given, the first set allograft rejection is delayed but if the irradiated recipient is given lymphocytes from a normal syngeneic donor first set rejection occurs normally. Injection of purified lymphocytes from a normal syngeneic donor brings about rejection of grafts in animals rendered tolerant to graft donor cells (Gowans and McGregor, 1965). However, lymphocytes from a tolerant animal fail to restore the capacity of a heavily irradiated syngeneic recipient to reject skin grafts from the donor strain. Thymectomized mice fail to reject skin grafts, but if they receive thymus tissue containing chromosomally marked cells, the subsequent proliferative mononuclear response to skin grafts may be seen to be largely due to division of marked cells which have migrated from the thymus. In passing, it may be noted that in these situations cells that can damage the graft *in vivo* are in a minority amongst the cells which infiltrate the graft, so that the ratio of attacker cells to target cells is probably very low. In contrast, in studies of target cell damage induced by cells *in vitro*, ratios of 10 or 100 cytotoxic lymphocytes to one target cell are usually necessary to achieve destruction of the majority. This raises the question whether some other cell or factor helps in the destruction of the graft. The phagocytic activity of macrophages is increased following exposure of lymphocytes to an antigen against which they are sensitized. Recent work indicates that macrophages may be recruited by sensitized lymphocytes in this way to recognize foreign antigens, and K-cell cytotoxicity also may play a part in the destruction of the target cell (see below).

Histopathology of Rejection

Serial examination of a transplanted organ or tissue of genetic type different from the host's reveals that for a short time its appearance may be similar to that of a graft of the same genetic type. First set renal allografts produce urine, and first set skin allografts heal in the same manner as a syngeneic graft. Subsequently signs of rejection develop but these vary greatly in time and severity.

There is an early cell mediated form—acute rejection—which is common and in clinical practice is usually reversible, and there is a later type which is mainly produced by antibody mediated mechanisms, and is uncommon and irreversible.

The macroscopic features of rejection are due to circulatory disturbances, oedema, cellular infiltration and destruction of the tissue. The circulatory disturbance may lead to pallor or cyanosis, swelling and haemorrhage. If the rejection process is very acute a transplanted kidney may become so swollen that it splits open (Fig. 3). If rejection occurs at a slower rate atrophy of the tissue accompanied by increasing fibrosis may be the main macroscopic manifestations.

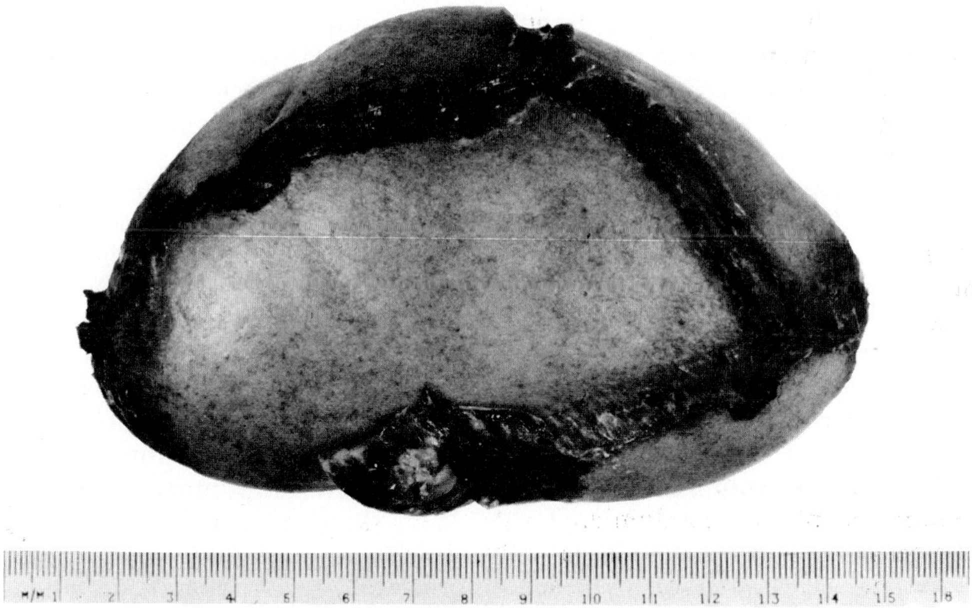

Fig. 3. Hyperacute rejection of kidney—macroscopic appearance. Spontaneous rupture of graft. (By courtesy of R. A. Sells.)

The microscopic features that develop during rejection of an allograft are, again, oedema, circulatory disturbances, cellular infiltration and destruction of the tissue of the graft. Mononuclear cell infiltration is a prominent feature of first set allograft rejection. Rejection begins within two to three days of transplantation if the allograft is in direct vascular communication with the recipient but in skin grafts the process takes longer and infiltration appears only after four to five days. In organ grafts the mononuclear cells at first cluster round the vessels but later extend into the parenchymal tissue. In some cases it has been reported that the number of mononuclear cells in lymph leaving allografts is increased within 24 hours of transplantation. A feature of the mononuclear cell infiltrate is the great morphological heterogeneity on light microscopy, but four types are recognizable: large mononuclear cells (which include both macrophages and blast cells), small lymphocytes and plasma cells. The majority of mononuclear cells present in the graft are undoubtedly derived from the recipient and carried to the graft by the blood stream. However some cells may be of donor origin and responsible for a graft versus host reaction. The pattern of migration of mononuclear cells into organ transplants initially consists of adherence to the endothelium of the vessels followed by migration into the surrounding tissue. Some cells migrate by passing between the cells of the vessel wall, but lymphocytes may pass through endothelial cell cytoplasm. Within a short time of arriving in the graft the mononuclear cells proliferate and mitotic figures can be observed. This proliferative activity is confirmed by studies on DNA synthesis which show that about 4% of mononuclear cells infiltrating an allograft four days after transplantation are synthesizing DNA.

The changes described so far are those observed in an unimmunized recipient. If, however, the graft is transplanted into an individual who is already immunized to donor antigen the rejection process may be much more severe and occur within a brief space of time. In a graft which is in vascular continuity with the recipient this process of rejection may occur within minutes or hours. For example, in hyperacute rejection of renal grafts changes may be apparent within minutes of vascular anastomosis. In this type of hyperacute rejection the major effect is severe endothelial cell damage and development of thrombi consisting of leucocytes, platelets, fibrin and red cells, leading to vascular obstruction. In less violent forms, mononuclear cell infiltration plays a predominant role. With skin grafts the process takes longer and may become apparent only after two or three days.

In the accelerated or hyperacute forms of organ allograft rejection, neutrophils play a more important role. In most organ transplants neutrophils are present immediately after transplantation and also in the later stages of rejection of the graft. However, in individuals already sensitized, large number of neutrophils may rapidly collect in the graft. These form aggregates with platelets and fibrin within the blood vessels and may play a role in damaging the vessel walls. Lysosomal enzymes liberated by neutrophils may also be responsible for damaging the internal elastic lamina in this type of rejection.

Vascular lesions develop in most allografts. In first set grafts focal mononuclear cell infiltration is seen in the vessel wall, associated with degeneration and necrosis of smooth muscle. If the rejection process is rapid, fibrinoid necrosis of the whole arterial wall may be seen, with immunoglobulin and complement deposits and neutrophils.

In the process of chronic rejection of a graft obliterative changes develop in vessels and substantial fibrous thickening of the intima of small arteries produces narrowing of the lumen of the vessel. In smaller vessels endothelial cell hypertrophy is sometimes a noticeable feature but in other cases leucocytes and monocytes may be seen adhering to the endothelial cells which appear later to undergo necrosis. Immunoglobulin and complement deposits have been demonstrated around these lesions. A significant feature of the vascular changes is the decrease in blood flow. Although seen most dramatically in hyperacute rejection this occurs in most organ or tissue grafts during any rejection process.

Mechanisms of Rejection

Acute rejection of a solid allograft depends upon cell mediated immunity, and the basic event is invasion by mononuclear cells producing destructive lesions in the graft. The predominant cells are those of the lymphocyte and macrophage series. Destruction of the vessels by humoral or cellular mechanisms is also a feature in rejection and may result in ischaemic infarction of the graft. In the destruction of a tissue in suspension, for example blood or bone marrow, humoral antibodies may play a more important role, destroying cells by means of complement mediated lysis, by coating donor cells, by causing uptake of the cells by the reticulo-endothelial system or by enhancing the mechanical fragility of the target cell. A wide variety of techniques is available to study the effects of these agents upon target cells:

i. release of isotopes from the target cell;
ii. release of radio-labelled nucleic acid or cytoplasmic protein;
iii. loss of ability to synthesize DNA or cytoplasmic protein;
iv. inhibition of colony forming cells or cytoplasmic protein;

v. use of dye exclusion techniques to estimate the percentage of non-viable cells;
vi. counting of surviving adhering cells;
vii. simple morphological observations.

The role of lymphocyte mediated cytotoxicity in the rejection of normal tissue allografts has been established. Cytotoxic cells have been found in the lymph from lymph nodes draining the graft three to five days after grafting and in the thoracic duct lymph three or four days later. Cytotoxic cells subsequently appear in the peripheral blood, the spleen, and even in more remote lymph nodes. Cells with lesser cytotoxic properties against target cells may be generated *in vitro* within 4–6 days of incubating competent lymphocytes with target cells in mixed lymphocyte culture, or by layering them on target cell monolayers. As well as cytotoxic T-cells, other cells are involved in allograft rejection. These are helper and suppressor T-cells, K-cells, B-cells and macrophages.

Cytotoxic T-Lymphocytes

Cytotoxic T-lymphocytes are generated by an allogeneic graft. Because these cells are present in greatly increased numbers at the time of graft rejection, it was suggested that they play an important role in the pathogenesis of rejection (Debray-Sachs *et al.*, 1973). Thus skin graft rejection may occur before the appearance of cytotoxic cells. Nevertheless, in mice the T-cell nature of these cytotoxic cells has been established by their sensitivity to anti-theta sera, and cell mediated lysis produced by cells generated *in vitro* by mixed lymphocyte culture is also abolished by pre-treatment of the cells with anti-theta serum. Furthermore, this type of cell is not present in nude athymic mice in which skin graft rejection is delayed. It therefore appears that this direct form of lymphocyte mediated cytotoxicity plays a major role in allograft rejection. The lymphocyte attaches via a uropod to a site on the target cell which is probably the SD antigen, and the end result is a permeability change leading to rupture of the cell.

Helper T-Cells

When donor thymus and lymph node cells are mixed prior to injection into a host animal, the graft versus host reaction is increased. Experimental work in the mouse suggests the existence of two thymic cell populations.

Adult mouse thymectomy depletes the spleen and thymus of theta-positive cells which are highly sensitive to azathioprine. Anti-lymphocyte serum, but not adult thymectomy, depletes blood and lymph node rosette-forming cells which are less sensitive to azathioprine. This suggests that there is a population of cells in spleen and thymus which is highly dependent on the thymic presence and which reverts to a more primitive stage after adult thymectomy, and a second population predominantly situated in the lymph node and blood which, having matured under thymic influence, has become less dependent on the thymus. The cells of this latter population are the classical long-lived recirculating T-lymphocytes. It has been shown that thymus and lymph node cells act synergistically in cell mediated lysis and mixed lymphocyte culture.

In addition to these two populations of T-lymphocytes, there are certain T-cells that have suppressor activity and control cell-mediated as well as humoral responses.

K-cell Cytotoxicity

T-lymphocytes are not the only cells involved in allograft immunity. Normal human lymphoid cells (K-cells) are capable of killing antibody-coated target cells. The sensitizing antibodies are of IgG class and only small amounts are necessary in order to induce a cytotoxic effect against the coated cells. Complement is not involved in the reaction. The nature of the cell responsible for the cytotoxic effect is not yet clear. It is thought that it lacks both T-cell markers and the abundant surface immunoglobulin of the B-cell. It is present in normal numbers in athymic nude mice, and the K-cell content of lymphoid cell suspensions is enriched by conditions which lead to the depletion of T-cells. Morphological studies indicate that the cytotoxic K-cell is probably not a typical monocyte or macrophage and it appears that it may either belong to a separate cell population or be an immature B-cell. The K-cell carries a receptor for the Fc part of the immunoglobulin molecule and is depleted by immunosuppressive agents, particularly azathioprine. Lymphocyte dependent antibodies which have been detected in allograft recipients have the ability to sensitize target cells to cytotoxic attack by K-cells.

Macrophages

These are found in large numbers in human renal grafts undergoing rejection and probably play a part in the process. Macrophages have been shown to become cytotoxic towards tumour cells after being armed by a soluble mediator secreted by activated T-lymphocytes and such macrophage arming has been demonstrated also after allogeneic stimulation. *In vitro*, macrophages can bring about specific lysis of target cells, and the cytophilic substance responsible for inducing this has been called "specific macrophage arming factor". The cytotoxic effect on the target cell is an induced membrane permeability which leads to the rupture of the cell. Cytotoxic macrophages appear to be capable of moving to other target cells, or reacting with several target cells at once. Apparently similar cytoxicity may be initiated when normal T-lymphocytes in close contact with potential target cells are activated by mitogens such as phytohaemagglutinin, concanavalin A, pokeweed mitogen, anti-lymphocyte serum or staphylococcal filtrate.

KIDNEY TRANSPLANTATION

The eleventh report of the Human Renal Transplant Registry (1973) states that 12,389 transplants were performed from 1951–72 of which 11,264 were first transplants, 1,019 were second and 106 third transplants. By far the greatest amount of experience in clinical transplantation has been gained in this field of renal transplantation.

Choice of Donors

The percentage of renal grafts from live related donors varies from one country to another. In more than 5,000 transplants in the United States 21% were parental kidneys, 21% were sibling kidneys and 51% were cadaveric non-related kidneys. On the other hand in Australia only 20 out of 1,148 renal allografts were from live related donors.

At present even mis-matched sibling and parent kidneys survive with better function than cadaveric kidneys well matched for HLA. With a sibling kidney there is a 1 in 4 chance of identity (Fig. 2). To this is to be added the certainty that a kidney removed from a live related donor will be in a better physiological state at the time of transplantation than a cadaveric kidney.

On the other hand there are hazards in subjecting a normal healthy person to investigation and nephrectomy. As results from cadaveric renal transplantation improve, the percentage of live related donor kidneys utilized is likely to fall, provided that effective means can be found to use the cadaveric kidneys potentially available for grafting.

The age of the donor of a kidney affects the result. Graft survival six months after transplant is 39% with 61–84 year donors and 57% with 6–50 year donors (Eleventh Report, Human Renal Transplant Registry, 1973).

Choice of Recipients

The age of the recipient is important. The survival rate of patients over 50 is significantly less than the survival rate of those under 50 years of age.

Renal transplantation has been carried out for almost every type of renal disease. Nearly three quarters of all transplants are in patients who have glomerulonephritis or pyelonephritis. Polycystic kidneys, congenital malformations, malignant hypertension and metabolic renal disease are among other diseases which have been treated by renal transplantation. The single universally recognized contra-indication to renal transplantation is primary oxalosis in which early and fatal involvement of the graft is common.

Changes Caused by Rejection of Kidney Transplants

Hyperacute Rejection

In the classic form of hyperacute rejection, the kidney becomes pink after the anastomoses are established but within a few minutes become cyanosed despite the fact that the large vessels are patent. It may be deep blue in colour, of blotchy appearance and flabby, or it may become distended, even to the point of rupture (Fig. 3). Histological examination at this time may reveal evidence of sequestration of platelets, neutrophils, complement components, fibrinogen and congulation factors II, IV and VIII. Occasionally the intravascular coagulation may be so severe that a consumptive coagulopathy with a bleeding diathesis is induced. Immunoglobulin and complement components may be localized along the glomerular and peritubular capillary walls. Platelets aggregate in the capillary lumen and neutrophils line the capillary wall. Fibrin appears in the capillary lumina and within a short time most of the intra-renal capillaries and arterioles are blocked by microthrombi. At a later stage cortical necrosis occurs and prominent masses of fibrin fill the glomerular capillaries and obstruct the arterioles and small arteries. Sometimes rejection may occur in a less hyperacute manner and renal function may not fail until a day or two after transplantation.

Antibody is incriminated in hyperacute rejection. It occurs most frequently in patients who have demonstrable cytotoxic antibodies directed against donor histocompatibility antigens, but the same histological picture may be found when there is ABO blood group incompatibility between host and donor, or when cold agglutinins are present in high titre in the recipient and the transplanted organ is still cool at the time of anastomosis to the host circulation. Antibody against donor antigen has been found in IgG, IgA and IgM classes. While these may be responsible for activating the complement pathway, this may also result from the effects of preformed antigen–antibody complexes or the presence of endotoxin in the transplanted kidney.

There is evidence of the participation of the complement, coagulation and kinin systems in this form of rejection. Complement consumption can be demonstrated by increased turnover of labelled complement components, or if the reaction is severe enough, by lowered plasma levels. In canine renal allografts, depletion of complement by administration of cobra-venom was found to reduce neutrophil infiltration but did not ameliorate hyperacute rejection. Hageman factor activation by antibody–antigen complexes may liberate kinins from kininogen. In hyperacute rejection, when anti-donor antibodies are present in the recipient's circulation, kallikreinogen levels have been seen to fall and this has also been observed experimentally. Not all recipients who reject renal allografts in this manner have cytotoxic antibodies reactive against donor tissue.

Patients who have been exposed to repeated blood transfusions and multiple pregnancies, or previous skin or kidney transplants, may become sensitized to transplantation antigens. In view of the uncertain role of antibodies to transplantation antigens and the association of anti-donor antibodies and hyperacute form of rejection, a negative cross-match between donor and recipient is an important requirement.

Acute Rejection

Although rejection of a primary (first set) allogeneic graft—the classic form of acute rejection—is regarded as mainly a manifestation of cell mediated immunity, the use of immunosuppressive agents may reduce this and give the humoral arm greater relative importance, with IgG and IgM, the first and third component of complement and fibrinogen (all demonstrable by immunofluorescence) deposited in the walls of arteries, arterioles, glomerular and peritubular capillaries. Clinical rejection under modern immunosuppressive therapy is not an all or none reaction. The majority of patients who receive a kidney transplant have at least one rejection episode during the first three or four months after transplantation. The first episode seldom progresses to complete renal destruction, and the functional changes produced by rejection appear to be in large part reversible if treated early enough. Early recognition and treatment of rejection is thus of great importance, especially as after each rejection episode detected clinically there remains a slight but permanent impairment of renal function.

Chronic Rejection

Chronic rejection is characterized clinically by slow deterioration in renal function. The vascular lesions which are so evident in chronic rejection were first noticed in a human kidney by Hume and his colleagues in 1955 in a renal allograft that had survived for 176 days. The intima of arteries and arterioles is thickened; ultrastructurally composed of fine collagen fibrils, smooth muscle cells and granular electron-dense material, the media is usually atrophic and the internal elastic lamina often ruptured. These lesions occur as the result of continual or intermittent formation of platelet and fibrin aggregates on the vessel walls which in time are covered by endothelium. Glomerulonephritis is also a manifestation of chronic rejection, glomerular lesions being seen in some grafts. The glomerular basement membrane is diffusely or segmentally thickened, there is a localized increase in mesangial cells and sometimes infiltration with polymorphs. Immunofluorescence shows granular deposits of IgM, IgG, C1 and C3 in the glomerular capillary walls and in the mesangium. By electron microscopy, deposits of amorphous material are seen on the subendothelial surface of the capillary basement membrane, and immunoglobulin and complement have also been identified. Antibodies to histocompatibility antigens have been eluted by acid buffer from a few grafts.

Biopsies from most long-term survivors, even those with apparently normally functioning kidneys, show fusion of glomerular foot processes and thickened basement membranes. From this the lesion may progress to proliferation of glomerular endothelial and mesangial cells with the basement membrane changes and intimal hypertrophy becoming more obvious.

Recurrent Disease

Human renal isogeneic grafts have been performed for more than 20 years. Recurrence of disease had been observed in these isografts. In rapid onset progressive glomerulonephritis, the graft may develop lesions at an early stage, but in slowly progressive glomerulonephritis lesions in the grafted kidney occur later and less frequently. The recurrent disease may resemble the late-onset glomerular lesions that develop during chronic rejection. Immunoglobulin, complement components and fibrinogen can be demonstrated in the basement membrane and mesangium.

Recurrence of disease processes appears less often in allografts than in isografts, possibly owing to the use of immunosuppressives.

Diagnosis of Renal Transplant Rejection

Rejection of the transplanted kidney is manifested by certain clinical changes but the non-specificity of the clinical features is well known and renal biopsy has become popular as a means of establishing the diagnosis. While biopsy reveals the presence of inflammatory changes in the kidneys rather than specifically indicating rejection of that organ, it confirms that the source of the inflammation is renal and not a systemic disturbance. Infiltration of the allograft by lymphocytes does not definitely prove the diagnosis of rejection as these cells may be found in a wide variety of abnormal conditions such as pyelonephritis, obstructive uropathy and interstitial nephritis, but peritubular focal mononuclear infiltration is regarded as specific for rejection.

Any significant episode of acute rejection is associated with impairment of renal function, and measurement of the plasma creatinine concentration gives a reliable indication of this. In patients with chronic renal failure treated by dialysis, the plasma creatinine level is rarely less than 4 mg per 100 ml, but with a well functioning renal allograft the serum creatinine should be less than 2 mg per 100 ml.

Improvement in renal function following therapy suggests that rejection has occurred, but is not definite evidence since steroids are well known anti-inflammatory drugs and may inhibit processes other than those of rejection.

The diagnosis of chronic rejection of a transplanted kidney is much more difficult. Increased plasma creatinine levels will result from severe lesions impairing renal function, but the process being by nature chronic allows time for hypertrophy to keep pace initially with the loss of nephrons. Eventually however, the plasma creatine begins to rise. Unlike acute rejection, there may be few, if any signs of inflammation. Ischaemia may lead to hypertension, and proteinuria may be present. Histologically the kidney may show the changes of tubular atrophy and fibrosis.

Some common causes of graft failure in the early post operative phase (i.e. within threc months of transplantation) are given below.

Acute Rejection

This is usually characterized by systemic disturbance with pyrexia and pain over the renal graft. The graft is enlarged and tender. There is fluid retention, decreased urinary output, decreased sodium excretion and proteinuria. The serum creatinine and urea rise. The peripheral blood white cell count rises and the platelet count usually falls. The onset of rejection is heralded by an increase in urinary fibrin degradation products. There may be an increase in peripheral lymphocyte DNA synthesis and macrophage inhibition factor production. Arteriography shows attenuation of small vessels. On a renal scan there is no excretory phase.

Venous Thrombosis

This is usually characterized by pain, and swelling over the renal graft, haematuria, a rise in blood pressure and an elevation of serum urea. The arteriogram is normal in appearance but the renal scan shows delayed excretion.

Arterial Obstruction

This is usually characterized by hypertension, with a graft normal on palpation. Microscopic haematuria heralds the sudden shut down of the graft. The arteriogram and renal scan show no flow to the graft.

Ureteric Obstruction

There is a slow fall-off in function but with good urinary urea and sodium concentration. An intravenous pyelogram shows dilation of the calyces.

Histocompatibility and Graft Survival

One of the most controversial topics in transplantation immunology today is the relationship of histocompatibility testing to the clinical results of transplantation. Although mixed lymphocyte culture of LD typing is now being used more, the major form of histocompatibility typing is still for serologically-defined HLA-antigens. The fact that a transplant between HLA-identical siblings has a greatly improved graft survival when compared to HLA-non-identical combinations has been thought a strong argument for the assumption that the serologically defined HLA-antigens are the important antigens in graft rejection. However, as may be seen from Fig. 2, the loci coding for HLA are only part of a major chromosomal histocompatibility region which controls a variety of other determinants. Since in HLA-identical siblings other areas of this major histocompatibility region are likely to be identical as well, the case for HLA is not proven. Discordant conclusions have been reached in different kidney transplant centres about the role of HLA-compatibility in kidney graft survival. The French and the London transplant groups found a clear correlation between SD matching and graft survival. Matching for the second locus (SD 2) appeared to be more important than matching for the first locus (SD 1). Analysis of patients in Europe by Van Rood and colleagues (1973) showed a correlation between HLA matching and graft survival only in patients with preformed antibody. On the other hand, in the United States, Belzer and colleagues (1974) found no association between SD matching and graft survival in either those with preformed antibodies or those without.

Certainly the results of renal transplantation in HLA-identical siblings have been very rewarding. There have been reports of 100% of such grafts functioning after three months and one year and 96% graft survival after two years (Descamps *et al.*, 1973). In addition, half the identical combinations had no detectable rejection episode during the first year. In semi-identical recipients, only 20% did not have a rejection crisis during the first year. Biopsy of kidney grafts in these combinations showed that 50% of HLA-identical siblings but only 9% of HLA semi-identical had normal biopsies two years after transplantation.

It is known that linkage disequilibrium exists between certain LD 1 determinants and some HLA-determinants and it has been postulated that the difference between the European and American results may be due to the fact that the linkage disequilibrium between LD 1 and SD 2 antigens is much less in the United States. Where strong linkage disequilibrium exists between SD 2 and LD and other antigens, indirect matching for the "true" histocompatibility antigens might be achieved by SD matching.

The correlation between LD compatibility and kidney graft survival indicates that LD 1 is probably important in determining graft survival. Several workers have examined mixed lymphocyte culture reactivity in unrelated donor transplants. Cochrum *et al.* (1973) found that MLC results could be divided into two groups; patients with an MLC in which DNA synthetic rates increased less than eight times the basal level, who had a one year graft survival rate of 86%; and patients in whom the DNA synthetic rate was greater than eight times the resting level who had a one year graft survival of only 22%. Minimal or no stimulation in MLC of HLA-identical sibs was associated with no episodes of rejection, whereas stimulation in MLC was associated with one or more episodes of rejection (Cochrum *et al.*, 1973).

The figures for patient and graft survival vary; those shown in Table 7 are derived from two large series.

TABLE 7
Survival

Donor		1 Year Patient (%)	1 Year Graft (%)	2 Year Patient (%)	2 Year Graft (%)	3 Year Patient (%)	3 Year Graft (%)
Live related	USA	84	73	81	70	75	65
	Europe	82	73	76	64	71	58
Cadaveric	USA	64	48	59	42	45	33
First graft	Europe	70	50	62	43	56	37
Cadaveric		—	36	—	27	—	23
Second graft	Europe	—	46	—	37	—	33

From figures given by Human Renal Transplant Registry, and European Dialysis and Transplant Association.

Immunosuppression in Renal Transplantation

Corticosteroids

Synthetic corticosteroids in large doses produce a rapid and profound decrease in circulating lymphocytes in the peripheral blood. They also have an anti-proliferative effect, hinder migration of white cells through endothelial barriers and stabilize lysosomal and cell membranes, preventing leakage of lysosomal enzymes.

In healthy volunteers the mixed lymphocyte response after administration of 100 mg or 1,000 mg of methyl-prednisolone intravenously was suppressed by both doses for at least 12 hours and the lymphopenia persisted for at least 24 hours (Cheigh *et al.*, 1975). When 16 mg of methyl-prednisolone was administered to volunteers every four hours over a period of five days, there was a sustained decrease (up to 50%) in the circulating IgG, the lowest immunoglobulin levels occurring during the second and third week after drug treatment. Thereafter there was a gradual rise towards pretreatment levels but even at three months the IgG levels were still depressed. However, ability to respond to primary and secondary antigenic stimulation was not decreased (Butler, 1975).

In acute rejection large doses of corticosteroids (e.g. one gram of methyl-prednisolone daily) given up to five days often reverses the rejection process. Such large doses can only be given for short periods of time because of hazardous side effects such as gastrointestinal bleeding. In general the usual practice following transplantation is to give initially one or two mg per kg

TABLE 8
Side effects of corticosteroids

Immunosuppressive	Infections by viruses, bacteria, fungi and protozoa.
Metabolic	Steroid-induced diabetes, lipidaemia, atherogenesis, sodium retention, negative nitrogen and potassium balance.
Gastrointestinal	Oesophageal, gastric, jejunal, ileal or colonic ulceration, pancreatitis.
Anti-inflammatory	Decreased wound healing.
Central nervous system	Psychosis.
Locomotor	Myopathy, osteoporosis and compression fractures, aseptic necrosis of bone.
Eye	Cataracts, glaucoma, exophthalmos.
Endocrine and other	Growth failure, Cushingoid appearance, steroid-dependence.

per day, or its equivalent, and during ensuing weeks to reduce the dosage to less toxic levels. There is less agreement on dosage during the later stages after transplantation. Some clinicians keep adult patients on 15–25 mg prednisolone a day, others continue to reduce until rejection threatens. Reduction during the year to less than 20 mg per day for a 70 kg individual is associated with a higher rate of rejection. Since large doses of steroid may be administered for a long period of time, attention must obviously be directed to side effects, some of which are illustrated in Table 8. Alternate day therapy maintains immunosuppression satisfactorily and lowers the risk of steroid complications.

Azathioprine

Since 1963, azathioprine has been the principal immunosuppressive agent in most renal transplant centres. Azathioprine is the imidazole derivative of 6-mercaptopurine. It can cause bone marrow depression and falls in white cell count occur suddenly. Because good renal function is needed for detoxication any marked decrease in the former may increase toxic effects unless the dosage is adjusted accordingly. Azathioprine is administered for the life of the graft.

Antilymphocyte Serum or Globulin (ALG)

In transplantation in animals ALG has markedly immunosuppressive effects. Antilymphocyte preparations have been used in human renal transplantation for several years by some units, but it is still not clear whether they improve the one or two year survival of the patient or the graft although some retrospective studies show improved patient and graft survival. It appears that patients with surviving kidney grafts have better renal function if they have received ALG. ALG also reduces the steroid requirement. A trial of ALG therapy under carefully controlled conditions is currently in progress. In reversing graft versus host disease after marrow transplantation it has been shown to be very effective.

Complications of Immunosuppressive Therapy

Recipients who do not develop episodes of graft rejection are generally less likely to suffer the major complications of immunosuppressive therapy.

Infection is the most serious of these. In the Human Renal Transplant Registry—Eleventh Report (1973) sepsis is one of the contributory causes of death in 45% of cases. The most common bacterial infections are with *Klebsiella*, *Pseudomonas* and *Staphylococcus*. Since the advent of penicillinase-resistant penicillins staphylococcal infections have become rare as a cause of death. Immunosuppressed patients are susceptible also to a variety of opportunistic agents, including fungi and viruses, and a high incidence of cytomegalovirus infection has been reported in renal transplant recipients (Lopez *et al.*, 1974). The clinical manifestations of the latter include hepatitis, pneumonia and heterophile antibody negative "glandular fever". Although cytomegalovirus has been frequently isolated from asymptomatic transplant recipients and in such cases is currently of little import it has been noted that symptomatic infections are associated with episodes of rejection. Lopez *et al.* found that in 61 renal transplant recipients only the viruses of the herpes group (that is cytomegalovirus, herpes simplex and herpes zoster) were consistently isolated. The onset of the virus infection was associated with clinical features of fever, leucopenia and renal allograft rejection. Renal biopsies performed when the serum creatinine level was elevated, revealed a classical histological picture of rejection. Most of the rejection episodes were reversed by an increased dose of steroids.

Other viral infections are common in recipients of renal transplants. Herpes zoster usually remains localized but herpes simplex may progress and lead to death.

Fungal infections occur, especially with *Candida* and *Aspergillus*, and cryptococcus infection, nocardiosis, histoplasmosis and mucormycosis have all been causes of fatal infection. Tuberculosis is also a hazard. Patients who develop one or more episodes of leucopenia are more likely to die from infection. Careful watch must therefore be kept upon the effect of immunosuppressants upon the bone marrow.

Development of Malignant Disease

An organ transplant recipient maintained on chronic immunosuppressive therapy has a 5% chance of developing cancer within the first few years after transplantation. The nature and incidence of the various types of tumours seen are discussed in Chapter 30.

The mean time after transplantation for the appearance of tumours is 28 months which makes the chances of transplantation of tumour from the donor being responsible very small.

LIVER TRANSPLANTATION

By 1974 more than 200 patients had received liver replacements. Starzl (1974) has reported that since the first hepatic transplant in 1963 he has transplanted 82 hepatic allografts, with 18 recipients surviving one year, and 9 surviving two years. A major problem in hepatic transplantation is the technical one of biliary duct reconstruction; this apart, graft rejection and systemic infection are the most important causes of failure.

Histopathology of Rejection

On the third or fourth day after transplantation mononuclear cells adhere to the portal veins and venules infiltrate around the portal tracts and central veins. Later, these cells infiltrate the parenchyma, and the liver cells in the central and middle zones begin to degenerate and undergo necrosis. The reticular framework subsequently collapses and bile pigment accumulates.

Hyperacute Rejection

Whether or not hyperacute rejection of liver grafts occurs is not certain. ABO mismatched livers have been transplanted into recipients whose conditions were grave enough to justify it and hyperacute rejection did not occur nor was there any obvious adverse consequence (Starzl, 1974). Livers have also been transplanted into patients who had anti-donor cytotoxic antibodies without evidence of hyperacute rejection. The liver appears to be more resistant to rejection than the kidney. In the heterograft model kidneys may be rejected within a few seconds of vascular anastomosis whereas the liver does not show signs for an hour or more.

Acute Rejection

This may be heralded by episodes of jaundice which develop from the sixth to eighth post transplant day and the serum bilirubin, transaminase and alkaline phosphatase levels rise. An increase in white cell count and erythrocyte sedimentation rate may be accompanied by a fall in platelet count. As with the kidney, the transplanted liver increases in size and shows decreased uptake of isotope on liver scan. Other forms of acute rejection occur; an anicteric form in which the serum transaminase and alkaline phosphatase levels increase but there is no increase in serum bilirubin; and a slower type in which the changes gradually appear between the second and fourth post-transplant week. In general however, serum bilirubin and pseudocholinesterase levels are the best signals of rejection.

Starzl (1974) has demonstrated that hepatic allograft rejection in dogs is delayed by immunosuppressive therapy, and in clinical hepatic transplantation the rejection process is of a low grade in immunosuppressed patients. In some recipients of liver grafts immunosuppressive therapy has been discontinued at times of severe infection without rejection supervening.

Immunosuppressive therapy for hepatic transplantation is essentially the same as for renal transplantation. Azathioprine and prednisone are the mainstays, but azathioprine is hepatotoxic as well as myelotoxic and its administration must be carefully controlled. Starzl (1974) uses, in addition, anti-lymphocyte globulin and cyclophosphamide if azathioprine induced hepatotixity is seen.

Infection is a major problem. Pulmonary infection with viruses and fungi, staphylococcus or pseudomonas has been reported, and oral moniliasis may follow broad spectrum antibiotic therapy. Biliary and abdominal infections may also develop and Starzl (1969) has described a syndrome of septic infarction in which gram-negative septicaemia and sudden marked elevation of the serum transaminase level are accompanied by the appearance on liver scans of large, persistent filling defects.

In the diagnosis of rejection the standard liver function tests are not helpful because they do not differentiate between rejection and other causes of jaundice after transplantation; e.g. hepatitis, azathioprine toxicity and hepatic obstruction. To assess whether or not rejection is occurring, the reactivity of lymphocytes has been examined; the leucocyte migration test and rosette inhibition test being used for this purpose (Eddleston, 1970).

BONE MARROW TRANSPLANTATION

The first successful human allogeneic marrow transplants were performed in 1958 on the victims of accidental total body irradiation. Earlier it had been found that mice could be protected from an otherwise lethal dose of X-ray by shielding the spleen with lead or by the intravenous injection of syngeneic and allogeneic marrow cells. The injected marrow cells lodged in various tissues but once equilibrium was reached, it was found that the recipients' haemopoietic and lymphopoietic compartments had been largely replaced by cells of donor type. Failed attempts at human marrow transplantation have been due to several causes: inadequate immunosuppression, administration of too few marrow cells, failure to recognize that transfusion before grafting may pre-sensitize to donor antigens, failure to adequately prevent or control the intensity of graft versus host reactions and failure to provide adequate supportive care of patients with marrow aplasia. Poor selection of patients, many of whom have been already grossly infected or moribund at the time of the procedure has added to the mortality.

Bortin (1970) reviewed the results of over 200 bone marrow grafts performed up to 1964 and found no survivors among patients with aplastic anaemia given allogeneic cells. At that time the importance of matching for the HLA and MLC system was not appreciated and many of the recipients in consequence experienced severe graft-versus-host or secondary disease. This is still a major problem in marrow transplantation. Even when donor and recipient are HLA-identical and MLC-unresponsive about half the recipients will develop graft-versus-host disease of varying severity (Storb *et al.*, 1974).

Manifestations of Graft versus Host Disease

Allogeneic bone marrow transplanted into patients is capable of being stimulated immunologically by the hosts' tissues. The grafted lymphoid tissue mounts an immunological rejection of host tissue and produces graft-versus-host disease. This is characterized by enlargement of the liver and spleen, rapid and progressive loss of weight, anaemia, diarrhoea, nausea and vomiting and exfoliative dermatitis.

Apart from loss of weight the development of a skin rash is a warning sign. In all 43 patients with proven graft-versus-host disease studied by Lerner *et al.* (1974), a maculo-papular skin rash was present. The rash was seen from the sixth day onwards, mainly involving the trunk but also present on the extremities and remainder of the body. The histological changes in the skin were classified in order of severity as: (1) local and diffuse vacuolar degeneration of the epidermal basal cells and acanthocytes, (2) focal diffuse spongiosis, i.e. a separation by intercellular oedema of the basal cells and acanthocytes, (3) changes similar to the latter, with occurrence of spaces and clefts after necrosis of the basal cells, and (4) frank loss of epidermis.

Variable mononuclear cell infiltration of the epidermis and papillary dermis was present, and contact between lymphocytes and degenerating epithelial cells observed. In this group of recipients the liver also showed evidence of graft-versus-host disease, namely degeneration and necrosis of hepatic parenchymal cells and of the epithelium of small bile ducts. Gastro-intestinal manifestations of graft-versus-host disease, i.e. diarrhoea, nausea and vomiting were also present. The degree of diarrhoea has been used as a means of assessing severity. Lesions occur in both large and small intestine but are most severe in the distal ileum, consisting of focal dilatation and degeneration of mucosal glands which may be diffuse or localized, mucosal oedema, mononuclear cell infiltration of the mucosa and submucosal flattening of villi and epithelial necrosis.

It may be difficult within the first ten days after grafting to distinguish between mild graft-versus-host disease and the effects of cyclophosphamide or irradiation, which can also produce oedema and mononuclear cell infiltration. Manifestations of graft-versus-host disease occur in the liver and may be difficult to distinguish from the viral hepatitis relatively common in patients who have received blood products frequently before transplantation.

Graft-versus-host disease may also be produced by giving blood products containing immunocompetent cells to immunodeficient individuals. To reduce the number of viable immunocompetent allogeneic lymphocytes transfused into such patients whole blood should be irradiated with 3,000 R in conditions of satisfactory oxygenation. Plasma can be frozen or thawed several times and then centrifuged to remove allogeneic cells. The use of stored blood does not obviate risk of graft-versus-host disease since lymphocytes in blood that has been stored 22 days are still capable of mitotic activity, and graft-versus-host disease has been observed after transfusion of blood stored for 12 days.

A major complication of graft-versus-host disease is infection, and the high incidence of fatal infections is probably related to the profound immunological depression that results from the graft-versus-host reaction and which to some degree may persist for up to $2\frac{1}{2}$ years after the graft.

Source of Donors

Marrow transplantation is used in the treatment of marrow aplasia, leukaemia and immunodeficiency. Patients with leukaemia or marrow aplasia can reject allografts and need to be conditioned by cytotoxic drugs, anti-lymphocyte preparations or irradiation in order to accept an allogeneic graft. On the other hand patients with T-cell immunodeficiency are susceptible to graft-versus-host disease and require immunosuppression to control this. It is thus of the utmost importance that the risk of graft rejection or graft-versus-host disease is reduced by seeking maximum histocompatibility between graft and donor. This in turn reduces the amount of immunosuppression required.

Compatible donors of marrow have until recently been found among siblings of the recipient. The chances of finding an HLA-identical sib are 1 in 4, whereas the chances of finding an unrelated identical donor are much less. Furthermore, the HLA, MLC and other loci are closely linked on the same chromosome and therefore these loci are more likely to match in HLA-identical siblings than in the unrelated HLA-identical donor. The best choice for a donor is an HLA-identical, MLC-identical sibling but even when the HLA and the MLC systems are matched, between 20 and 50% of recipients develop some form of graft-versus-host disease. In families where the parents share one HLA haplotype, it is possible to find a parent and child who are HLA- and MLC-identical and this parent can be selected as a bone marrow donor. Where there is no family member who is suitable, then unrelated HLA-identical and LD-identical donors may have to be used. The donor's LD compatibility can be determined either by identifying the LD determinants with known LD stimulator test cells and comparing this typing with the recipient's, or by using the recipient's lymphocytes in an MLC reaction against lymphocytes from the prospective recipient.

Transplantation of histoincompatible marrow is followed by graft-versus-host reactions, if the graft itself is not rejected. To avoid graft-versus-host disease, attempts have been made to selectively remove immunocompetent cells from the marrow grafts. One method of doing this is use albumin gradient separation of marrow cells (in animals the use of gradient separation is successful in reducing the severity of graft-versus-host disease when allo geneic cells are given). However, results of recent clinical transplants suggest that whole marrow is preferable to a stem-cell rich fraction obtained by this method.

When no HLA/MLC-identical donor is available foetal liver cells may be used as a source of stem cells. Bortin and Salstein (1969) revived interest in the use of foetal allogeneic liver cells for the treatment of immunodeficient individuals, and found moreover increased long-term survival of recipients when these were combined with thymus cells or thymic factors. The problems that beset attempts to use foetal liver cells as a source of stem cells in man have been due to technical difficulties in typing foetal cells, the storage of foetal tissue prior to transplantation, the problems of insufficient cell yields and the lack of information on optimal age for the foetal donor. The older the foetus the greater the cell yield but the more likely the graft to be immunocompetent. Successful transplants have been recorded with foetal tissue from nine, eleven and twelve week old donors given to infants with combined immunodeficiency. The cell yield from a foetal liver at 8–12 weeks is about $0{\cdot}6 \times 10^9$ cells but at 18 weeks increases to approximately $2{\cdot}7 \times 10^9$. Graft-versus-host disease has occurred after administration of cells from an 11-week foetus, and has been recorded in an infant with combined immunodeficiency who was given liver from a $9\frac{1}{2}$-week-old foetus. Ninety days later the recipient developed an erythematous exfoliative dermatitis accompanied by eosinophilia and diarrhoea. Skin biopsy revealed the lymphocyte infiltration characteristic of graft-versus-host disease.

With regard to optimal cell numbers, investigations in mice and monkeys show that where the donor is histoincompatible, four to ten times as many cells are needed as for a syngeneic graft. In matched sibling marrow transplants there are several reports of grafts which were unsuccessful initially but were successful when increased numbers of cells from the same donor were given.

With improving results in bone marrow transplantation and wider application of this form of treatment in marrow aplasia and acute leukaemia there is a need for HLA-matched donors to provide blood products in order to avoid sensitization against the HLA-antigens. There are more than 7,000 different HLA-phenotypes and this poses great problems in matching.

Methods of Pretreatment

To reduce the risk of graft rejection or graft-versus-host disease, various immunosuppressive regimes are used. Santos (1967) introduced an effective form of pretreatment in which 45 mg of cyclophosphamide per kg per day is given intravenously on each of the four days prior to the marrow infusion. Another method is to give 950 to 1,000 rads total body irradiation (mid-line tissue dose). Various combinations of these forms of pretreatment, together with antilymphocyte globulin and methotrexate are also used to encourage successful engraftment; for example one group (Storb *et al.*, 1974) have successfully used a regime of procarbazine, anti-thymocyte globulin and cyclophosphamide. Anti-thymocyte globulin has now been reported successful in reversing graft-versus-host disease. In 19 patients with moderately severe to severe GVH who were treated with this agent complete resolution of GVH occurred in 12 (Storb *et al.*, 1974).

Conditions in which Marrow Transplantation should be Considered

Aplastic Anaemia

Whether idiopathic or produced by drugs, viruses or radiation, this is a disease with high mortality. The proportion of patients who respond to conservative management varies from series to series, but less than a third survive 5 years (Williams *et al.*, 1973). In one series (Storb *et al.*, 1974) no patient treated by conservative means was alive after 3 years, while in the group in which marrow transplant was attempted there was 50% survival. The major problems as discussed above are finding a histocompatible donor, avoiding graft rejection and preventing graft-versus-host disease. In the regime of Santos (1972) intermittent methotrexate at a dosage of 10 mg/m^2 is given on days 1, 3 and 6 after the graft and thereafter 5 mg/m^2 weekly. This controls unwanted reactions well, but also delays recovery of the graft. Previous transfusions adversely affect the outcome of grafting so that in severe cases of marrow aplasia, early rather than late transplantation is advisable.

Immunodeficiency

Thymectomy in the new born mouse produces profound retardation of development of the immune system and in a normal environment neonatally thymectomized mice die. If such mice are grafted with intact thymus they have a normal life span and develop normal lymphoid tissue and normal immune mechanisms. Thymus extracts or thymus cell suspensions also restore such animals to normal immunological reactivity. The clinical equivalent of the thymectomized mouse is the congenital absence of thymus and parathyroid glands described by DiGeorge. Thymus rather than marrow transplants are the logical treatment for this condition and rapid restoration of delayed hypersensitivity and cell mediated immunity is seen in patients so treated.

Combined immunodeficiency is satisfactorily treated with HLA-identical marrow. The first successful allogeneic bone marrow transplant (Hong *et al.*, 1968) to correct severe combined deficiencies was performed in 1968. Since then many patients have been immunologically reconstituted with such transplants. Results show that a transplant from an HLA- and MLC-identical sibling donor is the method of choice. However, infants with combined immunodeficiency have been restored to immunological competence with marrows from related donors differing in the HLA but compatible in the MLC system, emphasizing the importance of MLC compatibility in bone marrow transplantation.

In mice which received histoincompatible marrows the development of graft-versus-host disease was mitigated by the induction of a germ-free state in the host. Germ-free isolation procedures have been used clinically in order to reduce the obvious risks of infection and have a possible role in graft-versus-host disease.

Acute Leukaemia

Marrow grafts from HLA-matched sibs are consistently achieved in patients with terminal leukaemia. Long-term control of leukaemia is a possibility with this procedure and a few long-term survivors are alive three years after grafting (Buckner *et al.*, 1974). Recurrence of disease and haemorrhage are particular problems and interstitial pulmonary infections and generalized sepsis following grafts are responsible for a significant mortality. Late infections occur in 60% of patients presumably as a consequence of immunological deficiency produced by graft-versus-host disease itself and by the use of immunosuppression to ensure graft acceptance. Cytomegalovirus and herpes virus are responsible for the interstitial pneumonitis seen in approximately 40% of the recipients. Recurrence of leukaemia after a successful bone marrow transplant from a sibling of the opposite sex has been shown to be due to leukaemic cells of donor origin (Fialkow *et al.*, 1971).

HEART TRANSPLANTATION

Since the first heart transplant in 1967, there have been at least 209 performed, nearly 30% of them at Stanford University Medical Centre. The overall actuarial survival for the Stanford patients is 43% at one year and 40% at two years. Since 1970 one year survival for all patients undergoing heart transplantation has been 50%.

As with other transplants, acute rejection and its complications are a major problem. In the Stanford series the incidence of acute rejection in the first three months following surgery has been one episode for every 20 patient days of follow-up, the first episode occurring within 10 days of transplantation. The most reliable diagnostic feature of acute rejection are electrocardiographic changes, the commonest being a decrease in the QRS voltage. Arrhythmias and conduction defects occur less frequently. Contrary to early expectation elevation of serum enzyme levels has not been a good indicator of rejection. Successful attempts have been made to diagnose acute rejection earlier by means of transvenous endomyocardial biopsy (Lower, 1974). Polymorphonuclear infiltration, interstitial oedema, cytolysis of myocardial fibres and mononuclear cell infiltration are features of the acute rejection process. There are also changes in the endothelium of larger coronary vessels, with intimal damage. Focal damage in the media resembles that in polyarteritis nodosa. Prednisolone, azathioprine or cyclophosphamide are used for immunosuppression. For acute rejection the dosage of prednisolone is increased, and for severe acute rejection methylprednisolone (one gram per day intravenously for three days) with or without addition of antithymocyte globulin, has been used.

A complication has been the development of graft coronary atherosclerosis between six months and three-and-a-half years after the transplantation. Acute rejection appears to be a significant factor in determining the occurrence of this change. With more effective immunosuppression, prompt treatment of rejection crises, the use of low cholesterol diets and treatment with oral anticoagulants, the frequency of these vascular changes appears to be less.

LUNG TRANSPLANTATION

At least 36 patients had received lung transplants by the end of 1974. One survived ten months, another six months and several one to two months after the operation, but no longer-term success has been achieved. The reason for transplantation in most of the recipients was severe pulmonary vascular disease although transplantation has been attempted in some cases of paraquat poisoning.

Following transplantation alveolar oedema and alveolar infiltrates develop in the transplanted lung, and increase in amount for three days after the operation, gradually regressing during the next three weeks. These changes lead to temporary impairment of ventilation of the transplant. The mechanisms of acute rejection affect both vascular and alveolar components of the lung homograft. Mononuclear cells infiltrate and form perivascular collections, there is thickening of the intima and narrowing of the lumen of small vessels which leads to increased vascular resistance in the transplant and a decreased blood flow. The alveolar changes consist of fibrinous exudates which contain pneumocytes, and are visible on X-ray as infiltrates. Their presence leads to decreased ventilation of the transplant. The signs of rejection are the sudden onset of dyspnoea, malaise and increased body temperature; increasing infiltration is seen on X-ray and the arterial oxygen tension is reduced. If due to rejection, these manifestations can be reversed by one gram intravenous injections of methyl-prednisolone given every 24 hours for a limited period, usually of 3–4 days.

Rejection is still a major unresolved problem in clinical lung transplantation. On immunosuppression it has been observed that the vascular phase of rejection is often decreased to a greater extent than the alveolar phase so that there is decreased ventilation but adequate perfusion. This ventilation-perfusion imbalance can result in large scale venous mixing, arterial hypoxaemia and death. More efficient immunosuppression might be helpful in reducing this imbalance. Membrane oxygenators have been successfully used to provide supplementary oxygenation for patients with acute respiratory insufficiency. Partial by-pass using oxygenators may be of help in supporting lung transplant recipients through critical phases of functional insufficiency of their grafts.

SKIN GRAFTS

Because of the ease of observation skin grafts have been a popular method of studying transplantation. The first attempts were made several thousand years ago, and successful full thickness autografts were performed at the beginning of the nineteenth century (see Rapaport and Converse, 1968). By the early 1900s the different behavior of autografts and allografts had been noted but it was only with the classic description of rejection of allografts by Medawar and his colleagues that the immunological basis of rejection became clear.

Acute Rejection

For several days after transplantation an allograft and an autograft look similar. After initial pallor the graft becomes pinker during the second day and the area around it also shows mild erythema. However, by the sixth day this surrounding pinkness has disappeared in an autograft but has become more marked and is accompanied by oedema in an allograft. The allograft subsequently becomes dep red, and a black eschar develops from fourteen days onwards. After an allograft has been rejected attempts to replace it with a second graft from the same donor may produce hyperacute rejection from the outset—a white graft. Delaying the application of the second graft from the same donor produces accelerated rejection with a black aschar at 7 or 8 days.

Skin grafting is one of the most difficult forms of transplantation, and prolongation of graft survival is more difficult to achieve than in renal transplantation. Batchelor and Hackett (1970) showed that HLA-matched skin grafts survived longer than grafts that were HLA-dissimilar.

Because of the possibility of being able to repeatedly harvest autografts from the patient at two-weekly intervals, the use of HLA-matched skin allografts has been advocated for the treatment of severely burned patients. The skin allograft reduces heat, fluid and protein loss and reduces the risk of infection while suitable autografts are harvested at intervals to replace allografts. Diethelm *et al.* (1974) have used parental skin allografts to treat children with 75% full thickness burns. Anti-thymocyte globulin was given and allograft survival of periods up to six weeks was achieved. Skin allograft transplantation may therefore have a place as a temporary measure in the treatment of severely burned patients.

CORNEAL TRANSPLANTATION

For more than a hundred years it has been known that corneal transplants do not suffer the usual fate of transplanted tissue. Medawar (1948) postulated that the success of corneal grafts might be explained by the normal avascularity and poor lymphatic drainage and by the low antigenicity of the graft. If for any reason these features are altered then the graft may be rejected. In rabbits the application of skin graft from the same donor during the immediate post-transplant period will cause a corneal graft to cloud.

REFERENCES

Bach, F. H. and Bach, M. L. (1973). Mixed lymphocyte culture and lympholysis assays. *In* "Immunological Aspects of Transplantation Surgery" (ed. Roy Calne), p. 112. M.T.P. Co.

Bain, B., Vas, M. R. and Lowenstein (1964). The development of large mononuclear cells in mixed lymphocyte cultures. *Blood* **23**, 108.

Batchelor, J. R. and Hackett, M. E. J. (1970). HL-A matching in treatment of burned patients. *Lancet* **1**, 581.
Belzer, F. O., Perkins, H. A., Fortman, J. L., Kounz, S. L., Salvatierra, O., Cochrum, K. C. and Payne, R. (1974). Is HLA typing of clinical significance in cadaver renal transplantation? *Lancet* **1**, 774.
Billingham, R. E., Brent, L. and Medawar, P. B. (1954). Quantitative studies of tissue transplantation immunity. II Origin, strength and duration of actively and adoptively acquired immunity. *Proc. R. Soc. B*, **143**, 58.
Bortin, M. M. (1970). A compendium of reported human bone marrow transplants. *Transplantation* **9**, 571.
Bortin, M. M. and Saltzstein, E. C. (1969). Graft versus host inhibition: foetal liver and thymus cells to minimize secondary disease. *Science* **164**, 316.
Buckner, C. D., Clift, R. A., Fefer, P., Lerner, G., Neiman, P. G., Storb, R. and Thomas, E. D. (1974). Marrow transplantation for the treatment of acute leukaemia using HL-A identical siblings. *Transplant. Proc.* **6**, 365.
Butler, W. T. (1975). Corticosteroids and immunoglobulin synthesis. *Transplant Proc.* **7**, 49.
Ceppellini, R. (1971). Old and new facts about transplantation antigens. *In* "Progress in Immunology" (ed. B. Amos), p. 973. Academic Press, London and New York.
Ceppellini, R., Bigliani, S., E. S. and Leigheb (1969). Experimental allotransplantation in man. II. Role of A_1, A_2 and B antigens. *Transplant. Proc.* **1**, 390.
Cheigh, J. S., Stenzel, K. H., Riggio, R. R., Katz, E. B. and Rubin, A. L. (1975). Effects of intravenous methylprednisolone on mixed lymphocyte cultures in normal humans. *Transplant. Proc.* **7**, 31.
Cochrum, K. C., Perkins, H. A., Payne, R. C., Kountz, S. L. and Belzer, F. C. (1973). The correlation of MLC with graft survival. *Transplant. Proc.* **5**, 391.
Debray-Sachs, M., Soucy, P. E. and Hamburger, J. (1973). A lymphocyte cytoxicity rebound phenomenon induced by enhancing sera. *J. Immunol.* **110**, 661.
Descamps, B., Hindlais, N. and Crosnier, J. (1973). Renal transplantation between 33 HL-A identical siblings. *Transplant. Proc.* **5**, 231.
Diethelm, A. G., Dimick, A. R., Shaw, J. F., Baker, H. J. and Phillips, S. J. (1974). Treatment of severely burned child with skin transplantation modified by immunosuppressive therapy. *Ann. Surg.* **180**, 814.
Eddleston, A. L. W. F. (1971). The leucocyte migration test in assessment of rejection. *In* "Immunology of the Liver" (eds M. Smith and R. Williams), Heinemann Medical Books, London.
Eijsvogel, V. P. (1974). Histocompatibility *in vivo* and *in vitro*. *In* "Progress in Immunology. II". Vol. 5 (eds L. Brent and J. Holborow), p. 107. North Holland Publishing Co., Amsterdam and Oxford.
Fialkow, P. J., Thomas, E. D., Bryant, J. I. and Nieman, P. E. (1971). Leukaemic transformation of engrafted human marrow cells *in vivo*. *Lancet* **1**, 251.
Ford, W. L. (1973). Lymphoid cell kinetics in graft-versus-host reactions and allograft rejection. *In* "Immunological Aspects of Transplantation Surgery" (ed. Roy Calne), p. 39. M.T.P. Co.
Gowans, J. L. and McGregor (1965). The immunological activities of lymphocytes. *In* "Progress in Allergy". Vol. IX (eds Kallow and Waksman), Karger, Basel.
Hong, R., Kay, H. E. M., Cooper, M. D., Meuwissen, H., Allan, M. J. G. and Good, R. A. (1968). Immunological reconstitution in lymphopenic immunological deficiency syndrome. *Lancet* **1**, 503.
Human Renal Transplantation Registry—Eleventh Report (1973). *J. Am. Med. Assoc*, **226**, 1197.

Joint Report of Fifth International Histocompatibility Testing Workshop in Histocompatibility Testing (1972). Munksgaard, Copenhagen.
Lerner, K. G., Kao, G. F., Storb, R., Buckner, C. D., Clift, R. A. and Thomas, E. D. (1974). Histopathology of graft-versus-host reaction in human recipients of marrow from HL-A matched sibling donors. *Transplant. Proc.* **6**, 367.
Lopez, C., Simmons, R. L., Mauer, S. M., Najarian, J. S. and Good, R. A. (1974). Association of renal allograft rejection with virus infections. *Am. J. Med.* **56**, 280.
Lower, R. R. (1974). Current status of clinical cardiac transplantation. *Transplant. Proc.* **4**, 107.
Medawar, P. B. (1958). Immunology of transplantation. *Harvey Lecture* **52**, 144.
Merrill, L. P., Murray, J. E., Hartwell Harrison, J. and Guild, W. R. (1956). Successful homotransplantation of the human kidney between identical twins. *J. Am. Med. Assoc.* **160**, 277.
Mitchison, N. A. (1954). Passive transfer of transplantation immunity. *Proc. R. Soc.* 3, **142**, 72.
Oliver, R. T. D., Sachs, J. A., Festenstein, H., Pegrum, G. D. and Moorhead, J. F. (1972). Influence of HL-A matching antigenic strength and immune responsiveness on outcome of 349 cadaver renal grafts. *Lancet* **11**, 1381.
Opeltz, G., Mickey, M. R. and Terasaki, P. I. Unrelated donors for bone marrow transplantation and transfusion support: pool sizes required transplant. *Transplant. Proc.* **6**, 405.
Park, B. H., Good, R. A., Gate, J. and Burke, B. (1974). Fatal graft-versus-host reaction following transfusion of allogeneic blood and plasma in infants with combined immunodeficiency disease. *Transplant. Proc.* **6**, 385.
Porter, K. A. (1974). Histopathology in clinical renal transplantation transplant. *Transplant. Proc.* **6**, 79.
Rapaport, F. and Converse, J. M. (1968). Skin transplantation. *In* "Human Transplantation" (eds F. Rapaport and J. Dauset). Grune and Stratton, New York and London.
Santos, G. (1967). *Exp. Haemat.* **14**, 32.
Santos, G. (1972). Application of marrow graft in human disease: its problems and potential. *In* "Contemporary Topics in Immunobiology". Vol. 1 (ed. M. G. Hanna, Jr.), Plenum Press, London.
Schrek, R. and Donnelly, W. J. (1961). Difference between lymphocytes of leukaemic and non-leukaemic patients with respect to morphologic features, motility and sensitivity to guinea-pig serum. *Blood* **18**, 561.
Snell, G. D. (1953). The genetics of transplantation. *J. Nat. Cancer Inst.* **14**, 691.
Starzl, T. E. (1969). "Experience in Hepatic Transplantation". W. B. Saunders, Philadelphia.
Starzl, T. E., Ishiwaka, M., Putnam, C. W., Porter, K. A., Picache, R., Husberg, B. S., Halgrimson, C. G. and Shroter, G. (1974). Progress in and deterrents to orthotopic liver transplantation with special reference to survival resistance to hyperacute rejection and biliary duct reconstruction. *Transplant. Proc.* **6**, Suppl. 1, 129.
Storb, R., Bluckman, E., Thomas, E. D., Buckner, C. D., Clift, R. A., Fefer, A., Glucksberg, H., Graham, T. C., Johnson, F. L., Lerner, K. G., Neiman, P. E. and Ochs, H. (1974). Treatment of established human graft-versus-host disease by antithymocyte globulin. *Blood* **44**, 57.
Veith, F. J. and Koerner, S. K. (1974). Present status of lung transplantation. *Arch. Surg.* **109**, 734.
Van Rood, J. J., Koch, C. T., Van Hooff, J. P., Van Leeuwen, A., Van Den Tweel, J. G., Fredericks, E., Shippers, H. M. A., Hendricks, G. and Van Den Steen, G. J. (1973). Graft survival in unrelated donor-recipient pairs matched for MLC and HLA. *Transplant. Proc.* **5**, 409.
Williams, D. M., Lynch, R. E. and Cartwright, G. C. (1973). Drug induced aplastic anaemia. *Sem. Haemat.* **10**, 195.

VII

Therapeutic Aspects

30

Drugs Affecting The Immune Response

ERIC R. HURD

In recent years it has become apparent that a large percentage of clinically useful drugs affect immune responses. Most of these agents suppress some part of the immune response, although the value of drugs that can enhance immunological processes is also recognized and it is likely that their clinical application will be more extensive in the future.

IMMUNOSUPPRESSIVE DRUGS: PHARMACOLOGICAL AND IMMUNOLOGICAL ASPECTS

Cytotoxic agents are being used more and more in the treatment of diseases mediated by immune processes such as the rheumatic and connective tissue diseases. Almost every anti-cancer drug has been shown to have immunosuppressive properties, as well as many of the other drug categories shown in Table 1. The most potent immunosuppressive effects, however, are obtained with the cytotoxic drugs. While many of these are loosely termed immunosuppressive, they differ widely in their mechanisms of action, toxicity and efficacy for treatment of non-neoplastic diseases.

The exact mechanisms of action of immunosuppressive drugs are difficult to determine partly because the physiology of the immune response has not yet been completely characterized. Possible target sites (Bach, 1971) are: (a) phagocytosis and antigen processing by macrophages; (b) antigen recognition by lymphocytes; (c) differentiation of lymphocytes; (d) mitosis of thymus-dependent (T) lymphocytes and bone marrow-dependent (B) lymphocytes; and (e) the so-called "final effect" which includes antibody production, secretion of delayed hypersensitivity mediators and lymphocyte cytotoxicity.

TABLE 1

Classes of commonly used agents with immunosuppressive activity

Alyylating agents	Cyclophosphamide (Cytoxan, Endoxana)
	Nitrogen mustard (Mustine)
	Chlorambucil (Leukeran, Chloraminophene)
	Busulfan (Myleran)
	Tri-ethylenethiophosphoramide (Thio-tepa)
	Uracil mustard (Uromustine)
Antimetabolites	
purine antagonists	6-Mercaptopurine (6-MP, purinethol)
	Azathioprine (Imuran)
	6-Thioguanine (Tabloid)
pyrimidine antagonists	5-Fluorouracil (5-FU)
	5-Fluorodeoxyuridine (FUDR, Floxuridine)
	Bromodeoxyuridine (BUDR)
	Cytosine arabinoside (Ara-c, Cytarabinose, Cytosar)
	Iododeoxyuridine (Idoxuridine, Stoxil)
	5-trifluoro-methyldeoxyuridine
	Azauridine (6-azauridine)
	6-azauridine-triacetate
	Azaribine
folic acid antagonist	Methotrexate
Antibiotics	Actinomycins C and D (Dactinomycin, Sanamycin)
	Puromycin
	Mitomycin C
	Rubidomycin (Daunorubicin, Cerubidin)
	Bleomycin (Blenoxane)
	Thiamphenicol
	Chloramphenicol (Chloromycetin)
	Adriamycin (Doxinibicin)
	Rifampicin (Rifadin, Rimactane, and other ansamycins)
	Distamycin A
	Alanosine
	Ovalicin
Hormes	Prednisone, prednisolone (Deltacortril, Precortisyl, Prednelan)
	Oestrogens
Enzymes	L-Asparaginase (Colaspase, Crasnitin)
	L-Glutaminase
	Papain
Vinca alkaloids	Vincristine (VCR, Oncovin)
	Vinblastine (VLB, Velban, Velbe)
Methyl hydrazine derivatives	Procarbazine (Matulane, Natulan)
Antifungal agents	Griseofulvin (Grifulvin, Fulvicin, Grisovin, Fulcin)
Anti-inflammatory drugs	Asprin
	Indomethacin (Indocin, Indocid)
	Phenylbutazone (Butazolidin)
	Gold Salts
	Alclofenac (4 allyloxy-3 chlorophenylacetic acid) (Prinalgin)
	Penicillamine (Distamine)
	Colchicine
Anti-parasitic Agents	Niridazole (Ambilhar)
Miscellaneous	Serotonin
	5-hydroxytryptophan
	Iproniazid (Marsilid)
	Hydroxyurea (Hydrea)

Modified from Mitchell and Bertino (1970).

Alkylating agents and Anti-metabolites

The concept that some of these drugs are *cycle-active* and others *non cycle-active* is helpful in understanding their actions. Bruce (1967) demonstrated that certain drugs, primarily alkylating agents (and also X-ray therapy), kill cells whether or not they are *in cycle*—i.e., in the process of replicating, while other agents, primarily anti-metabolites, are not able to kill if the cells are not in cycle (Fig. 1).

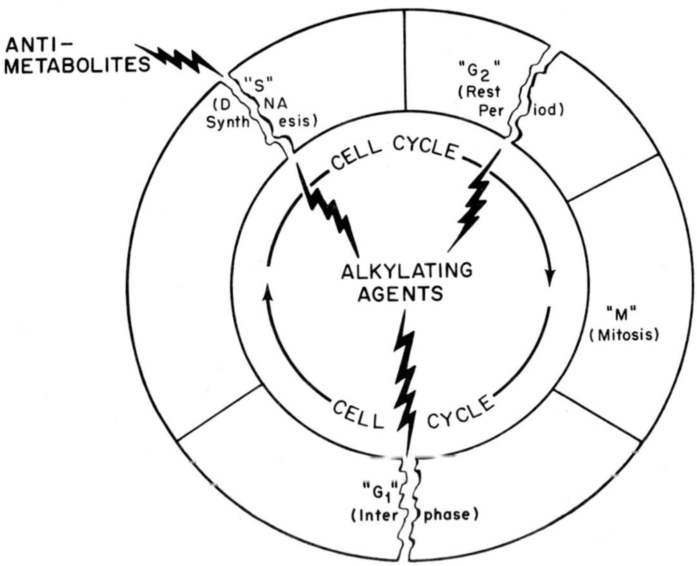

Fig. 1. The different sites of action during the cell cycle of the cytotoxic drugs. Modified from Starzl and co-workers (1972) and Andreis (1974).

The cell cycle may be divided into a G_1 (gap 1) or presynthetic phase, S (DNA synthesizing) phase, G_2 (gap 2) or premitotic resting phase and M phase (mitosis). Cycle active agents may kill by acting at different parts of the cycle, antimetabolites such as methotrexate, azathioprine and 6-MP appearing to act only on cells going through the S-phase. In a nonstimulated lymphocyte population, many of the cells are not in cycle, but in a prolonged G_1 or "G_0" state. These cells are not affected by exposure to cycle active agents, but may be killed by alkylating agents such as cyclophosphamide or by X-rays: although even these seem to kill cells in cycle to a greater degree than cells not in cycle.

Thus, methotrexate and azathioprine (or 6-MP) are *cycle-specific* S-phase inhibitors, while cyclophosphamide has both *cycle-specific* and *non cycle-specific* properties. Methotrexate, azathioprine and 6-MP kill primarily rapidly dividing cells; cyclophosphamide kills both dividing and non-dividing (resting) cells. The detailed pharmacology of these agents is described elsewhere (Calabresi and Parks, 1970; Bertino, 1973).

Of the alkylating agents, busulfan is at one end of a spectrum since it has a marked toxic effect on the bone marrow, primarily suppressing granulocytes and having little effect on lymphocytes. Cyclophosphamide is at the other end of the spectrum, with a very striking effect on circulating blood lymphocytes and a much lesser effect on granulocytes and the bone marrow. Chlorambucil lies in between, having more lymphocytotoxic effect but less bone marrow toxicity than busulfan.

Of the anti-metabolites 6-MP and azathioprine (which is an imidazole derivative of 6-MP) are the most commonly used for treatment of non-neoplastic disease. From the practical standpoint 6-MP and azathioprine are essentially the same although azathioprine is believed by some to have a better therapeutic index.

The three cytotoxic drugs, cyclophosphamide, azathioprine and methotrexate all suppress primary and secondary humoral immune responses, delayed hypersensitivity, skin graft rejection and auto-immune disease in animals. Unfortunately, few studies have compared the effects of these three drugs under the same experimental conditions. However, some striking differences in the mechanism of action of these three agents have become apparent, and are summarized below.

Anti-inflammatory Properties

If egg albumin is injected into the skin of a rabbit, polymorphonuclear leukocytes begin to arrive in the lesion during the first four hours, followed by mononuclear cells. If, however, the animals are pretreated with 6-MP, the polymorphonuclear leukocytes arrive in the lesion normally, but the numbers of mononuclear cells are markedly decreased. Neither cyclophosphamide nor methotrexate have this effect.

We have studied this phenomenon and have found that relative to control animals, animals treated with 6-MP have significantly decreased numbers of large lymphocytes and monocytes in the blood without a significant fall in numbers of polymorphonuclear leukocytes or small and medium lymphocytes. Concurrently, a significant decrease is seen in the percentage of tissue mononuclear cells in the inflammatory skin lesion. There is a highly significant correlation between the numbers of monocytes in the blood and the percentage of mononuclear cells in the lesion. These findings suggest that the anti-inflammatory effect of 6-MP results from suppression of a bone marrow response to local inflammation, affecting principally proliferating precursors of blood monocytes and the large lymphocytes. In agreement with these results other studies show inhibition of mononuclear cell exudation in patients taking 6-MP or methotrexate.

Cyclophosphamide, azathioprine and methotrexate are all effective in reducing the acute inflammation produced by thermal injury or a turpentine-induced pleurisy. There is a rough correlation between improvement and decrease in blood lymphocytes and monocytes but no correlation with polymorphonuclear leukocyte numbers. Comparison of the effects of these three agents on experimental adjuvant arthritis shows that the therapeutic/toxic ratio is most favourable with cyclophosphamide and least with azathioprine. Also, cyclophosphamide treatment brings about a much greater decrease in both lymphocytes and macrophages than either 6-MP or methotrexate in a glycogen-induced peritoneal exudate in the guinea-pig.

Effects on the Antibody-forming System

Studying the effects of cyclophosphamide, methotrexate and 6-MP on anti-typhoid antibody production in mice, Berenbaum and Brown (1964) compared the dose which killed 5% of the animals within one week (LD_5) with the dose required to reduce the antibody response of the mice by a factor of 2 (inhibitory dose—ID_2). They then calculated a therapeutic index which was defined as the ratio of the two doses (LD_5/ID_2). Cyclophosphamide had the highest therapeutic index followed by methotrexate and 6-MP (Table 2). These workers emphasize the fact that the toxicity and immunological effectiveness of these agents are highly dependent on their mode of administration, the nature and quantity of the antigen employed, its mode of administration and the species of animal tested. Results of studies comparing the effects of these three drugs on the primary antibody response to sheep erythrocytes in the rat were very similar, i.e., cyclophosphamide had the best therapeutic/toxic ratio, followed by methotrexate and azathioprine.

The differential effects of azathioprine and cyclophosphamide on humoral antibody production have been demonstrated in patients, with flagellin as test antigen. There was a significant suppression of humoral antibody to flagellin in cyclophosphamide-treated patients while the responses of azathioprine-treated patients did not differ significantly from those of non-treated control patients.

TABLE 2

Therapeutic indices of agents inhibiting antibody production

Agent	LD_5[a]	ID_2[b]	TI[c]
Cyclophosphamide	300·0	50·0	6·0
Methotrexate	6·3	1·25	5·0
6-Mercaptopurine	240·0	100·0	2·4

[a] LD_5 dose (in mg/kg) killing 5% of animals within one week.
[b] ID_2, dose (in mg/kg) lowering antibody titre to $1/2^2$.
c Therapeutic index—LD/ID.
From Berenbaum and Brown (1964).

Santos and Owens (1964) made a comparative study of cyclophosphamide, 6-MP and methotrexate at maximally tolerated doses on the primary agglutinin response in rats immunized with sheep erythrocytes (Fig. 2).

Antigen was given before, at the beginning or in the middle of a five-day course of treatment. Methotrexate and 6-MP were immunosuppressive only when the antigen was administered from two days before to the second day of the five-day course of drug treatment. Cyclophosphamide was immunosuppressive when the antigen was given from two days before to even two days after the end of the five-day course of therapy.

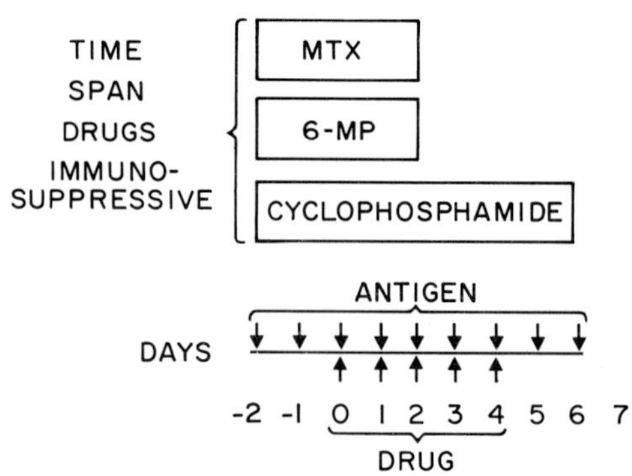

Fig. 2. Effects of methotrexate (MTX), 6-MP and cyclophosphamide on the primary agglutinin response in rats immunized with sheep erythrocytes. Modified from Santos and Owens (1964).

The antimetabolites 6-MP and methotrexate thus appear to suppress mainly an intermediate stage of the primary response, presumably the cellular proliferative phase, while cyclophosphamide suppresses all stages. It has been shown that 6-MP acts only on the so-called inductive phase. In our laboratory, we have shown that cyclophosphamide decreased both Coombs' antibody titre and amount of γ-globulin deposition in the glomeruli of NZB mice, while 6-MP had neither effect. This has recently been confirmed by others.

Cyclophosphamide treatment abolishes the immunoglobulin and complement deposits seen at the epidermal-dermal junction of the skin of NZB/NZW F1 hybrid mice while 6-MP therapy does not. Several workers have shown that cyclophosphamide can decrease anti-DNA antibodies, both in NZB mice and man. This suggests that cyclophosphamide can inhibit an ongoing immune response whereas 6-MP cannot. This is of course the situation that one faces in the treatment of patients, since the relevant immune responses are well established at the time that they are treated. It is of interest in this regard that in patients with systemic lupus erythematosus (SLE), cyclophosphamide treatment can reverse the findings on direct immunofluorescence of the skin whereas steroid therapy alone does not. There is also good correlation between positive skin findings and the presence of clinical or biopsy-proven renal disease and hypocomplementaemia (see Chapter 23).

Effects on Cellular Immunity

Studies of the effects of these drugs on cellular immunity have shown that all three in some circumstances depress cellular immunity. However, comparative studies show a greater effect with cyclophosphamide. For example, cyclophosphamide, but not 6-MP will delay dinitrochlorobenzene (DNCB) responses. A greater depression of the tuberculin reaction occurs with cyclophosphamide than with azathioprine. While both cyclophosphamide and methotrexate are more effective than 6-MP in suppressing a PPD skin test in guinea-pigs, only cyclophosphamide depletes thymus-dependent areas of the lymph nodes. The *in vitro* PHA response was likewise inhibited only by cyclophosphamide. One study showed that even when high doses of 6-MP had suppressed the tuberculin skin test, the animals' lymphocytes responded normally to *in vitro* stimulation by tuberculin, suggesting that what was observed was an anti-inflammatory effect. While both azathioprine and cyclophosphamide suppress immunoglobulin synthesis in patients, only cyclophosphamide suppresses the response of lymphocytes to mitogen. Complete suppression of passive transfer of cell mediated immunity with cyclophosphamide but little effect with methotrexate or azathioprine has been demonstrated. The donor lymphoid cell was shown to be a resting cell sensitive to cyclophosphamide. Tolerance production is much easier to achieve in mice treated with cyclophosphamide than with azathioprine or methotrexate.

Effects on Cell Populations

We have demonstrated that in NZB mice, cyclophosphamide decreases the numbers of recirculating small lymphocytes in the blood, whereas 6-MP preferentially reduces the numbers of polymorphonuclear leukocytes and large mononuclear cells. We have also noted eventual total depletion of small lymphocytes in the majority of our patients on cyclophosphamide. There is a marked decrease in blood lymphocytes with cyclophosphamide treatment, but no effect with either 6-MP or methotrexate. Recently we have demonstrated that in patients on cyclophosphamide, both the bone marrow-derived or B-lymphocytes and thymus-derived or T-lymphocytes are decreased, the reduction in total numbers of B- and T-cells occurring in parallel. This could explain the fact that cyclophosphamide decreases both humoral and cellular immunity. Others have demonstrated depletion of the B-cell compartment in animals on cyclophosphamide. It has also been shown that cyclophosphamide has a selective lymphotoxic action, while 6-MP and azathioprine have only mitostatic properties and no effect on non-dividing lymphoid cells.

Other Effects

In graft-versus-host disease in mice, cyclophosphamide suppresses the disease and prevents mortality, while neither methotrexate nor 6-MP have this effect. However, a study comparing methotrexate and cyclophosphamide treatment in canine graft-versus-host disease showed methotrexate to be superior. In experimental allergic encephalomyelitis cyclophosphamide is much more effective in suppressing the disease than either of the other two agents.

Cyclophosphamide, but not azathioprine, produces potentiation of suppression of anti-sheep red cell antibody and of homograft rejection in thymectomized mice. Small doses of cyclophosphamide produce a highly significant immunological defect in thymectomized animals not reproduced in intact animals.

It has been shown that cyclophosphamide and methotrexate achieve more antibody suppression with less haemopoietic cell suppression than 6-MP. Methotrexate and 6-MP profoundly affect actively proliferating transplanted hematopoietic and antibody-producing cells while cyclophosphamide affects all phases of the cells' proliferative cycle.

Some studies have suggested that azathioprine predisposes more to development of cancer than cyclophosphamide. However cyclophosphamide can also increase the incidence of neoplasia in the NZB/NZW mouse.

Conclusions

There are many discrepancies in the literature concerning the mechanism of action of these drugs. Table 3 is an attempt to summarize their known effects. All three drugs apparently suppress the primary immune response, although the effects of azathioprine and methotrexate are highly dependent on timing. Cyclophosphamide appears to be more effective in suppressing a secondary or ongoing immune response. It is for this reason, perhaps, that cyclophosphamide decreases deposition of immune complexes in the kidney of the NZB mouse whereas 6-MP does not. Azathioprine, 6-MP and methotrexate have more profound anti-inflammatory and mitostatic effects than cyclophosphamide.

TABLE 3

Summary of effects of drugs with alkylating and antimetabolite activity

Effect	Cyclo-phosphamide	Azathioprine and 6-MP	Metho-trexate
Reduced primary immune response	++	++	++
Reduced secondary immune response	++	±	+
Reduced immune complexes in NZB mice	++	0	0
Anti-inflammatory effect	+	++	+
Mitostatic effect	++	++	++
Reduced delayed hypersensitivity	++	+ (?Anti-inflammatory)	+
Suppression of passive transfer of cellular immunity	++	±	±
Lymphopenia	++	±	±
Facilitation of tolerance induction	++	+	+

From Hurd (1973).

Cyclophosphamide seems to have greater effects on delayed hypersensitivity and cellular immunity than either of the other two drugs; depletes small lymphocytes more effectively and produces tolerance much more easily. On the basis of these effects, certain differences in therapeutic indications become apparent.

For suppression of an ongoing immune response and immune complex formation such as occurs in rheumatoid arthritis and in systemic lupus erythematosus, an alkylating agent such as cyclophosphamide would be the drug of choice. It would also be the drug of choice for decreasing delayed hypersensitivity mechanisms or for situations in which elimination of clones of small lymphocytes is desired, since it has a lymphopenic effect.

For an anti-inflammatory effect, anti-metabolites such as azathioprine or 6-MP would be the best choices because these drugs have their greatest effect on dividing cells. It is presumably for this reason that they are effective in diseases such as psoriasis, where there is rapid cellular proliferation. They also affect the primary immune response, and this may be a factor in their known effectiveness in organ transplantation.

One could also postulate that the anti-metabolites may be able to impair the immune response by their ability to kill macrophages which are necessary for its elaboration. In diseases such as Wegener's granulomatosis, in which many macrophages are present in the lesions, anti-metabolites may be the agents of choice.

Methotrexate has immunosuppressive and anti-inflammatory properties which, in general, resemble those of azathioprine.

Pyrimidine antagonists such as azaribine, are effective in controlling moderate to severe psoriasis. Azaribine has practically no effect on the primary antibody response but in the guinea pig repeated administration significantly inhibits cellular immunity.

Antibiotics

The possible effects on the immune system of antibiotic therapy can be summarized as follows: interference with the various steps of protein synthesis, disturbance of processes such as translation, transcription and function of messenger RNA, elimination of antigen, and effects on macrophages and phagocytosis, and indirectly on the properdin system.

Actinomycin D inhibits antibody-forming precursor cells of bone marrow origin *in vivo* as well as *in vitro* anamnestic antibody responses. It inhibits

DNA-directed RNA synthesis, especially messenger RNA. In addition, it inhibits the primary response in rodents and chickens, when injected after the antigen and also impairs the *in vitro* primary response. Ongoing antibody synthesis is not affected. The antibiotic also blocks the lytic action of sensitized lymphocytes, and cell mediated reactions are impaired *in vitro*. Actinomycin C inhibits the primary response. Alanosine inhibits both antibody formation and delayed hypersensitivity in experimental animals if injected with, or prior to, antigen.

Mitomycin C at low doses affects DNA formation but not RNA or protein synthesis whereas at high doses the synthesis of all nucleic acids and proteins is affected. It inhibits the *in vivo* primary humoral immune response but does not affect ongoing antibody synthesis. The drug can cause lymphopenia and inhibits delayed hypersensitivity, and skin graft survival is prolonged in mice.

Puromycin inhibits ongoing protein synthesis *in vitro* and suppresses plaque forming cells. Rubidomycin has been shown to inhibit adjuvant arthritis in rats. Distamycin A produces complete inhibition of the primary immune response to sheep red blood cells *in vitro* when added to the culture within the first 24 hours. Adriamycin inhibits human lymphocyte transformation and is cytotoxic for lymphocytes. It also can suppress PHA-induced lymphocyte stimulation. Bleomycin selectively inhibits PHA responsive cells and thus may preferentially inhibit T-cell transformation *in vitro*. However, experimental studies have shown very little *in vitro* immunosuppressive effects on either the humoral or cellular immune systems. Thiamphenicol inhibits the primary immune response by impairing proliferation of antigen stimulated cells rather than by inhibiting immunoglobulin synthesis. This drug does not inhibit the secondary immune response. Chloramphenicol has neither effect but does inhibit protein synthesis. It also delays allograft rejection although not inhibiting delayed hypersensitivity.

Rifampicin is a commonly used anti-tuberculous agent. It is one of the rifamycins, in turn members of a larger group of substances, the ansamycins. These substances are able to suppress cell-mediated and humoral immunity in several animal species. Rifampicin has similar effects in man, and is the only one used clinically. This drug suppresses the skin test reaction to bovine serum albumin in rabbits, the PPD and DNCB skin tests in immunized guinea-pigs and the antibody response to sheep red blood cells in experimental animals. In man, conventional doses will suppress the PPD skin tests in tuberculous patients after several months of therapy. It also inhibits antibody to *Salmonella typhi* vaccine and keyhole limpet haemocyanin. It is known that rifampicin can inhibit PHA stimulated blast transformation of human peripheral blood lymphocytes.

Some interesting studies have demonstrated that in mice infected with rifampicin-resistant *M. tuberculosis*, both cortisone treated and rifampicin treated animals died sooner than untreated controls. Thus suppression of immunity caused by rifampicin treatment may predispose to bacterial infection and impair resistance to mycobacterial infection.

A major site of action of rifampicin is the macrophage. Phagocytic activity of macrophages and thus antigen handling by macrophages is impaired. The drug has no apparent effect on B- or T-lymphocytes. Concentrations of the drug within the limits used therapeutically do not suppress lymphocyte transformation.

Ovalicin is obtained from *Pseudorotum ovalis* and has been shown to reduce the primary immune response. It can prevent the onset of experimental autoimmune encephalomyelitis in rats and prolong skin allograft survival.

Hormones

The major agents in this group of substances are the glucocorticosteroid hormones of the adrenal cortex and their synthetic analogues prednisone and prednisolone. Oestrogens have weak immunosuppressive effects, particularly on cellular immunity.

Corticosteroids are known to have an anti-inflammatory action and decrease the number of mononuclear phagocytes at sites of inflammation. At certain dose levels treatment of mice or men with corticosteroids can produce a rapid and profound lymphopenia. However, there are considerable differences in susceptibility to glucocorticoids between various species (reviewed by Claman, 1972). The corticosteroid-sensitive species include the hamster, mouse, rat and rabbit while the resistant group includes the ferret, monkey, guinea pig and man.

Studies in patients (Fauci and Dale, 1975) show that four hours after the administration of prednisone, there is a profound lymphocytopenia and monocytopenia, with a differential depletion of thymus-derived lymphocytes. The lymphocytopenia is due primarily to a transient depletion of the recirculating portion of the intravascular lymphocyte pool. All these parameters return to normal by the following day (off prednisone) and remain normal. This drug-associated cyclic and transient monocytopenia and selective lymphocytopenia is probably due to redistribution of recirculating lymphocytes to other body compartments, particularly the bone marrow.

The reduction in mononuclear cells in an inflammatory site which occurs after treatment with glucocorticoids is apparently due to a diminished influx of mononuclear phagocytes from the peripheral blood. As with lymphocytes, corticosteroids apparently have no lytic action on mononuclear phagocytes.

In steroid-sensitive species, both primary and secondary antibody responses are impaired but very little inhibition occurs in steroid-resistant species, although in the latter, including man, steroids can suppress cell mediated immunity if large doses or prolonged treatment are used. For example, prednisone in a dosage of 40 mg per day orally will convert PPD skin tests from positive to negative after an average of 13·6 days.

In addition to the above effects, glucocorticosteroids inhibit chemotaxis of neutrophils and the movement of antigen–antibody complexes across the glomerular basement membrane, thereby diverting them from the capillary loop into the mesangium. They also inhibit release of active kinins from their substrates.

Specific corticosteroid receptors on lymphoid cells have recently been demonstrated. The interaction of these receptors with steroid leads to inhibition of cellular metabolism, including nucleic acid synthesis and glucose uptake.

In summary, corticosteroids in man have strong anti-inflammatory and weak immunosuppressive properties.

Enzymes

L-Asparaginase is an effective chemotherapeutic agent for treatment of human leukaemia. The enzyme catalyses the hydrolysis of asparagine to aspartic acid and ammonia and thus deprives the malignant cells of an essential amino acid, L-asparagine. Since most normal tissues synthesize their own L-asparagine and certain neoplastic tissues (e.g. the lymphoblast in acute lymphoblastic leukemia) do not, the malignant cell is killed.

By the same mechanism the enzyme interferes with activation and growth of lymphocytes inhibiting lymphocyte transformation without impairing cell viability.

L-asparaginase suppresses the primary immune response in mice and rabbits, the best immunosuppression occurring when drug and antigen are injected simultaneously. The drug may act on antigen recognition, before cellular multiplication. In experimental animals, other effects include prolongation of skin graft survival, decreased delayed hypersensitivity and production of lymphopenia with reduction in size of lymph nodes, thymus, and spleen.

It also inhibits the onset of experimental auto-immune encephalomyelitis.

In man, the enzyme suppresses antibody production and cellular immunity and inhibits PHA-induced stimulation of lymphocytes.

L-glutaminase is a glutamine antagonist and inhibits lymphocyte stimulation induced by PHA, streptolysin O and allogeneic antigens.

Anti-inflammatory Drugs

Salicylates have the capacity to suppress antigen–antibody reactions both *in vitro* and *in vivo*. Their effects include suppression of antibody production, interference with antigen–antibody aggregation *in vitro*, inhibition of antigen-provoked histamine release, inhibition of serum sickness and stabilization of capillary permeability following immunological insult. Aspirin can prevent the Schwartzman reaction. It also inhibits the action of complement *in vitro*. In *in vitro* lymphocyte cultures aspirin inhibits lymphocyte transformation. This effect may result from uncoupling oxidative metabolism which compromises energy stores available for mitogenic or antigenic responses. Salicylates also inhibit protein synthesis by PHA-stimulated lymphocytes *in vitro*.

Anti-inflammatory drugs such as aspirin, indomethacin and phenylbutazone have been shown to inhibit the release or activity of prostaglandins, stabilize lysosomal membranes or inhibit lysosomal enzyme activity. Recently these agents have been found capable of inhibiting lymphocyte mediated cytotoxicity in an *in vitro* target cell assay system.

Penicillamine and alclofenac, an arylacetic acid derivative, both significantly decrease levels of immunoglobulins in patients, particularly IgG and IgM. Both drugs may also depress the titre of rheumatoid factor in patients with rheumatoid arthritis.

Gold salts e.g. gold sodium thiomalate, gold sodium thiosulfate, aurothioglycamide or aurothioglucose inhibit the complement system, decrease lysosomal enzyme content or activity and decrease phagocytosis.

Colchicine can arrest plant and animal cell division *in vitro* and *in vivo*. It has a direct effect on cell division. Mitosis is arrested in metaphase due to failure of spindle formation. The drug thus has both anti-mitotic and anti-inflammatory properties. It inhibits phagocytosis and antibody production in mice and rats, and reduces the number of plaque-forming cells in the secondary immune response *in vitro*. Colchicine has no effect on delayed hypersensitivity. The drug inhibits onset of serum sickness in rabbits if it is injected before the antigen.

In general the anti-inflammatory drugs thus have weak immunosuppressive activity.

Anti-Parasitic Agents

Niridazole is an anti-parasitic which is at present the drug of choice for treatment of schistosomiasis. It can suppress manifestations of delayed hypersensitivity and retard allograft rejection in laboratory animals. In patients, it suppresses delayed dermal hypersensitivity to PPD, mumps and schistosome antigens and depresses PPD-induced lymphocyte transformation.

Miscellaneous Agents

The administration of either serotonin itself or drugs which increase serotonin concentration such as 5-hydroxytryptophan or iproniazid, exerts a depressive effect on the humoral immune system. The latent period of antibody production is prolonged, the intensity of the response is decreased, and the attainment of maximal titres is delayed. The secondary immune response is inhibited, and there may be impairment of immunological memory.

Hydroxyurea is a specific inhibitor of DNA synthesis. A single injection of hydroxyurea inhibits DNA synthesis in continuously dividing cells and in tissues stimulated to synthesize DNA by an appropriate stimulus. This drug prolongs graft survival and has weak suppressive effects on antibody production. It has recently been used for treatment of psoriasis.

CLINICAL USE OF IMMUNOSUPPRESSIVE DRUGS

Anti-inflammatory Agents

As noted previously, the anti-inflammatory agents have weak immunosuppressive properties. Their therapeutic efficacy is dependent primarily on their anti-inflammatory effects. Aspirin, indomethacin, phenylbutazone, gold salts, alclofenac and penicillamine all are agents commonly used for treatment of rheumatoid arthritis. The latter three drugs are used almost exclusively for this purpose except for penicillamine which is also used in treatment of

Wilson's disease. Aspirin, of course, is used for a wide variety of pain syndromes and inflammatory conditions. Indomethacin and phenylbutazone are commonly used for treatment of ankylosing spondylitis, Reiter's syndrome, psoriatic arthropathy and acute gouty arthritis. Colchicine is used almost exclusively for treatment of acute gout.

The major side effects seen in patients treated with aspirin include gastric intolerance, tinnitus and deafness. Salicylates also decrease platelet stickiness and prolong the prothrombin time. They should be used with caution in patients with a history of peptic ulcer disease or any bleeding diathesis.

Indomethacin may also produce gastrointestinal intolerance and should similarly be used with caution in peptic ulcer patients.

Phenylbutazone not only has gastrointestinal side effects but may also cause water and sodium retention and may produce an allergic dermatitis. The most serious side effect is that of bone marrow depression. Thus, this drug is contra-indicated in patients with a history of peptic ulcer disease, congestive heart failure and blood dyscrasias. It is also contra-indicated in patients taking oral anticoagulants.

The toxicity and side effects seen with gold salt therapy include (a) a pruritic dermatitis which can become exfoliative, (b) ulcerative stomatitis, glossitis and gingivitis, (c) bone marrow toxicity, especially neutropenia and thrombocytopenia and (d) toxic nephritis with proteinuria and haematuria.

Penicillamine may also cause dermatitis, nephritis and bone marrow depression. A unique form of toxicity is loss of taste which may be due to a deficiency of zinc, and possibly, copper.

The major side effect seen with colchicine treatment is gastrointestinal intolerance.

Corticosteroids

Corticosteroid treatment can bring about dramatic symptomatic improvement in a number of immunological disease states. However, as with the cytotoxic drugs, use of these agents has become extremely widespread in spite of a lack of controlled studies demonstrating that corticosteroids improve prognosis. For example, corticosteroids produce a dramatic response in many patients with rheumatoid arthritis. However, the disease may persist in spite of chronic corticosteroid therapy and the patient then has two diseases, rheumatoid arthritis and iatrogenic corticosteroid-induced complications. A second example is that of acute rheumatic fever. While many physicians use corticosteroids for treatment of the carditis, controlled studies have shown they do not improve prognosis. A third example is the use of steroids for treatment of lupus nephritis (see Table 4).

TABLE 4

Survival in patients with SLE glomerulonephritis treated with glucocorticosteroids

Author	Year	Daily dose and duration of Rx	No. of patients	Result
Bollet	1955	30 mg	7	"no effect"
Rothfield	1963	27 mg	7	5 of 7 dead
Pollack	1964	"low dose"	16	15 of 16 dead
		"high dose" = 50 mg × 6 months	32	16 of 32 dead
Lange	1965	60–100 mg	15	0 of 15 dead
Gary	1967	40–100 mg × 1–5 months	60	25 of 60 dead

From Gingler and Kaplan (1975) in Friedman (1975).

While corticosteroids bring about striking improvement in non-renal clinical features and some laboratory parameters, no adequately controlled studies have yet demonstrated prolongation of life or definite improvement of the glomerulonephritis.

Thus corticosteroids can bring about impressive symptomatic relief, but there is little evidence to show that they actually improve prognosis. When corticosteroids are used, attempts should be made to give the dose on alternate days since a decrease in incidence of side effects has been shown with this mode of therapy. A list of the most common toxic side effects of corticosteroids is shown in Table 5.

Fluid and electrolyte disturbances encountered consist primarily of hypokalaemic alkalosis. Sodium and fluid retention also may occur. Hyperglycaemia and glycosuria, i.e. steroid-induced diabetes mellitus, are also seen, particularly with large doses. In patients with diabetes mellitus, the need for insulin or oral hypoglycaemic agents may be increased.

An increased susceptibility to infection, whether bacterial, fungal, or viral is seen. Peptic ulceration is a quite common complication, and antacids should be given, particularly when large doses of corticosteroids are prescribed.

One of the most serious complications of corticosteroid therapy is the development of osteoporosis with resulting vertebral compression fractures. Pathological fractures of long bones similarly may occur and aseptic necrosis, usually of the femoral or humeral heads, is quite frequent.

Myopathy with muscle weakness and loss of muscle mass may be seen, and there is some evidence that fluorinated steroids e.g. triamcinolone may be more prone to produce this.

Steroid-induced psychosis can be a dangerous complication and the steroid dosage should be decreased if the underlying condition allows.

Many Cushingoid features are seen with chronic corticosteroid administration. The skin becomes very thin and fragile with loss of subcutaneous fat. In

TABLE 5
Toxicity of glucocorticosteroids

Fluid and electrolyte disturbances
Hyperglycaemia and glycosuria
Increased susceptibility to infections
Peptic ulcer
Osteoporosis and vertebral compression fractures
Myopathy
Psychosis
Cushingoid features
"Moon face"
"Buffalo hump"
"Central obesity"
Supraclavicular fat pads
Striae
Ecchymoses
Acne
Hirsutism
Posterior subcapsular cataracts
Aseptic necrosis
Impaired wound healing

addition menstrual irregularities may develop and in children growth may be suppressed.

Posterior subcapsular cataracts and worsening of glaucoma may occur. Hypertensive encephalopathy and pseudo-tumour cerebri may also develop. Alternate day therapy may decrease the incidence of side effects and degree of adrenal suppression. When steroids are tapered too rapidly, the patient may experience symptoms of a steroid withdrawal syndrome which consist primarily of fever, myalgias, arthralgias and generalized malaise.

Cytotoxic Agents

A list of the many non-neoplastic diseases which are either proven or presumed to be immunologically mediated diseases and have been treated with cytotoxic drugs is given in Table 6. Controlled studies are shown in Table 7.

Rheumatoid Arthritis (RA)

Steinberg (1973) has summarized the results of controlled trials using azathioprine or cyclophosphamide for treatment of rheumatoid arthritis or SLE (Table 8).

Several of the RA studies showed improvement in the active joint count, grip strength and morning stiffness and a reduction in synovial effusions with either azathioprine or cyclophosphamide. A significant reduction in the time taken to walk 50 feet has also been noted with both agents. Ability to withdraw corticosteroid therapy without an increase in disease activity has been observed with both drugs. It has been shown that more than 1 mg/kg per day of cyclophosphamide must be given to achieve a beneficial therapeutic response. A dosage lower than this is ineffective and toxicity is similar to that seen with higher dose therapy (1–2 mg/kg per day). In the 32-week study of the Cooperating Clinics Committee of the American Rheumatism Association (1970) high doses (100–150 mg/day) of cyclophosphamide were compared with low or placebo doses (5–15 mg/day). In the high-dose group, there was a significant improvement in grip strength, significant reduction in the number of painful joints and swollen joints and significant reduction in the time taken to walk 50 feet. There was a one-hour reduction in morning stiffness, not quite statistically significant. There was no change in the erythrocyte sedimentation rate. More of the high-dose patients had reductions of rheumatoid-factor titre and of serum IgG than did the placebo group. Of considerable importance was the finding that X-ray erosions were markedly reduced in the high-dose group as compared with the placebo group (Table 9).

A comprehensive review of clinical trials in which various immunosuppressive agents have been used for therapy of RA is that of Currey (1971).

In summary, results of controlled trials of azathioprine and cyclophosphamide in the treatment of severe RA suggest that both drugs, when given in sufficient quantity, are capable of suppressing disease activity. However, toxic effects were also observed.

Systemic Lupus Erythematosus (SLE)

In the controlled SLE studies in which azathioprine was used a number of beneficial effects were seen i.e. an increase in creatinine clearance, a decrease in proteinuria and a decrease in mortality. However, discontinuance of the azathioprine was associated with severe exacerbations of the disease. A decrease in glomerular cell proliferation has been noted in renal biopsies from SLE patients receiving azathioprine.

TABLE 6

Immunological conditions which have been treated with cytotoxic drugs

Haematological

- Autoimmune haemolytic anaemia
- Idiopathic thrombocytopenia purpura (ITP)
- Hyperglobulinaemic purpura
- Cryoglobulinaemia
- Erythroid aplasia
- Circulating anticoagulants

Rheumatological

- Rheumatoid arthritis
- Systemic lupus erythematosus
- Scleroderma
- Polymyositis and dermatomyositis
- Polyarteritis nodosa
- Wegener's granulomatosis
- Psoriatic arthropathy
- Behcet's syndrome
- Reiter's syndrome
- Felty's syndrome

Renal

- Allo-transplantation
- Chronic glomerulonephritis
- Goodpasture's syndrome
- Idiopathic nephrotic syndrome

Gastrointestinal

- Ulcerative colitis
- Regional enteritis
- Chronic active hepatitis
- Acute hepatitis
- Primary biliary cirrhosis

Dermatological

- Psoriasis
- Bullous pemphigoid
- Pemphigus
- Pyoderma gangrenosum
- Behcet's syndrome
- Sezary's syndrome

Ophthalmological
Uveitis
Sympathetic ophthalmia
Graves' ophthalmopathy
Keratoconjunctivitis sicca
Corneal graft failure
Neurological
Myasthenia gravis
Multiple sclerosis
Polyneuropathy
Pulmonary
Asthma
Goodpasture's syndrome
Pulmonary fibrosis
Sarcoidosis
Cardiological
Pericarditis

Modified from Steinberg *et al* (1972).

In a 10-week double-blind controlled trial comparing cyclophosphamide, azathioprine and placebo in the treatment of lupus glomerulonephritis (Steinburg and Decker, 1974) renal function, urine sediment, proteinuria, anti-DNA antibody, C3 and symptoms were assessed before and after therapy in 38 patients. Cyclophosphamide was significantly superior to both azathioprine and placebo for all six measures together and for the three renal measures alone. Cyclophosphamide was significantly better than placebo with regard to proteinuria, urinary RBC, and serum C3. Azathioprine was not significantly better than placebo in any individual measure.

Thus controlled studies suggest that both azathioprine and cyclophosphamide are efficacious in the treatment of SLE with perhaps some slight advantage with cyclophosphamide. However, more long-term information is necessary to determine whether the beneficial effects outweigh the toxic ones.

TABLE 7
Controlled clinical studies of cytotoxic therapy

Disease	Design	Result
Rheumatoid arthritis	corticosteroid-sparing effect	prednisone requirement lowered by azathioprine treatment
Rheumatoid arthritis	conventional vs. low doses of cyclophosphamide	cyclophosphamide ameliorated clinical and radiological signs of disease
Rheumatoid arthritis	cyclophosphamide vs. placebo (double-blind crossover)	cyclophosphamide effective
Rheumatoid arthritis	cyclophosphamide vs. placebo (double-blind)	small doses of cyclophosphamide ineffective
Rheumatoid arthritis	azathioprine vs. placebo (double-blind)	azathioprine effective
Psoriatic arthritis	methotrexate vs. placebo	skin and joint manifestations improved in methotrexate treated group
Psoriatic arthritis	azathioprine vs. placebo (double-blind)	azathioprine effective
Systemic lupus erythematosus	azathioprine plus prednisone vs. prednisone (prospective)	azathioprine effective
Regional enteritis	azathioprine vs. placebo	azathioprine ineffective
Regional enteritis	azathioprine vs. placebo	azathioprine diminished relapse rate
Chronic active hepatitis	azathioprine vs. prednisone	both agents effective
Chronic active hepatitis	chlorambucil vs. vitamins	chlorambucil ineffective
Nephrotic syndrome (children)	cyclophosphamide vs. no maintenance	cyclophosphamide effective in preventing relapse after induction of remission with prednisone
Nephrotic syndrome (children)	azathioprine vs. placebo	azathioprine ineffective
Nephrotic syndrome (adults)	azathioprine + prednisone vs. prednisone	either schedule ineffective
Glomerulonephritis	azathioprine or cyclophosphamide vs. no treatment	neither drug effective
Glomerulonephritis	azathioprine + prednisone vs. no treatment	no effect of treatment
Lupus nephritis	cyclophosphamide vs. placebo	cyclophosphamide may be effective
Multiple sclerosis	cyclophosphamide vs. no treatment	cyclophosphamide ineffective
Bronchial asthma	6-MP vs. conventional treatment	6-MP ineffective

From Skinner and Schwartz (1974).

TABLE 8

Summary of controlled trials in the treatment of rheumatoid arthritis and SLE with azathioprine (AZ) or cyclophosphamide (CY)

Disease	No. of patients	Drug	Dose[a]	Duration (months)	Result[b]
RA	49	AZ	High	12	+
	18	AZ	High	6	+
	10	AZ	High	4	+
	48	CY	High	8	+
	22	CY	High	9	+
	22	CY	Low	12	−
	54	CY	Low	8	−
SLE	35	AZ	High	6–48	+
	16	AZ	High	6	−
	13	AZ	High	38	+
	17	AZ	High	$2\frac{1}{2}$	0
	19	CY	High	$2\frac{1}{2}$	+
	13	CY	High	$2\frac{1}{2}$	+
	14	CY	Low	2–4	−

[a] High dose about 1·5–3·0 mg/kg per day; low dose about 0·7–1.4 mg/kg per day.
[b] +: favourable effect, −: no favourable effect, 0: uncertain.
Modified from Steinberg (1973).

TABLE 9

Number of joints with new or worse erosions

Group	No. of joints evaluated	Joints worse on initial film		Joints worse on final film	
		Observer A	Observer B	Observer A	Observer B
Low-dose (5–15 mg)	864	2	2	41	25
High-dose (100–150 mg)	648	0	0	3	2

From Cooperating Clinics Committee of American Rheumatism Association (1970).

Other Rheumatic Diseases

There appears to be little doubt that these agents (particularly azathioprine, 6-MP and methotrexate) are very effective in treatment of the classical type of psoriatic arthritis. Two controlled studies demonstrating improvement have been published, one using methotrexate and the other azathioprine. We have also observed striking improvement in all of 11 patients with classical psoriatic arthritis who were treated with 6-MP.

Although no controlled studies have been reported, beneficial effects of these agents have been reported for polymyositis, juvenile rheumatoid arthritis, Behcet's syndrome, Reiter's syndrome, Wegener's granulomatosis and scleroderma.

Gastrointestinal Diseases

In the treatment of chronic active hepatitis, both prednisolone and azathioprine have been found effective while chlorambucil has not.

Both azathioprine and 6-MP have been reported to be beneficial for treatment of inflammatory bowel disease but there are few controlled studies.

Haematological Diseases

Auto-immune haemolytic anaemia is best treated by use of corticosteroids and splenectomy. However, beneficial effects have been observed with 6-MP, thioguanine and chlorambucil.

Both azathioprine and cyclophosphamide have been reported to be effective for treatment of corticosteroid-refractory idiopathic thrombocytopenic purpura (ITP) but no controlled trials have been performed.

Cyclophosphamide, azathioprine and 6-MP have been reported as beneficial for controlling the haemorrhagic disorder associated with antibodies against factor VIII.

Neurological Diseases

Some patients with multiple sclerosis have improved with cyclophosphamide treatment and myasthenia gravis has been treated with both azathioprine and cyclophosphamide. The overall efficacy is difficult to evaluate in these studies.

The Problem of Toxicity

The differential toxicity of cytotoxic drugs has been compared by Decker (1973). The most common type of toxicity is, of course, due to effects on the bone marrow and haemopoiesis. All are capable of inducing bone marrow suppression. The degree of marrow suppression is usually dose related and can be modulated by dose changes, although rarely they cause idiosyncratic and irreversible marrow failure. In Table 10 a summary of the differential toxic effects of three agents is given.

TABLE 10

Relative frequencies of unwanted drug effects

	Cyclophosphamide	Azathioprine	Methotrexate
Oral ulcers	−	−	+
GI intolerance	+	−	+
Hair loss	++	−	+
Cystitis and bladder fibrosis	++	−	−
Infection	+	+	+
Teratogenesis	+	+	+
Hepatic damage	−	+	++
Aspermia	++	−	+
Anovulation	++	−	−
Neoplasia	+	++	+

Modified from Decker (1973).

Methotrexate can cause problems throughout the gastrointestinal tract Painful oral ulceration may occur, and with higher doses ulcerative lesions of the oesophagus, stomach and small bowel may produce a haemorrhagic enteritis. Nausea, vomiting and diarrhoea may occur even in the absence of ulcerative lesions. Nausea and, more rarely, vomiting, may complicate oral cyclophosphamide administration but, in controlled trials, the infrequency is only slightly greater than in placebo controls.

Alopecia occurs most commonly with cyclophosphamide and more rarely with methotrexate treatment. Total alopecia is uncommon and regrowth occurs upon drug withdrawal and usually, to some degree, even when the drug is continued.

A side effect which is unique for cyclophosphamide is cystitis which is produced by one of the metabolic breakdown products of the drug in the urine. Acute cystitis may occur with or without bleeding and may be associated with abnormal cytology. With time, the drug may slowly produce bladder fibrosis and telangiectasia of the mucosa wall. Uncontrollable bleeding from the bladder has been reported months after the drug has been stopped. The bladder fibrosis may prove to be a seriously disabling complication.

Transitional cell carcinoma of the bladder has been reported in cyclophosphamide-treated patients. Cyclophosphamide-induced cystitis in dogs can be ameliorated by bladder irrigation with acetyl cysteine but has not yet been used in humans. To minimize urinary bladder complications, large fluid intakes should be encouraged and instructions given to take the medication at bedtime.

The risk of infection is increased in patients treated with these agents, presumably because of suppression of immune mechanisms.

Virus infections such as measles and varicella may disseminate with a fatal outcome. The incidence of herpes zoster seems to increase but the course of the viral lesions is similar to that in otherwise normal individuals. Increased susceptibility to virus infections may be related to inhibition of interferon production, as has been shown for cyclophosphamide.

Tuberculous and fungus infections are much more likely to disseminate on these drugs than in the untreated individual and there are many reports of opportunistic infections such as cytomegalovirus or *Pneumocystis carinii* and fungal infections such as *Candida* and *Aspergillus*.

Teratogenic effects have been observed with all three agents, but mothers receiving these agents have also borne normal children. According to Decker (1973) the appropriate delay between stopping the drug and permitting conception is of uncertain duration; four months is sometimes suggested. Chromosomal changes have been described.

Hepatic damage is a serious and limiting factor in the chronic administration of methotrexate, whereas although azathioprine occasionally produces changes in liver chemistry these do not persist. Hepatitis and fibrosis resulting from methotrexate therapy are clearly related to total dose and duration of administration. With azathioprine or mercaptopurine, hepatotoxicity includes features of both intrahepatic cholestasis and parenchymal cell necrosis either of which may predominate. Irreversible liver damage has been reported with both azathioprine and 6-MP. Intermittent intravenous methotrexate may be less hepatotoxic than the orally administered drug.

The effects of cyclophosphamide and other alkylating agents upon gonadal tissues must be of major concern in younger patients. Ovulation stops, perhaps permanently, in a substantial proportion—probably 20–30%—of women maintained on effective doses of cyclophosphamide (2 mg/kg/day). Evidence from semen analyses, testicular biopsies and serum FSH levels shows even more profound effects on spermatogenesis, with permanent aspermia in men who receive as little as six months of treatment. The mechanism of the destruction of ova is unclear. It is of interest that neonatally thymectomized mice develop an identical ovarian pathology, since this raises the possibility that cyclophosphamide affects the ovary indirectly through its effect on the thymus and cellular immunity.

Probably the major concern in treatment with these agents is the possibility of inducing malignancy. Since one of the postulated roles of the immune system is surveillance and eradication of neoplastic clones, malignancies might be expected in patients on immunosuppressive drugs. Results of several studies are shown in Table 11. In 108 patients with rheumatoid arthritis treated with cyclophosphamide, two developed malignancies, one a reticulum cell sarcoma, another chronic lymphatic leukaemia. In 204 patients with psoriatic arthritis treated with methotrexate, seven patients developed neoplasms. In the Denver kidney transplantation group patients were treated with

TABLE 11

Incidence of neoplasms in patients on immunosuppressive drugs

Disease	No. of cases	Incidence (%) Cyclophosphamide	Azathioprine	Methotrexate
Rheumatoid arthritis	2/108	2·0%		
Psoriatic arthritis	7/204			3·4%
Transplant patients (Denver)				
including skin tumours			6·0%	
excluding skin tumours			3·8%	
Non-transplant	3/4000		0·07%	
Normal incidence			0·06%	

azathioprine and high dose steroids. A particularly worrying and peculiar lesion has been seen in the transplant group; 22 cases of lymphoma, of which 11 were intracerebral, occurred in a group of 5,000 recipients of kidney grafts. The foreign tissue in these patients may have acted as a chronic antigenic stimulus and this, with the corticosteroids given to all the patients, may be contributing to the development of the tumours. A more encouraging survey of 4,000 non-transplant patients treated with azathioprine revealed only three cases of neoplasm, approximately the normal expected incidence. It is of interest that in the NZB/NZW F1 mouse, 6-MP appears to be more likely to induce tumours than cyclophosphamide.

The American College of Surgeons Human Renal Transplant Registry (1973) reports that among 6,297 kidney-transplant recipients, the risk of developing lymphoma was 35 times higher than normal due almost entirely to reticulum-cell sarcoma, with an incidence 350 times greater than expected. Skin and lip cancers occurred four times more often than expected and other cancers, mostly soft-tissue sarcoma and hepatobiliary carcinoma, were 2·5 times more common. Other studies have also demonstrated an increased incidence of skin cancer in immunosuppressed patients.

Finally, a number of unusual and peculiar side-effects and reactions have occurred in patients taking these agents, e.g. meningitic reactions, fever, rash and headache, and acute renal insufficiency with azathioprine; pulmonary infiltrates with methotrexate; and pigmentation of the nails and teeth with cyclophosphamide.

Because 6-MP and azathioprine are degraded by xanthine oxidase and allopurinol is an inhibitor of xanthine oxidase, the dosage of azathioprine, or 6-MP should be reduced to one-third to one-fourth the usual dose, in patients on this drug.

Methotrexate is bound in part to serum albumin and toxicity may be increased by displacement by certain drugs, e.g. salicylates, sulphonamides, diphenylhydantoin, tetracycline, chloramphenicol, and para-amino-benzoic acid.

General Guidelines for Clinical Use

Guidelines for the use of cytotoxic drugs in the rheumatic diseases as set forth by Schwartz and Gowans (1971) are abstracted in Table 12 and should be followed in treatment of any patient with non-neoplastic disease. Both azathioprine and cyclophosphamide have been used at dosage levels between 0.7 mg/kg per day and 3·0 mg/kg per day (Table 8). It has been shown that less than 0·7 mg/kg per day of cyclophosphamide is clinically ineffective. In addition, the toxicity in the lower dosage range is similar to that of the higher

TABLE 12

Guidelines for use of cytotoxic drugs in non-neoplastic diseases

Life-threatening or seriously crippling disease
Reversible lesions must be present
Failure to respond to conventional therapy or intolerable side effects
No active infection
No haematological contraindication
Meticulous follow-up
Objective evaluation must be used
Informed consent
Protocol must be submitted for peer review

Modified from Schwartz and Gowans (1971).

dosage level. In the studies shown, the longest treatment period was 48 months. The exact length of time a patient should continue treatment with these agents is unknown. In general, however, attempts should probably be made to withdraw the drug if a patient has been in remission for 6 months to one year. It is probably wise to taper gradually the dosage level over a few weeks or months.

The dosage of 6-mercaptopurine is approximately 2 mg/kg per day. Methotrexate can be given in a variety of treatment schedules. With both drugs, liver function tests should be done frequently.

Differential Immunosuppression

Although cytotoxic drugs such as cyclophosphamide, methotrexate and 6-MP are generally used as non-specific immunosuppressive agents, under certain experimental conditions they can be used to suppress antibody production selectively without interfering with cell mediated immunity. Such a selective effect may be helpful in suppressing humoral blocking factors and allowing cell mediated immunity to be more fully expressed, for example in patients with solid tumours. Low doses of 5-fluorouracil, cytosine arabinoside and combinations of methotrexate and 5-fluorouracil will achieve the same results

When administered prior to antigen, amethopterin and 6-MP can enhance antibody formation, as studies on the production of splenic haemolysin plaque-forming cells in mice show (Table 13). The numbers of plaque-forming cells were increased by methotrexate and 6-MP but markedly suppressed by cyclophosphamide. When the drugs were given after antigen injection, there was suppression by all three drugs, but cyclophosphamide produced the greatest decrease. In earlier experiments along the same lines, it was shown that enhancement of antibody production results when antigen is administered five days after the last dose of a one-week course of 6-MP. Possibly this enhancement is due to the adjuvant effect of nucleic acids released from cells killed by the drug. Such an effect might explain the deterioration seen in some patients with SLE in whom azathioprine has been discontinued. Triggering of auto-immune haemolytic anaemia by X-irradiation and alkylating agents has been observed in patients with lymphosarcoma and chronic lymphocytic leukaemia.

Cyclophosphamide can suppress antibody formation and markedly enhance cellular immunity when given as a single injection 2 weeks after a BCG injection. The delayed hypersensitivity response may persist for as long as 6 months. It is also of interest that cyclophosphamide improves the environment for haemopoietic stem cell proliferation. Pretreatment with cyclophosphamide causes an increased rate of regeneration of transplanted stem cells in the marrow cavity of a lethally irradiated host.

TABLE 13

Action of immunosuppressants on the primary immune response to sheep RBC in mice

	Per cent of control response			
	Before antigen injection		After antigen injection	
Treatment	Increase	Decrease	Increase	Decrease
Amethopterin, 100 mg/kg	163	—	—	21
6-Mercaptopurine, 120 mg/kg	161	—	—	15
Cyclophosphamide, 200 mg/kg	—	1	—	1

From Uyeki (1967).

SUMMARY

A large number of therapeutic agents have some degree of immunosuppressive activity. The most potent is the cytotoxic group of drugs. The majority of the antibiotics, enzymes, anti-inflammatory drugs, anti-parasitic and the miscellaneous drugs listed in Table 1 have only weak immunosuppressive properties. Glucocorticosteroids have quite potent anti-inflammatory properties but weak immunosuppressive effects. This is particularly true in man, a relatively steroid-resistant species. Because of their potent immunosuppressive effects, the use of cytotoxic agents for the treatment of various types of non-neoplastic diseases has increased over the past several years.

Corticosteroids and three major types of cytotoxic drug have been the primary agents used. The latter are (1) alkylating agents, particularly cyclophosphamide (Cytoxan); (2) purine analogues such as 6-mercaptopurine (6-MP) (Purinethol) and azathioprine (Imuran) which is a derivative of

6-MP and (3) folic acid antagonists, e.g., methotrexate. These three groups of drugs have different mechanisms of action. In general, they all exert anti-inflammatory effects and decrease both humoral and cell mediated immunity. However, cyclophosphamide appears to be the best agent for killing small lymphocytes, decreasing circulating immune complexes, decreasing a secondary, or ongoing, immune response, decreasing cellular immunity and producing tolerance. The other drugs, 6-MP, azathioprine, and methotrexate, have more potent anti-proliferative and anti-inflammatory effects and, while able to decrease a primary immune response, have little effect on a secondary immune response. These agents predominantly kill monocytes and large lymphocytes.

For the above reasons, cyclophosphamide should be the drug of choice for treatment of diseases with circulating immune complexes or deposition of complexes such as one finds in systemic lupus erythematosus or rheumatoid arthritis. The other agents are most useful for their anti-proliferative effects, as in the treatment of psoriasis and psoriatic arthritis.

Although clinical results have been encouraging, the incidence of harmful side effects militates against widespread use of these agents.

In general, the major side effects include bone marrow toxicity, increased risk of infection of all types, possible increased risk of teratogenesis, increased incidence of sterility (particularly with cyclophosphamide), liver damage (6-MP and methotrexate), haemorrhagic cystitis and urinary bladder fibrosis (cyclophosphamide) and finally, the possibility of increased incidence of malignancy.

Use of these agents should be restricted to patients with life-threatening disease such as systemic lupus erythematosus with renal disease, or life-crippling disease such as severe chronic disabling rheumatoid arthritis which has failed to respond to conventional means of therapy.

More controlled trials and long-term follow-ups are necessary before a final assessment can be made of the proper use of immunosuppressive drugs in the treatment of patients with non-neoplastic diseases. Future studies may demonstrate combined therapy to be superior to the use of single agents without increasing toxicity. Intermittent therapy may also be of value. Other ways of manipulating immunological responses for therapeutic purposes are discussed in the next chapter.

REFERENCES

Andreis, M. (1974). Immunosuppression in the treatment of rheumatoid arthritis. Basic principles and available substances. *In* "Selected Therapeutic Problems in Rheumatoid Arthritis" (eds G. H. Fallet and T. L. Vischer), pp. 81–88. Urban and Schwargenberg, München-Berlin-Wien.

Bach, J. F. (1971). Immunosuppression by chemical agents. *Transplant. Proc.* **3**, 27.

Berenbaum, M. C. and Brown, I. N. (1964). Dose-response relationships for agents inhibiting the immune response. *Immunology* **7**, 65.

Bertino, J. R. (1973). Chemical action and pharmacology of methotrexate, azathioprine and cyclophosphamide in man. *Arth. Rheum.* **16**, 79.

Bruce, W. R. (1967). The action of chemotherapeutic agents at the cellular level and the effects of these agents on hematopoietic and lymphomatous tissue. *Can. Cancer Conf.* **7**, 53.

Calabresi, P. and Parks, R. E., Jr. (1970). Alkylating agents, antimetabolites, hormones, and other antiproliferative agents. *In* "The Pharmacological Basis of Therapeutics" (eds L. S. Goodman and A. Gilman, 4th ed. pp. 1348–1395. Macmillan Co., London, Toronto, New York.

Claman, H. N. (1972). Corticosteroids and lymphoid cells. *New Engl. J. Med.* **287**, 388.

Cooperating Clinics Committee of the American Rheumatism Association: A controlled trial of cyclophosphamide in rheumatoid arthritis. (1970). *New Engl. J. Med.* **283**, 883.

Currey, H. L. F. (1971). Immunosuppressive drugs in rheumatoid arthritis. *Mod. Trends Rheumatol.* **2**, 174.

Decker, J. L. (1973). Toxicity of immunosuppressive drugs in man. *Arth. Rheum.* **16**, 89.

Fauci, A. S. and Dale, D. C. (1975). Alternate day prednisone therapy and human lymphocyte subpopulations. *J. Clin. Invest.* **55**, 22.

Friedman, E. A. (ed.) (1975). Proceedings of the first international symposium on corticosteroids as immunosuppressive drugs, 1974. *Transplant. Proc.* **2**, 1.

Hurd, E. R. (1973). Immunosuppressive and anti-inflammatory properties of cyclophosphamide, azathioprine and methotrexate. *Arth. Rheum.* **16**, 84.

Mitchell, M. S. and Bertino, J. R. (1970). The pharmacology of immunosuppressive agents. *Conn. Med.* **34**, 843.

Santos, G. W. and Owens, A. H. (1964). A comparison of the effects of selected cytotoxic agents on the primary agglutinin response in rats injected with sheep erythrocytes. *Bull. Johns Hopkins Hosp.* **114**, 384.

Skinner, M. D. and Schwartz, R. S. (1972). Immunosuppressive therapy. *New Engl. J. Med.* **287**, 221.

Skinner, M. D. and Schwartz, R. S. (1974). Immunosuppressive therapy of immunoinflammatory diseases. *In* "Rheumatology" (ed. J. Rotstein), pp. 1–48. S. Karger, Basel.

Schwartz, R. S. and Gowans, J. D. C. (1971). Guidelines for the use of cytotoxic drugs in rheumatic diseases. *Arth. Rheum.* **14**, 134.

Starzl, T. E., Putnam, C. W., Halgrimson, C. G., Groth, C. G., Booth, A. S. and Penn, I. (1972). Renal transplantation under cyclophosphamide. *Transplant. Proc.* **4**, 461.

Steinberg, A. D., Plotz, P. H., Wolff, S. M., Wong, V. G., Agus, S. G. and Decker, J. L. (1972). Cytotoxic drugs in treatment of nonmalignant diseases. NIH Conference. *Ann. Int. Med.* **76**, 619.

Steinberg, A. D. (1973). Efficacy of immunosuppressive drugs in rheumatic diseases. *Arth. Rheum.* **16**, 92.

Steinberg, A. D. and Decker, J. L. (1974). A double-blind controlled trial comparing cyclophosphamide, azathioprine and placebo in the treatment of lupus glomerulonephritis. *Arth. Rheum.* **17**, 923.

Uyeki, E. M. (1967). Effects of several anti-tumor agents on spleen hemolysin plaque-forming cells. *Biochem. Pharmacol.* **16**, 53.

31

Therapeutic Manipulation of the Immune Response

W. G. REEVES

The previous chapter has discussed the role of drugs in the control of untoward immunological responses and as with most forms of drug therapy each individual agent is not wholly specific for the target at which it is aimed. Non-specific "immunosuppression" is now widely used for many diverse problems and is to date the only satisfactory way of controlling homograft rejection in man. Nevertheless, the hazards of such an immunological blitzkreig are great and opportunistic infection is still one of the commonest causes of death among renal transplant recipients.

On the other side of the chemotherapeutic balance sheet is the extraordinary success story of sodium cromoglycate which has transformed the management of atopic disease (notably extrinsic asthma) and so far has produced very little in the way of side-effects (see Chapter 22). It is hoped that further agents will appear for controlling other parts of the immunological system in such a localized and seemingly benign manner.

Much effort is currently directed toward discovering more sophisticated means of modulating immunological responses without disturbing other systems of the body. As further information is gained concerning the control mechanisms which operate during normal immunological responses then the manipulation of these positive and negative influences becomes more feasible (see Chapter 2). Cannon's concept of physiological homoeostasis (Cannon, 1932) is just as applicable to the immunological system and the notion of therapeutic immuno-regulation is now becoming a very attractive prospect for the management of a wide variety of disorders.

STATES OF HOST RESPONSIVENESS

Before manipulating a complex system it is necessary to be aware of the various states of activity or responsiveness which it can adopt. Few immunological events take place without some degree of untoward effect occurring within the host organism and Table 1 lists six patterns of responsiveness which may occur. *Specific reactivity* (in any of its three forms) occurs naturally and can also be induced experimentally or therapeutically in most situations where it is desired. *Specific non-reactivity* is currently a great challenge to immunological investigators and when successfully developed as a means of achieving graft acceptance will transform the management of organ-failure as well as the correction of various inborn errors of metabolism.

Non-specific reactivity is the least well documented category of all. It seems reasonable to postulate that failure or absence of the normal negative controlling influences e.g. suppressor cells, should result in a generally hyperactive state. Impaired suppressor cell activity has been described in patients with systemic lupus as well as their counterpart, the NZB/W hybrid mouse, and many studies have indicated the inordinately high levels of anti-

TABLE 1
States of host responsiveness

Response state	Examples
Specific reactivity: *Hetero-immunity* without host damage	Response to oral polio vaccine Graft rejection
Specific reactivity: *Hetero-immunity* with host damage	Post-primary tuberculosis Drug hypersensitivity
Specific reactivity: *Auto-immunity*	Idiopathic Addison's disease Auto-immune haemolytic anaemia
Specific non-reactivity:	"Enhancement" of renal allografts Response to some tumours
Non-specific reactivity:	Auto-immune disorders e.g. S.L.E. Some bacterial and viral infections Atopic disease
Non-specific non-reactivity: i.e. "anergy"	Primary immunodeficiency Sarcoidosis Hodgkin's disease Lepromatous leprosy

bodies that are present, reacting with a wide variety of antigenic material (Hollinger *et al.*, 1971). Certain microbial infections e.g. those due to EB virus, hepatitis B and various others, are associated with a variety of transiently positive auto-antibodies. Whether this is a positive adjuvant-like effect or represents an inhibition of the normal suppressor mechanisms is uncertain. Evidence from Tada *et al.* (1975) has demonstrated that the control of reaginic antibody production is conducted by a T-cell population which when absent allows an indiscriminate increase in this class of antibody. This may prove to be an important model for the events taking place in atopic disorders (see Chapter 22).

Non-specific non-reactivity occurs either as primary immunodeficiency or as a secondary phenomenon complicating various diseases such as those listed in the table. It is possible that the individuals who develop such anergic disorders may be constitutionally prone from the outset to respond in this particular way to microbial invasion and recent evidence suggests that the immune response to *Mycobacterium leprae* in man is associated with genes in the major histocompatibility complex (De Vries *et al.*, 1976). Immune response genes are recognized in various animal systems (see pp. 38–39) and several examples have been described in man. Non-specific non-reactivity or "anergy" is usually documented on the basis of absent delayed hypersensitivity skin reactions and impaired responses of peripheral blood lymphocytes to standard antigens. A reduction in numbers of reactive cells or their inordinate suppression is the most likely explanation for a generalized lack of responsiveness to a broad range of antigenic material. Where the impaired responsiveness is only seen against a single or localized group of antigen(s) it is possible that all the specifically reactive cells may already be fully preoccupied in the disease lesion. Evidence in support of this possibility comes from work on the inoculation of tumour cells into the afferent territory of draining lymph nodes (Alexander *et al.*, 1969) and also from studies on skin test negative patients with mycobacterial infections (Rook *et al.*, 1976).

The various immunological manipulations which are currently available or seem a near prospect will be discussed under the heading of the four broad categories of response as outlined in Table 2. Listed against these four categories are the various means of inducing each state of responsiveness. The ways in which the reverse or "corollary" state may be achieved are the same means by which the initial state of responsiveness can be corrected e.g. a state of *specific reactivity* to a particular antigen can be brought about by a process of active immunization, passive immunization or the reversal of specific suppression. On the other hand, the correction of a state of *specific reactivity* to one of *specific non-reactivity* may be achieved by inducing

TABLE 2

Manipulations of the immune response classified according to the state of host responsiveness that they produce

SPECIFIC REACTIVITY
(a) Active immunization
(b) Passive administration of specific antibody
(c) Reversal of specific suppression
SPECIFIC NON-REACTIVITY
(d) Clonal deletion or inactivation
Suppressor cells
Anti-idiotype reactivity
Antigen as "tolerogen"
(e) Peripheral blockade by antibody
(f) Specific immunoadsorption
(g) Competition between different classes of specific antibody
NON-SPECIFIC REACTIVITY
(h) Immunological reconstitution
Marrow transplantation
Thymus transplantation
Thymus extracts and hormones
Transfer factor
Leucocyte transfusion
γ-globulin administration
(i) Adjuvants and immunotherapy
(j) Levamisole
(k) Reversal of suppression
NON-SPECIFIC NON-REACTIVITY
(l) Lymphoid ablation
Irradiation
(m) Lymphocyte suppression
(n) Inhibition via G.V.H. response
(o) Plasma exchange

clonal deletion or inactivation, peripheral blockade by antibody or specific immunoadsorption and vice versa. The same corollary is applicable between *non-specific reactivity* and *non-specific non-reactivity*. Each manoeuvre is discussed in turn according to the sequence listed in Table 2. Some manoeuvres have specific as well as non-specific features e.g. transfer factor and suppressor cells, and these are listed in both situations as they arise.

SPECIFIC REACTIVITY

(a) Active Immunization

Inducing a mature immunological response to a pathogenic organism before the individual becomes naturally exposed to it, seems, at first sight, an eminently sensible way of preventing an infectious disease. That such a concept is often a naive simplification has become abundantly clear with increasing knowledge concerning the role of the host response in the pathogenesis of infectious disease (see Chapter 1) and the practical experience associated with the introduction of most forms of active immunization. The earliest form, variolation with smallpox crusts, had a mortality of 2–3% and was displaced by Edward Jenner's introduction of the alternative procedure of "vaccination" (*vacca*—a cow) utilizing material prepared from cowpox vesicles. Many successful regimes of active immunization against bacterial and viral diseases now form part of current practice but few have been entirely free from untoward effects. Vaccines are generally of two kinds: live attenuated organisms or inactivated "killed" material. *Bacillus Calmette-Guerin* (B.C.G.) is a live attenuated vaccine which has been used for inducing protection against *Mycobacterium tuberculosis* since the 1920s. The Lubeck disaster in 1930 provided a chastening example of the potential hazard underlying all live vaccines—that of admixture or contamination with more virulent material. In this case it led to the death of 77 out of a total of 251 neonates who had been given B.C.G. contaminated with a more pathogenic strain (Arbeiten aus dem Reichsgesundheitsamte, 1935).

Although the introduction of vaccines for tetanus, diphtheria, whooping cough, cholera, typhoid and yellow fever has been a considerable advance over the earlier method of passive immunization with immune sera, their efficacy is not 100% and they can give rise to unpleasant side-effects in a significant but small minority. The pertussis extract which forms part of the conventional "triple" vaccine is currently under meticulous scrutiny and there is a difficult balance to be found between the extremely rare but authenticated neurological sequelae (Kulenkampff *et al.*, 1974) and the prospect of a falling acceptance rate throughout the population with the inevitable consequence of outbreaks of a potentially serious paediatric illness (Warin, 1974). Frequent adverse reactions were described following the introduction of an inactivated measles vaccine (Fulginiti *et al.*, 1967) and unacceptable side-effects also occurred after the administration of a vaccine against respiratory syncytial virus (Kapikian *et al.*, 1969). In both instances immunized individuals developed a more severe illness after natural exposure to the wild virus than their non-immunized counterparts. The attenuated measles vaccines in current use are well tolerated and cause convulsions less often than the naturally acquired disease. Measles vaccination programmes are of particular importance in the Third World where it is one of the major causes of death in infancy. The acceptance rate for measles vaccination in the UK is only about 50% and this is undoubtedly connected with the adverse publicity surrounding the use of pertussus vaccine.

The use of oral polio vaccine is now well accepted and the protection it provides has been shown to correlate with the development of specific IgA in the gastrointestinal secretions (Ogra *et al.*, 1968). Although the parenterally administered vaccine produced reasonable levels of serum antibody this was not associated with a satisfactory level of immunity. Many other kinds of infectious disease are now susceptible to prevention by active immunization although some such as influenza present special problems associated with continuing change and "drift" in the antigenic nature of the prevalent virus.

Despite the trials and tribulations of vaccine production, a great deal of energy is currently being expended toward broadening their application to embrace such diverse and major problems as venereal disease, tropical diseases (notably malaria) and dental caries. Malaria still competes for being the major cause of death on a world wide basis and experimental studies in which active immunization has been used against sporozoites, as well as others concentrating on the merozoite stage of the parasite, hold out promise for a successful vaccine in the future (Cohen and Sadun, 1976). Recently, carious Rhesus monkeys have been shown to benefit from immunization with an inactivated *Strep. mutans* vaccine (Lehner *et al.*, 1976) suggesting that a programme of immunization may help to solve the problem of dental caries in man.

As a particular vaccination programme becomes increasingly successful in eradicating an infectious disease it is inevitable that the reasons for continuing such prophylaxis are increasingly questioned in view of the progressive rarity of the primary problem. If the acceptance rate falls significantly, the reappearance of epidemics of the disease in question can produce much more severe effects on the population concerned in view of the lack of herd or background immunity. Such a dilemma is currently posed by the smallpox eradication programme and various countries (including the UK) have elected to discontinue recommending smallpox vaccination as a routine procedure. If smallpox is not totally eradicated on a world-wide basis then there are grave risks of serious epidemics developing in the future.

(b) Passive Administration of Specific Antibody

The passive administration of hyperimmune sera has largely been replaced by the development of active vaccines. Nevertheless, anti-sera are available for the management of acute infections with *Clostridium tetani*, *Cl. welchii* and *C. diphtheriae*. These antisera are usually raised in the horse and their administration has the attendant problem of adverse reactions developing against the foreign protein. This possibility has encouraged the development of preparations of human anti-tetanus immunoglobulin derived from out-dated bank blood. Other preparations of human globulin are available for the treatment and prophylaxis of infections with hepatitis B, rubella, small-pox, mumps, and varicella zoster virus.

Several workers have endeavoured to conjugate anti-tumour antibody with noxious materials in an attempt to inhibit tumour growth. Ghose and co-workers demonstrated that the administration of ^{131}I labelled antibody can inhibit the growth of the Ehrlich ascites tumour in mice (Ghose *et al.*, 1967) and *in vitro* studies with daunomycin conjugated anti-tumour antibody have shown toxicity for mouse lymphoid tumour cells (Levy *et al.*, 1975). In a human study, chlorambucil conjugated antibody has given rise to clinical regression of cutaneous melanoma metastases although the intravenous administration of this heterologous anti-serum had to be discontinued because of anaphylactic reactions (Ghose *et al.*, 1975). It is possible that modifications of this technique will offer a novel approach to the control of malignant disease and the incorporation of such material into liposomes may enhance its effect (Gregoriadis, 1976).

Rhesus Iso-immunization

Rhesus iso-immunization is one of many undesirable forms of specific reactivity and paradoxically the administration of anti-D antibody during the post-natal period (Clarke *et al.*, 1963) has been a major advance in its prevention. There may be special facets of the Rhesus system and the mode of natural immunization which have favoured the success of this enterprise.

It does not rely on the "blindfolding" of Rhesus antigens *per se* for if Rhesus positive cells that are also Kell positive are given to Rhesus negative volunteers followed by anti-Kell antibody then immunization against the Rhesus phenotype is still prevented. The mechanism for this effect is obscure but seems likely to be a form of antigen sequestration rather than specific unresponsiveness.

(c) Reversal of Specific Suppression

The possibility of reversing the effect of suppressive influences on the immune response is discussed in more detail under non-specific effects in section (k) below. The use of cyclophosphamide to inactivate suppressor B-cells in the guinea-pig (Polak and Turk, 1974) and the development of antisera specific for the suppressor subpopulation of T-cells in the mouse suggest that similar manoeuvres may become possible in man.

SPECIFIC NON-REACTIVITY

The classical experiments of the 1950s on the induction of "actively acquired tolerance" (Billingham *et al.*, 1956) held out great promise for human organ transplantation. Further work in animals showed that "low" or "high" zone tolerance could be induced by the administration of widely differing doses of antigen and adoptive transfer studies demonstrated the differential susceptibility of T- and B-lymphocytes to the tolerizing stimulus (Chiller *et al.*, 1971). It soon became clear that the tolerant state was very difficult to maintain over a long period. Significant prolongation of allogeneic skin grafts has been achieved by treating recipient mice with a short course of anti-lymphocyte serum (ALS) in conjunction with a high dose of F1 hybrid spleen cells (Lance and Medawar, 1969). A similar effect has been observed in cyclophosphamide treated mice injected with sheep red blood cells (Many and Schwarz, 1970) and these effects may well be caused by the destruction of antigen-stimulated cells. The mechanisms which may apply when specific unresponsiveness can be induced in adult animals have been recently reviewed (Brent and Kilshaw, 1976). Deletion of a specifically reactive clone of cells fitted the clonal selection theory of immunity most aptly but various other intriguing explanations have since appeared to challenge this view (Dresser, 1976).

The discovery of other phenomena, such as suppressor cells and anti-idiotype reactivity, has further complicated the classical explanations for the tolerant state and it is preferable to maintain the term "immunological tolerance" for most kinds of specific unresponsiveness without implying any particular underlying mechanism (Dresser, 1976). Three possible mechanisms by which such a state may be achieved will now be discussed with additional comment concerning the role of suppressor cells and anti-idiotype reactivity in their operation. Competition between different classes of specific antibody (category (g)) is not strictly an example of "tolerance" but is included at the end of this section in view of its ability to modulate the effect of an immune response. The prevention of Rhesus iso-immunization by the administration of anti-D antibody post-natally is not, strictly speaking, an example of specific unresponsiveness and is discussed further on pp. 685 and 1107.

(d) Clonal Deletion or Inactivation

There is still a considerable body of evidence in support of clonal absence, in a functional sense, as the explanation for neonatally induced tolerance in experimental animals (Brent *et al.* in Dresser, 1976). Most of the work opposing this view, comes from studies using the micro-cytotoxicity test developed by Hellstrom *et al.* (1971). The mechanism of killing in this test is still unclear and may not have an absolute requirement for T-cells. Furthermore, the animals that were used in their studies may well have been only partially tolerant.

Even when there is convincing evidence of absent reactivity to a particular specificity in a truly tolerant animal it is still very difficult to distinguish between the genuine absence of specifically reactive cells i.e. clonal deletion, and the presence of specifically non-reactive cells i.e. clonal inactivation (Brent *et al.* in Dresser, 1976). Neonatally induced tolerance may well be associated with an irreversible deletion of reactive cells but various other models of the tolerant state—especially those in which the unresponsiveness is transient or capable of reversal by immunization regimes—are more likely to be due to clonal inactivation. Whether such an effect is achieved by anti-idiotype reactivity or specific suppressor cells or a combination of both is debated.

Suppressor Cells

Evidence for the existence of cells which can specifically suppress rather than augment or "help" an immune response has been accumulating since the description of "infectious tolerance" in 1972 (Gershon and Kondo, 1972). This model demonstrated that lymphoid cells taken from mice rendered tolerant to sheep erythrocytes could suppress the response of normal cells challenged with an immunogenic dose of this antigen. The enhanced antibody production demonstrated following thymectomy or the administration of anti-lymphocyte globulin (Baker *et al.*, 1973) could be explained on this basis, as also could the immunosuppressive effect of graft-versus-host reactions (Katz, 1972). A model of allotype suppression in the mouse has also been shown to be mediated by suppressor T-cells (Herzenberg *et al.*, 1973) and a similar phenomenon relating to idiotype suppression is described below. Various animal studies have demonstrated the specific nature of the suppression and that it is usually mediated by a subpopulation of T-lymphocytes (Zembala and Asherson, 1973; Taussig, 1974).

Animals have been shown to develop an increased incidence of autoimmune disorders when T-cell depleted and there is good evidence for impaired suppressor T-cell function in the New Zealand mouse (NZB/W) hybrid when it develops its lupus-like disease (Talai and Steinberg, 1974). Evidence of suppressor cell activity in man includes a non-specific suppressive effect of T-cells taken from patients with variable hypogammaglobulinaemia (Waldmann *et al.*, 1974) and erythroid-colony suppressing lymphocytes in aplastic anaemia (Hoffman *et al.*, 1977). The suppressor subpopulation of T-lymphocytes has unique surface properties (Taylor and Basten, in Dresser, 1976) and in man it is preferentially stimulated *in vitro* by concanavalin A (Hubert *et al.*, 1976). The role of suppressor cells in the production of tolerant responses is discussed by Taylor and Basten and the possibility that they may express anti-idiotype activity is both an economical and an attractive one. This brings the transplantation story full circle and experiments by Brent's group have demonstrated their role in at least one model of specific unresponsiveness to histo-compatibility antigens (Kilshaw *et al.*, 1975).

Anti-idiotype Reactivity

The unique and specific chemical configuration of an antibody combining site—known as the "idiotype"—can itself be immunogenic when injected into a suitable host. The same is true of the antigen receptor on lymphoid cells and Ramseier and Lindenmann (1972) were the first to demonstrate the production of anti-idiotype antibodies when parental strain mouse cells were injected into an F1 hybrid. Although the parental strain cells are not rejected by the F1 hybrid, some of them do contain specific receptors for the histo-compatibility antigens of the other parent. These idiotypic determinants, not being found in the hybrid animal, are recognized as foreign and induce the production of anti-idiotypic antibody (previously described as aliotypic). If such reactivities gave exact mirror-images then one might expect the configuration of the anti-idiotype combining site to be identical with the original antigenic determinant itself. As the antigen-combining site is a cleft-like structure it becomes difficult to envisage an antibody reacting with it as a total fit and it seems more likely that anti-idiotypic antibodies react against individual determinants located towards the more complex edge of the combining site. It then becomes possible to envisage a progressive series of anti-idiotypic reactivities extending from the original combining site and these intriguing possibilities have caused several authors to propose "network theories" of the immune response by which most established phenomena can be explained (Raff, 1977).

At a more practical level, the prospect of raising antibodies specific for the idiotype or receptor of a clone of reactive cells suggests that there may be exciting possibilities for the highly specific manipulation of the immune response with particular reference to immunosuppression. As with most forms of operationally defined tolerance, this should allow the specific inhibition of an individual response with preservation of an otherwise intact immunological apparatus. This has already been realized at an experimental level. Long lasting unresponsiveness can be induced in neonatal mice by the administration of anti-receptor antibody although mice treated as adults were only suppressed for several weeks and their cells responded normally in culture (Strayer *et al.*, 1974). Work by Wigzell's group has shown that significant prolongation of allogeneic skin grafts can be achieved in the rat by treatment with anti-idiotype antibody (Binz and Wigzell, 1976). There may be important limiting conditions determining the efficacy of anti-idiotype reagents e.g. the concentration of the idiotype present in the recipient animal, and it is too early to tell whether this approach will provide the answer for antigen-specific immunosuppression in man. Anti-idiotype reagents have been used to identify monoclonal cells in B-cell lymphomas and lymphocytic leukaemias (Hough *et al.*, 1976) and they may have a wider application to auto-immunity and infection in addition to malignant disease (Lewis *et al.*, 1976). A further development of interest is that the administration of a low dose of anti-idiotype antibody can give rise to chronic specific suppression which can then be adoptively transferred by a subpopulation of T-lymphocytes—by definition "suppressor cells" (Eichmann, 1975).

Antigen as "Tolerogen"

In the preceding part of this section on specific non-reactivity little mention has been made of the role of antigenic structure in its elicitation. It has been known for many years that specific unresponsiveness to contact sensitizers can be induced in animals by the prior administration of hapten, orally or intravenously, and much of the evidence points to the role of suppressor cells in this phenomenon (Polak and Geleick, 1975). Attempts have also been made to modulate or inhibit auto-immune reactivity by the introduction of antigenic material and complete reversal of experimental allergic encephalomyelitis (EAE) has been achieved in the Rhesus monkey by giving daily injections of encephalitogenic antigen daily for 12 days after the onset of clinical signs of EAE (Eylar *et al.*, 1972). This is probably brought about by the direct effect of antigen on sensitized lymphocytes as also seems to be the case in the process of "densitization" to contact sensitivity and is often a short-lived phenomenon.

Other work has shown that haptenic determinants can readily induce specific unresponsiveness when coupled to non-immunogenic carrier molecules e.g. host immunoglobulin or a random synthetic polymer of D-glutamic acid and D-lysine. Borel *et al.* (1976) and Chiorazzi *et al.* (1976) have in this way induced specific and long-lasting tolerance to the benzyl penicilloyl (BPO) hapten which is responsible for most of the reactivity in reaginic hypersensitivity to penicillin. They were also able to reverse established sensitivity to this material. Whatever the mechanism for this phenomenon may be it holds considerable promise for the prevention and modification of untoward reactivity in man once the relevant antigenic determinants have been defined.

(e) Peripheral Blockade by Antibody

The phenomenon that prior immunization with non-viable tumour extracts could promote the subsequent growth of a tumour inoculum was first described in 1907. Casey later coined the term "enhancement" and Kaliss first showed that the effect was mediated by antibody (Feldman, 1972). Various animal studies demonstrated that this principle could be used to encourage the acceptance of foreign grafts and prolonged survival has been observed with kidney, heart, skin, ovary, testis and lymphoid tissue. Skin is the most difficult tissue to enhance and the survival time of any graft is more readily prolonged if the histocompatibility difference is a minor one. Under these conditions renal allografts have maintained function indefinitely in the rat (French and Batchelor, 1969) and some success has been achieved in man (Batchelor *et al.*, 1970).

Various observers have suggested that renal grafts may do better when their recipients have previously received blood transfusions (Opelz and Terasaki, 1976) although whether the administration of blood stored by freezing has an even greater effect is debated (Fuller *et al.*, 1977). Such blood, although largely free of granulocytes, still contains its lymphocyte population and other work shows that kidney grafts do well in the presence of incompatibility of the B-lymphocyte alloantigen system (Ettinger *et al.*, 1976). This system of antigens comparable to the Ia system in the mouse (see p. 39) is now considered to be of particular importance in the production of enhancing effects (Batchelor and Welsh, in Dresser, 1976). The phenomenon of "graft adaptation" is also of interest here, for, under certain defined circumstances, grafts that have already survived in a host can be accepted by another host which simultaneously rejects a fresh graft of similar origin. This phenomenon is not widely applicable and established grafts transferred into unmodified secondary hosts usually undergo a slow process of rejection.

Although the administration of donor specific antibody can suppress allograft rejection it is likely that other mechanisms operate to achieve a steady state beyond the stage of induction (Batchelor and Welsh, in Dresser, 1976). Recipient animals bearing "enhanced" kidney allografts show a progressive decline in cellular immunity against donor antigens and it is not possible to transfer non-reactivity with serum from graft-bearing animals. Such animals are able to accept further tissue of identical donor origin without any other immunological manipulation whereas untreated animals of recipient strain reject such tissue in the normal way. Various attempts to abrogate this state of specific unresponsiveness such as active or adoptive immunization fail to cause rejection. Experiments in which animals bearing long-surviving "enhanced" kidney grafts are maintained in parabiosis with syngeneic immunized partners show that the latter develop a weakened capacity to reject renal allografts (Bowen *et al.*, 1974). This indicates the presence of an active inhibitory process and a model of unresponsiveness developed by Brent's group suggests that a suppressor cell population may be active in the steady state phase of graft enhancement (Kilshaw *et al.*, 1975).

There is thus good evidence to show that the initial phase of passive enhancement is readily achieved by antisera directed against recipient histocompatibility antigens particularly of Ia specificity (Batchelor and Welsh, in Dresser, 1976). To arrive at a permanent or steady state of enhancement requires the functional inactivation of the killer subpopulation of T-cells (T_1) which may be achieved via the suppressive activity of another T-cell subset.

(f) Specific Immunoadsorption

The *in vitro* technique of affinity chromatography or solid-phase immunoadsorption has been widely used in recent years for the removal and/or purification of individual molecules including antigen and antibody (Cuatrecasas, 1972). The presence of specific antibody in the circulation of patients during the active phase of various immunological disorders has prompted experimentation aimed at utilizing this technique in the form of an on-line immunoadsorption module connected directly to the circulation. Initial experience with a bovine serum albumin immunoadsorbent connected to the circulation of immunized rabbits achieved partial depletion of antibody and this system has been improved by the use of protein-substituted nylon catheters inserted into the inferior venae cavae of heparinized dogs (Lyle *et al.*, 1974). Accurate information about the chemical nature of the relevant antigen is required for comparable studies in man and Goodpasture's syndrome, Rhesus haemolytic disease and systemic lupus are obvious candidates. *In vitro* and *in vivo* studies have been performed with a DNA system (Terman *et al.*, 1976) and a 65% reduction in the DNA binding level of human serum was achieved by using a DNA-cellulose immunoadsorbent incorporated into agar gel. Other work has explored the possibility of removing tumour associated antigen from the serum of two patients with malignant disease (hypernephroma and carcinoma of the colon, respectively) using $F(ab)_2$ tumour antibody fragments conjugated to the surface of a polymethyl methacrylate immunoadsorption chamber (Langvad *et al.*, 1975).

Although intensive and non-specific plasmaphoresis is being applied to an ever-increasing number of clinical situations (see p. 1131) it is relatively crude in concept and makes considerable demands on materials necessary for plasma replacement. The possibility of specific removal suggests that the efficient depletion of antibody or antigen from the circulation of patients may become a practical method of treatment. The success of such manoeuvres will depend very largely on the chemical characterization of the relevant antigenic material; the investigation of which has been a Cinderella area of immunology for too long. The removal of specific antibody is usually associated with increased *in vivo* production due to positive feedback effects consequent upon the reduced circulating level (Schenkein *et al.*, 1971) and the combination of administering a cytotoxic drug or anti-lymphocyte reagent at the time of maximal response may augment the effect of specific removal. Those patients with Goodpasture's syndrome who have been successfully treated by intensive non-specific plasmaphoresis have also received such therapy (Lockwood *et al.*, 1976).

Specific immunoadsorption has also been achieved experimentally at the cellular level by continuous drainage of the efferent lymphatic of an antigen-stimulated lymph node in the sheep (McConnell *et al.*, 1974) and a situation more akin to clonal deletion follows the administration of sufficient radioactive antigen in the mouse (Willcox *et al.*, 1975). Neither of these approaches seem readily applicable to man but the trapping of specific cells has been demonstrated in antigen-coated columns and the recently developed fluorescence-activated cell sorter (Julius *et al.*, 1974) is capable of separating lymphocytes according to their surface immunochemistry—provided that an appropriately specific fluorescein-conjugated antiserum is available. Extensions of such methods may aid the search for practical methods of clonal inhibition or removal in the future.

(g) Competition Between Different Classes of Antibody

Amelioration of the untoward effects of a specific antibody response can be achieved by tilting the balance between biologically active and biologically inactive antibody molecules bearing the same specificity. This has often been alleged to be the basis for "desensitization" of reaginic hypersensitivity (see p. 772) where IgG "blocking" antibody favourably competes for IgE antibody. Complement fixation of IgG anti-dengue antibody can be blocked by the concomitant appearance of antibody of IgM class (Scott and Russell, 1972) and non-complement fixing IgG_1 can favourably compete with complement fixing IgG_2 allo-antibody in the mouse (Harris and Harris, 1972). Of more clinical relevance is the finding that non-neutralizing IgG antibody can inhibit the neutralizing effect of IgA antibody in herpes simplex keratitis (Centifanto and Kaufman, 1971). Undoubtedly there are many other examples of inter-class competition between antibody molecules and this phenomenon may be of especial importance in the modulation of the final pathways of the immune response.

NON-SPECIFIC REACTIVITY

(h) Immunological Reconstitution

Marrow Transplantation

Severe combined immune deficiency (S.C.I.D.—see pp. 515–519) is the primary immunological indication for marrow transplantation although success has also been achieved in chronic granulomatous disease (The Westminster Hospitals Bone-marrow Transplant Team, 1977). Much more experience has been gained in the use of marrow transfer in the management of leukaemia and aplastic anaemia (Thomas, 1975). Marrow transplantation presents formidable problems when both donor and recipient are immunologically competent. Immunosuppressive "preconditioning" is necessary to prevent rejection of even a histocompatible sibling graft. This is usually achieved by giving high dose cyclophosphamide or other cytotoxic agents before grafting and a greater effect may be achieved by preceding this with a sensitizing transfusion of donor cells to activate the relevant clones of cells prior to administration of the cytotoxic drug. The use of marrow transplantation in leukaemia is based on an aggressive programme of whole body irradiation usually in combination with cyclophosphamide and "immunotherapy" with irradiated autologous leukaemic cells. It is also possible that a degree of graft-versus-host response may help to augment the anti-leukaemic effect (Bortin, 1974).

In S.C.I.D. little in the way of immunosuppressive treatment is required if a compatible sibling donor can be found. These patients are particularly prone to develop serious graft-versus-host reactions and the closeness of the match is critical, especially where unrelated donors are being considered. A fatal graft-versus-host reaction can occur following transfusion of a single unit of unirradiated blood and prior irradiation will functionally eliminate any lymphocytes contained therein. In one instance an incompatible bone marrow graft was successfully used in S.C.I.D. by utilizing the presence of an antibody in the mother's blood showing specificity for both the father's and the patient's lymphocytes (Buckley *et al.*, 1971). This was shown to block one-way (maternal→ paternal) MLC responsiveness. The patient was then given marrow cells from her mother with infusions of maternal plasma both before and for some time after this procedure to achieve a form of "enhancement" (see page 1112) of host acceptance by the graft. This helps to illustrate the difficulties surrounding the location of compatible donors on the one hand and the means of abrogating the specific immune response on the other; both of which have encouraged the search for other tissue which may be able to reconstitute patients with S.C.I.D.

Initial experience with foetal thymus or foetal haematopoietic (liver) tissue were unsuccessful even when both sources of material were given together. A recent report (Buckley *et al.*, 1976) demonstrates that it is possible to reconstitute with foetal liver alone and other work (Hong *et al.*, 1976) demonstrates that transplantation with thymic epithelium obtained from short-term culture of normal human thymus can reconstitute both T- and B-lymphocyte function in S.C.I.D. The period of *in vitro* culture was associated with the loss of host lymphocytes. This controversial finding suggests that combined immunodeficiency may result from a primary defect of the thymus. Whatever the explanation for this may be it is clear that the development of foetal tissue banks will greatly assist this means of reconstituting patients with various forms of immunodeficiency (Markowski and Lawler, 1977). Reconstitution of patients with aplastic anaemia or lethally-treated leukaemia has a much greater requirement for haematopoietic cells and it is likely that the establishment of large panels of carefully matched prospective marrow donors will continue to be necessary for these other purposes.

Thymus Transplantation

Primary T-cell deficiencies in the presence of normal B-cell function are readily corrected by the grafting of foetal thymus tissue. Thymus grafts continue to produce their beneficial effect when enclosed within a millipore chamber and this is a useful way of reducing the chances of a graft-versus-host reaction. It also confirms that potent soluble factors generated in thymic tissue are responsible for most of its immunopoietic effect.

Thymus Extracts and Hormones

Miller's classical observation that the thymus had a key role in immunological maturation has been followed by increasing interest in the nature of the differentiation factors involved (Friedman, 1975). Several soluble materials have been extracted from thymus tissue and have been shown to be effective in nanogram quantities on cells of the T-lymphocyte series (White, in Friedman, 1975). The two main contenders are thymopoietin (previously called thymin) and thymosin, each having a protein structure with a molecular weight of the order of 10,000. These materials promote the maturation of T-lymphocytes from stem cells and are able to restore various functional impairments associated with T-lymphocyte deficiency i.e. numbers of E-rosettes, responsiveness to T-cell mitogens, MLC responsiveness and graft-versus-host reactivity. It has been suggested that one of the target cells for the activity of these thymus derived factors may be the "null" cell. Certainly it would seem to belong to a subset of T-cells or their immediate precursors (Bach, 1976).

Sensitive assays have been developed for these materials including radioimmunoassay and a rosette bioassay. These methods have revealed the presence of thymic hormones in the blood of man and animals and have shown that their levels are significantly reduced in the presence of deficiencies of the T-cell compartment. The increase in numbers of peripheral blood lymphocytes which form rosettes with sheep red blood cells can be used as an *in vitro* assay for the thymic hormone effect. An impressive increase in seen *in vitro* when cells are taken from patients with most forms of T-cell deficiency and this may prove to be a useful way of deciding whether thymosin replacement is likely to be successful in an individual case *in vivo*. Daily administration of thymosin to a child with thymic hypoplasia gave rise to improvement in T-cell rosettes as well as delayed hypersensitivity skin tests although *in vitro* responses to T-cell mitogens remained unchanged (Wara *et al.*, 1975). Other work has shown that the acquired T-cell deficiency manifest in New Zealand hybrid (NZB/W) mice can be corrected by the administration of thymosin and that the *in vitro* incubation of peripheral blood lymphocytes from patients with active SLE corrects the T-cell lymphopenia and reduces the number of "null" cells (Scheinberg *et al.*, 1975). Another study has shown that the T-cell lymphopenia which follows the administration of influenza virus can be reversed *in vitro* in the presence of thymosin as evidenced by the increase in E-rosettes (Scheinberg *et al.*, 1976). It is likely that the administration of purified thymic extracts will obviate the necessity for thymus grafting once sufficient quantities of the material become available and that its use may be extended to other anergic states including malignant disease.

Transfer Factor

This material was discovered by Lawrence when he observed that the passive transfer of cellular immunity could be achieved by using non-viable lymphocytes instead of intact cells (Lawrence, 1955). He also showed that leukocyte homogenates could perform the same function. Since then transfer factor has been used in many experimental and clinical situations, yet the finer points of its chemical structure and biological activity remain controversial (Ascher *et al.*, 1976). Transfer factor is usually prepared by taking buffy-coat cells from a unit of blood. These are frozen and thawed and then dialysed against water or culture medium. The dialysate is concentrated and checked for sterility prior to administration. Lyophilization is the preferred method of storage. Variations in the method of preparation have given rise to different forms of transfer factor designated by different subscripts i.e. TF_D is a generic symbol for all dialysed preparations; TF_W and TF_{DM} indicating that the starting material has been dialysed against water and medium respectively. TF_C and TF_G denote that further purification has been performed by chromatographic separation. Other designations such as TF_Z (indicating its origin in Zurich) add to the potential confusion.

It has been customary to prepare TF from cells taken from a donor who exhibits marked reactivity to the antigen to which the recipient shows only poor or absent reactivity. Much of the experimental work has been done within the tuberculin or PPD system and it has become clear that the degree of reactivity transferred does not necessarily correlate with the level of donor reactivity and can follow the administration of TF prepared from PPD-negative sources. The use of such a complex antigen as PPD may well have blurred the edges of the specificity of transfer and studies using donors recently sensitized to keyhole limpet haemocyanin (KLH) have demonstrated more convincing evidence of specificity of transfer as well as a degree of correlation between the level of donor reactivity and the degree of subsequent responsiveness of the recipient (Zuckerman *et al.*, 1974). Other workers (Ascher and Andron, in Ascher *et al.*, 1976) have emphasized the importance of using reciprocal controls in any specificity studies of the activity of transfer factor and have also found that antigens other than PPD usually give a reasonable correlation between the level of donor sensitivity and the degree of sensitivity achieved in the recipient. Various investigations have shown that the augmenting effect of transfer factor on lymphocyte transformation of recipient cells to antigen is often antigen dependent rather than antigen specific and is only seen when pre-committed, antigen-reactive cells are present within the recipient lymphocyte population (Hamblin *et al.*, and Cohen *et al.*, in Ascher *et al.*, 1976). Augmentation of recipient lymphocyte transformation has been rarely observed in the absence of antigen and it is likely that the antigen dependent effects have both specific and non-specific features, the former relating to the specificity of donor reactivity (Arala-Chaves *et al.*, in Ascher *et al.*, 1976).

The vagaries of the different methods of preparation and the different sources of starting material, in addition to uncertainty about its mode of action, demonstrate the need for satisfactory *in vitro* methods for assay and quantitation of transfer factor preparations prior to their use in animal and human situations. Lymphocyte stimulation has been used in various ways as well as an effect on leukocyte migration inhibition. Important optima to define include the dose of transfer factor added as well as the dose of antigen and the duration of the culture. The narrow dose range for TF effectiveness *in vitro* and the marked influence of the degree of recipient responsiveness to antigen emphasize the importance of defining optimal conditions in these assays although their exact relevance to the transfer of an *in vivo* factor is still uncertain (Ascher and Andron, in Ascher *et al.*, 1976). An increase in the number of E-rosettes is not detectable *in vitro* in the presence of TF unless the cells are previously trypsinized when an increase in both the absolute as well as the relative numbers of E-rosettes can be detected during the first three hours of incubation although no net increase is seen after 24 hours (Holzman *et al.*, in Ascher *et al.*, 1976). However, a significant increase in the number of E-rosettes detectable *in vivo* has been seen in some immunodeficient patients treated with TF and it may be that a greater effect would be seen *in vitro* if the lymphocyte population was enriched with immature T-cells. Thymosin on the other hand has an effect on untreated lymphocytes (see above).

Transfer factor is a low molecular weight material ($\leqslant 10{,}000$) and probably consists of a polypeptide/polynucleotide complex. Certainly it is not immunoglobulin-like and, being non-immunogenic, it has not been possible to raise specific antisera. Its lack of immunogenicity may of course, be a considerable advantage when contemplating its administration to recipients who are not genetically identical with the sources from which it has been prepared.

Clinical Application

Transfer factor preparations have been used with greatest success in those conditions where there is well-documented T-cell deficiency. Patients with the Wiskott–Aldrich syndrome (W–A) have benefitted from repeated injections of TF with a reduction in the severity of their eczema, thrombocytopenia and recurrent infections (Spitler *et al.*, 1972). It is of interest that it is the subpopulation of patients with W–A who have a defect in monocyte IgG receptors that respond to TF whereas those without this defect rarely seem to benefit. A few patients with thymic aplasia (e.g. the DiGeorge and Nézelof syndromes) may show slight improvement with TF administration but this may be confined to the conversion of skin test reactivity (Ballow and Good, in Ascher *et al.*, 1976). A few other patients with less marked and possibly more distal T-cell defects may respond quite dramatically to TF therapy (Valdimarsson *et al.*, 1974) and it is suggested that the success of TF therapy correlates with a certain critical level of T-cell differentiation. There are some children who respond poorly to thymus transplantation or transfer factor alone but who respond well to the administration of TF after thymus transplantation and this has even been observed in severe combined immunodeficiency (Amman *et al.*, 1973).

Other conditions associated with impaired cellular responses have been improved by TF therapy e.g. lepromatous leprosy, coccidioidomycosis and chronic muco-cutaneous candidiasis. The latter forms a very mixed group and it is the type II or granulomatous variety that is responsive to transfer factor (Valdimarsson *et al.*, 1973). Some virus infections have been improved but although TF restores an *in vitro* defect to measles virus observed in patients with multiple sclerosis (Utermohlen and Zabriskie, 1973) there is no convincing data in support of a beneficial clinical effect as yet.

A double blind cross-over trial in rheumatoid arthritis failed to detect any significant clinical improvement although a mild increase in skin test positivity and *in vitro* responses was observed (Maini *et al.*, 1976). Remissions have been recorded in Behçet's syndrome and in major aphthous ulceration and previous reports of improvement of Behçet's disease following fresh blood transfusion may be explained on the basis of a transfer factor effect. So far, there is very little objective evidence of improvement following TF in the treatment of malignant diseases such as carcinoma of the breast, malignant melanoma and osteogenic sarcoma although in the last two instances significant alteration in *in vitro* tests has been achieved.

Therapeutic Regime and Side-effects

A preparation of transfer factor prepared from the lymphocytes derived from one or two units of blood are given as a subcutaneous injection of the dialysed and lyophilized material. The choice of donor will vary with the clinical indication and injections are usually repeated at between one and six monthly intervals. The injections themselves may be transiently painful. The risk of transmitting hepatitis virus seems negligible. There is always the theoretical possibility of exacerbating hypersensitivity reactions to microbial or other antigens (Bullock *et al.*, 1971) and concomitant treatment with steroids or other inflammatory drugs may be necessary during the early stages. There are circumstantial suggestions that uncontrolled lymphoid cell proliferation may occur when TF is used in immunodeficiency disorders (Gelfand *et al.*, 1973) and that auto-immune disease may be induced or exacerbated (Ballow *et al.*, 1973).

As well as a clearer definition of what transfer factor is, and does, there is a very great need for large double blind controlled trials of TF in those disorders in which there is any suggestion that it may have therapeutic merit. Some are now in progress and the results are awaited with great interest.

Leukocyte Transfusion

While this may not feature strictly as a form of immunological reconstitution, it is now being used in various centres to support patients with severe neutropenia complicated by infection that is poorly responsive to antibiotics. It is only with the advent of specific means of collecting granulocytes that this procedure has become a practical reality: the two chief methods being centrifugation and filtration. Centrifugation is achieved by the use of a specifically designed cell separator (IBM or Aminco) which can collect any of the chief blood fractions while connected on-line to the donor or patient. A discontinuous system (Haemonetics) is less efficient for collecting granulocytes and causes greater intermittent changes in blood volume. The relative merits of these various devices have been recently reviewed (Russell and Powles, 1976). Granulocyte yields can be increased by adding a red cell sedimenting agent such as hydroxyethyl starch (HES) to the donor blood which makes for a cleaner separation between the red cell and granulocyte layers in the centrifuge bowl. The administration of prednisolone or dexamethasone also helps to increase the circulating granulocyte count in the donor although many people find that a brief period of muscular exercise prior to leukocyte donation is sufficient to increase the circulating count in order to provide yields of the order of $1\text{–}5 \times 10^{10}$ granulocytes from a single run. Leukophoresis can also be achieved by filtration of donor blood through nylon fibres (Leukopack/Fenwal) followed by elution of the granulocytes from the nylon by washing through with a solution of ACD/plasma/saline. Yields tend to be higher with filtration although a much higher incidence of febrile transfusion-type reactions is seen after the administration of leukocytes prepared by this method in contrast to those prepared by centrifugation (Goldman and Lowenthal, 1975).

Although the half-life of granulocytes is only of the order of six hours, there is evidence to suggest that the transfusion of $1\text{–}5 \times 10^{10}$ leucocytes can prove beneficial to neutropenic patients with life-threatening infections (Goldman and Lowenthal, 1975). A neutrophil count of less than $0{\cdot}5 \times 10^{9}$/litre in conjunction with severe infection is usually taken as the indication for such treatment. ABO compatibility of the cells is essential and although HLA compatibility is desirable it is not necessary for a beneficial effect to be produced. The most frequent patients requiring such treatment are those with aplastic anaemia or depressed marrows following cytotoxic therapy for leukaemia. Patients undergoing marrow transplantation also require granulocyte transfusions to cover the period of "pre-conditioning" immunosuppression as well as tiding them over until the graft begins to function. The problem of finding sufficient suitable donors for leukophoresis is a real one and warrants special study. Strict attention has to be paid to donor selection to reduce any possible hazard to a minimum. Donors should be less than 50 years of age and without any history of a medical condition which might contra-indicate anticoagulation or blood donation. The use of ABO compatible relatives is often convenient but may be contra-indicated if marrow transplantation is to be attempted later on as it may prejudice the acceptance of a graft. Cells harvested from patients with chronic granulocytic leukaemia can be a useful source of material and their functional activity has been shown to approximate to that of normal cells (Russell and Powles, 1976). It is essential to irradiate granulocytes prior to infusion whenever they are to be given to immunosuppressed individuals, and a case of fatal graft-versus-host disease has recently been described following leukocyte transfusion in a patient with myeloid leukaemia (Ford *et al.*, 1976). A dose of 1,500 rad is usually sufficient.

Although there is considerable circumstantial and some statistical evidence in favour of the beneficial effect of granulocyte transfusion (Higby *et al.*, in Goldman and Lowenthal, 1975) there is still a need for adequate controlled trials to define the best criteria for their use. It is also possible that further developments will allow the selective collection and administration of peripheral blood lymphocytes in the management of immunodeficiency disorders. Leukophoresis by the methods described above is also a very efficient means of obtaining cells for the preparation of transfer factor.

γ-Globulin Administration

Purified preparations of non-specific human γ-globulin are available for replacement therapy in patients who show significantly depressed levels of serum immunoglobulins in association with recurrent infection. The commonest indication is in the management of primary hypo-γ-globulinaemia (see pp. 509–511) although patients with secondary deficiencies in association with disorders such as myelomatosis may also benefit. The administration of whole plasma may be necessary in severe infection complicating hypo-γ-globulinaemia and this can be speedily administered by the use of an on-line cell separator (Oon and Hobbs, 1975).

(i) Adjuvants and "Immunotherapy"

A variety of materials are known to augment immunological responses when given in association with antigen. The use of such adjuvants has been common practice for many years in the development of potent antisera; the material most often used is Freund's complete adjuvant consisting of dead mycobacteria added to a water-in-oil emulsion of soluble antigen (Freund, 1951). Antibody production can be increased by using emulsion alone but significant enhancement of cellular responses requires addition of a mycobacterial extract. Detailed studies have shown that it is the peptidoglycan fraction of the mycobacterial membrane which has adjuvant properties but that this effect is further enhanced if "cord factor" (trehalose-6, 6-dimycolate) is also present (Lederer *et al.*, 1975). Most clinical studies have used whole mycobacteria in the form of B.C.G. and have been applied to the treatment of malignant disease. Other materials which have been widely used as adjuvants,

TABLE 3
The differential action of adjuvants on T- and B-lymphocytes

Adjuvant	T-cells	B-cells
Mycobacterial extracts	+ +	
Corynebacterium parvum	−	+
Bordetella pertussis	+ +	+

Modified from Allison, in Ciba Symposium, 1973

particularly in experimental animals, include killed *Corynebacterium parvum* and *Bordetella pertussis* (Ciba Symposium, 1973). Certain helminth extracts show a predilection for enhancing IgE responses to co-administered antigen (Orr *et al.*, 1972). Although most of the experimental data is derived from the mouse, there is good evidence to indicate that the mechanism of action of different adjuvants varies in terms of their primary cell target (Table 3). It should be noted that both the effects of *C. parvum* i.e. B-cell stimulation and T-cell inhibition are likely to be mediated via a primary action on macrophages (Howard, in Ciba Symposium, 1973).

Quite apart from the more formal approach to "immunotherapy" outlined below there is also a closely argued case for the modification of poor quality immunological responses which have been incriminated in the pathogenesis of both hetero-immune and auto-immune disease (Peters and Lachmann, 1974; Soothill, 1976). It has been demonstrated that the avidity of antibody produced in response to test antigen is correlated with the tendency for a particular strain of mice to develop glomerulonephritis—presumably as a consequence of natural exposure to virus infection (Soothill and Steward,

1971). The avidity of antibody produced can be increased to "normal" levels by the co-administration of adjuvant but, as yet, these studies have not found practical application in the management of human auto-immune disease.

Hitherto, the term, "immunotherapy", has become almost synonymous with the use of adjuvant-like materials in the treatment of malignant disease (see pp. 1014–1017). Initial studies using B.C.G. in the treatment of acute lymphoblastic leukaemia gave promising results (Mathé *et al.*, 1969) although further studies have failed to confirm this beneficial effect. B.C.G., either alone or in conjunction with tumour cells or extracts, has been used in the treatment of a variety of human malignancies e.g. lymphatic and myeloid leukaemia, malignant melanoma and carcinomas of breast and skin (Bast *et al.*, 1974). Despite the large number of studies there is a grave lack of randomized controlled investigations from which satisfactory conclusions can be drawn. This problem is compounded in diseases such as malignant melanoma which have an inherently unpredictable course. A recent study incorporating a randomized and controlled protocol revealed a complete absence of benefit in the treatment of stage II B malignant melanoma with contact immunotherapy utilizing B.C.G. and irradiated tumour cells (McIllmurray *et al.*, 1977). This in conjunction with experience of intralesional immunotherapy of cutaneous melanoma suggests that, where feasible, the local administration of adjuvant may have a greater effect.

A retrospective study of patients who had undergone pneumonectomy for bronchial carcinoma showed that those who developed a post-operative empyema had a lower recurrence rate (Ruckdeschel *et al.*, 1972) and intrapleural instillation of B.C.G. has given encouraging results in resectable bronchial carcinoma (McKneally *et al.*, 1976).

Corynebacterium parvum causes more unpleasant and potentially serious side-effects than B.C.G. but does seem to promote survival in human metastatic disease originating from breast and lung cancers (Israel and Edelstein, 1975). Attempts are being made to purify extracts of *C. parvum* in the hope that its unpleasant endotoxin-like effects may be separable from its adjuvanticity. Enthusiasm for adjuvant immunotherapy is currently waning although it is possible that greater benefit may be realized when more is known about the important chemical structures involved and the optimal conditions for their administration e.g. size and number of doses, timing, route of administration and combination with appropriate tumour extracts. The incorporation of both antigen and adjuvant into liposomes may offer an improved method of administration without granuloma formation at the site of injection (Gregoriadis, 1976). Initial attempts to combine immunotherapy with chemotherapy have not yielded consistent improvement and this approach seems less logical than the combination of immunotherapy with an augmenting agent such as levamisole.

(j) Levamisole

This agent was introduced in 1965 as an anthelmintic for the treatment of nematode infections in man and a variety of other animals. Incidental observations suggested a state of enhanced resistance to various kinds of infection in animals that had received such treatment. Specific experimentation soon confirmed its potency in augmenting the process of active immunization e.g. against *Brucella*, as well as its ability to reduce the effect of direct inoculation of pathogenic material. Animal studies also suggested a stimulatory effect on tumour immunity.

Clinically, the most marked effect is seen on delayed hypersensitivity skin tests in patients who develop anergy in association with malignancy and other diseases. Restoration of normal numbers of circulating T-lymphocytes (E-rosettes) has been observed and enhanced *in vitro* responses to both phytohaemagglutinin and concanavalin A occur when otherwise poorly responsive lymphocytes are cultured in the presence of levamisole. B-lymphocytes do not seem to be affected and there is little change in total antibody levels although a switch from IgM to IgG production has been observed (Renoux *et al.*, 1976). Treated animals also show an enhanced clearance of colloidial carbon and phagocytosis can be enhanced *in vitro*. It is likely that the effect of levamisole on T-cell immunity is mediated via macrophage stimulation or via a direct effect on T-cell activation or recruitment (Renoux *et al.*, 1976). Its effect has been compared to the activity of thymosin and both these agents produce a decrease in the "null" cell population (Rosenthal *et al.*, 1976).

Clinical Applications

Levamisole has been shown to be of benefit in various forms of recurrent infection associated with immunodeficiency, particularly of neutrophil or T-cell function. Anergic delayed hypersensitivity responses following infection with influenza or measles virus have been reversed by the administration of levamisole. Largely anecdotal evidence suggests that levamisole may have a beneficial effect in the management of rheumatoid arthritis as well as other arthropathies such as ankylosing spondylitis and Reiter's syndrome. Certainly, levamisole seems to be at least as effective as penicillamine in rheumatoid arthritis and is probably better tolerated (Huskisson *et al.*, 1976). However, one of its important potential side-effects, neutropenia, may possibly be a more frequent problem in patients with rheumatoid disease.

A double blind study in recurrent aphthous ulceration showed improvement in 64% of patients after the drug had been administered for two or more months (Lehner *et al.*, 1976) and a beneficial effect has been observed in Crohn's disease (Bertrand *et al.*, 1974).

There is considerable circumstantial evidence for its use in human cancer although very few adequately controlled studies have yet appeared. As with adjuvant immunotherapy (described above) there is no evidence to suggest that levamisole can be of benefit in patients with advanced malignancy. In those who have been rendered clinically tumour-free it is possible to show a measure of improvement as evidenced by prolongation of both disease-free intervals as well as survival in patients treated for breast cancer (Rojas *et al.*, 1976). This study also showed an increase in the percentage and intensity of delayed hypersensitivity skin reactions as well as in the absolute lymphocyte count. A controlled study of its use in the management of resectable carcinoma of the lung has also given encouraging results (Study group for bronchogenic carcinoma, 1975). There are suggestions that levamisole and B.C.G. may be additive in their effects but this possibility has yet to be fully tested.

Side Effects

Gastrointestinal symptoms e.g. nausea, vomiting, diarrhoea and abdominal cramps, are not uncommon. Feelings of general malaise also occur and occasionally a 'flu-like syndrome develops. Skin rashes and neutropenia seem to develop more commonly in patients with rheumatoid arthritis and the latter is usually reversible if the drug is stopped fairly promptly. Leukocyte agglutinins have been demonstrated in several patients developing a neutropenia on levamisole and the tendency for white cell antibodies to develop in rheumatoid arthritis (i.e. as part of Felty's syndrome) may explain the increased incidence of neutropenia in rheumatoid patients treated with this drug. Indeed, one might expect a drug which stimulated T-cell activity to aggravate various auto-immune conditions and it should be noted that clinical exacerbation was noted following the treatment of a small group of patients with multiple sclerosis (Dau *et al.*, 1976). Levamisole has been shown to aggravate gingivitis and we have observed clinical deterioration of a chronic but stable trichophyton dermatitis in association with considerable improvement in *in vitro* lymphocyte responses.

The appearance of a drug which has potent effects on all or part of the T-subpopulation of lymphocytes is a promising development for the clinical manipulation of immunological diseases. As the identity and function of different lymphocyte subpopulations becomes more clear in man it is hoped that further agents will be developed that have a more restricted cellular target. An interesting parallel might be drawn between such developments and the way in which progressively more refined and specific adrenergic stimulating and blocking agents have been elaborated following the acquisition of more detailed knowledge of the autonomic nervous system and its receptors.

(k) Reversal of "Suppression"

Various infective and inflammatory diseases are associated with a clinical state of "anergy" (Bryceson, 1974) and this is often a feature of some forms of malignant disease, notably Hodgkin's disease. Evidence for the inordinate activity of suppressor cell populations is accumulating and may in some instances reflect a state of antigenic competition (Taussig, 1973). Over-exuberant suppressor cell activity has been described in patients with myelomatosis (Broder *et al.*, 1975), aplastic anaemia (Hoffman *et al.*, 1977), hypo-γ-globulinaemia (Waldmann *et al.*, 1974) and in association with fungal infection (Stobo *et al.*, 1976). In most of these situations it is likely that a subpopulation of T-cells is involved but the stimuli for their hyper-reactivity are poorly understood. Concanavalin A can activate suppressor cell activity when incubated with peripheral blood lymphocytes *in vitro* (Hubert *et al.*, 1976) but a specific anti T-cell suppressor reagent has yet to be described in man. In other situations there is evidence that a B-cell population may be active in the suppression of delayed hypersensitivity responses and such effects can be abrogated by the administration of cyclophosphamide to experimental animals (Polak and Turk, 1974). Once "over-suppression" has been identified in a particular clinical situation agents such as this may be of use in the future in reversing the suppressed state. This makes an intriguing comparison with the traditional role of cytotoxic drugs as "immunosuppressive" agents.

NON-SPECIFIC NON-REACTIVITY

(I) Lymphoid Ablation

Adenotonsillectomy has not been strikingly associated with immunological sequelae although specific studies have indicated that the nasopharyngeal level of specific IgA antibody can fall after this procedure and as little is known about the primary role of such lymphoid tissue it seems reasonable to discourage removal unless this is clinically imperative. Splenectomy is, undoubtedly, associated with more hazard on the basis of deficient responses to certain bacteria e.g. *Strep. pneumoniae*, *N. meningitidis* and *H. influenzae*. Infections usually take the form of septicaemia or meningitis and may be fulminating. The risk is greatest in children under five years of age although this continues into adult life. The abnormal propensity to infection is associated with the defective clearance of particulate antigens, impaired production of IgM antibodies and reduced C3 and alternative pathway component levels. A non-specific opsonin, tuftsin, is normally produced in the spleen and its absence both after splenectomy as well as in those patients who have an inherited deficiency is associated with an increased tendency to infection (Constantopoulos *et al.*, 1973).

Immunological indications for splenectomy include idiopathic thrombocytopenic purpura and auto-immune haemolytic anaemia. It has also been recent practice to perform splenectomy during staging laparotomy for Hodgkin's disease but there is, as yet, no convincing proof that splenectomy improves the outlook and it increases the hazard of infection. In other situations, when splenectomy is inevitable, a piece of spleen should be left behind (subcutaneously or in the rectus sheath) for there is evidence that this can prevent serious infection in experimental animals. When children under five have their spleens removed they should be placed on prophylactic oral penicillin for at least three years and also given weekly intramuscular injections of γ-globulin. Any potential infection with the relevant organisms should be treated extremely promptly in an asplenic patient even if pyrexia and leukocytosis are the only manifestations.

Thymectomy in adults does not seem to cause any detectable deficiency and its chief immunological indication is in the management of myasthenia gravis particularly when the disease is of recent onset. A good response to thymectomy has been correlated with the presence of active germinal centres within the thymus tissue.

The piecemeal removal of lymph nodes is often performed as part of block dissection for malignant disease and in itself is not obviously associated with any immunological deficit. The main concern in the minds of those who remove regional nodes as part of radical surgery for malignant disease is whether the individual nodes contain metastatic disease or whether they are playing an important part in the host response to the tumour.

Chronic drainage of thoracic duct lymph is associated with impaired immunological reactivity and can produce significant prolongation of graft survival. The effect is a very non-specific one and patients are prone to opportunistic infection. The development of relatively non-toxic preparations of anti-lymphocyte serum and its fractions has removed the necessity for such a procedure.

Irradiation

Whole body irradiation was used as a means of immunosuppression prior to renal transplantation but fell into disfavour because of the dangers of marrow aplasia. Extra-corporeal irradiation of the blood has been shown to prolong graft survival but other forms of immunosuppression are more commonly used. Recent work indicates that suppressor T-cells are particularly radio-sensitive and this may explain the abrogation of tolerance, as well as the exacerbation of auto-immunity that can follow irradiation (Anderson and Warner, 1976).

(m) Lymphocyte Suppression

Anti-lymphocyte serum (ALS) and its purified fraction anti-lymphocyte globulin (ALG) are powerful agents capable of blotting out T-cell reactivity without affecting many of the other cell systems that are subject to the effects of cytotoxic drugs. Toxic reactions include pain at the site of injection, urticaria, itching, fever and thrombocytopenia. Some patients have developed immune complex renal disease and, as most therapeutic preparations are raised in the horse, adverse reactions to the horse serum or globulin can occur. Tolerance can be induced to equine IgG prior to the commencement of ALG therapy (Jones *et al.*, in Roussell and Hoffbrand, 1976). Such a manoeuvre enhances the effect of the ALG and reduces the risk of hypersensitivity reactions. The more refined preparations in current use are raised against thoracic duct lymphocytes or cultured lymphoblasts and a more selective effect can be achieved by using membrane fractions of the latter. Anti-thymocyte globulin (ATG) has also been used with a similar degree of success in the suppression of cell-mediated responses. The major use of these materials has been in renal transplantation programmes where there is convincing evidence of an additive effect when given in conjunction with conventional immunosuppressive therapy. However, the use of ALG or ATG in a variety of other disorders is still largely anecdotal (Roussel and Hoffbrand, 1976) and properly conducted trials are needed before any judgement can be made. Conditions in which these agents have been used include multiple sclerosis, myasthenia gravis, systemic lupus, polyarteritis nodosa, dermatomyositis and the more aggressive forms of nephritis. ALG and ATG are an established part of the management of bone marrow transplantation and are particularly useful for combating graft-versus-host reactions (G.V.H.).

More sophisticated lymphocyte antisera may become available in the future which could specifically affect individual T- or B-lymphocyte subpopulations subserving particular functional activities e.g. suppression or cytotoxicity, without interfering with other lymphocyte functions.

(n) Inhibition via G.V.H. Response

The induction of graft-versus-host disease is an effective means of suppressing both humoral and cellular immune responses. When induced in New Zealand (NZB/W) hybrid mice it diminished the severity of their disease and reduced antibody responses to both exogenous and endogenous antigens (Lehman *et al.*, 1976). High dose cyclophosphamide was even more effective in this study and it is unlikely that the induction of a graft-versus-host reaction will prove useful in the control of human disease.

(o) Plasma Exchange

Manual plasmaphoresis has been a stand-by measure in the treatment of severe paraproteinaemia with hyperviscosity or cryoglobulinaemia for some years. With the development of cell separators, initially for leukophoresis (see p. 1122), it soon became possible to exchange larger volumes of plasma by use of on-line techniques (Oon and Hobbs, 1975). As with the manual technique, plasma substitutes have to be given e.g. purified protein fraction, dried plasma or fresh frozen plasma, and this can create problems of supply.

An important application of intensive plasmaphoresis has been in the management of severe Rhesus iso-immunization. This condition is becoming progressively less common following the introduction of prophylactic anti-D post-partum but there are still a few patients who became sensitized before this programme began or who nevertheless escape such prophylaxis. Plasma exchange is the only means of treatment before intra-uterine transfusion (IUT) becomes feasible and some authorities now feel that the risks of IUT are sufficiently great to put the onus on plasma exchange for as long as it can maintain the maternal antibody level low enough to protect the foetus from severe involvement (Pole *et al.*, 1974 and Fraser and Tovey, 1976). Ideally, four litre exchanges should be performed twice weekly although maintaining venous access may present problems in some patients. Figure 1 illustrates thc Aminco celltrifuge in use to treat a patient with severe Rhesus iso-immunization and Fig. 2a indicates the progressive reduction in anti-D level that is seen during the course of a four litre exchange in such a patient. During the procedure the patient's blood is anticoagulated extracorporeally. This is best achieved with heparin as the administration of acid citrate dextrose (A.C.D.) can cause untoward effects. Adverse reactions to the procedure are

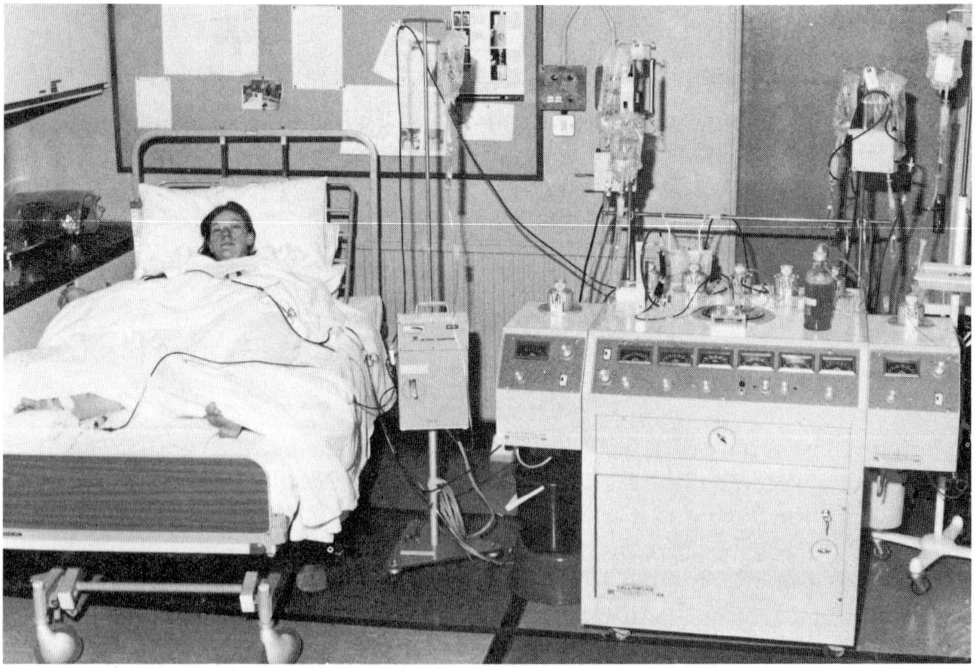

Fig. 1. A patient with severe rhesus iso-immunization being treated by intensive plasmaphoresis in the Nottingham Cell Separator Unit.

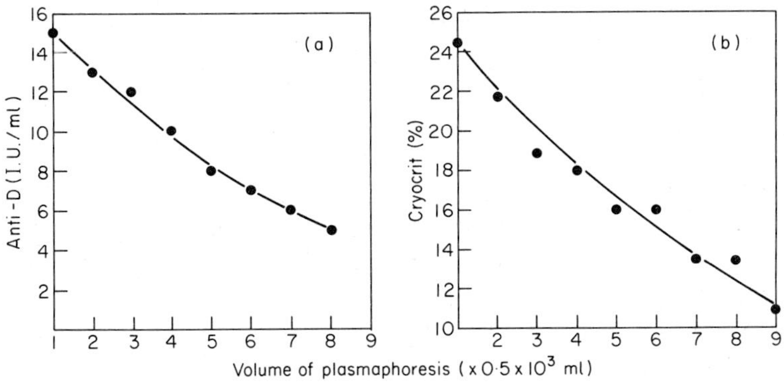

Fig. 2. Graphs demonstrating the progressive decline in serum parameters during plasmaphoresis: (a) the reduction in serum anti-D level during a 4,000 ml plasma exchange for severe Rhesus iso-immunization; (b) the reduction in percentage cryoglobulin or "cryocrit" during a 4,500 ml plasma exchange for severe mixed cryoglobulinaemia.

significantly reduced by placing a blood warmer in the recipient line and the prevention of hypocalcaemic symptoms is achieved by the continual addition of calcium gluconate to the replacement fluids.

The application of this technique to the management of renal disease was instituted in a group of patients with Goodpasture's syndrome in conjunction with corticosteroids and cytotoxic drugs (Lockwood *et al.*, 1976). Lung haemorrhage and renal function improved and in some of the patients the anti-GBM antibody failed to return to its previously high level. Plasma exchange has also been performed in a patient with Goodpasture's syndrome following renal transplantation and this in conjunction with immunosuppressive therapy has enabled the graft to function well for 18 months despite significantly high levels of anti-GBM antibody at the time of transplantation which would otherwise have been expected to produce recurrent disease (Cove-Smith *et al.*, 1977). More recently plasma exchange in conjunction with immunosuppression has been applied to the treatment of fulminating immune-complex crescentic nephritis (Lockwood *et al.*, 1977). Many of the patients had clinical features suggestive of widespread vasculitis and it is relevant that the majority who responded favourably had detectable circulating immune complexes. In the renal work, purified protein fraction has been used as the replacement material and it is argued that part of the beneficial effect may be achieved via depletion of complement and coagulation factors which would otherwise be expected to contribute to the antibody-mediated disease. Another study has shown improvement in a group of patients with systemic lupus and here again the most favourable results were found in those patients who showed high levels of circulating complexes and reduced serum complement levels (Jones *et al.*, 1976).

Hyperviscosity and cryoglobulinaemia respond even more dramatically to plasmaphoresis and such treatment is of particular value in tiding the patient over until chemotherapy is able to control the primary disorder. Figure 2 also shows the progressive fall in the percentage cryoprecipitate or "cryocrit" during a 4,500 ml plasma exchange of a patient with severe mixed cryoglobulinaemia complicating rheumatoid arthritis. Increased extracorporeal anticoagulation is required in these circumstances and a warming coil has to be placed in the donor line to prevent the abnormal protein from precipitating out and obstructing flow through the narrow ports in the centrifuge bowl and seal. Plasma exchange has also been used to administer large quantities of fresh plasma to patients with hypo-γ-globulinaemia complicated by severe infection or patients with complement or other protein deficiencies that require prompt correction.

Other applications of this technique will undoubtedly follow but it should be emphasized that it is relatively crude in principle and specific immunoadsorption (see p. 1114) may provide a more economical solution to the removal of specific antibody in the future.

CONCLUSION

This chapter has reviewed a motley collection of ways in which the immune response can be manipulated at both experimental and clinical levels. The various manoeuvres have been discussed against a framework of host responsiveness in an attempt to display important similarities and differences of approach. Certain paradoxes are apparent e.g. the use of cyclophosphamide to enhance responsiveness (p. 1128) the induction of specific reactivity to promote graft acceptance (p. 1112) and the exacerbation of auto-immune disease by irradiation (p. 1130). Their existence serves to emphasize the great changes that have taken place in immunological thinking in recent years. The previously crude means of stimulating and inhibiting immunological responses are increasingly giving way to sophisticated methods of modulating the part rather than the whole. Some of the most exciting developments lie in the area of specific unresponsiveness and when this becomes a readily applicable manoeuvre across a wide range of antigenic systems then the management of many immunological and non-immunological disorders will change dramatically.

Cell transfers to correct inborn errors of metabolism such as haemoglobinopathies, lipidoses, mucopolysaccharidoses, etc., will be possible, and initial studies have already given encouraging results with tissue transplants in several disorders of this kind (Groth *et al.*, 1971, Good and Bach, 1974, Dean *et al.*, 1975).

The production of specific non-reactivity as well as subtle forms of immunological reconstitution are likely to be an increasing preoccupation of the clinical immunologist in the near future.

REFERENCES

Alexander, P., Bensted, J., Delorme, E. J., Hall, J. G. and Hodgett, J. (1969). The cellular immune response to primary sarcomata in rats. II Abnormal responses of nodes draining the tumour. *Proc. Roy. Soc. London* B. **174**, 237.

Ammann, A. J., Wara, D. W., Salmon, S. *et al.* (1973). Thymus transplantation. Permanent reconstitution of cellular immunity in a patient with sex-linked combined immunodeficiency. *New Eng. J. Med.* **289**, 5.

Anderson, R. E. and Warner, N. L. (1976). Ionizing irradiation and the immune response. *Adv. Immunol.*, **24**, 215.

Arbeiten aus dem Reichgesundheitsamte (1935). "Die Säuglingstuberkulose in Lubeck". Springer, Berlin.

Ascher, M. S., Gottlieb, A. A. and Kirkpatrick, C. H. (Eds) (1976). "Transfer Factor: Basic Properties and Clinical Applications". Academic Press, New York and London.

Bach, J.-F. (1976). The mode of action of thymic hormones and its relevance to T-cell differentiation. *Trans. Proc.* **8**, 243.

Baker, P. J., Stashak, P. W., Amsbaugh, D. F. and Prescott, B. (1974). Regulation of the antibody response to type III pneumococcal polysaccharide. II Mode of action of thymic-derived suppressor cells. *J. Immunol.* **112**, 404.

Ballow, M., Dupont, B. and Good, R. A. (1973). Autoimmune hemolytic anaemia in Wiskott-Aldrich syndrome during treatment with transfer factor. *J. Pediat.* **83**, 772.

Bast, R. C., Zbar, B., Borsos, T. and Rapp, H. J. (1974). B.C.G. and cancer. *New Eng. J. Med.* **290**, 1413 and 1458.

Batchelor, J. R., Ellis, F., French, M. E., Bewick, M., Cameron, J. S. and Ogg, C. S. (1970). Immunological enhancement of human kidney grafts. *Lancet*, **II**, 1007.

Bertrand, J., Renoux, G., Renoux, M. and Palat, A. (1974). Maladie de Crohn et levamisole. *Nouv. Presse Med.* **3**, 2265.

Billingham, R. E., Brent, L. and Medawar, P. B. (1953). "Actively acquired tolerance" of foreign cells. *Nature* **172**, 603.

Binz, H. and Wigzell, H. (1976). Successful induction of specific tolerance to transplantation antigens using auto-immunisation against the recipients own natural antibodies. *Nature* **262**, 294.

Bortin, M. M. (1974). Graft versus leukaemia. *in* "Clinical Immunobiology" Vol. 2 (ed F. H. Bach and R. A. Good). Academic Press, New York and London.

Bowen, J. E., Batchelor, J. R., French, M. E., Burgos, H. and Fabre, J. W. (1974). Failure of adoptive immunisation or parabiosis with hyperimmune syngeneic partners to abrogate long-term enhancement of rat kidney allografts. *Transplantation* **18**, 322.

Brent, L. and Kilshaw, P. J. (1976). Humoral factors in specific unresponsiveness to transplantation antigens. *Trans. Proc.* **8**, 209.

Broder, S., Humphrey, R., Durm, M., Blackman, M., Meade, B., Goldman, C., Strober, W. and Waldman, T. (1975). Impaired synthesis of polyclonal (non-paraprotein) immunoglobulins by circulating lymphocytes from patients with multiple myeloma. Role of suppressor cells. *New Eng. J. Med.* **293**, 887.

Bryceson, A. (1974). Anergy and suppressed cellular immunity in disease. *Prog. Immunol.* II **3**, 161.

Buckley, R. H., Amos, D. B., Kremer, W. B. and Stickel, D. L. (1971). Incompatible bone-marrow transplantation in lymphopenic immunologic deficiency: Circumvention of fatal graft-versus-host disease by immunologic enhancement. *New Eng. J. Med.* **285**, 1036.

Buckley, R. H., Whisnant, J. K., Schiff, R. I., Gilbertsen, R. B., Huang, A. T. and Platt, M. S. (1976). Correction of severe combined immunodeficiency by fetal liver cells. *New Eng. J. Med.* **294**, 1076.

Bullock, W. E., Fields, J. and Brandriss, M. (1971). Transfer factor therapy in lepromatous leprosy: an evaluation. *J. Clin. Invest.* **50**, 16a.

Cannon, W. B. (1932). "The Wisdom of the Body". W. W. Norton and Co., New York.

Centifanto, Y. M. and Kaufman, H. E. (1971). *In* "The Secretory Immunologic System". (Eds D. H. Dayton, P. A. Small, R. M. Chanock, H. E. Kaufman and T. B. Tomasi), N.I.C.H.H.D., Bethesda.

Chiller, J. M., Habicht, G. S. and Weigle, W. O. (1971). Kinetic differences in unresponsiveness of thymus and bone marrow cells. *Science* **171**, 813.

CIBA Symposium 18 (New series) (1973). "Immunopotentiation", Elsevier, Amsterdam.

Clarke, C. A., Donohue, W. T. A., McConnell, R. B., Woodrow, J. C., Finn, R., Krevans, J. R., Kulke, W., Lehane, D. and Sheppard, P. M. (1963). Further experimental studies on the prevention of Rh haemolytic disease. *Brit. Med. J.* **1**, 979.

Cohen, S. and Sadun, E. (1976). "Immunology of Parasitic Infections". Blackwell, Oxford.

Constantopoulos, A., Najjar, V. A., Wish, J. B., Necheles, T. H. and Stolbach, L. L. (1973). Defective phagocytosis due to tuftsin deficiency in splenectomised subjects. *Am. J. Dis. Child.* **125**, 663.

Cove-Smith, J. R., McLeod, A. A., Blamey, R. W., Knapp, M. S. and Reeves, W. G. (1977). Transplantation, immunosuppression and plasmaphoresis in Goodpasture's syndrome. (In press.)

Cuatrecasas, P. (1972). Affinity chromatography of macromolecules. *Adv. Enzymol.* **36**, 29.

Dau, P. C., Johnson, K. P. and Spitler, L. E. (1976). The effect of levamisole on cellular immunity in multiple sclerosis. *Clin. Exp. Immunol.* **26**, 302.

Dean, M. F., Muir, Benson, P. F., Button, L. R., Batchelor, J. R. and Bewick, M. (1975). Increased breakdown of glycosaminoglycans and appearance of corrective enzyme after skin transplants in Hunter syndrome. *Nature* **257**, 609.

Dresser, D. W. (Ed.) (1976). Immunological tolerance. *Brit. Med. Bull.* **32**, No. 2.

Eichmann, K. (1975). Idiotype suppression. II Amplification of a suppressor T cell with anti-idiotypic activity. *Eur. J. Immunol.* **5**, 511.

Ettinger, R. B., Terasaki, P. I., Opelz, G., Malekzadeh, M., Pennisi, A. J., Uittenbogaart, C. and Fine, R. (1976). Successful renal allografts across a positive cross-match for donor B-lymphocyte alloantigens. *Lancet* **II**, 56.

Eylar, E. H., Jackson, J., Rothenberg, B. and Brostoff, S. W. (1972). Suppression of the immune response: reversal of the disease state with antigen in allergic encephalomyelitis. *Nature* **236**, 74.

Feldman, J. D. (1972). Immunological enhancement: A study of blocking antibodies. *Adv. Immunol.* **15**, 167.

Ford, J. M., Lucey, J. J., Cullen, M. H., Tobias, J. S. and Lister, T. A. (1976). Fatal graft-versus-host disease following transfusion of granulocytes from normal donors. *Lancet* **II**, 1167.

Fraser, I. D. and Tovey, G. H. (1976). Observations on Rh iso-immunisation: past, present and future. *Clin. Haematol.* **5**, No. 1.

French, M. E. and Batchelor, J. R. (1969). Immunological enhancement of rat kidney grafts. *Lancet* **II**, 1103.

Freund, J. (1951). The effect of paraffin oil and mycobacteria on antibody formation and sensitization. *Am. J. Clin. Path.* **21**, 645.

Friedman, H. (Ed.) (1975). Thymus factors in immunity. *Ann. N.Y. Acad. Sci.* **249**, 1–547.

Fulginiti, V. A., Eller, J. J., Downie, A. W. and Kempe, C. H. (1967). Altered reactivity to measles virus. Atypical measles in children previously immunized with inactivated measles virus vaccine. *J. Am. Med. Ass.* **202**, 1075.

Fuller, T. C., Delmonico, F. L., Cosimi, A. B., Huggins, C. E., King, M. and Russell, P. S. (1977). *Trans. Proc.* (In press.)

Gelfand, E. W., Baumal, R., Huber, J., Crookston, M. C. and Shumak, K. H. (1973). Polyclonal gammopathy and lymphoproliferation after transfer factor in severe combined immunodeficiency disease. *New Eng. J. Med.* **289**, 1385.

Gershon, R. K. and Kondo, K. (1972). Tolerance to sheep red cells: breakage with thymocytes and horse red cells. *Science* **175**, 996.

Ghose, T., Cerini, M., Carter, M. and Nairn, R. C. (1967). Immunoradioactive agent against cancer. *Brit. Med. J.* **1**, 90.

Ghose, T., Norvell, S. T., Guclu, A. and Macdonald, A. S. (1975). Immunochemotherapy of human malignant melanoma with chlorambucil-carrying antibody. *Europ. J. Cancer* **11**, 321.

Goldman, J. M. and Lowenthal, R. M. (Eds) (1975). "Leucocytes: Separation, Collection and Transfusion." Academic Press, New York and London.

Good, R. A. and Bach, F. H. (1974). Bone marrow and thymus transplants: cellular engineering to correct primary immunodeficiency, *in* "Clinical Immunobiology" Vol. 2. (Eds F. H. Bach and R. A. Good), Academic Press, New York and London.

Gregoriadis, G. (1976). The carrier potential of liposomes in biology and medicine. *New Eng. J. Med.* **295**, 704 and 765.

Groth, C. G., Hagenfeldt, L., Dreborg, S., Lofstrom, B., Ockerman, P. A., Samuelsson, K., Svennerholm, L., Werner, B. and Westberg, G. (1971). Splenic transplantation in a case of Gaucher's disease. *Lancet* **I**, 1260.

Harris, T. N. and Harris, S. (1972). Effect of anti-mouse IgG, on some complement-requiring alloantibodies of the mouse. *J. Immunol.* **109**, 1096.

Hellstrom, I., Hellstrom, K. E. and Allison, A. C. (1971). Neonatally induced allograft tolerance may be mediated by serum-borne factors. *Nature* **230**, 49.

Herzenberg, L. A., Chan, E. L., Ravitch, M. M., Riblet, R. J. and Herzenberg, L. A. (1973). Active suppression of immunoglobulin allotype synthesis. III Identification of T cells as responsible for suppression by cells from spleen, thymus, lymph node, and bone marrow. *J. Exp. Med.* **137**, 1311.

Hoffman, R., Zanjani, E. D., Lutton, J. D., Zalusky, R. and Wasserman, L. R. (1977). Suppression of erythroid-colony formation by lymphocytes from patients with aplastic anaemia. *New Eng. J. Med.* **296**, 10.

Hollinger, F. B., Sharp, J. T., Lidsky, M. D. and Rawls, W. E. (1971). Antibodies to viral antigens in systemic lupus erythematosus. *Arth. Rheum.* **14**, 1.

Hong, R., Santosham, M., Schultze-Wisserman, H., Horowitz, S., Hsu, S. H. and Winkelstein, J. A. (1976). Reconstitution of B and T lymphocyte function in severe combined immunodeficiency disease after transplantation with thymic epithelium. *Lancet* **II**, 1270.

Hough, D. W., Eady, R. P., Hamblin, T. J., Stevenson, F. K. and Stevenson, G. T. (1976). Anti-idiotype sera raised against surface immunoglobulin of human neoplastic lymphocytes. *J. Exp. Med.* **144**, 960.

Hubert, C., Delespesse, G. and Govaerts, A. (1976). Concanavalin A-activated suppressor cells in normal human peripheral blood lymphocytes. *Clin. Exp. Immunol.* **26**, 95.

Huskisson, E. C., Scott, J., Balme, H. W., Dieppe, P. A., Trapnell, J. and Willoughby, D. A. (1976). Immunostimulant therapy with levamisole for rheumatoid arthritis. *Lancet* **1**, 393.

Israel, L. and Edelstein, R. (1975). A phase II study of daily Corynebacterium in 33 disseminated cancers. *Proc. Am. Assoc. Canc. Res.* **16**, 67.

Jones, J. V., Cumming, R. H., Bucknall, R. C., Asplin, C. M., Fraser, I. D., Bothamley, J., Davis, P. and Hamblin, T. J. (1976). Plasmaphoresis in the management of acute systemic lupus erythematosus. *Lancet* **1**, 709.

Julius, M. H., Sweet, R. G., Fatham, C. G. and Herzenberg, L. A. (1974). Fluorescence activated cell sorting and its applications. Mammalian cells: Probes and Problems. Proceedings of First Los Alamos Life Science Symposium. Atomic Energy Commission Series. (CON573–1007). 107.

Kapikian, A. Z., Mitchell, R. H., Chanock, R. M., Shvedoff, R. A. and Stewart, C. E. (1969). An epidemiological study of altered clinical reactivity to respiratory syncytial (R.S.) virus infection in children previously vaccinated with an inactivated R.S. virus vaccine. *Am. J. Epidemiol.* **89**, 405.

Katz, D. H. (1972). The allogeneic effect on immune responses: model for regulatory influences of T lymphocytes on the immune system. *Transplant. Rev.* **12**, 141.

Kilshaw, P. J., Brent, L. and Pinto, M. (1975). Suppressor T cells in mice made unresponsive to skin allografts. *Nature* **255**, 489.

Kulenkampff, M., Schwartzman, J. S. and Wilson, J. (1974). Neurological complications of pertussis inoculation. *Arch. Dis. Child.* **49**, 46.

Lance, E. M. and Medawar, P. B. (1969). Quantitative studies on tissue transplantation immunity. *Proc. Roy. Soc. London* B. **173**, 447.

Langvad, E., Hyden, H., Wolf, H. and Kroeigaard, N. (1975). Extra-corporeal immunoadsorption of circulating specific serum factors in cancer patients. *Brit. J. Cancer* **32**, 680.

Lawrence, H. S. (1955). The transfer in humans of delayed skin sensitivity to streptococcal M substance and tuberculin with disrupted leucocytes. *J. Clin. Invest.* **34**, 219.

Lederer, E., Adam, A., Ciorbaru, R. *et al.* (1975). Cell walls of mycobacteria and related organisms. Chemistry and immunostimulant properties. *Mol. Cell. Biochem.* **7**, 87.

Lehman, D. H., Wilson, C. B. and Dixon, F. J. (1976). Increased survival times of New Zealand hybrid mice immunosuppressed by graft-versus-host reactions. *Clin. exp. Immunol.* **25**, 297.

Lehner, T., Challacombe, S. J., Wilton, J. M. A. and Caldwell, J. (1976). Cellular and humoral immune responses in vaccination against dental caries in monkeys. *Nature* **264**, 69.

Lehner, T., Wilton, J. M. A. and Ivanyi, L. (1976). Double blind crossover trial of levamisole in recurrent aphthous ulceration. *Lancet* **II**, 926.

Levy, R., Hurwitz, E., Maron, R., Arnon, R. and Sela, M. (1975). The specific cytotoxic effects of daunomycin conjugated to antitumour antibodies. *Cancer Res.* **35**, 1182.

Lewis, M. G., Phillips, T. M. and Jerry, L. M. (1976). Immunising against receptors for antigen. *Lancet* **II**, 858.

Lockwood, C. M., Rees, A. J., Pinching, A. J., Pussell, B., Sweny, P., Uff, J. and Peters, D. K. (1977). Plasma exchange and immunosuppression in the treatment of fulminating immune-complex crescentic nephritis. *Lancet* **1**, 63.

Lockwood, C. M., Rees, A. J., Pearson, T. A., Evans, D. J., Peters, D. K. and Wilson, C. B. (1976). Immunosuppression and plasma-exchange in the treatment of Goodpasture's syndrome. *Lancet* **1**, 711.

Lyle, R., Parker, B. M. and Parker, C. W. (1974). The use of protein-substituted nylon catheters for selective immunoadsorption *in vivo*. *J. Immunol.* **113**, 517.

Maini, R. N., Scott, J. T., Roffe, L. M., Hamblin, A. S. and Dumonde, D. C. (1976). Preliminary experience of transfer factor in rheumatoid arthritis: clinical and immunological studies, *in* "Infection and Immunity in the Rheumatic Diseases". (Ed. D. C. Dumonde), Blackwell Scientific Publications, Oxford.

Many, A. and Schwartz, R. S. (1970). On the mechanism of immunological tolerance in cyclophosphamide-treated mice. *Clin. Exp. Immunol.* **6**, 87.

Markowski, B. and Lawler, S. D. (1977). Use of early fetal tissues obtained from suction termination of pregnancy. *Lancet* **1**, 186.

Mathé, G., Amiel, J. L., Schwarzenberg, L., Schneider, M., Cattan, A., Schlumberger, J. R., Hayat, M. and Devassal, F. (1969). Active immunotherapy for acute lymphoblastic leukaemia. *Lancer* **1**, 697.

McConnell, I., Lachmann, P. J. and Hobart, M. J. (1974). Restoration of specific immunological virginity. *Nature* **250**, 113.

McIllmurray, M. B., Embleton, J., Reeves, W. G., Langman, M. J. S. and Deane, M. (1977). A controlled trial of active immunotherapy in the management of stage IIB malignant melanoma. *Brit. Med. J.* **1**, 540.

McKneally, M. F., Maver, C. and Kausel, H. W. (1976). Regional immunotherapy of lung cancer with intra-pleural B.C.G. *Lancet* **1**, 377.

Ogra, P. L., Karzon, D. T., Righthand, F. and MacGillivray, M. (1968). Immunoglobulin response in serum and secretions after immunisation with live and inactivated polio vaccine and natural infection. *New Eng. J. Med.* **279**, 893.

Oon, C. J. and Hobbs, J. R. (1975). Clinical applications of the continuous flow blood separator machine. *Clin. Exp. Immunol.* **20**, 1.

Opelz, G. and Terasaki, P. I. (1976). Prolongation effect of blood transfusions on kidney graft survival. *Transplantation* **22**, 380.

Orr, T. S. C., Riley, P. A. and Doe, J. E. (1972). Potentiated reagin response to egg albumin in *Nippostrongylus brasiliensis* infected rats. III Further studies on the time course of the reagin response. *Immunology* **22**, 211.

Peters, D. K. and Lachmann, P. J. (1974). Immunity deficiency in pathogenesis of glomerulonephritis. *Lancet* **1**, 58.

Polak, L. and Geleick, H. (1975). Differing mechanisms of tolerance and desensitisation to dinitrochlorobenzene in guinea pigs. *Europ. J. Immunol.* **5**, 94.

Polak, L. and Turk, J. L. (1974). Reversal of immunological tolerance by cyclophosphamide through inhibition of suppressor cell activity. *Nature* **249**, 654.

Pole, J. R., Donald, I., Barr, W. and Willoughby, M. L. N. (1974). Plasmaphoresis in Rhesus iso-immunisation. *Lancet* **II**, 1459.

Raff, M. C. (1977). Immunological networks. *Nature* **265**, 205.

Ramseier, H. and Lindenmann, J. (1972). Aliotypic antibodies. *Transplant Rev.* **10**, 57.

Renoux, G., Renoux, M., Teller, M. N., McMahon, S. and Guillaumin, J. M. (1976). Potentiation of T-cell mediated immunity by levamisole. *Clin. Exp. Immunol.* **25**, 288.

Rojas, A. F., Mickiewicz, E., Feierstein, J. N., Glait, H. and Olivari, A. J. (1976). Levamisole in advanced human breast cancer. *Lancet* **1**, 211.

Rook, G. A. W., Carswell, J. W. and Stanford, J. L. (1976). Preliminary evidence for the trapping of antigen specific lymphocytes in the lymphoid tissue of "anergic" tuberculosis patients. *Clin. Exp. Immunol.* **26**, 129.

Rosenthal, M., Trabert, U. and Muller, W. (1976). The effect of levamisole on peripheral blood lymphocyte sub-populations in patients with rheumatoid arthritis and ankylosing spondylitis. *Clin. Exp. Immunol.* **25**, 493.

Roussell, R. H. and Hoffbrand, B. I. (Eds) (1976). Anti-lymphocyte globulin in clinical practice. *Postgraduate Med. J.* **52**, Suppl. 5.

Ruckdeschel, J. C., Codish, S. D., Stranahan, A. and McKneally, M. F. (1972). Postoperative empyema improves survival in lung cancer. *New Eng. J. Med.* **287**, 1013.

Russell, J. A. and Powles, R. L. (1976). A practical guide to granulocyte transfusion therapy. *J. Clin. Path.* **29**, 369.

Scheinberg, M. A., Cathcart, E. S. and Goldstein, A. L. (1975). Thymosin-induced reduction of "null" cells in peripheral blood lymphocytes of patients with systemic lupus erythematosus. *Lancet* **1**, 424.

Scheinberg, M. A., Blacklow, N. R., Goldstein, A. L., Parring, T. A., Rose, F. B. and Cathcart, E. S. (1976). Influenza: response of T-cell lymphopenia to thymosin. *New Eng. J. Med.* **294**, 1208.

Schenkein, I., Bystryn, J.-C. and Uhr, J. W. (1971). Specific removal of in vivo antibody by extracorporeal circulation over an immunoadsorbent in gel. *J. Clin. Invest.* **50**, 1864.

Scott, R. M. and Russell, P. K. (1972). Complement fixation blocking activity of anti-dengue IgM antibody. *J. Immunol.* **109**, 875.

Soothill, J. F. (1976). Some intrinsic and extrinsic factors predisposing to allergy. *Proc. Roy. Soc. Med.* **69**, 439.

Soothill, J. F. and Steward, M. W. (1971). The immunopathological significance of the heterogeneity of antibody affinity. *Clin. Exp. Immunol.* **9**, 193.

Spitler, L. E., Levin, A. S., Stites, D. P., Fudenberg, H. H., Pirofsky, B., August, C. S., Stiehm, E. R., Hitzig, W. H. and Gatti, R. A. (1972). The Wiskott-Aldrich syndrome. Results of transfer factor therapy. *J. Clin. Invest.* **51**, 3216.

Stobo, J. D., Paul, S., Van Scoy, R. E. and Hermans, P. E. (1976). Suppressor thymus-derived lymphocytes in fungal infection. *J. Clin. Invest.* **57**, 319.

Strayer, D. S., Cosenza, H., Lee, W. M. F., Rowley, D. A. and Kohler, H. (1974). Neonatal tolerance induced by antibody against antigen-specific receptor. *Science* **186**, 640.

Study group for bronchogenic carcinoma (1975). Immunopotentiation with levamisole in resectable bronchogenic carcinoma: a double-blind controlled trial. *Brit. Med. J.* **3**, 461.

Talal, N. and Steinberg, A. D. (1974). The pathogenesis of auto-immunity in New Zealand Black mice. *Curr. Topics Microbiol. Immunol.* **64**, 79.

Tada, T., Taniguchi, M. and Takemori, T. (1975). Properties of primed suppressor T-cells and their products. *Transplant. Rev.* **26**, 106.

Taussig, M. J. (1973). Antigenic competition. *Curr. Topics Microbiol. Immunol.* **60**, 125.

Taussig, M. J. (1974). Demonstration of suppressor T cells in a population of "educated" T cells. *Nature* **248**, 236.

Terman, D. S., Stewart, I., Robinette, J., Carr, R. and Harbeck, R. (1976). Specific removal of DNA antibodies in vivo with an extracorporeal immunoadsorbent. *Clin. Exp. Immunol.* **24**, 231.

Thomas, E. D., Storb, R., Clift, R. A., Fefer, A., Johnson, F. L., Neiman, P. E., Lerner, K. G., Glucksberg, H. and Buckner, C. D. (1975). Bone marrow transplantation. *New Eng. J. Med.* **292**, 832 and 895.

Utermohlen, V. and Zabriske, J. B. (1973). Suppressed cellular immunity to measles antigen in multiple sclerosis patients. *Lancet* **2**, 1147.

Valdimarsson, H., Hambleton, G., Henry, K. and McConnell, I. (1974). Restoration of T-lymphocyte deficiency with dialysable leucocyte extract. *Clin. Exp. Immunol.* **16**, 141.

Valdimarsson, H., Higgs, J. M., Wells, R. S., Yamamura, M., Hobbs, J. R. and Holt, P. J. L. (1973). Immune abnormalities associated with chronic mucocutaneous candidiasis. *Cell. Immunol.* **6**, 348.

De Vries, R. R. P., Lai, A., Fat, R. F. M., Nijenhuis, L. E. and Van Rood, J. J. (1976). HLA-linked genetic control of host response to Mycobacterium leprae. *Lancet* **II**, 1328.

Waldmann, T. A., Durm, M., Broder, S., Blackman, M., Blaese, R. M. and Strober, W. (1974). Role of suppressor T cells in pathogenesis of common variable hypogammaglobulinaemia. *Lancet* **II**, 609.

Wara, D. W., Goldstein, A. L., Doyle, N. E. and Amman, A. J. (1975). Thymosin activity in patients with cellular immunodeficiency. *New Eng. J. Med.* **292**, 70.

Warin, J. F. (1974). Immunization: balancing the risks. *Proc. Roy. Soc. Med.* **67**, 374.

Westminster Hospitals Bone-marrow Transplant Team (1977). Bone-marrow transplant from an unrelated donor for chronic granulomatous disease. *Lancet* **I**, 210.

Willcox, H. N. A., Humphrey, J. H. and Cross, A. M. (1975). Recovery of B lymphocyte responsiveness after complete radioactive antigen suicide, and the affinity of antibody made after incomplete suicide. *Cell. Immunol.* **16**, 348.

Zembala, M. and Asherson, G. L. (1973). Depression of the T cell phenomenon of contact sensitivity by T cells from unresponsive mice. *Nature* **244**, 227.

Zuckerman, K. S., Neidhart, J. A., Balcerzak, S. P. and Lobuglio, A. F. (1974). Immunologic specificity of transfer factor. *J. Clin. Invest.* **54**, 997.

Subject Index

Entries in bold type indicate important basic terms. The page numbers in bold type refer to the fullest description of their meaning.

C

H

I

J

K

M

N

O

P

R

U